Neuro-Ophthalmology

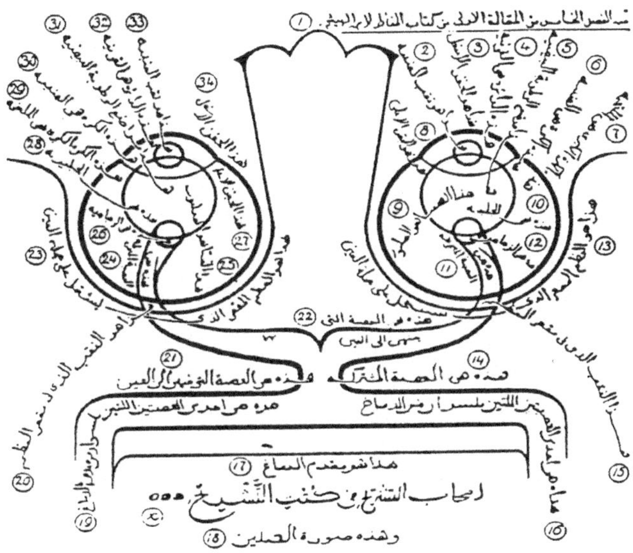

- more recent diagnostics and therapies
- modern etiopathomechanisms
- current rehabilitation of people with impaired vision

Judit Somlai • Tibor Kovács
Editors

Neuro-Ophthalmology

Springer

Editors
Judit Somlai
Unit of Neuro-Ophthalmology
Department of Neurology and Stroke
Military Hospital
Budapest
Hungary

Tibor Kovács
Department of Neurology
Semmelweis University
Budapest
Hungary

ISBN 978-3-319-28954-0 ISBN 978-3-319-28956-4 (eBook)
DOI 10.1007/978-3-319-28956-4

Library of Congress Control Number: 2016939129

Printed on acid-free paper

This Springer imprint is published by Springer Nature
The registered company is Springer International Publishing AG Switzerland

Dedicated to:
László Remenár, M.D.†
(National Neurosurgical Scientific Institute, Budapest, Hungary)

Márta Hajda, M.D.
(National Neurosurgical Scientific Institute, Budapest, Hungary)

Prof. Yochanan Goldhammer †
(Tel Hashomer Medical Center, Tel Aviv, Israel)

Prof. Josef Flammer
(University Eye Clinic, Basel, Switzerland)

Preface

Medical specialties are becoming more and more complex. The knowledge of experts covers more and more circumscripts. Together with several other factors, this phenomenon enhances the importance of teamwork. Our book also aims to meet this need. Neuro-ophthalmology falls in a niche between the two specialties combining their knowledge concerning the sense of sight. Vision is the most important system which links us to the outside world. Its complexity in itself requires the expertise of several specialties, not to mention the visual symptoms of numerous diseases of not neurological origin.

Judit Somlai, who has become a household name in Hungarian neuro-ophthalmology, managed to win over almost 50 experts to cooperate in the explanation and education of this field.

This book has some antecedents, as since its first publication (1996) it has already been revised twice. Both revisions (2007 and 2010) incorporated substantially updated and supplemented content, written by an increasing number of authors. You can get an idea of the dynamic development of the field just by considering the shortened time between two revisions and the expansion of the book; the present publication has twice as many pages as the previous one.

Similarly to the previous book, the rehabilitation of chronic visual impairment and the available aids get extensive coverage.

This book is also an excellent example of integration and work based on a complex conceptual base, which is frequently lacking in today's health care.

I would like to congratulate the authors of this book for providing us with this consistent and trustworthy knowledge, and I would also like to recommend it to experts working in the field of ophthalmology, neurology, neurosurgery, traumatology, radiology, as well as cardiovascular medicine and rehabilitation.

Péter Halász, M.D.

Contents

Part III Conventional, Novel and Complementary Examinations in Ophthalmology

Functional Tests of the Visual Pathway System

Neuro-Ophthalmological Examinations of the Eye Movements

Contributors

Klára Aczél, M.D. Outpatient Department of Ophthalmology, Military Hospital, Budapest, Hungary

Csaba Balázs, M.D. Department of Internal Medicine–Endocrinology, Budai Hospital of Hospitaller Brothers, Budapest, Hungary

Péter Barsi, M.D., PhD, Habil Szentâgothai Knowledge Center – MR Research Center, Semmelweis University, Budapest, Hungary

Unit of Neuroradiology, Department of Neurosurgery, University of Pécs, Pécs, Hungary

György Benedek, M.D., PhD Faculty of Medicine, Institute of Physiology, Albert Szent-Gyòrgyi Clinical Center, University of Szeged, Szeged, Hungary

Béla Csákány, M.D., PhD Department of Ophthalmology, Semmelweis University, Budapest, Hungary

Márta Tolnay Csattos, M.D. Head of National Institution for Blind People Tiflopedagogist, Rehabilitation Instructor, National Institution for Blind People, Budapest, Hungary

Andrea Deák, M.D. Orthoptic Unit, Department of Ophthalmology, Albert Szent-Györgyi Clinical Center, University of Szeged, Szeged, Hungary

Patricia Domsa, M.D. Ophthalmologist, Pediatric Ophthalmologist, Madarâsz Street Pediatric Hospital, Budapest, Hungary

Department of Ophthalmology, Semmelweis University, Budapest, Hungary

Rubrica Health Center, Budapest, Hungary

Csaba Ertsey, M.D., PhD Department of Neurology, Semmelweis University, Budapest, Hungary

Agnes Farkas, M.D., PhD Department of Ophthalmology, Semmelweis University, Budapest, Hungary

László Fornádi, M.D. Department of Neurology, Jahn Ferenc South Pest Hospital, Budapest, Hungary

Gyula Gács, M.D., PhD Outpatient Department, Budapest City Council Péterfy Sândor Street Hospital, Budapest, Hungary

Ildikó Gádor, M.D. Unit of Otoneurology, Department of Otorhinolaryngology, National Institute of Neurology, Budapest, Hungary

György Geréby, M.D. Department of Neurology and Stroke Center, Budapest City Council Saint John Hospital and United Hospitals of North Buda, Budapest, Hungary

Szilvia Gulyás, M.D., PhD Electrophysiology Unit, Department of Neurology, Faculty of Medicine, Semmelweis University, Budapest, Hungary

Zoltan Harkányi, M.D., PhD Department of Radiology, CT Laboratory, Heim Pál Pediatric Hospital, Budapest, Hungary

Zsolt Illés, M.D. Department of Neurology, University of Pécs, Pécs, Hungary

Márta Janáky, M.D., PhD, habil. Electrophysiological Unit, Department of Ophthalmology, Faculty of Medicine, University of Szeged, Szeged, Hungary

László Joszt Social Worker, Rehabilitation Instructor of Visually Impaired Patients Physical Accessibility Expert, National Institution for Blind People, Budapest, Hungary

József Kenéz, M.D., PhD MR Laboratory, Székesfehérvár, County Hospital, Székesfehérvár, Hungary

Department of Radiology, Semmelweis University, Budapest, Hungary

Department of Radiology, National Traumatology Institute, Budapest, Hungary

Department of Neurology, Semmelweis University, Budapest, Hungary

Department of Neuroradiology, Haynal Imre Postgraduate University of Health Sciences, Budapest, Hungary

Vera Klein, M.D. Ophthalmologist, Neuro-ophthalmologist, Health Care Nonprofit Ltd., Budapest, Hungary

Katalin Korányi, M.D. Neuro-Ophthalmology Section, Hungarian Ophthalmological Association, National Institute of Oncology, Budapest, Hungary

Tibor Kovács, M.D., PhD, Habil. Department of Neurology, Faculty of Medicine, Semmelweis University, Budapest, Hungary

Cerebrovascular and Dementia Unit, Department of General Neurology, Budapest, Hungary

Dementia and Dystonia Outpatient Department, Semmelweis University, Budapest, Hungary

Lajos Rudolf Kozák, M.D., PhD Bolyai Research Fellow, MR Research Center, Semmelweis University, Budapest, Hungary

Gábor Lovas, M.D., PhD Department of Neurology, Délpesti Jahn Ferenc Hospital, Budapest, Hungary

Mária Judit Molnár, M.D., PhD, med. habil Department of Molecular Neurology and Research Center, Center for Rare Neurological Diseases, Semmelweis University, Budapest, Hungary

Zita Morvay, M.D., PhD Diagnoscan, Szeged, Hungary

Zita Snagy Nagy Department for Multiprofile Rehabilitation of Locomotor Diseases, National Medical Rehabilitation Institute, Budapest, Hungary

Institute of Psychology, Eötvös Lóránd University, Budapest, Hungary

László Nemes, M.D., PhD National Hemophilia Center and Hemostasis Outpatient Unit, Military Hospital, Budapest, Hungary

János Németh, M.D. Department of Ophthalmology, Faculty of Medicine, Semmelweis University, Budapest, Hungary

Éva Nieszner, M.D., PhD Unit Head, Head Physician Internist, Cardiologist, Diabetology Specialist, Angiology Specialist, Military Hospital, Budapest, Hungary

Ernő Pálfia, M.D. Ophthalmologist, Pediatric Ophthalmologist, Budapest, Hungary

Judit Pálfia, M.D. Ophthalmologist, Pediatric Ophthalmologist, Pálfia Ltd., Budapest, Hungary

Gyula Pánczél, M.D., PhD Department of Neurology, Budapest City Council Péterfy Sándor Street Hospital and Outpatient Department, Budapest, Hungary

György Pfliegler, M.D., med.habil Department of Rare Diseases, 2nd Department of Internal Medicine, Institute for Internal Medicine, Medical and Health Center, University of Debrecen, Debrecen, Hungary

György Pulay, M.D. Outpatient Department, Accident Center, Budapest City Council Péterfy Sándor Street Hospital, Budapest, Hungary

Zsuzsa Récsán, M.D., PhD Department of Ophthalmology, Faculty of Medicine, Semmelweis University, Budapest, Hungary

Bernadett Salomváry, M.D. Head of Department, Head Physician Ophthalmologist, Neuro-ophthalmologist, Orbital Surgeon, National Institute of Neurology, Budapest, Hungary

Neuro-Ophthalmology Section, Hungarian Ophthalmological Association, Budapest, Hungary

Magdolna Simó, M.D., PhD Department of Neurology, Faculty of Medicine, Semmelweis University, Budapest, Hungary

Gábor Márk Somfai, M.D., PhD Department of Ophthalmology, Faculty of Medicine, Semmelweis University, Budapest, Hungary

Judit Somlai, M.D. Head of Unit of Neuro-Ophthalmology, Department of Neurology and Stroke, Military Hospital, Budapest, Hungary

Unit of Neuro-Ophthalmology, Hungarian Ophthalmological Association, Budapest, Hungary

Trustee, NOSZA Foundation (for the Prevention and Screening of Ocular Storke), Budapest, Hungary

Anna Soproni, M.D. Ophthalmologist, Pediatric Ophthalmologist, Private Medical Office, Budapest, Hungary

Péter Szatmári "Informatics for People with Visual Injury" Foundation, Budapest, Hungary

György T. Szeifert, M.D., med. habil Unit for Neurosurgical Injuries, Péterfy Accident Center, Semmelweis University, Budapest, Hungary

Jenő Szeifert, M.D. Faculty of Education and Psychology, Institute of Health Promotion and Sport Sciences, Eötvös Lóránd University, Budapest, Hungary

Zsuzsa Szepessy, M.D., PhD Department of Ophthalmology, Faculty of Medicine, Semmelweis University, Budapest, Hungary

István Szikora, M.D., PhD Neurointerventional Unit, National Institute of Neurology, Budapest, Hungary

Ildikó Szilvássy Districts 2 and 14 Outpatient Department, Budapest, Hungary

Ágnes Szirmai, M.D., PhD Department of Otorhinolaryngology, Head and Neck Surgery, Faculty of Medicine, Semmelweis University, Budapest, Hungary

Mihály Szuhaj "Informatics for People with Visual Injury" Foundation, Budapest, Hungary

Erika Tátrai, M.D., PhD student Department of Ophthalmology, Faculty of Medicine, Electrophysiologist, Budapest, Hungary

Szabolcs Tóth, M.D. University Professor, DMSC Neurosurgeon, Electrophysiologist, Budapest, Hungary

János Vajda, M.D., PhD Head Physician Neurosurgeon, National Institute of Neurology, Budapest, Hungary

György Várallyay, M.D. Head Physician Radiologist, Neuroradiologist, Szentagothai Knowledge Center – MR Research Center, Semmelweis University, Budapest, Hungary

Anna Verseghi, M.D. Rehabilitation Unit for Patients with Skull and Brain Injury, National Medical Rehabilitation Institute, Budapest, Hungary

The eternal dilemma concerning which is harder:
to imagine a world one has never seen
or
to lose a world that has once been familiar with
and
to accept that it will never return?
We must never decide, just let empathy guide us.

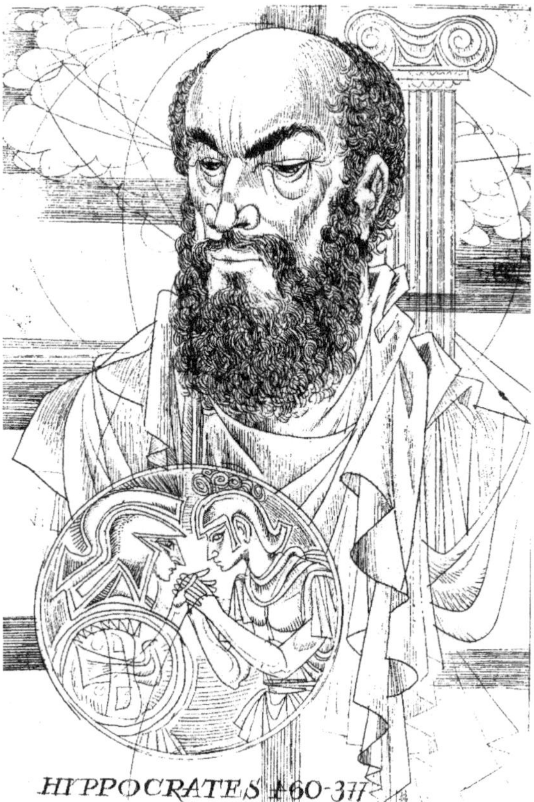

Hippocates graphic illustration was created by †János Kass (1927–2010), Hungarian Graphic Sculptor

Part I

The Importance and Role of Neuro-Ophthalmology

1 The Importance and Role of Neuro-ophthalmology in Ophthalmological Clinical Practice

Judit Somlai

Neuro-ophthalmology (NO) is a new diagnostic sub-specialty on the periphery between neurology and ophthalmology that encompasses the ophthalmological symptoms of internal diseases with neurological or neurosurgical complications. The visual pathways (between the retina and the visual cortex) and the oculomotor system (between the eye muscles and the cortical centers) have direct contact with almost the whole length of the central nervous system. Therefore, if we note any disorder in these functions, we can draw conclusions regarding the extent and the location of the damage with the help of neuro-ophthalmological assessment. Our empirical knowledge will probably inform us of the etiology of the disorder as well. The tests will give us information about:

- the localization
- the extent of the damage
- disorders that cause only loss of function at the onset without morphological changes detectable on CT or MRI scans
- the efficiency of the treatment and the progress of the disease
- the qualitative and objective assessment of care and rehabilitation.

J. Somlai, M.D.
Head of Unit of Neuro-Ophthalmology, Department of Neurology and Stroke, Military Hospital, Budapest, Hungary

Unit of Neuro-Ophthalmology, Hungarian Ophthalmological Association, Budapest, Hungary

Trustee, NOSZA Foundation (for the Prevention and Screening of Ocular Stroke), Budapest, Hungary
e-mail: dr@somlaijudit.hu; http://somlaijudit.hu

J. Somlai, T. Kovács (eds.), *Neuro-Ophthalmology*, DOI 10.1007/978-3-319-28956-4_1

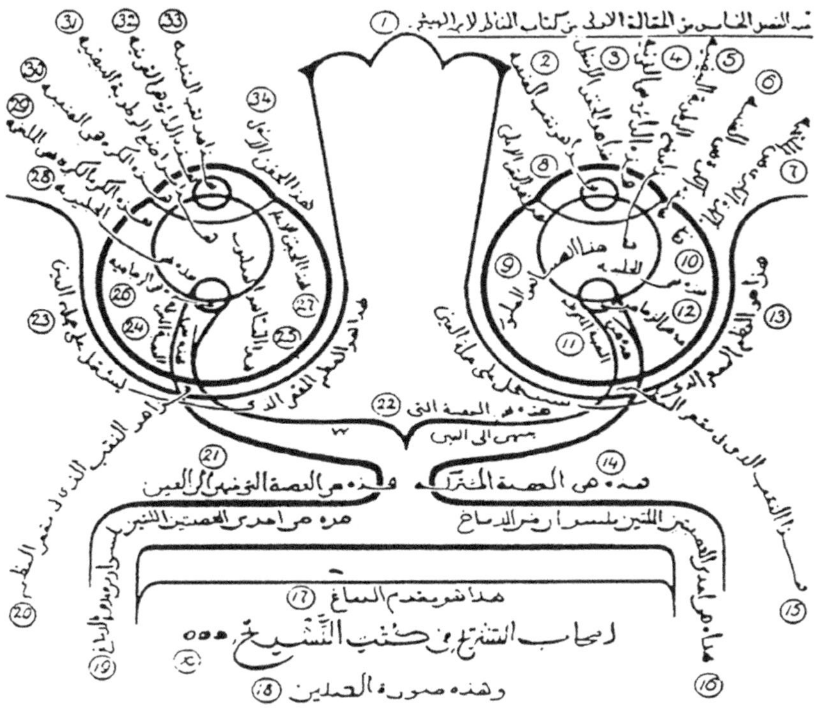

Drawing from the era of Islamic medicine. Their ideas of the visual pathways were not far from reality, especially regarding the chiasmatic region

Topography, a.k.a. 'localization diagnostics' can help us to identify the location and extent of pathological changes anywhere in the visual and oculocomotor pathways, e.g., in the case of loss of visual field or paralytic strabismus. Examinations enable us to quantify the extent of the abnormality, but they can also help us to exclude pathological processes.

Disease processes that result in loss of vision can evade even the most modern diagnostic tools for a relatively long period of time. On the other hand, some functional disorders, such as transient loss of vision and/or diplopia can indicate or herald an imminent or actual disease process. The results of conservative and surgical treatments can be evaluated using neuro-ophthalmological tests, e.g., an increased visual field defect can indicate relapse or progression of the disease. If necessary, patients should be followed up for life by experts from the affected and related fields on regular consultations.

Similar to almost all fields of clinical medicine, cutting-edge diagnostic techniques are at the forefront of neuro-ophthalmology.

This feature can be explained by the fact that the earlier a disease is diagnosed, the more efficient the appropriate therapy and the lower the chance of residual symptoms will be.

Medical treatment is complemented by comprehensive rehabilitation performed by our assistants with special qualifications. This way we can not only alleviate patients' symptoms, but we can also assist their recovery and resumption of regular activities with the help of modern diagnostic techniques and useful advice.

The Importance of Neuro-ophthalmology in Neurology

2

Tibor Kovács

Content

The eye is the mirror of the soul, or it is rather a mirror of the brain, a window to the brain, at least for neurologists. In neurology, the examination of the optic nerve and eye movements are part of the physical examination. Fundoscopy is vital in emergency neurology. Visual field testing is performed both during neurological and ophthalmological examinations, but its most accurate assessment is best performed with ophthalmological devices. Eye movement and pupil reaction tests are also carried out by both specialties; however, the criteria for these evaluations might be the most different in these tests.

The interdependence of neurology and ophthalmology is justified by the complexity of the visual system. The eyes are ultimately part of the brain, the retina develops from the diencephalon, and the layers of the eyeball are related to the meninges. The retina and the brain are supplied by a common artery. The orbits and the intracranial structures feature strong anatomical connections. The visual system has some contact with all regions of the brain from the retina to the occipital cortex. The anatomy and the vestibular connections of oculomotor regulation constitute some of the most difficult topics both in medical and specialty training. Structures related to vision can be found almost everywhere in the nervous system (one-third of supratentorial structures plays a role in vision); thus, they can be affected by nearly all neurological diseases; the description of the disorder can help to identify the trigger factor (Newman et al. 2003).

As a result, it is easy to understand why ophthalmologists and neurologists often point at each other when faced with several diseases of the visual and oculomotor system. In our everyday practice, most of us have seen patients with anterior ischemic optic neuropathy pushed to and fro by neurological and ophthalmological wards and outpatient clinics. Neuro-ophthalmology is a field where the specialist has to be an ophthalmologist and a neurologist at the same time, which is, of course, not achievable. As a result of the system of education, everybody qualifies as an ophthalmologist or a neurologist first, which means that we are going to have neurologists who are good at ophthalmology and ophthalmologists who are good at neurology; a

T. Kovács, M.D., PhD, Habil.
University Associate Professor, Department of Neurology, Faculty of Medicine, Semmelweis University, Budapest, Hungary

Cerebrovascular and Dementia Unit, Department of General Neurology, Semmelweis University, Budapest, Hungary

Dementia and Dystonia Outpatient Department, Semmelweis University, Budapest, Hungary
e-mail: tibor@neur.sote.hu

J. Somlai, T. Kovács (eds.), *Neuro-Ophthalmology*, DOI 10.1007/978-3-319-28956-4_2

situation which has both advantages and disadvantages. The most significant consequences of this separation are apparent in the case of rare diseases. In 1992, a child was admitted to the Department of Neurology in Boston, USA (Engle 2007) with bilateral ptosis and downward gaze. Investigations for myasthenia, mitochondrial disease, and congenital myopathy yielded no results. The result of ophthalmological consultation was somewhat surprising for the neurologists as the ophthalmologists diagnosed the case as congenital fibrosis of the extraocular muscles. This disease entity was unknown for the neurologists in spite of the fact that it had been first described in ophthalmology in the 1800s, as belonging to the group of ocular fibroses, the most well-known manifestation of which is Duane syndrome. In ophthalmological literature, the cause of this group of diseases was thought to be the primary fibrosis of the extraocular muscles. Nowadays the group has extensive neurological literature as well, as the cause of oculomotor disorders has proved to be a developmental disorder of cranial nerve motor neurons (congenital cranial dysinnervation disorders) rather than fibrosis. There are many other 'surprising' diseases like this; therefore, this book might serve to decrease the number of such surprises for both ophthalmologists and neurologists.

References

Engle EC. Oculomotility disorders arising from disruptions in brainstem motor neuron development. Arch Neurol. 2007;64:633–7.

Newman NJ et al. Neuro-ophthalmology update. Continuum Am Acad Neurol. 2003;9:11–78.

Part II

Objectives and Recent Results in the Neuro-Ophthalmological Clinical Practice

3 Mechanisms of Parallel Information Processing in the Visual System

György Benedek

Contents

Visual information encoded on the retina is processed in two anatomically independent pathway systems in the central nervous system. This parallel character of the structure and functioning of the visual system has long since been known, however, researchers have only recognized its physiological and clinical importance in the past years.

The original concept of Aristotle has matched the five senses: sight, sound, smell, taste and touch with independent sensory organs. In 1844, Volkmann suggested that the different sensory modalities perceived through the skin (touch, vibration, cold, warm, pain) are transmitted by distinct populations of neurons in the central nervous system. This idea has founded the principle of parallel, independent processing of somatic sensations.

As a pioneer of the principle of parallel processing in the visual system, Bishop made an observation in 1933 about distinct groups of optic fibers of frogs and rabbits based on their conduction speed. This has led him to the conclusion that these different fiber groups transmit different components of visual perception similarly to somatosensory pathways. However, while it was quite easy to recognize the submodalities processed in a parallel fashion in the somatosensory system, the differentiation of the visual submodalities in the visual system has been shown to be significantly more difficult. The main reason for this was that none of the fiber groups could be linked to the receptor populations known at that time (cones and rods).

The publication of Enroth-Cugell and Robson was considered as a breakthrough, as they described two different types of ganglion cells in the retina of the cat: the Y and the X cells. The authors found that the stimuli on the relatively big receptive field of the Y-cells are not summed linearly, while X cells added stimuli linearly in their small receptive field. X cells were in the majority around the central area, while Y cells were mostly found in the peripheries (Fig. 3.1). The importance of the two different cell groups were particularly highlighted when a great difference was discovered in the conduction speed of the axons pertaining to these two cell types.

G. Benedek, M.D., PhD
Faculty of Medicine, Institute of Physiology, Albert Szent-Györgyi Clinical Center, University of Szeged, Szeged, Hungary
e-mail: benedek@phys.szote.u-szeged.hu

J. Somlai, T. Kovács (eds.), *Neuro-Ophthalmology*, DOI 10.1007/978-3-319-28956-4_3

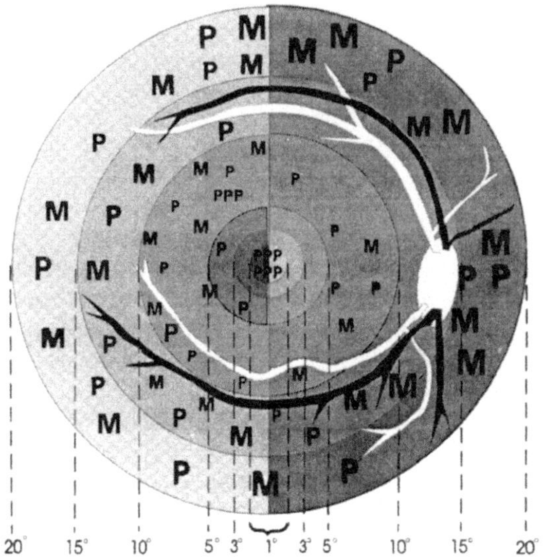

Fig. 3.1 Schematic diagram of the spatial distribution of M-and P-cells in the retina. Font size represents the ratio of the soma/dendritic (receptive) field. After Lennie

Y cells have fast conduction fibers (30–40 m/s), while the fibers of the X-cells conduct considerably slower (18–25 m/s). Apparently, the X cells may play a role in the processing of fine details, while Y cells may participate in motion perception. In 1972, Stone and Hoffmann described a third cell type in the retina, the W-cells. These cells have a large receptive field, a characteristically prolonged firing pattern, direction selectivity and axons with a remarkably low- 4–12 m/s conduction speed. (The role of W-cells in visual perception has not been clarified yet.)

The primate and human homologues of the X/Y cells were identified as the P ganglion cells (X cell, α-cell) that send projecting axons to the parvocellular layers of the lateral geniculate body (CGL) and the M cells (Y cell, β-cell) projecting to the magnocellular part of the CGL. Eighty percent of the retinal ganglion cells are P-cells, 20% of them are M cells.

A further cell type was described in the primate retina, the koniocellular (K) cells. The role of these cells and the koniocellular pathway (K) originating from them in visual perception is little known, therefore, it is not discussed further. The pathways originating from the M and P cells typically retain their character, thus the conduction speed of the axons as well, even after making connections in the CGL and the cortical areas.

Characteristics of the retinal P ganglion cells

- small soma and small dendritic field
- greater cell density around the central fovea
- axons of moderate diameter
- projection to the parvocellular area of the CGL

Characteristics of the retinal M ganglion cells:

- big soma with moderate dendritic field
- evenly distributed in the retina
- thick axons
- projection to the magnocellular area of the CGL

It is a general characteristic of both cell types that the size of the dendritic and receptive fields increases towards the periphery of the retina (Fig. 3.1).

The distinct characteristics of cortical projections mainly have been detected by cytochrome oxidase enzyme staining in the monkey brain and by labeled 2-deoxi-glucose determination. Based on these studies, the existence of a P-cell pathway running to the temporal cortex via the CGL and the primary visual cortex, and an M-cell pathway running via the CGL and the primary visual cortex to the parietal cortex is also possible in humans (Fig. 3.2).

Considering the physiological characteristics of the parallel optic pathways, they show variable sensitivity to low and high spatial frequencies. Their temporal sensitivity to frequencies is also different. It seems that the M pathways are particularly sensitive to rapid changes in low and moderate spatial frequencies, while the P pathways are particularly sensitive to slowly changing high spatial frequencies. In humans these pathways can be investigated primarily by the critical fusion frequency, and the temporally and spatially changing contrast sensitivity methods. The M-cell pathway prefers low spatial frequency stimuli modulated by frequencies of 5–10 Hz.

The P pathway originating mainly from the foveal area is sensitive to the considerably slower changing but finer spatial frequencies. The

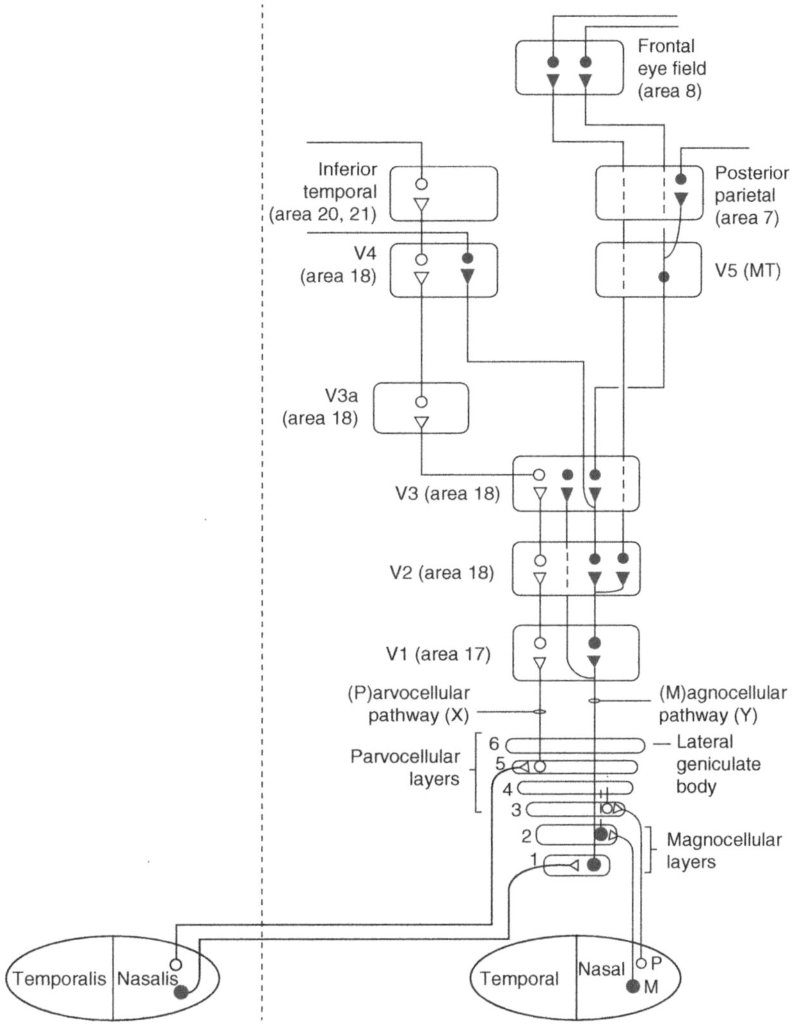

Fig. 3.2 Schematic diagram of the structure of the visual pathway

existence of the two pathways allows the visual image projected on the retina to provide two distinct pieces of information via the two different information processing systems. The M-cell pathway provides early information on changing forms affecting a greater area of the retina, irrespective of the finer details. Signals of the finer details reach the cortex later via the P-cell pathway, that is, the visual system receives general, global information before local information primarily about focal details could reach it. The M-cell pathway provides a rapid insight mainly about the part of the field of vision where some changes take place. This information facilitates the functioning of the P-cell pathway by enabling the tuning mechanism of the fovea, and promotes the integration of the focal information transmitted by the P-cell pathway into the background provided by the M-cell pathway. One of the first pieces of behavioral evidence of the parallel processing in the visual system is the observation that in splitbrain monkeys deprived from interhemispheric connections two types of visual signals can be distinguished based on the learning process. There are stimuli that can be learned separately by both hemispheres of the monkeys, and there are stimuli that do not allow duplicate learning. The so called split signs are those that are composed of well distinguishable, easily defined pairs of stimuli, for example, a cross for one hemisphere and a circle for the other. However, there are also pairs of stimuli that can be most simply characterized as being globally different from each other. For example, five stars in the field of vision against six stars, or dimming of the field of vision against a bright one, or orange color against the complementary color of blue.

It is true for all non-split stimulus complexes that they can be inverted into their pair by means of a simple function transformation. This may be equivalent to the behavioral situation, when related to the spatial movement of the animal, the apparent structure of a stimulus is altered due to the motion related change in the direction, brightness and perspective.

This experiment led Trevarthen to the description of the two distinct aspects of visual behavior. According to his assumption, the organization of the visual system primarily corresponds to the structure of the visuomotor system. The visuomotor system serves two basic functions. Locomotor displacements change the relationship between the body and the contours of the spatial configurations, e.g., surface objects. Global vision stands in the background of the visual coordination of these movements.

Opposingly, during manipulative behavior to change the environment, both vision and motor actions are directed to one point in space. Vision is concentrated on one spot, on one special object and its details, while our motor mechanisms are also focused on this. This type of visual activity is named focal vision, a form of visual function that subserves fine discriminative functions.

Characteristics of global vision:

- very sensitive to motion that is changes in the visual image
- mainly influenced by events in the lateral part of the field of vision
- sensitive in case of low brightness levels as well
- generally remains an unconscious process

Characteristics of focal vision:

- preference to detect spatial differences
- excessive representation of the central part of the field of vision
- preference to photopic intensity level
- requires attention, becomes conscious

Interrelations of Focal and Global Vision

1. Low-definition peripheral mechanisms sensitive to high speed adapt early by fixed head position, leading to rapid extinguishment of the peripheral picture. As opposed to this, movement in the peripheries leads to suppression of the central, focal vision. Focal vision is also inhibited during rapid position changing motion.
2. Low light intensity environment promotes environmental vision, while photopic environment helps focal vision.
3. A third possibility of interaction is based on the different operation speed of the two systems. The latency of the oculomotor responses evoked by changes in the visual space is considerably shorter than a saccadic response following a certain single focal characteristic. This may be in association with the fundamentally different conduction speed of the X and Y systems. Earlier arriving Y discharges contain different information and may induce different responses.

Clinical Evidence

The differentiation between global and focal vision is also possible in such pathological processes, where the two parallel systems are not equally damaged.

The largest amount of available data is available on glaucoma, Alzheimer's disease and amblyopia ex anopsia. There are data on the involvement of the magno- and parvocellular pathway systems and accordingly the various involvements of focal and global vision, and also in behavioral disorders following severe cerebral hypoxia and Parkinson's disease. Knowledge on the M- and P-cell pathways may also contribute to the understanding of certain dyslexias.

The latest updates on the three most frequent disorders are discussed in the following.

Glaucoma

Histological studies have shown that in glaucoma it is mainly the large ganglion cells that are damaged along with the thick optic nerve fibers. Electrophysiological and psychophysical abnormalities also refer to damage of the M-cell pathway. Differences have been found on electroretinography performed by patterned stimulation and in the visual evoked potential in glaucoma patients. These differences were more prominent in case of rapidly changing stimuli with low spatial frequency. Atkin et al. have found decreased high frequency flicker sensitivity in glaucoma patients. Towle et al. have reported increased latency of the main component of the VEP in glaucoma patients in case of rapidly alternating big checkerboard pattern stimulation.

Price et al. have similarly found increased VEP latency in glaucoma. These data refer to the relative sparing of the P-cell pathway and dominant damage to the M-cell pathway in glaucoma patients. Specially designed psychophysical experiments are needed to interpret the changes in the visual information accompanying these damages.

Alzheimer's Disease

Alzheimer's disease is of unknown etiology, and it leads to dementia. Retinal and optic nerve damages have been described in patients with Alzheimer's disease. In advanced Alzheimer's disease 30–60% of the ganglion cells are dysfunctional. Histological studies have shown that initially, these changes affect mainly the M-cells of the retinal ganglion cells. Functional evidence also refers to the dominance of the M-cell pathway damage. Earlier visual evoked potential examinations in the visual cortex have not indicated such abnormalities, however, these examinations were performed with sharp contrast, low temporal frequency stimulation, primarily activating the P-cell pathway. Trick et al. showed damage to pattern electroretinography (PERG), if they tested patients with Alzheimer's disease with high frequency stimuli. Hutton et al. have found connections between disorders of the slow pursuit eye movement and Alzheimer's disease. Similar symptoms were detected in monkeys after damage to the cortical areas of the M-cell pathway.

Amblyopia

Amblyopia ex anopsia (deprivation amblyopia) is a functional deterioration in vision not accompanied by abnormalities of the fundus or the retina, and it cannot be corrected optically. Amblyopia has several animal models. Amblyopia can be induced by eyelid suture at a certain early developmental stage (as this eliminates pattern viewing, but the animal still notices changes in luminescence). Artificially induced anisometropia has similar consequences. Two types of amblyopia can be distinguished both in animal studies and clinical amblyopia: sensitivity may be decreased to only high or all kinds of spatial frequencies. This raises the possibility that two distinct kinds of damage are in the background of the clinical presentation of amblyopia. It is possible that the P-cell pathway is selectively damaged, or dysfunction of both the M-cell and P cell pathways together causes the clinical symptoms and signs of amblyopia.

In human amblyopia the decrease of temporal definition is not always accompanied by impairment of the sensitivity to low spatial frequencies, thus, it cannot be directly linked to the damage of the M-cell pathway. Experiments on monkeys have shown specific dysfunction of the P-cell pathway in anisometropic amblyopia. Experimental induction of anisometropia is possible by causing continuous paralysis of accommodation by the administration of atropine. This is followed by characteristic behavioral and histological signs if the sensitivity to high spatial frequencies is decreased, and cellular damage can be detected in the parvocellular layer of the lateral geniculate body. Human anisometropic amblyopia is also accompanied by decreased sensitivity to high spatial frequencies. These results show that anisometropic amblyopia selectively involves the P-cell pathway. This corresponds to the clinical observation that the vision of children with amblyopia is only poorer in photopic circumstances; there is no difference between the normal and the amblyopic eye in scotopic circumstances not requiring focal vision. Therefore, amblyopia can be considered as a selective disorder of focal vision.

The above mentioned morphological, physiological, psychophysiological and clinical observations bring up a new aspect of vision tests. The theory that considers vision primarily as focal vision by full contrast should be abandoned. Abnormalities that cause disorders of global vision by intact focal vision should be recognized.

Currently, contrast sensitivity testing and certain kinds of evoked potentials provide some information on the selective disorder of M-cell pathways. It would be necessary to selectively examine the two pathways, and objective methods should be elaborated to better understand the physiological and pathological processes in the visual system.

Further Readings

Atkin A, Bodis-Wollner I, Wolkstein M. Abnormalities of contrast sensitivity in glaucoma. Am J Ophthalmol. 1979;88:205–13.

Bassi CJ, Lehmkuhle S. Clinical implications of parallel visual pathways. J Am Optom Assoc. 1990;61:98–110.

Bishop GH. Fiber groups in optic nerve. Am J Physiol. 1933;106:460–74.

Bradley AF, Freeman RD. Contrast sensitivity in anisometric amblyopia. Invest Ophthalmol Vis Sci. 1982;21:467–76.

Cleland BG, Levick WR. Brisk and sluggish concentrically organized ganglion cells in the cat's retina. J Physiol (Lond). 1974;240:421–56.

Enroth-Cugell C, Robson JG. The contrast sensitivity of retinal ganglion cells of the cat. J Physiol (Lond). 1966;187:517–52.

Hess RF. Contrast sensitivity assessment of functional amblyopia in humans. Trans Ophthalmol Soc UK. 1979;99:391–7.

Hutton JT, Shapiro J, Loewenson RB. Abnormal eye movements in dementia and aging. Trans Am Neurol Assoc. 1981;106:320–3.

Lennie P. Parallel visual pathways: a review. Vision Res. 1980;40:561–94.

Lovegrove WJ, Carzia RG, Nicholson SB. Experimental evidence for a transient system deficit in reading disabled children. J Am Optom Assoc. 1990;61:98–110.

Quigley HA, Sanchez RM, Dunkelberger GR. Chronic glaucoma selectively damages large optic nerve fibers. Invest Ophthalmol Vis Sci. 1987;28:913–20.

Rashbass C. The relationship between saccadic and smooth tracking eye movements. J Physiol (London). 1961;159:326–38.

Sestokas AK, Lehmkuhle S. Visual response latency of X- and Y-cells in the dorsallateral geniculate nucleus of the cat. Vision Res. 1986;26:1041–54.

Stone J, Dreher B. Parallel processing of information in the visual pathways. A general principle of sensory coding. Trends Neurosci. 1983;5:441–6.

Stone J, Hoffmann KP. Very slow conducting ganglion cells in the cat's retina:a major, new functional type. Brain Res. 1972;43:610–6.

Towle VL, Moskowitz A, Sokol S. The visual evoked potential in glaucoma and ocular hypertension: effects of check-size, field-size, and stimulation rate. Invest Ophthalmol Vis Sci. 1983;24:175–83.

Trevarthen CB. Two mechanisms of vision in primates. Psychol Forsch. 1968;31:299–337.

Trick GL. Retinal potentials in patients with primary open-angle glaucoma: physiological evidence for temporal frequency-tuning defects. Invest Ophthalmol Vis Sci. 1985;26:750–9.

Van Essen DC. Visual areas of the mammalian cerebral cortex. Annu Rev Neurosci. 1979;2:227–63.

Volkmann AW. Handwörterbuch der Physiologie (Handbook of physiology). Wagner R, editor, vol 2. Braunschweig; 1844. P. 521–26.

A New Direction: Neuro-endocrino-immunology

4

Csaba Balázs

Content

One of the unexpected and highly important biological discoveries of the last decade was that the psycho-neuroendocrine and the immune systems are not only in interaction, but also use common biochemical signals. The decoding of this common "language" was made possible with the help of the latest results of molecular biology and genetics. Not all details of this complex interaction are known today, but our current knowledge is satisfactory to state that it is not a separated, but an integrated psycho-neuroendocrino-mmune system that is responsible for the maintenance of the homeostasis in the body. Loss of this delicate balance may lead to various pathological conditions, thus to development of autoimmune diseases. It is known that the immune system is composed of a complicated network of cells with controlled interactions. The recognition of antigens is performed by monocytes, macrophages and dendritic cells (DC). This recognition is a complex process, consisting of the degradation of the substances taken up by the cells, the evaluation of the epitopes of the degraded substances, and transmission of the information gathered from these substances. The molecules of the so-called major histocompatibility complexes (MHC) have an important function in the recognition and presentation of antigens. The recognized information is transmitted to the thymus- and bursadependent cells (T and B lymphocytes). The former ones can also be divided into two groups. The Th1 (T helper 1) cells are responsible for the delayed type immune reactions, the Th2 (T helper 2) cells regulate the humoral immunological processes. T cells divide in the presence of activating agents (mitogenes) and antigens; they undergo the so-called blast transformation. During this process, they produce biologically active substances, part of which may be cytotoxic. B lymphocytes take effect via structurally and functionally different antibodies. Part of the antibodies bind to their own individual immunoglobulins (idiotype) and create the so-called idiotype–anti-idiotype network, which has an important role in the fundamental task of the immune system to preserve individual integrity. Other antibodies are cytotoxic or capable of inhibiting or stimulating the function of cells (e.g., anti-TSH receptor stimulating autoantibodies increasing thyroid function, or inhibitory autoantibodies in patients with Graves' disease). Lymphokines produced by these cells were thought to be responsible for the interactions of the immune system. However, it has been recognized in the recent years that lymphokines are

C. Balázs, M.D.
Department of Internal Medicine–Endocrinology,
Budai Hospital of Hospitaller Brothers,
Budapest, Hungary
e-mail: drbalazscsaba@gmail.com

J. Somlai, T. Kovács (eds.), *Neuro-Ophthalmology*, DOI 10.1007/978-3-319-28956-4_4

produced not only by the cells of the immune system, but by other cells, such as cells of the neuroendocrine system as well, therefore, nowadays these information transferring substances are rather called cytokines. Cytokines are polypeptide-type molecules binding specifically to cell surface proteins (receptors) and alter their function. The structure of cytokines and cytokine receptors is already known, some of them have also been successfully cloned. In contrast to hormones, cytokines deliver their effects dominantly in a paracrine or an autocrine fashion. However, it also has to be mentioned that sometimes there are overlaps between the effects of hormones and cytokines. This means that cytokines can be detected in the peripheral circulation, and they may act as hormones (e.g., interleukin-6 stimulates the hypothalamic–pituitary axis the most intensively), on the other hand, some hormones (e.g., prolactin, ACTH, TSH) are known to act as cytokines in the tissues (Fig. 4.1). Cytokines bind to specific receptors and may transmit inhibitory or stimulating signals. Cytokine receptors may detach from the surface of the cells and be present in a soluble form. These soluble cytokine receptors may be important partly in the regulation of cytokine production and partly in the effect of cytokines as well. Cytokine agonists and antagonist take effect in a different way, and they are expected to gain increasing therapeutic importance in the future. The basis of the holistic view of medicine is that it studies the physiological and pathological regulatory operations of the body in a unified way. The decoding of the integrative language summarizing the regulation of the human body has opened a new direction in medicine. The essence of this interaction is that the cells of the neuroendocrine system are capable to produce cytokines, while lymphocytes and macrophages produce neurotransmitters and hormones. The most recent results show that certain areas of the brain differentially coordinate the maturation and function of immune cells, and the "humunculus" model based on this indicates which brain regions regulate the maturation and activity of the immune system (Fig. 4.2).

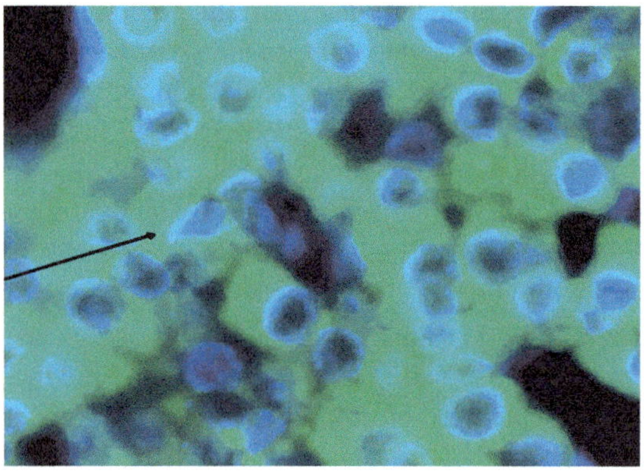

Fig. 4.1 Detection of prolactin mRNA by in situ hybridization in lymphocytes (*green* fluorescence indicates prolactin, *blue stain* depicts the nucleus)

Several examples can be mentioned from the general practice for interactions between systems formerly have been thought to be autonomic. Hormones (steroids, prolactin, thyroid hormones) may influence both physiological and pathological functions of the immune system. Monoclonal antibodies against cytokines are already suitable in the daily routine for the treatment of endocrine diseases with autoimmune pathomechanism. Although neuro-ophtalmological autoimmune diseases belong to the group of organ-specific pathologies that affects "only" a single organ, to understand the pathomechanism, diagnostics and management of these diseases, a broader outlook on the above only roughly described regulatory processes based on multidirectional interactions and affecting the whole body is needed.

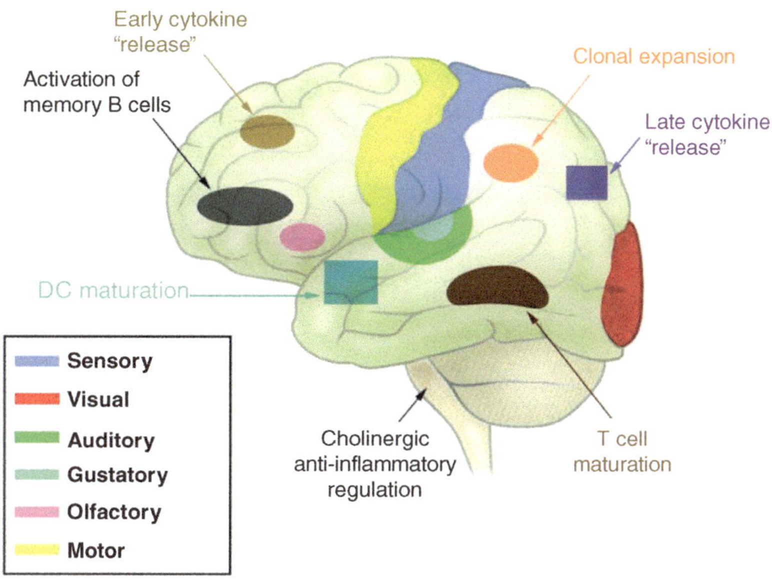

Fig. 4.2 Map of the cerebral regulation of the immune system. *DC* dendritic (antigen presenting) cells

Further Readings

Nathan C. Points of control in inflammation. Nature. 2002;420:846–52.

Paridaens D, et al. The effect of etanercept on Graves' ophthalmopathy: a pilot study. Eye (Lond). 2005;19: 1286–9.

Romagnani P, et al. CXCR3 mediated opposite effects of CXCL10 and CXCLA in Th1 or Th2 cytokine production. J Allergy Clin Immunol. 2005;116:1372–9.

Rotondi M, et al. Role of chemokines in endocrine autoimmune diseases. Endocr Rev. 2007;10:2006–44.

Sternberg EM. Neuroendocrine regulation of autoimmune/inflammatory diseases. J Endocrinol. 2001;169: 429–35.

Tracey KJ. Physiology and immunology of the cholinergic anti-inflammatory pathway. J Clin Invest. 2007; 117:289–96.

Visual and Oculomotor Disorders in Internal Diseases

5

György Pfliegler

Contents

'The eye is the mirror of the soul', this old saying is true for the whole body as there are several diseases affecting other organs or sometimes the whole body that can cause changes to the eyes as well; moreover, they are often detected during an ophthalmological examination. Therefore, ophthalmologists have a huge responsibility (just like doctors working in other fields of medicine) to consider the whole person when examining just one organ (the eye). In this chapter, we provide a non-exhaustive review of the most important internal conditions where ophthalmological changes are of extraordinary diagnostic and therapeutic importance, reflecting a recent change in attitude.

Vascular Diseases

The recognition of the unity of the vascular system has recently come to the forefront in medicine again. While historically cerebrovascular, cardiovascular and peripheral vascular diseases were considered to be separate disease entities, nowadays the vascular system is considered undivided. This is also true for small blood vessels; thus, vascular diseases of the retina can be the result of *generalized atherosclerosis* or the consequence of embolisation. The source of embolism may be a thrombus in the left atrium (auricle) or a plaque in the carotid arteries. The most common result is the obstruction of blood vessels in the ocular fundus. In *hypertension,* the circulation of the retina, choroid and optic nerve is also affected. The condition of the fundus depends on the duration and control of hypertension. Grade 1 hypertension is characterised by twisted, sclerotic arterioles that resemble silver or copper wiring, while grade 2 features arteriovenous crossing abnormalities and lipid

G. Pfliegler, M.D., med. habil.
Department of Rare Diseases,
2nd Department of Internal Medicine,
Institute for Internal Medicine,
Medical and Health Center, University of Debrecen,
Debrecen, Hungary
e-mail: g.pfliegler@gmail.com

J. Somlai, T. Kovács (eds.), *Neuro-Ophthalmology*, DOI 10.1007/978-3-319-28956-4_5

exudates. Malignant hypertension (diastolic blood pressure over 110 mmHg) is fortunately becoming less frequent. Grade 3 and 4 retinal changes include hemorrhages, cotton wool spots and papilledema. Contrary to the previous practice, it has recently been realized that fast and dramatic reduction of blood pressure can lead to the development of stroke and loss of vision. Vision can also be affected if the area damaged by ischemic or hemorrhagic stroke includes the visual cortex or the visual pathway, or if the paralysis of cranial nerve 7 leads to inability to close the eyes, thereby resulting in drying of the cornea and infection.

Endocrine and Metabolic Diseases

Diabetes mellitus is associated with the development of retinopathies, glaucoma and cataract. In developed countries, the most frequent cause of blindness is retinopathy. Glaucoma is mostly attributable to retinopathy, while cataracts are usually the result of a direct damage to the structure of the lens hyperglycemia or protein kinase C activation. Most ophthalmological parameters (e.g., visual acuity, central vision, foveolar thickness, etc.) show strong correlation with HbA1c levels. The visual complications of diabetes used to be considered incurable; however, as a result of a recent change in attitude, aiming to achieve normoglycemia, physiological changes in glucose levels, active ophthalmological care (e.g., early assessment with digital photos taken in mydriasis, measurement of intraocular pressure, grid- or panretineal photocoagulation, cryotherapy, etc) progression may be slowed down significantly or can even be stopped. It is true for background retinopathy, preproliferative and proliferative retinopathy. In proliferation, increased angiogenesis can be indicated by increased levels of vascular endothelial growth factor (VEGF) in peripheral blood samples and abnormal von Willebrand factor (vWF), which suggest endothelial dysfunction. If these observations are confirmed by larger studies, the more convenient blood-based monitoring of the disease may soon become available. Vitreoretinal surgery may yield promising results for the most advanced cases.

Diseases of the thyroid gland. Graves' ophthalmopathy is one of the diseases in which the relationship between an internal disease and ophthalmological symptoms was detected first. However, it has to be noted that these symptoms can occur in euthyroidism and hypothyroidism as well, and they can also precede the development of endocrine disorders. The initial, inflammatory stage lasts for about a year, and it is followed by scarring. The stages of the disease are distinguished according to the NOSPECS system (N=No signs or symptoms, O=Only signs, no symptoms S=Soft tissue involvement, P=proptosis, E=extraocular muscle involvement, C=corneal involvement, S=Sight loss), yet in practice the eyes and the surrounding tissues can give us good guidance as well (free of infection, or swollen and inflamed). Contrary to the previous practice, patients with ophthalmopathies are no longer treated surgically because steroids, irradiation, and other conservative methods have proved to be effective even in serious cases. Patients with Hashimoto's thyroiditis sometimes report visual field deficits.

Pituitary gland adenomas larger than 10 mm in size press on the optic chiasm causing bitemporal hemianopsia. In other cases or anatomical situations, they can cause visual field deficits by pressing on other parts of the optic tract. Other hormonal diseases can have ophthalmological manifestations as well, such as cataract, tetany of ocular muscles, calcium precipitation in the conjunctiva and cornea in *(pseudo)hypoparathyroidism.* Keratitis has been reported in *autoimmune polyendocrine deficiency.*

- Kayser–Fleischer rings are well-known diagnostic signs in *Wils*on's disease; however, they can be absent in children and when there are no neurological symptoms. Sunflower cataracts (radiating opacities that do not influence vision) are also visible. Recently, beside d-penicillamine zink substitution has been widely used. Zink can also be given in pregnancy.
- In amyloidosis, amyloid deposits in the eye and its suspensory apparatus can cause several non-specific changes (purpura, retinal hemorrhage, nodules in the eyelids, exophthalmus, disordered pupil reactions, etc).

- Hemorrhage and thrombosis in the fundal veins can occur in cystic fibrosis.
- Amino acid metabolism disorders have partly overlapping, partly different ophthalmological symptoms of various severities. In homocystinuria lens dislocation, glaucoma, retinal detachment, optic nerve atrophy and cataract can be seen. In cystinosis cystin crystals can precipitate in the cornea, conjunctiva and lens, photophobia, retinal blindness can develop and pigmented, peripheral retinal degeneration is also characteristic. The symptoms of tryptophan metabolism disorder (Hartnup-disease) can be diplopia, photophobia, convergence disorder, nystagmus, and blepharitis. Bright light usually triggers or aggravates the symptoms.
- In one of the lipid metabolism disorders, in congenital hypercholesterolemia, 'fish-eye disease' may appear as bilateral corneal opacity resembles the eyes of fish.
- The various forms of porphyrin metabolism dis*orders* are uniformly characterized by increased photophobia.

Hematological Diseases

In multiple myeloma and Waldenström macroglobulinemia, it is the high viscosity that causes retinal damage and, consequently, visual impairment. Its acute management is apheresis, but in the long run the treatment of the underlying disease is necessary. *Myelodysplastic syndrome, acute myelogenous leukemia and other malignant hematological diseases* are mostly associated with retinal hemorrhage due to severe thrombocytopenia, but the infiltration of pathological cells has also been reported in some cases (I had a patient with Prof. András Berta where the first manifestation of mantle cell lymphoma was in the left orbit). Simultaneous fundal thrombosis and bleeding can develop in essential thrombocythemia, polycythemia vera and paraproteinemia. Sjögren's syndrome and, ultimately cataract can develop following *allogenous bone marrow transplant,* presumably as the combined result of radiation damage, chemotherapy, high-dose steroids and graft-versus-host disease.

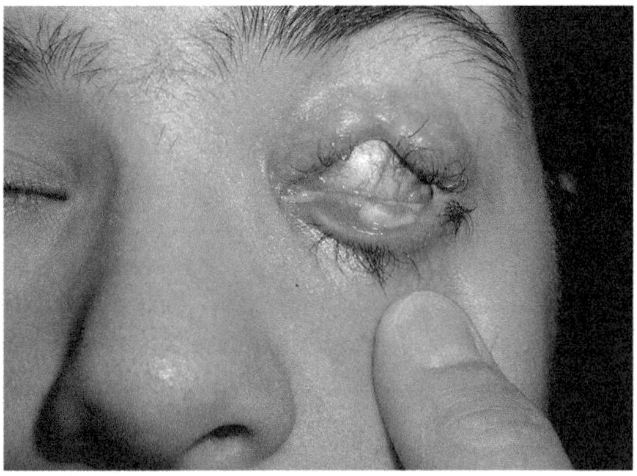

Fig. 5.1 Ligneous conjunctivitis in compound-heterozygous plasminogen deficiency (photo by Valéria Nagy, M.D., University of Debrecen, Department of Ophthalmology)

Of non-malignant hematological diseases, *Osler's disease* might be associated with conjunctival and retinal telangiectasis. Congenital *plasminogen deficiency* can cause *ligneous conjunctivitis* (Fig. 5.1). Bilateral proliferative retinopathy can develop in *sickle cell anemia;* in severe cases, allogenous bone marrow transplant can prevent the loss of vision. *Fanconianemia* is characterized by strabismus, ptosis, nystagmus and microophthalmopathy. Severe cases of *thalassemia* feature thin, rod-like vascularisation of the conjunctiva. In *sickle cell anemia,* the above mentioned symptoms can be accompanied by angioid streaks and avascular areas in the retina. *For fundal thrombosis and ischemic optic neuropathy see the relevant chapter.*

Autoimmune Diseases

Autoimmune disorders constitute a large and widely investigated group. A classic example is *Sjögren's syndrome,* which leads to keratoconjunctivitis sicca as a result of decreased tear production. In *ankylosing spondylitis* iritis, photophobia, red eyes and visual impairment usually precede arthritis; these symptoms normally respond to corticosteroids and pupil dilation. In *rheumatoid arthritis,* we should note the presence of scleritis, keratoconjunctivitis, episcleritis and ulcers on the corneal margin; the latter symptom can indicate very poor prognosis as it can herald fatal systemic vasculitis. *Systemic lupus erythematosus* (SLE) features the above mentioned symptoms, but the retinal blood vessels and the optic nerve may also be affected. As a result, hemorrhage, cotton bud spots, microaneurysm, exudate, vascular disorders and retinal thrombosis can develop. In *juvenile rheumatoid arthritis* ophthalmological symptoms (iritis, cataract, and band keratopathy) do not show a strong correlation with the severity of systemic symptoms. Secondary glaucoma develops in about 15 % of the cases. *Polyartertis nodosa* is also characterized by ocular inflammation. *Giant – cell arteritis* is also worth mentioning as it has a special predilection for the arteries of the eye. Ischemic optic neuropathy is associated with sudden loss of vision, ptosis caused by the paralysis of a third cranial nerve branch, and the outward turning of the affected eye (while the pupil stays in the middle). High-dose corticosteroids administered immediately can prevent spread to the other eye.

Congenital Immune Deficiency Syndromes

DiGeorge syndrome (congenital thymic aplasia) is characterised by hypertelorism and slanting palpebral fissures. *Chediak–Higashi syndrome* is associated with pigment deficiency, photophobia, nystagmus, papilledema, decreased tear production and lymphocytic infiltration of the optic nerve.

Gastrointestinal Diseases

Episcleritis and uveitis are more frequent in inflammatory bowel diseases *(ulcerative colitis, Crohn's disease)*, while scleritis, which is usually more severe, occurs less frequently. Conjunctivitis is also listed among the extraintestinal symptoms of these diseases, yet it is not a specific phenomenon. Genetic factors play an important role in the development of the disease, and also in the development of extraintestinal symptoms. The most common HLA constellations are HLA-A2, DR1, DQw5, DRB1*0103, B*27 and B*58. In *Plummer–Vinson syndrome,* keratoconjunctivitis sicca, canthus ragades and marginal blepharitis may develop as a result of iron and multiple vitamin deficiencies.

Hypo- and Hypervitaminosis

Symptoms of avitaminosis and hypovitaminosis can be detected with low levels of vitamins *A, B, C, D, E and K,* while overdose usually occurs with *vitamins A, B and D.* Overdose is mostly the result of alternative therapy and self-healing.

Vitamin overdose (*hypervitaminosis*) rarely causes ophthalmological symptoms; the main symptoms usually develop in other organs. Vitamin A overdose can cause visual disorders and characteristic double vision in children; however, it is the result of increased intracranial pressure (pseudotumor cerebri). Excessive intake of vitamins D and E can hinder the absorption of vitamin A, thereby leading to the development of the typical symptoms of vitamin A deficiency (see Table 5.1).

Genetic Disorders

Several genetic disorders belong to the heterogenous group, and the majority of these diseases are already diagnosed in childhood. Major criteria of *Marfan's syndrome* include ectopia lentis, while minor criterias are flat cornea, increased axial length, hypoplastic iris and ciliary muscles. *Neurofibromatosis* can affect the eyelids, iris, orbit, and the optic nerve; however, the leading symptom is the development of Lish nodules, which are caused by the accumulation of melanocytes in the iris. Storage diseases tend to affect the eyes as well, e.g., retina degeneration and corneal opacity develop in mucopolysaccharidosis, cherry-red central spots occur in the retinae in

Table 5.1 Ophthalmological symptoms of hypovitaminosis and avitaminosis

Water-soluble vitamins	Ophthalmological symptoms
Vitamin B_1 deficiency	Paralysis of oculomotor nerves, optic neuritis, dichromatism, visual field deficits
Vitamin B_2 deficiency	Blepharoconjunctivitis, keratitis, corneal vascularization, retinal hemorrhage
Vitamin B_3 (niacin, nicotinic acid) deficiency	Conjunctivitis, keratitis, papilledema, photophobia, hemeralopia
Vitamin B_{12} deficiency	Optic nerve disorders, retinal hemorrhage
Vitamin C deficiency	Hemorrhage in various parts of the eye, cornal ulcer, paralysis of ocular muscles
Fat-soluble vitamins	**Ophthalmological symptoms**
Vitamin A deficiency	Xerophthalmia → infection → corneal ulcers, nyctalopia, foamy (Bitot's) sports appear in the conjunctiva
Vitamin D deficiency	Zonular cataract, orbital ossification disorders, optic nerve atrophy, phlyctenular keratitis
Vitamin E deficiency	Keratitis, cataract
Vitamin K deficiency	Bleeding in the fundus of the eye

gangliosidosis, while mucolipidosis type 4 features strabismus, and Fabry disease is associated with cornea verticillata.

Nowadays, in several cases, patients' life can be prolonged and the quality of life can be improved by enzyme replacement and occasionally by bone marrow transplantation. Anterior uveitis frequently develops in HLA-B27 positive patients in *ankylosing spondylitis*. *Hermansky–Pudlak syndrome* (a rare, hereditary disease) is characterized by periocular albinism, disordered platelet function, anemia, and nystagmus. The eyes and their suspensory apparatus are also affected in muscular atrophy, connective tissue diseases, osteogenesis imperfecta, amyloidosis, etc. See relevant chapters.

Infectious Diseases

HIV-induced *acquired immune deficiency syndrome* affects the eyes in 75 % of the patients. The causes can be opportunistic or viral infections, tumors and drug toxicity. In patients whose immune system is compromized for other reasons, the eyes and the retina can be infected with cytomegalo virus (CMV) or herpes simplex (HSV) virus, and systemic fungal infections (e.g., candidiasis) can develop as well. Toxocariasis and trichinosis develop as a result of consuming, e.g., raw, infected boar meat. The eyes can also be affected in several other infectious diseases, such as Lyme disease, brucellosis, leptospirosis, tuberculosis, syphylis, or endocarditis.

Iatrogenic Diseases of the Eyes: Adverse Effects of Medications

They involve an increasing number of patients. A significant number of people take anticoagulants (acenocoumarol, warfarin, or the new, targeted oral FXa-, or FIIa-inhibitors; new oral anticoagulants/NOAC-s/) for primary or secondary prophylaxis. However, in case of overdose, bleeding occurs at the most diverse sites, e.g., in the fundus of the eye, subconjunctival suffusion or in the eyelids. If the anticoagulant is vitamin K antagonist it is of utmost importance to determine INR levels immediately should any kind of bleeding (including ophthalmological) or the suspicion of an overdose arises. It is strictly forbidden to use any other, previously used ranges (e.g., rate, per centage, or index); only INR is accepted (the therapeutic range is usually between 2 and 3). However, with NOACs INR is of no value and should never be used. For screening the presence of NOAC in a patient prothrombin time (PT with Xa inhibitors) or thrombin time (TT with IIa-inhibitor) can be used but only totally normal value means that there is no drug effect. The time of the last drug intake is also essential due to the relatively short half lives of these anticoagulants. There are several other, frequently used medications in internal medicine that have ophthalmological side effects – this is something we have to remember when taking the patient's history or evaluating the symptoms. Here there are some examples for illustration: calcium channel blockers (e.g. *nifedipine, amlodipine), nitrates (nitroglycerin)* can cause visual disorder, periorbital edema, eye irritation; *non-steroidal anti-inflammatory drugs* are associated with cornea deposits, disordered color vision, visual field deficits, nystagmus, toxic maculopathy; *tamoxifen* used in the treatment of breast cancer can lead to the development of retinopathy, dichromatism, visual field deficits; *digoxin, propranolol, amiodarone* (cardiovascular drugs) can trigger cornea and lens opacities, dry eyes, papillitis; *furosemide, ACE-inhibitors might also* induce visual disorders and conjunctivitis, and *anticholesterol medications* (e.g., atorvastatin, simvastatin) can cause lens opacity and visual impairment, cataract. *Antibiotics* mostly induce allergic reactions and sensitivity to light. *Barbiturates, hydantoinderivatives* may cause nystagmus. *Corticosteroids* can lead to the development of papilledema, increased intraocular pressure and toxic cataract. The *antituberculotic drug,* PAS may provoke exophthalmus, streptomycin can impair accommodation, ethambutol can damage the optic nerve, and isoniazid (INH) may cause amblyopia. It is well-known that *chloroquine* can be associated with maculopathy, cornea impregnation, ptosis, corneal opacity, retina degeneration, central scotoma and photophobia, while *amiodarone* can cause optic neuropathy as well. The anti-epileptic *carbamazepine* has been reported to cause blurred and double vision. *Digitalis* has been used less frequently in recent decades, so we might not have to consider it when trying to find the trigger factor of dazzling, miosis, disordered color vision and blurred vision. *Interferon-alpha treatment* may cause temporary blindness. Several *chemotherapeutic agents* may damage the eyes as well, e.g., methotrexate can cause cataracts and blepharitis, while vinca alkaloides (vincristine, vinblastine) are associated with the paralysis of the eye muscles and optic nerve atrophy.

This list, which is by no means complete, draws our attention to the fact that we always have to obtain information of all the medicinal products a patient takes, and unless we can find the obvious cause of the complaints, these preparations have to be considered as pathogenic agents, too. There are some examples of the opposite happening as well: if steroid eyedrops are administered without monitoring for a long time, they can induce Cushing's disease, and in our practice a patient has attempted to commit suicide with pilocarpine drops.

Apart from the internal diseases mentioned above, there are several other syndromes that are associated with ophthalmological changes, such as sarcoidosis, multiple sclerosis, phacomatosis, myasthenia gravis, etc. Besides malignant hematological conditions, breast, lung, kidney, colon and genital tumors can metastasize to the orbit. Following the short, more or less etiological review, we will try to illustrate the various function of an ophthalmological examination (and also that of the ophthalmological way of thinking) by summarizing several clinical pictures that should be considered when diagnosing a cataract. Similar sections can be found in other chapters of the book, e.g., in connection with *papilledema, sudden loss of vision, oculomotor disorders and their potential causes.*

Cataract

Its various types are characteristic of different age groups, and the underlying diseases are different as well. In the elderly, when the disease develops gradually, we have to consider *senile cataract,* fast progression suggests *diabetes,* muscle jerks and coexisting characteristic symptoms can be the result of *hypoparathyroidism,* the simultaneous development of bilateral cataract raises the suspicion of *poisoning,* or if it follows trauma to the skull, we should think of *traumatic origin.* Cataracts can also develop as a result of *lightning, electric shock, irradiation, intrauterine toxoplasmosis, or rubella.* They can be the feature of several diseases that have skeletal and neurological manifestations (e.g., spinocerebellar ataxia) or dermatological symptoms (e.g., Fabry disease, congenital ichthyosis, etc). The development of a cataract is also typical in types *1* and *2 galactosemia*. The diseases listed above (and several other syndromes) belong to the group of rare diseases, which means that their prevalence is lower than 5/10,000. Naturally, we do not want to suggest that these disease entities should always be considered on setting up the first diagnosis; however, if there is no comforting 'frequent' explanation for the patient's symptoms (cataract or other), we should consider the possibility of some disease that is unknown to us. If we have this approach and refer the patient to the appropriate center, we can shorten the frequently prolonged diagnosis of rare cases and fasten the initiation of the proper therapy.

Bibliography

Afandi B, Toumeh MS, Saadi HF. Cushing's syndrome caused by unsupervised use of ocular glucocorticoids. Endocr Pract. 2003;9:526–9.

Balázs E, Rózsa L, Pfliegler G, Berta A. Amit a Hippel-Lindau szindrómáról jelenleg tudunk. Újabb eredmények a szemészetben. [What we should know about Hippel-Lindau syndrome. Recent advances in ophthalmology]. Módszertani Levél. 1998;1:63–80.

Bautista Juanes JA, Theischen M, Beelen DW, et al. Ocular complications of long-term survival of bone marrow transplantation. A prospective study with 21 patients. Klin Monatsbl Augenheilkunde. 1993;202: 110–5.

Betkó J. Szemészeti határterületek, szindrómák. [Interdisciplinary fields and syndromes in ophthalmology] Medicina Budapest. 2006.

Carpineto P, Ciancaglini M, DiAntonio L, et al. Fundus microperimetry patterns of fixation in type 2 diabetic patients with diffuse macular edema. Retina. 2007;27:21–9.

Cojocaru VM, Ciurtin C, Pop M, et al. Ophthalmological involvement in rheumatic disease. Oftalmologia. 2006;50:56–61.

Kezuka T, Usui N, Suzuki E, et al. Ocular complications in myelodysplastic syndromes as preleukemic disorders. Jpn J Ophthalmol. 2005;49:377–83.

Lakatos L, Pandur T, Dávid G, et al. Association of extraintestinal manifestations of inflammatory bowel disease in a province of western Hungary with disease phenotype: results of a 25-year follow up study. World J Gastroenterol. 2003;9:2300–7.

Mencucci R, Rossi Ferrini C, Volpe R, et al. Ophthalmological aspects in allogenic bone marrow transplantation: Sjögren-like syndrome in graft-versus-host disease. Eur J Ophthalmol. 1997;7:13–8.

Mohammadpour M, Javadi MA. Keratitis associated with multiple endocrine deficiency. Cornea. 2006;25: 112–4.

Mohan JS, Lip PL, Blann AD, et al. The angiopoietin/Tie-2 system in proliferative sickle retinopathy: relation to vascular endothelial growth factor, its soluble receptor Flt-1 and von Willebrand factor, and to the effects of laser treatment. Br J Ophthalmol. 2005; 89:815–9.

Pfliegler G. Haemoglobinopathiák [Hemoglobinopathies]. In: A belgyógyászat alapjai (szerk. Tulassay Zs.). Budapest: Medicina; 2007a. p. 1276–7.

Pfliegler G. Tárolási betegségek [Storage diseases]. In: A belgyógyászat alapjai (szerk. Tulassay Zs.). Budapest: Medicina; 2007b. p. 1634–46.

Pfliegler G, Palatka K. Attempted suicide with pilocarpine ophthalmic drops. Am J Ophthalmol. 1995;120: 399–400.

Primary Care Committee, Clin. Care Group, Am. Optometr. Assoc. Quick reference to ocular manifestations of commonly prescribed systemic medications.

Rákóczi É, Pfliegler G, Maródi L. A diagnosztika útvesztői Fabry-kórban [Diagnostic puzzles in Fabry disease]. Háziorv Tképző Szle. 2004;9:40–2.

Zile M. Vitamin A deficiences and excess. In: Kliegman RM, Behrman RE, Jensen HB, Stanton BF (szerk.), editors. Nelson textbook of pediatrics. 18th ed. Philadelphia: Saunders-Elsevier; 2007. P. 335.

Genetic Aspects of Neuro-ophtalmological Diseases

6

Mária Judit Molnár

Contents

There are several neuro-ophthalmological disorders that have genetic abnormalities in the background. Part of these diseases has monogenic, that is, autosomal dominant, recessive or maternal inheritance, while others pertain to the polygenic and multifactorial disease categories. This section summarizes the most frequent monogenic neuro-ophtalmological diseases in clinical practice.

Monogenic Neurological Diseases with Ophthalmological Relevance

Myasthenia syndromes

- Congenital myasthenia syndromes (CMS)

Muscular dystrophies

- Myotonic dystrophy type 1 (DM1)
- Oculopharyngeal muscular dystrophy (OPMD)
- Congenital muscular dystrophies (CMD)

Hereditary neuropathies

- Congenital cataracts facial dysmorphism neuropathy (CCFDN)

Mitochondrial diseases:

Developing due to defects of mtDNA

- Leber's Hereditary Optic Neuropathy (LHON)
- Neuropathy, ataxia, retinitis pigmentosa (NARP)
- Chronic progressive external ophthamoplegia (Kearns-Sayre syndrome) CPEO (KSS)

Developing due to defects of nuclear DNA

- Progressive external ophthalmoplegia (PEO)
- Optic atrophy Type 1 (OPA1)
- Neuropathy caused by mitofusin mutations

In this section the characteristics of the above mentioned diseases and the genetic abnormalities in their background are summarized.

Congenital Myasthenia Syndromes (CMS)

Depending on the affected part of the neuromuscular junction, congenital myasthenia syndromes can

M.J. Molnár, M.D., PhD, med. habil.
Department of Molecular Neurology and Research Center, Center for Rare Neurological Diseases, Semmelweis University, Budapest, Hungary
e-mail: molnarmj@neur.sote.hu;
http://molneur.eoldal.hu

J. Somlai, T. Kovács (eds.), *Neuro-Ophthalmology*, DOI 10.1007/978-3-319-28956-4_6

be divided into presynaptic, synaptic and postsynaptic forms. The presynaptic form accounts for 5 % of the congenital myasthenia syndromes. Cholinacetyltransferase deficiency, synaptic vesicle and quantal release defects pertain to this group. The other group contains the diseases related to the damage of the synaptic basal lamina; these pathologies are responsible for 15 % of the CMSs. In this group, clinical symptoms are caused by abnormalities of the end plate AChE (Acetylcholinesterase). Most frequently, in 70 % of the cases, CMS is caused by postsynaptic damage. For the latter, the pathological AChR (Acetylcholin Receptor) kinetics with or without AChR deficiency (slow and fast channel syndromes) may be responsible, or it may be a result of AChR deficiency with or without minor kinetic defect, or may be due to rapsyn and plectin deficiency.

Although several genetic defects may stand in the background of CMS, clinical symptoms are very similar. Certain forms already begin in infancy. In these cases the weak crying and sucking, the frequent dysphagia, or maybe the respiratory disturbance of the newborn or the infant call the attention to the disease. In diseases with childhood onset, the muscle weakness after physical exertion and the delay in motor development refer to the disorder of the neuromuscular junction. On physical examination often ptosis, fixed or fluctuating ophthalmoplegia can be detected, spinal deformities and diffusely decreased muscle mass are also not rare findings.

Diagnostics: If CMS is suspected, routine laboratory tests including serum CK are followed by repetitive stimulation, which shows decreased amplitude of the motor unit potentials in many cases. Importantly, repetitive stimulation should not only be performed at 3 c/s. Either maximal strain or 10, 20, 30 c/s stimulation should be attempted. Since children hardly tolerate high frequency stimulation, 10 c/s stimulation with longer than usual, that is, 30- or 60-s intervals may be tried. In certain forms doublets can be elicited on stimulation of individual motor nerves. The diagnosis of CMS can be established with high confidence based on the abnormal repetitive stimulation, the AChR and anti-MUSK antibody negativity, the clinical symptoms, and family history. Genetic testing of the certain forms is carried out by international laboratories specialized to this testing.

Therapy: in most cases anti-cholinesterase drugs have a positive effect, but this is not a general observation. In such cases diaminopyridine therapy may be attempted. This drug is not available in Hungary. Immunosuppressive therapy is never administered in CMS, since the disease is has no autoimmune etiology, therefore no effect of such treatment can be expected.

Muscular Dystrophies

Myotonic Dystrophy

This is the most frequent neuromuscular disease in adulthood. The prevalence of the disease is 13.5/100 000 newborns. The onset of the disease varies greatly; it may start at any time from the neonatal period until advanced age. In cases with childhood-onset, mental retardation is more frequent, often accompanied by delay in the motor skills. The most characteristic symptom is myotonia, a disturbance of muscle relaxation. In most cases this is discovered as the patient cannot release the tightly closed water tap. The appearance of the face may be characteristic due to the weakness of the mimic muscles (ptosis, masseter atrophy), the speech may be peculiar due to weakness of the tongue and gothic palate. Ophthalmoplegia does not accompany this disease. Severe atrophy and paresis of the skeletal muscles may be present. Lower limbs muscles distant from the trunk also weaken, therefore the patient's ankle is often becomes sprained. Pelvic muscles, thigh flexors, soleus and gastrocnemius muscles generally remain unaffected. This is a multisystemic disease, cataract, gynecomastia, endocrine dysfunction and cardiomyopathy may be often present besides involvement of the muscular system. EMG, which detects characteristic myotonic discharges in the muscles, is indispensable in the diagnostics of this disease. Myotonic dystrophy is a trinucleotide repeat disorder, in the DM1 form there is a CTG repeat expansion in the myotonin kinase gene, while in case of the DM2, which has a very similar clinical phenotype, a CCTG repeat can be found in the KCNBP zinc finger protein gene (ZNF9).

Oculopharyngeal Muscular Dystrophy (OPMD)

The prevalence of the disease is variable. The prevalence in French-Canadians is 1:1000, and 1:600 in Bukharan Jews in Israel. The frequent occurrence of the two founder mutations is due to the frequent marriage of relatives in both populations. The European prevalence is: 1:100,000. Clinical symptoms begin in the second to sixth decade. It is the ptosis that calls the attention to the disease. Weakness of the oculomotor muscles may be of variable extent. During the progression of the disease, the ocular symptoms are often accompanied by dysphagia and weakness of the muscles in the tongue. In more severe forms proximal weakness of the limbs may also develop. The disease is caused by a trinucleotide repeat expansion of the PABPN1 gene. The repeat expansion is transcribed into the PABPN1 protein and thus a toxic protein is produced, forming characteristic intranuclear inclusions by accumulating in the nuclei of the cells. These inclusions can be detected by electron microscope and may also help in the diagnostics of the disease.

Congenital Muscular Dystrophies (CMD)

Congenital muscular dystrophies are muscular diseases with symptoms already developing in infancy or even in newborn age. Characteristic symptoms are generalized hypotonia and delayed motor development. Abnormality of the extracellular matrix proteins, abnormal glycosylation of the alpha dystroglycan or other proteins expressed in the muscle cells stand in the background of the clinical symptoms. All these diseases have poor prognosis, beside the severe muscle weakness and hypotonia, symptoms of central nervous system, epileptic seizures and ocular malformations often complicate the clinical picture. From neuro-ophthalmological aspect, the glycosylation defects of the alpha dystroglycan are of particular importance. These are the Walker-Warburg Congenital MD, the Muscle-Eye-Brain Disease (MEB), the Fukuyama Congenital MD, and the Fukutin-Related Protein (FKRP) MD. These diseases are rare, but we provide a detailed description of them because of their characteristic clinical appearance.

- *Muscle-Eye-Brain Disease (MEB):* the ocular malformation is striking already in newborns, and it is accompanied by generalized hypotonia. This may be associated in infancy with epileptic seizures and slow psychomotor development. Abnormal neuronal migration is detected by brain MRI. Histological examination reveals myogenic damage in the muscle fibers and uneven merosin expression. The expression of glycosylated alpha dystroglycan is also deficient. The disease is caused by a mutation of the POMGnT1 (protein- mannosyl-b1,2 N-acetyl-glucoseamynil-transferase).
- Walker–Warburg syndrome: multiplex anomalies of the anterior and posterior ocular compartment may be associated with hypotonia, epileptic seizures and mental retardation. The disease is lethal in fetal or newborn age. On histological examination of the muscle biopsy specimen the lack of glycosylated alpha dystroglycan expression can be detected. The disease is inherited in an autosomal recessive fashion and it is caused by a mutation in the O-Mannosyltransferase 1 (POMT1) gene.
- Fukuyama muscular dystrophy: This disease is frequent in Japan due to the presence of a founder mutation, but it could be successfully identified in the Caucasian population as well. Symptoms begin in childhood in the form of limb girdle muscular dystrophy, accompanied by cardiomyopathy, eye-related symptoms and involvement of the central nervous system (epilepsy, mental retardation, cerebellar and cerebral cortical dysplasia). The genetic defect is in the fukutin gene, which also plays a role in the construction of the carbohydrate chain of the alpha dystroglycan.

Hereditary Neuropathy

Congenital Cataracts Facial Dysmorphism Neuropathy Syndrome (CCFDN)

The disease is characteristic to the Gypsy population, as it is caused by a IVS6+389C→T founder mutation in the C-Terminal Domain Phosphatase 1 (CTDP1) gene of the RNA Polymerase II gene.

Based on the facial dysmorphism and the congenital cataract the disease can already be suspected at birth. The hereditary neuropathy is generally only diagnosed in infancy or in early childhood. The Charcot Marie Tooth (CMT) denomination encompasses hereditary neuropathies. Type 1 and 2 can be differentiated. CMT 1 indicates the demyelinating forms, while CMT2 the axonal forms. Severe optic neuropathy was reported in several patients suffering from axonal forms caused by mutations of mitofusin. The mitofusin gene pertains to genes influencing mitochondrial dynamics, therefore, the diagnostic algorithm of the disease is described in that section.

Mitochondrial Diseases

Mitochondrial cytopathies form a heterogeneous group of multisystemic diseases, mainly resulting in diseases of the central nervous system and the skeletal muscles, but they may also cause dysfunction of several other organs. Primarily tissues with high energy demand, like the central nervous system, skeletal muscle, cardiac muscle, endocrine organs, liver, kidney and eyes are affected. Clinical signs are specific but greatly varied. Mutations of maternally inherited mitochondrial DNA (mtDNA) and nuclear DNA (nDNA) determining the function of mitochondria may lead to the development of mitochondrial disease. Mutations of the DNA may result in nucleotide substitution affecting an RNA, rRNA or a structural gene and lead to gene rearrangement due to deletion/duplication. In certain cases, depletion of the mtDNA results in severe symptoms. According to our current knowledge, the average prevalence of mitochondrial diseases (mtDNA and nDNA-linked) can be estimated to 1:5000. Some mitochondrial mutations are markedly frequent, among these the most frequent is the A3243G point mutation, the prevalence of which is 16.3/100,000 in the Finnish adult population. Until now approximately 500 pathogenic mtDNA mutations have been identified in the background of nearly 200 diseases (www.mitomap.org). Due to the acceleration of the nDNA research, there is a growing number of nuclear mitochondrial gene mutations that can be linked to some of the clinical phenotypes. Classification of mitochondrial diseases into subgroups raises several problems due to the specialties of mitochondrial biology. These specialties are: the different mitochondrial content of certain tissues and cells, the simultaneous presence of wild type and mutant mtDNA in the cells (heteroplasmy); the threshold effect (a certain heteroplasmy ratio is necessary to the dysfunction of the cells), the same mtDNA mutation may lead to variable clinical presentations, and there is no obvious phenotype-genotype correlation. According to these, the purely clinical picture-based classification is the most useful in clinical diagnostics, even though many patients do not fit into either category. In many cases beta-oxidation disorders represent a difficulty, but in these cases myopathological diagnostics may help the clinician.

Diseases of the mtDNA Linked to Protein Coding Genes

Approximately 80 proteins take part in the construction of the mitochondrial respiratory transport chain. From these only 13 coding genes can be found in the mitochondrial genome, all coding certain subunits of the respiratory transport chain. In the protein coding genes of the mtDNA more than 200 pathogenic mutations are known (www.mitomap.org). Most mutations can be found in the genes encoding various subunits of the NADH dehydrogenase and the cytochrome c oxidase. Besides these a smaller number of mutations can be found in the genes encoding the cytochrome oxidase b and 6th and 8th subunits of the ATPase. One of the most frequent mutations of the protein coding genes is the Leber's optic neuropathy (LHON).

Mitochondrial diseases causing neuro-ophthalmological symptoms may also develop due to mutations of the mitochondrial genes in the nuclear DNA, since mitochondrial function is determined by the coordinated operation of the nuclear and mitochondrial DNA molecules. Nuclear genes influencing mitochondrial function are those encoding the subunits of the respiratory transport chain, playing a role in the intergenomial signalization, influencing mitochondrial dynamics, being responsible for the lipid milieu, and other genes encoding proteins affecting mitochondrial function. The mitochondrial translational machinery contains multiple polypeptides determined by the nucleus and rRNA and tRNA encoded in the mitochondria, and the big respiratory complexes consist of subunits encoded by both genomes. The nDNA encodes approximately 1000 mitochondrial proteins, only 67 of which play a role in the functioning of the respiratory chain. Mitochondrial proteins encoded by the nDNA are synthesized in the cytoplasm and are imported to the mitochondrium by a specific transport system. Besides playing a basic role in the energy metabolism of the cells, mitochondria participate in several other cellular processes as well. Interaction between the nuclear and mitochondrial genomes is fundamental in their biogenesis and functioning. Disturbances in the intergenomial communication between nuclear and mitochondrial DNA may affect mtDNA both quantitatively (mtDNA depletion) and qualitatively (multiple mtDNA deletion syndromes). Diseases with multiple mtDNA deletions are generally associated with neuro-ophthalmological symptoms. In the clinical practice progressive external ophthalmoplegia (PEO) with autosomal dominant (AD) inheritance is encountered most frequently. In 50 % of the cases with AD-PEO syndromes mutations of the POLG1 gene, in 30 % mutations of the Twinkle gene, and in 7–8 % mutation of the ANT1 gene stand in the background of the clinical symptoms. Other diseases associated with multiple mtDNA deletions may cause optic atrophy with autosomal inheritance and severe deterioration of vision. The most frequent mutation in the background of the autosomal dominant optic atrophy (ADOA) is in the gene of the dynamin-like OPA1 located in the inner membrane of the mitochondrium.

Possibilities of Molecular Genetic Diagnostics in Mitochondrial Diseases

In some cases the clinical presentation is already characteristic to the respective mitochondrial disease, and molecular genetic testing of the DNA isolated from the blood is enough to establish the diagnosis. However, in many cases the situation is not that simple, and multiple diagnostic procedures have to be involved before genetic testing, such as for example ENG examination, multimodal electrophysiological tests, blood/cerebrospinal fluid lactate level evaluation, imaging studies, cardiologic examination, histological, histochemical and biochemical processing of the muscle biopsy and DNA analysis. Molecular genetic tests comprise quantitative mtDNA determination with real-time PCR, SNP screening, and sequencing of the whole mitochondrial genome or the suspicious nuclear gene. Morphological examinations reveal the accumulation of mitochondria with pathological structure in the muscle; the disease is characterized by "ragged red" fibers with modified trichrome Gömöri-stain, "ragged-blue" fibers in modified SDH preparations, and COX-negative fibers with cytochrome oxidase stain. Ultrastructural examination finds mitochondria with abnormally organized cristae, frequently containing paracrystalline inclusions. The suspicion of mtDNA-linked diseases is suggested if the inheritance is maternal, and accompanying diseases on the maternal side refer to mitochondrial disease. In such cases the so-called mtDNA hot spots are investigated during routine diagnostics. In case of Leber's hereditary optic neuropathy, the basic pathogenic mutations to which other phenotype-modifying mutations may be associated are known. The latter ones alone do not cause LHON. If mitochondrial disease of nuclear origin is suspected, the clinician's choice of nuclear mitochondrial genes is directed primarily by the clinical symptoms. For example, in case of progressive ophthalmoplegia with autosomal dominant inheritance, we recommend the evaluation of mtDNA deletions in muscle tissue as first diagnostic step. If a multiple mtDNA deletion causing disturbance in the intergenomial communication is revealed, sequencing of the POLG1, Twinkle, ANT1 or RRM2B genes is recommended. If severe deterioration in vision and optic atrophy are detected, the OPA1 or the mitofusin genes should be tested of the regulatory genes of the mitochondrial dynamics. Mutations of mitofusin may result in axonal neuropathy as well. Since there are no mutation hot spots in these genes, sequencing of the whole gene is necessary.

Currently this solution has high costs and most laboratories only examine the sequence of the coding exons, focusing on single nucleotide polymorphisms. This technique does not find the smaller-larger deletions and duplications, furthermore intronic mutations also remain undetected.

However, the rapid development of molecular biological methods gives us hope, that the diagnostic facilities will be explosively improved already in the near future.

References

Karpati G, Hilton Jones D, Bushby K, Griggs R. Disorders of voluntary muscle. Cambridge/London: Cambridge University Press; 2010.

Molnár MJ, Karpati G. Az izombetegségek alapjai és modern szemlélete [Principles of muscular diseases and modern approach]. Budapest: Springer; 2001.

Molnar MJ. A neuromuscularis betegségek diagnosztikája, kezelési és rehabilitációs lehetőségei. Neurorehabilitáció [Diagnostics, treatment and rehabilitation options of neuromuscular diseases. Neurorehabilitation]. Ed.: Zs.Vekerdy, MD Medicina; 2010.

Recent Knowledge in the Neurosurgical Practice Regarding the Visual System

7

János Vajda

In the Book of Neuro-Ophthalmology (Literatura Medicina Publishing, 1996) the 2nd section of chapter "Neurosurgical aspects of the diseases of the visual pathway" summarized the vascular neurosurgical diseases of the visual pathway. Since then, the literature and our own experience with cavernomas in the parenchyma of the optic nerve and the chiasm – less frequently the oculomotor cranial nerves -only seen on MR images with high accuracy has been growing, and it could not be included in the volume published 10 years earlier. The clinical presentation of the optochiasmatic cavernoma mainly consists of sudden deterioration in vision, loss or restriction of the visual field depending on the location of the cavernoma and the fresh hemorrhage, acute headache depending on the size of the hemorrhage, and general malaise. Its incidence is low compared to the total number of cerebrovascular events, but it is important among the newly recognized diseases due to its specific appearance and suitability to surgical treatment. It is worth mentioning those cases, where the optochiasmatic cavernoma is an additional finding, that is, when the abnormality has not bled before or the hemorrhage did not cause any symptoms, or no imaging study was performed because of visual pathway-related complaints. Cavernomas belong to the group of arteriovenous malformations, their characteristic feature is that the direct connection(s) between the arterial and venous system does not exceed the level of the arterioles, and the veins are intraparenchymal vascular segments. For this reason, we can understand the considerably milder clinical symptoms compared to the angiomas, since hemorrhage from the cavernoma occurs by low pressure, and its damaging effect is much smaller than that of the bleeding angioma. It is also related to the fact that the hemorrhage most frequently remains within the lesion, and the blood is taken up by the cavernous veins of the lesion during the absorption of the hematoma. Through this mechanism, each hemorrhage may increase the diameter of the cavernoma. The patchy remnants of the successive hemorrhages and the vessels of the cavernoma together result in a characteristic MR image that consists of black (hemosiderin) and white (thrombus) details, while the CT scan is only positive in case of a large, newly developed hematoma, and angiography has no diagnostic value due to the small size of abnormal vessels.

Due to its clinical and neurosurgical importance corresponding to its increasing recognition, the literature on it is also growing and describes its etiology. The theories of persisting abnormalities from the early stage of vascular development or developmental variants are supported by the fact that in at least one third of the cases it coexists

J. Vajda, M.D., PhD
National Institute of Neurology, Budapest, Hungary
e-mail: janosvajda@gmail.com; http://www.oiti.hu

J. Somlai, T. Kovács (eds.), *Neuro-Ophthalmology*, DOI 10.1007/978-3-319-28956-4_7

with a focal variation of the cerebral venous system (developmental venous anomaly, DVA). At the same time it is also known that by follow-up examinations, formation and growth of cavernomas can be revealed in formerly intact regions as well. (Of course the question remains whether this is only about the size limitations of visibility, while the malformation has been there the whole time.) It has been suggested also from other impacts affecting the cerebrovascular system that they may play a role in the formation of cavernoma(s) after the development of the vascular system is completed. One of the most recent cases from the National Neurosurgical Institute is an example for this: after subtotal resection of her craniocervical malignant ependymoma, the young female patient received radiotherapy with simultaneous and successive multiple follow-up MRI scans. After 10 years, because of clinical and CT signs of brainstem hemorrhage, an MR examination was performed showing two extensive pontine cavernomas in a DVA environment, which was also not present on the previous examinations.

The multiplex appearance of optochiasmatic cavernomas is similarly characteristic to other cerebral locations, where further lesions may occur in the same or in different cerebral structures (Figs. 7.1 and 7.2). In these cases optimal timing of the treatment needs consideration based on the aspects of clinical emergency, as the individual bleeding risk of each location is unknown. The yearly risk of repeated hemorrhage of cavernomas is 1–2 % and it is accumulating, thus every surgical resection is justified, being its risk smaller than the risk of hemorrhage extrapolated on the expected life span. In most locations this means that under the age of 60, preventive surgery is also justified. In those optochiasmatic cavernoma cases that have already been published and those we have encountered in our institute, surgery was even more recommended as it was not only preventive, but also therapeutic due to the compression of the visual pathway exerted by the bleeding (Fig. 7.3). This active tendency is further supported by the fact that optochiasmatic cavernomas can be easily accessed, and they broadly reach the surface, their surgery belongs to the topic of suprasellar and temporomedial microsurgery. Our cases carry the message that cavernous vessels and venous sinuses – the characteristic of which is that they can easily be disentangled as a bunch of grapes from the gliosis – in contrast to other cerebral locations, can be shrunk by bipolar coagulation, and optochiasmatic cavernomas are anchored with a surprising amount of scar tissue in the surrounding parenchyma. The manipulation required by the necessary radicality represents higher risk, of which the surgeon should be aware. To avoid the slightest loss, the vessels should be followed even closer. All of the known and published cases improved in the optochiasmatic functions, no mortality was detected.

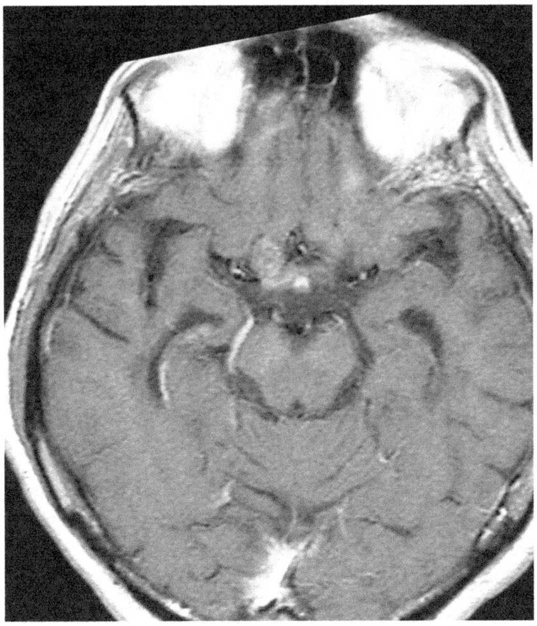

Fig. 7.1 CT scan revealing subacute hemorrhage of the left optochiasmatic cavernoma

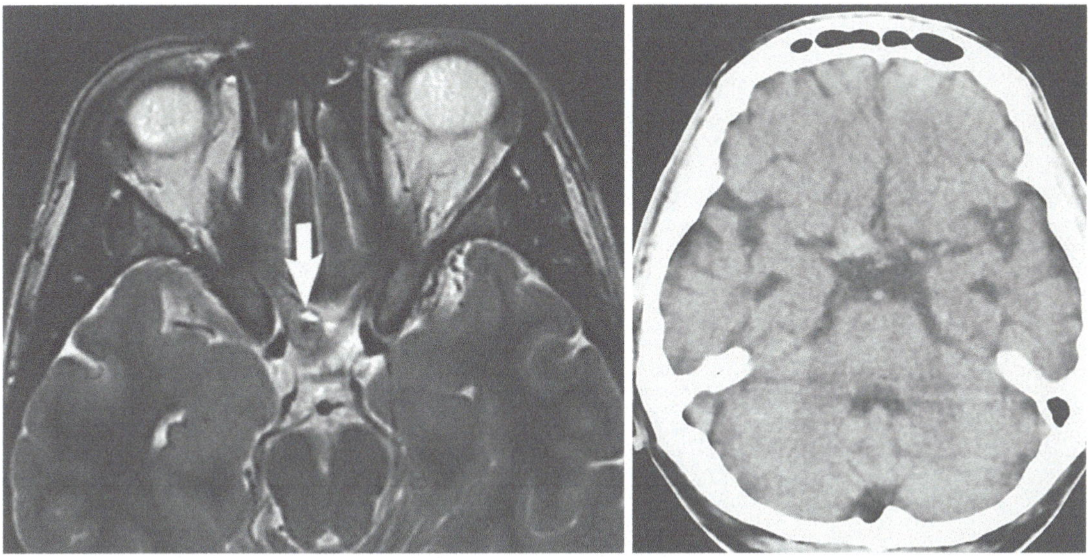

Fig. 7.2 MRI scan showing locational relationships of the cavernoma As the CT scan only proves the presence of hemorrhage, MRI scan is recommended, as the T1 and T2 scans confirm presence of the hemorrhage and provide information on its size as well, furthermore detect the consequent bleeding in the appropriate structure of the central nervous system

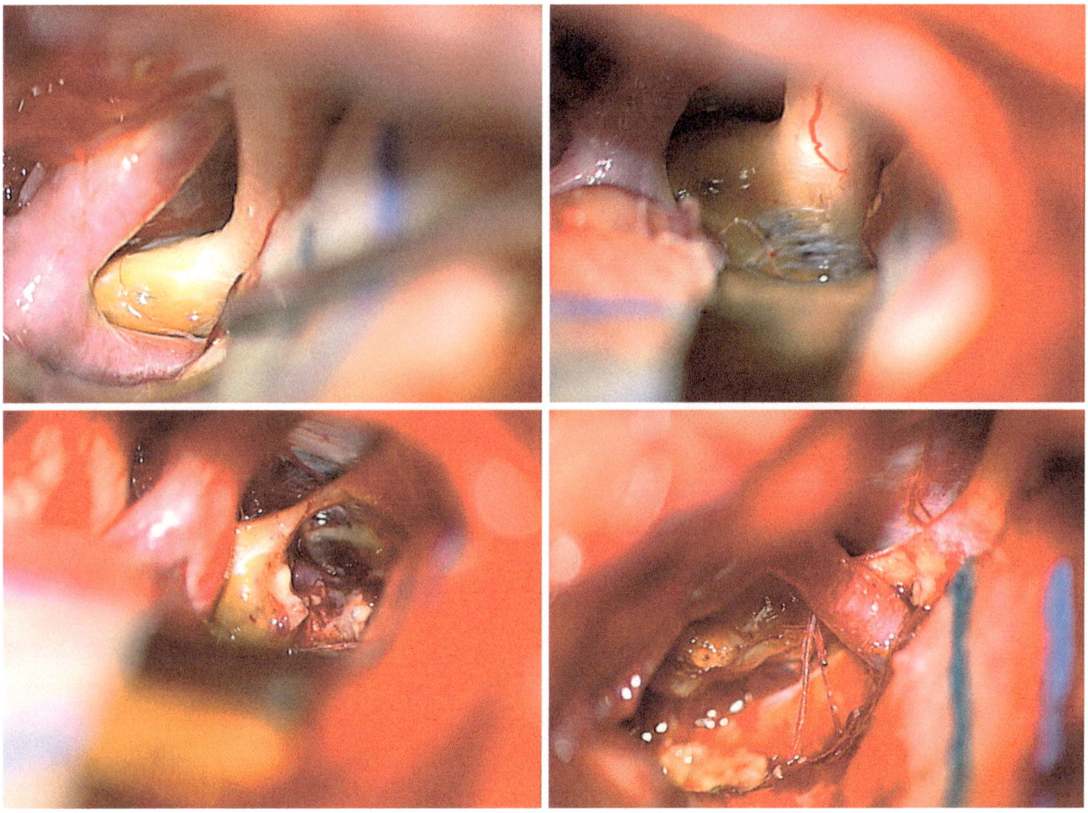

Fig. 7.3 The intraoperative image shows the stages of disentangling of the cavernoma from the fibers of the visual pathway

The Role of Gamma Knife Stereotactic Radiosurgery in the Treatment of Neuro-ophthalmological Diseases

8

György T. Szeifert and Jenô Szeifert

Contents

The terminology and principles of stereotactic radioneurosurgery were elaborated in 1951 by Professor Lars Leksell, successor of Herbert Olivecrona at the Department of Neurosurgery of the Karolinska Institute. The aim of radiosurgery is to "completely and precisely destroy the determined target volume containing pathological or normal cells, by a single, high-dose (radiotherapy) irradiation, without damaging the surrounding tissues" This effect can be achieved by the precise focusing of multiple low-energy beams to the target. Three different techniques can be applied to reach this goal: the linear accelerator (LINAC), the Bragg peak (or proton beam) and gamma knife radiosurgery. The Leksell gamma knife® (LGK) is a device specially dedicated to neurosurgical purposes, capable to destroy the desired tissues without opening the skull. It exerts its biological effect through the ionizing gamma rays of 201 pieces of cobalt-60 isotope sources positioned on a hemispheric surface and focused to the center.

Among the methods available so far, LGK has proven to be the most precise, its <0.5 mm accuracy makes it particularly suitable for delicate neurosurgical interventions. Radioneurosurgery was originally developed for the treatment of functional neurological diseases (drug-resistant pain), but soon brain tumors and arteriovenous malformations (AVM) became the main target of the procedure. It has acquired a significant role in the treatment of neuro-ophthalmological diseases as well. The prototype of the gamma knife was installed in 1967 in Stockholm at the Sophiahemmet Hospital (Figs. 8.1 and 8.2), and since then more than 600,000 patients were treated with this device in the currently functioning nearly 300 LGK centers of the world.

Based on the clinical experience gained so far, LGK became the "gold standard" in radioneurosurgery. The C-model of the LGK, the main technical novelty of which is a computer-guided robot, the automatic positioning system (APS), was installed in 1999 at the Erasmus Hospital in Brussels. With the help of the robot, the target of the successive (radio pulses) irradiation shots can be automatically altered during the treatments, in

G.T. Szeifert, M.D., med. habil. (✉)
Unit for Neurosurgical Injuries,
Péterfy Accident Center, Semmelweis University,
Budapest, Hungary
e-mail: gszeifert@yahoo.co.uk

J. Szeifert, M.D.
Faculty of Education and Psychology,
Institute of Health Promotion and Sport Sciences,
Eötvös Lóránd University, Budapest, Hungary

J. Somlai, T. Kovács (eds.), *Neuro-Ophthalmology*, DOI 10.1007/978-3-319-28956-4_8

contrast to the earlier mechanical settings. Furthermore, such an integrated digital chain was configured, starting from the imaging to the planning and the emission of the radiation, which further increased the targeting accuracy. The latest development, LGK Perfexion (Fig. 8.3) is capable to treat the cervical region in addition to the skull, and automation of the diameter (alteration) modification of the radiation collector tubes (collimators) significantly shortened treatment time.

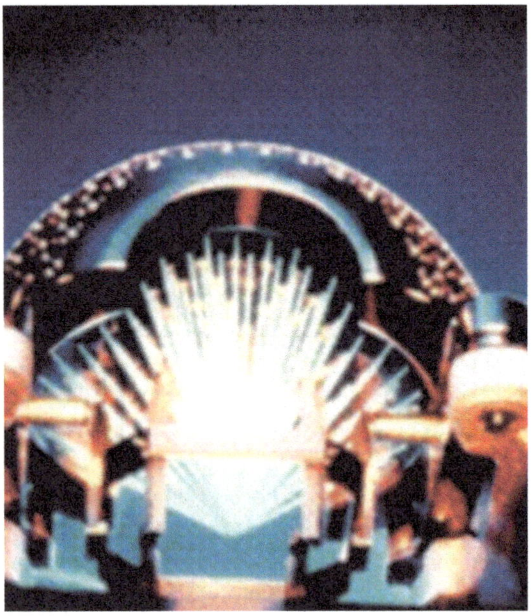

Fig. 8.1 Operating principle of the gamma knife: the hemispheric collimator helmet containing the ray collector tubes with the γ-rays focused to the center

The first model of this system started its operation in 2006 in Marseilles (Hôpital La Timone). The gamma knife has not been accepted in Hungary yet, even though it can be found in all of the neighboring countries. In Hungary the cooperation (of) between the National (Neurosurgical) Institute of Neurosurgery and the National Oncological Institute began in 1991, in Budapest with LINAC-based (radioneurosurgery) radiosurgery. Later, stereotactic radiosurgical interventions were launched with linear accelerators at the University of Pecs, in Miskolc and in Szombathely, and with a Chinese development of a rotational gamma system at the University of Debrecen.

Fields of Application

Neurosurgery has used the technical advancements of the past decades to seek the least invasive methods to be able to approach deep brain regions and pathologies while preserving the surrounding healthy tissues to the greatest possible extent. Thanks to high performance computers, advanced surgical microscopes and modern imaging techniques, neurosurgical interventions today can be planned in advance on three dimensional brain reconstructions. The *"image-guided" neuronavigation systems* help to precisely localize

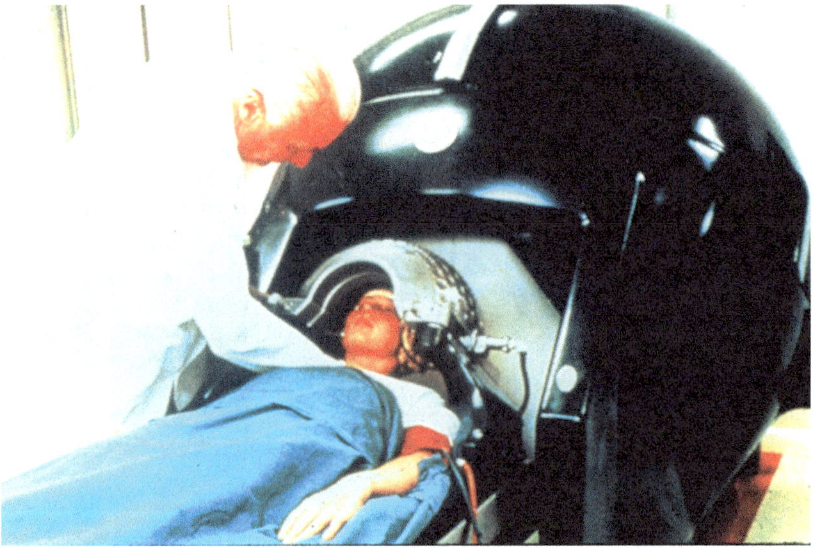

Fig. 8.2 The prototype of the gamma knife with its (creator) inventor Professor Lars Leksell

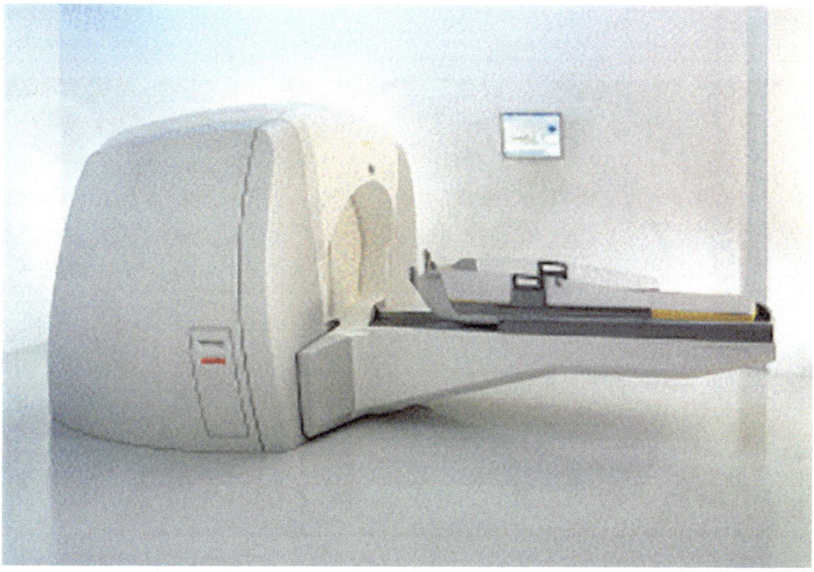

Fig. 8.3 The latest development: the Perfexion gamma knife

and find the lesion during surgery. The availability of endoscopic techniques has contributed to the better visualization of structures and their lesions in the ventricles and on the skull base. The development of electrophysiology has helped in differential diagnostics. These techniques altogether have made possible the significant decrease in the extent and invasiveness of craniotomies.

Further developing the concept of "minimally invasive neurosurgery", radiosurgery and gamma knife are now enabling surgery without general anesthesia and craniotomy, with computer-guidance and through the intact skull. Its original mission was to relieve drug-resistant pain of tumorous patients by thalamotomy. However, its indications have been significantly (widened) extended to date, and they are continuously (broadened) developing by the treatment of new diseases. The technique can be applied as primary surgery, as an alternative to conventional craniotomy to eradicate hardly accessible pathologies with high surgical risk. It can be used as secondary intervention as well, in case of recurrent or residual tumors, as complementary therapy to other procedures, for example in malignant glioma cases as a "booster" to chemotherapy or fractionated radiotherapy. Considering that radiosurgery operates by the effect of radiation, it works safely by lesions smaller than 3–3.5 cm in diameter and a volume of 10–15 cm^3. In case of greater tissue masses, possible undesirable side effects of radiation have to be taken into (account) consideration, therefore, in such cases the treatment may be performed in several fractions called "staged radiosurgery". Nowadays **indications** basically cover three main fields: tumors, vascular malformations and functional diseases. ***Brain tumors*** make up two thirds of the procedures, within this single and multiple carcinoma metastases take the first place (Fig. 8.4).

A great advantage of the technique over the former surgeries with craniotomy is that it can be successfully applied in one session in case of tumors located distant from each other in different brain regions. Newly developing tumor foci can also be eradicated by further treatments. Reactivity to treatment is good (independent) irrespective of the histological type, and the treatment is also successful in case of metastases formerly considered radioresistant and unresponsive to conventional fractionated radiotherapy. Malignant astrocytomas take the second place among malignant tumors; the technique can be applied as primary treatment in hardly accessible tumor locations, for example, in case of brainstem gliomas, or additional to conventional chemotherapy as a booster. Out of benign tumors, it can be beneficial in the surgery of meningeomas (primarily at the skull base), vestibular schwannomas, pituitary tumors and the solid part of craniopharyngi-

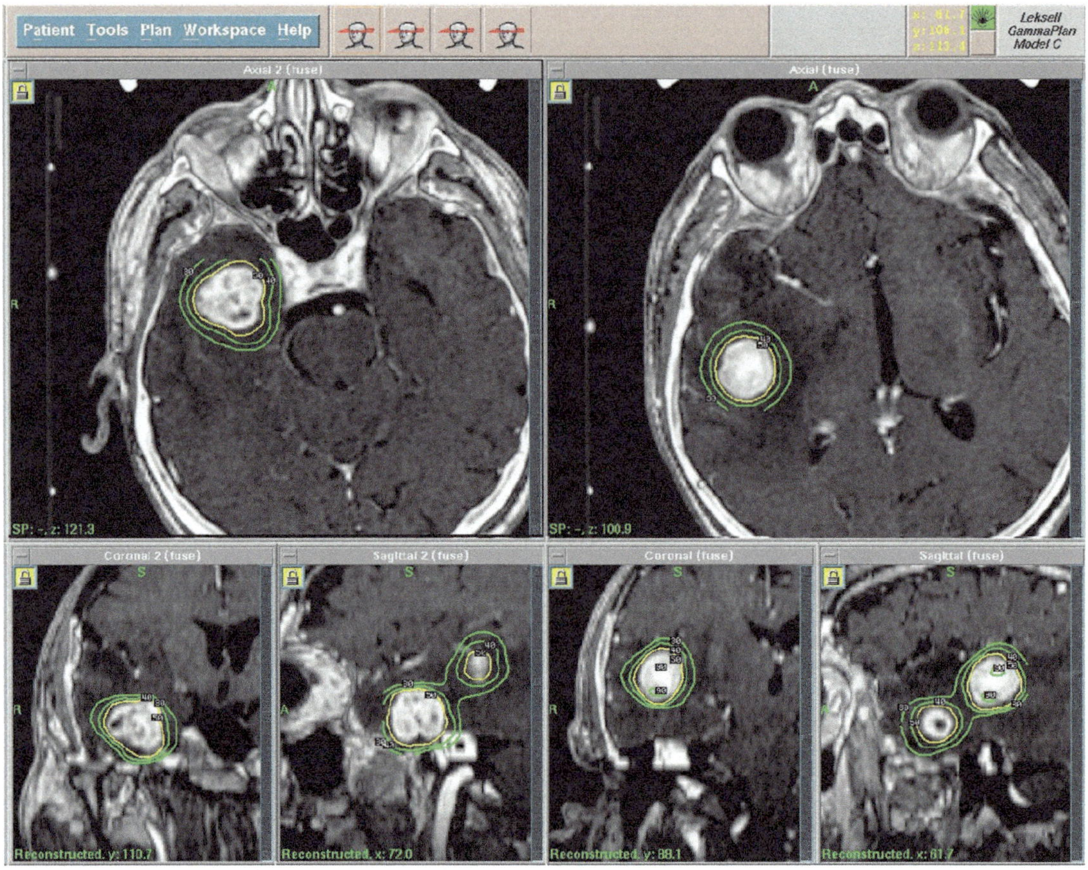

Fig. 8.4 Treatment plan of double cerebral metastases

omas. In (Of) cerebrovascular pathologies, arteriovenous malformations (AVM) were among the earliest indications, and they still constitute up (amount) to 20 % of the interventions. MRI and follow-up angiography examinations revealed that 65–87 % of the AVMs become obliterated and 75 % shrink in 2–5 years following the treatment. However, until the end of obliteration process, during the so-called latency-period, the risk of hemorrhage is still 2–4 % each year, according to the natural history of the disease. Results are contradictory regarding cavernomas, publications supporting and disapproving the treatment effect both exist, further long-term international follow-up studies are (needed) required to see its effects clearly. The treatment of venous anomalies (DVA) is contraindicated, since these malformations are part of the physiological venous drainage and have to be considered as a developmental variant. It cannot be applied for aneurysm surgery; there were some attempts, but the results are not convincing. Regarding the importance of the task, it is one of the big future challenges of gamma-neurosurgery, and it awaits to be solved.

In ***functional diseases,*** it is applied with excellent results to cease or relieve trigeminal neuralgia. Considering the high success rate (of the treatment) and the low risk of the intervention, in many centers it is recommended as first-line treatment. In other functional diseases, thalamotomy and pallidotomy were performed to decrease tremor, and capsulotomy by gamma knife was successfully made in obscessive-compulsive disorders. In drug-resistant epilepsies lesionectomy and selective amygdalo-hippocampectomy were also performed, but this technique has not become widely used in these cases because of the side effects. In pediatric neurosurgery, it is functioning with similarly good results as in the above mentioned cases. The ossification of the skull limits

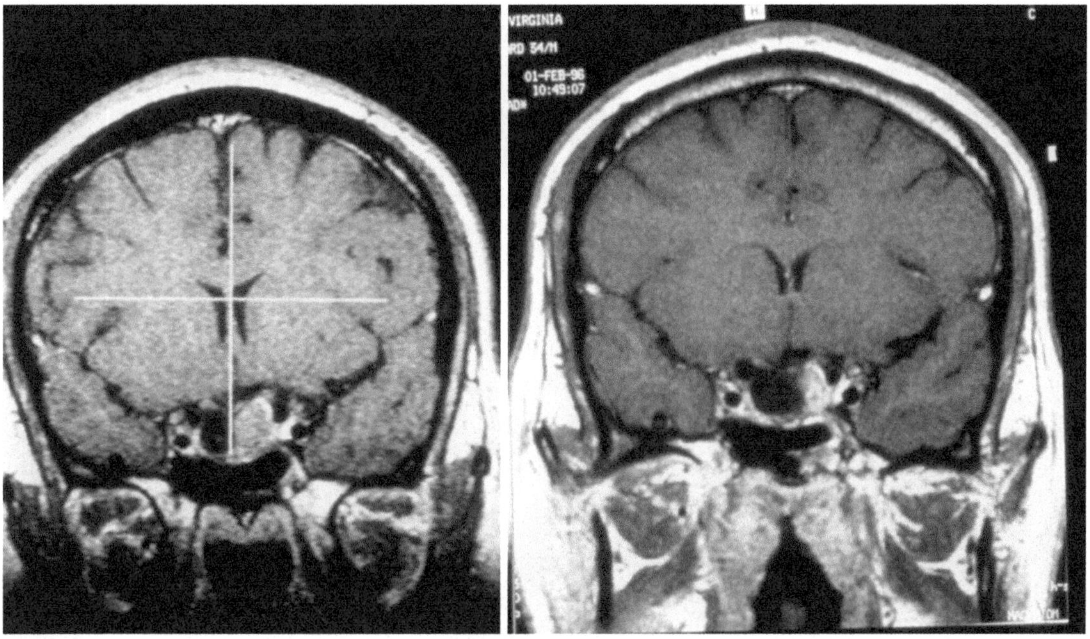

Fig. 8.5 Pituitary tumor reaching the chiasm during GK treatment (*left side*). Shrinkage can be seen at 1-year follow up (*right side*)

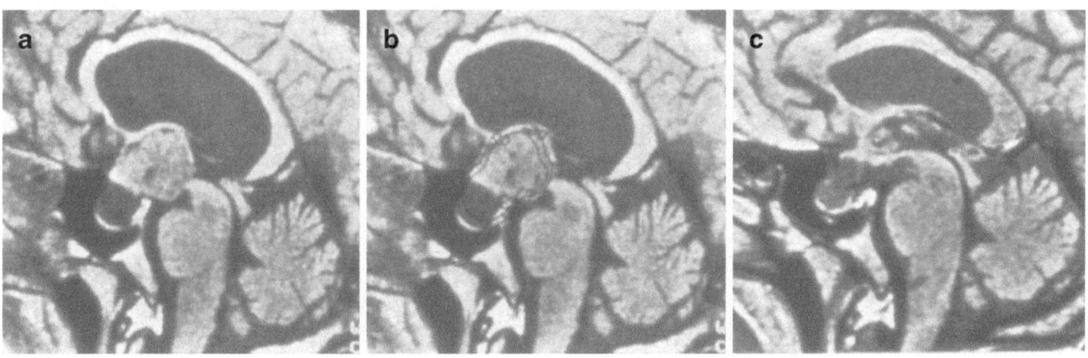

Fig. 8.6 Regression due to radiosurgery of intra-suprasellar craniopharyngeoma causing a chiasm lesion

the age of applicability (approximately 2 years), as the frame has to be attached. General anesthesia is necessary in case of small children with difficulty in cooperation.

Its ***application in neuro-ophthalmology*** may be necessary in special locations of the above mentioned pathologies, which may affect the eyes, the orbit, and any part of the visual pathway. Ocular indications comprise uveal melanomas, ocular metastases, advanced-stage glaucoma, age-dependent macular degeneration, hemangioblastomas, angioreticulomas, pseudotumors and autonomic pain. The treatment of ocular diseases requires special manipulations, considering that the eyes move, and they have to be fixated before the intervention, and because of the eccentric position, the irradiation is performed in prone position, that is while lying with the abdomen down. In diseases of the orbit, the gamma knife can be used for the treatment of different tumors. From the pathologies affecting the various segments of the visual pathway, it is most frequently used to eradicate tumors of the sellar, suprasellar and parasellar regions, that is, pituitary tumors, craniopharyngiomas, meningeomas and metastases (Figs. 8.5, 8.6 and 8.7).

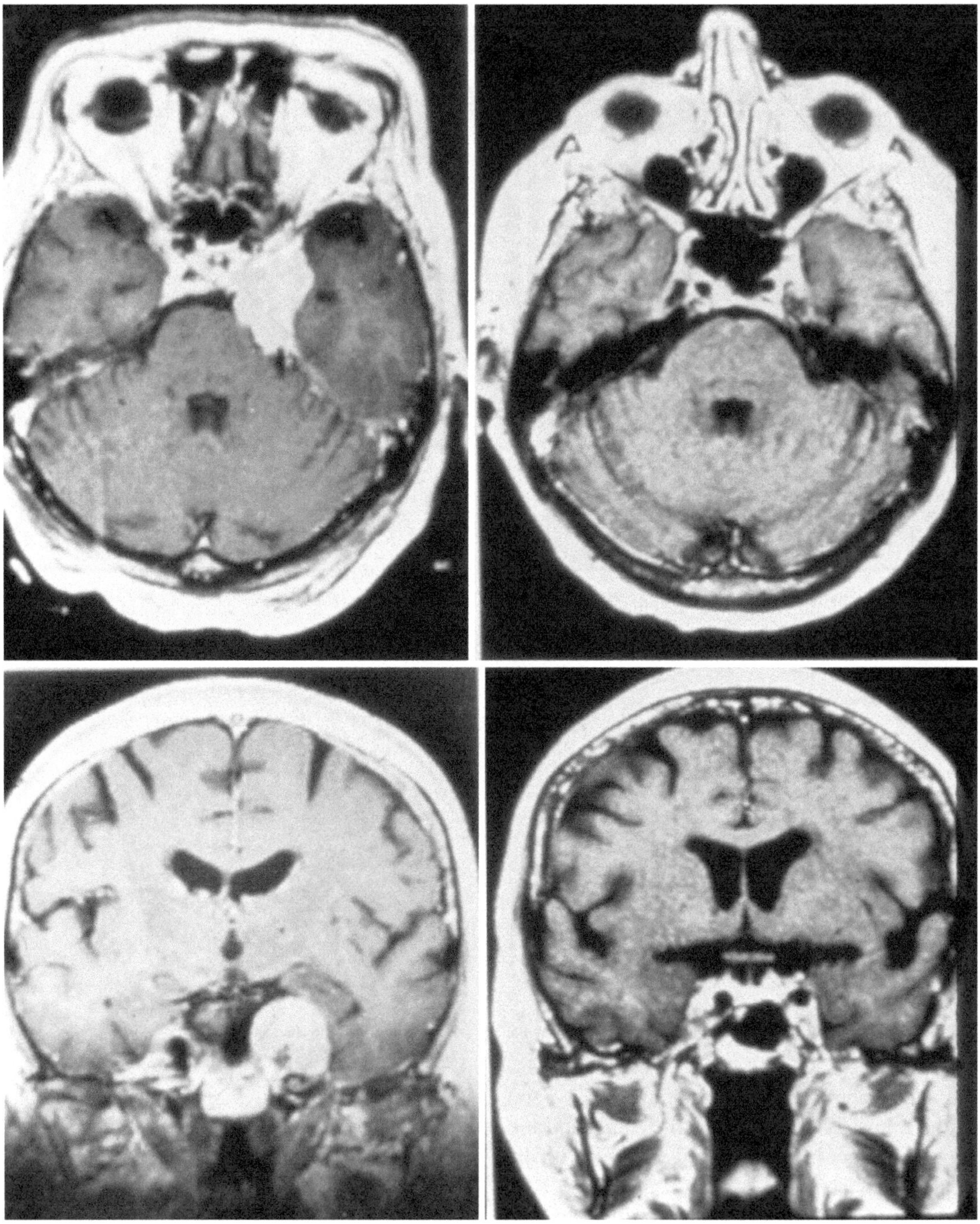

Fig. 8.7 Parasellar meningeoma (*left side*) causing eye movement disorder. One year after the gamma radiosurgery, the tumor has vanished

Because of the proximity of the optic nerve, oculomotor nerves and optic chiasm, these interventions require very cautious and careful planning, since the structures mentioned above are considerably sensitive to radiation, therefore, the rays of irradiation that would possibly cross and damage them are eliminated by an exclusion program. Hemispheric, parenchymal

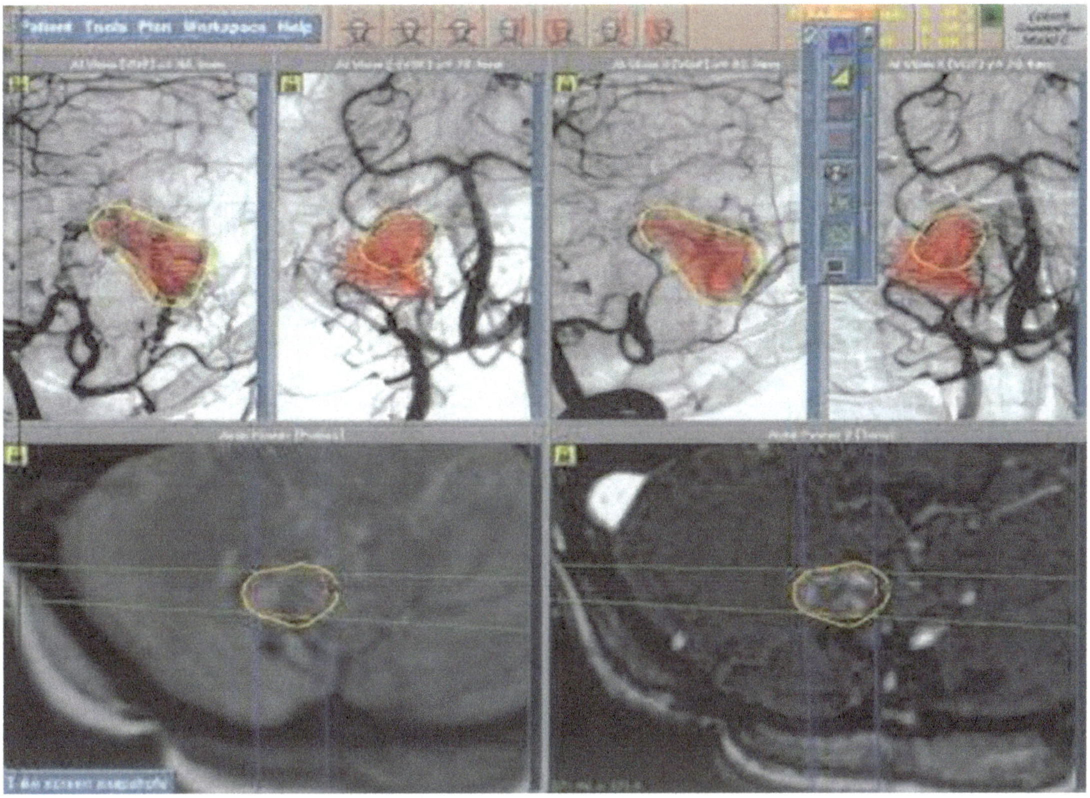

Fig. 8.8 Treatment plan of gamma knife radiosurgery in a case of an arteriovenous malformation (AVM)

(focal gliomas), and extraparenchymal (metastases, meningeomas) tumors and arteriovenous malformations (Fig. 8.8) damaging the fibers of the optic radiation and the occipital visual cortex make up a significant portion of gamma knife radiosurgical interventions.

Phases of Gamma Knife Radiosurgery

The procedure can be performed as 1-day surgery; on the first day the patient is admitted for the treatment, usually the next day the patient can be discharged to his/her home, there is no need for intensive care. Surgical intervention begins with the attachment of the stereotactic frame (Leksell Frame G-Model, Elekta) to the patient's head (Fig. 8.9), generally under local anesthesia (children or restless patients may require general anesthesia).

A basic part of the procedure is that the target volume desired to be destroyed within the brain, the eyeball or the orbit has to be positioned in the center or its proximity of the X, Y, Z coordinate system determined by the frame. This is followed by the stereotactic targeting by imaging procedures, based on an MRI examination in most centers. Although the resolution of the MRI is sensitive to brain tissue and its pathologies, it is susceptible to spatial distortion(s), which is compensated by the fusion of the MR images to CT scans. For the treatment of vascular malformations, MR and CT examinations are completed by angiography. Out of functional imaging techniques, positron emission tomography (PET) examinations may be of substantial help in determining the target volume in case of lesions with poorly defined border, for example gliomas. Visualization of the different metabolic activity of normal and pathological brain regions greatly contributes to the

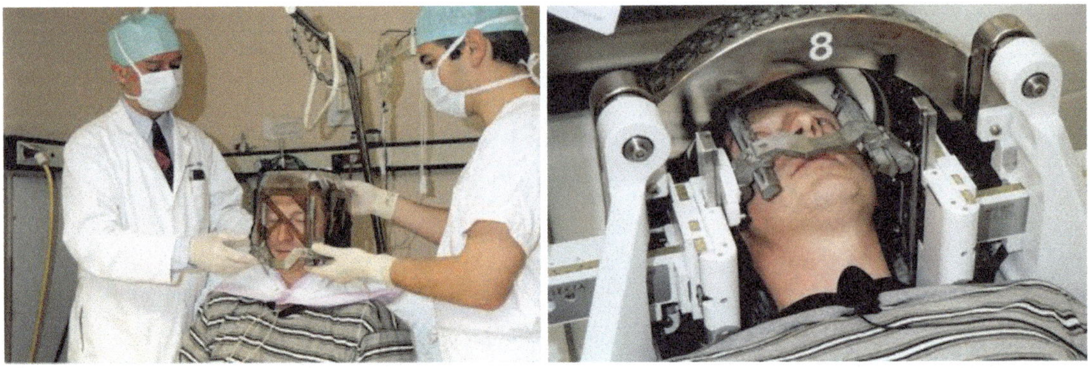

Fig. 8.9 Attachment of the stereotactic frame (*left side*), and fixation of the patient's head with APS for gamma knife radiosurgery (*right side*)

differentiation of neurological, neuro-ophthalmological and also neurosurgical diseases, (even in) cases, when conventional imaging techniques do not show obvious morphological abnormality. The resulting metabolic data make it possible to perform sophisticated planning by integrating them into the static anatomy derived by the MRI and CT scans. The image-transfer to the planning computer is possible via internet or intranet. This helps to perform the most important operation of the procedure requiring high (the most) expertise: the definition and anatomical delineation of the target volume desired to destroy, and the planning of the radiosurgery. This process evolves as a result of teamwork, with the cooperation of a neurosurgeon, a radiologist, an oncologist and a physicist. The treatment plan is made by setting the diameter, spatial position and dosing of the different shots of radiation. High performance computers make it possible to perform three dimensional simulation of the dose distribution on the stereotactic CT, MR and DSA images. The aim is to create a spatial formation that fits best to the shape of the target volume and covers it completely ("high conformity"), while the neighboring normal tissues receive only minimal radiation ("high selectivity"). The planning is finished by determining the dosing of the radiation influenced by the volume of the lesion, its histological type, relation to surrounding eloquent structures and prior radiotherapy. Next, the data are digitally transferred to the controlling computer. During gamma knife radiosurgery, the patient's head is fixed to the automatic positioning system via the stereotactic frame (Fig. 8.9).

During the treatment, for each shot of radiation, the APS changes the stereotactic coordinates based on the data of the computer to bring the different parts of the target volume in the center of the radiation unit. The frame is removed after the end of radiation surgery. The patient is under observation for one night, and can usually be discharged the next day being in the same condition as on admission, without being restricted in basic activities necessary for self-care. Irritating symptoms, general malaise, headache, nausea and cranial nerve symptoms may develop as rare side effects, but they are mostly transient and relieved after a few days of medical treatment.

Limitations of the Technique

According to its original purpose and construction, gamma knife has limitations in the aspects of anatomy and indications. The anatomical restriction of the C model used in two thirds of the centers is the skull base, it cannot reach lesions located caudal to the level of the foramen magnum. The nowadays expanding gamma knife Perfexion can be applied for pathologies of the cervical region as well. Limitations of its indication may be mainly represented by diffuse and infiltrating pathologies greater than 3 cm (for example astrocytomas). In case of arteriovenous malformations, risk of hemorrhage is present until the complete obliteration (2 years on average) and the treatment has to be repeated in certain cases. Since the source of radiation is the radioactive cobalt-60, with the decay of the isotope, the radiation energy of the gamma knife is decreased, resulting in proportionate elongation of the treatment time. The half-life of the Co-60 is 5.26 years, and according to the general practice, (refill) reloading necessary in a 7–10 years period.

Possibilities of Further Development

Regarding the minimally invasive character and the low cost-effectiveness of radiosurgery compared to conventional surgical interventions with craniotomy, the demand for radiosurgical techniques is considerably increasing worldwide. The treatment of neuro-ophthalmological disorders may be one of the most dynamically developing fields, as currently there are many unexploited possibilities. This question may be especially prominent in Hungary, where the capacity in operating rooms and intensive care beds available for neurosurgical interventions is 50 % lower than the European average. The number of gamma knife interventions has shown a fourfold yearly increase in the last 10 years, the number of the newly installed centers has duplicated in each year. A great advantage of gamma knife over other radiosurgical techniques is that a uniform system has been created worldwide with a central database, to which each center is connected. More than 1500 publications have reported on the experience of the past four decades. Thanks to the scientific activity and the (uniformed) unified system, treatments are performed based on similar principles and with similar results worldwide. The straightforwardness and accessibility of data have greatly increased confidence in the technique. As CT, MRI and DSA have become a standard procedure in neurosurgical practice, radiosurgery also has to be an integrated part of the neurosurgical armamentarium in the twenty-first century. This is demanded above all by the aspects of the patients in need, and not at least by the interests of the health care financing as well.

Further Readings

Bagó A, Fedorcsák I, Nyáry I. A neuronavigáció és szerepe a modern idegsebészetben. Új módszer ismertetése, elso hazai tapasztalatok [Neuronavigation and its role in modern neurosurgery. Review of the new method, first Hungarian experience]. Clin Neurosci/ Ideggy Szle. 2000;53:20–7.

Czirják S, Szeifert GT. Surgical experience with frontolateral keyhole craniotomy through a superciliary skin incision. Neurosurgery. 2001;48:145–50.

Fedorcsák I, Kontra G, Horváth A, Szabó L. Agyi stereotaxiás sugársebészet. A módszer ismertetése és az elso hazai sugársebészeti rendszer bemutatása [Stereotactic radiosurgery of the brain. Review of the method and presentation of the first radiosurgical system in Hungary]. Orv Hetil. 1992;133:289–92.

Lunsford LD, Sheehan JP, editors. Intracranial stereotactic radiosurgery. New York: Thieme; 2009.

Langmann G, Pendl G, Müllner K. Gamma knife radiosurgery for uveal melanomas: an 8-year experience. J Neurosurg. 2000;(Suppl 3):184–9.

Larsson B, Leksell L, Rexed B, et al. The high-energy proton beam as a neurosurgical tool. Nature. 1958;182: 1222–3.

Leksell L. The stereotactic method and radiosurgery of the brain. Acta Chir Scand. 1951;102:316–9.

Szeifert GT, Kondziolka D, Levivier M, Lunsford LD, editors. Radiosurgery and pathological fundamentals. In: Lunsford LD, editor. Progress in neurological surgery, vol 20. Karger: Basel; 2007.

Steiner L, Leksell L, Greitz J, et al. Stereotaxic radiosurgery for cerebral arteriovenous malformations. Acta Chir Scand. 1972;138:459–64.

Gildenberg PL, Tasker RR, editors. Stereotactic and functional neurosurgery. New York: McGraw-Hill; 1998.

Neurointerventional Treatment of Diseases Causing Neuro-ophthalmological Symptoms

9

Istvan Szikora

Contents

I. Szikora, M.D., PhD
Neurointerventional Unit,
National Institute of Neurology, Budapest, Hungary
e-mail: szikora@oiti.hu; http://www.oiti.hu

Introduction

Due to the rapid development of Digital Subtraction Angiography (DSA) and endovascular treatment techniques, interventional neuroradiology (or in short neurointerventional therapy) has gained an outstanding role in the treatment of a significant proportion of cerebrovascular diseases in the past decades. Due to the anatomical relationships, several cerebrovascular diseases cause neuro-ophthalmological symptoms directly or indirectly. Vascular pathologies in the background of these diseases or being located right in the orbit can generally be approached well with the tools of neurointervention, furthermore, they often represent the first-choice technique.

Aneurysms in the cavernous sinus (CS), in the supraclinoid segment of the internal carotid artery (ICA) and arteriovenous shunts within or on the surface of the CS, cause symptoms in an indirect fashion. Thrombosis or embolism of the central retinal artery (CRA) developing in association with the stenosis or embolism of the ICA causes symptoms in a direct way. Of neoplastic diseases, neuorinterventional therapy may have a role in the treatment of retinoblastoma.

In the followings we review the pathology, pathomechanism, imaging diagnosis, the technique and expected results of neurointerventional therapy of intracranial and intraorbital diseases treatable by neurointerventional methods.

J. Somlai, T. Kovács (eds.), *Neuro-Ophthalmology*, DOI 10.1007/978-3-319-28956-4_9

Aneurysms of the Extradural and Supraclinoid Internal Carotid Artery

Pathology and Pathomechanism

Rupture of the Aneurysm

There are two mechanisms by which aneurysms of the ICA may cause symptoms. Following rupture of smaller aneurysms, mechanical pressure of the hemorrhage and chemical irritation may both cause damage to the cranial nerves running in the neighborhood. This occurs mainly in case of aneurysms located in the junction of the ICA – Posterior Communicating Artery (PCom). Sudden growth of the aneurysm located there frequently causes headache and partial oculomotor nerve palsy, even without subarachnoid hemorrhage (SAH). However, these symptoms are worth to be regarded as alarming signs, because the SAH may often occur in a few days or maybe weeks. SAH after rupture of the PCom aneurysm is often associated with complete or partial oculomotor nerve palsy (Fig. 9.1a–c).

Compression of Cranial Nerves Due to Aneurysm

ACI aneurysms within the CS do not cause SAH because of their extradural location. Thus, they

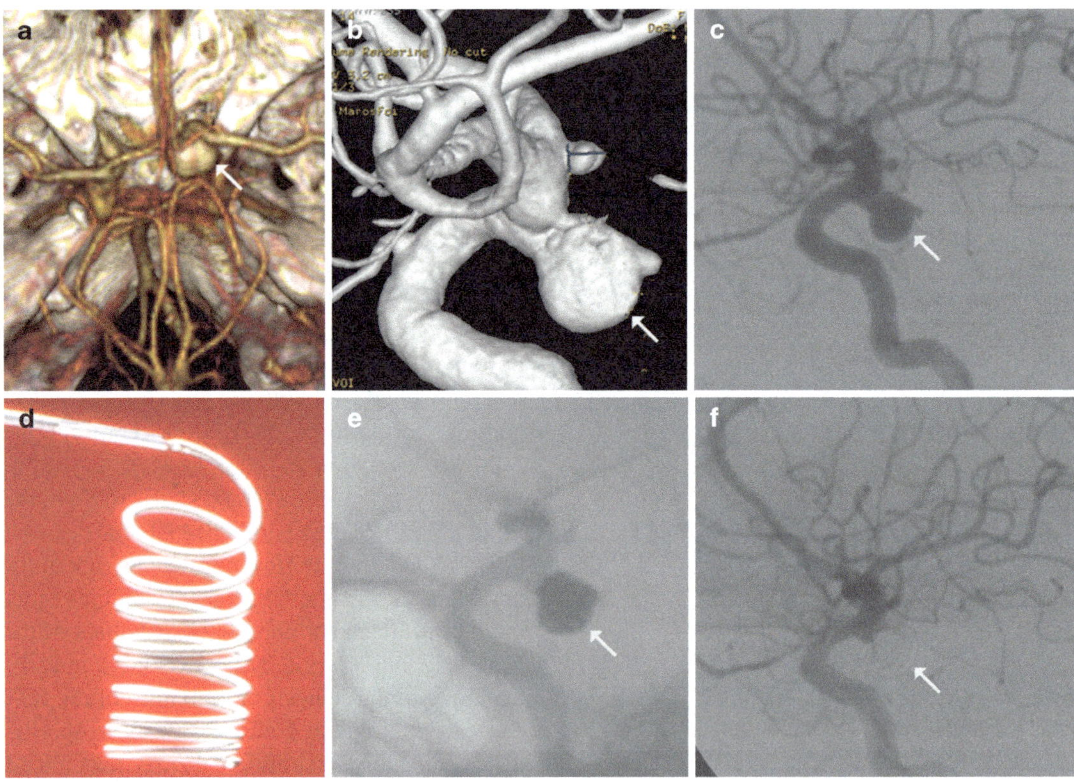

Fig. 9.1 Aneurysm of the Internal Carotid Artery (ICA) – Posterior Communicating Artery (PCom) and its neurointerventional treatment with microcoils (**a**) CT angiography (CTA). The aneurysm in the posterior wall of the ICA is indicated by an *arrow*. (**b**) Digital Subtraction Angiography (DSA): left ICA contrast angiography, 3D reconstruction. The aneurysm is indicated by an *arrow*. (**c**) DSA left ICA contrast angiography, lateral 2D image of the angiography. The aneurysm is indicated by an *arrow*. (**d**) Detachable microcoil for the occlusion of aneurysms (GDC microcoil, Boston Scientific Neurovascular, Fremont, CA, USA). (**e**) The shadow of the microcoils inserted in the aneurysm is indicated by an *arrow* in the fluoroscopic image. (**f**) Lateral DSA image after the treatment, left ICA contrast angiography. There is no enhancement in the aneurysm. The subtraction artifact of the inserted microcoils is indicated by an *arrow*

can reach quite big size (2–3 cm) in a symptom- and complaint-free state, while they are increasingly bending the lateral wall of the CS in a lateral direction. Subsequently, diplopia and frequently a severe hemicranial headache develop, often with a sudden onset and accompanied by nausea. It is the compression of the abducens nerve that is responsible for the diplopia, which is often accompanied by irritation of the 1st and 2nd branches of the trigeminal nerve as well (Fig. 9.2a, b).

Of supraclinoid ICA aneurysms, those located near the origin of the ophthalmic artery (OA), that is the paraophthalmic aneurysms, also frequently reach a remarkable size due to their hemodynamic characteristics, before they rupture. Larger paraopthalmic aneurysms may expand the optic nerve, causing progressive deterioration in vision (Fig. 9.3a, b).

Imaging Diagnosis

After SAH, the fastest and most effective imaging diagnostic algorithm is to perform cranial computer tomography (CT) and computer tomography-angiography (CTA) in a single session (Fig. 9.1a). The latter is usually also sufficient to determine the treatment method (neurointervention or open surgery) of the detected aneurysm. The most frequently used imaging techniques to detect aneurysms without hemorrhage are magnetic resonance imaging (MRI) (Fig. 9.3b) and

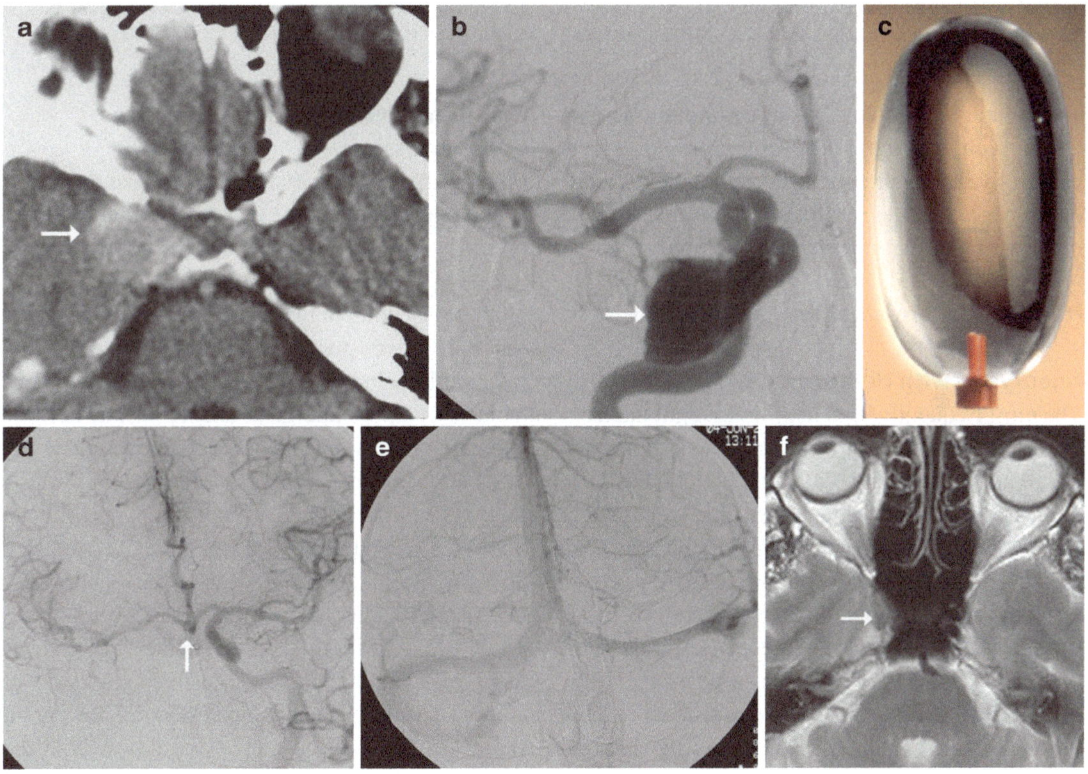

Fig. 9.2 Permanent balloon occlusion of the Internal Carotid Artery because of intracavernous giant aneurysm. (**a**) Postcontrast cranial CT. The right cavernous sinus is inflated, the inhomogeneous contrast enhancement indicates the giant aneurysm within it (*arrow*). (**b**) DSA, the right ICA contrast angiography depicts the giant aneurysm (*arrow*). (**c**) Detachable microballoon used for vascular occlusion (DSB balloon, Boston Scientific, Fremont, CA, USA). (**d**) Test occlusion. DSA, left ICA contrast angiography and right ICA balloon occlusion, arterial phase. The intracranial branches of the right ICA are also filled completely through the anterior communicating artery (*arrow*). (**e**) Test occlusion. DSA, left ICA contrast angiography and right ICA balloon occlusion, venous phase. The right and left hemispheric venous systems are depicted simultaneously and symmetrically, proving satisfactory cross-circulation. (**f**) Axial, T2-weighted spin echo MR scan made half year after the occlusion of the ICA, showing the collapsed right cavernous sinus (*arrow*). The aneurysm cannot be seen

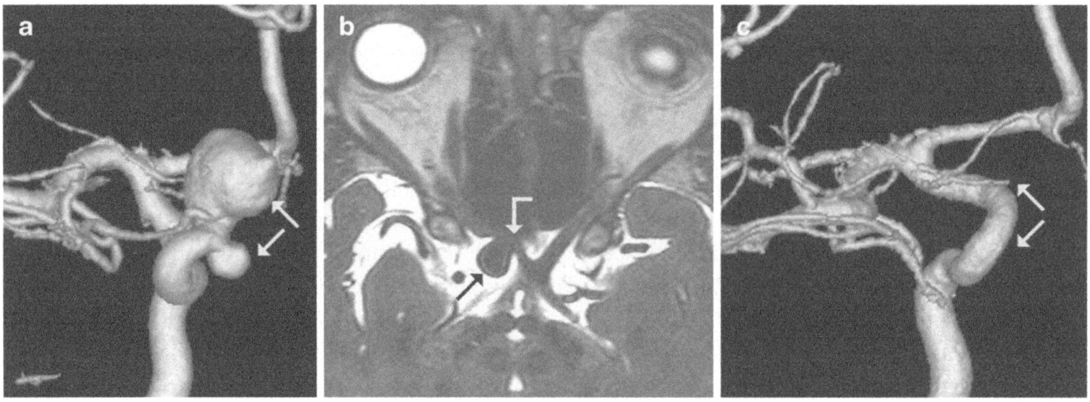

Fig. 9.3 Aneurysm of the Internal Carotid Artery (ICA) – Ophthalmic Artery junction. (**a**) DSA, right ICA contrast angiography, 3D reconstruction, PA direction. The double aneurysms of the paraophthalmic segment of the ICA are indicated with *arrows*. (**b**) Heavily T2-weighted (cisternography) spin echo MR image, axial plane. The aneurysm of the right ICA (*arrow*) bends the right optic nerve medially and anteriorly (*broken arrow*) (**c**) DSA, 3D reconstruction, right ICA contrast angiography 6 months after the insertion of the flow diverter stent. The aneurysms cannot be seen, the *arrows* indicate the reconstructed lumen of the ICA

angiography (MRA). These examinations can detect well the mass and compression effects caused by the aneurysm. However, catheter angiography (DSA) is mostly indispensable for the making of the treatment plan.

Neurointerventional Therapy

Aneurysms with Hemorrhage

The most frequently used neurointerventional technique for the treatment of aneurysms is filling the aneurysm sac with embolic material, which is most often a controlled-release detachable platinum microcoil. In case of aneurysms with hemorrhage, the advantages of this technique has been proven by a randomized comparative trial, therefore, this is the intervention of choice in these cases, if the morphology of the aneurysm makes it possible. Under continuous fluoroscopy, the aneurysm sac is filled through a microcatheter inserted via the femoral artery (FA) with microcoils of various sizes and configurations, until the contrast filling of the sac disappears (Fig. 9.1b–f). Although the volume of the aneurysms treated this way is not reduced after the treatment, the oculomotor nerve palsy, which develops after the rupture, generally disappears or considerably improves in a few weeks or maybe months. This speaks for that symptoms are rather caused by the chemical irritation of the hemorrhage, than the physical compression.

Giant Aneurysms Causing Symptoms of Compression

First of all, it is important to emphasize that since aneurysms located in the CS are of extradural location, they are only to be treated in symptomatic cases. As they have no risk of causing SAH, it is unnecessary to treat them in an asymptomatic state for preventive purposes. The above described microcoil occlusion is less successful in the treatment of symptomatic giant aneurysms, as in these cases symptoms are unequivocally caused by the mass effect of the aneurysm. The thorough filling of the sac may reduce its pulsation resulting in improvement, but the mass effect cannot be relieved this way. Besides, recurrence is quite frequent after microcoil occlusion of giant aneurysm sacs. Therefore, two methods are suitable for the treatment of giant aneurysms causing symptoms of compression: permanent occlusion of the parent vessel (ICA) or modifying of the flow within the parent vessel causing thrombosis of the aneurysm. Earlier only the first one of the two methods was available. The occlusion of the parent vessel is a feasible procedure even nowadays. Obviously, its criterion is that the function of the ICA to be occluded has to be substituted by the Willis circle through the contralateral ICA or the posterior circulation. The collateral circulation can be examined with DSA. A simple method is the filling of the contralateral carotid or vertebral artery during

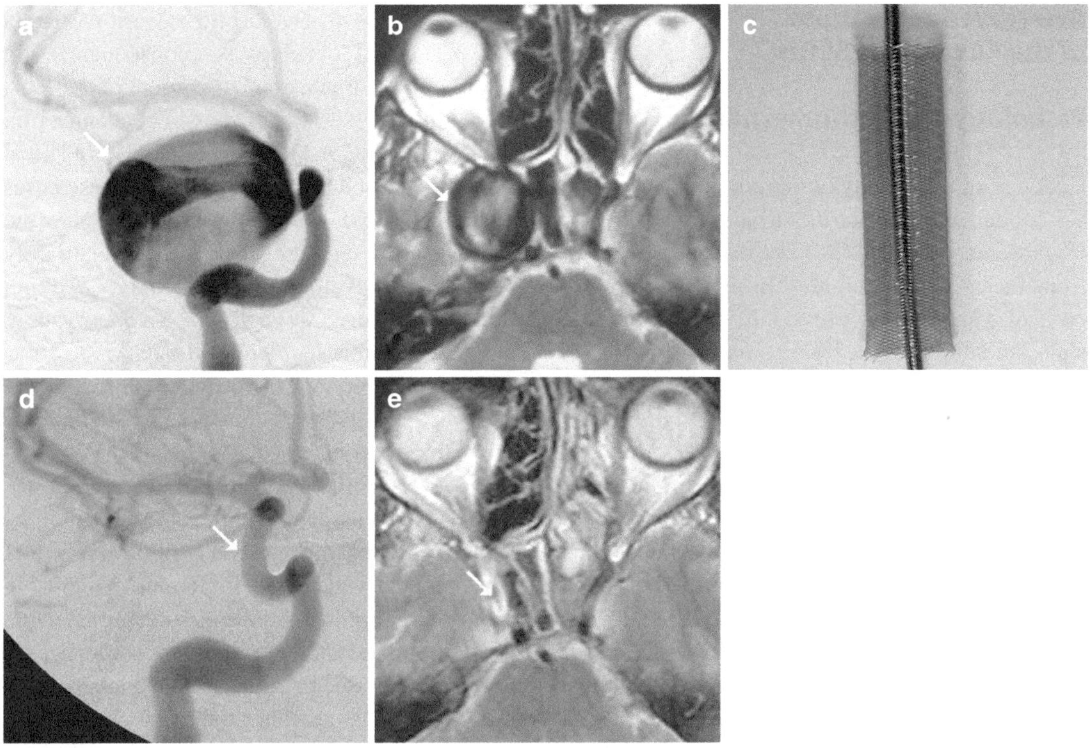

Fig. 9.4 Intracavernous giant aneurysm of the Internal Carotid Artery (ICA) and its neurointerventional treatment with flow diversion. (**a**) DSA, right ICA contrast angiography, image in oblique PA direction. The giant aneurysm is indicated by an *arrow*. (**b**) Axial T2-weighted spin echo MR image. On the right side the lateral wall of the cavernous sinus is laterally bent, the giant aneurysm within it can be seen as a flow void signal (*arrow*). (**c**) Flow diverter stent with high metal coverage (Pipeline stent, EV3, Irvine, CA, USA). (**d**) DSA, right ICA contrast angiography, 6 months later. The aneurysm cannot be seen, its location is indicated with an *arrow*. The lumen of the ICA is completely reconstructed. (**e**) Axial, T2-weighted spin echo MR image 2 years after the treatment. The aneurysm has disappeared, the inflated cavernous sinus has collapsed (*arrow*)

the manual compression of the common carotid artery to be occluded. In this case, the examination of the venous filling is particularly important besides the evaluation of the arterial cross circulation. If the venous phase occurs simultaneously on both sides, or there is no delay longer than 2 s on the side to be occluded, the ICA can be sacrificed. In this case, the ICA carrying the aneurysm is occluded with a detachable microballoon (Fig. 9.2). The reliability of the method can be increased with simultaneous transcranial Doppler examination.

However, the occlusion of the ICA carries approximately 5 % risk of ischemic side effect, even after the thoroughest examination of cross circulation, its long-term results are uncertain, but it is known to increase the risk of the development of a novel aneurysm in the contralateral ICA or the anterior communicating artery (ACom). Therefore, given the currently available technical options, it seems more feasible to modify the flow in the ICA with the application of flow-diverter stents, so that this would lead to thrombosis of the aneurysm. These internal vascular prostheses are adequately flexible to be inserted through the carotid artery into the appropriate position, but their metal coverage is sufficient to slow down the flow between the parent vessel and the aneurysm to the extent that it induces thrombosis of the aneurysm. With this method it is possible to achieve in almost 100 % of cases the complete occlusion of aneurysms causing symptoms of compression, and their collapse, that is the cessation of mass effect, is also confirmable by MRI (Figs. 9.3 and 9.4), in rare cases (<1 %), however, hemorrhagic side effects may occur.

Arteriovenous Shunts of the Cavernous Sinus

Pathology and Pathomechanism

Under normal hemodynamic circumstances, the CS collects blood from the orbit via the superior (SOV) and inferior (IOV) ophthalmic vein, and from the middle cerebral vein and the cerebral cortical venous system via the sphenoparietal sinus, and drains to the internal jugular vein (IJV) via the inferior petrosal sinus (IPS). If an arterio-venous shunt drains into the CS, the flow is reversed due to the increased pressure. Independent from the direction and source of the inward-flow, the outward-flow will be directed in a retrograde direction toward the facial venous system and the external jugular vein (EJV) via the SOV and toward the IJV via the IPS, and significantly less frequently toward the cerebral cortical venous system via the sphenoparietal sinus, obviously at a much higher than physiological pressure and flow velocity (Fig. 9.5a). All of the developing symptoms are due to the above mentioned hemodynamic changes. This is the reason for the development of clinically virtually identical symptoms in pathologically completely different diseases.

One of these is the carotid-cavernous fistula (CCF). The CCF develops as a consequence of a rupture of the intracavernous segment of the ICA, accordingly it serves as a direct connection between the ICA and the CS (Fig. 9.5). It is most frequently caused by head trauma. In these cases the injury of the skull base virtually tears the intracavernous segment of the ICA. Very rarely CCF may develop spontaneously, without trauma. It is caused by rupture of an aneurysm in the intracavernous segment of the ICA.

The more frequent form of AV shunts of the CS always develops "spontaneously". This form is the dural AV fistula of the CS (DAVF). The pathogenesis of the DAVF is not exactly known, but it is suggested that it develops during the recanalization of a former sinus thrombosis. It is most frequently detected in female patients in advanced age and with diabetes (in contrast to the mostly traumatic CCF, which is rather the disease of young males due to the traumatic background). Its essence is that an abnormal connection develops between the arteries supplying the wall of the affected dural sinus and the cavity of the sinus. Therefore in case of CS-DAVF there is no direct connection between the lumens of the ICA and the CS. The AV shunt is formed between the countless minor arteries and the cavity of the

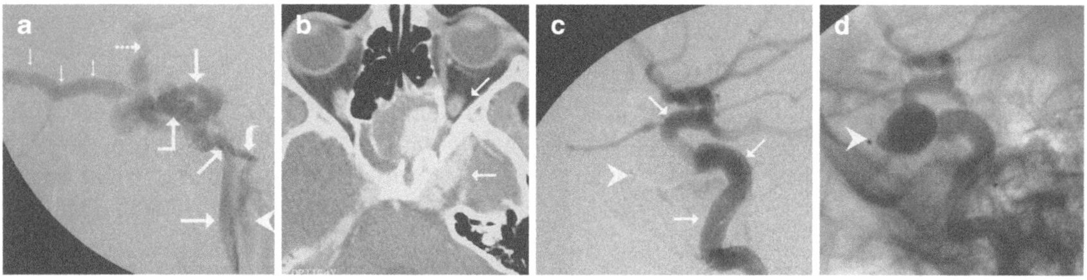

Fig. 9.5 Carotid-cavernous fistula and its neurointerventional treatment. (**a**) DSA, ICA contrast angiography, image in oblique direction. The *arrows* indicate the distal cervical and intracavernous segments of the ICA. There is no filling in the intracranial segment due to the stealing effect of the fistula. The cavernous sinus (*broken arrow*) is filled in the early arterial phase due to the fast-flow shunt. From here, venous drainage is directed toward the orbit via the superior ophthalmic vein (*small arrows*), toward the medial cerebral vein via the sphenoparietal sinus (*dashed arrow*) and toward the internal jugular vein (*arrowhead*) via the inferior petrous sinus (*tilted arrow*). (**b**) Postcontrast cranial CT. The left cavernous sinus (*arrow*) is dilated, it shows inhomogeneous enhancement. The superior ophthalmic vein is thickened (*oblique arrow*). (**c**) DSA, ICA contrast angiography, image in oblique direction. The artifact of the detached microballoon (*arrowhead*) can be seen in the cavernous sinus. The lumen of the internal carotid artery is normal, after the cessation of the steal effect its intracranial segment is filling also well (*arrows*). The filling of the fistula has disappeared, the cavernous sinus, the superior ophthalmic vein, the sphenoparietal sinus and the inferior petrous sinus cannot be seen

sinus. The supplying branches may origin from one or both external carotid arteries (ECA) and from the ICA as well (Fig. 9.6b, c). However, venous drainage is performed via the same routes as in case of the CCF. Accordingly, clinical symptoms do not differ either, at the most, the difference is that in case of the DAVF symptoms develop slowly and gradually, while in CCF suddenly. The clinical presentation is quite characteristic: exophthalmus, chemosis, ptosis, eye movement disorder aggravating frequently to complete ophthalmoplegia, in case of longer persistence progressive deterioration of vision, and continuous "locomotive" murmur (Fig. 9.6). The chemosis and the exophtalmus are caused by the intraorbital venous congestion as a consequence of the increased venous pressure; the paralysis of the oculomotor nerves is explained by the compression exerted by the elevated pressure in the CS, and the deterioration in vision is partially due to the venous congestion and partially to the compression. The objective "locomotive" murmur that can be heard with auscultation above the eye is a consequence of the arterial flow in the SOV, while the subjective murmur in the IPS is caused by blood flowing with arterial velocity. Besides the ophthalmological consequences, the disease carries the risk of SAH as well, if the venous drainage is also directed towards the cerebral cortical veins. The fast-flow CCF frequently

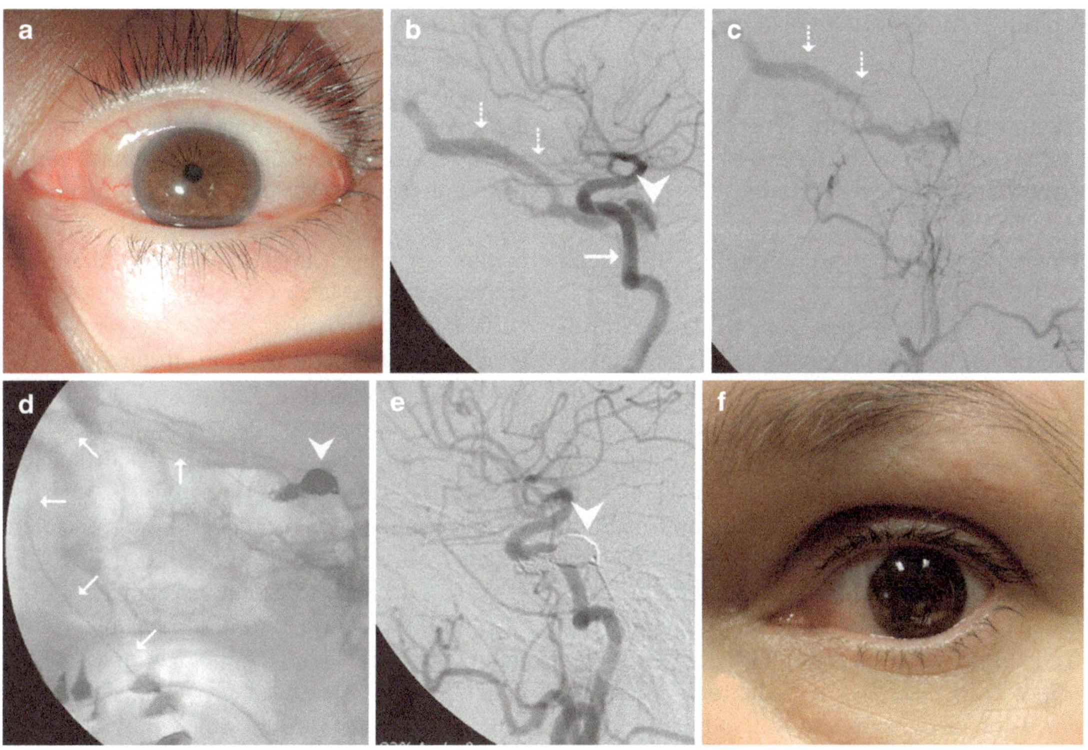

Fig. 9.6 Dural fistula of the cavernous sinus (DAVF) and its neurointerventional treatment. (**a**) "Red eye": conjunctival injection, chemosis. (**b**) DSA, ICA contrast angiography, image in oblique direction. The cavernous sinus (*arrowhead*) draining toward the superior ophthalmic vein (*dashed arrows*) is filled from the ICA (*arrow*) via its minor dural branches in the arterial phase. (**c**) DSA, external carotid artery contrast angiography, image in oblique direction. The cavernous sinus (*arrowhead*) draining toward the superior ophthalmic vein (*dashed arrows*), is also filled from the numerous minor branches of the external carotid artery. (**d**) Microcoils (*arrowheads*) are inserted in the cavernous sinus via the cubital vein, the external jugular vein, the facial vein and the superior ophthalmic vein (*arrows*). (**e**) Common carotid artery DSA image in an oblique direction made after microcoil filling of the affected cavity of the cavernous sinus. There is no filling either in the cavernous sinus or the superior ophthalmic vein. (**f**) The external ocular symptoms have disappeared 2 weeks after the intervention

causes significant steal effect (Fig. 9.5a) and it may provoke severe ipsilateral cerebral blood circulation disorder.

Imaging Diagnosis

The simplest way of establishing the imaging diagnosis of both the CCF and the CS DAVF is to perform contrast-enhanced CT examination, which detects well the broadening of the cavernous sinus and dilation of the SOV (Fig. 9.5b). This can be visualized with more details by MR, and MRA provides information on the character of the shunt as well. The dynamics of the arteriovenous flow decisive regarding the therapeutic options, can only be assessed with DSA, thus this is mostly inevitably performed.

Neurointerventional Therapy

Carotid-Cavernous Fistula

Whereas the clinical presentation is identical, the CCF and the CS DAVF are decisively different from therapeutic aspect. The carotid-cavernous fistula is mostly well and easily accessible from the arterial side via the ICA. The orifice of the fistula can be occluded (Fig. 9.5) in the most simple and effective way by inserting a microcatheter from the ICA to the CS via the orifice, with a microballoon attached to the catheter, but detachable after the filling (Fig. 9.2c). Frequently this intervention can be performed quite quickly and effectively. If it is unsuccessful to get across the orifice of the fistula with the balloon, microcoil occlusion of the fistula may also be attempted, but it has considerably higher costs and lower efficacy. In some of the cases the orifice of the fistula is so broad, that it cannot be occluded in itself. In such cases we may be constrained to occlude the ICA. Naturally, its criteria have to be assessed the same way, as it was already detailed in the discussion of the aneurysms. Finally, the fistula may be approached from the venous side as well, even from the femoral vein via the IJV and the IPS, or via the SOV by its direct opening (see below). After the occlusion of the fistula, the "locomotive" murmur immediately disappears, the external ocular symptoms relieve quickly, but the eye movement disorder may long persist, and it is not always resolved completely. The damaged vision also improves mostly quickly, but in most cases there is no regeneration after complete loss of vision.

Cavernous Sinus Dural Arteriovenous Fistula

Treatment of the CS DAVF considerably differs from the above mentioned therapies. As there is no direct connection between the lumen of the ICA and the CS, approach from the arterial side would only be possible via numerous minor branches, most of which generally originate from the ICA. It is not only difficult to approach the latter and to perform embolization through them, but also carries the risk of cerebral embolism and stroke. Therefore it is almost always the venous approach that is the only effective method in these cases. As already described above, in favorable cases, if the IPS can be penetrated and reached, it can be performed via puncture of the femoral vein, through the IJV and the IPS. Inserting a microcatheter on this route into the appropriate compartment of the CS, it can be occluded with detachable microcoils. This requires mostly a big amount of microcoils, which renders the procedure expensive. At the same time, the flow in the DAVFs is characteristically relatively slow, therefore, in contrast to the fast-flow CCFs, microcoil occlusion is quite effective in this case. If the IPS cannot be visualized or penetrated, in some of the cases the cavity of the CS may be accessible via the EJV through the facial vein and the SOV (Fig. 9.6). If it is not possible, the SOV can be opened surgically through the upper eyelid and the fistula can be occluded by directly inserting a catheter in it (Fig. 9.7). In successful cases, similarly good results can be expected as described above by the CCF. As the DAVF generally occurs in advanced age, due to its slow flow there is almost no risk of intracranial

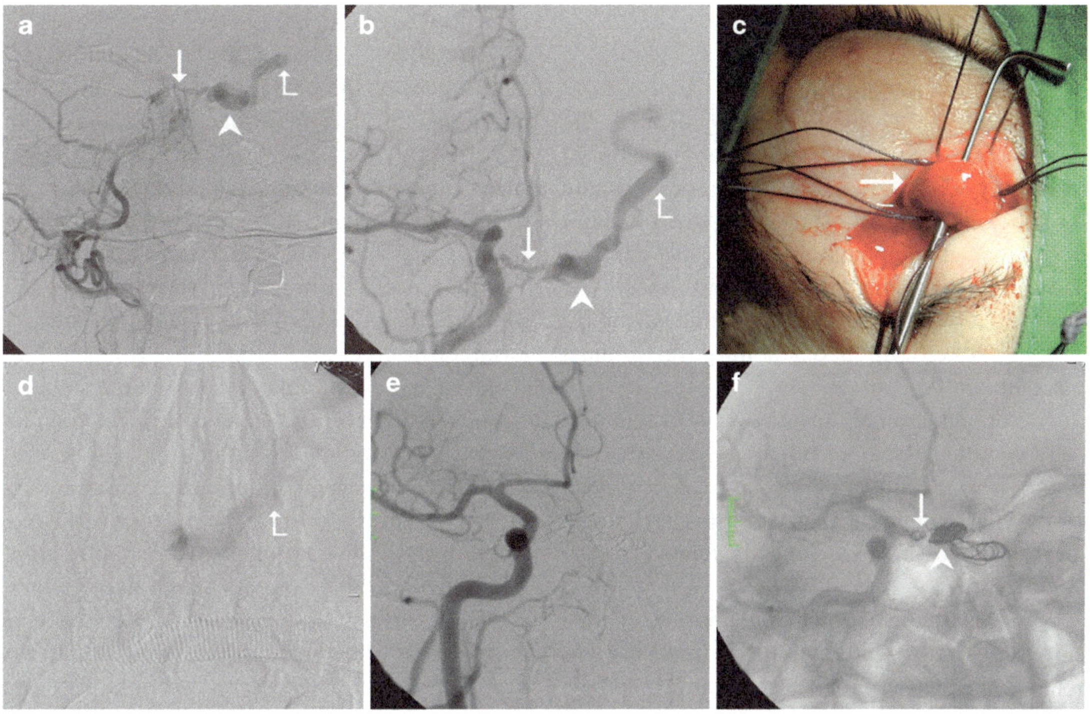

Fig. 9.7 Neurointerventional treatment of a cavernous sinus DAVF with direct access to the superior ophthalmic vein. DSA, filling of the external (**a**) and internal (**b**) carotid artery, PA direction The external carotid artery fills the contralateral cavernous sinus (*arrowhead*) via the medial meningeal artery, the minor dural branches of the internal carotid artery, via the intracavernous sinus and it fills the contralateral superior ophthalmic vein (*broken arrow*) via the contralateral cavernous sinus. (**c**) The surgically opened superior ophthalmic vein in the upper eyelid (*arrow*). (**d**) A superselective venogram is made from the superior ophthalmic vein (*broken arrow*) via a microcatheter inserted in the superior ophthalmic vein. (**e**, **f**) After embolization no filling can be seen on the angiographies of the common carotid artery either via the external or the internal carotid artery. (**e**) Microcoils inserted into the cavernous sinus (**f**: *arrowhead*) and the intercavernous sinus (**f**: *arrow*) occlude the fistula

hemorrhage or steal effect, and it may even resolve spontaneously in 10–15 % of the cases, invasive treatment is not necessarily constrained, taking its risks also into account. Spontaneous regression may be promoted by manual compression of the ipsilateral common carotid artery several times daily, and the eye-related symptoms may be relieved by diuretic treatment.

Central Retinal Artery Occlusion

Pathology and Pathomechanism

Central retinal artery occlusion (CRAO) is detected on average in 1 out of 10,000 ophthalmological examinations in the United States. The leading risk factors are diabetes, hypertension, and valvular heart disease. Under the age of forty it is mostly of cardiac origin, while above the age of 40 it is mainly caused by atherosclerosis. At this age 45 % of patients with CRAO suffers from stenosis in the carotid artery. Besides this, less frequent causes may be arteritis, coagulopathies or polycythemia.

Imaging Diagnosis

The CRAO is an ophthalmological diagnosis, imaging examinations are only suggested if neurointerventional treatment is chosen, and in this case naturally DSA is performed.

Neurointerventional Therapy

There are no established standards of CRAO treatment. Several publications evaluated the possibilities of systemic as well as intraarterial thrombolysis. A great advantage of systemic thrombolysis is that it can be performed without delay, special equipment and expensive devices. There is no comparative study in this aspect. The available results suggest that systemic thrombolysis performed within 6.5 h improves clinical outcome.

Direct intraarterial thrombolysis is theoretically significantly more effective than systemic lysis. The ophthalmic artery can be catheterized easily via the femoral artery approach, thus the local thrombolysis is technically relatively easy to perform.

Similarly to the findings of numerous separate case series, a recently published metaanalysis found some extent of improvement in 93 % of the examined 158 cases, and in 13 % complete regeneration of the vision. However, the procedure requires a 24-h available complete emergency service with angiography and neurointervention, like the neurointerventional treatment of acute stroke. This explains that although sporadic reports have been published in this topic, there is no unequivocal proof of the efficacy of either the intravenous or the intraarterial thrombolysis. In our opinion, this can only be expected if the neurointerventional treatment of acute stroke will become part of the clinical routine. In this case, in addition to patients with stroke, the treatment of patients with CRAO would also be manageable. As far as we know, today none of the institutions in Hungary perform routinely intraarterial treatment of CRAO.

Retinoblastoma

Neurointerventional Therapy

The application of neurointerventional techniques in the treatment of retinoblastoma has arisen very recently. The ophthalmic artery can be effectively catheterized with the help of the currently used microcatheters (see above). It can be understood based on the circulatory circumstances of the orbit and the bulb, that chemotherapeutic agents can be delivered in remarkably high concentrations with local superselective infusion, and due to the relatively slow flow and the lack of collateral blood supply, the rinse-off effect is also minimal. This has provided the theoretical background for the attempt to apply superselective intraarterial chemotherapy as primary treatment in children with retinoblastoma to avoid enucleation. The intervention can be performed on an outpatient basis and it can be repeated several times if necessary. Although the case numbers of early studies are low, results are impressive. According to the data of the latest publication, 3.2 superselective infusion treatments were applied on average per patient in 23 children (3 months to 8 years) with different combinations of melphalan, topotecan and carboplatin. From the 27 treated eyes, enucleation was only necessary in one case and there was no need for radiotherapy and systemic chemotherapy. On low total dose no systemic side effects occurred, apart from neutropenia not requiring treatment, and locally only banal side effects were detected. For the present, having only scarce initial experience, the value of the method cannot be safely assessed, but based on the results it can be regarded by all means as a promising perspective.

Further Readings

Abramson DH, et al. A phase I/II study of direct intraarterial (ophthalmic artery) chemotherapy with melphalan for intraocular retinoblastoma initial results. Ophthalmology. 2008;115(8):1398–404, 1404 e1.

Abramson DH, et al. Superselective ophthalmic artery chemotherapy as primary treatment for retinoblastoma (chemosurgery). Ophthalmology. 2010;117(8):1623–9.

Andreou A, Ioannidis I, Psomas M. Transvenous embolization of a dural carotid-cavernous fistula through the contralateral superior petrosal sinus. Neuroradiology. 2007;49(3):259–63.

Biousse V. Thrombolysis for acute central retinal artery occlusion: is it time? Am J Ophthalmol. 2008;146(5):631–4.

Fattahi TT, et al. Traumatic carotid-cavernous fistula: pathophysiology and treatment. J Craniofac Surg. 2003;14(2):240–6.

Graham R, Shehab A. Central retinal artery occlusion. EMedicine; 2009.

Guglielmi G, et al. Electrothrombosis of saccular aneurysms via endovascular approach. Part 2: preliminary clinical experience. J Neurosurg. 1991;75(1):8–14.

Hattenbach LO, et al. Intravenous thrombolysis with low-dose recombinant tissue plasminogen activator in central retinal artery occlusion. Am J Ophthalmol. 2008;146(5):700–6.

Irie K, et al. Transvenous embolization of traumatic carotid cavernous fistula with mechanical detachable coils. Minim Invasive Neurosurg. 1996;39(1):28–30.

Kam CK, Alvarez H, Lasjaunias P. Treatment of carotid cavernous fistula secondary to rupture of a giant intracavernous carotid aneurysm. Transarterial coiling of aneurysm and carotid compression. A case report. Interv Neuroradiol. 2003;9(3):293–8.

Komiyama M, et al. Indirect carotid-cavernous sinus fistula: transvenous embolization from the external jugular vein using a superior ophthalmic vein approach. A case report. Surg Neurol. 1990;33(1):57–63.

Larson JJ, et al. Treatment of aneurysms of the internal carotid artery by intravascular balloon occlusion: long-term follow-up of 58 patients. Neurosurgery. 1995;36(1):26–30. discussion 30.

Lylyk P, et al. Curative endovascular reconstruction of cerebral aneurysms with the pipeline embolization device: the Buenos Aires experience. Neurosurgery. 2009;64(4):632–42. discussion 642–3; quiz N6.

Martin EM, Hummelgard AB. Detachable balloon occlusion of carotid-cavernous sinus fistula. J Neurosci Nurs. 1987;19(3):132–40.

Michels KS, et al. Transvenous embolization of a dural carotid-cavernous sinus fistula via the inferior ophthalmic vein. Ophthal Plast Reconstr Surg. 2007; 23(6):480–2.

Molyneux A, et al. International Subarachnoid Aneurysm Trial (ISAT) of neurosurgical clipping versus endovascular coiling in 2143 patients with ruptured intracranial aneurysms: a randomised trial. Lancet. 2002; 360(9342):1267–74.

Molyneux AJ, et al. International Subarachnoid Aneurysm Trial (ISAT) of neurosurgical clipping versus endovascular coiling in 2143 patients with ruptured intracranial aneurysms: a randomised comparison of effects on survival, dependency, seizures, rebleeding, subgroups, and aneurysm occlusion. Lancet. 2005;366(9488):809–17.

Mounayer C, et al. Superior petrosal sinus catheterization for transvenous embolization of a dural carotid cavernous sinus fistula. AJNR Am J Neuroradiol. 2002;23(7):1153–5.

Noble J, et al. Intra-arterial thrombolysis for central retinal artery occlusion: a systematic review. Br J Ophthalmol. 2008;92(5):588–93.

Rosso D, Hammond RR, Pelz DM. Cavernous aneurysm rupture with balloon occlusion of a direct carotid cavernous fistula: postmortem examination. AJNR Am J Neuroradiol. 1999;20(5):771–3.

Sorteberg A, et al. Angiographic balloon test occlusion and therapeutic sacrifice of major arteries to the brain. Neurosurgery. 2008;63(4):651–60. discussion 660–1.

Szikora I, et al. Intracranialis aneurysmák kezelése elektrolitikusan leválasztható mikrospirálokkal [Treatment of intracranial aneurysms with electrolytically detachable microcoils]. Cli Neurosci (Ideggyógyázsati Szemle). 1995;48:409–16.

Szikora I, et al. Dural arteriovenous malformations. In: Intracranial vascular malformations and aneurysms. New York/Heidelberg: Springer; 2008.

Szikora I, et al. Treatment of intracranial aneurysms by functional reconstruction of the parent artery: the Budapest experience with the pipeline embolization device. AJNR Am J Neuroradiol. 2010;31(6): 1139–47.

Turowski B, et al. Early fatal hemorrhage after endovascular cerebral aneurysm treatment with a flow diverter (SILK-stent): do we need to rethink our concepts? Neuroradiology. 2011;53(1):37–41.

van der Schaaf IC, et al. Endovascular treatment of aneurysms in the cavernous sinus: a systematic review on balloon occlusion of the parent vessel and embolization with coils. Stroke. 2002;33(1):313–8.

Wang ZG, et al. HydroCoil occlusion for treatment of traumatic carotid-cavernous fistula: preliminary experience. Eur J Radiol. 2009;71(3):456–60.

Xin-Ya Qian C, et al. Rupture of an aneurysm of the persistent trigeminal artery presenting as a carotid-cavernous sinus fistula. Orbit. 2009;28(5):275–80.

Recent Results in Neuropathology: Demyelinating and Conformational Diseases

10

Tibor Kovács

Contents

Neuropathology is the field of pathology specialized to the nervous system, it involves almost all sections of general pathology, but several groups of diseases are known that are unfamiliar for professionals proficient in general pathology. It is impossible to provide a brief review of the entire topic, instead of this I would like to summarize the new discoveries of two groups of diseases: the most frequent group of the diseases of the visual system in the neurological practice, the demyelinating diseases, and by the regulation of eye movements, the recent classification of degenerative neurological diseases, the conformational diseases, with Parkinsonian syndromes as examples.

T. Kovács, M.D., PhD, habil.
Department of Neurology, Faculty of Medicine, Semmelweis University, Budapest, Hungary

Cerebrovascular and Dementia Unit, Department of General Neurology, Semmelweis University, Budapest, Hungary

Dementia and Dystonia Outpatient Department, Semmelweis University, Budapest, Hungary
e-mail: tibor@neur.sote.hu

Demyelinating Diseases

The primary damage of the myelin along with relatively intact axons is a characteristic of demyelinating diseases, thus diseases of the myelin sheet and the cell types producing it belong to this group. Cases of impaired myelin synthesis have to be differentiated from demyelinating diseases. According to one of the numerous classifications, inflammatory, viral, metabolic, hypoxic-ischemic and compression-related forms exist. Multiple sclerosis is the most frequent inflammatory form, its pathological types are classic (Charcot type), acute (like Marburg's disease, Balo concentric sclerosis), and neuromyelitis optica (Devic disease), the classification of which has become ambiguous nowadays. The differentiation of acute disseminated encephalomyelitis often represents a difficulty both clinically and pathologically.

The pathology of classic multiple sclerosis is characterized by plaques of various size and shape. Besides damage to the periventricular white matter, the corpus callosum, the optic nerve and the spinal cord, cortical plaques are characteristic. The following plaque types can be differentiated with histological methods:

1. Active plaques: periventricular lymphocyte infiltration and lipid-laden macrophages can be found in the entire area of the plaque.
2. Inactive plaques: gliotic plaques containing a few cellular components, the axon-density is also reduced within them.

J. Somlai, T. Kovács (eds.), *Neuro-Ophthalmology*, DOI 10.1007/978-3-319-28956-4_10

3. Chronic active plaques: plaque inactive in the center, having active characteristics on the periphery.
4. "Shadow" plaques: sharply circumscribed plaques, where fibers with thin myelin sheet can be detected due to remyelination. The simultaneous presence of different plaque types is a diagnostic characteristic of multiple sclerosis.

Neuromyelitis optica (Devic) is the combination of uni- or bilateral retrobulbar neuritis and acute transverse myelitis. Besides foamy macrophages and perivascular granulocyte infiltration, IgM and complement deposits can be detected in the acute lesion. More recently, the disease has been explained by IgG antibodies against the aquaporin-4 water channels. Pathology reflects its clinical heterogeneity by classifying it into subgroups, which have been already widely accepted recently.

Type 1 and 2 are the consequence of immune-mediated damage. In Type 1, demyelination is the consequence of T cell and macrophage-dependent mechanisms. In Type 2, T cells can also be detected, but the role of B cell-derived IgG and the complement system is also significant. Type 2 is the most frequent: it comprises approximately half of the abnormalities.

In Type 3 and 4 abnormalities of the oligodendrocytes are predominant. In Type 3, the amount of myelin-associated glycoprotein decreases before the morphology of the oligodendrocytes is damaged. According to data of animal studies, this causes degeneration of the distal projections of the oligodendrocytes, presumably via apoptosis. The mechanism of the least frequent Type 4 is currently unknown; primary damage to the oligodendrocytes is likely. The above mentioned types may be mixed inter- and intraindividually, and temporally as well (during the course of the disease), although the latter two are doubted by many scientists (Table 10.1).

Table 10.1 Subgroups of multiple sclerosis based on pathogenesis

Type	Phenotype	Mechanism
I		T cell and macrophage-related
	Autoimmune demyelination	
II		Antibody- and complement-dependent
III		Distal oligodendropathy and apoptosis
	Dystrophy of oligodendrocytes	
IV		Primary degeneration of oligodendrocytes

The pathological classification may be associated with therapeutic consequences, particularly if the *in vivo* markers of the subgroups will be successfully identified.

It has also become widely accepted in the recent years that axonal damage is also significant in the cortical plaques, thus, it plays an important role in the development of cognitive damage (Fig. 10.1).

Conformational Diseases

One of the most important discoveries of the last decade has become part of the curriculum. According to the theory, the damage of the

Fig. 10.1 The pathology of multiple sclerosis. (**a**, **b**): Demyelinating focus in the optic nerve (*arrow*). (**c**, **d**) Extensive demyelination of the optic chiasm (*arrow*). (**e**, **f**) Periventricular demyelination (**g**) Plaques in the pons. (**h**) Chronic active plaque (magnified framed part of F, 400×). In the *upper right corner* the hypocellular central part can be seen, in the *bottom left corner* myelinated fibers are colored *blue*. On the border between the two areas the great number of lymphocytes and macrophages indicates the ongoing demyelination. (**i**) The structure of neurons is intact within the plaque (a few neurons are indicated by *arrows*) (magnification of the framed part of G, 200×). (**j**) Active plaque with extensive infiltration of CD68 positive macrophages (*brown color*) from a biopsy specimen. (**a**, **c**, **g**, **h**, **i**) Luxol fast blue-Nissl stain (Klüver-Barrera): the cells are *violet*, the myelin is *blue*. (**b**, **d**, **e**) Gallyas silver impregnation for astroglia (gliosis is colored *brown*). (**f**) Hematoxylin-eosin. (**j**) CD68-immunohistochemistry

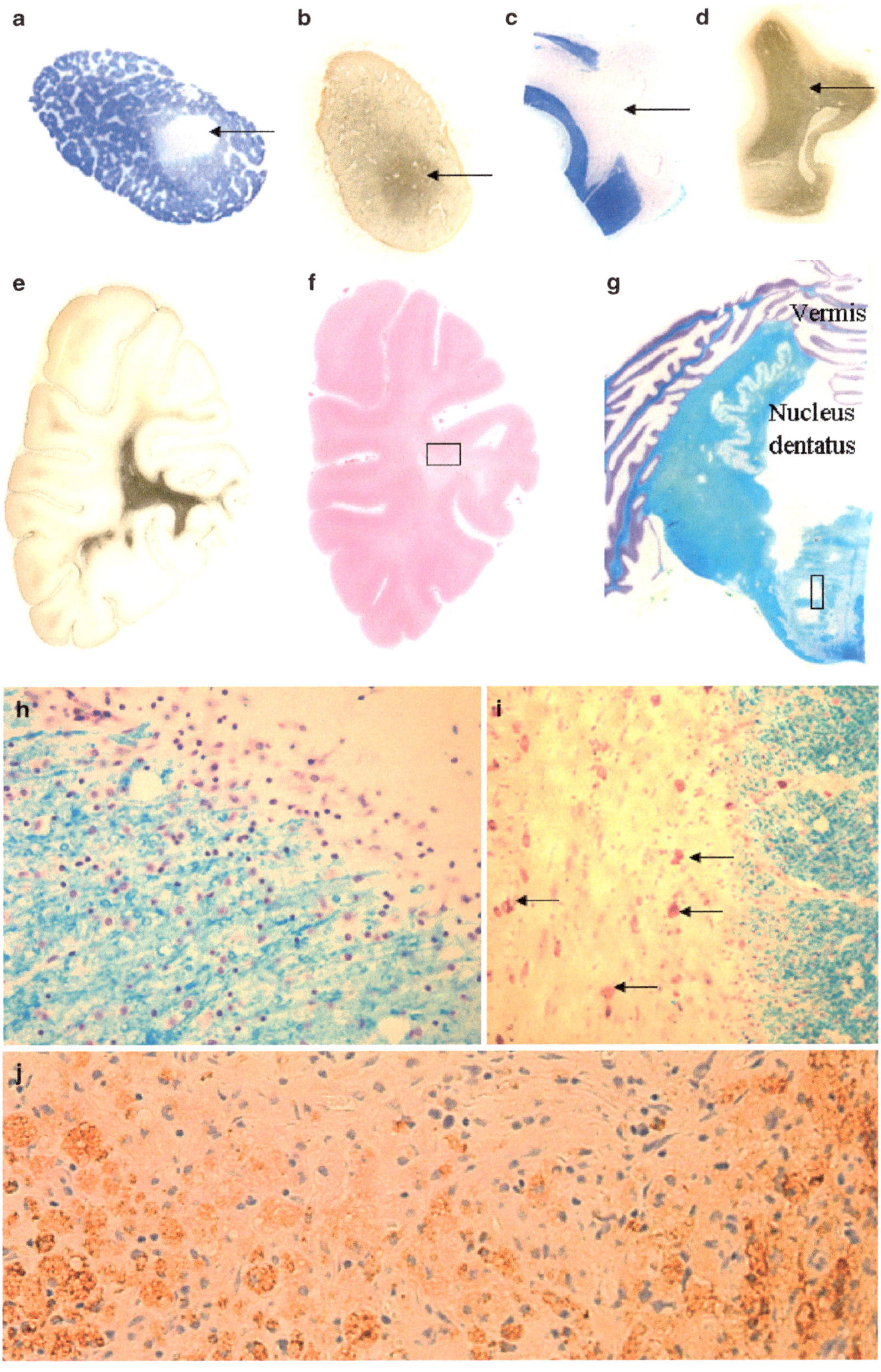
a
b
c
d
e
f
g
Vermis
Nucleus dentatus
h
i
j

neurons and glia cells is caused by inclusions of proteins with abnormal structure. Alteration of the secondary structure (conformation) of the normal protein leads to the aggregation of protein molecules, and the compacted protein is not accessible for the catabolic cellular processes, thus it is further accumulated, forming inclusion bodies. Extracellular inclusions occur in prion diseases and Alzheimer's disease and in some other, rare forms of amyloidosis. Intracellular and intranuclear inclusions are characteristic to trinucleotide repeat diseases, for example Huntington disease, but it is important to mention the inclusion bodies with distinctive morphology found in progranulin mutations recently detected in frontotemporal dementia.

According to the characteristic protein of the cytoplasmic inclusions, we can speak about synucleinopathies, tauopathies, and ubiquitin diseases. In the latter group, the yet unknown protein deposited in the inclusions is tagged by ubiquitination for the protein degradation mechanisms of the cell, thus ubiquitin is a non-specific protein. Typical representatives of synucleinopathies are Parkinson's disease and multiple system atrophy (MSA). The most frequent tauopathy is Alzheimer's disease, whereas progressive supranuclear palsy (PSP) and corticobasal degeneration (CBD) are tauopathies presenting as Parkinsonian syndrome. Of these diseases MSA has to be highlighted, as its specific histological abnormalities, the glial cytoplasmic inclusions (Fig. 10.2) were described by Professor Má-tyás Papp and Professor Peter Lantos in 1989.

The importance of this discovery is similar to that of the Lewy bodies or neurofibrillary bundles characteristic to Parkinson's disease, the inclusions are even called Papp-Lantos-bodies. In addition to this, the MSA was the first neurological disease in that the primary abnormalities are found in the glia cells and not in the neurons. This observation has started the transformation of neuropathology: it has turned out that several oligo- and astroglial inclusion bodies exist, many of them have become diagnostic criterion: besides the Papp-Lantos bodies in MSA, the tufted astrocytes in PSP and the astrocytic plaques in CBD.

The confident diagnosis of Parkinsonian syndromes is provided by histological examination

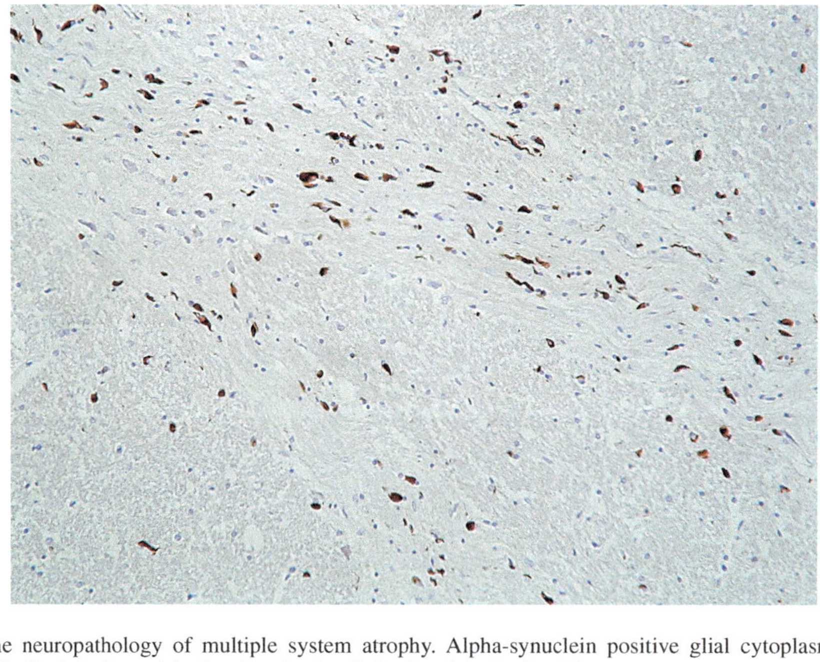

Fig. 10.2 The neuropathology of multiple system atrophy. Alpha-synuclein positive glial cytoplasmic inclusions (Papp-Lantos bodies) (in *brown*) in the oligodendroglial cells of the basis of the pons

of the brain. Clinical recognition is often difficult, primarily in the initial phase of the disease. Neuro-ophthalmology can help in this aspect, more exactly the electrophysiological evaluation of eye movements and the description of the characteristic abnormalities.

In MSA abnormal cillations (macro square wave jerks) appear on fixation, caused by dysfunction of the pontine reticular formation. The abnormal smooth pursuit, the optokinetic nystagmus and the nystagmus are consequences of cerebellar and pontocerebellar dysfunction. In PSP the vertical eye movement disorder is due to the damage of the mesencephalic connections, the square wave jerks are due to damage of the connections of the pontine reticular formation, and the hypometric saccades are due to damage of the pontocerebellar connections. In CBD damage to the parietal (Brodmann 39-40) and frontal (Brodmann 8) eye fields stands in the background of the increased saccade latency and the oculomotor apraxia. Nystagmography is a well applicable method in the clinical practice in the diagnostics of Parkinsonian syndromes.

Further Readings

Brück W. Clinical implications of neuropathological findings in multiple sclerosis. J Neurol. 2005;252 Suppl 3:III/10–4.

Brück W. New insights into the pathology of multiple sclerosis: towards a unified concept? J Neurol. 2007;254 Suppl 1:I/3–9.

Carrell LW, et al. Conformational diseases. Lancet. 2000;350:134–8.

Galetta SL, et al. Neuromyelitis optica is a variant of multiple sclerosis. Arch Neurol. 2007;64:901–3.

Gulyäs S, et al. Szemmozgäsok elektrofiziolögiai vizsgälata Parkinson-szindrömäban [Electrophysiological examination of eye movements in Parkinsonian syndrome]. Conference of the Hungarian Scientific Parkinson Society, abstract, 2006.

Jellinger KA. Neuropathological spectrum of synucleinopathies. Mov Disord. 2003;18 Suppl 6:S2–12.

Komori T. Tau-positive glial inclusions in progressive supranuclear palsy, corticobasal degeneration and Pick's disease. Brain Pathol. 1999;9:663–79.

Lassmann H. Recent neuropathological findings in MS - implications for diagnosis and therapy. J Neurol. 2004;251 Suppl 4:IV/2–5.

Lennon VA, et al. IgG marker of optic-spinal MS binds to the aquaporin 4 water channel. J Exp Med. 2005; 202:473–7.

Love S. Demyelinating diseases. J Clin Pathol. 2006;59: 1151–9.

Mackenzie IRA, et al. The neuropathology of frontotemporal lobar degeneration caused by mutations in the progranulin gene. Brain. 2006;129:3081–90.

Papp MI, et al. Glial cytoplasmic inclusions in the CNS of patients with multiple system atrophy (striatonigral degeneration, olivopontocerebellar atrophy and Shy-Drager syndrome). J Neurol Sci. 1989;94: 79–100.

Peterson JW, et al. Transected neuritis, apoptotic neurons, and reduced inflammation in cortical multiple sclerosis lesions. Ann Neurol. 2001;50:389–400.

Prineas JW, et al. Demyelinating diseases. In: Graham DI, Lantos PL, editors. Greenfield's neuropathology. 7th ed. London: Arnold; 2002. p. 471–550.

Rottach KG, et al. Dynamic properties of horizontal and vertical eye movements in parkinsonian syndromes. Ann Neurol. 1996;39:368–77.

Tolnay M. Review: tau protein pathology in Alzheimer's disease and related disorders. Neuropathol Appl Neurobiol. 1999;25:171–87.

Weinshenker BG. Neuromyelitis optica is distinct from multiple sclerosis. Arch Neurol. 2007;64:899–901.

Part III

Conventional, Novel and Complementary Examinations in Ophthalmology

29. The Role of the EMG-ENG in Diagnosing Neuro-ophthalmologic Diseases
30. Computed Tomography Examinations
31. Neuroradiology, Functional MRI
32. Novel Information Regarding the Visual and Eye Movement Systems in Otoneurology
33. Electro-Oculography (EOG) Examination of Eye Movements
34. The Importance of Familiar Thrombophilias in the Clinical Practice. Novel Ways in Anticoagulant Therapy
35. Novel Consideration Regarding the Role of Evoked Potential in Confirming the Diagnosis of Eye Movement Disorders of Brainstem Origin

11 Algorithm of the Neuro-ophthalmological Examination Used in the International Practice

Judit Somlai

Contents

A neuro-ophthalmological examination is usually required for patients with severe or chronic and/or multiple injuries. This is why the first encounter with the patient is so important. A key part of it is making contact with the patient before the neuro-ophthalmological examination, that is, taking *the past medical history, anamnesis*. The practical importance of taking the past medical history in neuroophthalmological patients is as high as in any field of clinical medicine. In addition to the conventional ophthalmological examination procedures (e.g., visual acuity, accurate fundoscopy, etc.), patients must always be asked about their visual symptoms. A detailed assessment of the visual symptoms often orients the examiner already in this phase as to which disease group the patient should be investigated for, and it helps clarify the symptoms and determine immediate actions. Unilateral loss of vision, for example, may present with various subjective symptoms, the type and intensity of which may be important information. The history of systemic diseases is just as important, since an underlying medical disease may often be the cause of unilateral loss of vision or sudden-onset double vision. Even with the results of the latest test procedures, the principle is that the test results of dysfunctions due to eye symptoms must be evaluated together, in synthesis, i.e., clinical and test results must be assessed together with the symptoms reported by the patient and the supplementary consultation results, taking their evolution into account, and the patient must always be guided and examined in a target-oriented way during the differential diagnostic process.

Modern neuro-ophthalmological examination procedures and the conventional methods available to the majority of the colleagues working in the clinical practice provide together an objective measurement tool for the assessment of the dysfunctions of both the visual pathway system and the oculomotor system.

Our examinations require a special, ***reverse thinking***. The reason for it is that the eye symptoms,

J. Somlai, M.D.
Unit of Neuro-Ophthalmology, Department of Neurology & Stroke, Military Hospital, Budapest, Hungary

Neuro-Ophthalmology Section, Hungarian Ophthalmological Association, Budapest, Hungary

Trustee, NOSZA Foundation (for the Prevention and Screening of Ocular Storke), Budapest, Hungary
e-mail: dr@somlaijudit.hu; http://somlaijudit.hu

J. Somlai, T. Kovács (eds.), *Neuro-Ophthalmology*, DOI 10.1007/978-3-319-28956-4_11

visual complaints lead us towards systemic diseases, that is, a minor abnormality may indicate (or predict) a significant disorder. For example, anisocoria is a pupil symptom only, which may be due to a life-threatening increase in intracranial pressure or an aneurysm that serves as a source of bleeding.

An objective evaluation of the symptoms reported by the patient is not always easy.

- ***Cooperation issues*** *and* ***severe general condition*** are known phenomena in neurological and neurosurgical patients. Despite these, a quick examination of the visual functions is important for determining both the necessary investigations and the required treatment. Therefore, quick but accurate testing procedures have been introduced and are intended to be improved to meet the requirements of our patients and our times.
- In the ***examination of pediatric patients***, modern examination procedures have allowed us to get around not only the difficulty in cooperation due to the age of these patients but also the mental dysfunctions caused by the underlying disease. Computer perimetry, for example, can be performed in most of our patients, with the help of an assistant, already from the ages of 4–5 years.
- Antechiasmal lesions, especially those developed in the intraorbital segment, are difficult or impossible to access even with the latest **neuroradiological procedures**. The only assessment option for dysfunctions due to retrochiasmal optic nerve lesions, especially in their early phase when they do ***not yet cause*** morphological, neuroradiological changes, is an accurate neuro-ophthalmological examination. For example, a visual field test which may be decisive also as to the height of the lesion at the same time.
- Neuro-ophthalmological methods may help us in objectifying cortical blindness or marked bilateral loss of vision by determining the residual islands of vision, to evaluate the ***further quality of life and occupation options of the patient***.
- At the beginning of the examination of the eye movement system, the patient reports sudden-onset, intolerable diplopia and marked image displacement. They often cause space perception and fixation disorders, inability to read, dizziness, and inability to get about. In certain groups of diseases, it may be accompanied by diurnal variation and, in certain severe cases, by severe neurological and systemic symptoms, e.g., difficulty swallowing or breathing, which may even be life-threatening. Severe complications can be prevented if the patient is given adequate treatment already at the beginning of the occurrence of the eye symptoms, following a proper examination.

Examination of Visual Acuity (Near Vision, Distant Vision, Sciascopy if Required)

The complex neuro-ophthalmological examination always starts with a ***visual acuity test***. *Distant vision* is measured from a distance of 5 m, using correction, whereas at the bedside, current visual acuity is assessed based on counting fingers, hand motion and light perception. It is recommended to always perform this monocularly and with adequate correction, and a lack of correction should be temporarily compensated with a pinhole occluder. The examination of distant vision is completed with chart reading using both eyes to determine if the patient has diplopia.

Near vision is also tested first separately on the two eyes, and then the two eyes are examined together, using adequate correction. The degree of near visual acuity is measured using the standard Csapody near visual acuity chart or reading cards with numbers (see Table 11.1). Visual acuity can be quantified from the largest to the smallest font size (Csapody XIII. – V).

When near vision is examined monocularly, the accommodation ability of the lens can be assessed, whereas with a binocular reading test, the accommodation reflex (near triad – convergence, miosis and lens accommodation) can be evaluated. If a monocular decrease in visual acuity is detected, which patients mostly consider amblyopia ex anopsia and nothing abnormal can be found with objective refractive error measurement (sciascopy), then thorough examination of the optic nerve and detailed analysis of the visual functions are required not only with basic methods but also with supplementary procedures such as electrophysiology, neuroradiology, etc.

For example, the first and, for a long time, only symptom of childhood optic gliomas is a decrease in visual acuity; exophthalmus is a late symptom. The

Table 11.1

Examination of the optic nerve – measurement of the visual functions	
History (auto- and heteroanamnesis)	
Basic methods: Visual acuity (VA) – VA distant vision – VA near vision - reading distance Color vision Afferent pupillomotor reflex Critical fusion frequency (CFF) (figure)	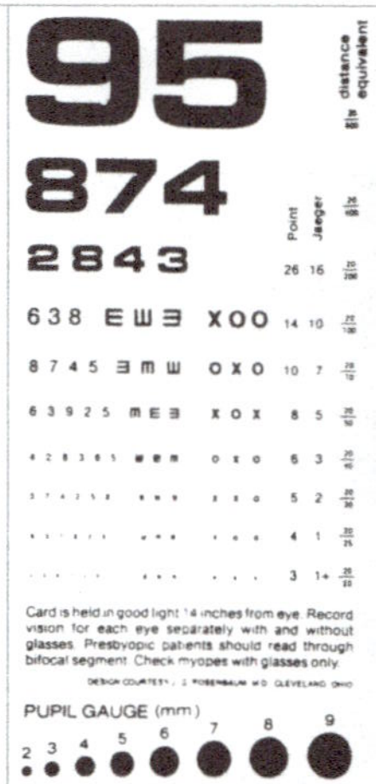 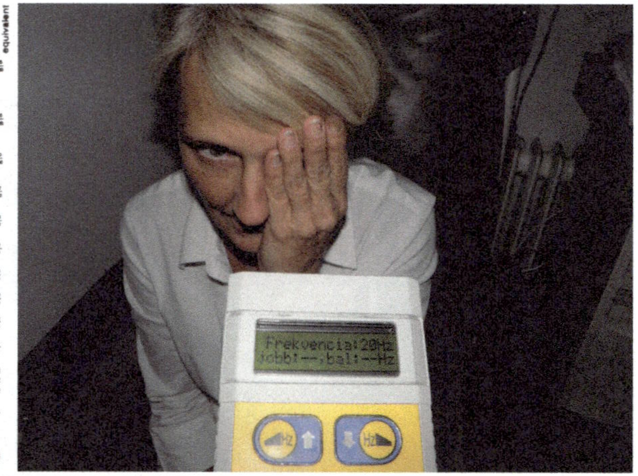
Measurement of the conduction capacity of the optic nerve: Electrophysiology Electroretinography (PERG, mfERG) Visual Evoked Potential test (VEP)	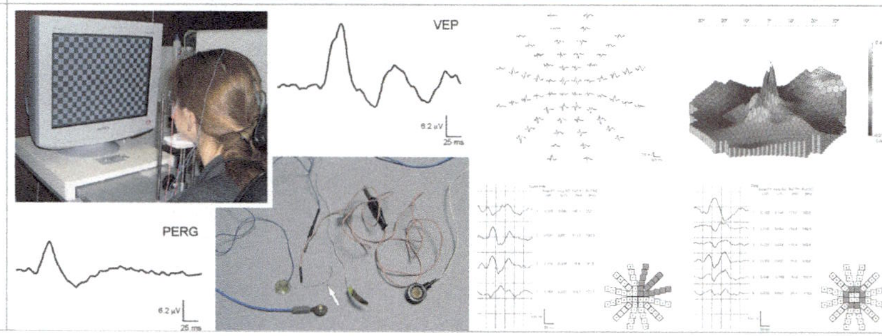

(continued)

Table 11.1 (continued)

Examination of the optic nerve – measurement of the visual functions	
Examination of the visual field: Confrontation—at the bedside Bjerrum screen (campimetry) (figure) center of vision, blind spot Projection perimetry (static, kinetic) (figure) central and peripheral visual field together	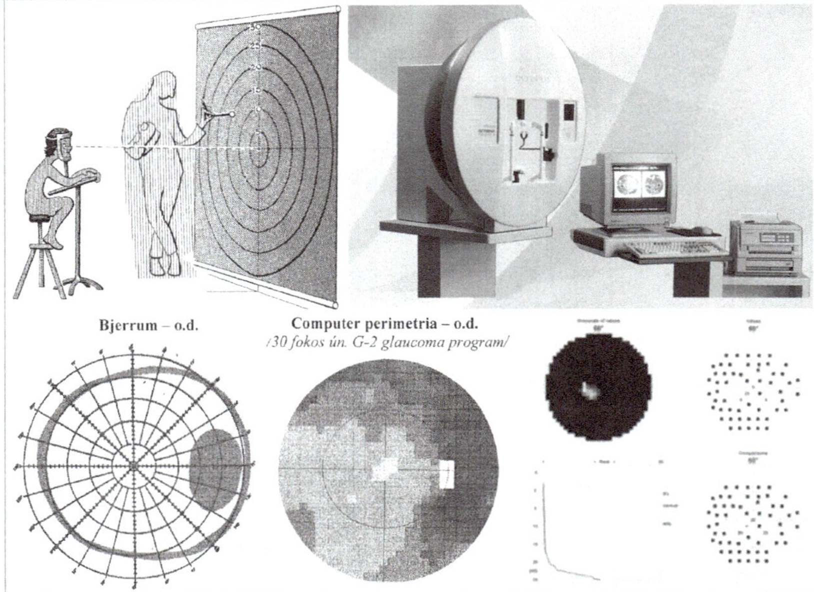
Examination of blood flow in the retina and the optic disc: Heidelberg Retina Flowmeter (HRF) Fluorescein angiography (FLAG)	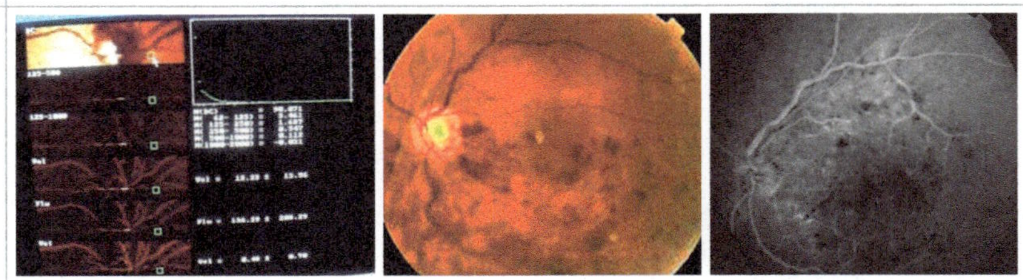

residual damage, however, will be considerably less if it is recognized and treated in a timely manner.

Examination of Color Vision

The early recognition of and screening for congenital and acquired color vision abnormalities is performed with the use of *pseudoisochromatic plates*. Further differentiation can be achieved with color arrangement tests, such as the *Farnsworth–Munsell 100 hue test* and *anomaloscopy*. The latter indicates even the mildest abnormality in hue discrimination. An acquired color vision abnormality or blindness may be of any origin, such as inflammation, trauma, or circulatory disorder, and it indicates damage to the antechiasmal segment of the optic nerve. *(For the details of color vision tests and disease types, see* Chap. 14 *on pages 89-95).*

Measuring the Conduction Capacity of the Retina and the Visual Pathway

The *critical fusion frequency (CFF) value* quantified on both eyes separately determines the conduction capacity of the visual pathway system. The vibrating signal of increasing frequency is perceived by the patient as a single signal above a critical frequency value. The quick examination can be performed even at the bedside, and since only minimal cooperation of the patient is required, it is a quick but adequate screening test also in the case of patients in severe condition. In addition, the progression or regression of the disease and, not least, the efficacy of the therapy can be assessed with it (*see* Table 11.1). The procedure that examines the early, functional damage of the retina is *electroretinography (ERG)*, which may be performed simultaneously with the *visual evoked potential (VEP) test* that assesses the nerve conduction of the visual pathway system, and which provides useful information not only about the degree of damage but also about its location between the retina and the visual cortex (*see* Table 11.1). For the most modern methods available and the clinical indications, *see* Chaps. 15 and 16 *on pages 97 and 111, respectively.*

Examination of the Pupils

The pupils are examined with an ophthalmoscope or a penlight, in a dark room. If a local cause of anisocoria is possible, slit-lamp examination is recommended. With the examination of the direct and indirect light responses, the involvement of the afferent and efferent pupillomotor pathway and the degree of damage can also be determined. The afferent pathway, in the antechiasmal segment, runs together with the afferent pupillomotor nerve fibers. Therefore, a sign that indicates damage to the afferent pupillomotor pathway is the Marcus–Gunn sign, which predicts or indicates a lesion of the afferent–antechiasmal optic nerve fibers that run together with the afferent pupillomotor pathway. The lesion of the efferent nerve fiber, its eye symptom is anisocoria, is the marker of a very important neurological condition. In most cases, it may be a result of increased intracranial pressure and intracranial aneurysm. If required, in case of anisocoria of unknown origin, the dysfunction of the sympathetic or parasympathetic nerve fibers is confirmed or ruled out with **pharmacological tests**. For the pupillomotor examination tests and the clinical syndromes, *see* Chaps. 23 and 52 *on pages 207 and 463, respectively.*

Examination of the Fundus

The most important and most frequently used examination performed by ophthalmologist and neurologists is the examination of the fundus with *direct ophthalmoscopy or an indirect method.* Ophthalmoscopy is used to assess the edges and color of the optic disc, as well as the excavation of its surface, and in case of increased intracranial pressure, the prominence of the surface can be measured in diopters and monitored. It is important to carefully describe the ratio and condition of the vessels that enter and leave, as well as the macula and the parafoveal belt, and to record the consequences of the circulatory disorder in case of pathological conditions. In case of circulatory disorders of "major blood vessels" that enter at the optic disc, *fluorescein angiography (FLAG) and indocyanine green angiography (ICGA)* are performed. The blood flow in the end arteries and capillaries that run near the optic disc and supply the optic disc itself is assessed with a *Heidelberg*

Retina Flowmeter (HRF), a not-widely used but useful method, which performs *scanning laser Doppler flowmetry*. (For the details of FLAG and ICGA, *see* Chap. 19 *on page 145, and for a photograph of the HRF device, see* Table 11.1 *on page 69*.) The examination method called *Ocular Coherence Tomography (OCT)* is more and more extensively used in the clinical practice because it provides numerical and digitally, multiply processed information not only about the changes of the macular and perimacular layers but also about the morphological changes of the nerve fiber bundle that radiates into the optic nerve, the papillomacular region (for details about its use in clinical practice, *see* Chap. 20 *on page 157 and* Table 11.2 *at the end of this Chapter)*.

Examinations of the Visual Field

Severe visual field deficits can be screened for with a *confrontation visual field exam* already at the bedside, assessing the peripheral perception of hand motion separately in both eyes. If this method is used binocularly, attention hemianopias can be ruled out. A thorough examination of the peripheral part of the visual field can be performed with the conventional *Goldmann perimeter* or with *computer perimetry*. The latter enables us to use this examination method even in the case of poor patient cooperation or a severe condition. During the examination of the central visual field, i.e., the central 30° of the visual field or the central region, an enlargement of the optic disc may indicate its dysfunction early. In lack of a computer perimetry, the innermost part, i.e., the central 10° of the visual field can be assessed accurately with a *Bjerrum screen* and target set (*for the visual field testing methods and their practical importance, see* Chap. 17 *on page 119, and see* Table 11.2 *for illustrations)*.

Examination of the Eye Movements

In case of eye movement disorders, the first complaints of the patient are intolerable diplopia when looking in the distance and an inability to read. Besides, patients report dizziness and spatial perception disorder. The examination of both the peripheral and the central oculomotor systems, even at the bedside, starts with establishing whether the palpebral fissures are identical (e.g., ptosis) and describing the eye alignment in straight gaze (primary position).

The next step is to observe, with the suspension of fusion, the *monocular* eye movements and then, with *alternating cover*, the movement to take up fixation. This is important because the movement direction of the paretic eye is the same as that of the paretic ocular muscle, i.e., it "points at the direction of the paresis." It is followed by observing the *smooth pursuit eye movements* in the nine gaze directions. We assess whether the eye movements are conjugate and unrestricted, and whether there is nystagmus, and if so, of what type and direction it is. After that, the *slow-continuous* pursuit supranuclear gaze system is tested with the examination of smooth pursuit eye movements. (See also Chap. 21 on page *171* for the method and importance of the cover–uncover test.) The *saccadic oculomotor system* that allows fast macular refixation is examined by instructing the patient to look at alternating fixation points (see Part 5.4 on page *461*).

The assessment of the *pupillomotor reflexes* (afferent and efferent parasympathetic and sympathetic pupillomotor pathways) is of diagnostic and differential diagnostic value in the everyday practice with regard to pupillary disorders such as anisocoria, miosis, mydriasis, and afferent and efferent reflex dysfunctions. The task of ophthalmologists and, especially, neuro-ophthalmologists is to assess the type and degree of image displacement, as well as its objective change, with double image analysis. The type and degree of the eye movement disorder, and its change, can be assessed quickly and with little cooperation from the patient with the help of the *Hess screen*, instructing the patient to fixate at the far point. The examination tools of diplopia that occurs also during reading are the prism bar and the Maddox rod. The questionable results of the conventional methods are confirmed by the latest otoneurological and electrophysiological methods applicable in case of eye movement disorders, which are of differential diagnostic value (*see* Table 11.3 *and for further details, see* Chaps. 21, 23 and 24 *on pages 171, 207 and 217, respectively)* (Table 11.4).

Table 11.2

Examination of the optic nerve – morphological examination	
Examination of the fundus Direct ophthalmoscopy Indirect examination	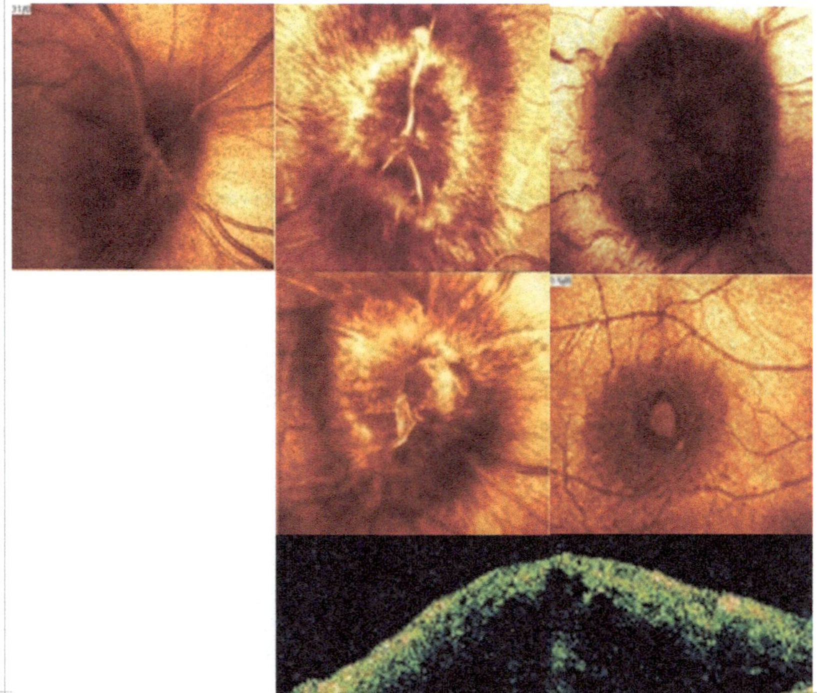
Measurement of nerve fiber loss of the optic disc Octopus perimetry Heidelberg Retina Flowmeter (HRF) Optical Coherence Tomography (OCT)	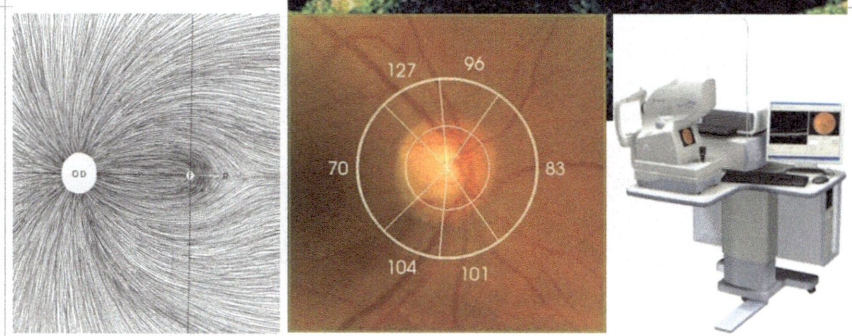

(continued)

Table 11.2 (continued)

Examination of the optic nerve – morphological examination	
Examination of the macular and the papillomacular regions (measurement of retinal nerve fiber layer thickness/its change) Optical Coherence Tomography (OCT)	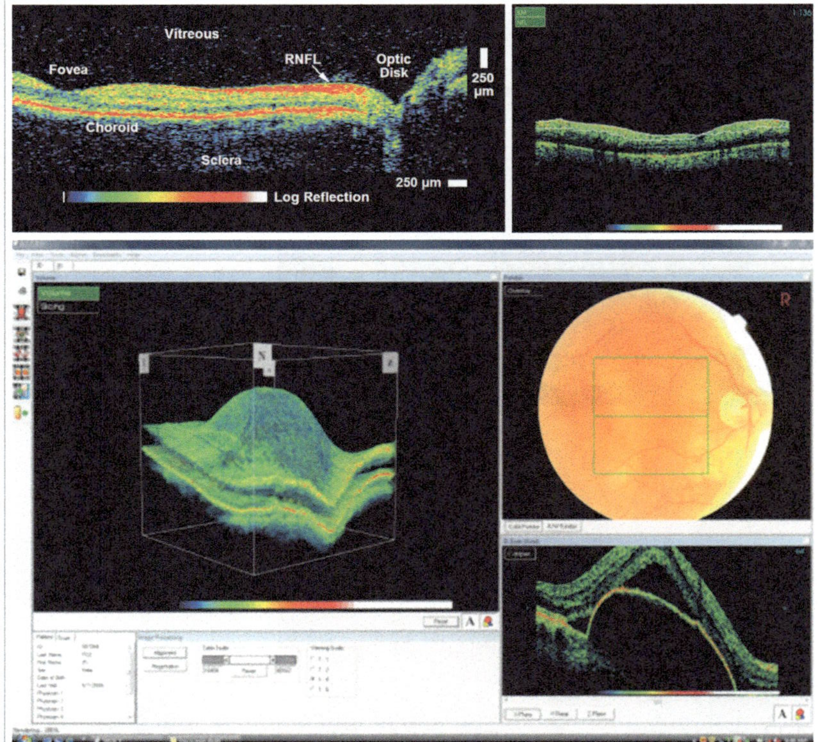

Table 11.3

Diagnostic options of eye movement disorders in unconscious patients	
Primary eye alignment, "primary position" Palpebral fissure Pupillomotor reflexes	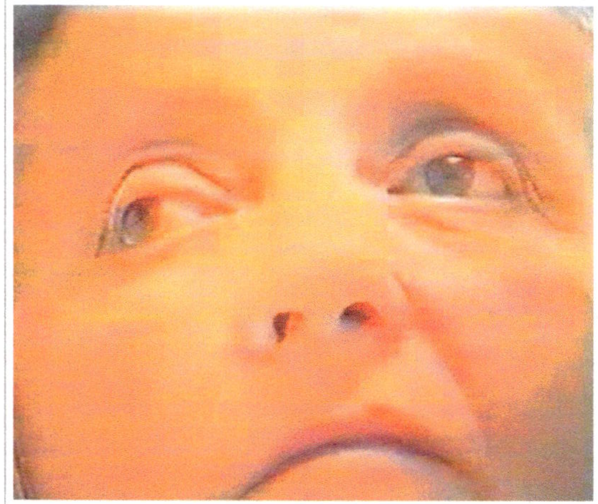

(continued)

Table 11.3 (continued)

Diagnostic options of eye movement disorders in conscious patients	
Basic eye movement examinations: Primary eye alignment,"primary position" Movement to take up fixation Pupillomotor reflexes Smooth pursuit: in 9 directions Double image analysis: near, far	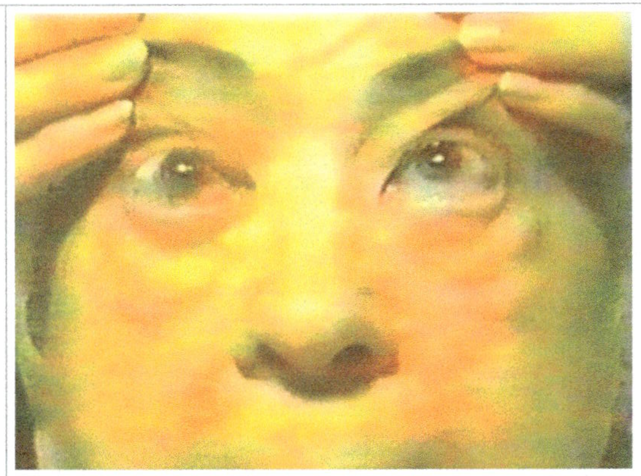 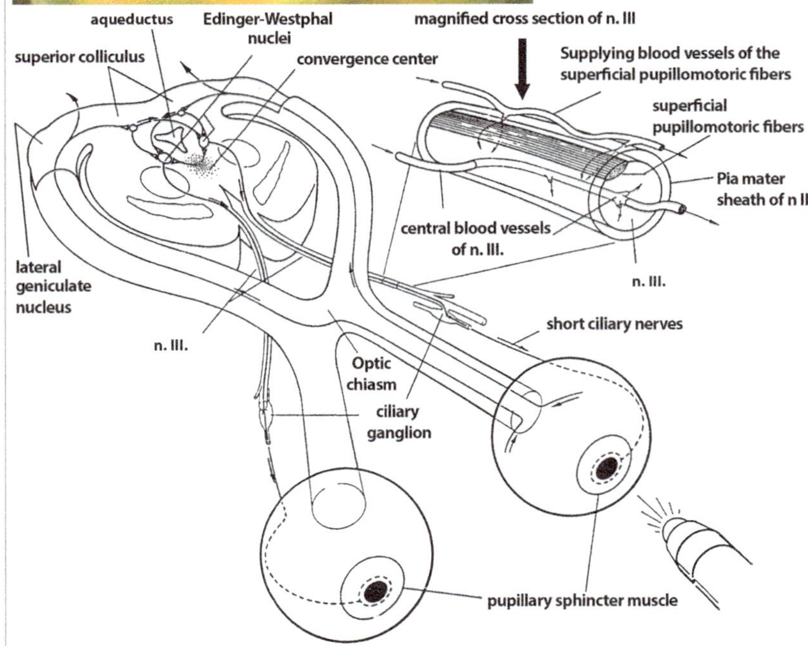

Measurement of near double image Maddox rod Prism bar	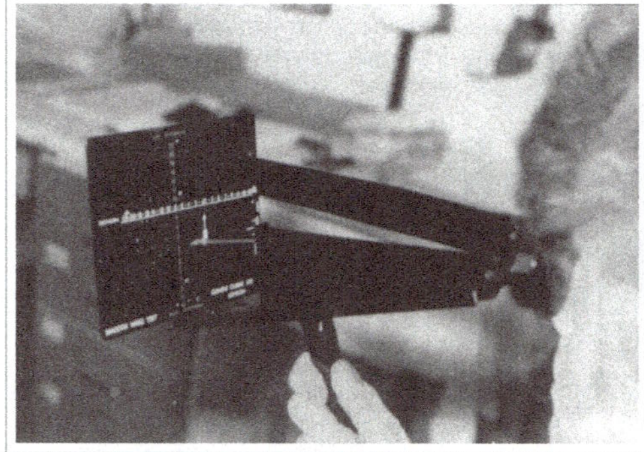 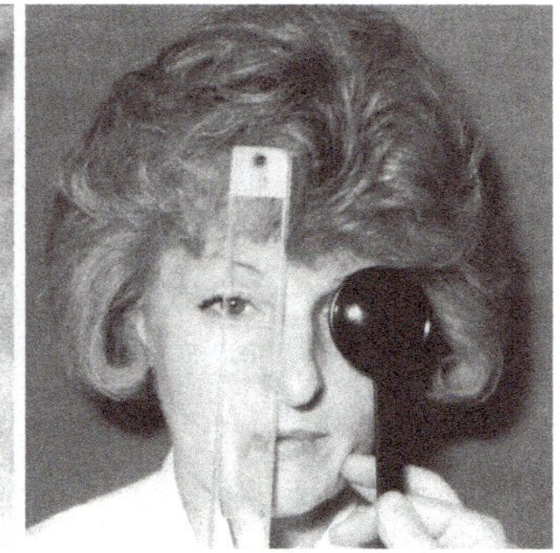
Examination of far double image: Hess screen Polatest Treatment of double image With prism glasses With ocular muscle surgery	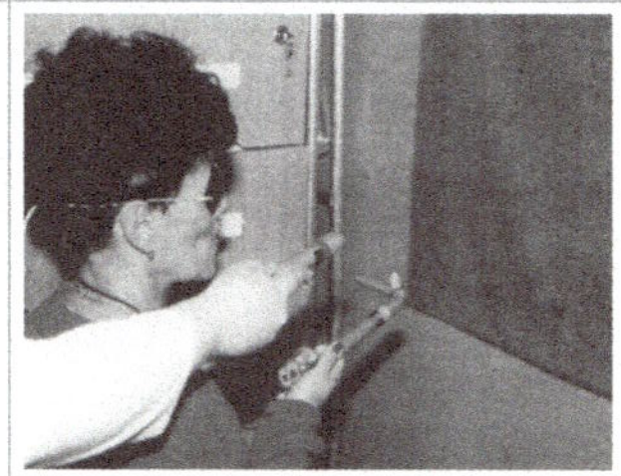 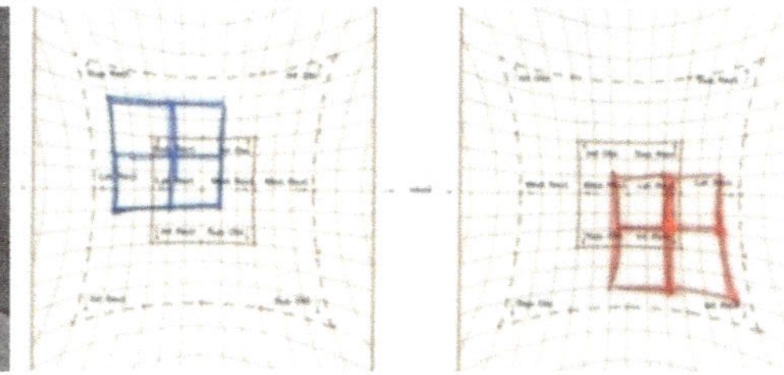
Supplementary tools Video recording (documentation, teaching) Fundus photography series (rotational nystagmus – angle measurement) Differential diagnostics: EMG (± edrophonium test)	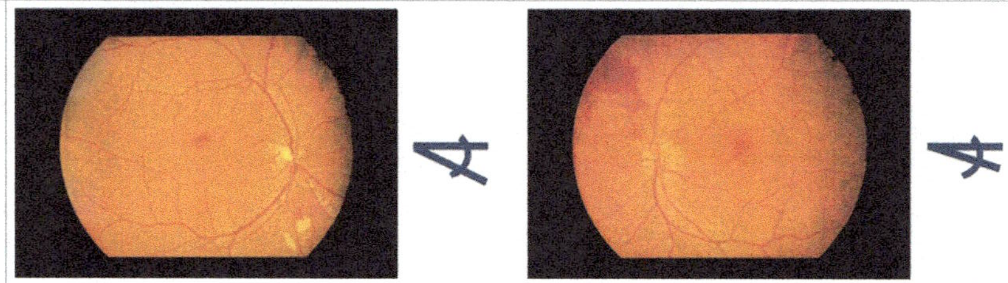

Table 11.4

Diagnostic options of eye movement disorders – otoneurology, neurology and neuro-ophthalmology	
Vestibuloocular reflex (VOR) diagnostics: Examination of semicircular canals, otoliths, utricular functions: SVV Electrophysiological methods: Electrooculography (EOG, IRD, scler-SC-EOG, video-EOG) Optokinetic nystagmus (OKN) (simultaneous examination of smooth eye movement [SEM] and fast eye movement [FEM] phases)	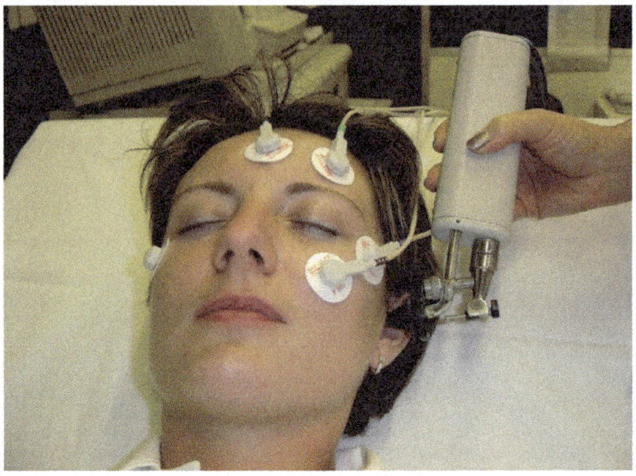 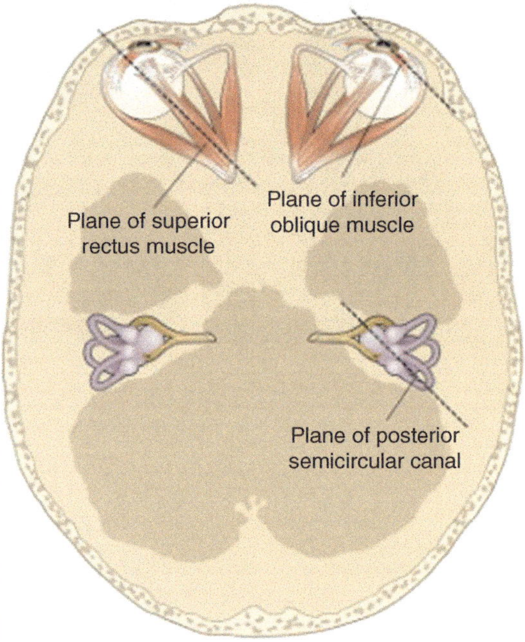

12 Objective and Subjective Examination Methods of Visual Acuity

Márta Janáky

Contents

One of the most important functions of the eyes is object vision. Its two components are central (focal) vision, which is measured with the examination of visual acuity, and peripheral vision, which can be measured with the assessment of the visual field. The examination of visual acuity has objective and subjective methods.

Subjective examinations:

- assessment of distant vision,
- assessment of near vision.

Objective methods:

- vision estimation based on optokinetic nystagmus,
- FPL (Forced choice Preferential Looking) test,
- VEP (visual evoked potential: examination of response evoked in the visual cortex).

M. Janáky, M.D., PhD, habil.
Electrophysiological Unit, Department of Ophthalmology, Faculty of Medicine, University of Szeged, Szeged, Hungary
e-mail: janaky@opht.szote.u-szeged.hu

The use and applicability of each method are determined by the age and mental status of the patient, and the purpose of the examination.

Subjective Examination Methods of Visual Acuity

To assess subjective distant visual acuity, reading charts have been designed for use in routine clinical practice. Based on international agreement, the unit of visual acuity is the recognition of a symbol (optotype) that contains details of a visual angle of 1 min of arc in size. This visual angle of 1 min of arc is considered to be the resolution capability of the intact eye. On the charts used for the measurement of distant vision, the line thickness of each symbol is 1 min of arc from a specified distance (5 m in Hungary), and the size of the whole symbol is 5 min of arc.

The symbols may be numbers, letters, Snellen E symbols, Ammon symbols, Landolt C symbols or Ferre–Rand symbols. In Hungary, the decimal vision chart of Kettesy is the accepted, standardized reading chart. The chart is illuminated evenly from the two sides, but charts illuminated from behind are also used. The disadvantage of the reading chart method is that in case of repeat examinations, the repeating symbols are easier to recognize. The Zeiss visual acuity testing device projects different symbols and, therefore, its symbols cannot be learned. The ETDRS visual acuity examination is not a routinely used method yet,

J. Somlai, T. Kovács (eds.), *Neuro-Ophthalmology*, DOI 10.1007/978-3-319-28956-4_12

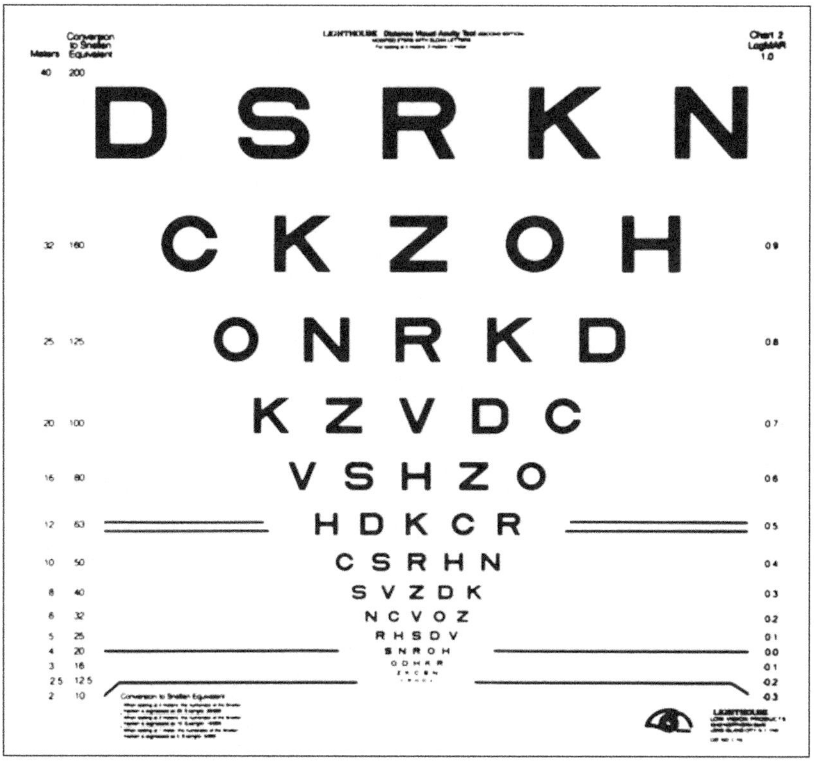

Fig. 12.1 ETDRS visual acuity chart

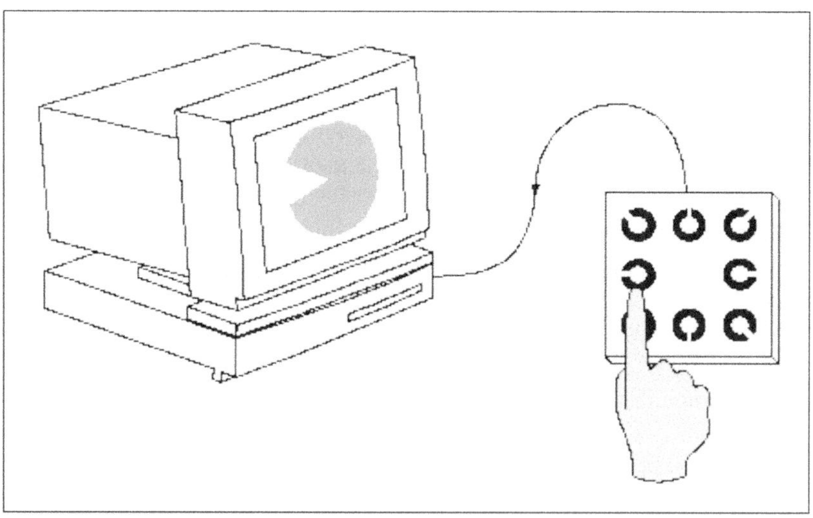

Fig. 12.2 Freiburg visual acuity test

but its use is now required in scientific publications (Fig. 12.1). Nowadays, more and more frequently, computers are used for testing visual acuity. Based on the recognition of various random (unpredictable) symbols (e.g., Landolt C symbols) displayed on the screen, the computer calculates the visual acuity with a precision to one hundredth (e.g., Freiburg vision test) (Fig. 12.2).

To assess the visual acuity in small children, simple charts have been designed, which contain images of objects (house, car, glass), circles, squares (Hyvarinen), Snellen E symbols (Albini's test), or black hands (Sjögren's hand test). During the STYCAR test (Sheridon and Cordiner), children choose the symbol that is asked for from similar symbols given to them (A, V, H, T, X, O, U, L). The vision of infants and persons with intellectual disability can be assessed based on the fixation and pursuit of objects shown. A decisive test to rule out blindness may be the examination of pupillary light reflex. This method is suitable for the diagnosis of blindness due to antechiasmal optic nerve lesions only. Naturally, these latter methods only allow for a rough assessment of the vision.

Of the charts that are used to assess near visual acuity, the Csapody charts are used routinely in Hungary. The texts of different font sizes are to be read from a distance of 30–50 cm. The size of the font is indicated by a Roman numeral from I to XIII. Visual acuity is indicated by the number at which the patient can no longer see the text. The text of different font sizes is available in nine languages. Besides the continuous text, there are other annexes: sheet music for musicians, slide rule for technical workers, and telephone book or timetable for others. In case of vision-related complaints, pocket-size cards can be used to assess vision at the bedside. Based on the font size recognized, distant vision may be estimated as well.

Objective Examination Methods of Visual Acuity

The first objective examination methods of visual acuity were based on the observation of optokinetic nystagmus (OKN). Nystagmus is a rhythmic, involuntary, biphasic eye movement triggered by moving stripes. The subject is looking at a revolving cylinder that has light and dark vertical stripes on it. The evoked nystagmus depends on the distance between the stripes (the width of the stripes), which is seen under a certain angle of vision from a given distance. The nystagmus also depends on the movement speed of the symbols, and its direction depends on the direction of the movement (the direction of the slow phase corresponds to the revolution direction of the cylinder, whereas that of the fast phase is the opposite). Changing the stripe width (i.e., the angle of vision corresponding to the stripe pattern) provides the basis for the estimation of visual acuity. The disadvantage of the method is that it is difficult for the examiner to observe the nystagmus and hold the cylinder at the same time. This method was mainly used in children. The accuracy of the examination is affected by the fact that children are usually moving, and many times they do not look at the stripes, especially if their vision is reduced.

The measurement of optokinetic nystagmus is based on the combination of the sensory and a motor function. Therefore, the reason for the lack of nystagmus or the reduced nystagmus amplitude that can be recorded may be not only a sensory cause but also a dysfunction of the supranuclear pathways. The examination may also be used to unveil hysterical blindness.

The basis of the forced choice preferential looking (FPL or PL) test is that it is easier for an infant to fixate at a patterned screen or object than at a similar-sized and evenly illuminated homogeneous field. Specific Snellen-equivalent stripes are displayed on a screen, while the examiner is observing the direction of the eyes and head of the child from behind a hole. The examiners themselves do not see what patterns are displayed. The visual acuity is determined by the smallest pattern that is still looked at by the child. The result is given in spatial frequency, i.e., cycles per degree. The FPL test includes at least 100 separate stimulus presentations. This test lasts for more than one hour (it is hard, almost impossible, to maintain the attention of a child or an infant for such a long time). The test has versions that require less time. The disadvantage of these methods is that they require the assistance of two or more adults, they are also time consuming, and an alert and attentive child is needed for a successful test. The visual evoked potential (VEP) test is based on the fact that the electrical activity of the visual cortex changes in response to light stimulus. Since the macula is represented by a large area on the surface of the visual cortex, the functional status of the fovea (the part of the macula that is responsible for sharp vision) can be well characterized by the pattern VEP (PVEP) test. The size of the squares in the black and white checkerboard pattern used during the test represents a specific visual angle from a given distance, i.e., checkerboard patterns of different square sizes are visible under different visual angles from the given distance.

The basis for the measurement of visual acuity is the recognition of symbols representing specific visual angles. Therefore, changing the square size of the checkerboard pattern could serve as a basis for the objective measurement of visual acuity. If the patient sees the pattern, its changes in contrast evoke changes in the electrical activity of the visual cortex. If the patient does not see it, the changes in the pattern are not perceived, and therefore the VEP test will be inevaluable. The visual angle of the square size that just evokes response in the visual cortex is the resolution capability, i.e., the visual acuity, of the given eye. During the examinations, however, the age-related accommodation ability must be taken into account, which may have a fundamental effect on the estimation of the actual visual acuity. Accommodation can be blocked by dilating the pupils but in this case, the pattern will not be sharp.

Therefore, an objective examination of visual acuity is available, and only minimal cooperation is required. Its use, however, requires not only good and expensive equipment but also an experienced examiner who can interpret the complex waveform, i.e., the obtained results, correctly. Since accommodation is blocked when the pupils are dilated, which decreases contrast sensitivity based on the square wave, i.e., hinders the recognition of the symbols, this method has not been able to gain ground in the clinical practice yet.

Further Readings

Boros B, Kettesy A, Kukán F. Szemészet [Ophthalmology]. Budapest: Medicina; 1980. p. 54–7.

Csapody J. Látáspróbák [Vision tests]. Budapest: Medicina; 1979. p. 11–6.

Fodor F, Péterffy P. Szemészeti funkcionális vizsgálatok [Ophthalmological functional examinations]. Budapest: Medicina; 1989. p. 11–2.

Friendly DS. Visual acuity assessment of the preverbal patient. In: Isenberg SJ, editor. The eye in infancy. Chicago/London: Year Book Medical Publishers. INC; 1989. p. 48–56.

Haner MR, White CT. Evoked conical responses to checkerboard patterns: effect of check size as a function of visual acuity. Electroenceph Clin Neurophysiol. 1970;28:48.

Hoyt CS, Ickel BL, Billson FA. Ophthalmological examination of the infant. Developmental aspects. Surv Ophthalmol. 1982;26:177.

Nelson LB. Techniques for testing for visual acuity. In: Pediatric ophthalmology. Philadelphia: WB Saunders; 1984. p. 21–5.

Radnót M, Follmann P. Szembetegek vizsgálata [Examination of ophthalmological patients]. Budapest: Medicina; 1974. p. 91–106.

Sokol S. Measurement of infant visual acuity from pattern reversal evoked potentials. Vision Res. 1978;18:33.

Examination of Contrast Sensitivity

13

Márta Janáky

Contents

A very important ability of ours is that we can recognize relatively small objects. An ability of no less importance is that we can perceive little differences in brightness without a sharp edge. The first ability is measured with the examination of visual acuity, whereas the second one, with that of contrast sensitivity. The examination of contrast sensitivity is not yet in general use in the clinical practice. It is often considered an insignificant complaint if a patient with intact visual acuity sees the objects flatter or darker. An isolated decrease in contrast sensitivity is a characteristic symptom in certain diseases and, many times, it bothers the patient more than decreased visual acuity.

M. Janáky, M.D., PhD, habil.
Electrophysiological Unit, Department of Ophthalmology, Faculty of Medicine, University of Szeged, Szeged, Hungary
e-mail: janaky@opht.szote.u-szeged.hu

Contrast Sensitivity

Campbell and Green were the first to report the measurement of contrast sensitivity in 1965. Their procedure consisted of using sinusoidal grating fringe patterns which differed in the degree of brightness (contrast) and in the distance between the fringes of the pattern used (spatial frequency). In this pattern, the difference in light intensity and brightness between the adjacent areas changes in a sinusoidal way. The contrast of the fringe pattern is determined by the sum of the brightness waves above and below the mean level. The size of the image on the retina also has a role in the recognition of details. If an object is moving away from us, it seems smaller. The distance between the fringes of the pattern is the cycle. Spatial frequency is expressed by the number of cycles seen under 1° from a specific distance. Its unit of measurement is cycle per degree.

When an object is moving away from us and, therefore, getting smaller, the perception of details with lower contrast becomes harder. The reason for this is not only that the angle under which we see the object is getting smaller but also that the visual system is less sensitive to contrast if the distance between the contrasting areas becomes shorter. The visible parts of objects often contain areas with regular and irregular spatial frequency.

J. Somlai, T. Kovács (eds.), *Neuro-Ophthalmology*, DOI 10.1007/978-3-319-28956-4_13

The Contrast Sensitivity Curve

The visual system is more sensitive to certain spatial frequencies than to others. The normal contrast sensitivity curve is bell-shaped and its peak is between 1.6 and 3.2 cycles per degree (Fig. 13.1).

The abscissa represents the spatial frequency and the visual acuity value that corresponds to the spatial frequency (at a contrast of 100 %). The ordinate represents the contrast on a logarithmic scale. On the logarithmic scale, the full, 100 % contrast is the 0 value. The just perceivable contrast (contrast threshold) is between 2 and 3.

Robson demonstrated that in case of low contrast, the human visual system is most sensitive to a spatial frequency of about three cycles per degree. As the frequency of the pattern increases above or decreases below this value, contrast sensitivity decreases too. The highest spatial frequency perceived by humans is approximately 40 cycles per degree.

If the graph shown on Fig. 13.1 is continued towards the higher spatial frequencies, the curve intersects the abscissa. Such spatial frequency can be seen only at a contrast of 100 %. Patterns with a spatial frequency above this cannot be distinguished from homogeneous gray. Therefore, this value equals the maximal visual acuity. The upper limit of perception (contrast sensitivity) is 30–40 cycles per degree, lower than the maximal visual acuity. The reason for this is that in practice it is difficult to create a 100 % sinusoidal pattern. (Instead of a sinusoidal pattern, a square pattern is used on the visual chart.)

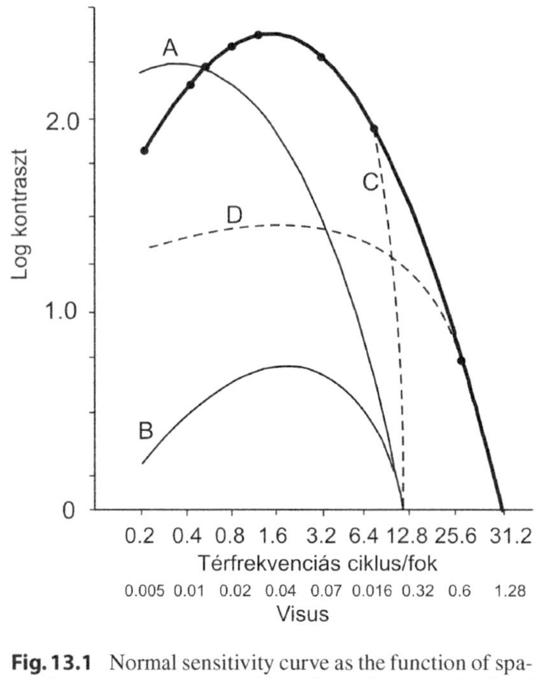

Fig. 13.1 Normal sensitivity curve as the function of spatial frequency and contrast (*thick line*). Curves *A*, *B*, *C* and *D* indicate different types of contrast sensitivity disorders (see the text)

The clinical measurement of visual acuity focuses on a single point of contrast sensitivity, where the curve intersects the abscissa. The entire spectrum of vision can be measured with the examination of contrast sensitivity.

Different diseases may be associated with different shapes and positions of the contrast sensitivity curve, as well as different points of intersection. For example, a curve that is shifted to the left and intersects the abscissa at, e.g., 10 cycles per degree, corresponds to a visual acuity of 5/20, i.e., 0.25. This type of change is characteristic to amblyopia (curve A). The entire curve may be shifted downwards, for example a visual acuity of 0.25. This condition evidently indicates a different, more severe decrease in vision (curve B). Curve C represents a case where the decrease in vision is restricted to high spatial frequencies only. This curve can be seen in case of refractive errors. Curve D indicates that the contrast sensitivity of the patient is impaired with regard to low spatial frequencies. The visual acuity may be 1.0 but there is still vision impairment.

Methods

The examination of contrast sensitivity has been used in psychological and clinical research for a long time, but it has just started to gain ground in the clinical practice. The first devices that were designed displayed the electrically generated pattern on an oscilloscope. The subject was looking at the screen that displayed a pattern of a specific spatial frequency from an accurately specified distance. The patient had to decrease the contrast with a knob until the pattern disappeared. Others used patterns of different spatial frequencies that were displayed in succession to establish the contrast sensitivity curve. The disadvantages of this method are that the examination is time-consuming, and the equipment is expensive and immobile. Because of these disadvantages, the method has not been used extensively in the practice. For similar reasons, the sinusoidal pattern displayed on a television screen has not been used for routine clinical examinations either.

To get around the above problems, charts and then books (modeled after the Ishihara book) with different spatial frequencies and contrasts were designed. Such a book has 6 pages and, when viewed from a distance of 57 cm, the spatial frequency of each page is 0.2, 0.4, 0.8, 1.6, 3.2, and 6.4 cycles per degree. The contrast changes in a logarithmic way.

The disadvantage of the method is that the quality of the book changes over time, and that the result depends on the illumination and inclination of the book.

Currently, a wall-mounted chart is used for routine examinations (Ginsburg test). The evenly illuminated chart, which shows stripe patterns of different spatial frequencies and contrasts, is viewed from a distance of 3 m or 1 m (depending on the Snellen visual acuity). The spatial frequency of the patterns changes in the vertical dimension, whereas their contrast changes horizontally. The patient's task is to recognize the inclination of the stripe patterns. In our practice, the VCTSR 6500 chart (VCTS stands for Vision Contrast Test System) manufactured by Vistech Consultants Inc. (USA) is used for routine examinations (Fig. 13.2).

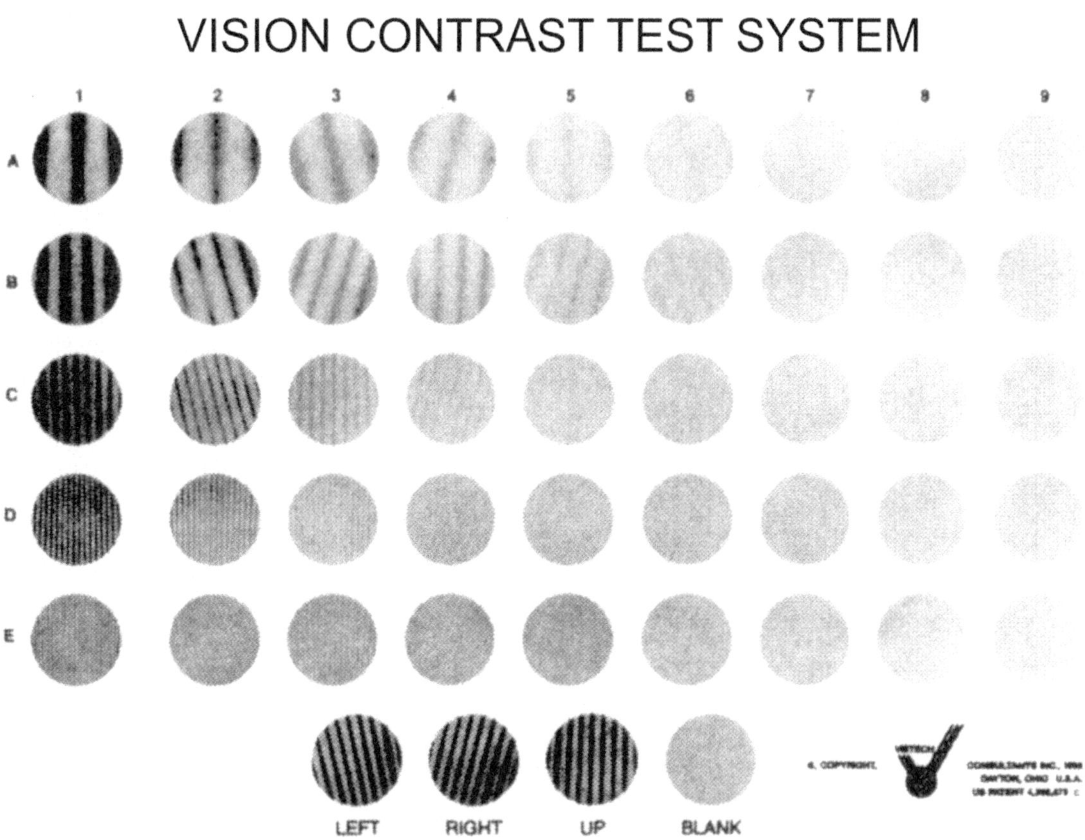

Fig. 13.2 Test chart used for the examination of contrast sensitivity

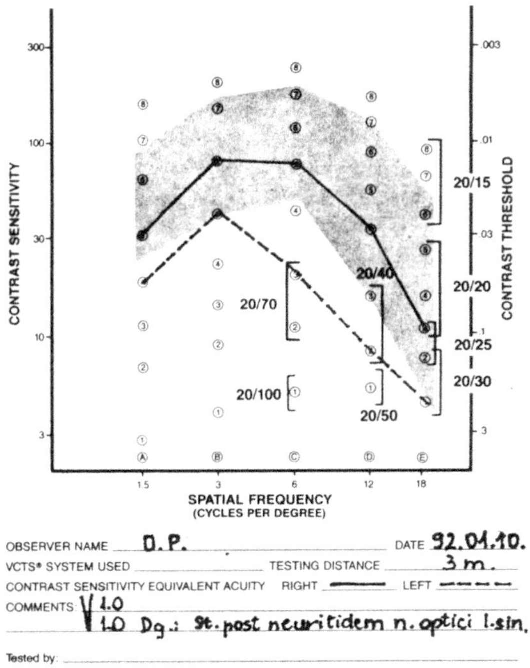

Fig. 13.3 Following optic neuritis, there is a visible difference between the two eyes despite the intact (1.0) visual acuity (the *gray band* represents the normal range)

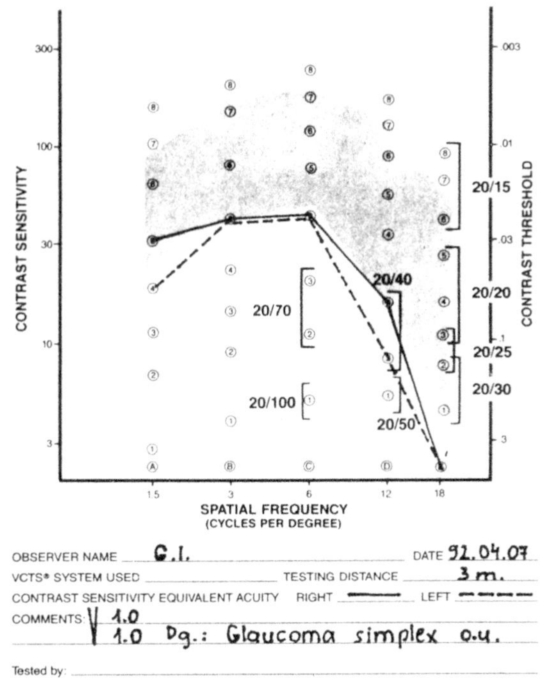

Fig. 13.5 The method is suitable for detecting impairment due to glaucoma even in the case of intact (1.0) visual acuity

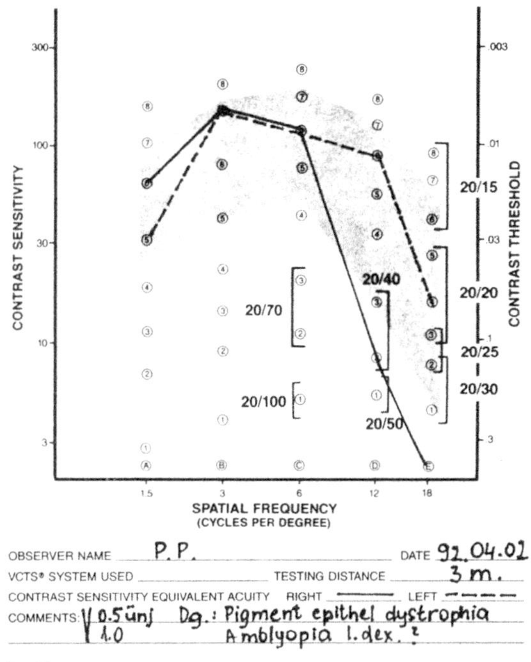

Fig. 13.4 The cause of the vision impairment was not pigment epithelial dystrophy but amblyopia. There is a marked difference between the two sides

Use in the Practice

A change in contrast sensitivity has been described as the first symptom of numerous conditions. It is to be assessed especially in the following neurological diseases: multiple sclerosis, Parkinson's disease, intracranial space-occupying lesions, and retrobulbar neuritis. This method may be sensitive already in the subclinical phase of the diseases. As to ophthalmological diseases, an abnormal value may be indicative of macular conditions, amblyopia or glaucoma. Although the examination similarly to other routine examinations is not of disease-specific value when used alone, it has a place among ophthalmological and neuro-ophthalmological examinations. It reveals a visual function that cannot be approached with other methods. It enables the detection of a difference in functional impairment between the two eyes, and it is also suitable for the monitoring of healing. (Figs. 13.3, 13.4, and 13.5 show some of our own cases.)

Further Readings

Arden GB. The importance of measuring contrast sensitivity in cases of visual disturbance. Br J Ophthalmol. 1978;62:198–209.

Arden GB, Gucukoglu AG. Grating test of contrast sensitivity in patients with retrobulbar neuritis. Arch Ophthalmol. 1978;96:1626–9.

Beck RW, Ruchman MC, Savino JP, Schatz NJ. Contrast sensitivity measurements in acute and resolved optic neuritis. Br J Ophthalmol. 1984;68:756–9.

Bodis-Wollner I, Diamond SP. The measurement of spatial contrast sensitivity in cases of blurred vision associated with cerebral lesions. Brain. 1976;99:695–710.

Bulens C, Meerwaldt JD, Van der Wildt GJ, Keemink CJ. Visual contrast sensitivity in drug induced Parkinsonism. J Neurol Neurosurg Psychiatry. 1989;52:341–5.

Campbell FW, Green DC. Optical and retinal factors affecting visual resolution. J Physiol (Lond). 1965;181:576–83.

Németh J, Ágoston G. Kontrasztérzékenység vizsgálata Ginsburg-teszttel [Examination of contrast sensitivity with the Ginsburg test]. Szemeszet. 1990;127:29–34.

Robson JG. Spatial and temporal contrast sensitivity functions of the visual system. J Opt Soc Am. 1966;56:1141–59.

Ross JE, Bron AJ, Clarke DD. Contrast sensitivity and visual disability in chronic simple glaucoma. Br J Ophthalmol. 1984;68:821–7.

Wolkstein M, Atkin A, Bodis-Wollner I. Contrast sensitivity in retinal disease. Ophthalmology. 1980;87:1140–9.

14 Examination of Color Vision

Klára Aczél

Contents

Color vision is a feature of visual perception that makes differentiation based on wave length possible. Trichromatic color vision characteristic to the human eyes appeared in primates, and it meant a great evolutionary advantage by making the distinction between ripe fruit and green leaves possible. The verbal description of color sensation is far from representing the range of colors that our eyes are able to distinguish. Color sensation can be described with three physical properties:

- *Hue:* determined by the location within the spectrum (wave length);
- *Saturation (colorimetric purity)*: the quantitative ratio of the given hue relative to the white mixed to it;
- *Brightness (luminosity)*: the amount of emitted or reflected light energy in the perceived color.

The three-dimensional system of color sensations is the Munsell's color system, where each color sensation can be described mathematically (Fig. 14.1).

According to the trichromatic color vision theory of *Young* and *Hemlholtz*, there are three kinds of photopigments with different absorption maximums in the cones, and all color sensations can be achieved with the additive mixing of these three primary colors in different ratios (Fig. 14.2).

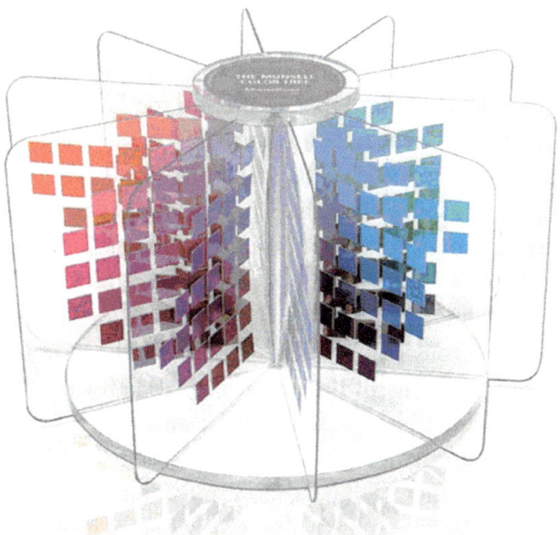

Fig. 14.1 Schematic picture of Munsell's three-dimensional color space *(redrawn)*

K. Aczél, MD
Outpatient Department of Ophthalmology, Military Hospital, Budapest, Hungary
e-mail: klara_aczel@yahoo.com

J. Somlai, T. Kovács (eds.), *Neuro-Ophthalmology*, DOI 10.1007/978-3-319-28956-4_14

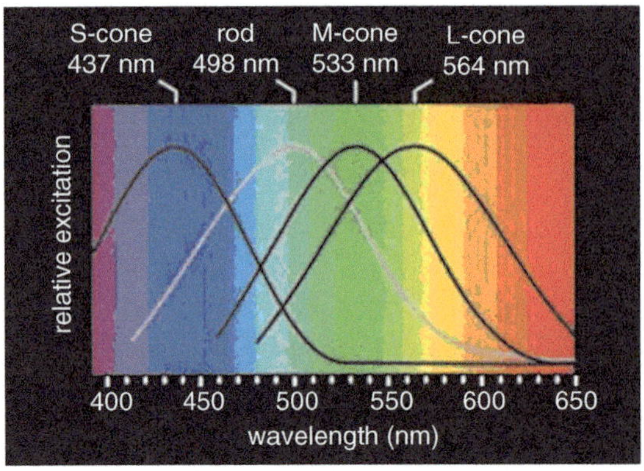

Fig. 14.2 Absorption spectra of the photopigments (*redrawn*)

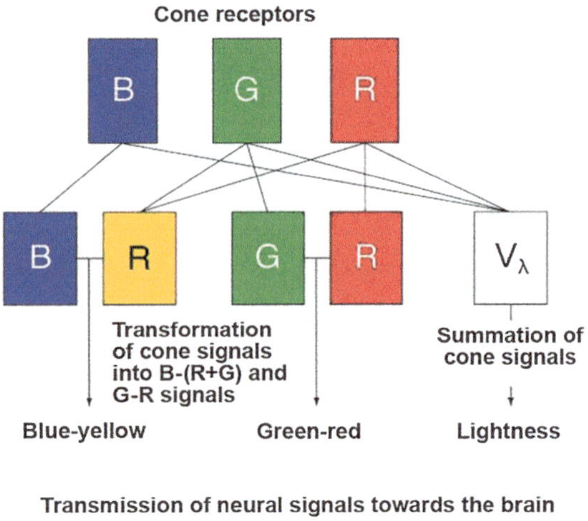

Fig. 14.3 Simplified model of the process of color perception

Contrary to this, the theory of Hering derives the formation of color sensation from three opponent encoding processes (red–green, blue–yellow, and black–white). Based on our current knowledge, the trichromatic theory is correct at the level of receptors, cones contain three different photopigments, each with a different spectral sensitivity: the absorption maximum of the S pigment is 426 nm, that of the M pigment is 530 nm, and the L pigment has 2 variants, one with an absorption maximum of 552 nm, and another with 557 nm. At the post-receptor level, the trichromatic information from the cones is further encoded by opponent neurons, at the level of the bipolar cells: in the L–M (red–green) opponent cells, the stimuli from the L and M cones are opposed, in the S-(L+M) (blue–yellow) opponent cells, the additive stimulus from the L and M cones with the stimulus from the S cones, and in the achromatic opponent cells, the stimuli from the L and M cones (Fig. 14.3). These opponent neurons can also be demonstrated in subsequent segments of the retinocortical pathway, and of the three main pathways, the encoding of red-green information is processed in the parvocellular pathway, that of blue-yellow information, in the koniocellular pathway, and that of achromatic information, in the magnocellular pathway.

Color Vision Defects

There are congenital and acquired color vision defects. The cause of *congenital* color vision defects is that the protein part of one of the photopigments in the cones has a genetically encoded defect. Changes in the amino acids of opsin result in a shift in the absorption maximum of the photopigment and, therefore, the perception of the given primary color is reduced or completely missing. Since the overall majority of hereditary color vision defects affect the M (green) and L (red) photopigments that have just recently been separated during evolution, the discrimination ability of persons with a congenital color vision defect is usually impaired in the red-green range. *Acquired* color vision defects result from different eye diseases, ophthalmo-neurological conditions and toxicities, and therefore cannot be explained with a single pathomechanism.

Color vision defects due to a change in the refractive media are caused by that part of the light that reaches the retina is absorbed in the refractive media; in case of changes in the external retina layers, the trichromatic system is affected, whereas in case of alterations in the internal retina layers, the optic nerve, and the visual pathway, the explanation should be looked for in the opponent neural channels. According to Köllner's rule, the involvement of the refractive media and the external retina layers usually leads to blueyellow defects, whereas damage to the internal retina layers or the optic nerve rather results in red-green color vision defects. In the clinical practice, it may be problematic to determine whether we are faced with a congenital or

Table 14.1

Congenital	Acquired
Usually red–green type	Red–green, blue–yellow or mixed
Mostly affects men	Men and women are equally affected
Both eyes are equally affected	The eyes are often affected to different degrees
Object colors are named correctly, or the error is typical	Many object colors are named erroneously
Does not change over time	Progression or regression is possible
Standard klinikai tesztekkel jól klasszifikálható	Varying or contradictory results with standard clinical tests
Other visual functions are not affected	Often associated with other vision problems (decreased visual acuity, visual field defect)

an acquired color vision defect. The main differential diagnostic points are summarized in Table 14.1. A subjective experience of deterioration in color perception occurs mostly in the case of acquired color vision defects, but often the worsening of visual functions that are more important in everyday life (visual acuity, visual field) is in the foreground. The detection of color vision defects and the monitoring of their progression and regression are of high importance especially in the case of optic nerve diseases, since, as *Linksz* observed, color vision is the first function that is affected, and it is the last one that is restored in optic neuritis.

Examination Methods of Color Vision

The examination methods of color vision are classified into three main groups, which are described below.

Pseudoisochromatic Plates

The principle of pseudoisochromatic tests is that the background and the figure formed by dots of different colors on the plate can be distinguished based on hue discrimination only. The color pairs used on the color diagram are selected based on the confusion axis (protan, deutan or tritan) of persons with congenital color vision defects and, therefore, typical errors are encountered in case of congenital impairment only. Plate sets of numerous different makers and designs are available in printed form: Ishihara, AO Color Vision Test, AOH-H-R, Dvorine, Rabkin, Farnsworth F2, and Velhagen. In Hungary, the Ishihara or the Velhagen plate set is used in most of the ophthalmology offices. It must be noted that the Ishihara plate set does not include a figure for the detection of the tritan-type color vision defect, but it can be found in the Velhagen plate set. Based on the principle of pseudoisochromatic tests, electronic test sequences that can be displayed on a monitor have also been developed, which are also suitable for the quantitative assessment of color discrimination, since the threshold of hue discrimination can be measured by decreasing the saturation of the color pair used. Its disadvantage is that the color display of the monitor requires regular calibration.

Color Mixing Methods

Persons with normal color vision are able to produce any color that matches the test color with trichromatic additive color mixing from the three primary colors. Anomaloscopes used in the clinical practice employ dichromatic color mixing. The subject's task is to find a match for the test color by mixing two suitably selected primary colors. Anomaloscopes designed for finding the Rayleigh match (Nagel anomaloscope and its improved versions) have the highest practical importance. The Rayleigh match is a match of the 589-nm yellow test color of specified brightness with a suitable-ratio mixture of 545-nm yellowish-green and 670-nm red. It is suitable for the screening and differential diagnostics of *protan* and *deutan* color vision defects. In case of the Nagel anomaloscope, the person with *normal color vision* (normal trichromat) finds a single match of a specific mixture of the primary colors red and green with a yellow color of specified brightness. *Dichromats* (patients with protanopia or deuteranopia) find a match for all redgreen mixtures (including the end positions): those with *deuteranopia* by using a yellow color with the same lightness, whereas those with *protanopia*, since the long-wavelength part of the spectrum is shorter for them, by using a darker yellow for the red end position and a lighter yellow for the green end position. *Anomalous trichromats* choose an abnormal red-green mixture ratio for the standard yellow test color: those with *protanomaly* use more red, and those with *deuteranomaly* use more green in their mixture. To assess *tritan color vision defects*, the *Pickford–Nicholson anomaloscope* can be used to find the Engelking–Trendelenburg match (by mixing 470-nm blue and 517-nm green to match the 490-nm test color). Since congenital tritan color vision defects are quite rare, this anomaloscope rather has a role in the examination of *acquired* blue-yellow *color vision defects*.

The use of the Nagel anomaloscope in the diagnostics of acquired color vision defects is of low importance because matchings characteristic to congenital color vision defects are not encountered. This is because as the hue discrimination ability decreases, the absolute and relative matching ranges increase, i.e., the range of different mixture ratios within which the subject finds a match with the test color widens. A typical defect in conditions associated with macular edema is *pseudoprotanomaly,* when the disorientation of photoreceptors results in a shift in their spectral sensitivity. In this case, a matching range that is widened and shifted towards red can be observed. In severe optic nerve conditions, a matching range that extends to the extreme ends (characteristic to dichromates) can be found.

Color Arrangement Tests

The various color arrangement tests consist of suitably selected sets of pigment colors. The task of the subject is to arrange these in the correct order according to hue. Each sample set consists of elements from the *Atlas of the Munsell Color System* that can be clearly characterized, have the same brightness and chroma value (colorfulness),

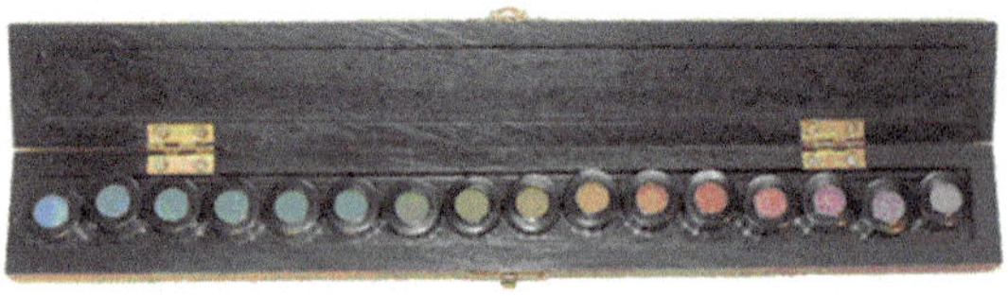

Fig. 14.4 Farnsworth-Munsell Panel D-15 test

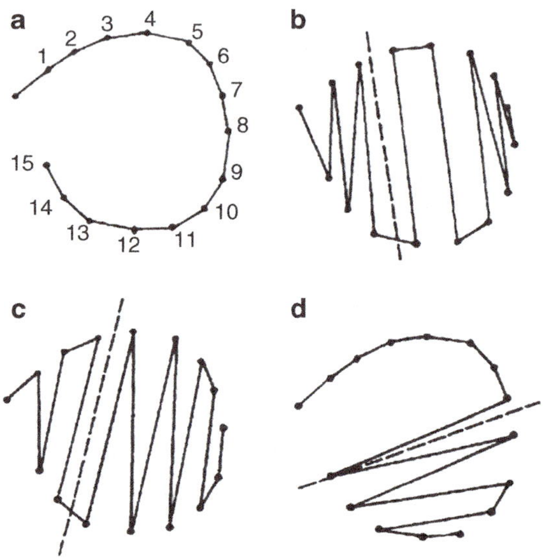

Fig. 14.5 Evaluation diagram of the Farnsworth Panel D-15 test in case of normal color vision (**a**), and protan (**b**), deutan (**c**) and tritan (**d**) color vision defect

and are of different hue. Based on the location of the chromaticity points of the sample elements on the color diagram, the confusion axes theoretically calculated for each color vision defect can be used in the evaluation (Fig. 14.4). These examinations are most appropriate for the detection of quantitative and qualitative changes in the hue discrimination ability and, therefore, the examination of acquired color vision defects.

Farnsworth Panel D-15 Test

The task is to arrange fifteen Munsell color samples of the same brightness and chroma value in the correct order, starting from a reference color. The result can be plotted on a circle diagram, and the alignment of the characteristic direction of errors and the confusion axes visible on the color diagram gives the type of the color vision defect (protan, deutan, tritan) (Fig. 14.5). It is also suitable for quantitative evaluation, the degree and alignment of the color vision defect can be characterized by a vector.

Lanthony Desaturated Panel D-15 Test

A more difficult and, therefore, higher-sensitivity version of the Farnsworth Panel D-15 test, which consists of a series of colors with lower chroma values (closer to gray).

Lanthony New Color Test

It includes four colored series with different chroma values (8-6-4-2) and one gray series. The test consists of two phases: in the separation phase, the task is to separate the gray caps and the colored caps, whereas in the classification phase, the subject must arrange the gray caps in the correct order based on lightness, and the colored caps based on hue. The evaluation is based on the location of the gray caps mixed among the colored ones or the colored caps mixed among the gray ones.

Farnsworth-Munsell 100-hue Test

This is the most widely used examination method of acquired color vision defects. It includes 85 Munsell color samples of the same brightness and chroma value, sorted into four boxed for an easier overview (Figs. 14.6 and 14.7). The subject must arrange the samples in each box, always making sure that the difference in hue between adjacent samples is the lowest possible. The error score is determined for each plate by the sum of the absolute values of the difference in order number between adjacent plates. The sum of scores greater than two will be the total error score. The degree of the color vision defect will be given numerically by the total error score. The upper limit of normal increases somewhat with age, and generally a score above 100 is considered abnormal. The distribution of error scores by plate on the circle diagram is characteristic and allows for a qualitative assessment of the color vision defect (Figs. 14.8, 14.9, 14.10, 14.11,

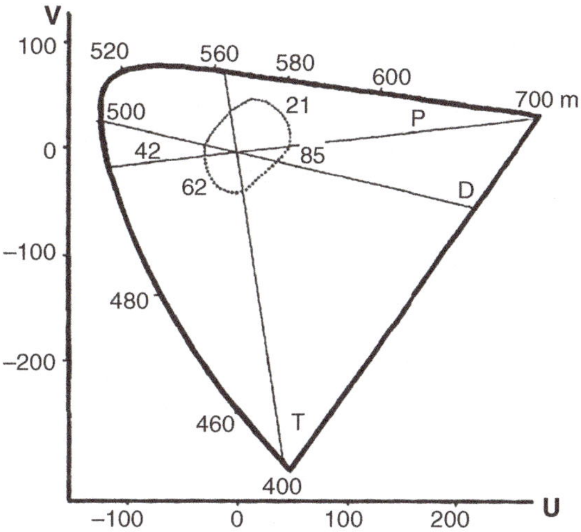

Fig. 14.7 Location of the chromaticity points of the Farnsworth–Munsell 100-hue test sample elements on the CIE(*U*, *V*) color diagram, with the protan (*P*), deutan (*D*) and tritan (*T*) main confusion axes *(redrawn)*

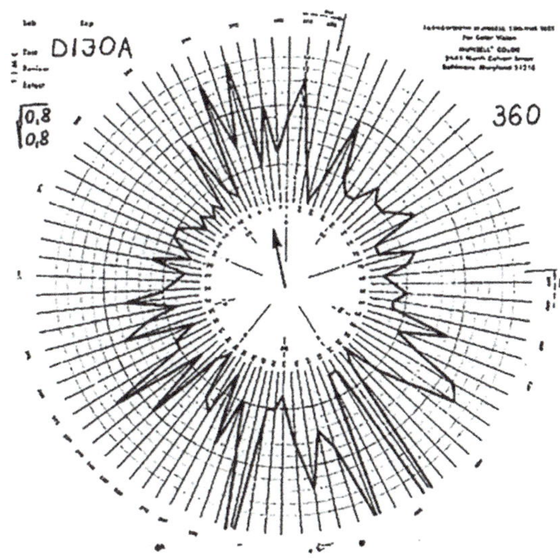

Fig. 14.8 Findings of the Farnsworth–Munsell 100-hue test in mild form of dominantly inherited juvenile optic atrophy (DIJOA): normal visual acuity and marked discrimination disorder along the blue–yellow axis

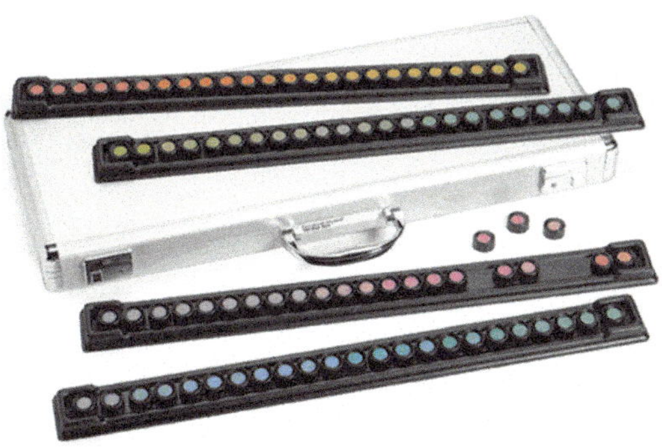

Fig. 14.6 Farnsworth–Munsell 100-hue test

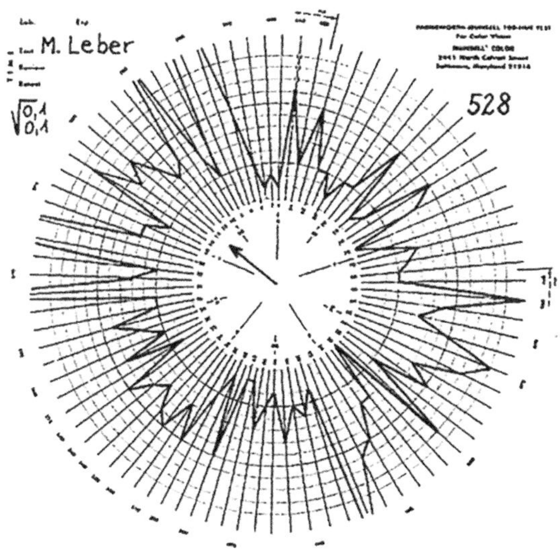

Fig. 14.9 A Farnsworth–Munsell 100-hue test showing severe red–green discrimination defect in Leber optic atrophy

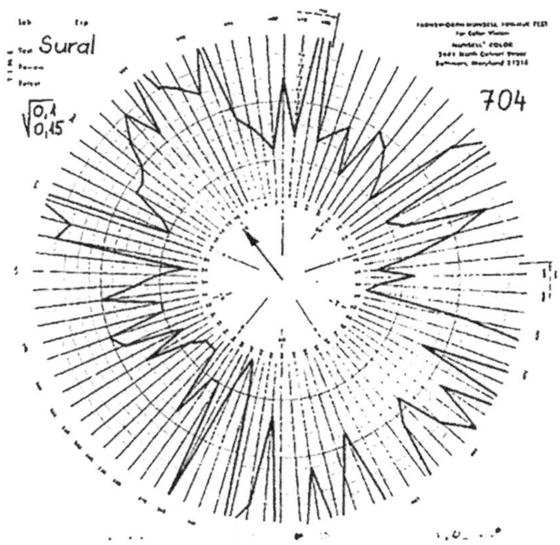

Fig. 14.11 Very severe red–green discrimination defect in ethambutol-induced optic neuropathy

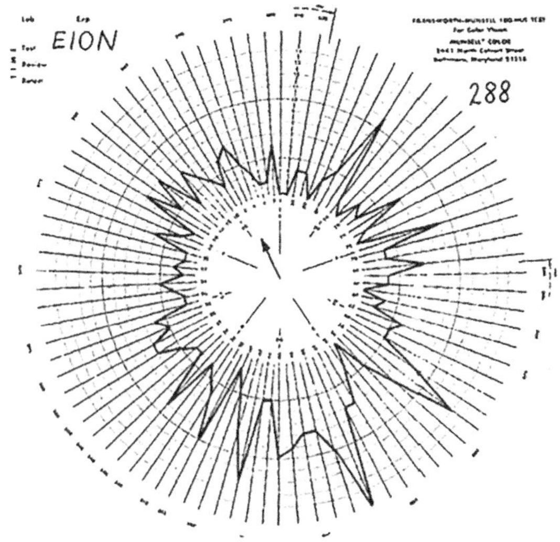

Fig. 14.10 Discrimination defect with a transient axis between red–green and blue–yellow on the Farnsworth–Munsell 100-hue test in anterior ischemic optic neuropathy

and 14.12). The alignment resulting from the accumulation of errors and its significance can also be expressed numerically via mathematical processing.

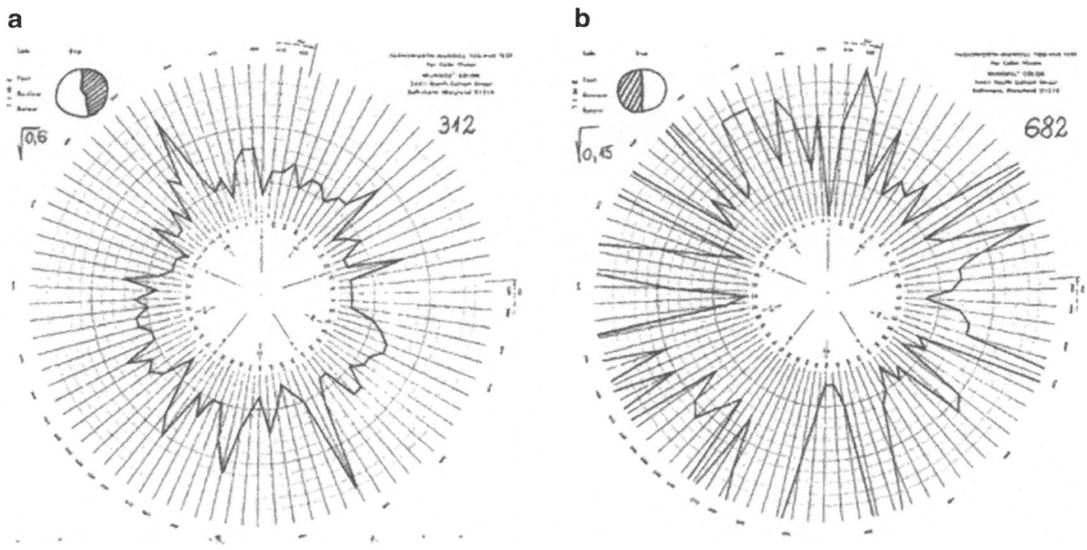

Fig. 14.12 In addition to bitemporal visual field loss due to a hypophyseal adenoma, the eye where the involvement of the center is less (**a**) shows mild, blue–yellow defect, whereas the one with a higher center involvement shows severe, diffuse discrimination defect

Further Readings

Aczel G. A szintevesztes elmeletenek mai dlldsa. Újabb eredmenyek a szemeszetben [Current status of the theory of color vision defects. Recent results in ophthalmology]. 1971. 1:1–68.

Aczel K. A szin-diszkrimindcio kvantitativ ertekelese a Farnsworth-Munsell 100-hue teszt alapjdn. [Quantitative evaluation of color discrimination with the Farnsworth-Munsell 100-hue test]. Szemeszet. 1990;127:97–104.

Allan D. Fourier analysis and the Farnsworth-Munsell 100-hue test. Ophthal Physiol Opt. 1985;5(3):337–42.

Farnsworth D. The Farnsworth-Munsell 100-hue test for the examination of color discrimination. Manual. Baltimore: Munsell Color Company; 1957.

Griffin JF, Wray SR. Acquired color vision defects in retrobulbar neuritis. Am J Ophthalmol. 1978;86:193–201.

Grigsby SS, Vingrys AJ, Benes SC, King-Smith PE. Correlation of chromatic, spatial and temporal sensitivity in optic nerve disease. Invest Ophthalmol Vis Sci. 1991;32(13):3252–62.

Hart WM. Acquired dyschromatopsias. Surv Ophthalmol. 1978;32(1):10.

Jaeger W. Die diagnostische Wert der Pseudoprotanomalie für die Differentialdiagnose zwischen Netzhaut- und Optikuserkrankungen. Klin Mbl Augenheilk. 1987;191:427–9.

Lugo M, Tiedman JS. Computerized scoring and graphing of the Farnsworth-Munsell 100-hue color vision test. Am J Ophthalmol. 1986;101:469–74.

Gy L. Szinmeres [Colorimetry]. Budapest: Muszaki Könyvkiado; 1982.

Nishimuta M, Kitahara K. Color discrimination in optic nerve diseases. Neuroophthalmology. 1985;5(4):253–8.

Pokorny J, Smith VC, Verriest G, Pinckers AJLG. Gongenital and acquired color vision defects. New York: Grune and Stratton; 1979.

Procedures for testing color vision. Report of Working Group. 41. National Academy Washington, DC, 1981.

Schwartz SH. Visual Perception. A clinical orientation. 4th ed. New York: McGraw-Hill; 2009.

Smith VC, Pokorny J, Pass AS. Color axis determination in the Farnsworth-Munsell 100-hue test. Am J Ophthalmol. 1985;100:176–83.

Verriest G, Van Laethem J, Uvijls A. A new assessment of the normal ranges of the Farnsworth-Munsell 100-hue test scores. Am J Ophthalmol. 1982;93:635–42.

Victor JD. Evaluation of poor performance and asymmetry in the Farnsworth-Munsell 100-hue test. Invest Ophthalmol Vis Sci. 1988;29(3):476–81.

Vingrys AJ, King-Smith PE. A quantitative scoring technique for panel tests of color vision. Invest Ophthalmol Vis Sci. 1988;29(1):50–63.

Winston JV, Martin DA, Heckenlively JR. Computer analysis of Farnsworth-Munsell 100-hue test. Doc Ophthalmol. 1986;62:61–72.

Wyszecki G, Stiles WS. Color science: concepts and methods, quantitative data and formulae. New York: Wiley and Sons; 1982.

15 Electroretinography (ERG): Electrophysiological Examination of the Retina

Ägnes Farkas

Contents

Electrophysiological examination of the retina is, currently, the only objective, non-invasive method that provides information about the functional status of the retina. It is suitable for the differentiation of the functions of the rod and cone systems, the diffuse and local, hereditary and acquired diseases of the retina, and the conditions accompanied by damage to the retina and the optic nerve. It also provides useful information for the diagnosis of visual losses of unknown origin. This group of assessments includes time-consuming examinations with special equipment needs, and they require qualified and experienced personnel to order, perform and evaluate them. A general principle is that electrophysiology should not be the first diagnostic method, and it should be performed based on the results of psychophysical tests only. The exceptions for this principle are patients that are unable to cooperate and pediatric patients. Comparison of the results (between institutions, within a country and internationally) is feasible only if the tests are performed in accordance with a uniform protocol, but even such a protocol does not eliminate the need for the establishment of age-specific reference ranges at each examination site. The reliability of the results is confirmed by reproducibility. The International Society for Clinical Electrophysiology of Vision (ISCEV) issues and regularly updates guidelines summarizing standard examination conditions for each method (www.iscev.org).

Electroretinography

History of the Development of the Method

In 1849, du Bois-Reymond measured a potential of 6 mV between electrodes placed on the posterior surface and the cornea of a removed fish eye,

Ä. Farkas, M.D., PhD
Department of Ophthalmology, Semmelweis University, Budapest, Hungary
e-mail: faragnes@gmail.com

J. Somlai, T. Kovács (eds.), *Neuro-Ophthalmology*, DOI 10.1007/978-3-319-28956-4_15

discovering thus the existence of the standing potential of the eye. He found that the cornea is positive compared to the posterior pole of the eye. In 1865, Holmgren measured an electrical response to light in removed frog eye, and then in 1880, by removing the anterior segment of the eye and placing the electrode directly onto the surface of the retina, he established that the response comes from the retina itself. Almost at the same time, but independently from Holmgren, Dewar and McKendrick reported an 'action current' measured on the illuminated eye, and they found a relationship between the amplitude of the electrical response and the logarithm of the intensity of the stimulus. Responses with the highest amplitude were triggered by stimuli that seemed to be the brightest for the human eye. In 1877, Dewar demonstrated that an electrical response can be measured on the intact animal eye if a reference electrode is placed on the cleaned skin surface. He reported the first successful human electroretinogram. In 1880, Kuhne and Schneider, who were working with isolated frog and fish eyes, found that action currents in response to light originate from the receptor layer, rather than the ganglion cell layer. The electrical measurement instruments of that time were not suitable for the measurement of rapid changes in potential. Brücke and Garten demonstrated that similar electric responses can be measured on the eyes of different vertebrates. Gotch used a special electrometer and was the first to observe, in frog eyes, that a response can be measured both at the beginning and at the end of the light stimulus. He used the term 'off-effect' for the latter. Einthoven and Jolly measured detailed responses on frog eyes with a galvanometer, and were the first to report the different components of the retinogram: the initial negative wave, which is followed by a larger, positive reponse (*b*) and then later by a slower, positive potential, the *c* wave. When the light stimulus stops, the *d* wave or off-effect can be seen. The authors were of the opinion that the potential measured on the eye is actually the integrated mass response of numerous independent components. Kahn and Löwenstein reported the first human electroretinography (ERG) in a scientific journal in 1924, and considered it part of the clinical examination of the human eye but concluded that the practical difficulties make their method unsuitable for use in the clinical practice. Due to the technological advance of electrodes and the amplifying, averaging and recording devices, the research of Granit (conducted between 1933 and 1947) led to the study of the origins of the retinogram components and the analysis of the waves still used today. According to him, the rapid-onset cornea-negative wave is the a-wave, the subsequent, considerably larger cornea-positive wave is the b-wave, and the third, slow-onset positive component is the c-wave. He thought that the a-wave comes from the receptors themselves and the *b* wave originates from the part of the visual pathway between the receptors and the ganglion cells (according to Bartley, the bipolar cells). The studies of Noell indicated that the c-wave comes from the pigment epithelium (and he found that the a-wave that comes from the receptors has an early and a late component). Tomita (1950) and Brindley (1956) were the first to use intraretinal microelectrodes for the study of the origin of retinogram components (De Rouck 2006). Recently, transport processes and pharmacological studies based on the blockage or stimulation of ion channels have been the preferred examination methods, performed mostly in apes (rhesus monkeys). Thanks to these, we know today that the electrical response to light stimulus that can be measured on the cornea is generated directly in the neurons of the retina or, as a consequence of the change in the extracellular potassium concentration, in the retinal glial cells (Frishman 2006). Each cell type can be specifically stimulated by deliberately choosing the quality (structure [light or pattern, such as checkerboard], intensity, wavelength, frequency) of the stimulus and the adaptation state of the eye (photopic, scotopic, mesopic).

Conventional or Ganzfeld ERG

The examination consists of stimulating the eye with a single (or repeated) flash of light through a dilated pupil. The responses from the photosensitive cells add up and a summed electrical reponse can be measured. The best and most widely used method of the diffuse (Ganzfeld, full-field or flash diffuse as known in the United States) light stimulation of the retina is with the use of the Ganzfeld stimulator (Hogg 2006). The stimulator is a sphere of 500 mm in diameter, the with specially formed hole, which receives the head of the patient (resting on a chin support). Different light sources can be operated in the interior of the sphere to achieve the desired adaptation state, and then they ensure the illumination of the background, the light stimulus and its optimal effect during the examination. For the light stimulation of patients in lying position (or under general anesthesia) or children, the 'mini' Ganzfeld stimulator can be used, which can be placed on the eye.

Components of the Ganzfeld ERG (GfERG) Examined in the Clinical Practice and Their Origin

Early receptor potential (ERP): in case of a high-intensity light stimulus, an immediate negative response can be measured, which comes from the photopigment embedded in the cell membrane, in the outer segment of the photoreceptors. The negative a-wave (late receptor potential) follows the standard light stimulus with a measurable latency, and its formation is related to the hyperpolarization of the photoreceptors. According to studies, the scotopic a-wave corresponds to the activity of the rods only, whereas besides the cones, elements proximal to them also have a role in the formation of the photopic a-wave. The tall positive b-wave mostly comes from the activity of the depolarizing on-bipolar cells but the participation of the Müller cells is also confirmed by several observations. The low positive c-wave is generated by the hyperpolarization of the apical surface of the pigment epithelium and the distal part of the Müller cells.

Oscillatory potentials: When a strong light stimulus is used, low-amplitude, high-frequency waves appear on the upslope of the b-wave, the number of which (normally 4–10) depends on the quality of the stimulus, the species, etc. They are present in both the scotopic and the photopic adaptation statuses, and their formation involves both the rod and the cone system. Their cellular origin is not fully known but they likely come from the inner retina (amacrine cells and/or inner plexiform layer) supplied by the central retinal artery. Their number and amplitude decrease or they disappear in ischemic conditions of the retina (e.g., occlusion of the central retinal artery, diabetic retinopathy).

30-Hz flicker response: If a high-frequency (30-Hz) stimulus is applied during photopic adaptation, sinusoidal, flicker responses can be observed, which were previously considered to be originating from the cones but according to recent studies, a postreceptor origin is likely (Bush et al. 1996).

Photopic negative response (PhNR): The negative wave following the b-wave, which is considered to be coming from the ganglion cells, was described both in animal and human studies at the turn of the millennium. Several pieces of data support that PhNR and component N95 of the pattern-ERG may correspond to the same electrical response of the retina. This observation has high clinical importance because if the above equation is true, PhNR is a better indicator of ganglion cell dysfunction because with an adequate stimulus, it is easier to evaluate and a bigger response can be measured, which is independent from the refractive error and less affected by the opacity of refractive media (Frishman 2006).

GfERG in the Everyday Clinical Practice

ERG was introduced into clinical practice by Karpe (1945). According to the clinical guideline revised in 2004, the GfERG protocol includes the following five types of examination:

In dark-adapted state (adaptation time: 20 min):

1. Examination of the rod response with weak light stimulus;
2. Examination of the mixed (rod+cone) response with strong light stimulus;

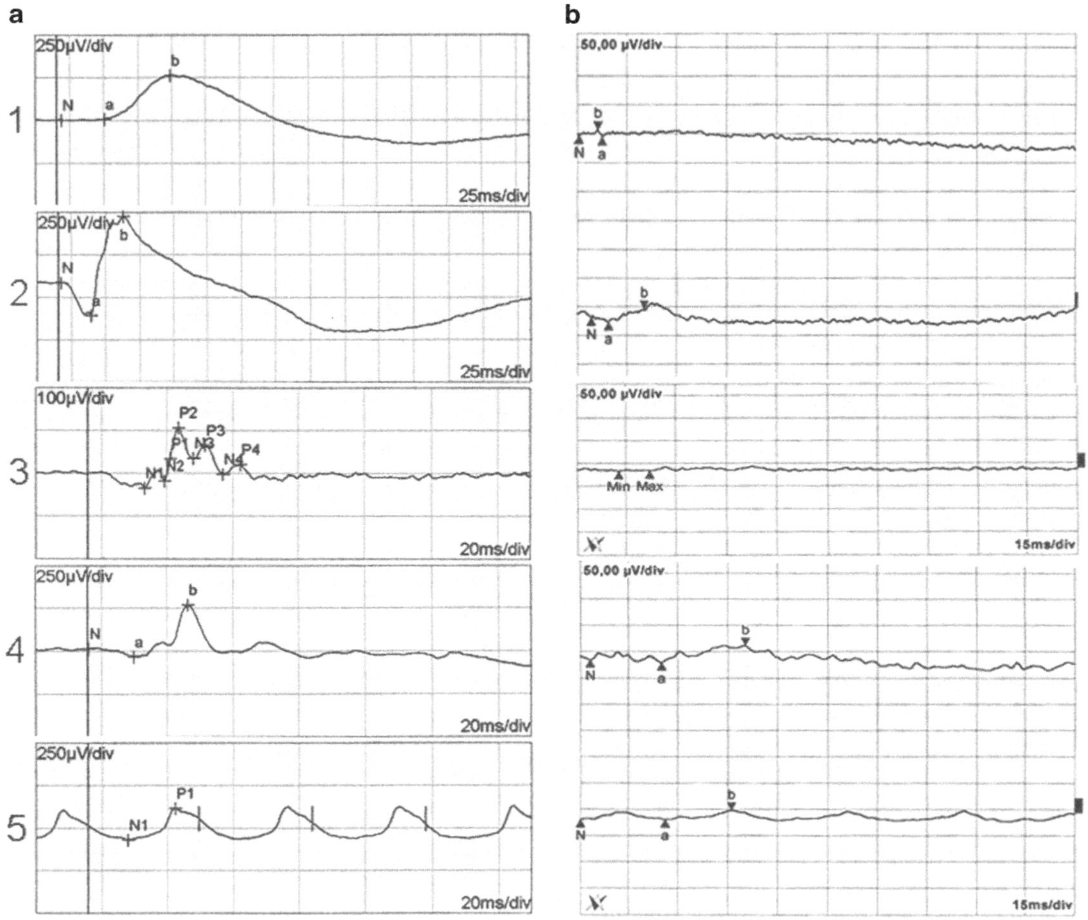

Fig. 15.1 GfERG examination protocol in intact eye (**a**) and in advanced retinitis pigmentosa (**b**). Only residual cone function can be measured in the affected eye (waves 2, 4 and 5)

3. Examination of oscillatory potentials (in both adaptation states, although it is used more often in the dark; the adaptation time in light-adapted state is about 10 min);
4. Examination of the cone response with strong light stimulus;
5. Examination of the flicker response to a frequent (most often 30-Hz) stimuli.

Figure 15.1a and 15.3a shows responses (De Rouck 2006; Frishman 2006; Hogg 2006; Bush et al. 1996; Marmor et al. 2004) measured on a healthy eye in accordance with the above protocol. Figure 15.1b shows the examination results of a patient with advanced retinitis pigmentosa (rod-cone dystrophy), where very weak residual cone function can be observed only (waves 2, 4 and 5). The recommended strength of the light stimulus (standard flash, SF) at the surface of the Ganzfeld bowl is 1.5–3.0 photopic cd-s-m^{-2}. The photostimulator is suitable for the examination if it is capable of emitting a light stimulus that is lower than SF by 3 logarithmic units. The duration of the light stimulus usually does not exceed 5 ms. If a stimulus that is considerably longer than this (150 ms) is used, ON and OFF responses can also be measured. For the additional technical details of the examination, see the ISCEV guideline (Marmor et al. 2004). Besides the technical background (amplification, recording and averaging, if required), an important requirement of the examination is an active electrode placed on the cornea or on the surface of the eye near the cornea that provides good contact even in the case of eye movements. The recommended application site of the reference electrodes is the temple or the earlobe, and that of the grounding electrode is the forehead.

Active electrodes: Riggs was the first to use a silver electrode filled with physiological saline solution and built into a scleral contact lens for an ERG examination in 1941. Karpe placed a thin tube facing the eyeball into the plastic sclera shell, and led the rod-like silver chloride electrode through it to the eye, which was in contact with it in one point. The Burian-Allen electrode is a metal ring built into the PMMA lens that keeps the interpalpebral space open. (Ring electrodes ensure a more reliable contact). Over time, numerous other types of active electrodes have been developed, e.g., a gold foil 'hooked' over the lower lid (Arden), a fiber electrode floating on the corneal tear film (named DTL after Dawson, Trick and Litzkow), a loop electrode made of a noble metal wire that can be hooked into the lower fornix (Hawlina-Konec), which provide lower quality waves than contact lens electrodes but are still useful in certain cases.

ERG-Jet electrode: corneal floating lens with a narrow gold foil ring attached to its inner surface. It provides a good and stable contact.

Measuring the Parameters of the ERG Components

Amplitudes: the amplitude of the a-wave is measured from the baseline to the negative peak of the wave, whereas that of the b-wave is measured from the peak of the a-wave to the peak of the b-wave. The ERG response can also be characterized with the *b/a* ratio. In healthy eyes, the amplitude of the b-wave is higher than that of the a-wave.

Time course

Time to peak (implicit time): the time from the start of the light stimulus to the peak of the wave. In practice, the implicit time of the a- and b-waves is evaluated most often.

Latency: the time between the start of the stimulus and the start of the response (not individual waves but the electrical response as a whole that has a latency) (Fig. 15.2).

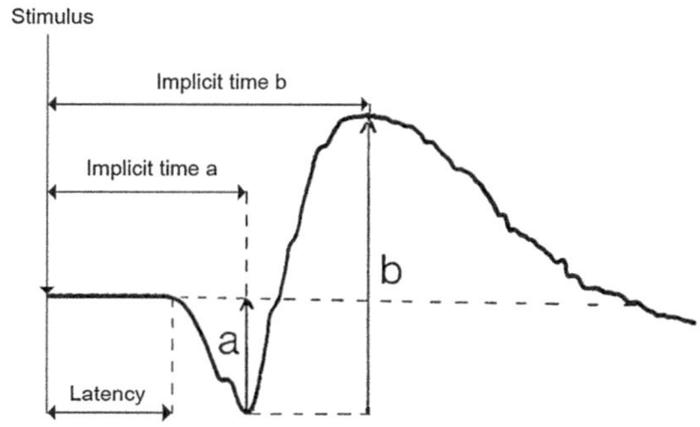

Fig. 15.2 Measurement of the amplitude and time parameters of GfERG components

Electronegative ERG (or negative ERG): the above ratio may be reversed in different abnormal conditions (Nagy et al. 2005; Weleber 2006). According to the classical definition, a negative ERG means that a normal-amplitude a-wave is accompanied by a b-wave with a severely decreased amplitude that is lower than that of the a-wave (Fig. 15.3b), such as in X-linked juvenile retinoschisis and congenital stationary night blindness.

In the past two decades, the term 'negative ERG' has been applied to all cases where the amplitude of the b-wave is lower that of the *a*-wave, even if the *a*-wave itself is subnormal (e.g., certain forms of retinitis pigmentosa). Figure 15.3a shows the GfERG examination protocol characteristic to complete color blindness with intact scotopic and extinguished photopic activity.

Electroretinography with Pattern (Reversal) Stimulation

Pattern (Reversal) ERG (PERG)

If stimulation during the ERG examination is performed with a black and white checkerboard pattern (alternating the elements between black and white with a specified frequency), the electrical response provides information about the ganglion cells of the retina and, due to central fixation, about the macular function as well. (These structures

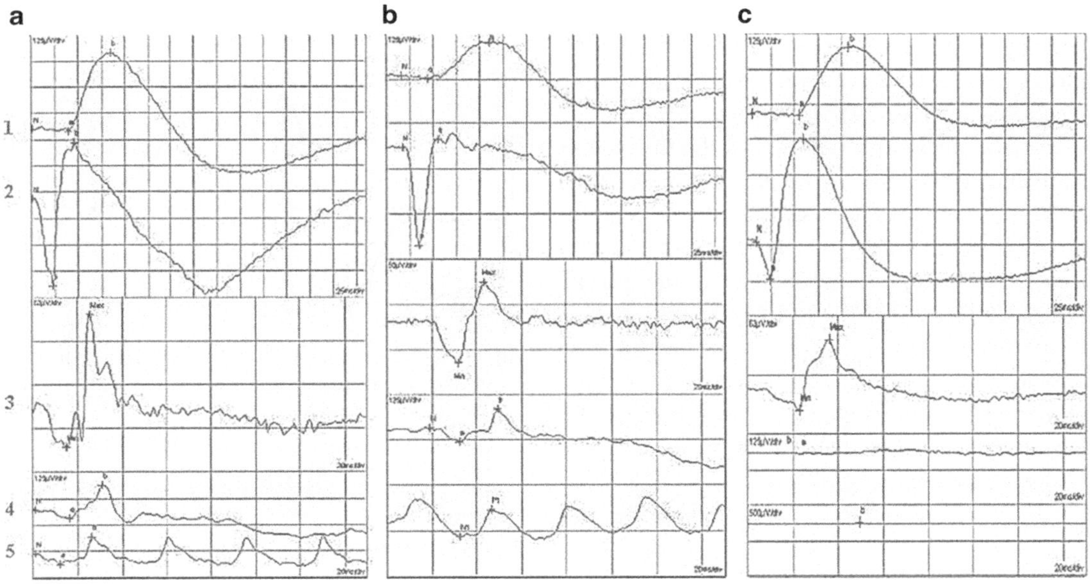

Fig. 15.3 GfERG examination protocol in an intact eye (**a**), X-linked juvenile retinoschisis (**b**) and congenital acromatopsia (**c**)

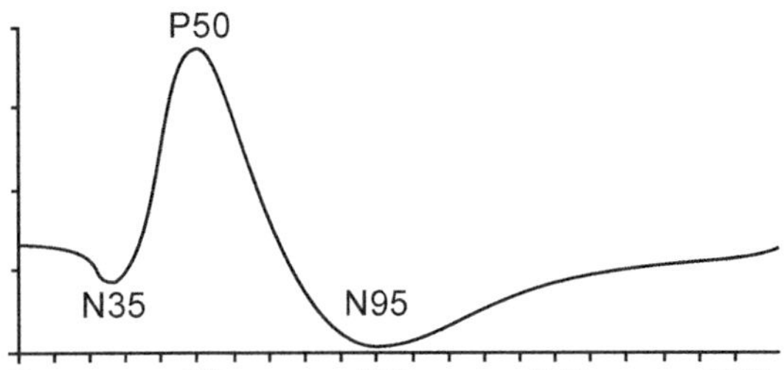

Fig. 15.4 Schematic illustration of the Pattern ERG curve

cannot be examined with GfERG.) For example, if the result of the VEP test is abnormal, PERG helps find out if the abnormal VEP finding is caused by a lesion of the macula or the optic nerve. (Multifocal ERG examination is also suitable for the assessment of the macular function.) The transient examination mode (six pattern changes per second, which corresponds to a frequency of about 3 Hz) enables the independent assessment of the following components (Fig. 15.4):

- N35: a small negative wave with a time to peak of 35 ms
- P50: a positive component with considerably higher amplitude
- N95: a negative wave with even higher amplitude

Waves P50 and N95 have clinical importance. The fact that the responses are very low (in a healthy eye, the amplitude of P50 is between 2 and 4 μV, and that of N95 is somewhat higher) makes the examinations more difficult. The current hypothesis as to the origin of the waves is that P50 characterizes the condition of the macula, whereas N95 indicates that of the optic nerve (Holder et al. 2007). According to a new hypothesis (Bach), P50 corresponds to the input activity of the ganglion cells, and N95 to the output ('spiking') activity (Bach et al. 2006).

Focal and Multifocal Electroretinography (mfERG)

Conventional electroretinography performed with the Ganzfeld method (GfERG) characterizes the summed electrical activity of the outer (and middle) retina, and the impairment of up to about half of the photoreceptors is required for an about 50 % decrease in amplitude on the retinogram (Armington et al. 1980; Schuurmans et al. 1978). Focal (or foveal) electroretinography was developed for the diagnostics of local diseases of the retina, primarily of those affecting the posterior pole (Arden et al. 1966). Of the various technical solutions, the method of Sandberg (Sandberg et al. 1977) has become the most popular, which involves the stimulation of an area of interest of about 3° in diameter with a stimulator built into an ophthalmoscope. Although the method has been employed successfully by some work groups (Miyake et al. 1988), it has not been used extensively in the clinical practice due to the technical difficulties. A significant advance in the field of electroretinography is multifocal electroretinography (mfERG) developed by Sutter and Tran (Sutter et al. 1992) and published in 1992. The method has been used in Hungary since 2000 (Farkas et al. 2005). With the use of a special stimulus and the mathematical analysis of the results, the new method enables the functional topographical examination of a defined area (of 50–60° in diameter) of the retina. The numerous small retinograms recorded under photopic conditions quasi map the retina and show even small areas of abnormal/extinguished or intact function.

Method: The special stimulus pattern consists of different numbers (61 and 103 in the clinical routine and 214 for scientific study purposes) of aligned black and white hexagons, where the size of the hexagons changes from the center to the periphery in inverse proportion to cone cell density. (If the hexagons forming the stimulus pattern were identical in size, recording the high central curves in case of intact macular function would be difficult.) The elements of the stimulus pattern change their color from black to white and vice versa in a seemingly unsystematic sequence, which is actually an almost random/pseudo-random M (maximum length) sequence (Sutter et al. 1992). The color of each hexagon changes according to the above algorithm, in the same sequence but joining the sequence in different phases. The changes in color are experienced as a vibrating visual effect by the person fixating at the stimulus pattern. Since the number of white and black elements is almost the same in every moment of the stimulation, the lightness of the stimulus is stable. The actual stimuli are the white hexagons, the display density of which can be controlled with the insertion of black hexagons in changing numbers. If the display interval of the white hexagons is sufficient for the completion of the simulation process, and the subsequent stimulus reaches the retina in its resting status, a first order kernel (FOK) retinal response can be recorded, which basically characterizes the linear function of the outer retina. This method is used routinely for clinical-purpose examinations. When the stimuli follow each other so frequently that the next stimulus reaches the retina in its activated status, the recorded electrical response characterizes the non-linear function of the retina and, second, third and higher order responses can be recorded (Sutter et al. 1992) which are still subjects of scientific research.

In the everyday practice, there are three ways to plot the results. As a result of the examination, a number of small retinograms (kernels) corresponding to the number of hexagons in the stimulus pattern are plotted. The sum of these is the trace array (or plot) that provides information in a similar way to the result of the visual field test. The individual waves of the trace array cannot be thought of as directly recorded potentials from the areas stimulated by the appropriate hexagons. The elements of the multifocal reponse are mathematical extracts obtained with cross-correlation from the continuously recorded, summed electrical activity, which are characteristic to the functioning of the given area.

Figure 15.5 shows the schematic illustration of the formation of the multifocal response. According to Hood et al. (2000), the first two waves (the lower negative N1 and the higher positive P1) of the mfERG currently used in the clinical practice and the photopic *a*- and b-waves of the GfERG are mostly generated in the same retinal cells. Similarly to the conventional ERG examination, the amplitude (μV) and time to peak value (implicit time, ms) of the waves are measured. In the clinical practice, the P1 wave is evaluated, whereas the N1 wave is of limited clinical importance due to the low value of its parameters. Because of the different sizes of the stimulus hexagons, the electronic activity of a unit of area, the response density (in nV/degree^2) should be used instead of the amplitude (in μV)

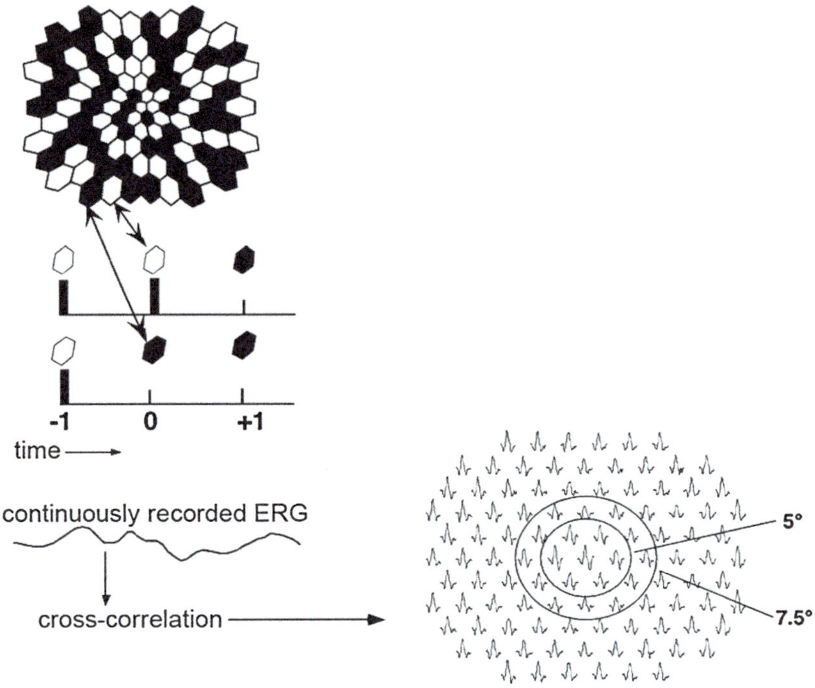

Fig. 15.5 Process of formation of the multifocal electroretinogram: A stimulus pattern consisting of 103 hexagons, with two selected hexagons below it (their color at the given time, as well as in the previous and next phases), and the trace array calculated with cross-correlation from the continuously recorded retinogram, with the central areas of 5° and 7.5° in radius marked

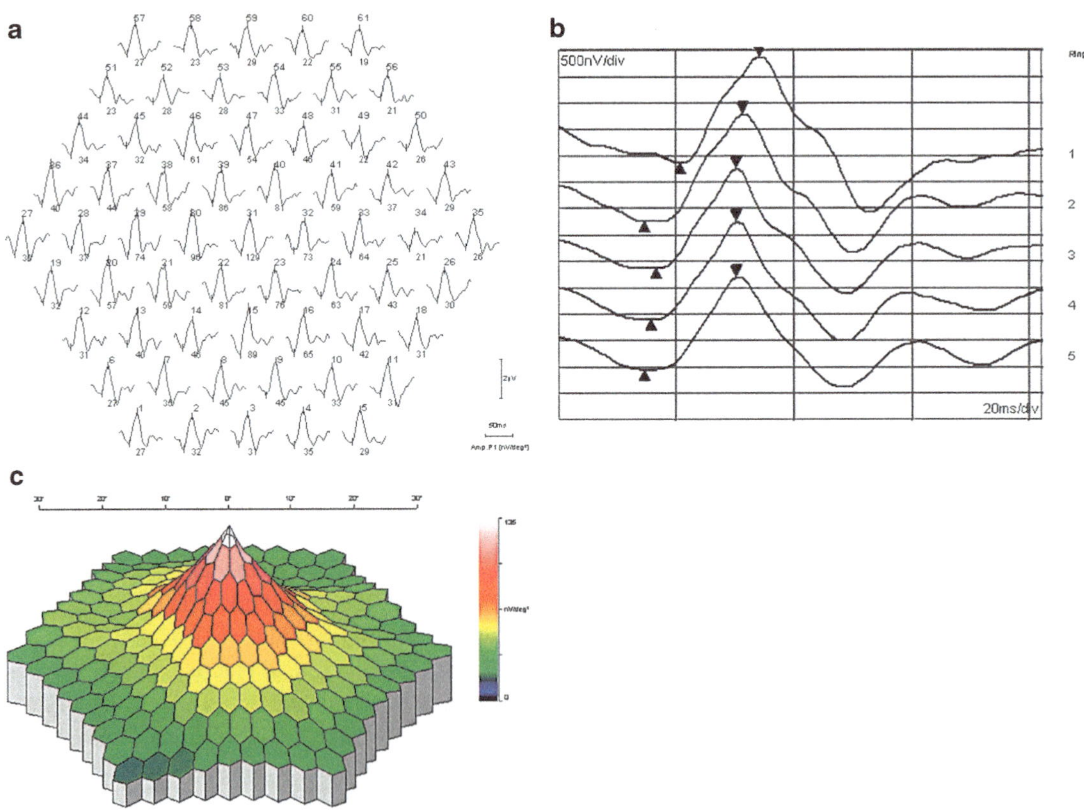

Fig. 15.6 (**a**) mfERG: intact trace array obtained during the examination of the right eye with a stimulus pattern of 61 hexagons. Trace No. 21 with a subnormal-amplitude wave indicates the location of the optic disc. (**b**) mfERG: ring display of an intact eye. The amplitude of the waves decreases in the downward direction (from the center towards the periphery). (**c**) mfERG: 3-dimensional display of an intact eye (related to the normal for the age group [135 nV/degree^2])

of the waves to characterize the examination results. In the area of the optic disc, not a complete loss of function but one (or more) wave(s) with decreased amplitude can be recorded (since it is never only one stimulus hexagon but several ones that are projected on the optic disc). If the blind spot can be identified on the trace array, it is an important, indirect proof of proper fixation (Fig. 15.6a). In the evaluation of concentric dysfunctions, the ring display is useful, which shows the average electrical activity of hexagons that are at the same distance from the center (Fig. 15.6b). The results can also be displayed in a 3-dimensional view, which is quite spectacular, especially in color, but its evaluation is recommended only in conjunction with the trace array (Fig. 15.6c).

Practical implementation of the method: There are numerous differences between the first equipment that was designed for the multifocal technique (United States, VERIS) and the German device (Retiscan) used in many European countries, which makes it impossible to compare the results numerically (Bock et al. 1999). In 2007, an ISCEV standard was created also for this examination (Hood and et al. 2007).

The Most Important Elements of the Examination Protocol

Preparation: The mfERG is recorded after 15 min of adaptation in a room with artificial illumination that provides stable light conditions. Since the diameter of the pupil has an effect on the results, the pupils are dilated for the examination (usually 1 drop of cyclopentolate is sufficient), and the diameter is recorded. The best optical correction for the examination distance is recommended.

Electrodes: All types of electro des used for the ERG examination are suitable. The best contact and, therefore, the highest amplitude values are provided by the types that are in contact with the cornea and the bulbar conjunctiva next to the cornea (contact lens, e.g., 'ERG-Jet', DTL). (An important requirement is that the contact lens must be transparent in the area that corresponds to the pupil.) The reference electrodes are placed on the temple, near the lateral corner of the eye, whereas the grounding electrodes are placed on the skin of the forehead. Stimulation: The stimulator is usually a CRT display or an LCD projector (or an array of LEDs). The refresh rate is 75 or 60 Hz. To achieve an optimal contrast of about 90 % for the white and black stimulus hexagons, the average luminance of the stimulus pattern must be 50–100 cd/m^2 during the examination. The examination distance must be determined so that the patient can see the entire stimulus pattern under an angle of vision of 20–30°. The examination is usually performed monocularly. The fixation of the patient must be checked (preferably with suitable monitor). The fixation symbol displayed at the center of the stimulus pattern must be chosen based on the visual acuity and age of the patient so that it covers the smallest possible area of the central hexagon. The stimulus pattern that consists of 61 hexagons is used in the everyday practice. The stimulus pattern that consists of 103 elements and is of greater 'resolution capability' provides more accurate information in case of macular lesions, but the amplitude-noise ratio is worse than in the previous case. The examination does not mean a burden for the patients, and usually children above the age of 5 years also tolerate it well. (It is not continuous but performed in 8 phases, with pauses of a few seconds, and takes a total of about 4–8 min depending on the compliance of the patient.)

Contraindication: it cannot be performed in narcosis, and it is contraindicated or to be considered in case of epilepsy. Origin of the mfERG waves: pharmacological studies have confirmed that, under standard conditions, implicit time and amplitude are primarily influenced by the functioning of the receptors (cones) and the bipolar cells, respectively (Birch 2001). In the typical form of retinitis pigmentosa (in a not markedly advanced stage), there is usually no difficulty fixating. Typically, the central electrical activity is maintained to varying degree. Retinitis pigmentosa is primarily a disease of the receptors. In the initial phase, a decrease in amplitude is less typical than the prolongation of the implicit time (Seeliger et al. 1998).

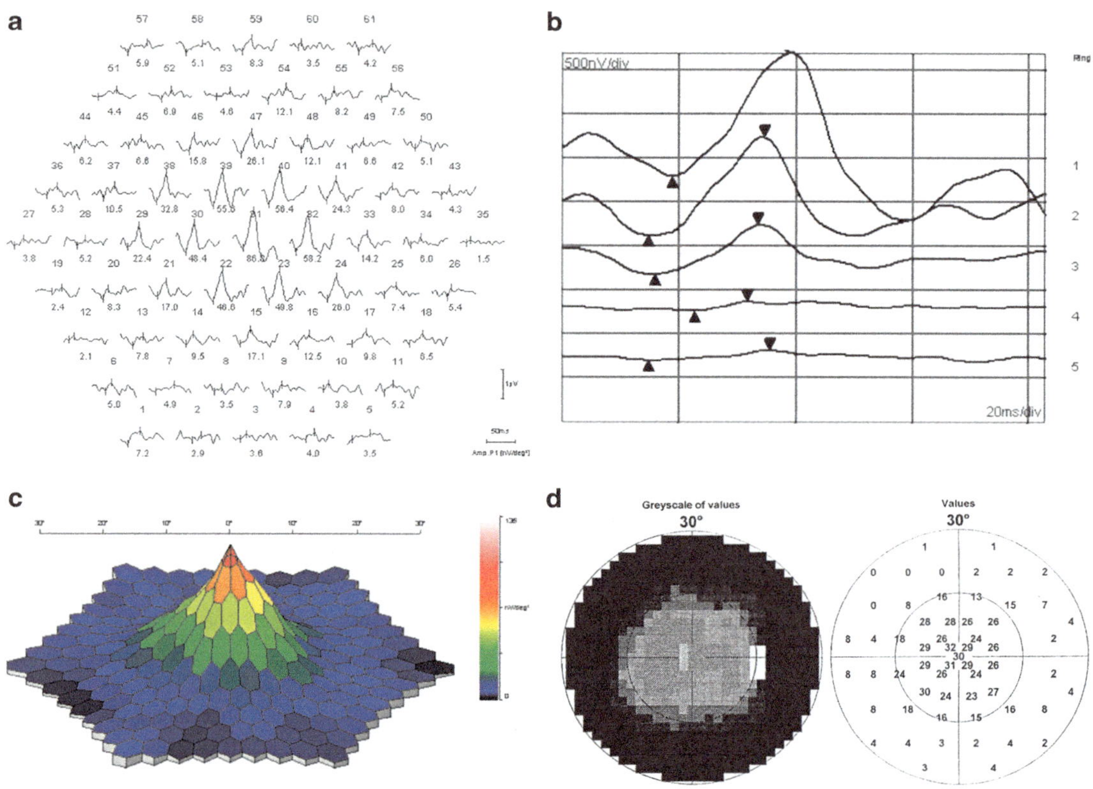

Fig. 15.7 (**a**) mfERG: Retinitis pigmentosa, trace array. The amplitude of the central wave is within the normal range. Subnormal potentials in the second ring, markedly subnormal potentials in the third ring, and residual potentials in the two peripheral rings. (**b**) mfERG: Retinitis pigmentosa, ring display. There is no measurable electrical activity in the two peripheral rings. (**c**) mfERG: Retinitis pigmentosa, 3D display. The central peak is visible in accordance with the functioning area of the retina (the relation is based on the normal for the age group, 135 nV/degree^2) but the periphery is markedly 'flat. (**d**) Visual field test results of the eye presented on **a**, **b** and **c**

Figure 15.7a–d shows the trace array, the ring and 3D display of the examination results, and the result of the visual field test for a patient in a moderately advanced stage.

In Stargardt macular dystrophy (Fig. 15.8a), the location of the dysfunctioning area, due to the difficulty fixating, is usually noncentral, which is visible also on the trace array (Fig. 15.8b). The amplitudes are subnormal at the center, and they are closer and closer to normal as we go towards the periphery (Kretschmann et al. 1998). Correspondingly to the decreased function, the center is sunken on the 3-dimensional image (Fig. 15.8c). It is important to emphasize that electroretinography performed with the conventional method is still indispensable in cases where the lesion is not clearly acquired.

Electrooculography

History: The existence of the standing potential of the eye and that its amplitude depends on the light conditions, have been known since the observations made by du Bois-Reymond (1849) and Holmgren (1865), respectively. The origin of the potential was investigated by several scientists in the nineteenth century, and it was assumed that it comes from the pigment epithelium of the retina. Due to the unmet technical requirements, it was only in 1940 when a recording system with properly stable direct current was developed, which was suitable for tracking also the slow changes (c-wave) in the retina.

The resting standing or base potential measured between the anterior and posterior poles

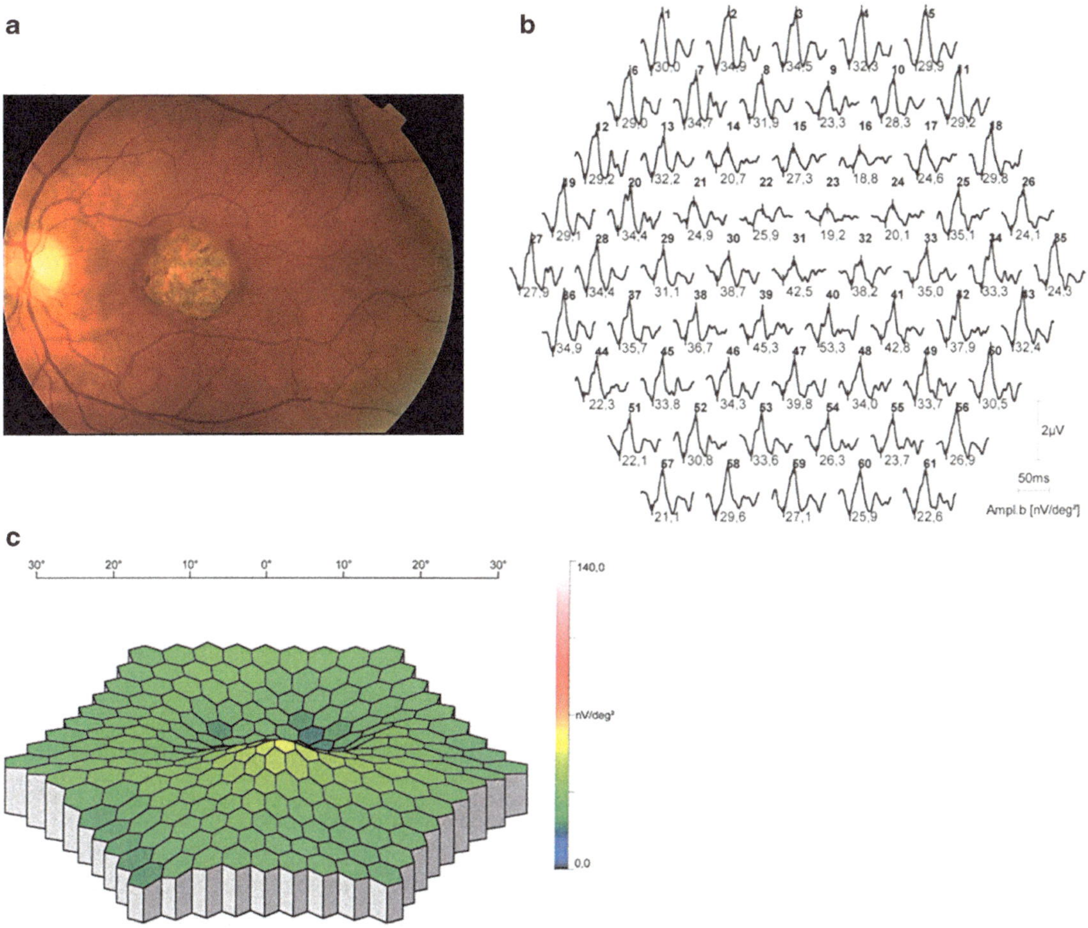

Fig. 15.8 (**a**) Stargardt disease, marked macular dystrophy. (**b**) On the trace array of the presented eye, the area of abnormal waves is slightly shifted upwards due to improper fixation. The periphery shows good function. (**c**) mfERG, 3D display: the area of impaired function is 'sunken' compared with its surroundings

of the eye mostly comes from the pigment epithelium of the retina, and changes in accordance with the light conditions of the eye. Marg was the first to use the term electrooculography (EOG) for the measurement of the base potential in 1951. Since the first description of the human EOG, the studies conducted on animal eyes, isolated eyes and isolated pigment epithelium preparations have provided numerous pieces of data about the ion channels between the inner and outer surfaces of the pigment epithelium, the ion transport mechanisms and ion pumps, as well as the relationship between these and the electrooculogram (Arden 2006a).

Components of the EOG and their origin: The electrooculogram has two components, a light-insensitive and a light-sensitive one (Arden 2006b).

- The first component depends on the integrity of the pigment epithelium, as well as on extra-retinal factors (cornea, lens, ciliary body). It is responsible for the 'dark trough' (the minimum value measured in dark), and it is independent of previous light conditions and the status of the photoreceptors. In dark, the base potential decreases for about 8–10 min.
- The second, light-sensitive component is generated by the depolarization of the basal

membrane of the pigment epithelium (and does not depend directly on the potassium concentration of the retina). This depolarization of the basal membrane results in the increased potential of the pigment epithelial cells (transepithelial potential). The remaining part of the process requires functioning photoreceptors. In response to light, photoreceptors lose sodium and take up potassium from the subretinal space (where the potassium concentration decreases). After the light is switched on, the EOG shows an initial decrease lasting for 60–75 s ('rapid oscillation,' hyperpolarization of the basal membrane of the pigment epithelium, related to the transport of chloride ions), and then a slow increase with a 'light peak' (maximum value measured in light) lasting for 7–14 min, which is followed by sinusoidal oscillations that can be recorded for about 2 h.

According to animal experiments and observations in humans, the standing potential increases in case of hypoxia, and shows a sudden drop in response to oxygen. These changes are related to the change in the potassium concentration of the subretinal space, and are likely the consequences of the current activity of the sodium-potassium pump in the inner segment of the photoreceptors.

Theoretical principle of the recording of the EOG: Recording during eye movements, which is widely used, is based on the following theoretical consideration: since the corneo-retinal base potential of the eye spreads symmetrically around the optical axis in every direction, if the eye that can be considered a dipole, moves from right to left and vice versa, the voltage recorded with electrodes placed relatively far away changes depending on the rotation angle. In 1962, Arden and Fojas found that the comparison of the potentials measured on the light-adapted and dark-adapted eye (light peak/dark trough=Arden ratio) provides more useful information than the absolute value of the resting potential (Arden 2006b).

Examination procedure:

- Prior adaptation is required with average room illumination, for the time needed for placing the electrodes and providing the patient with information about the examination. (If the eyes were illuminated previously, a waiting period of about 1 h is recommended.)
- Electrodes: small, non-polarizing, usually silver chloride skin electrodes are placed near the medial and lateral canthi of both eyes, symmetrically. (The grounding electrode is placed on the forehead.)
- During the examination, the patient is sitting in front of a Ganzfeld bowl, which provides proper diffuse light adaptation during the light phase, and the LEDs located to the right and left of the fixation points in the center of the bowl (correspondingly to a 30° angle of vision), which are flashing in alternation, control the saccadic eye movements in both phases of the examination. (In case of a dilated pupil, the recommended illumination of the bowl is 100 cd/m^2, and without dilation, it is 400–600 cd/m^2.)
- The examination takes approximately 30 min (15 min for each of the dark and light phases). For 10 s in every minute (10×), the subject is looking rhythmically from one light source to the other, each of which is visible under a visual angle of 15° to the right or left of the center (without moving the head).
- During the evaluation of the examination, the EOG amplitudes (average value of the 10-s active periods; an amplitude of 150 μV is the lower limit of normal) and the Arden ratio (light peak/dark trough; the normal value is above 1.65–1.8) must be determined (Brown et al. 2006).

Clinical utility of EOG: The examination is essentially simple but also time-consuming, and therefore it is usually dispensable in case of diseases where the retina is abnormal based on the ophthalmoscopic picture and the ERG (rod dystrophies, chorioretinal atrophies, inflammatory conditions and vascular lesions).

In most cases, the EOG and ERG findings are in accordance with each other. Best disease is an exception. It has been observed that the light

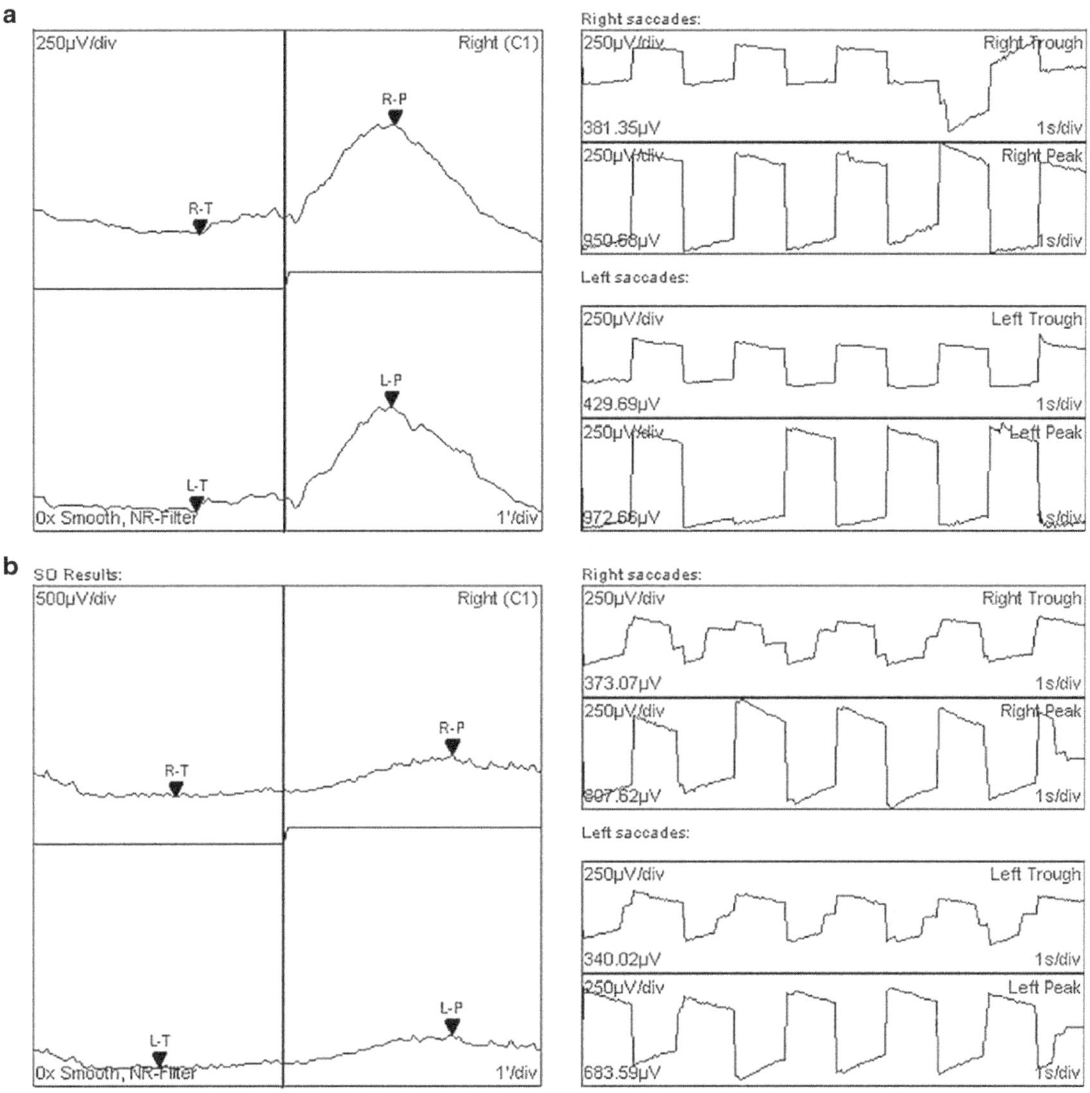

Fig. 15.9 (**a**) EOG findings of a healthy person. On the left, the dark trough and the light peak can be recognized well in both eyes. (On the right, the traces recording the eye movements are shown.) (**b**) EOG findings in Best disease. The light peak is not visible in either eye, and there is only a minimal rise during the light phase compared with the traces recorded during the dark phase

peak is present if there is physical contact between the pigment epithelium and the photoreceptors (e.g., the response is absent in retinal detachment). This may be the mechanism of the absence (of differential diagnostic value) of the EOG light peak with normal ERG findings in Best vitelliform dystrophy. Figures 15.9a, b show the EOG examination results of a healthy subject and a patient with Best disease.

References

Arden GB. Chapter 2: History of the electro-oculogram. In: Heckenlively JR, Arden GB, editors. Principles and practice of clinical electrophysiology of vision. Cambridge: MIT Press; 2006a. p. 11–3.

Arden GB. Chapter 11: Origin and significance of the electro-oculogram. In: Heckenlively JR, Arden GB, editors. Principles and practice of clinical electrophysiology of vision. Cambridge: MIT Press; 2006b. p. 123–38.

Arden GB, et al. Foveal electroretinogram as a clinical test. Br J Ophthal. 1966;50:740.
Armington JC, et al. Summation of retinal potentials. J Opt Soc Am. 1980;51:877–86.
Bach M, et al. Chapter 13: The origin of the pattern electroretinogram. In: Heckenlively JR, Arden GB, editors. Principles and practice of clinical electrophysiology of vision. Cambridge: MIT Press; 2006. p. 185–96.
Birch DG. The focal and multifocalel electroretinogram. In: Fishman GA, editor. Electrophysiologic testing in disorders of the retina, optic nerve and visual pathway. San Francisco: The Foundation of the American Academy of Ophthalmology; 2001. p. 177–95.
Bock M, et al. A comparison of two multifocal systems. Doc Ophthalmol. 1999;97:157–78.
Brown M, et al. ISCEV standard for clinical electro-oculography (EOG). Doc Ophthalmol. 2006;113:205–12.
Bush RA, et al. Inner retinal contributions to the primate photopic fast flicker electroretinogram. J Opt Soc Am A. 1996;13:557–65.
De Rouck AF. Chapter 1: History of the electroretinogram. In: Heckenlively JR, Arden GB, editors. Principles and practice of clinical electrophysiology of vision. Cambridge: MIT Press; 2006. p. 3–10.
Farkas A, et al. Multifokdlis elektroretinogrdfia: a retinafunkcio objektiv topogrdfiai vizsgdlata [Multifocal electroretinography: objective topographical examination of the retinal function]. Szemeszet. 2005;142:83–8.
Frishman LJ. Chapter 12: Origins of the electroretinogram. In: Heckenlively JR, Arden GB, editors. Principles and practice of clinical electrophysiology of vision. Cambridge: MIT Press; 2006. p. 139–83.
Hogg C. Chapter 19: Stimulus devices, calibration, and measurement of light. In: Heckenlively JR, Arden GB, editors. Principles and practice of clinical electrophysiology of vision. Cambridge: MIT Press; 2006. p. 265–83.
Holder GE, et al. ISCEV standard for clinical pattern electroretinography, 2007 update. Doc Ophthalmol. 2007;114:111–6.
Hood DC. Assessing retinal function with the multifocal technique. Prog Ret Eye Res. 2000;19:607–46.
Hood DC, et al. Standard for clinical multifocal electroretinography. 2007. PDF.
Kretschmann U, et al. Multifocal electroretinography in patients with Stargardt's macular dystrophy. Br J Ophthal. 1998;14:267–75.
Marmor MF, et al. Standard for clinical electroretinography. Doc Ophthalmol. 2004;108:107–14.
Miyake Y, et al. Local macular electroretinographic responses in idiopathic central serous retinopathy. Am J Ophthalmol. 1988;106:546–50.
Nagy N, et al. Negativ tipusu elektroretinogrammal jdro korkepek. Szemeszet. 2005;142:167–70.
Sandberg MA, et al. A hand-held, two-channel stimulator-ophthalmoscope. Arch Ophthalmol. 1977;95:1881–2.
Schuurmans RP, et al. Photocoagulation and the electroretinogram. Doc Ophthalmol Proc Ser. 1978;15:297–301.
Seeliger M, et al. Multifocal electroretinography in retinitis pigmentosa. Am J Ophthalmol. 1998;125:214–26.
Sutter EE, et al. The field topography of ERG components in man – I. The photopic luminance response. Vis Res. 1992;32:433–46.
Weleber RG. Chapter 72: Differential diagnosis of the electronegative electroretinogram. In: Heckenlively JR, Arden GB, editors. Principles and practice of clinical electrophysiology of vision. Cambridge: MIT Press; 2006. p. 809–22.

Functional Examinations of the Visual Pathway System with Electrophysiological Methods

16

Márta Janáky

Contents

A fundamental task of neuro-ophthalmology is to demonstrate the integrity or detect the impairment of the visual pathway. Determining the nature of the impairment and precisely localizing it is very important, since these may have therapeutic consequences, and a wrong diagnosis has an impact on the entire life of the patient and fundamentally influences their lifestyle. A broad range of electrophysiological methods are available for the assessment of the functional status of the visual system. The proper selection and application of these methods help localize the lesion from the retina to the visual cortex. Information about the functional integrity of the pigment epithelium is provided by electrooculography (EOG). Standardized electroretinography (ERG) is suitable for the precise measurement of the rod and cone function, as well as the function of the bipolar Müller cells, the amacrine cells and the cells in the inner retinal layers. The central, 30° area of the retina – especially the function of the cones – is assessed with multifocal ERG (mfERG). The function of the central ganglion cells sensitive to contrast changes is shown with pattern electroretinography (PERG). The axons of the retinal ganglion cells send the visual information through the lateral geniculate body to the visual cortex, of which the visual evoked potential (VEP) test provides information. Damage to the ganglion cells results in ascending optic atrophy; a lesion of the optic nerve, in turn, has an impact on the functioning of the ganglion cells through descending atrophy. It is, therefore, obvious that the PERG and VEP examinations must always be used in conjunction. The development of the multifocal technique (multifocal ERG and multifocal VEP) has enabled the functional assessment of localized areas of the visual field with regard to the retina and the visual cortex. The entire range of the electrophysiological methods is rarely used by the clinical physician. The many types of examinations would take a lot of time and would be burdensome for the patient. The most necessary examinations that may lead closer to the accurate diagnosis or to answering the questions raised must be chosen based on the clinical symptoms.

M. Janáky, M.D., Ph.D., habil.
Electrophysiological Unit, Department of Ophthalmology, Faculty of Medicine, University of Szeged, Szeged, Hungary
e-mail: janaky@opht.szote.u-szeged.hu

Pattern Electroretinography (PERG)

During the PERG examination, the visual stimulus is the black and white checkerboard

J. Somlai, T. Kovács (eds.), *Neuro-Ophthalmology*, DOI 10.1007/978-3-319-28956-4_16

pattern displayed on the computer screen. It is recommended to use the standard method of the International Society for Clinical Electrophysiology of Vision (ISCEV) because it enables the comparison of the results and experiences. According to the standard method, the contrast of the pattern must be close to 100 % (but never lower than 80 %). The size of the stimulating field is 10–16°, and the checkquare size used is 0.8° ± 3° (for special cases, such as glaucoma, larger squares can also be used). The applied filter is 1–100 Hz. PERG can be triggered with low- or high-frequency stimulation. The low-frequency stimulation (of 1 o 3 Hz) results in a transient response, whereas a steady-state response is obtained above a stimulation frequency of 16 Hz. The latter one is primarily used in scientific research, since this evoked response is suitable for mathematical processing.

In clinical routine examinations, the transient response is evaluated because individual trace components can be measured and assessed well in this case. The examination of the VEP and PERG recordings, the normal traces and the electrodes used are shown on Fig. 16.1.

Previously, the recommended recording electrode was the bipolar Burian–Allen lens electrode but nowadays, other types are also recommended by the standardization committee. These include the Arden gold foil electrode, the DTL fiber electrode, the HK-loop electrode that can be hooked over the lower lid, or the conventional gold cup electrode used for EEG examinations that can be attached to the skin of the lower eyelid.

Each electrode has advantages as well as disadvantages. For a long time, it was thought that contact lens-type electrodes provide the most reliable response.

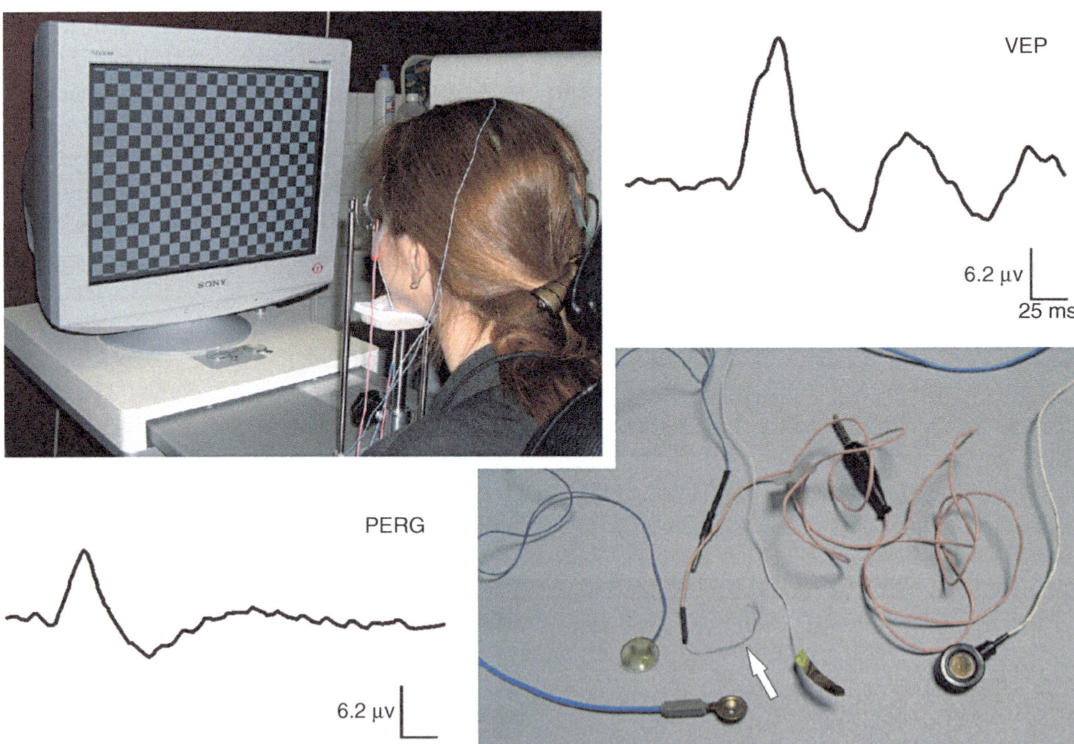

Fig. 16.1 Examination setup (*upper left*), intact VEP recording (*upper right*), intact PERG recording (*lower left*), ERG electrodes (*lower right*). The *white arrow* is pointing at the DTL electrode (the electrode recommended by the 2007 ISCEV guidelines)

This electrode, however, is expensive, hard to place, and inconvenient during and, therefore, unsuitable for longer examinations (e.g., for repeat procedures due to the requirement of reproducibility). It is fragile and its sterilization is a difficult. It is difficult to wear the corrective device in addition to the contact lens for the pattern ERG. Children are afraid of the discomfort and pain associated with the placement. These factors have set back the spreading and routine use of ERG examinations. According to the 2007 guidelines, it also decreases the quality of the image projected onto the retina, and therefore its use is no longer recommended. The Arden gold foil is placed in the palpebral fissure in the midline of the lower eyelid (like the paper strip for Schirmer's test), and is secured with an adhesive bandage on the outside. It is easier to wear and sterilize, compared with the contact lens. The HK-loop electrode made of silver wire that can be hooked over the lower eyelid is based on a similar principle. The DTL or fiber electrode is a plastic fiber coated with silver chloride and attached to a conductive wire. It is placed near the lower eyelid, parallel to it, at the corneal limbus, and secured with an adhesive bandage to the skin at the lateral orbital edge. The DTL electrode is so thin that anesthetic drops are required only in the case of positively sensitive patients. The electrode can be placed by a trained assistant. It is cheap, single-use (i.e., there is no need for sterilization), there is no risk of infection, and it is suitable for longer examinations as well. It can be used simultaneously on both eyes and, therefore, the total examination time is shorter. Because of the above advantages, it is more and more popular, and it is the electrode recommended by the ISCEV in its 2007 guidelines. The gold cup electrode that can be attached to the skin in the midline of the lower eyelid is used for the examination of infants and young children. It does not injure the eye, and it needs no sterilization, but its disadvantage is that the recorded signal is weaker than in the case of an electrode placed directly onto the anterior surface of the eye. The reference electrode can be placed on the temple, on the earlobe, or behind the ear, on the mastoid process. There are no strict requirements as to the placement site. The grounding electrode is placed on the middle of the forehead (gold cup electrode). The examination must be performed with normal-diameter pupils and under mesopic illumination. After determining the refractive error, stimulation is performed binocularly, with near correction (the eye with better vision helps the fixation of the other one). If a simultaneous VEP examination is performed, the stimulation must be monocular, after covering the non-stimulated eye. The average of 200 individual responses is evaluated. Due to the criterion of reproducibility, the stimulation must be repeated.

Examination of the Visual Evoked Potential (VEP)

A diffuse light stimulus can be used to evoke the cortical response. This can be the flash of a stroboscope or the light of a lightemitting diode (LED). Each retinal ganglion cell (X, Y, or W) takes part in the response evoked by the diffuse light stimulus. Through the axons of different conduction velocity, the stimuli reach the cortex at different time points, and therefore, a multiple-peak curve is obtained. Since the reponse is highly variable, this method is rarely used.

In infants and in case of not fully transparent refractive media, the LED stimulation method can be used because the red light emitted by the LED penetrates the eyelid of the sleeping child or the cloudy refractive media, and some amount of information can be obtained about the function of the retina and the visual pathway. Pattern onset/offset stimulation can also be used in pediatric patients. These responses are also highly variable. If the visual acuity permits, VEP is examined in routine clinical practice using the phase changes of the black and white checkerboard pattern as stimuli (Fig. 16.1).

The recommended square size is 1° and 15 min (at least two patterns with different square sizes are to be used). If the contrast of the pattern approaches 100 %, and the frequency of the stimulation is between 0.5 and 2 Hz, the transient response (transient VEP, see Fig. 16.1) is obtained, which can be used in routine clinical examinations. The steady-state response is obtained when using a higher stimulating frequency (above 16 Hz). Filtering: at 1–100 Hz, 100 responses each time must be averaged and evaluated. The recording electrode (gold cup electrode) can be placed at the Oz point (10 % of the inion–nasion distance above the external occipital protuberance, in the midline) in accordance with the international 10/20 system. The fovea and the perifovea are represented on the surface of the cortex, and the response evoked by the stimuli from both sides can be recorded well at this site. In case of visual field defects due to optic tract lesions, the recording electrode may be placed at the O1 and O2 points, and the half-field stimulation may also be used. In this case, the temporal or the nasal half of the visual field is stimulated with the checkerboard pattern from the fixation point, while the other half remains dark. This method has not been used widely in the clinical practice. The reference electrode, in accordance with the ISCEV guidelines, is placed at the Fz point, and the grounding electrode at the Fpz point. With the refractive error corrected, monocular stimulation must be applied (after covering the nonstimulated eye). If amblyopia is suspected, binocular stimulation must also be performed to assess binocular facilitation.

Multifocal Technique

Multifocal visual evoked potential (mfVEP) response is a series of potentials evoked by the stimulation of well-defined areas of a 30° area of the retina and recorded over the visual cortex. The cortical activity can be recorded with electrodes (gold cup electrodes) placed over the occipital region of the scalp. Although the procedure is very similar to that used during conventional VEP examinations, the stimulus and the response are displayed in a very different way. The active recording electrode, in case of monopolar recording, is placed on the scalp in the midline, 4 cm above the external occipital protuberance. In case of multiple-channel recording, electrodes are placed 1 cm above the inion and 2 cm to the right and 2 cm to the left of it. The indifferent or reference electrode is placed at the inion, and the grounding electrode at the middle of the forehead. The stimulating (dart-board) pattern is displayed on the computer screen.

The dart-board pattern is divided to 60 sectors. Each sector contains 16 squares (a checkerboard pattern of eight black and eight white squares). The size of each sector and the squares within them were designed taking the cortical representation of the retina into account. The size increases from the center outwards for a stimulation of areas of almost the same size on the cortical surface. Therefore, the innermost sector is of 1.2°, and the outermost one is of 7° in width (Fig. 16.2).

In the multifocal technique, each sector may change independently from each other every 12.3 ms. The change of the checkerboard pattern within them is random, where each element is displayed according to a predefined, m-sequence. The result of this is that the average lightness of the screen is constant in time. The refresh rate of the screen is 60 Hz, and the sampling frequency is 1200 Hz. Gain: 100,000; filtering: set to 3 and 35 Hz. The stimulation consists of rounds, with pauses during which the patient may blink, to maintain fixation. Each round lasts for 27 s. The stimulation results in a summed response recorded from the surface of the visual cortex, from which a total of 60 cortical responses (as the pattern contains 60 sectors) corresponding to specific areas of the retina can be obtained with a mathematical method known as cross-correlation. These responses are called kernels. The multifocal VEP test works with second-order kernels, which show the derivatives or differences of the cortical responses given to the stimuli coming in fast succession. One response curve (one kernel) represents a time frame of 200 ms. The standardization committee has not yet created guidelines for the multifocal VEP test.

Evaluation of the Evoked Responses

During the evaluation of the PERG, the implicit time of the N35, the P50 and the N95 wave components (implicit time is the time between the appearance of the stimulus and the appearance of the given peak, whereas latency is the time between the two peaks), and the N35–P50 and

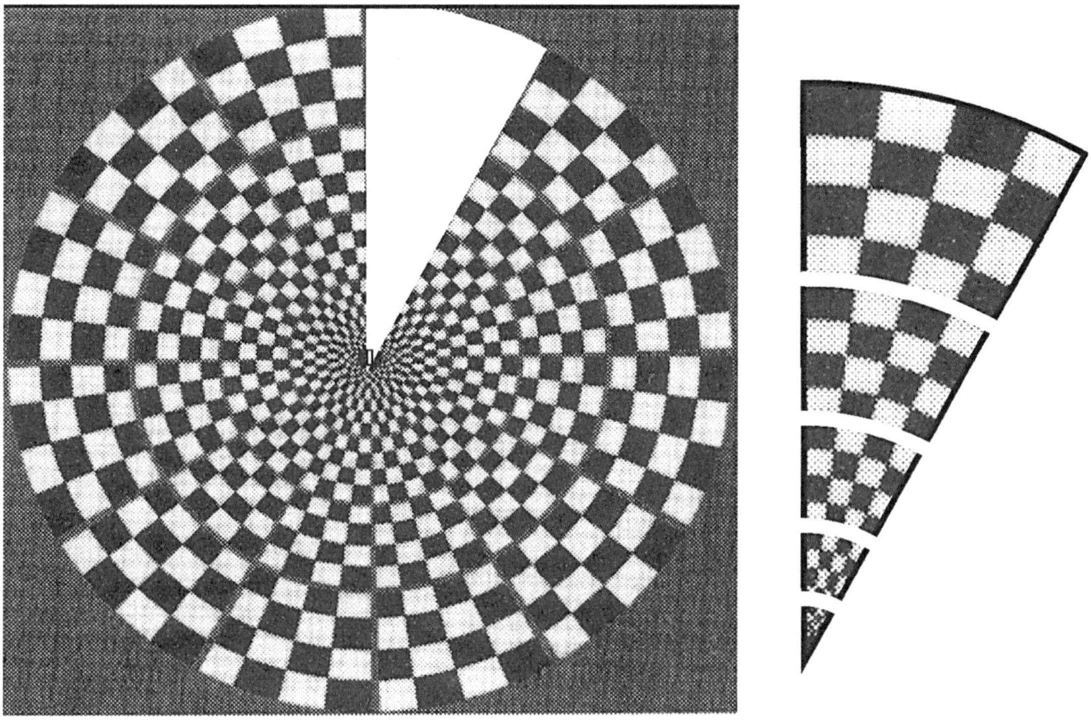

Fig. 16.2 On the *left*: black and white dart-board pattern used to evoke multifocal VEP. On the *right*: Enlarged view of the missing, 'cut out' sector

P50–N95 amplitude values are determined. The ratio of the amplitude values P50/N95 and N35/P50 is also calculated to determine selective amplitude reduction. Although the exact locations of generation of the PERG wave components are not yet fully known, the N95 wave component is proven to be specific to the stimulation pattern and to originate from the ganglion cells. Therefore, a selective reduction of the P50/N95 wave component indicates impairment of the ganglion cells or the optic nerve. The selective impairment of the N35/P50 wave, in turn, is characteristic to macular diseases. The ratio of amplitudes P50/N95 and N35/P50 (which is normally greater than 1) does not depend on visual acuity, and indicates and localizes impaired function in an early stage, even in cases where there is no decreased visual acuity. The N35/P50 amplitude reduction is often accompanied by P50/N95 amplitude reduction, and the ratio is unchanged in this case: it indicates a macular disease (Fig. 16.3).

During the evaluation of the VEP test, the peak latency of waves N75, P100 and N135, and the amplitude of waves N75/P100 and P100/N135 are measured. (The term latency is used instead of implicit time in the literature on VEP.) In the waveform analysis, normal, W-shaped and low prolonged waveforms are distinguished. For this latter, the difference between the N135–N75 peak latencies is determined to express the degree of prolongation objectively. The retinocortical time (RTC) is measured, which is the latency difference between the PERG P50 and the VEP P100 peak (in ms) and expresses the time elapsed between the activation of the retinal ganglion cells and the arrival of the stimulus in the visual cortex (Fig. 16.4).

During the processing of mfVEP recordings, the individual traces are evaluated as a whole (trace array), and each individual trace can be selected to calculate its amplitude and latency. To analyze the waveform of individual traces, the scalar product is used, which gives the differences between corresponding points of the ideal trace and the recorded trace.

A ring analysis is also available, which is the evaluation of the results obtained by averaging the cortical responses to the stimulation of concentric areas of the retina. Quadrant analysis

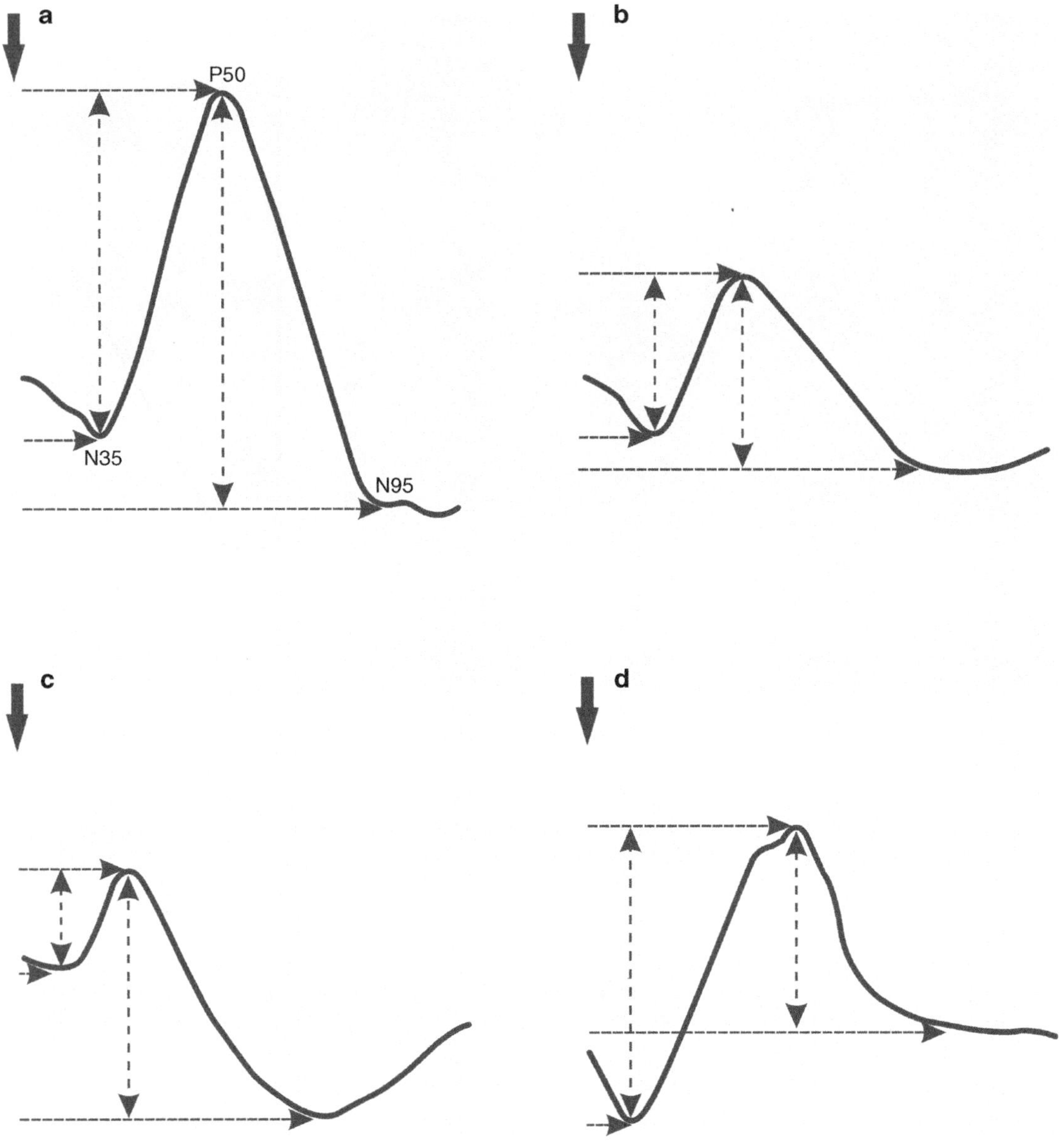

Fig. 16.3 Schematic view of PERG abnormalities. (**a**) intact PERG response. The *dotted lines* mark the peak parameters. (**b**) Reduced-amplitude response. (**c**) Selective N35/P50 wave amplitude reduction. (**d**) Selective P50/N95 wave amplitude reduction

means the evaluation of cortical responses obtained by summing the responses evoked in each of the four retinal quadrants. The three-dimensional view of the trace array is the most spectacular but it cannot be used in itself for any conclusion (Fig. 16.5).

The multifocal visual evoked potentials are very similar in the two eyes of a given patient because the corresponding points of the two retinas are projected to the same points of the visual cortex. Comparison of the responses from the two eyes therefore helps the assessment of a unilateral visual field defect. The comparison of responses on the horizontal and vertical recordings also helps evaluate abnormal responses more accurately.

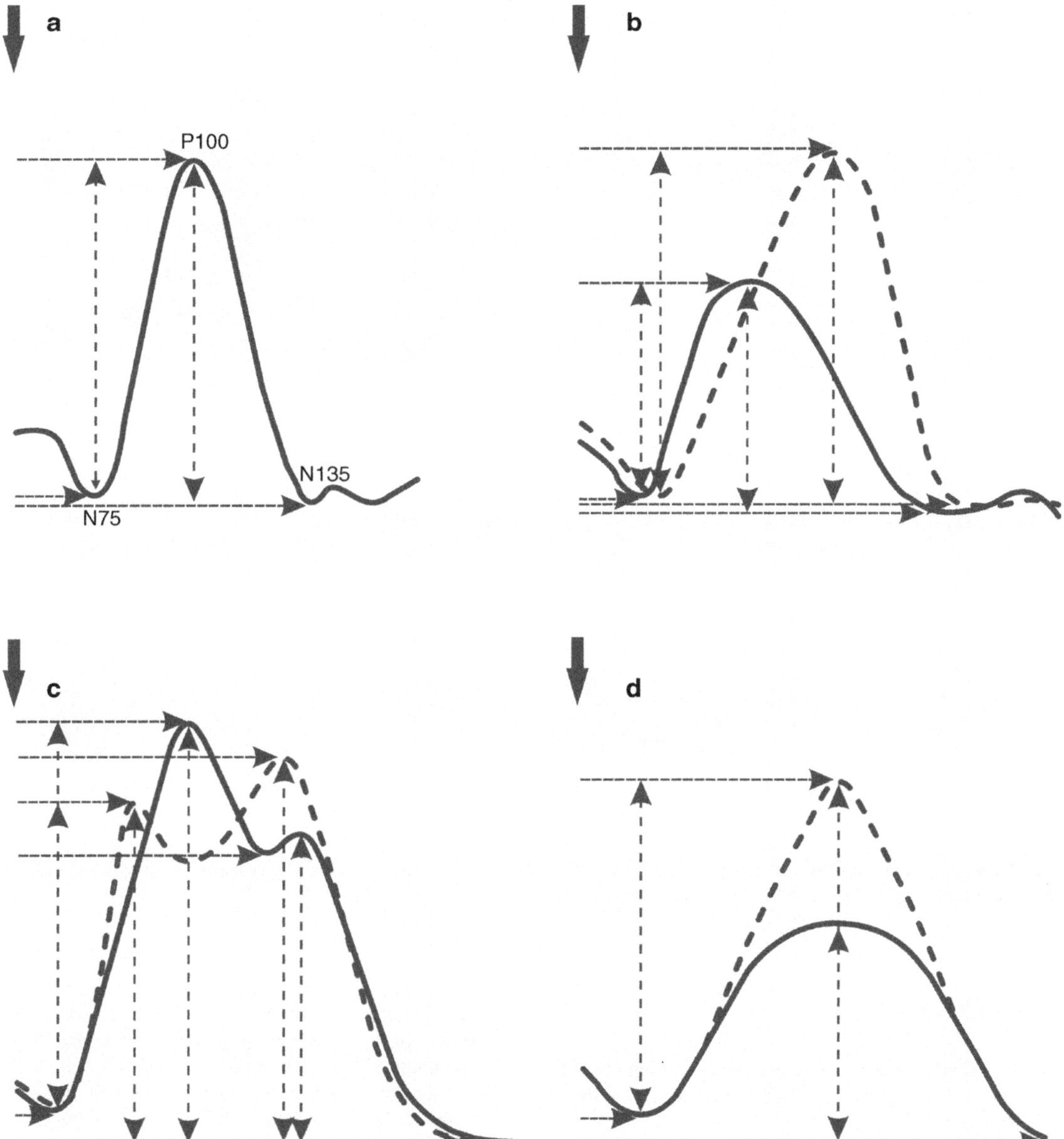

Fig. 16.4 Schematic view of VEP abnormalities. (**a**) Intact response. (**b**) *Solid line*: reduced-amplitude, normal-latency response curve. *Dotted line*: prolonged-latency, normal-amplitude response curve. (**c**) W-waveform (doubled) VEP response types. *Solid line*: the P1 amplitude is higher than the P2. *Dotted line*: the P2 amplitude is higher. (**d**) Reduced-amplitude, prolonged-waveform response. The *thick black arrows* indicate the start of the stimulation

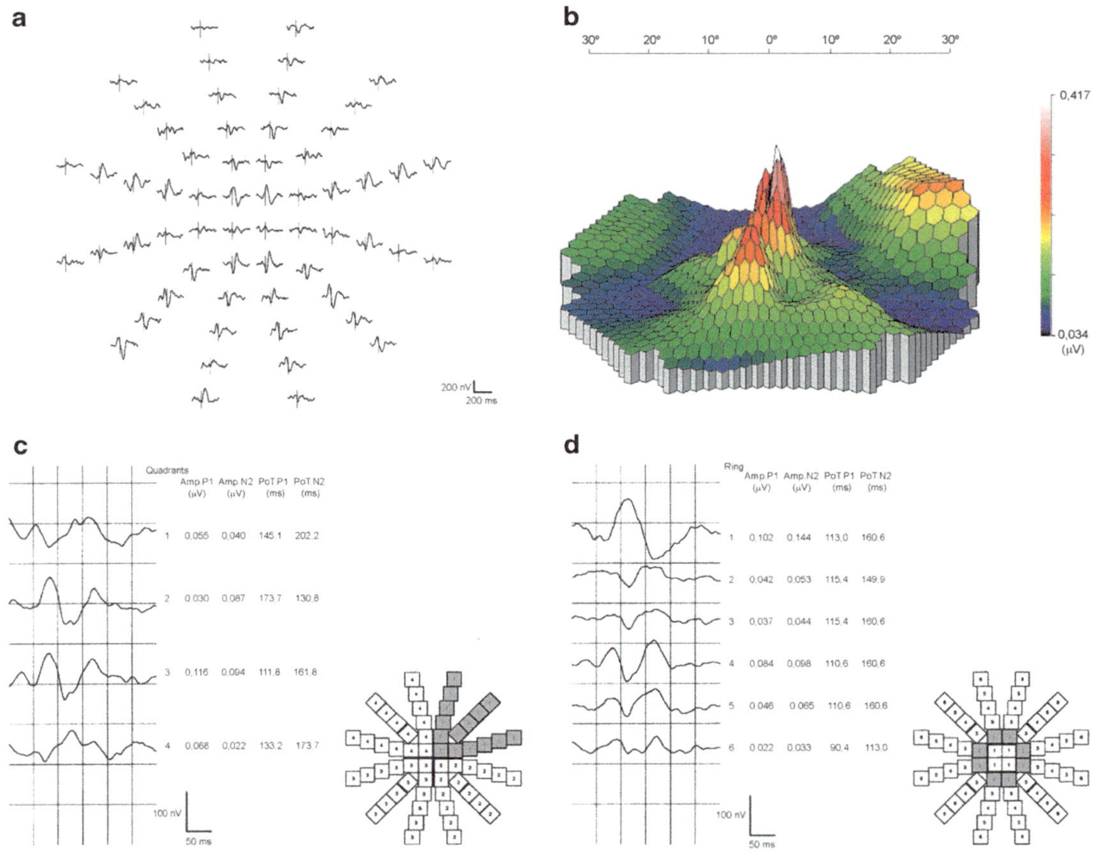

Fig. 16.5 Multifocal visual evoked potentials (mfVEP). (**a**) Trace array. (**b**) Three-dimensional view. (**c**) Quadrant analysis of the responses. (**d**) Ring analysis of the responses

Further Readings

Arden GB, et al. A gold foil electrode: extending the horizons for clinical electroretinography. Invest Ophthalmol Vis Sci. 1979;18:421–6.

Dawson WW, et al. Improved electrode for electroretingrapy. Invest Ophthalmol Vis Sci. 1979;18:988–91.

Hawlina M, et al. New noncorneal HK-loop electrode for clinical eletroretinography. Doc Ophthalmol. 1992;81:253–9.

Holder GE, et al. For the International Society for Clinical Electrophysiology of Vision: ISCEV standard for clinical pattern electroretinography 2007 update. Doc Ophthalmol. 2007;114:111–6.

Janáky M és mtsai. Új fejezet a látókérgi kiváltott válasz vizsgálatok történetében: a multifokális módszer klinikai alkalmazása [A new chapter in the research of evoked responses of the visual cortex:the use of a multifocal method in clinical medicine]. Clin Neurosci/Idegseb Szeml. 2004. 57(11–12):377–83.

Odom JV, et al. Evoked potentials standard. Doc Ophthalmol. 2004;108:115–23.

17 Clinical Importance of Conventional and Modern Visual Field Tests in the Topographical Diagnostics of Visual Pathway Disorders

Judit Somlai

Contents

Since the visual pathway travels across almost the entire central nervous system, if a dysfunction is developed in any location, the neuro-ophthalmological examination methods enable us to assess the entire visual system from the photoreceptors of the retina to the visual cortex. The visual field test is a method for assessing function and may provide information about the following:

- the degree of visual pathway dysfunction
- the anatomical height of the lesion, i.e., topographical localization
- confirmation or exclusion of lesions that do not yet show morphological changes (e.g., MRI findings that do not show a morphological change)
- the efficacy of the systemic treatment, and the objective result of rehabilitation

Traquair wittily described the visual field as an island of vision surrounded by a sea of blindness. The peak of the island corresponds to the site of sharp vision, the macula. The blind spot, which is the connection point between the optic nerve and the eyeball, forms a small crater, whereas the height lines of the island are the isopters, which represent the spatial projections of the points of the retina that have the same sensitivity to light.

J. Somlai, M.D.
Unit of Neuro-Ophthalmology, Department of Neurology & Stroke, Military Hospital, Budapest, Hungary

Neuro-Ophthalmology Section, Hungarian Ophthalmological Association, Budapest, Hungary

Trustee, NOSZA Foundation (for the Prevention and Screening of Ocular Storke), Budapest, Hungary
e-mail: dr@somlaijudit.hu; http://somlaijudit.hu

J. Somlai, T. Kovács (eds.), *Neuro-Ophthalmology*, DOI 10.1007/978-3-319-28956-4_17

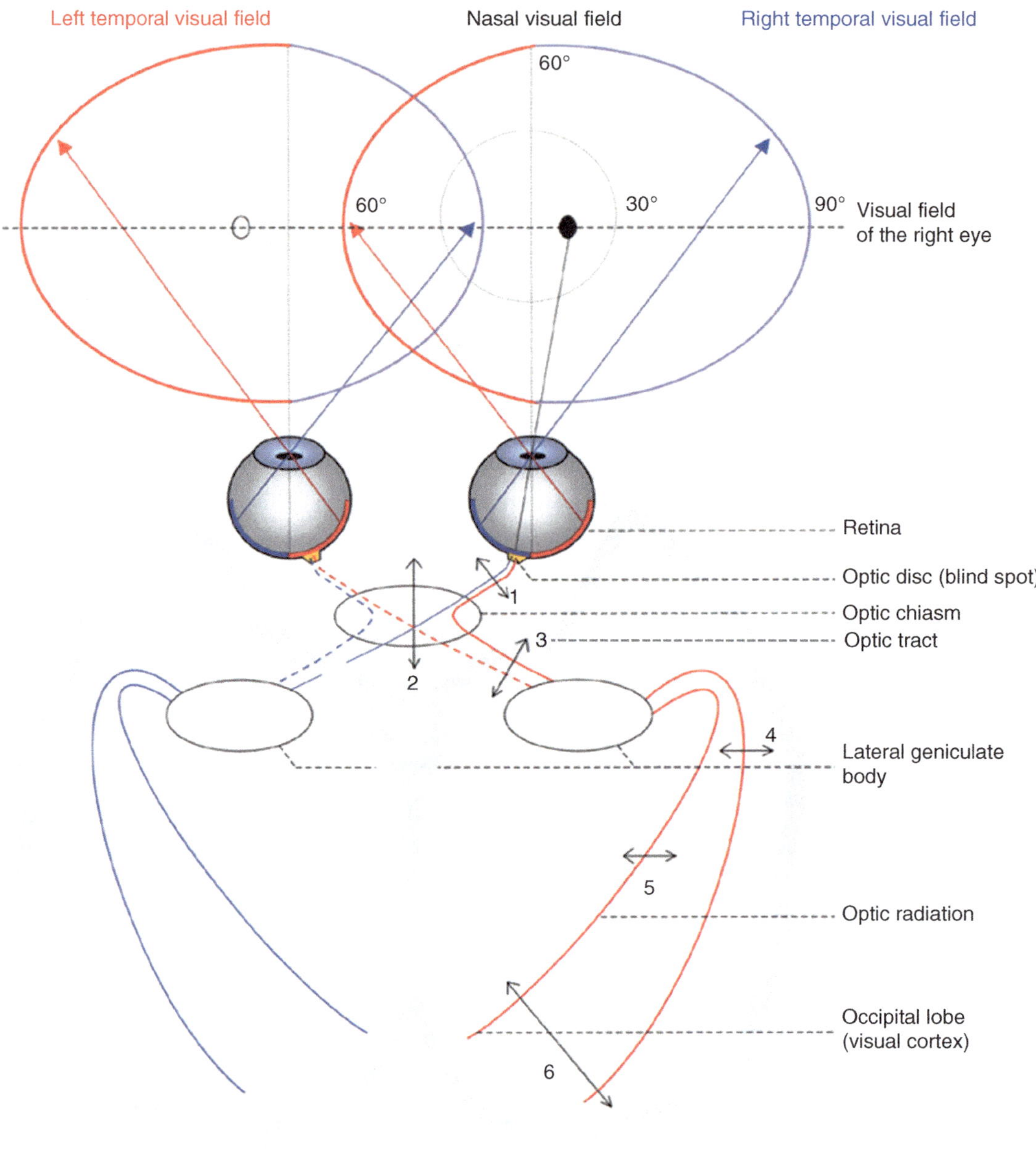

Fig. 17.1 Projection of the image of an object projected onto the nasal and temporal areas of the retina in the visual pathway system (Redrawn after Josef Flammer et al.: *Automated Perimetry, Visual Field Digest*, Fifth Edition, 2004, HAAG-STREIT AG)

During the visual field test, a relatively small and well-defined area of the retina (called visual field point) is stimulated. The visual field is examined with devices designed for this purpose and basically in two ways:

1. The ***kinetic perimetry*** shows the edges of the visual field using a small-sized, moving target of varying intensity. A visual field limit traced with a specific stimulus value is called an *isopter*. The higher the intensity and the size of the target are, the greater the isopter. With the moving target, the edges of vision and, besides, the location of the blind spot and the vision field defects can be detected. This is a cross-section of the Traquair's island of vision.

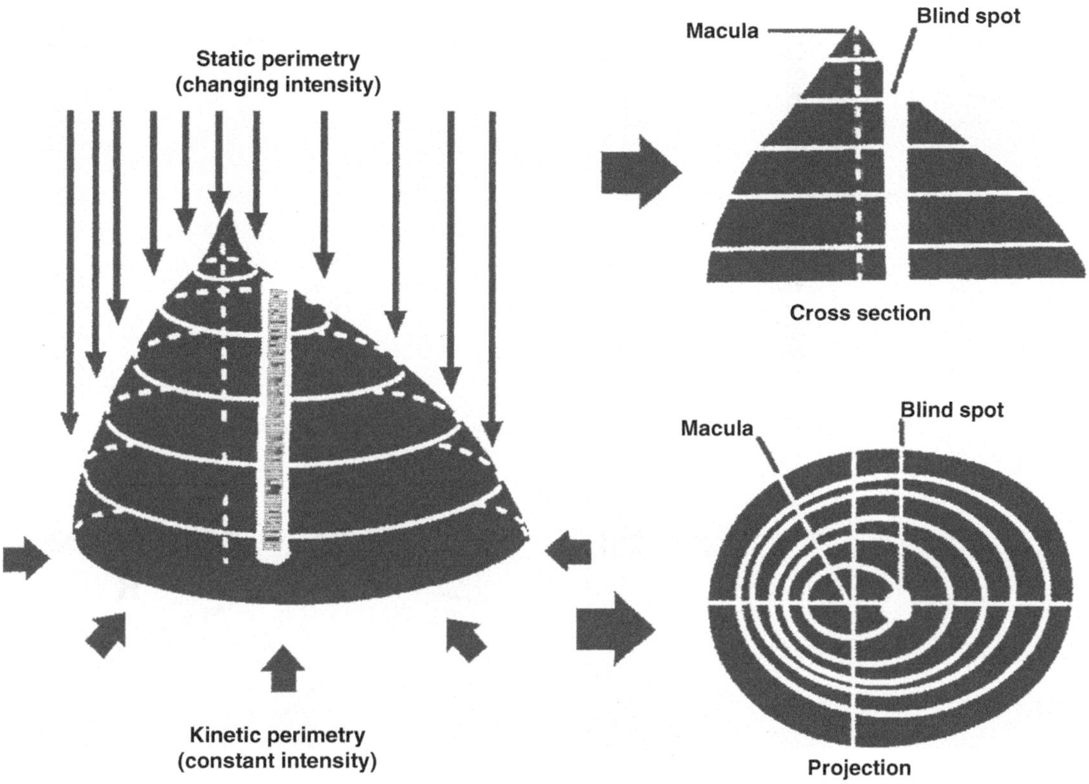

Fig. 17.2 Schematic overlooking view of the Traquair island; side-view section: schematic static perimetry; top-view section: schematic kinetic perimetry (Redrawn after J.S. Barton et al.: *Field of Vision*, (*A Manual and Atlas of Perimetry*) Springer, 2003)

2. ***Static or light perception (quantitative) perimetry*** uses a still target of varying intensity for the visual field test. The threshold values of light stimuli are determined using this method. The curve obtained is the second cross-section of the Traquair's island. The contrast is determined by the light density of the target and that of the background. The smallest difference in light density that can be still detected by the subject is the light density difference threshold (see Figs. 17.1 and 17.2).

Confrontation Visual Field Test

If the visual field test can be performed at the bedside only, due to the general condition of the patient, this conventional procedure may detect significant visual field losses. The examiner stands or sits facing the subject and covers the eye that is not being examined. The patient is instructed to fixate at the face of the examiner on the side to be examined, and they must detect the finger of the examiner moving at/approaching from different points of the periphery. A small object (such as an eye drop dispenser) can also be used, approaching from different points of the visual field periphery. With a minimal cooperation from the patient, the degree of severe hemianopias and the size of residual peripheral visual fields can also be determined this way. The method can be used also in patients returning from a prolonged loss of consciousness and in severe general condition, who have difficulty cooperating.

Campimetry with Tangent (Bjerrum) Screen

During the test, the patient is fixating at the center of a flat, black or gray surface (Bjerrum screen), and gives a sign if they think that a white, circle-

Fig. 17.3 Schematic view of the Traquair island of vision of the kinetic and static perimetries (Redrawn after J.S. Barton et al.: *Field of Vision (A Manual and Atlas of Perimetry)* Springer, 2003)

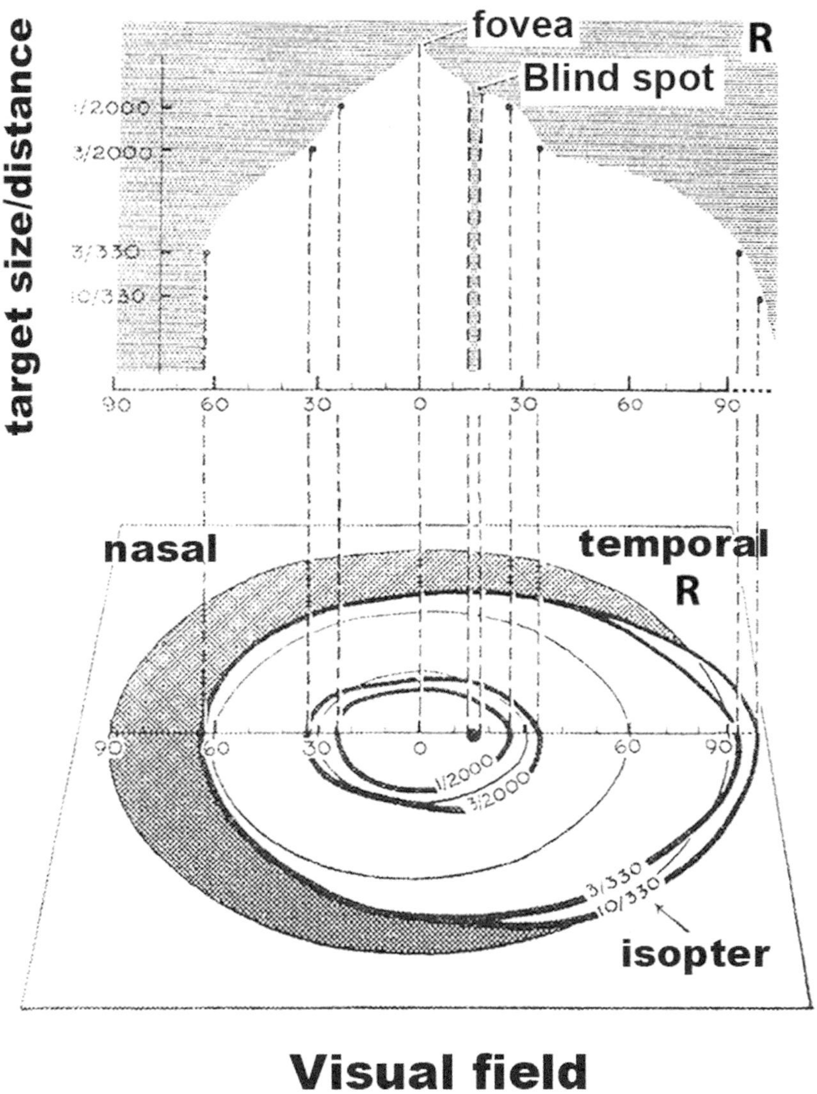

shaped object attached to a black stick is approaching from any point of the periphery. The size of the target (between 1 and 30 mm in diameter) is chosen in accordance with the visual acuity of the patient. This examination method that has been popular for a long time is very useful in detecting central (i.e., within 30°) visual field defects, since lesions of the area representing the central, i.e., macular region and the blind spot i.e. papilla region can be observed magnified on the flat examination surface.

The clinical importance of the method is the detection of optic disc and/or macular lesions and the early dysfunction of the papillomacular bundle. It indicates a visual field defect in its early stage, when there are no morphological changes yet or they are questionable (Figs. 17.3 and 17.4).

The Advantages of Campimetry

- The equipment is relatively cheap.
- It can be performed even in patients with low compliance or in severe general condition. It is exploratory but provides valuable information.
- It can be used as a screening tool in the early phase of the disease, e.g., in the case of incipient papillary edema causing episodes of

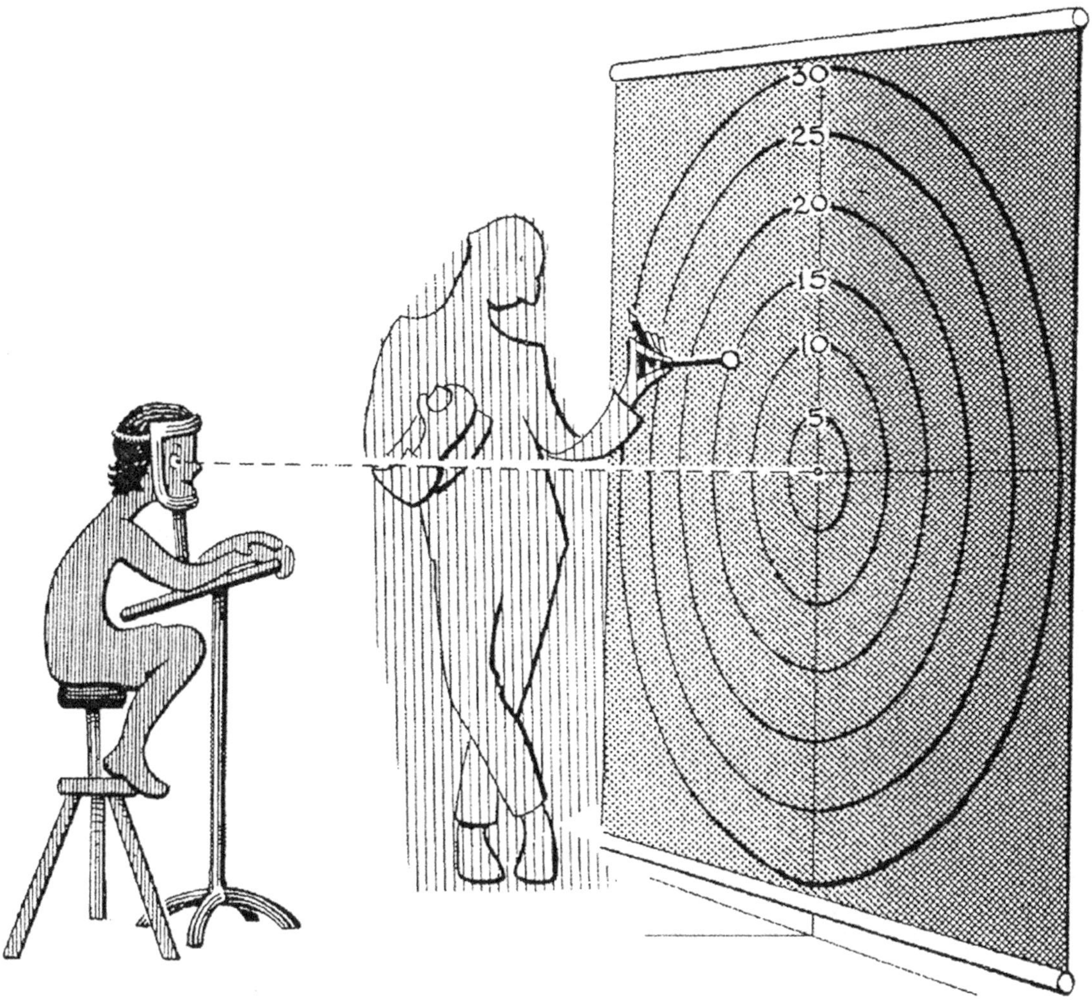

Fig. 17.4 Visual field exam with Bjerrum screen (Redrawn after J.S. Barton et al.: *Field of Vision (A Manual and Atlas of Perimetry)* Springer, 2003)

amaurosis fugax, an enlarged blind spot may confirm or rule out subjective symptoms.

- Since the spherical visual field is projected onto a flat surface, the central lesions (e.g., central scotomas, blind spot enlargements), within 20°, can be detected with a multifold magnification, and the changes can also be followed with proportional scale.

The Disadvantages of Campimetry

- The procedure establishes the limits of the visual field within 30° only; peripheral defects between 30° and 80° cannot be examined.

Kinetic Perimetry

During the examination, targets of a light density that differs from that of the background are moved in the visual field, and points that are just perceived by the subject are recorded. It is the Goldmann perimeter only that is used in today's practice.

Kinetic Perimetry with Goldmann Screen

It is a manual examination procedure. During the examination, a target of constant brightness is projected into an evenly illuminated metal bowl. First

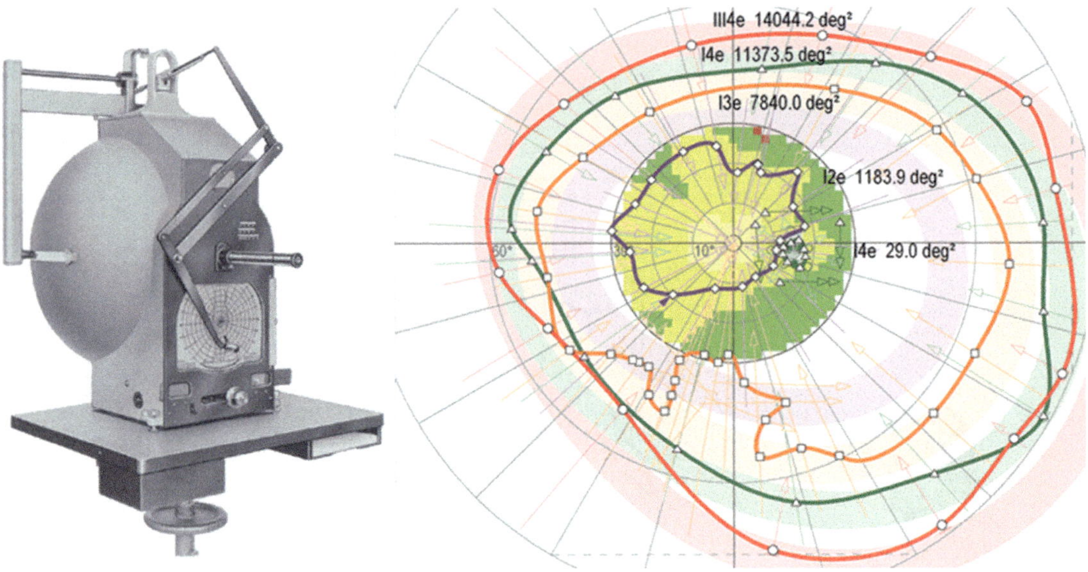

Fig. 17.5 (**a**) Visual field exam with Goldmann perimetry. (**b**) Results obtained with a Goldmann perimetry

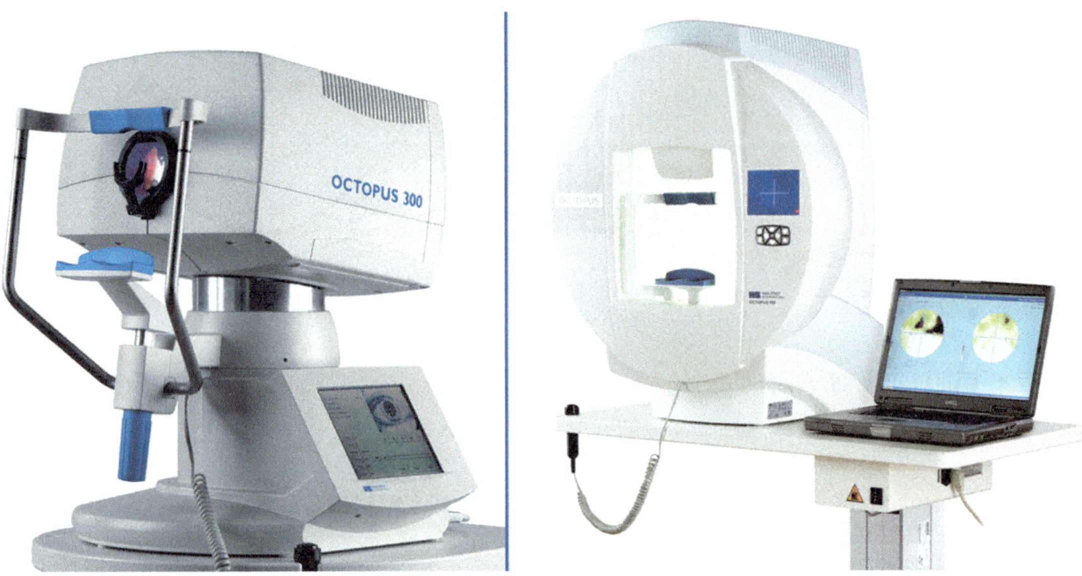

Fig. 17.6 (**a**) Octopus-300 perimeter (**b**) Octopus-900, the latest computer perimeter

larger, and then smaller targets, stimulus lights (moved from the periphery towards the center) are flashed to establish the limits of the visual field. The blind spot, as well as the absolute and relative scotomas can also be detected with the smallest target. It is important to observe the requirements of the examination; otherwise, false positive or negative visual field defects may be detected. Defects within the limits of the visual field are scotomas, which are caused by conduction problems of the retinal photoreceptors or the fibers of the optic nerve (Figs. 17.5 and 17.6).

The Advantages of Goldmann Perimetry

- The peripheral and central visual fields can be assessed simultaneously.

- The peripheral defects most frequently seen in visual pathway lesions can be quickly detected and followed.
- It is an inexpensive examination tool.
- It is an accurate and fast examination tool with low maintenance needs in the long run.

The Disadvantages of Goldmann Perimetry

- Plots a visual field contour but does not map the degree or type of the defects.
- It cannot indicate the depth of the scotomas within the defects, and cannot detect the changes of relative or absolute scotomas.
- It is difficult to document the examination results.

Computer Perimetry: Projection Perimetry

It was in 1960 when Dubois–Poulsen and Magis first attempted to automate the Goldmann perimeter, and then, in 1975, Lynn and Tate proposed the introduction of computerization. During computer perimetry (CP), the flash (location, time, duration, brightness, order) of target and the recording of the results are controlled by a computer, and the information obtained is stored in its memory. The method, based on the principles of raster perimetry, involves stimuli of varying brightness appearing at specific points (determined by the program of the computer) in the hemisphere of the device. The order of the light flashes at the test points changes randomly.

The Two Basic Examination Principles of Raster Perimetry

During the '*threshold testing*,' the light stimulus threshold of the retina is determined at the test points examined. Starting with a dim target, the device displays brighter and brighter targets until the subject perceives them. At a single test point, in case of an intact eye, 3 targets of different brightness are required, whereas this number is between 4 and 6 in case of a scotoma (4–2 algorithm). During '*suprathreshold testing*,' the device displays a target that is slightly brighter (typically by 5 dB) than the expected stimulus threshold at each test point, which can be perceived by a subject with intact visual field. Since the stimulus threshold of the retina increases towards the periphery, the device displays brighter and brighter targets in the peripheral field. In case of a scotoma that causes a visual field defect, the device determines the degree of the defect by flashing brighter and brighter targets. In case of an absolute scotoma (a sign of complete loss of function), the device makes another attempt, whereas in case of a relative scotoma (that indicates partial dysfunction), 2 or 3 attempts are made. The programs combine the two strategies, i.e., the test begins with suprathreshold targets, and in case of visual field defects, the device switches to threshold testing in the area of the scotomas. A false positive result is when the subject responds to the auditory stimulus only, and a false negative result is when the subject does not respond to a light stimulus detected earlier.

Display Modes of the Results Obtained During Computer Perimetry

- mean sensitivity (MS; mean sensitivity of the retina in dB)
- dB scale: numerical display of the light sensitivity threshold values at each test points
- comparison table: numerical values (in dB) of the (positive or negative) deviations from the control values
- the 'gray scale:' the defects are marked with different shades of gray based on the obtained test point values.

Table Values of the Computer Perimetry Results

1. mean sensitivity (MS): mean sensitivity of the entire visual field in dB
2. mean defect (MD): decrease in sensitivity of the entire visual field, compared with the normal value

3. short term fluctuation (SF): sensitivity during the test period, determining the mean difference between two measurements
4. loss variance (LV): the difference in sensitivity between the points of the visual field is the variance of sensitivity loss, and after the subtraction of its corrected value, the corrected LV is obtained, which is a consequence of the physiological fluctuation.
5. Bebie's cumulative defect curve: the curve indicates the loss of sensitivity by displaying the normal value range and if the curve is below the normal, it means a diffuse sensitivity loss. If the curve runs within the normal value range, and then shows a sudden drop, it predicts a local/unilateral retinal defect. If the curve runs below the normal value range, parallel to it, and then shows a sudden drop, it is a combined diffuse and local defect, with a more pronounced local involvement.

Classification of the defects based on the decrease in retinal sensitivity:

- normal fluctuation: 1–2 dB
- early relative defect: 3–5 dB
- relative defect: 5–19 dB
- absolute defect: >20 dB.

The computer perimeter (CP) tests the entire visual field, mapping not only the location of the defects but also their degree (indicating relative or absolute scotoma). Of the 12 available programs, 6 are used in the everyday clinical practice, depending on the type of the disease. For example, in case of optic neuritis, the field within 30° and 10° is mapped, whereas if a lesion of the retrochiasmal segment of the optic nerve is suspected, the device detects the degree and type of the peripheral (30–60°) homonymous loss with accessory programs. In case of complete blindness or incomplete amaurosis (e.g., due to cortical blindness), two programs may be used that help testing with the largest target and a 6° fixation target that is suitable also in case of difficulty fixating (these are the 'low vision peripheral' [LVP] and the 'low vision central' [LVC] programs). The map of the obtained results can be printed and evaluated immediately, and stored in the high-capacity memory of the computer, which enables comparisons to be made at any time in case of repeat tests. In neuro-ophthalmological patients, computer perimetry has its highest clinical importance in topographical diagnostics, as it will be seen in the clinical chapters.

The Most Frequently Used Computer Perimetry Tests Include

Glaucoma program: used for detecting the size of the blind spot within 30°, and lesions within the central 15°. Of the neuro-ophthalmological diseases, retinal prethrombosis or incipient papilla oedema indicates enlarged blind spot syndrome with high sensitivity.

Macular program: suitable for the detection and monitoring of central (within 10° and 5°) relative and absolute scotomas, e.g., in retrobulbar neuritis.

Diabetes program: detects homonymous and heteronymous quadrantanopias or hemianopias within 60°. In addition, in such visual field defects, the halving or intactness of the macular, i.e., the central region that is so important in regard to the visual functions of the patient can be assessed. The changes of the absolute and relative scotomas within the hemianopias accurately reflect the changes in the function of the retrochiasmal segment of the visual pathway system in the long term.

Low vision peripheral (LVP): tests the residual islands of vision at the periphery, between 30° and 85°, with the largest targets and the highest brightness, e.g., in case of incomplete cortical blindness.

Low vision central (LVC): has the same purpose as the previous one, within 30°.

The Advantages of Computer Perimetry

The target to be detected can be projected at any point of the hemisphere, and the size and intensity of the target can be adjusted rapidly and on a wide scale. The fixation of the patient is constantly monitored by a camera, and it can be followed on the side of the device during the examination, and in case of inaccurate fixation, the examination is paused. The variety of programs can be selected in accordance with the visual field defects due to the different diseases, tailored to the given subject and their current condition. The assistant may perform the examination independently—after training—, and prepare the results for evaluation. In possession of the quick and accurate numerical data, the obtained result can be evaluated immediately and, at the same time, compared with previous results, with the help of the 'gray scale.' It is one of the most important examination tools of incomplete cortical blindness, malingering, hysterical blindness and dissimulation. All information can be saved in the gigabytes of computer memory available, and stored on cassettes (previously) and the latest data storage media, to be compared at any time. It accurately indicates the changes in optic system functions and, thus, the clinical progression or regression of the underlying disease (Figs. 17.7 and 17.8).

The Disadvantages of Computer Perimetry

- Artifacts, e.g., due to difficulty in eye opening, fixation disorder, etc.
- Expensive equipment, high maintenance and service costs.

Diagnostic Importance of Visual Field Tests in the Topographical Localization of Optic Nerve Lesions

In the Intraocular and Intraorbital Segments of the Optic Nerve

- distinguishing between the ophthalmological and neurological diseases of the antechiasmal optic nerve segment
- detection and finding the cause of vision losses not accompanied by neuroradiological–morphological changes (e.g., CT signs)
- recognition of the condition, prevention of its progression and adequate treatment after finding the cause of eye symptoms developed as the first sign of systemic medial illnesses (e.g., immune vasculitis)
- detection, etiology-specific treatment and follow-up of blood flow deficits of the retina and/or the optic disc developed in any phase of a cerebrovascular disease
- screening for the neuro-ophthalmological signs of systemic neurological conditions, testing the efficacy of the treatment, providing treatment and care for the patient together with the neurologist, the neurosurgeon and other specialties (Fig. 17.9).

Modern Diagnostic Options for Neurological and Neurosurgical Conditions That Affect the Chiasm and the Parasellar Region

- The earliest and practically the most effective diagnostic tool of dysfunctions caused by lesions of any origin that affect the antechiasmal, the chiasmal and the parasellar regions is the visual field test (Bjerrum screen and computer perimetry).
- Preoperative and postoperative assessment of neurosurgical conditions that also affect the optic system, and long-term follow-up of the patient's visual functions
- It provides a close monitoring of visual pathway functions in case of hypophyseal conditions (e.g., hypophysis microadenoma) and other central endocrinological lesions that do not require surgical intervention (Figs. 17.10, 17.11 and 17.12).

Importance of the Examination of Optic Tract and Optic Radiation Dysfunctions

- In the clinical practice, visual field defects (quadrantanopias, hemianopias) may be the only eye symptoms of, for example, multiple

INTERZEAG OCTOPUS 1-2-3 V 2.19a
Seven-in-One

Name:		Eye / Pupil[mm]:	**Left (OS) / 5.3**
First name:		Date / Time:	28.08.1995 13:27
ID #:		Test duration:	8:28
Birthdate:	21.04.1926	Program / Code:	G1X / 3
Age:	69	# Stages / Phases:	4 / 1
Sex:	male	Strategy / Method:	Normal / Normal
Refr. S / C / A:	/ /	Test target / duration:	III / 100 ms
Acuity:	20/20	Background:	31.4 asb
IOP:	17	# Questions / Repetitions:	288 / 0
Diagnostics:		# Catch trials:	pos 0 / 19, neg 0 / 19

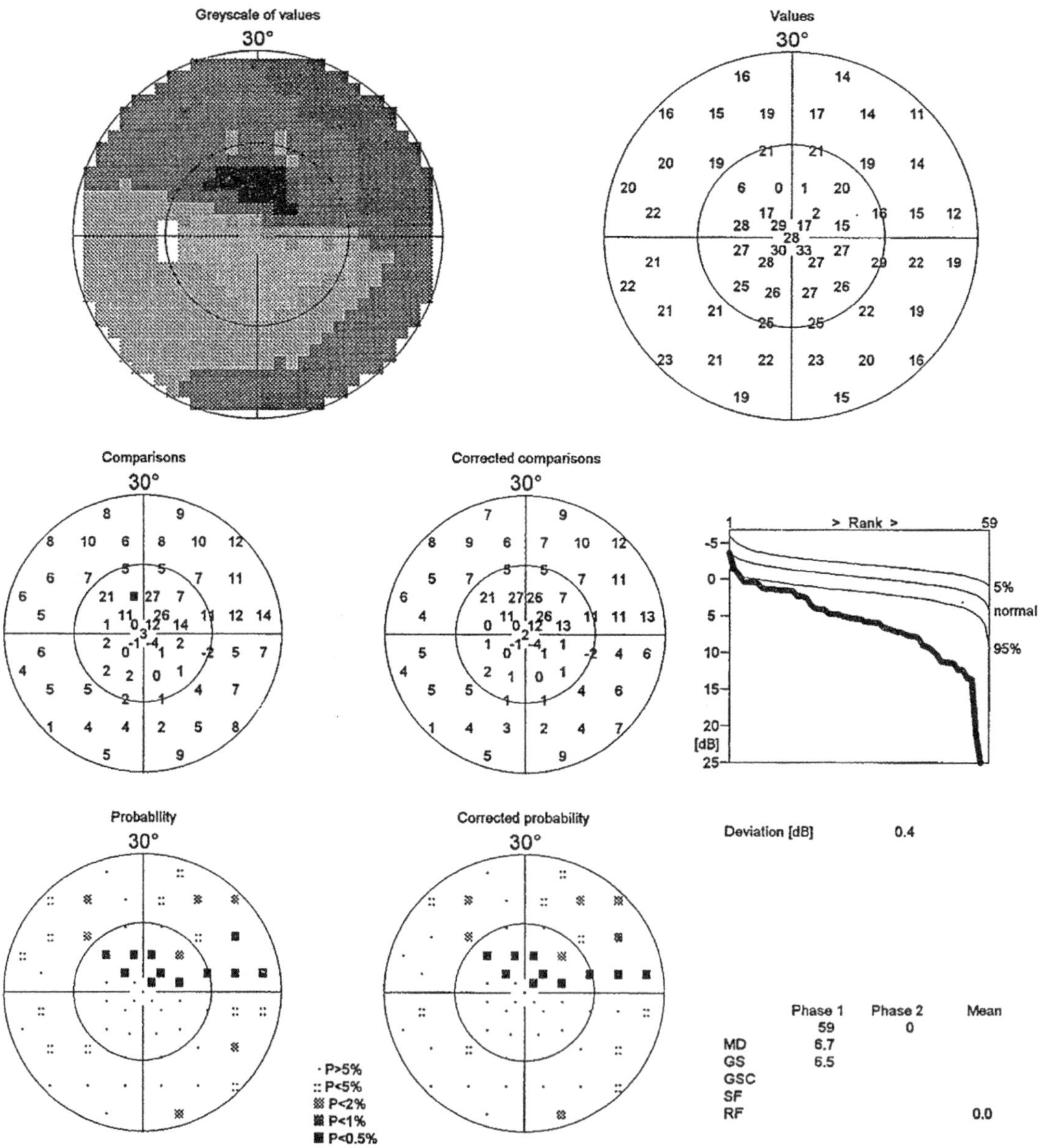

Fig. 17.7 Results of the Octopus perimetry test with numbers and the 'gray scale' result maps

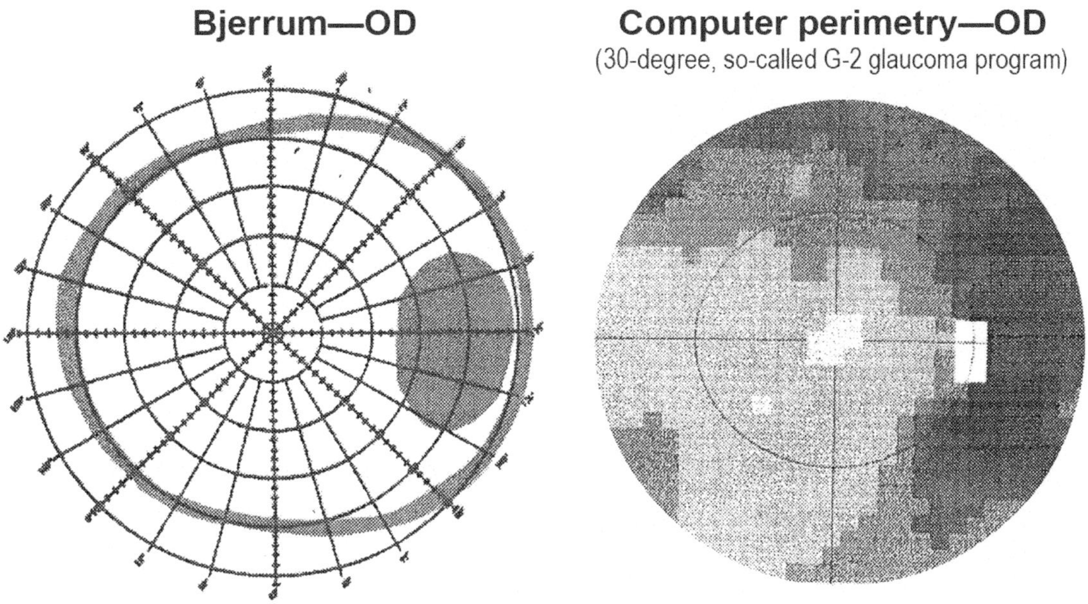

Fig. 17.8 Representation of the visual field on the Bjerrum screen and with the G2 program of computer perimetry in 'enlarged blind spot syndrome'

cerebrovascular lesions or involvement of the optic pathway in demyelination processes. The long-term follow-up enables the simultaneous monitoring of therapeutic efficacy and the progression of the condition.

- The preoperative and postoperative assessment of supratentorial neurosurgical conditions is a considerable help in longterm treatment, also in the case of acute decompensation.
- It may help in the topographical diagnostics of traumatic optic neuropathy injuries due to head trauma and, with the examination of polytraumatized patients, not only in the assessment of injuries but also in the reorganization of living conditions and the establishment of the final status that affects future work possibilities as well.

Practical Importance of the Modern Assessment of Visual Cortex Injuries

- Testing the degree of incomplete cortical blindness with the LVC and LVP programs of computer perimetry
- During the investigations of amaurosis developed at a young or adult age, the assessment determines the lifestyle and working possibilities by establishing the residual peripheral visual field.
- The most difficult task is to diagnose cortical blindness not accompanied by morphological–MRI changes (e.g., cortical hypoxia after cardioversion).

With the examination of the visual field, the dysfunction of the visual pathway system can be detected in almost every neuroophthalmological

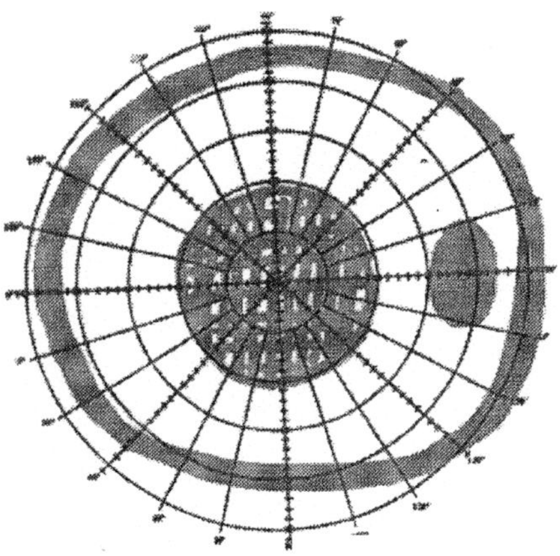

Bjerrum screen—OD
(10-degree central absolute scotoma)

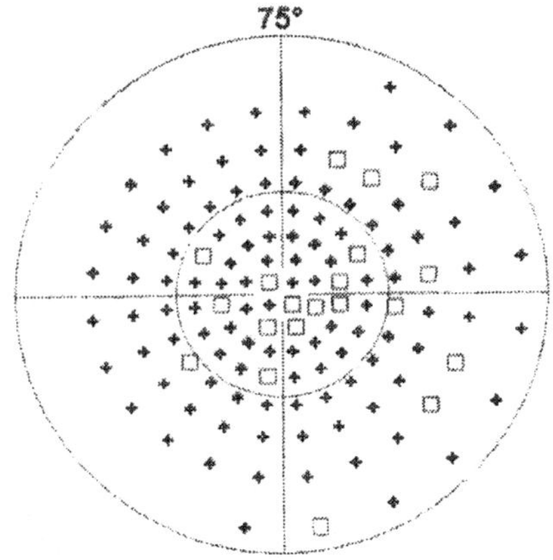

Computer perimetry—OD
(75-degree filtering program No. 07)

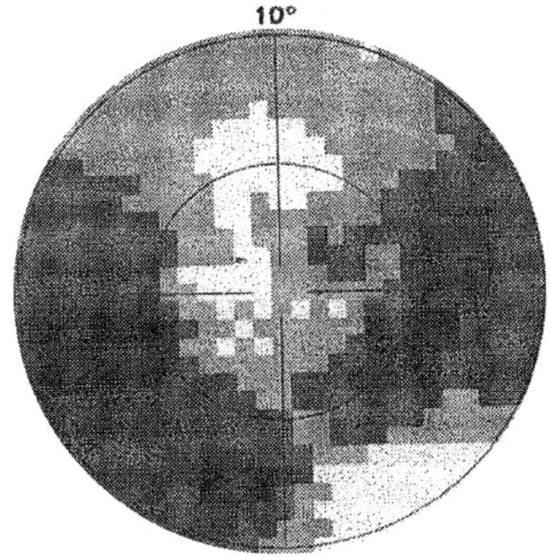

Computer perimetry—OS
(so-called M2-macula program that tests the center within 10 degrees)

Fig. 17.9 Detection of the 'central absolute scotoma' with the Bjerrum screen and computer perimetry – program No. 07 (within 75°) and the central macular region program (within 10°)

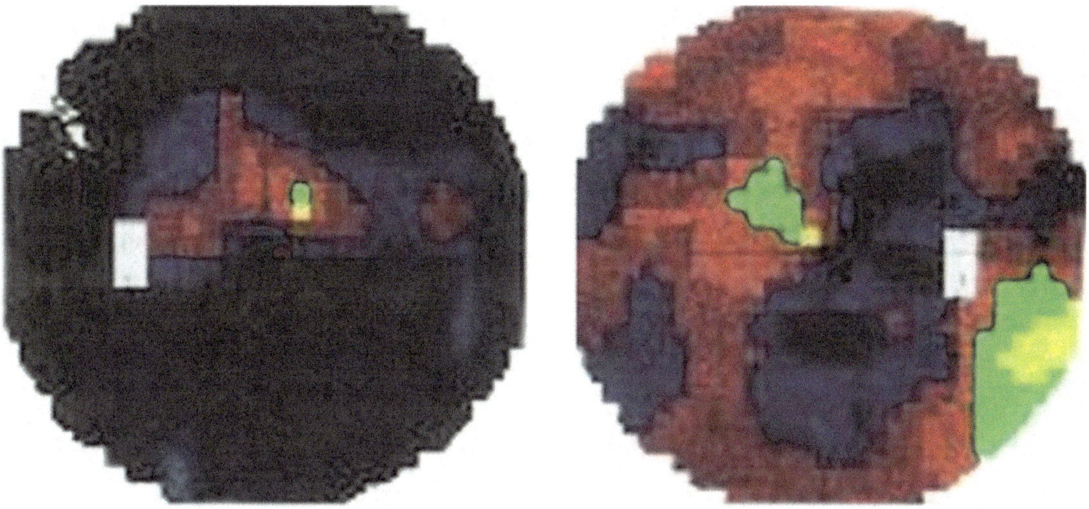

Fig. 17.10 Computer perimetry picture (glaucoma program) of a severe visual field defect due to bilateral, nonarteritic anterior ischemic optic neuropathy developed in the optic disc, at the beginning of the intraorbital segment of the optic nerve

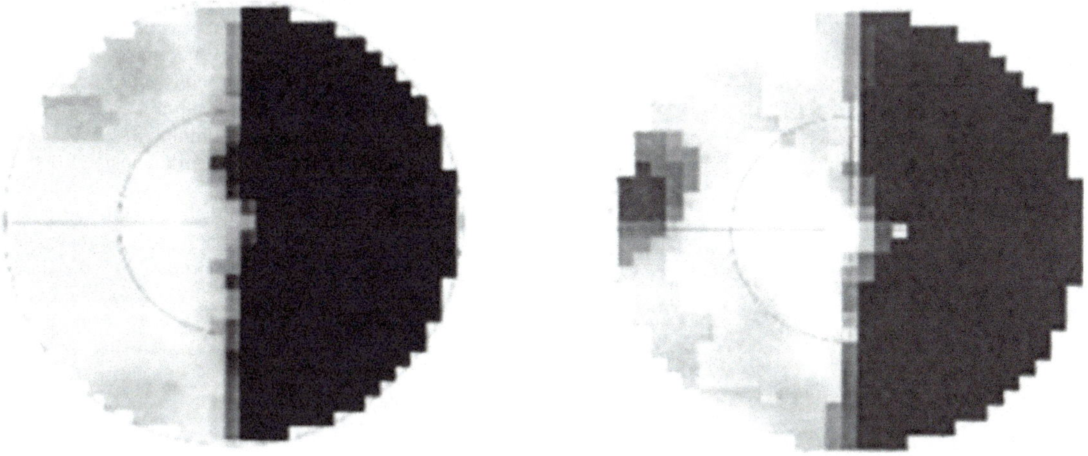

Fig. 17.11 Right-sided homonymous hemianopia due to a supratentorial spaceoccupying lesion, which spares the central region up to 3°. (The diabetes program (D1) performs the test up to 60°)

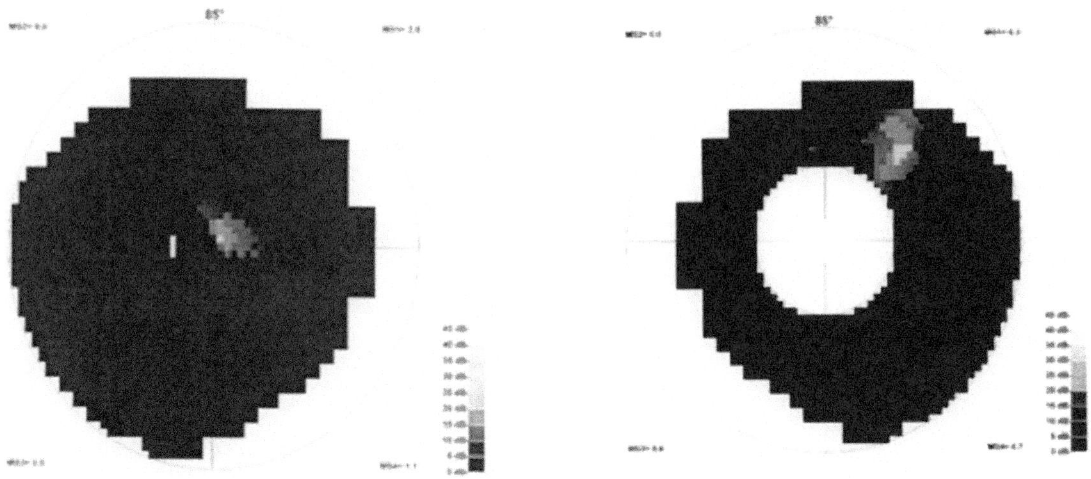

Fig. 17.12 Test performed in cortical blindness: On the *right*, the LVP program shows an almost complete amaurosis between 30° and 85°. On the *left*, the combined LVC and LVP programs, testing between 0° and 85°, show a residual island of vision of a few degrees only, even with the largest target

patient, in any segment of the pathway, and it helps in the long-term follow-up of the patient's visual functions and in checking the course of the disease.

Further Readings

Folmann P. Kinetikus perimetria: alapelv, gyakorlat, értékelés, hibalehetőségek [Kinetic perimetry: principle, practice, evaluation, possible errors]. SOTE Tömő utcai füzetek. 2000.

Holló G. Korszerű automata perimetria 2000. Elméleti alapok és klinikai gyakorlat [Modern automated perimetry 2000. Theoretical principles and clinical practice]. SOTE Tömő utcai füzetek. 2000.

Klein V. A látótérvizsgálatok fiziológiai alapelvei, módszerei, gyakorlati jelentőségük [Physiological principles, methods and practical importance of visual field tests]. Neuroophthalmologia. 1996.

Németh J. A komputerperimetria módszere és gyakorlati jelentősége [Method and practical importance of computer perimetry]. Neuroophthalmologia. 1996.

Patten J. Neurological differential diagnosis. London: Springer; 1995.

Somlai J. A legújabb neuroophthalmologiai metodikák jelentősége a látópálya és a látókéreg megbetegedéseinek lokalizációjában [Importance of the latest neuro-ophthalmological methods in the localization of visual pathway and visual cortex conditions]. Ideggyógyászati szemle. 2000;52(5–6):178.

Weijland A, Fankhauser F, Bebie H, Flammer J. Automated perimetry. Visual field digest. Köniz/Bern: Haag-Streit AG; 2004.

18 The Differential Diagnosis of Visual Field Deficits at the Bedside

Gyula Gács and Ildikó Szilvássy

Contents

In this chapter we wish to present the diagnostic significance of visual field deficits with the help of case presentations. We would like to focus primarily on aspects that are best suited to facilitate everyday diagnostic practice, at least according to our experience. We are not going to cover the appropriate technique of visual field testing and potential mistakes that can be made, although in some cases we are going to highlight them.

When trying to determine the location of the injury, we have to consider the characteristic features of the visual field deficit, as well as the findings of the following examinations: vision test, color vision test, and assessment of the optic disc. Course books written in Central Europe frequently mention Wernicke's hemianopic pupil reactions as a way to differentiate between lesions of the optic tract and those of more distant parts of the optic pathway. Anglo–Saxon literature hardly mentions these reactions, and we are not fully convinced of their diagnostic value either.

However, we have to emphasize the significance of the Marcus-Gunn phenomenon (in the Anglo–Saxon literature: relative afferent pupillary defect). This sign is characteristic of partial injuries to the optic pathway in front of the lateral geniculate body. If we shine a bright light into the unaffected or less affected eye and elicit the appropriate pupil reaction (constriction), and then shine the light suddenly into the other eye, the pupil of the unaffected eye will dilate. Normally, the sudden transition of the light should not affect the size of the pupil. However, in case of a partial injury to the chiasm or the optic tract if you change the location of the light, not as much light energy will be conducted through the injured afferent visual system; therefore, the consensual light reflex of the pupil will result in the dilation of the contralateral pupil. The most important considerations of the differential diagnosis are shown in Table 18.1.

G. Gács, M.D., PhD (✉)
Outpatient Department, Budapest City Council Péterfy Sándor Street Hospital, Budapest, Hungary
e-mail: gacs.gyula@peterfykh.hu

I. Szilvássy
Districts 2 and 14 Outpatient Department, Budapest, Hungary
e-mail: gacs.gyula@peterfykh.hu

J. Somlai, T. Kovács (eds.), *Neuro-Ophthalmology*, DOI 10.1007/978-3-319-28956-4_18

Table 18.1

	Optic nerve	Optic chiasm	Optic tract	Temporal lobe	Parietal lobe	Occipital lobe
Vision	Normal or decreased	Normal or decreased	Normal or decreased	Normal	Normal	Normal
Color vision	Normal or decreased	Normal or decreased	Normal or decreased	Normal	Normal	Normal
Field of vision	Central scotoma	Bitemporal scotoma	Incongruent Homonymous Hemianopsia	Homonymous upper quadrant hemianopsia	Homonymous lower quadrant hemianopsia	Homonymous lower, upper or complete congruent hemianopsia
Marcus-Gunn phenomenon	+	±	±	–	–	–
Optic disc atrophy	±	±	±	–	–	–

Henceforward, we are going to use case presentations to illustrate the differential diagnosis of symptoms detected in patients who had injuries to different parts of the visual pathway. We do not aim at completeness as there are separate chapters in this book that deal with the different segments, including one on the chiasm as well.

Pituitary Gland Tumor with Long-Standing Negative Results on Visual Field Testing

A 55-year-old male patient had had sella turcica enlargement for years (skull image taken due to his physical features that suggested hypopituitarism). At the time of the diagnosis, transsphenoidal pituitary surgery was not available in Hungary, so he was regularly monitored with visual field tests at a neurosurgery unit. On each examination, he had a full visual field. At one point, transsphenoidal pituitary surgery was introduced in Hungary as well, and the patient had to undergo a pre-operative assessment. During the visual field test typical bitemporal loss of visual field was detected when the patient was shown size II and III targets; however, with increased target sizes the results were normal (Fig. 18.1). When the findings of the previous tests were reviewed, it turned out that only size IV and V targets were used on all occasions. On the basis of this case, we wish to draw the attention to the fact that it is impossible to conclude on neuro-ophthalmological conditions if the techniques of the visual field test are not appropriate (small target size, correction, correction or consideration of astigmatism).

Bitemporal Visual Field Narrowing Imitating a Chiasmatic Lesion: Tilted Disc

A 25-year-old female patient with myopia was examined for an eyeglass prescription. During the visual field examination bitemporal loss of vision was detected. However, she had no complaints and her visual acuity was normal (1.0). (For field of vision see Fig. 18.2, for findings of funduscopy see Fig. 18.3.)

Considerations: As you can see in the figure illustrating the visual field, the temporal deficits spread only to the medial part of the blind spot, and they do not reach the midline. In real chiasmal syndrome the visual field deficit always reaches the midline. The funduscopic image corresponds to a phenomenon which is called 'tilted disc' in the Anglo–Saxon literature. The visual field deficit is characteristic of this congenital abnormality. Naturally, there are no congenital abnormalities that could prevent the development

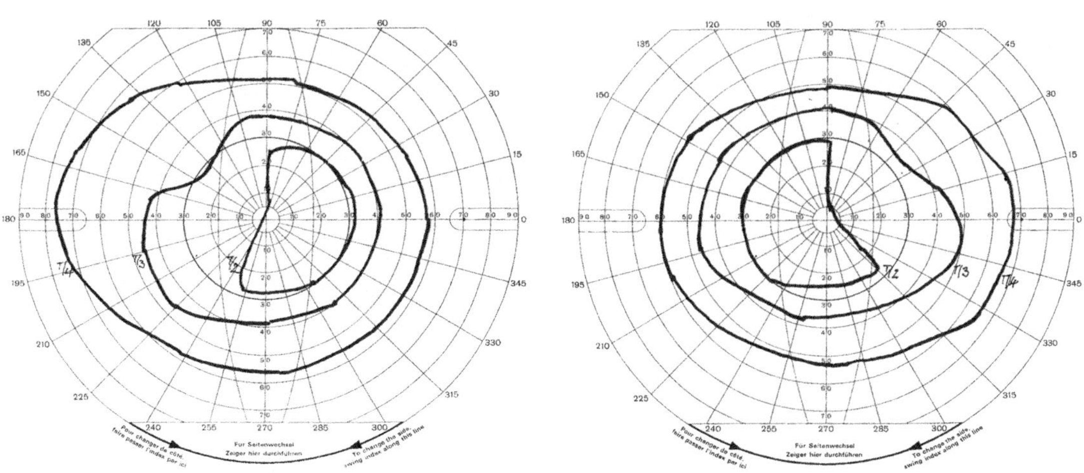

Fig. 18.1 Bitemporal loss of visual field (detected with small targets) due to a pituitary gland tumor (when examined with bigger targets, the field of vision was found to be full)

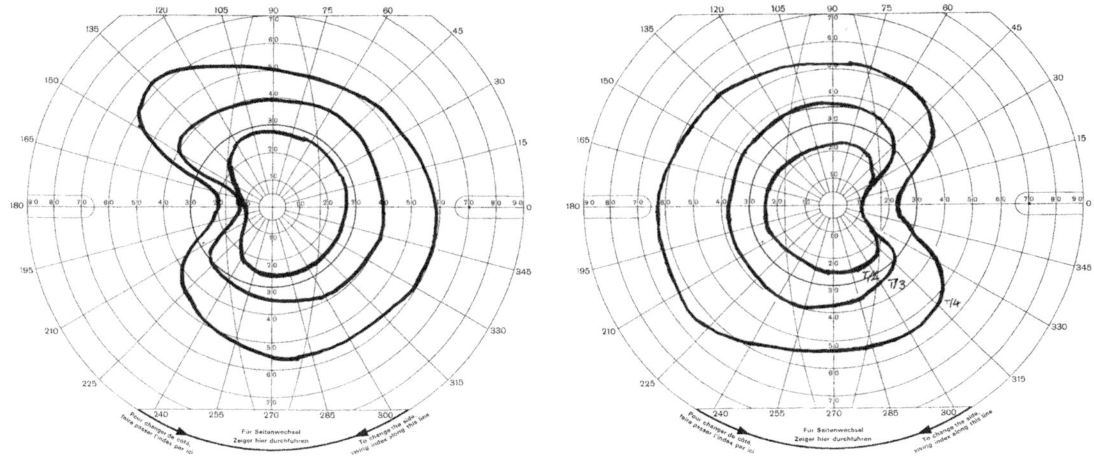

Fig. 18.2 Bitemporal visual field depression that does not reach the midline

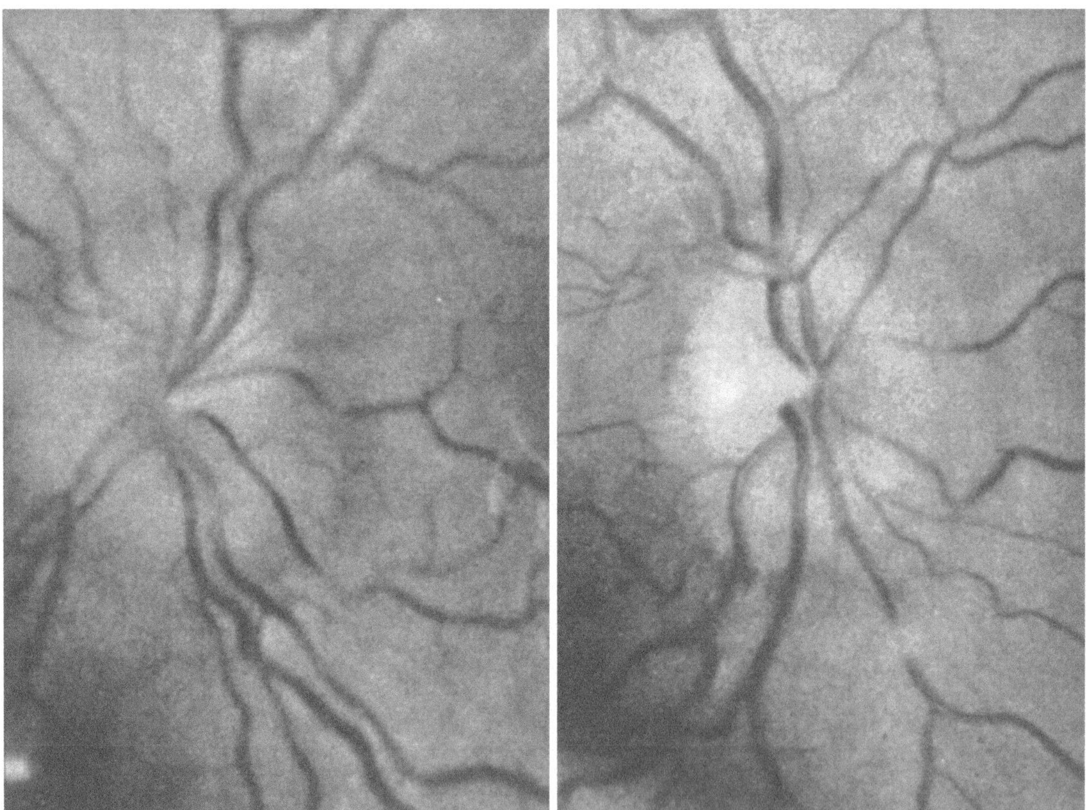

Fig. 18.3 Fundoscopic image of a tilted disc with hypoplasia of the nasal side of the optic discs, which causes depression of various extents on the temporal side of the visual field

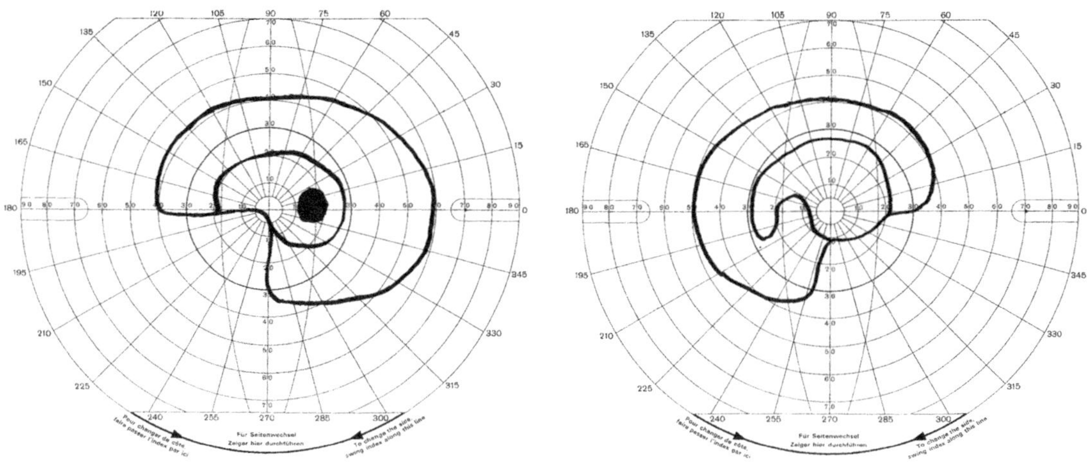

Fig. 18.4 Binasal loss of visual field in a patient with glaucoma

of a central nervous system disease, so if this incidental finding had been associated with any other symptom, further investigations should have been performed. There are also other scotomas the location of which can be bitemporal, e.g., an enlarged blind spot associated with prolonged congestion or scotomas caused by retinitis pigmentosa. However, they either do not reach the midline or spread over it, and this feature makes them fundamentally different from bitemporal hemianopsia caused by tumors of the pituitary gland or the region of the sella turcica.

Binasal Loss of Visual Field

A 58-year-old female patient complained of dazzling and blurred vision that she experienced during reading and knitting. Earlier she had no complaints and had not been examined by an ophthalmologist. Vision: 1.0 on both sides. Binasal lower quadrant hemianopsia was detected in the field of vision (Fig. 18.4).

Intraocular pressure: 24/23 mmHg.

Considerations: Intracranial pathologies practically never give rise to binasal hemianopia. Course book suggestions that list bilateral carotid aneurysms and carotid siphon sclerosis as possible pathogenic factors are not based on actual case presentations. The only neurological relevance is that binasal deficits can develop as a result of prolonged papilledema, but it is easily detectable based on fundoscopic image. In other cases, we have to look for a retinal or other ophthalmological cause. Further examinations and clinical course: Slightly excavated optic discs are visible on both sides. Further recording of the patient's intraocular pressure unambiguously revealed glaucoma.

We wish to emphasize that apart from the well-known patterns of visual field deficits in glaucoma (enlarged blind spot, Bjerrum's scotoma, Roenne's nasal step, central tunnel vision with a temporal island), some bilateral nasal losses are also rather common, so further investigations to look for intracranial lesions are not warranted.

Optic Tract Syndrome

A 54-year-old male patient had a myocardial infarction 5 years ago. For 18 months, he had had vague visual complaints that had intensified in the last month. He had no headache or other complaints. A CT scan performed 1 year ago was normal. Vision on the left side was 0.8, on the right side 1.0. Marcus–Gunn phenomenon was detected on the left side. The visual field test showed incongruent, homonymous hemianopsia on the right side (Fig. 18.5). The fundus was intact.

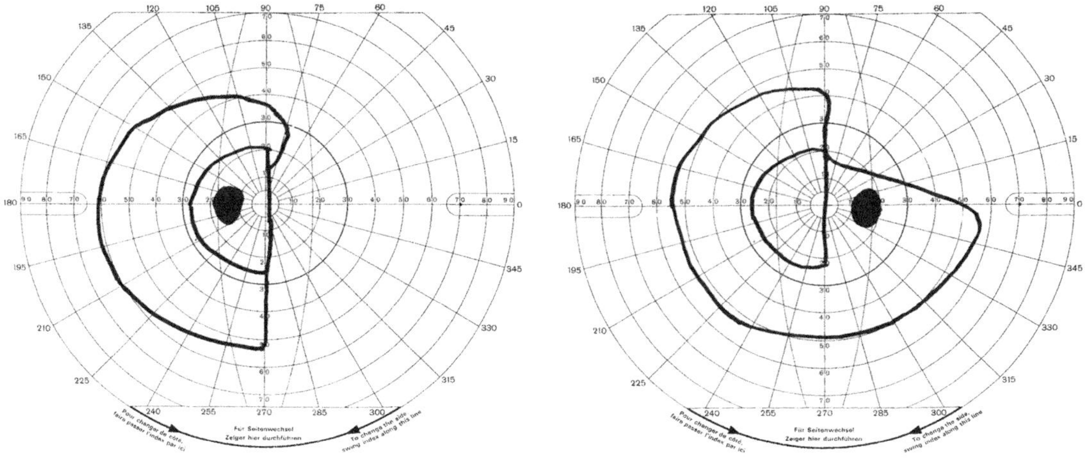

Fig. 18.5 Incongruent homonymous hemianopsia in optic tract syndrome caused by craniopharyngeoma

Considerations: Obviously incongruent hemianopsia with slight visual impairment and Marcus–Gunn phenomenon support optic tract syndrome. Marcus–Gunn phenomenon mostly develops on the side affected by the temporal loss of vision as more fibers are damaged here; therefore, more afferent stimuli are lost. However, if the visual field deficit is greater nasally (as is the case here), the Marcus–Gunn phenomenon develops there. The optic tract is rarely the only structure to be affected; in most cases the changes also affect the chiasm and the optic nerve(s). That's why it is more appropriate to call it optic tract syndrome than optic tract lesion.

The most common causes of this rare syndrome:

(a) craniopharyngeoma,
(b) pituitary tumor
(c) aneurysm in the carotid artery
(d) demyelinization.

Based on the probability of frequency and the lack of other symptoms and signs (including endocrinological), the most likely diagnosis was craniopharyngeoma.

Further examinations and clinical course: Another CT scan was performed following the administration of intrathecal contrast agent, and it showed a suprasellar cystic space-occupying mass. It has to be noted that without the administration of intrathecal contrast agent, suprasellar cystic lesions may not be detected on CT scans. MRI examinations, naturally, do not have this disadvantage.

Transient Optic Tract Syndrome with Other Neurological Symptoms

A 28-year-old female patient had had transient double vision for 2 years. For a year she had also felt clumsiness in the left hand. She presented at our clinic complaining of vague visual disturbance. Her vision was 0.6 on the right side, and 1.0 on the left side. Marcus–Gunn phenomenon was detected on the right side. No other neurological signs were detected. Figure 18.6 shows a right sided, highly incongruent homonymous hemianopsia in her field of vision.

Considerations: Visual impairment associated with visual field deficit and Marcus–Gunn phenomenon suggest left sided optic tract syndrome. Her previous symptoms that presented at various times and neurological locations raised the likelihood of a demyelinization process.

Further examinations and clinical course: Oligoclonal gammopathy was detected in the agar electrophoresis of the cerebrospinal fluid. T2 weighted MRI images (Fig. 18.7) showed several hyperintense periventricular foci in the

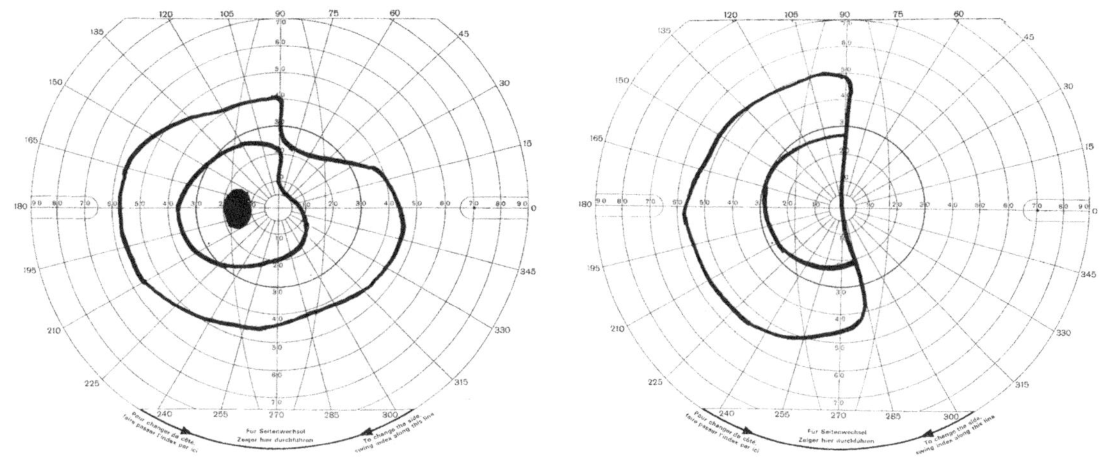

Fig. 18.6 Optic tract syndrome in multiple sclerosis

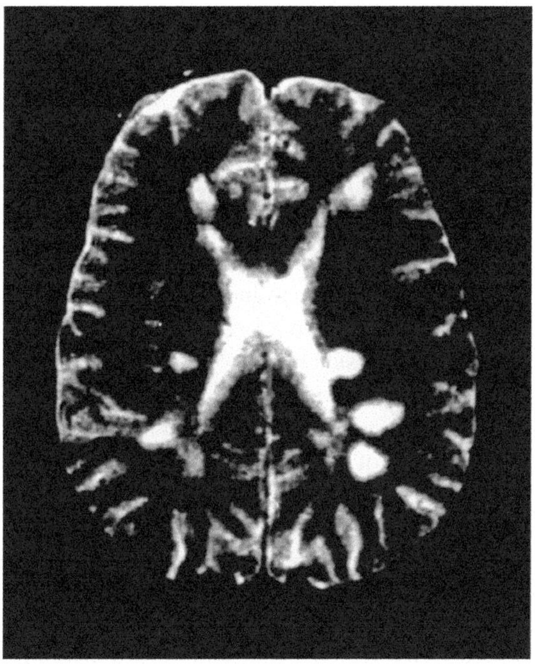

Fig. 18.7 T_2 weighted MRI shows hyperintense white matter foci

white matter. Although optic tract lesions are rare in multiple sclerosis, in this patient it was obviously the case. Her symptoms of visual impairment and visual field deficit disappeared following aggressive, high-dose dexamethasone therapy.

Hemianopsia Associated with a Parietal Lesion

A 35-year-old male, whose sibling was treated for superior sagittal sinus thrombosis, suddenly developed weakness and numbness in his left extremities and he became spatially disoriented. On examination, we found latent paresis in the left upper extremity, mild apraxia and left sided hypesthesia. His vision was normal, and the fundus intact. Visual field test revealed left lower quadrant visual field deficit (Fig. 18.8).

Considerations: Lower quadrant visual field deficit can be the result of a lesion in the parietal white matter or damage to the upper bank of the calcarine sulcus. In this case, the accompanying symptoms (hemihypesthesia, apraxia) suggest a parietal location. The sudden onset of the disorder suggests a vascular pathology.

Further examinations and clinical course: Angiography revealed obstruction in the parietal branches of the medial cerebral artery (right side) (Fig. 18.9). The young age of the patient and the family history raised the suspicion of a hereditary clotting disorder. Coagulation tests revealed antithrombin III deficiency. Contrary to the occipital origin, when lower quadrant hemianopsia originates from the parietal lobe, it is almost always associated with other neurological symptoms. Damage to the right, non-dominant hemisphere is

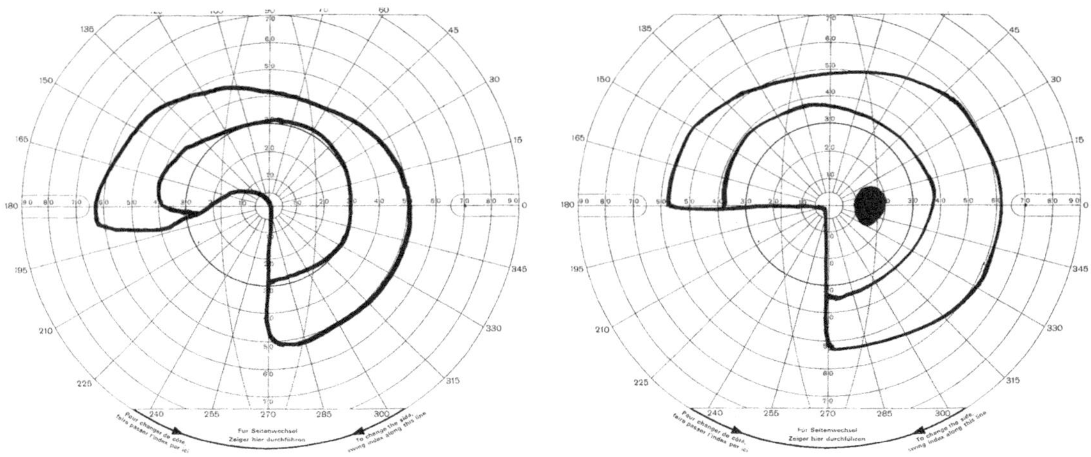

Fig. 18.8 Lower quadrantanopsia in case of a parietal lesion due to branching of the middle cerebral artery

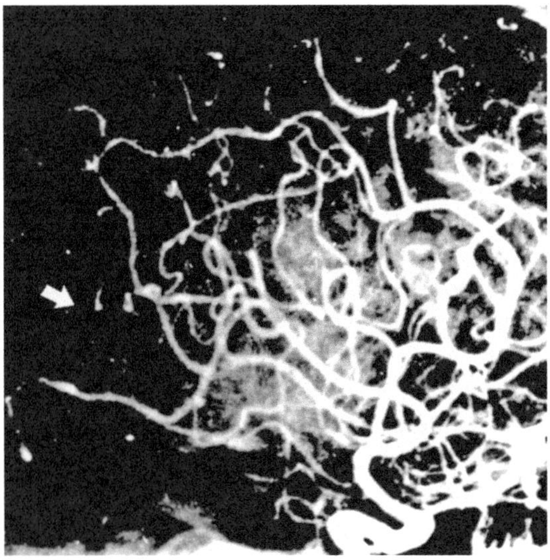

Fig. 18.9 Angiogram of the right carotid artery. The *arrow* indicates the area of the missing posterior parietal artery

mostly accompanied by hemihypesthesia, apraxia and neglect phenomena in the left side of the body. Damage to the dominant parietal lobe is associated with sensory symptoms (including loss of visual field) as well as speech disorder, finger agnosia, right–left confusion, agraphia, acalculia, which frequently render the detection of quadrantanopsia extremely difficult or even impossible. Quadrant or complete homonymous hemianopsia that have no other symptoms and can be investigated easily mostly originates from the occipital cortex and not from the optic radiation.

Transient Cortical Blindness, Followed by Quadrantanopsia

A 70-year-old male patient had a history of myocardial infarction 3 years ago and recurrent paroxysmal atrial fibrillation. 10 days earlier, he experienced sudden loss of vision in both eyes, accompanied by malaise. Some hours later he regained his vision gradually, but noticed that he could not see objects in the left side of his visual field. Over the course of some days, this latter complaint also improved; however, he had difficulty orientation, which meant he needed the assistance of street names to orient himself even in a known area.

His vision was 1.0 with left upper quadrant loss of visual field (Fig. 18.10). He also had mild spatial disorientation.

Considerations: Although homonymous upper quadrant visual field deficits can be the result of both temporal white matter lesions and damage to the lower bank of the calcarine sulcus, the lack of other symptoms and the phenomena experienced during the development of the symptoms suggest occipital origin.

Sudden bilateral loss of vision without fundal symptoms is mostly characteristic of cortical blindness, but rarely it can also occur in severe,

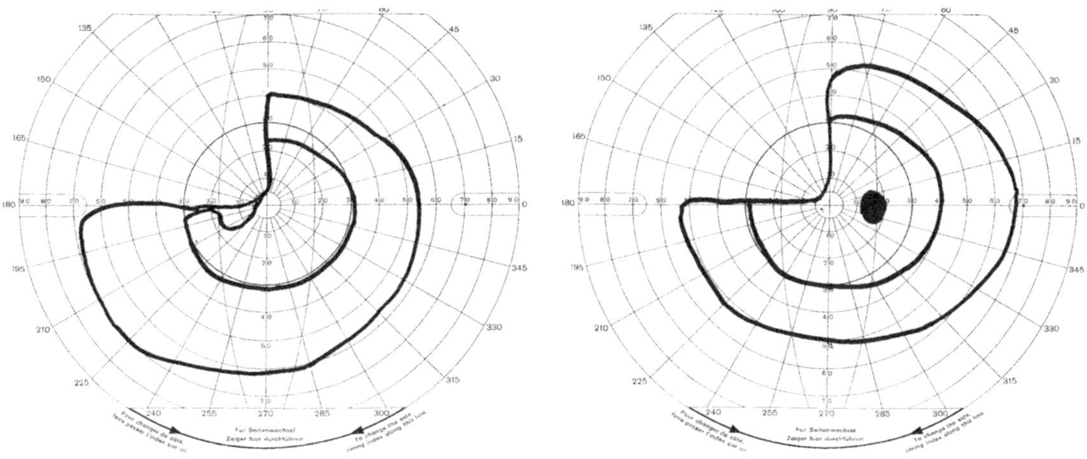

Fig. 18.10 Upper quadrantanopsia as a result of slight occipital malacia

bilateral retrobulbar neuritis or can be psychogenic as well. Cortical blindness is the result of a simultaneous circulatory disorder in both posterior cerebral arteries, which can be caused by an embolism occluding the tip of the basilar artery when there is insufficient supply from the posterior communicating artery. Caplan called it 'top of the basilar' syndrome. Apart from cortical blindness Hertwig–Magendie sign, loss of voluntary eye abduction, (pseudoabducens palsy), blind spot anomalies and memory disorders can develop. The symptoms of our patient must have been caused by the 'top of the basilar' syndrome with the direct trigger, the embolus, coming from the heart (atrial fibrillation in the history). The permanent damage to the right occipital lobe is likely to have been caused by the fragmentation and migration of this embolus (see the image of the CT scan, Fig. 18.11).

Further clinical course: The patient was put on anticoagulant therapy. Disorientation problems ceased after some time.

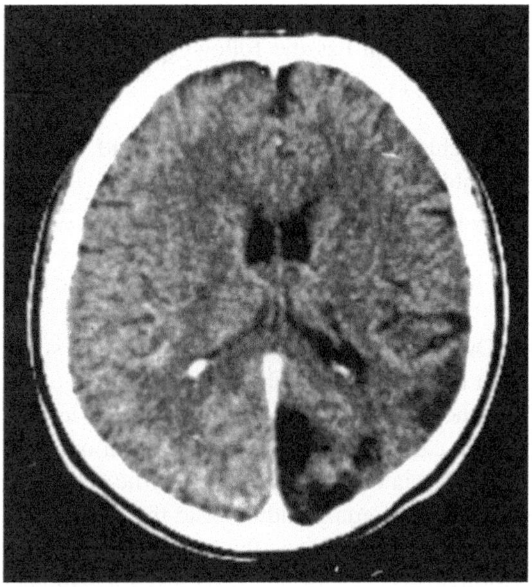

Fig. 18.11 Slight occipital malacia following transient complete cortical blindness

Homonymous Hemianopsia in Case of an Occipital Lesion

A 34-year-old man developed a sudden, mild frontal headache, and then he realized he could not see objects on his left. Later he found out that he could not read either. He had no other diseases or preceding symptoms. On examination his vision was 1.0 with mostly congruent, homonymous hemianopsia on the left. The field of vision was intact in the middle and another sickle-shaped intact area was detectable in the left temporal region (Fig. 18.12). No other neurological signs were detected. Optokinetic nystagmus could be elicited with all-direction drum rotation.

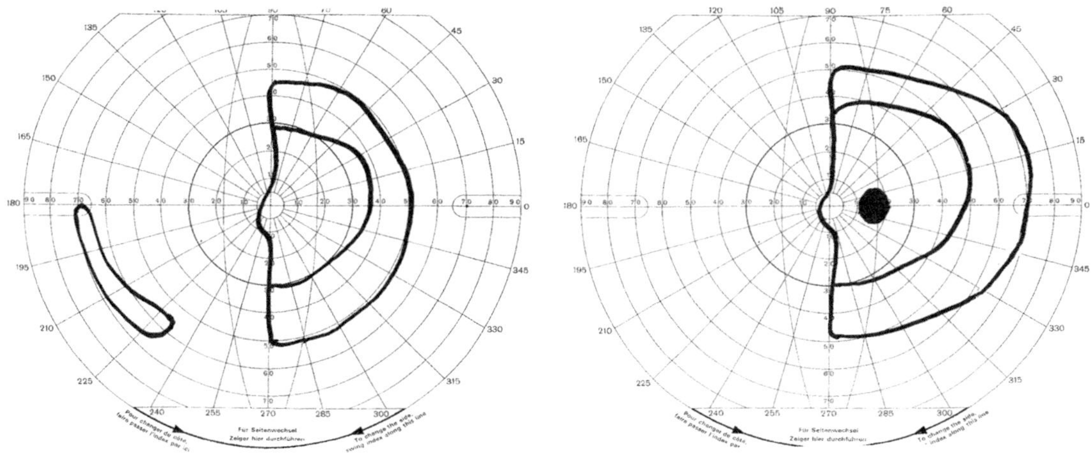

Fig. 18.12 Highly congruent occipital homonymous hemianopsia with intact central area and temporal sickle

Considerations: Hemianopsia caused by an occipital lesion has the following characteristic features:

(a) highly congruent loss of visual field,
(b) intact central vision,
(c) a potentially intact temporal sickle or its isolated loss,
(d) lack of other symptoms in most of the cases.

Our patient matched all these criteria, so he must have had an occipital lesion. In spite of his age, the sudden onset suggests a vascular lesion.

The cause of intact central vision in occipital hemianopsia was the topic of scientific debate for a long time. Certain authors said that it is a fixation disorder that keeps the area of the macular vision intact in case of hemianopsia. Another explanation was the multiple blood supply of macular fibers. However, there is no unambiguous evidence to prove this suggestion. The bilateral representation of maculae has been suspected for some time, and present-day animal models, as well as surgical and electrophysiological observations seem to prove it as well.

This sickle-shaped temporal region is located between 60° and 90° of the visual field, and it belong to the most nasal area of the retina. Obviously, it has no nasal counterpart in the visual field of the other eye. It has been known for a long time that this temporal area may remain intact in 10% of occipital hemianopsia. Nowadays we know for a fact that it happens when the lesion does not affect the outermost area of the striate cortex, as it is this region where the most nasal retinal areas are represented. The opposite of this phenomenon can also occur when the lesion affects only the most frontal occipital region: in such cases only this sickle-shaped temporal area will be lost. However, we have to be very cautious when assessing such a visual field, as areas beyond 60° are not easy to illustrate, and such narrowing of the visual field is usually due to retinal causes. Optokinetic nystagmus is also worth mentioning. Some authors consider the loss of optokinetic nystagmus as evidence of an occipital lesion. However, according to other observations, optokinetic nystagmus is most likely to change or be lost in parietal lesions. In such lesions, it is sometimes impossible to elicit even when there is no loss of visual field. Overall, we can state that optokinetic nystagmus is of not much assistance when trying to differentiate between various types of homonymous hemianopsia.

Further examinations and clinical course: CT examination revealed occipital infarction on the right side. Cerebral angiography showed a normal vascular network with no stenosis or obstruction. Both posterior cerebral arteries were normal. The young age of the patient and the normal angiogram raised the possibility of a cardiac

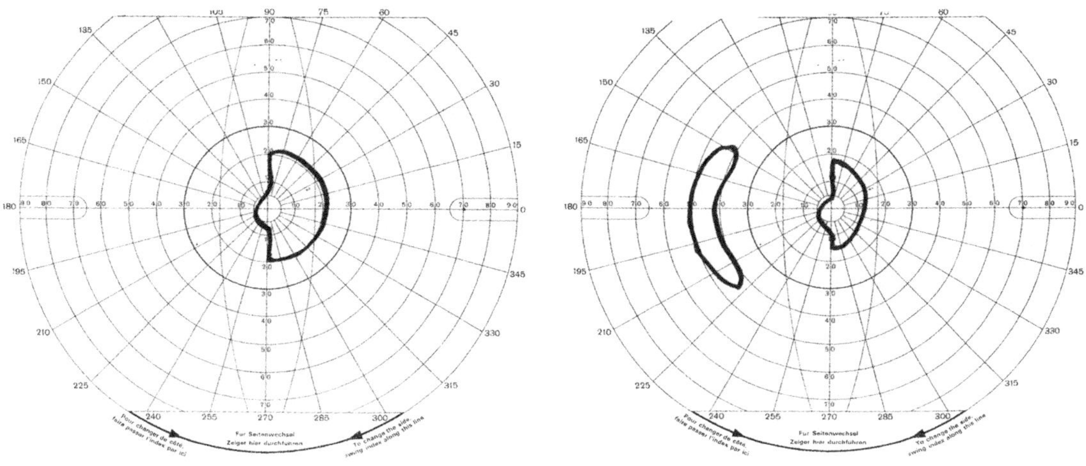

Fig. 18.13 Bilateral homonymous hemianopsia

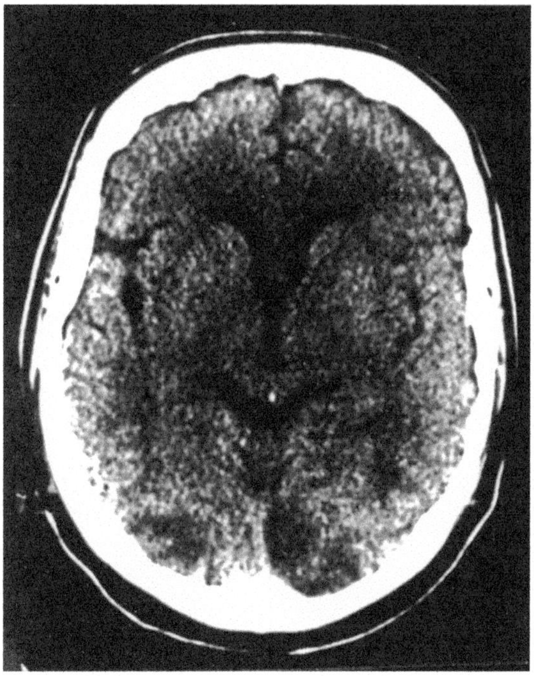

Fig. 18.14 Bilateral occipital lobe infarction with high intensity areas at the edges

embolism. The findings on Holter monitoring were normal. Echocardiography revealed mitral prolapse. Mitral prolapse is relatively common, and in most patients it is an incidental finding. However, in cerebrovascular events of patients under 40, its incidence is 6 times as high as in the same age group of the general population. Therefore, even if the incidental, asymptomatic mitral prolapse justifies no treatment, anticoagulants might be considered in vascular events. The patient's loss of visual field did not change; 3 years after its development it was the same, although his reading and orientation skills improved significantly through learning. Unfortunately, the loss of visual field caused by occipital infarction is frequently permanent.

Bilateral Homonymous Hemianopsia

A 54-year-old male patient experienced sudden visual impairment. On examination his vision was 0.4 on both sides, and his orientation was very poor (for field of vision see Fig. 18.13). There were no other neurological signs or symptoms, the fundus was intact.

Considerations: Visual impairment and the narrowing of the visual field would suggest a retinal cause; however, the rest of the examination shows that what remained of the central field of vision respect the vertical axis, and the two sides are highly congruent. The intact temporal half-moon also supports the presence of an occipital lesion. The findings of the visual field test and the course of development suggest an occipital vascular lesion.

Further examinations: CT examination (Fig. 18.14) showed subacute malacia in both occipital lobes with high intensity areas at the edges. Angiography revealed obstruction in the left posterior cerebral artery and severe arteriosclerosis in the other arteries. The primary obstruction is likely to have occurred at the peak of the basilar artery or in both posterior cerebral arteries, and one of them probably recanalized before the angiography. Such cases could be called partial cortical blindness, but most authors differentiate between cortical blindness and cases that are associated with some remaining field of vision and refer to the latter type as bilateral homonymous hemianopsia. Obviously, the difference is only about the degree. In our case the CT suggests that the bilateral occipital ischemic lesions developed at the same time, and it also supports the primary obstruction of the basilar peak. Another group of 'bilateral homonymous hemianopsia' cases is the combined result of visual field deficits that developed at various times.

Further Readings

Bell RA, Thompson HS. Relative afferent pupillary defect in optic tract hemianopsia. Am J Ophthalmol. 1978;85:538–43.

Benton S, Levy J, Swash M. Vision in the temporal crescent in occipital infarction. Brain. 1980;103:83–97.

Bunt AH, Minckler DS. Foveal sparing. Arch Ophthalmol. 1977;95:1445–7.

Frontera AT, et al. Bilateral homonym hemianopsia with preservation of central vision. Mt Sinai J Med NY. 1974;41:480–5.

O'Connor PS. The Marcus–Gunn pupil in experimental optic tract lesions. Ophthalmology. 1982;89:1690–8.

Spector RH, et al. Occipital lobe infarctions: perimetry and computed tomography. Neurology. 1981;31:1098–106.

Walsh TJ. Temporal crescent or half-moon syndrome. Ann Ophthalmol. 1974;6:501–5.

19 The Role of Fluorescein Angiography and Optical Coherence Tomography in the Examination of Circulatory Disorders of the Optic Disc

Zsuzsa Récsán and Zsuzsa Szepessy

Contents

The retina is supplied by a double circulatory system: the outer layers of the retina (the photoreceptors and the pigment epithelium) are avascular and supplied by the choriocapillary network via diffusion. The inner layers of the retina are supplied by the central retinal artery. An anastomosis between the two circulatory systems is rare. The submacular and the peripapillary regions are supplied by the short posterior ciliary arteries. Both circulatory systems belong to the system of the ophthalmic artery. The blood from the choroidea is drained through the vortex veins. The vortex veins open into the inferior and the superior ophthalmic veins. The inferior ophthalmic vein ends in the pterygoid venous plexus, whereas the superior ophthalmic vein opens into the cavernous sinus. There is collateral circulation between the inferior and superior ophthalmic veins. The central retinal vein drains blood from the retina and the prelaminar part of the optic nerve, and opens into the cavernous sinus. Therefore, on the venous side, there is communication between the retinal and the choroidal circulation.

Occlusion of the retinal vessels selectively affects the inner retina. The occlusion is central if it is developed within the optic disc, and therefore, the occlusion site itself cannot be visualized with the ophthalmoscope. A branch occlusion is an occlusion distal to the lamina cribrosa. A circulatory disorder in the short posterior ciliary arteries leads to ischemic optic neuropathy.

Trunk and Branch Occlusion of the Central Retinal Artery

The pathomechanism of the arterial occlusion may be either thrombosis or embolism. Embolism is the cause in more than twothirds of branch occlusion cases, and in only one-third of trunk occlusions. The most widely accepted view is that trunk occlusions are most often caused by a thrombus developed in the area of the lamina cribrosa or immediately behind it, in the proximal direction. Thrombus formation is usually due to atherosclerosis, but it may also be caused by malformation, inflammation, trauma or coagulopathy. Sixty percent of patients with trunk occlusion have hypertension, and 25 % of them have diabetes mellitus. A potential source of embolism is detected in only 40 % of the cases (Table 19.1).

Z. Récsán, M.D., PhD (✉) • Z. Szepessy, M.D., PhD
Department of Ophthalmology, Faculty of Medicine, Semmelweis University, Budapest, Hungary
e-mail: zsrecsan@gmail.com; szepzsu@yahoo.com

J. Somlai, T. Kovács (eds.), *Neuro-Ophthalmology*, DOI 10.1007/978-3-319-28956-4_19

Table 19.1 Conditions associated with the occlusion of the central retinal artery

Cardiovascular diseases of arteriosclerotic origin	Plaque, stenosis, dissection in the ophthalmic artery, the cervical arteries, the aorta or the branches of the aortic arch
Heart diseases	Arrhythmia, valvular or ventriculoseptal conditions, mural thrombus, subacute bacterial endocarditis
Coagulopathies	Presence of antiphospholipid antibodies, protein C, S or antithrombin III deficiency, elevated platelet factor 4 levels
Tumor	Metastatic tumor, leukemia, lymphoma
Medical interventions	Angiography, angioplasty, chiropractic manipulation of the neck, depot corticosteroid injection
Systemic vasculitises	Systemic lupus erythematosus, polyarteritis nodosa, temporal (giant cell) arteritis
Infectious diseases	Syphilis
Traumatic injury to the eye or the orbit	Direct pressure on the eyes, penetrating eye injury, retrobulbar injection, retrobulbar hematoma, Purtscher's syndrome
Non-traumatic eye disorders	Prepapillary arterial loop, optic disc drusen, necrotizing herpetic retinitis, orbital mucormycosis, toxoplasmosis
Other diseases, conditions	Amniotic fluid embolism, pancreatitis, cocaine abuse, intravenous drug use

In case of *arterial trunk occlusion*, the patient reports pain-free, sudden loss of vision, the fundus shows signs of diffuse ischemia, and the macula is cherry-colored. The clinical picture is usually unambiguous. In uncertain cases, fluorescein angiography may be of help. It is typical that the 'occluded' vessels almost always show blood flow, and complete occlusion is very rare. The arm-to-retina time is prolonged, and the arterial filling is considerably slower than normal. The flow of the dye, the advancing peak is characteristic. The arteriovenous transit is also very slow. The late-phase images often show a stained optic disc. The optical coherence tomography supports the observation that in case of arterial occlusion, it is primarily the inner retina that is damaged, intracellular edema occurs because of the ischemia.

The retina is thickened. Since the edema is intracellular, there are no low-reflectivity cystoid spaces on the topogram. The layers of the inner retina, supposedly because of coagulation necrosis, are strongly reflective, and cast a shadow over the photoreceptor layers and the pigment epithelium–choriocapillary complex. Since the area of the fovea lacks the inner retinal layers, there is no shadowing effect here, and the base of the choriocapillary–pigment epithelium complex shows higher reflectivity than its surroundings (Fig. 19.1). During the follow-up of the patient, thinning of the retina is observed in case of chronic vessel occlusion. The macular volume decreases, and in case of trunk occlusion, the peripapillary nerve fiber layer also becomes thinner. A useful indicator for the follow-up of the patient is the change in macular volume, foveal thickness and peripapillary nerve fiber layer (RNFL) measured with OCT.

The emboli causing *branch occlusion* can be divided into three main groups: cholesterol (Hollenhorst plaque), platelet fibrin and calcific emboli. Less frequent forms are emboli that contain tumor cells, emboli from a septic source, and fat emboli formed in case of large-bone fractures. Similarly to trunk occlusions, branch occlusions may also be caused by local, ophthalmological lesions. Systemic hematological or coagulation disorders may even lead to recurrent occlusions. The patient reports a painfree, sudden-onset loss of vision in the visual field segment that corresponds to the affected branch, and central vision is intact in most of the cases. The milk-white retinal area on the fundus corresponds to the ischemic area supplied by the occluded artery. The edge of the lesion is determined by the drainage area of the neighboring vein branch. The FLAG shows a circulatory block and a considerably decreased flow of the dye in the affected artery branch, and as a consequence, the circulation in the neighboring vein branches is also slower. On the OCT images, the inner retinal layers are considerably and diffusely thickened and hyperreflective in

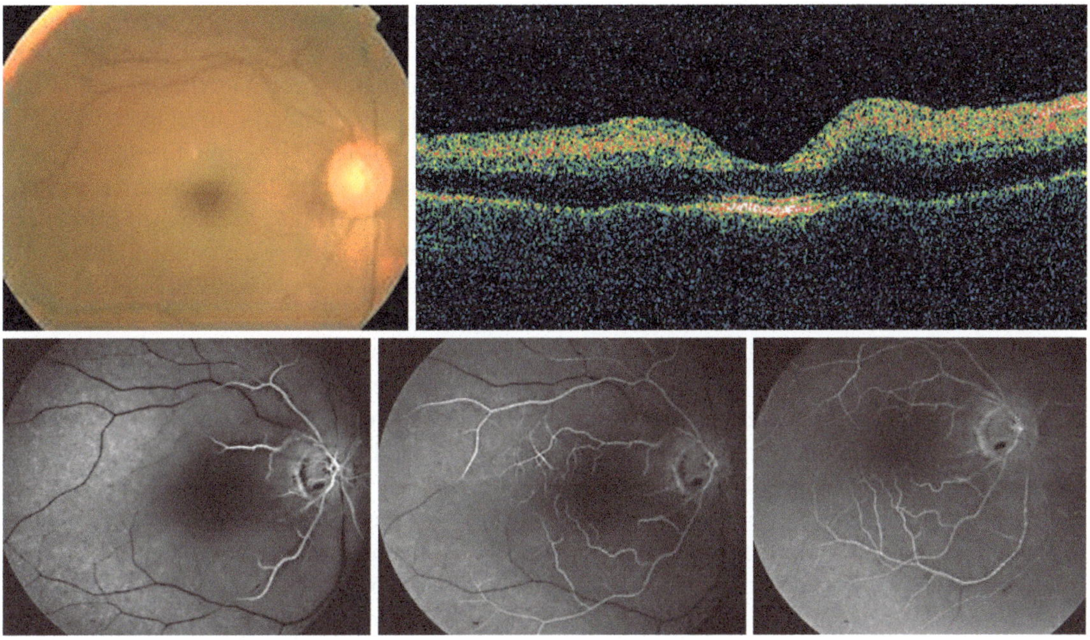

Fig. 19.1 Central retinal artery occlusion with a small flame-shaped hemorrhage on the optic disc. The inner retinal layers are thickened and hyperreflective and cast a shadow over the photoreceptors and the pigment epithelium–choriocapillary complex. The FLAG images show the slow arterial filling, and the advancing peak of the dye can be followed well

the area that corresponds to the occluded artery branch, there is a consequential shadow over the photoreceptors and the pigment epithelium–choriocapillary complex, and the cystoid spaces characteristic to extracellular edema are absent.

Trunk and Branch Occlusion of the Central Retinal Vein

Venous occlusions can be sorted into three groups based on location. Trunk (central), hemicentral and branch occlusions are distinguished. In case of a trunk occlusion, the entire central retinal vein is occluded. Hemicentral occlusion means the occlusion of one trunk of the congenitally dual-trunk central retinal vein. About 20 % of the population have a dual-trunk central retinal vein. Branch occlusion is most commonly seen in the superior temporal vein branch. Retinal venous circulatory disorders are relatively common. The incidence of venous trunk occlusion is second to that of diabetic retinopathy. The most common predisposing conditions are diabetes mellitus, arterial hypertension and atherosclerotic cardiovascular lesions. It is known that it is five times more common in patients with open-angle glaucoma, presumably due to the damage to the structure of the lamina cribrosa caused by the elevated intraocular pressure. Acute closed-angle glaucoma may also provoke venous trunk occlusion.

The pathomechanism of *venous trunk occlusion* is not fully clarified. There is a theory according to which the occlusion is caused by a thrombus formed in the area of the lamina cribrosa or directly behind it. The adjacent artery has a role in the formation of the thrombus because its wall is thickened due to arteriosclerosis and, by exerting pressure on the wall of the vein, it leads to turbulent flow and, consequentially, endothelial cell damage in it. Endothelial cell proliferation is also assumed to occur in the process of thrombus formation. According to another theory, the thrombosis of the vein trunk is an end stage caused by numerous possible primary factors, e.g., compression or inflammation of the optic nerve, conditions of the orbit, structure abnormalities of the lamina cribrosa, or hemodynamic factors. Since the already slow blood flow in the veins is against a relatively high resistance, the venous circulation is especially sensitive to changes in hematological factors (increased erythrocyte sedimentation rate, increased blood viscosity, elevated hematocrit, antithrombin III, fibrinogen and homocysteine levels, presence of antiphospholipid antibodies or lupus anticoagulant, activated protein C deficiency). In case of venous circulatory disorders developed by young patients, the hematological assessment may find antiphospholipid syndrome or Leiden point mutation.

Some opine that the two forms of venous trunk occlusion, the ischemic type and the non-ischemic type are manifestations of different severity of the same disease. Others think that the two types differ in their pathogenesis. In the ischemic form, there is also a severe arterial circulatory disorder. In the non-ischemic form, the thrombus is located behind the lamina cribrosa, in a more distal position.

The clinical presentation of the ischemic and non-ischemic venous trunk occlusion is similar. There are dilated veins of deformed course on the fundus and dot- or puddle-like hemorrhages in all four quadrants of the retina, cotton wool spots characteristic to infarcts may appear in the nerve fiber layer, the macula is edematous, the capillaries around the optic disc are markedly dilated and the optic disc also shows edema. Making a distinction between the two forms is important. In the non-ischemic form, the prognosis is more favorable, there is a higher chance of vision improvement, and neoangiogenesis is less common. It is known, however, that in one-third of the cases, the non-ischemic form may transform into ischemic form over the first 3 years. In one tenth of these patients, the transformation into the ischemic form occurs in the first 4 months.

It is not easy to tell the two forms apart in the acute phase. Examination of the pupils is considered to be very important. In the non-ischemic type, there is usually no or only a very mild afferent pupillary defect. Less bleeding can be seen on the fundus. If there are cotton wool spots, they are low in number and mainly located around the optic disc. On the fluorescein angiogram, staining can be observed along the dilated retinal veins that have deformed course, there is a slow, continuous leakage of dye from the dilated capillaries around the optic disc, and microaneurysms can be seen. The retinal capillary bed is intact. In the long term, vision is determined by the cystoids macular edema caused by the chronic circulatory disorder in the capillaries. The process resolves within 6–12 months, leaving a pigment disorder in the area of the macula behind, but an epiretinal membrane or subretinal fibrosis may also occur at the posterior pole. All of this can be followed well with OCT.

In the ischemic form, there is marked vision loss, and the number and extension of bleedings and cotton wool spots is increased. A considerable cystoid edema can be observed in the macula, although covered with hemorrhages. In 60 % of the cases, neoangiogenesis occurs in the anterior segment (iris, chamber angle) in the first 9 weeks, and neovascular glaucoma is developed within 3 months. (In case of venous trunk occlusion, neoangiogenesis is possible but not typical in the posterior segment, on the optic disc and in other areas.) The fluorescein angiogram is hard to evaluate because the extensive hemorrhages block the macular edema and cover the non-perfused areas. There are studies according to which in case of a non-perfused area the size of 10 or more optic discs, the risk of neoangiogenesis in the anterior segment is very high and therefore such forms should be considered as ischemic. Other studies are more permissive and consider a visual acuity of lower than 0.1 or a non-perfused retinal area the size of 30 or more optic discs to be the threshold. Despite the bleedings, OCT is suitable for the early detection of macular edema. Both fluorescein angiography and optical coherence tomography have a role not primarily in making the diagnosis or distinguishing between the ischemic and the non-ischemic form but rather in monitoring the course of the disease. Non-perfused areas are easier to detect with fluorescein angiography once the hemorrhages are resorbed. (It is worth taking photos not only of the posterior central areas but, with directed view, also of the periphery.)

Neoangiogenesis is easier to detect or, if suspected based on the ophthalmoscopic picture, confirm. The condition of the macula can be followed well with OCT (Figs. 19.2 and 19.3). In case of venous occlusions, OCT provides information also about the optic disc. In the acute phase, sector-like peripapillary nerve fiber layer (RNFL) thickening may occur in case of branch

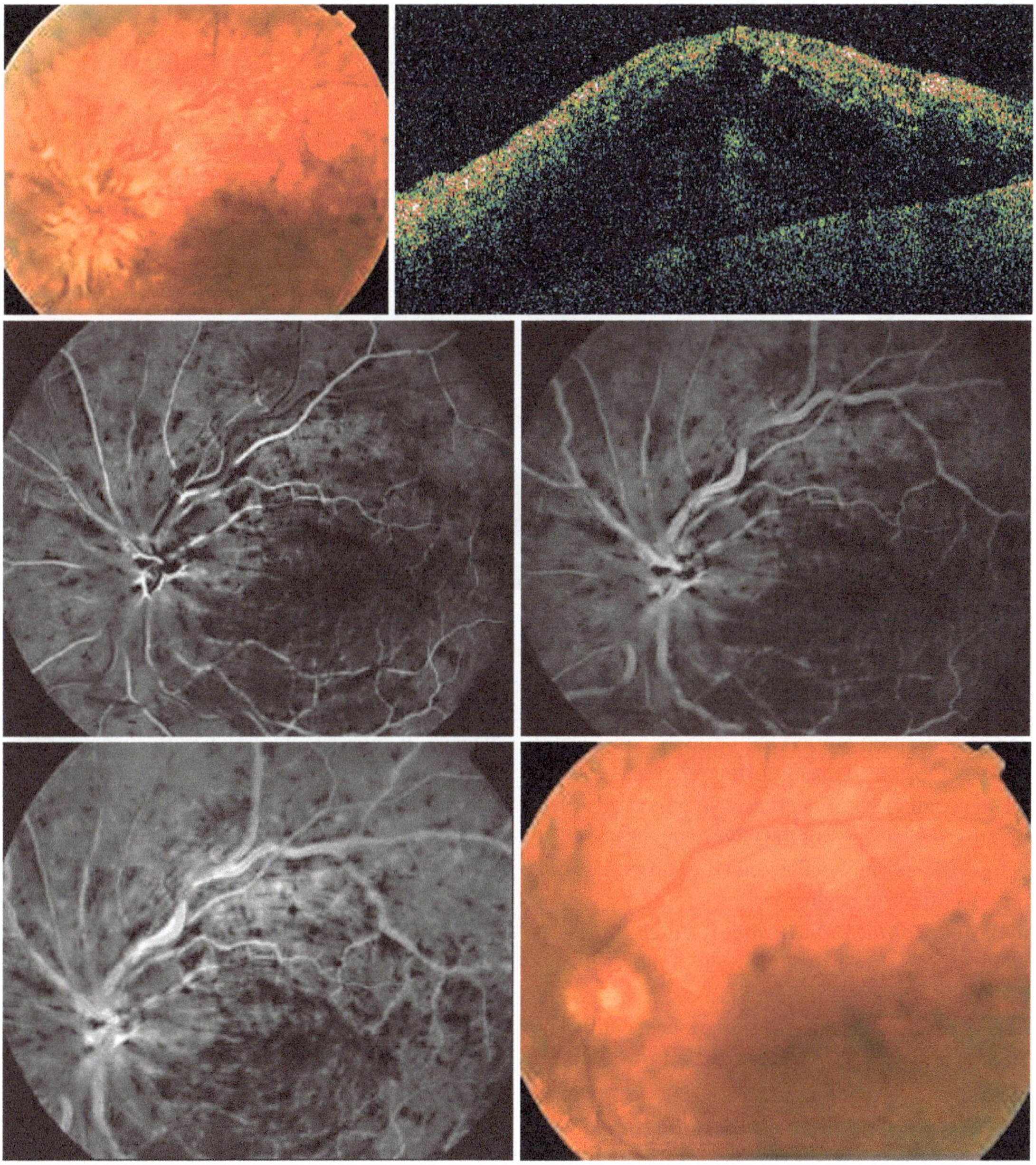

Fig. 19.2 Central retinal vein occlusion. *Upper images*: In the acute phase, dilated veins of deformed course, hemorrhages and numerous cotton wool spots around the optic disc can be seen. OCT shows macular edema, and thickening, increased reflectivity and shadowing effect of the inner retinal layers. On the fluorescein angiograms, staining along the dilated vein branches of deformed course and mild dye leakage along the superior temporal venous branch can be observed. *Lower images*: 9 months later, the hemorrhages are almost completely absorbed, and there is cystoid edema in the macula. Circulation in the large vessels is almost completely restored but the superior temporal vein branch is still thickened and of deformed course, and there is late filling in it

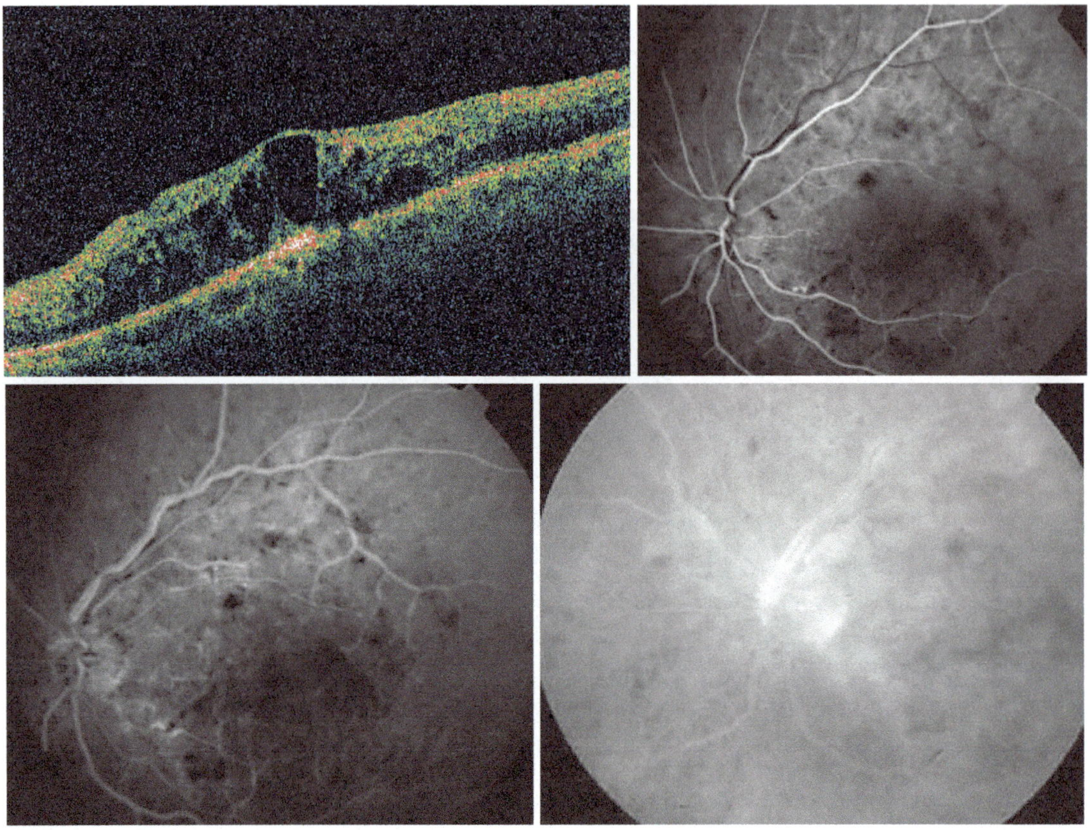

Fig. 19.2 (continued)

occlusion, whereas concentric RNFL thickening can be measured around the optic disc in case of trunk occlusions. During follow-up, the edema of the nerve fiber layer decreases in an average of 2 months, and atrophy of the RNFL and its decrease below the normal value can be observed 6–8 months after the occlusion.

Venous branch occlusion is three times as common as trunk occlusion. It almost always occurs in the arteriovenous crossing, where the artery and vein run in a common sheath. The artery is on the top, in the direction of the vitreous body. The artery, which is rigid because of arteriosclerosis, compresses the wall of the vein. Therefore, turbulent flow and, consequentially, endothelial cell damage and thrombus formation start within the vein. The majority of branch occlusions are superotemporal. The likely reason for this is that the highest number of arteriovenous crossings is found here. Rarely, branch occlusion is caused by a local eye condition, e.g., inflammation such as toxoplasmosis, or Eales disease. It may accompany Coats' disease, macroaneurysm, papillary drusen, retinal capillary drusen and other systemic diseases (sarcoidosis, Behçet's syndrome). Glaucoma is a known risk factor.

The clinical picture is characteristic. Patients report sudden-onset blurred vision and a defect in the visual field that corresponds to the occluded vessel. In the acute phase, flame-like hemorrhages can be observed along the occluded vein branch on the fundus. The number of hemorrhages reflects the degree of the occlusion. FLAG is an efficient tool in the confirmation of the diagnosis and planning the therapy. Arterial filling is generally normal, and the capillaries are dilated and show a deformed course. The circulation in the occluded vein branch is considerably slower and late. Hypofluorescence can be seen because of the hemorrhages and the nonperfused areas. As the hemorrhages are resorbed, the extension

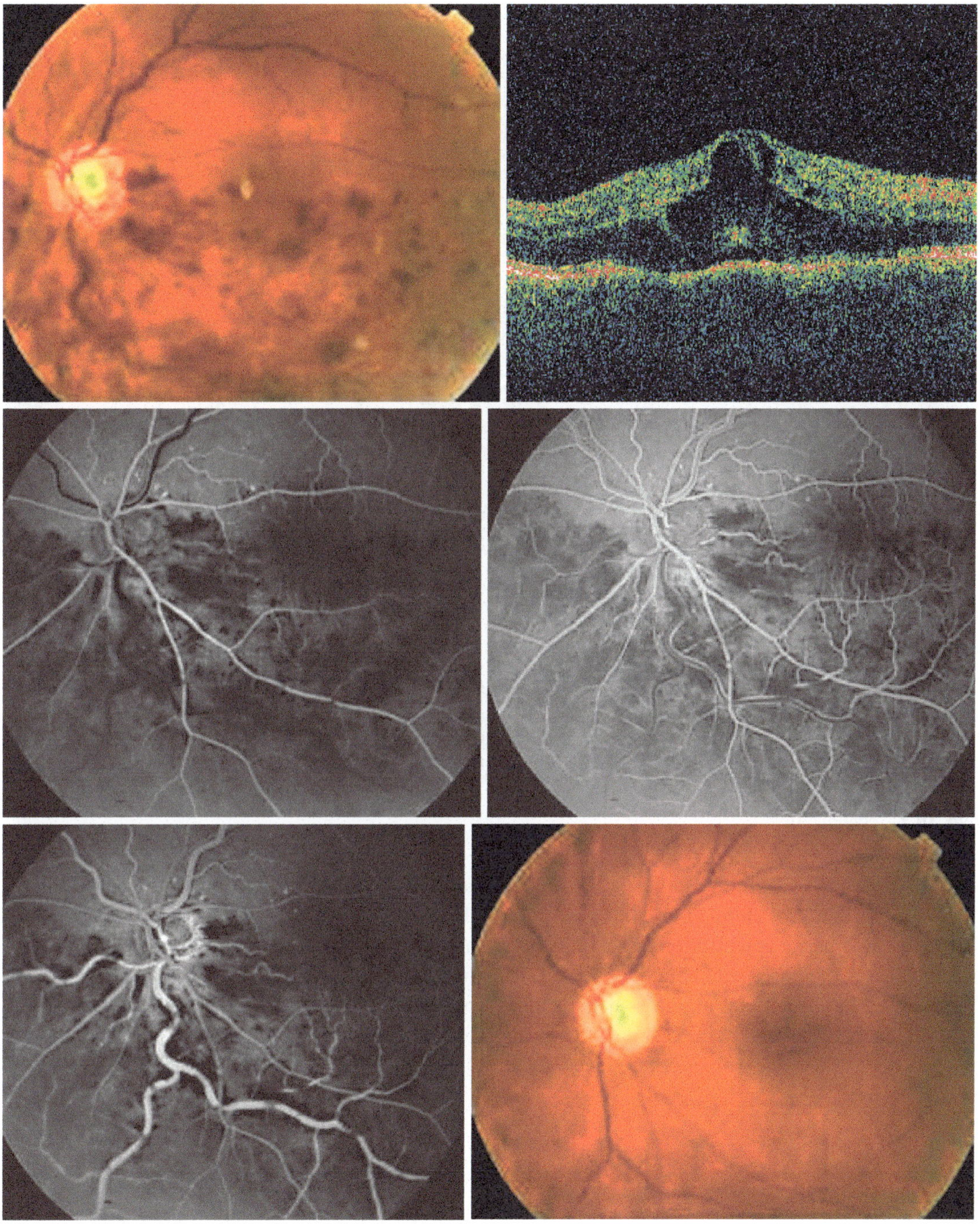

Fig. 19.3 Hemispheric occlusion in the inferior central vein branch. The *upper images* show the acute phase and the *lower images* the status 9 months later. Despite the hemorrhages, the OCT shows the cystoid edema of the macula already in the acute phase. The FLAG makes it clear that filling is late both in the inferior nasal and the inferior temporal vein branches. Nine months later, the cystoid macular edema, although decreased, is not yet resolved. Edema can be observed beneath the papillomacular zone. The foveal avascular zone is broadened. There are dilated collaterals between the inferior and superior temporal vessel arches. Temporal to the macula, and nasally in the mid-periphery, severe damage to the capillary network can be seen. Especially in the nasal periphery, circumscribed neoangiogenesis is possible

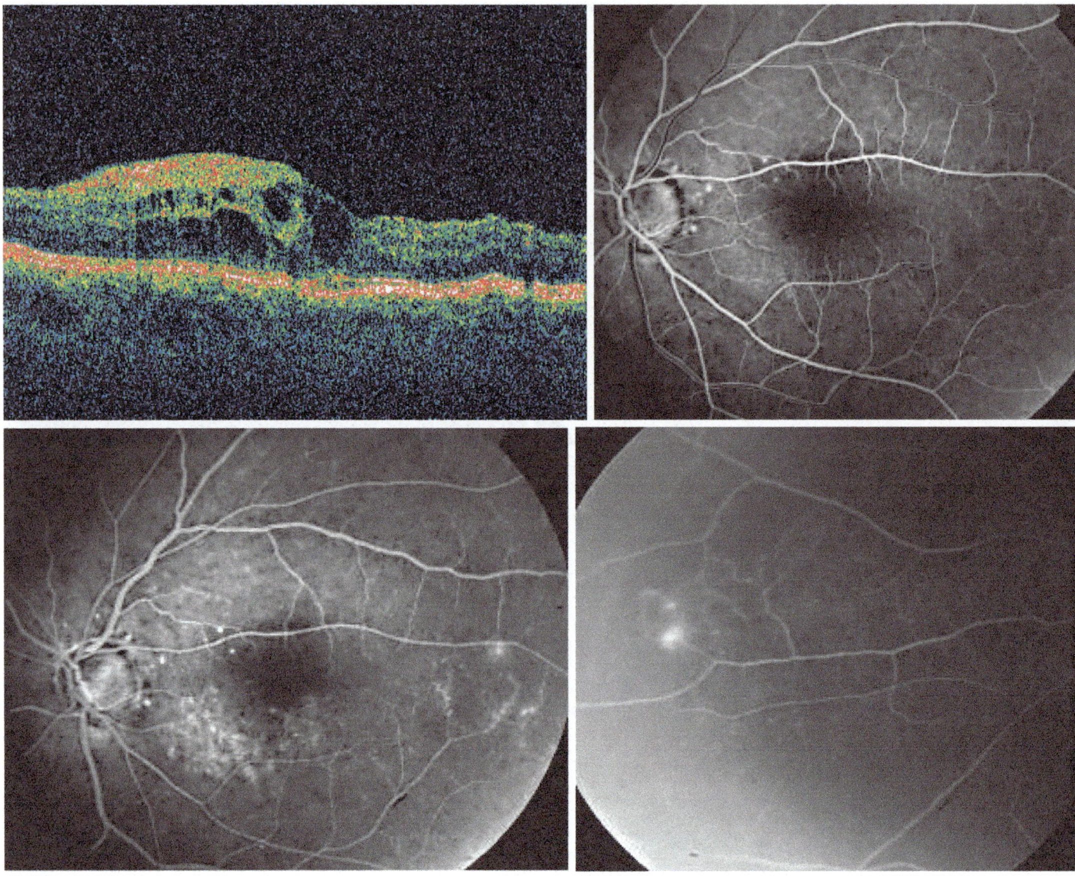

Fig. 19.3 (continued)

of the damage to the retinal capillary bed is more and more visible. Collateral circulation is formed between the superior and inferior vessel branches, and it crosses the horizontal boundary. In case of any doubt, fluorescein angiography helps safely distinguish between collateral vessels and neoangiogenesis on the optic disc or other places of the retina. Optic coherence tomography is good for the detection of cystoid macular edema, as well as the monitoring of its slow absorption (taking 6–12 months) and the development of any complications (epiretinal, subretinal fibrosis) during follow-up.

Anterior Ischemic Optic Neuropathy (AION)

Ischemia of the optic nerve, owing to its structure, most commonly occurs in the area of the optic disc. As a result of the impaired blood supply of the optic disc, the perfusion in the tightly packed nerve fibers may drop below a critical level. The most common manifestation form of optic nerve ischemia is anterior ischemic optic neuropathy but a similar picture can be seen in diabetic papillopathy, hypertensive papillopathy and optic neuropathy associated with migraine, which are also likely to be of ischemic origin. Ischemia of the intraorbital segment of the optic nerve (posterior ischemic optic neuropathy, PION) is a rare condition.

Anterior ischemic optic neuropathy has two forms. In giant cell arteritis, arteritic AION is caused by the vasculitis in the short posterior ciliary arteries. The medical history ('temporal arteritis': headache, sensitivity of the scalp, masticatory pain) and the significantly increased erythrocyte sedimentation rate (70–120 mm/h) are characteristic. In non-arteritic AION, the circulatory disorder affects the branches that directly supply the optic disc and that are distal to the short posterior ciliary arteries. Risk factors include hypertension, diabetes, ischemic heart disease, and hypercholesterolemia, as well as increased bleeding tendency and perfusion impairment due to elevated intraocular pressure.

The clinical picture is dominated by the deterioration of vision. It is characterized by a relative afferent pupillary defect and a curved scotoma most often developed in the inferior half of the visual field, which is connected with the center. On the fundus, initially there is an edematous optic disc with blurred edges and striped hemorrhages around it, and then sectors and, finally, the whole area of the optic disc becomes atrophic.

With the localization of the circulatory disorder, FLAG may help in the distinction of the two types. In case of arteritic AION, filling is considerably late in the optic disc and the neighboring choroidea (30–70 s, Fig. 19.4). In case of non-arteritic AION, there is late filling in the optic disc but the dye appears earlier than in AION of vasculitic origin. In non-arteritic AION, filling in the peripapillary choroidea is not late, and the flow is not or only slightly different from that seen in healthy control subjects of the same age. The change in the thickness of the retinal nerve fiber layer can be monitored with optic coherence tomography (Fig. 19.5). Thickening of the nerve fiber layer can be detected already in the early phase, and it increases further when an infarct occurs in the optic disc. Simultaneously with the atrophy of the optic nerve, the nerve fiber layer gets thinner and the cup/disc (C/D) ratio increases.

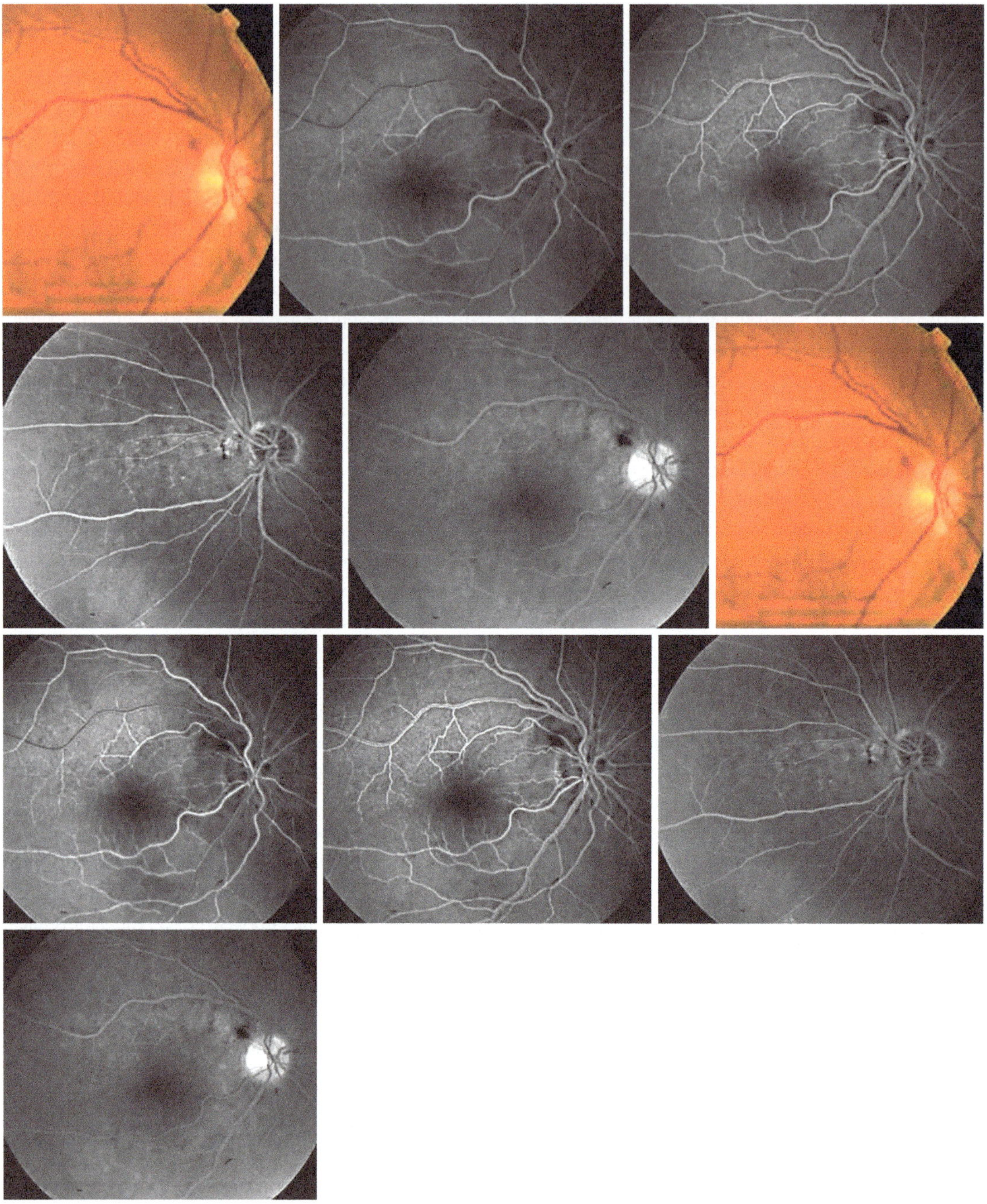

Fig. 19.4 AION developed by a patient with histologically confirmed giant cell arteritis (filling in the optic disc and the peripapillary region is considerably late)

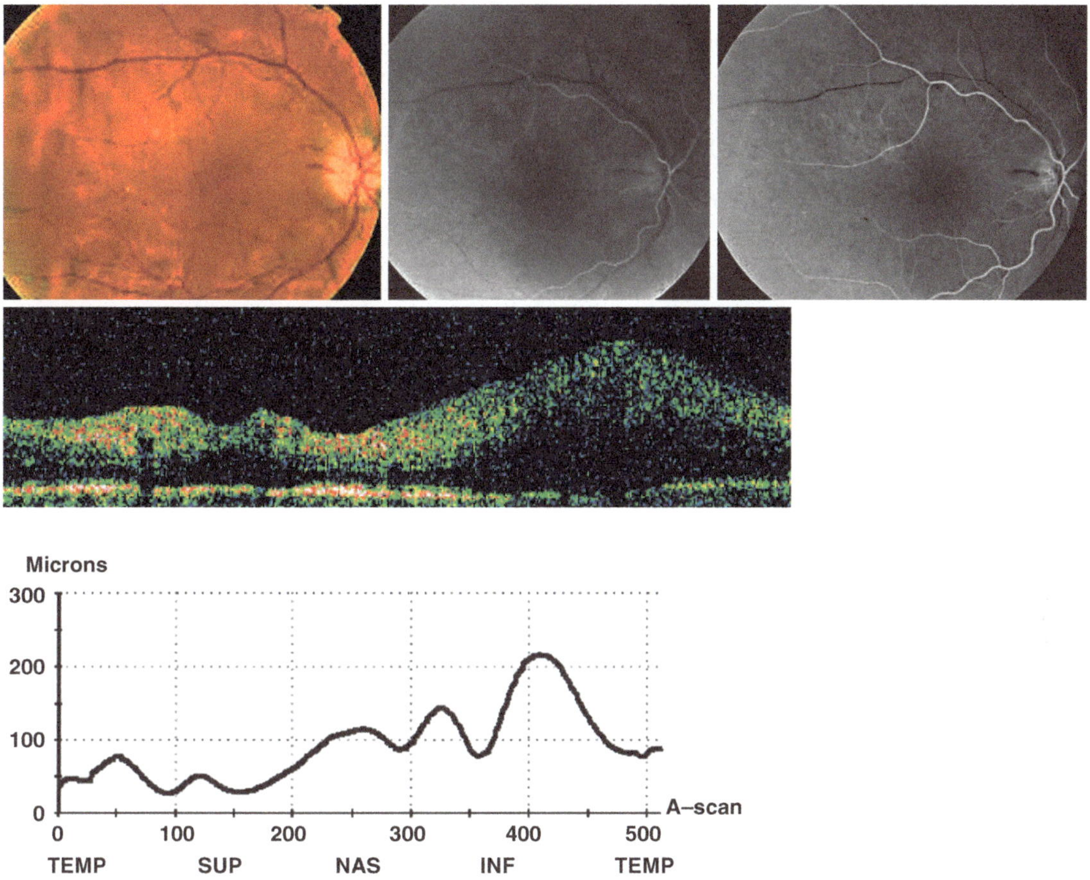

Fig. 19.5 Non-arteritic AION, the filling in the optic disc and the peripapillary region is not late; dye leakage from the dilated capillaries of the optic disc can be seen already on the early images. OCT: the retinal nerve fiber layer is thickened in the acute phase

References

Arnold AC, Hepler RS. Fluorescein angiography in acute anterior ischemic optic neuropathy. Am J Ophthalmol. 1994;117:222–30.

Asefzadeh B, Ninyo K. Longitudinal analysis of retinal changes after branch retinal artery occlusion using optical coherence tomography. Optometry. 2008;79:85–9.

BCSC Retina and Vitreous. 2004, Section 12. P. 136–45.

Contreras I, Rebolleda G, Noval S. Optic disc evaluation by optical coherence tomography in nonarteritic anterior ischemic optic neuropathy. Invest Ophthalmol Visual Sci. 2007;48:4087–92.

The Central Retinal Vein Occlusion Study Group. Natural history and clinical management of central retinal vein occlusion. Arch Ophthalmol. 1997;115:486–91.

DeLeon-Ortega J, Carroll KE, Arthur SN. Correlations between retinal nerve fiber layer and visual field in eyes with nonarteritic anterior ischemic optic neuropathy. Am J Ophthalmol. 2007;143:288–94.

Duker JS, Sivalingam A, Brown GC, Reber R. A prospective study of acute central retinal artery obstruction. Arch Ophthalmol. 1991;109:339–42.

Hayreh SS, Zimmermann MB, Podhajsky P. Incidence of various types retinal vein occlusion and their recurrence in demographic characteristics. Am J Ophthalmol. 1994;117:429–41.

Hayreh SS. Ischemic optic neuropathy. Progr Retinal Eye Res. 2009;28:34–62.

Hayreh SS. HCRVO: pathogenesis, clinical features, and natural history. Arch Ophthalmol. 1980;98:1600–8.

Hayreh SS, Jonas JB. Optic disc morphology after arteritic anterior ischemic optic neuropathy. Ophthalmology. 2001;108:1586–94.

Johnson TM. El-defrawy: prevalence of factor V Leiden and activated protein C resistance in central retinal vein occlusion. Retina. 2001;21:161–6.

Jonas JB, Xu L. Optic disc morphology in eyes after non-arteritic anterior ischemic optic neuropathy. Invest Ophthalmol Visual Sci. 1993;34:2260–5.

Leung CK, Tham CC, Mohammed S, Li EY, Leung KS, Chan WM, Lam DS. In vivo measurements of macular and nerve fibre layer thickness in retinal arterial occlusion. Eye (Lond). 2007;12:1464–8.

Siatkowski RM, Gass JDM, Glaser JS. Fluorescein angiography in the diagnosis of giant cell ateritis. Am J Ophthalmol. 1993;115:57–63.

Schuman JS, Puliafito CA, Fujimoto JG. Optical tomography of ocular diseases. Thorofare: Slack Inc.; 2004.

20 Optical Coherence Tomography of the Optic Disc and the Macula in Neurodegenerative Diseases

Gábor Márk Somfai, Erika Tátrai, and Magdolna Simó

Contents

Optical coherence tomography (OCT) was introduced in the beginning of the 1990s as a new imaging tool that enables the high-resolution in vivo examination of biological tissues. It was first used in ophthalmology where the OCT technology revolutionized the diagnostics of the conditions of the macula and the vitreo-retinal interface. Today, there is intensive research on the possible applications of OCT in other specialties, e.g., angiology, oncology, gastroenterology, dermatology, and dentistry. In the future, OCT may play an important role in the diagnosis and monitoring of neurodegenerative diseases, owing to the fact that the retina is such a unique place of the nervous system where nerve fibers without myelin sheath forming direct synapses with the central nervous system can be found. These nerve fibers come from the ganglion cells of the retina, leave the eyeball through the lamina cribrosa, and then run towards the lateral geniculate body forming the optic nerve. According to recent studies, a pathological impairment of the retinal nerve fiber layer (RNFL) can be observed in numerous neurological conditions. Measuring the thickness of the nerve fiber layer with OCT may therefore be a reliable and accurate non-invasive method for the detection and monitoring of neurodegeneration, which, besides accurate diagnostics, may become an invaluable tool to assess the efficacy of neuroprotective substances.

The principle of OCT is similar to that of the ultrasound, with the difference that instead of a sound wave, a low-coherence light beam is projected onto the tissue to be imaged. Currently, there are two types of commercially available OCT devices. For a detailed operation of OCT devices, please see the abundant literature; to summarize, third-generation time-domain OCT (TD-OCT) devices enable the examination of the light beam backscattered from the eye with the help of a moving reference arm, whereas newer, fourth-generation devices do this using a mathematical principle, analyzing the wave length spectrum of the backscattered light beam with Fourier transformation. The elimination of the moving part resulted in an almost 70- fold increase in imaging speed, and further technological innovations led to an improvement of

G.M. Somfai, M.D., PhD (✉) • E. Tátrai, M.D.
M. Simó, M.D., PhD
Department of Ophthalmology, Faculty of Medicine, Semmelweis University, Budapest, Hungary
e-mail: somfaigm@yahoo.com

J. Somlai, T. Kovács (eds.), *Neuro-Ophthalmology*, DOI 10.1007/978-3-319-28956-4_20

depth resolution from 10 to 5 µm. Commercially available third-generation OCTs can generate about 400 A-scans in 1 s, whereas in the case of fourth-generation Fourier-domain OCT (FD-OCT) devices, this number may reach 26,000, which enables a quicker and more accurate rendering but increases the computational capacity required for the analyses. Taking into account that third-generation OCT devices are currently more widespread on the market, we will primarily describe the examination results that can be obtained with these devices. Figure 20.1 shows the OCT image of a healthy macula—owing to the high resolution, the retinal layers of different optical density can be well distinguished. When scanning the optic disc, it is possible to guide the imaging around the optic disc, the result of which is 'spread' on Fig. 20.2. Since the highly reflective layer of the nerve fibers is well distinguished from the moderately reflective layer of the ganglion cells (see Fig. 20.1), the peripapillary RNFL is well mea-

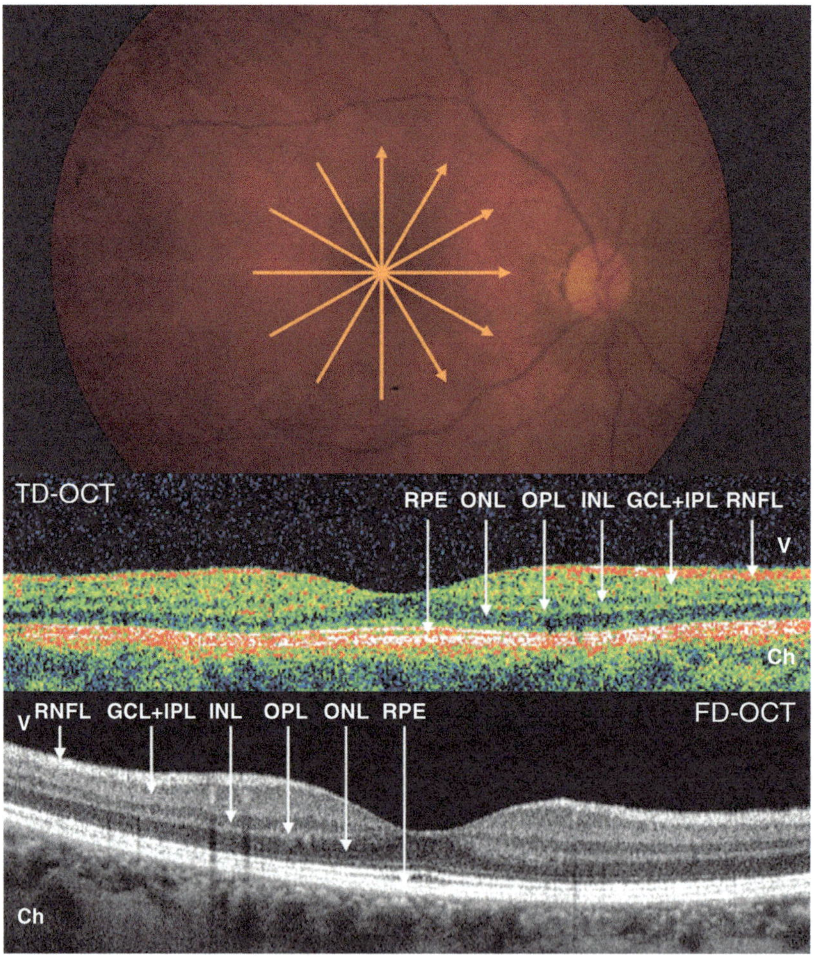

Fig. 20.1 Healthy fundus (*top*); the yellow arrows are pointing in the direction of the rendering planes of the time-domain OCT. OCT image of the macula of the same healthy eye acquired with a time-domain device (*middle*, falsecolor image) and a Fourier-domain OCT device (*bottom*, grayscale image). In the middle of the OCT images, the foveola can be recognized, where the photoreceptors are the only neuroretinal cells present, and the cones have the highest density in this area of the retina. *V* vitreous body, *RNFL* retinal nerve fiber layer, *GCL* ganglion cell layer, *IPL* inner plexiform layer, *INL* inner nuclear layer, *OPL* outer plexiform layer, *ONL* outer nuclear layer, which includes the photoreceptor layer, *RPE* retinal pigment epithelium, *Ch* choroidea. On the FD-OCT image, the spaces in the choroidea correspond to the choroidal vessels

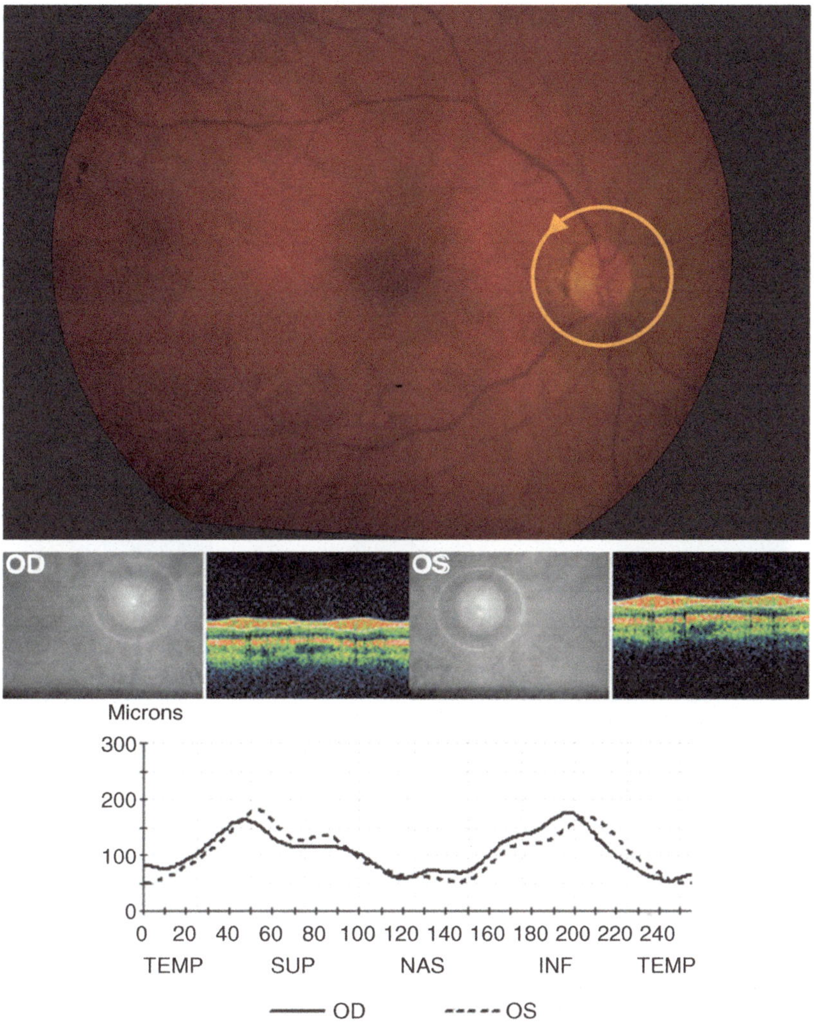

Fig. 20.2 Peripapillary RNFL curve acquired with a TD-OCT device. During the examination, the retina is scanned around the optic disc along a circle of 3.4 mm in diameter (*yellow arrow*). After tracing the vitreo-retinal boundary and the outer boundary of the innermost (closest to the vitreous body) hyperreflective layer, the distance between these two gives the thickness of the RNFL. Bottom: the RNFL thickness curve for the two eyes, the parallel course of the two curves is well visible

surable, and the thickness curves of the two eyes typically run parallel to each other.

The above two scanning modes, i.e., the examination of the macula and the optic disc, are used most often in the clinical practice. It is important during both examinations to try and reach the highest signal strength (SS) possible. In practice, it means that only images acquired with a signal strength of at least 6 on the scale of 10 of third-generation OCT devices are worthy of evaluation, because in case of lower signal strengths, the algorithm that measures the thickness of the retina and the nerve fibers may determine the boundary of the retina incorrectly when examining the nerve fiber layer or the macula, and thus false low or high values may be measured. If the refractive media are cloudy, we may not be able to perform a scan with good signal strength, and in this case, we should be cautious when analyzing thickness data. Figure 20.3 illustrates the measurement errors due to weak signal during the measurement of the macula and the peripapillary RNFL.

As already mentioned, measurement of the retinal nerve fiber layer thickness may become important in the case of neurological conditions, but it is also indispensable in the monitoring of damages due to glaucoma. The most general measure to describe the peripapillary RNFL is the average RNFL thickness, which is suitable for general orientation, characterizing the total mass of nerve fibers, but it does not show local

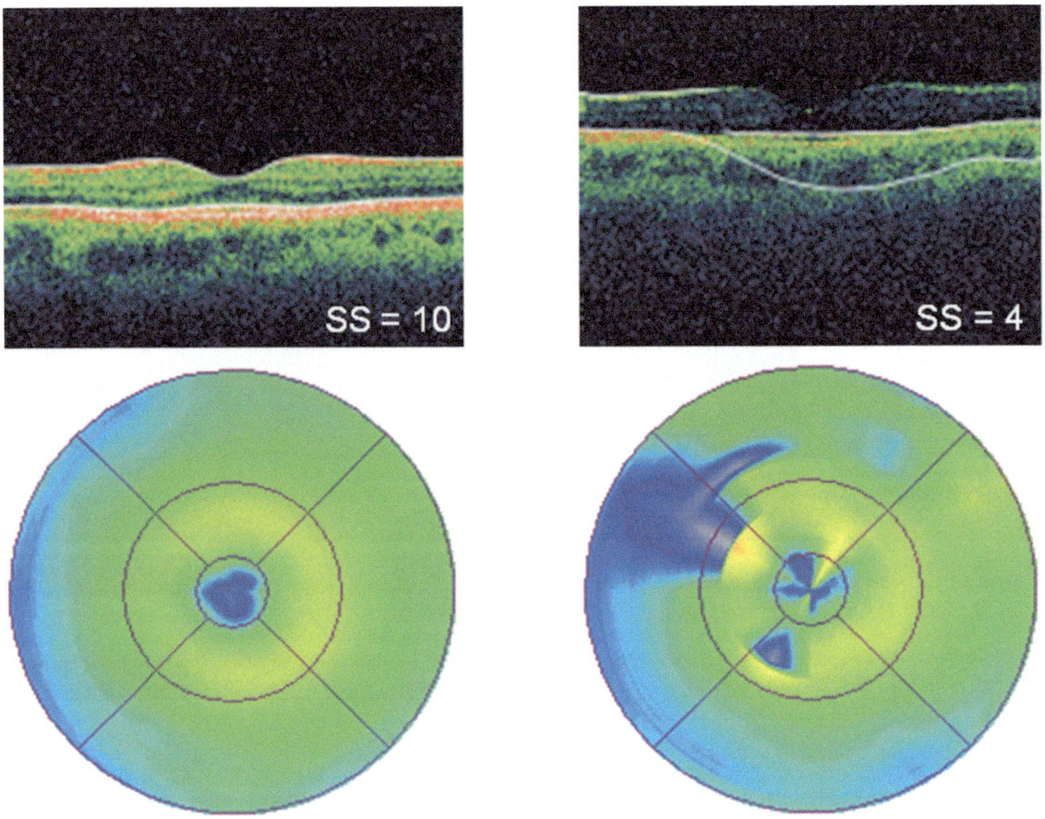

Fovea vastagság	149 ± 4 μm
Teljes macula térfogat	6,56 mm^3

Fovea vastagság	187 ± 50 μm
Teljes macula térfogat	6,38 mm^3

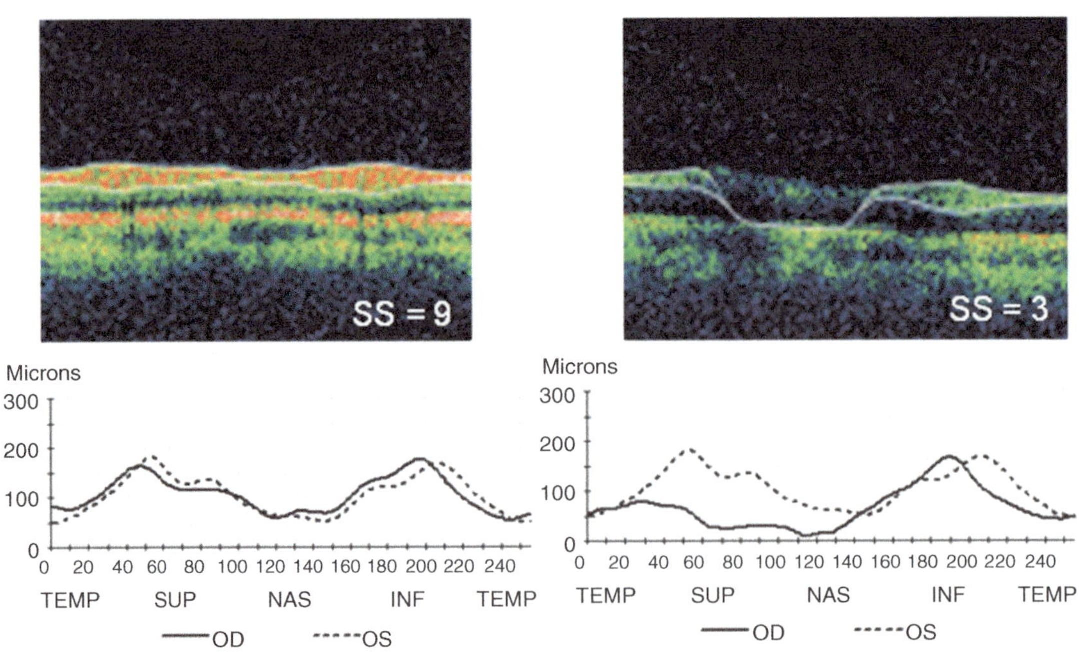

changes. For a more accurate analysis and to determine the location of the lesion, it is indispensable to assess the RNFL thickness in each quadrant or in even smaller areas, in the sectors within the quadrants. It is known that damages due to glaucoma manifest as a characteristic vertical increase in the depression of the optic disc, which is caused by nerve fiber loss in the inferior and superior quadrants; in neurodegenerative diseases, however, the decrease in nerve fiber thickness is higher in the temporal quadrant, which corresponds to the papillomacular bundle. A deviation from the normal nerve fiber layer thickness can be detected with the help of the normal value database supplied with most OCT devices, which serves as a reference to which the measured data of the subject are compared, identifying the areas where the RNFL thickness is abnormal (see Fig. 20.4). When analyzing the numerical values, however, it must be taken into account that nerve fiber layer thickness may show high individual variations, and that it decreases with age even in healthy eyes. If our OCT device does not contain a normal value database, the starting point may be that in the age group between 20 and 60 years, the normal value of the mean peripapillary RNFL thickness is 105 ± 10 μm when measured with a third-generation OCT device. We should be cautious, however, when comparing thickness data mea-

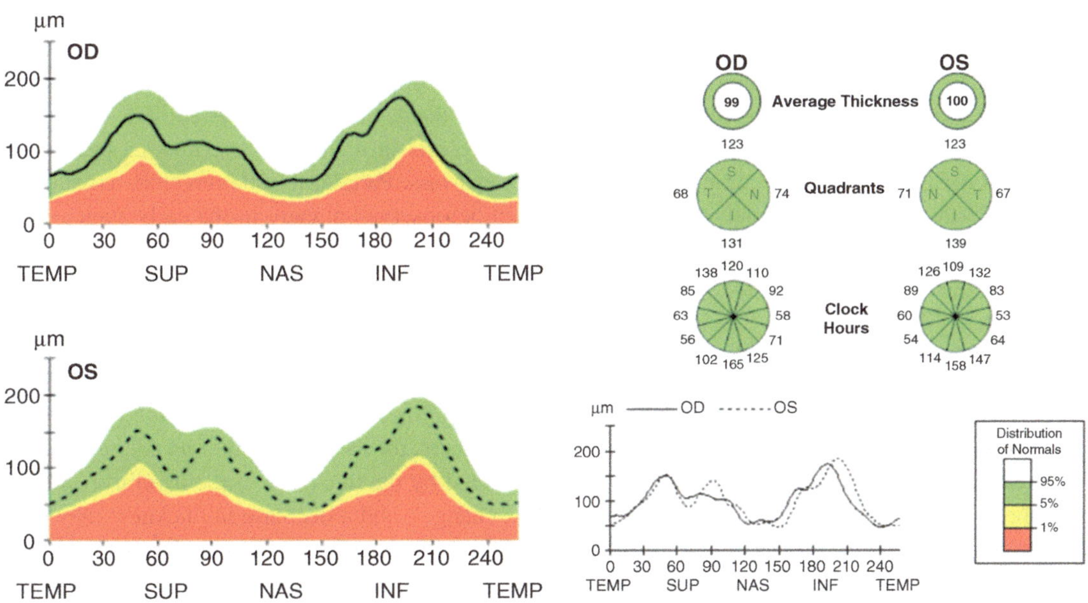

Fig. 20.4 Peripapillary nerve fiber layer thickness curves of healthy eyes; thickness values measured in each point are shown in relation to the normal value database of the device. The scanning and analysis were performed with a fourth-generation OCT device. In the *bottom right* part of the figure, it can be observed that the nerve fiber thickness curves of the two eyes are almost parallel to each other. The *top right* part shows the mean nerve fiber layer thickness, as well as the thickness values measured in each quadrant and sector

Fig. 20.3 Examples of boundary tracing errors due to low signal strength during examinations performed on the same subject. The *top* images show the TD-OCT picture of the same macula, with appropriate settings and high signal strength on the left and with inappropriate settings and, consequently, weak signal on the right. It is well visible on the false-color macular maps that in case of low signal strength, incorrect tracing of the retinal boundary may lead to incorrect macular thickness and volume values. The *bottom* images show the peripapillary scan of the same eye in case of high and low signal strength. When the signal is strong, the thickness curves of the peripapillary nerve fibers in the two eyes are parallel to each other in case of a healthy subject. If the signal is weak, a considerably smaller nerve fiber layer thickness may be measured due to the boundary tracing errors, which may implicitly lead to incorrect conclusions sured with different OCT devices because newer, fourth-generation OCT devices measure different peripapillary nerve fiber layer thickness values than third-generation OCT devices, and there are differences in the measurements even between the different fourth-generation OCT devices.

OCT devices also enable the measurement of macular volume and thickness. About 34–38 % of macular thickness is given by the ganglion cell complex (GCC), which includes the nerve fiber layer, the ganglion cell layer and the inner plexiform layer, and which therefore includes the body and the proximal and distal parts of the ganglion cells and, thus, its measurement can be used to assess the integrity of the ganglion cells. In a retrograde way, the loss of optic nerve fibers due to different diseases leads to the loss of ganglion cells, and therefore GCC thickness and, consequentially, the thickness and volume of the entire retina, decreases. Although certain fourth-generation OCT devices now enable the measurement of GCC thickness and comparison of the measured values with the normal value database (Fig. 20.5), measurement of the macular volume is also suitable for monitoring the changes in thickness. The normal value of macular volume in the age group of 20–60 years is approximately 7.0 ± 0.4 mm^3 when measured with a third-generation OCT device. Since Fourier-domain OCT devices trace the outer boundary of the retina in a different way than third-generation OCT devices, and there is a difference in the established location of the retinal boundary even between the different fourth-generation devices, this normal value does not apply to newer devices, and caution must be exercised when comparing thickness values measured with different devices.

Based on the above, the OCT device may be an excellent tool for the detection of neurodegeneration at the levels of both nerve fibers and ganglion cells. If the natural course of neurodegeneration can be described for diseases such as Alzheimer's disease, Parkinson's disease and multiple sclerosis, OCT may help not only to make a more accurate diagnosis but also to measure the change in the degree of axonal damage in response to the applied therapy, or other, more expensive procedures (e.g., MRI) for the quantitative detection of neurodegeneration may be replaced.

The Role of OCT in the Examination of Multiple Sclerosis

Multiple sclerosis (MS) is an inflammatory disease of the central nervous system, in which the immune system attacks the myelin sheath that covers the neuronal axons, simultaneously at various sites of the central nervous system. The inflammation results in damage to the myelin sheath and axonal loss. Parallel to inflammation, axonal loss can be observed already in the early stage of the disease, and since this leads to irreversible changes, it is of high importance to detect and treat the disease as early as possible. Measurement of the retinal nerve fiber layer thickness is a unique possibility to detect axonal damage in vivo. Since the retinal nerve fiber layer consists of unmyelinated fibers, the measurement of its thickness is not affected by the thickness of the myelin sheath (or its change), and a decrease in thickness may only result from a decrease in the number of nerve fibers. The measurement of the nerve fiber layer thickness with OCT in patients with multiple sclerosis has gradually moved to the focus of interest in the past decade since the objective measurement of axonal damage may have an important role not only in the examination of patients but as already

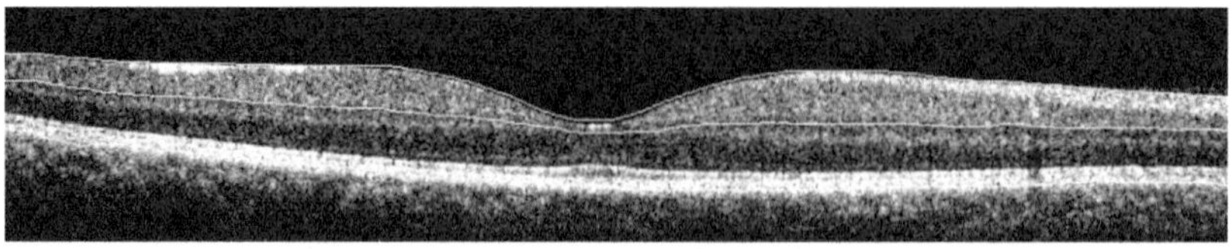

Fig. 20.5 Measurement of the ganglion cell complex (GCC) thickness on the OCT image of a healthy eye acquired with an FD-OCT device. The GCC includes the RNFL, the GCL and the IPL (see Fig. 20.1)

mentioned several times also in the monitoring of drug effects. Another suitable, objective method for the monitoring of the degree of axonal loss is the measurement of the decrease in cerebral volume with MRI, the results of which correlate well with the measurement of nerve fiber layer thickness with OCT, but the OCT scan is way faster, more accessible, simpler and cheaper than MRI and, therefore, it seems to be more suitable for the monitoring of axonal damage. Naturally, OCT does not replace MRI, which is indispensable for making the diagnosis of the disease, but it may be a useful tool for ophthalmologists and neurologists in the assessment and monitoring of the degree of axonal damage.

The first symptom in about 20 % of MS patients is optic neuritis (ON), which is characterized by monocular deterioration in vision developed in a few days, and which is accompanied by pain on eye movements. In one-third of the cases, optic neuritis is accompanied by the inflammation of the optic nerve head, which is called optic papillitis. In case of acute papillitis, an increased peripapillary nerve fiber layer thickness can be measured, the degree of which correlates with the prolongation of VEP latency. Surprisingly, the degree of the increase in RNFL thickness does not depend on the location of the lesion, i.e., it is more characteristic not in the case of inflammations closer to the optic disc, but is affected by the size of the lesion. Supposedly, larger lesions play a role in the development of papilledema by inhibiting venous drainage and axonal transport. In the remaining two-thirds of the optic neuritis cases, fundoscopy shows no abnormalities, and we are speaking of retrobulbar neuritis in these cases. Once optic neuritis is over, the thickness of the nerve fiber layer exponentially decreases, regardless of the initial thickening of the nerve fiber layer. A decrease in RNFL thickness can be detected already after 3 months in about 10 % of the patients, it appears between months 3 and 6 in 85 % of them, and rarely occurs after 6 months. The loss of nerve fibers retrogradely affects the ganglion cells as well, which results in decreased macular volume after optic neuritis (Fig. 20.6).

Steroid therapy results in the complete restoration of visual acuity in most of the patients, but other components, such as color vision and contrast sensitivity, often remain impaired, probably because of axonal loss. It is supported by the observation that the thickness of the nerve fiber layer measured with OCT correlates with visual acuity, contrast sensitivity, color vision and the degree of visual field defect. A relationship between morphological and functional defects is further indicated by the fact that the thickness of the nerve fiber layer correlates with the amplitude and latency of the electrical response obtained during an mfVEP examination in eyes previously affected by optic neuritis.

Axonal damage, however, occurs not only in the eye previously affected by optic neuritis; the eye of MS patients that has not been affected by optic neuritis also shows a decrease in mean peripapillary nerve fiber layer thickness and macular volume, the degree of which however does not reach the thinning observed in the eyes previously affected by ON. The exact cause of the decrease in nerve fiber layer thickness observed in the contralateral eyes is not yet known but it supposedly involves subclinical inflammations and slow, continuous axonal loss. It is logical that in case of a continuous thinning of the nerve fiber layer, there should be a linear negative relationship between peripapillary RNFL thickness and the duration of the disease, but this is not unequivocal as it has been confirmed by certain studies but refuted by others. The atrophy of the nerve fiber layer in the eye not affected by optic neuritis is the result of the axonal loss accompanying the disease, and therefore its degree may be indicative of the axonal loss occurring in the entire brain. The above are supported by the observation that the thickness of the nerve fiber layer measured in the unaffected eye correlates with the physical impairment of the patient measured on the Expanded Disability Status Scale (EDSS), which is also caused by the axonal damage. The purpose of the interferon therapy is to prevent the development of inflammatory foci, and decrease the degree of axonal loss and, thus the residual symptoms. As of the writing of this chapter, the authors know of only one study, where the mean and temporal RNFL thickness showed a lower decrease in patients treated with immune-

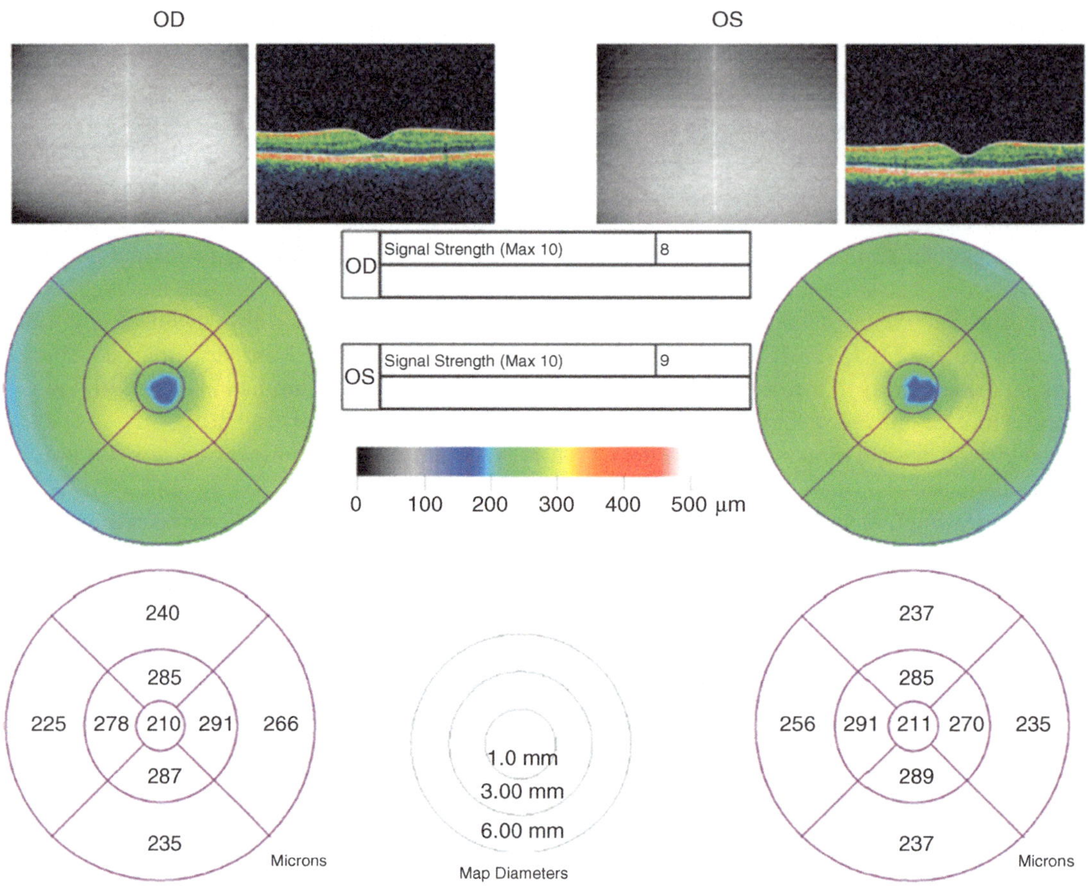

OD	Foveal Thickness	154+/-1 microns
	Total Macular Volume	7.1 mm^3
	Scans used	1, 2, 3, 4, 5, 6

OS	Foveal Thickness	162+/-7 microns
	Total Macular Volume	7.08 mm^3
	Scans used	1, 2, 3, 4, 5, 6

Fig. 20.6 Comparative analysis of the examination of the two maculae of a healthy subject performed with a TD-OCT device. It is visible both on the falsecolor image and in the thickness values that there is high-degree symmetry between the two eyes. On the thickness map, the central part that corresponds to the foveolar depression is the thinnest (*blue*), whereas the clivus around it is the thickest part of the macula (*yellow*), and from here towards the periphery, the retina gets gradually thinner and, correspondingly, the color-coded thickness map turns into blue in the peripheral parts

modulator therapy than in untreated patients; however, it also supports the potential role of OCT in the monitoring of the treatment.

It is known that, based on its course, multiple sclerosis can be classified into four subtypes, and distinguishing between these is important because of the difference in prognosis and for choosing the appropriate treatment. The majority of patients belong to the relapsing-remitting form at the beginning of the disease. In this group, sudden deteriorations (shubs) and longer or shorter symptom-free periods are alternating. The most common symptoms include sensory deficits, optic neuritis, weakness, coordination problems and autonomic symptoms. Initially, a shub is usually followed by complete resolution but with the progression of the disease and the increase in the number of shubs, residual symptoms also appear. In a few years or one or two decades, the relapsing–remitting form may transform into the secondary progressive form, where the status of the patient is determined by the residual symptoms, and a slow progression can be observed. The prognosis of this form is worse, and the patient has increasing physical disability. In the primary progressive form, nervous system functions gradually worsen, and there is no improvement in the condition. Optic neuritis is not a characteristic symptom in this form. A few percent of the patients have the relapsing-progressive disease form. The nerve fiber loss characteristic to each subtype may be assessed in the eye unaffected by optic neuritis because there is no fiber loss due to inflammation in addition to the fiber loss caused by axonal damage. In the relapsing–remitting form, the loss is less marked than in the progressive forms. Although the optic nerve is unaffected in the primary progressive disease form, there is still nerve fiber loss, which confirms that axonal damage may occur even without an active lesion in this disease. In the progressive forms, more residual symptoms are accompanied by a higher degree of axonal loss (Figs. 20.7 and 20.8).

Neuromyelitis Optica (Devic's Syndrome)

Neuromyelitis optica (NMO) was previously considered a subtype of multiple sclerosis but there are several evidences now that it is a separate disease. Distinguishing it from multiple sclerosis is not always easy but it is important because of the worse prognosis and the difference in therapeutic protocols. In Devic's syndrome, primarily the optic nerve and the spinal cord are affected, and the involvement of the spinal cord is not restricted to the maximum two segments seen in MS but extends to at least three segments. Initially, the

a

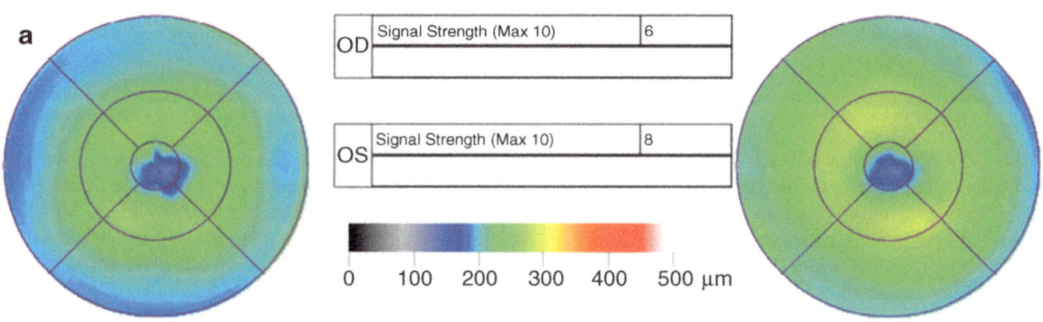

OD	Foveal Thickness	148+/-9 microns
	Total Macular Volume	6.07 mm^3
	Scans used	1, 2, 3, 4, 5, 6

OS	Foveal Thickness	142+/-2 microns
	Total Macular Volume	6.62 mm^3
	Scans used	1, 2, 3, 4, 5, 6

b

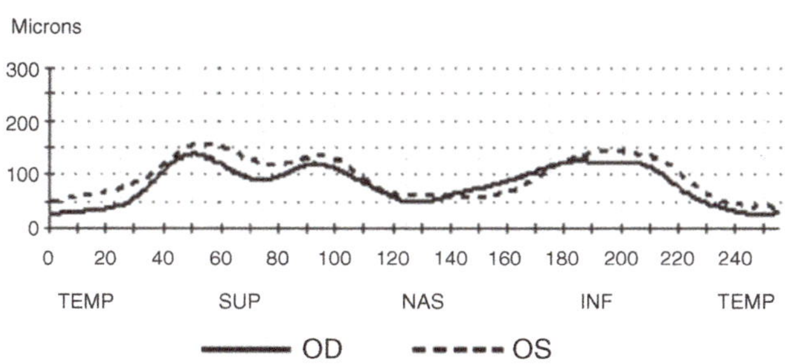

	OD	OS
RNFLavg	82,75	96,41

Fig. 20.7 The figure summarizes the OCT examination results of the macula and optic disc of a patient with relapsing-remitting multiple sclerosis. The patient previously had optic neuritis in the right eye. (**a**) It is well visible on the false-color maps and also in the thickness results that, correspondingly, the right macular volume is smaller compared with the left one, which is on the lower limit of the normal range. (**b**) Mean peripapillary nerve fiber layer thickness is also decreased in the eye previously affected by ON but it is on the lower limit of normal in the other eye too

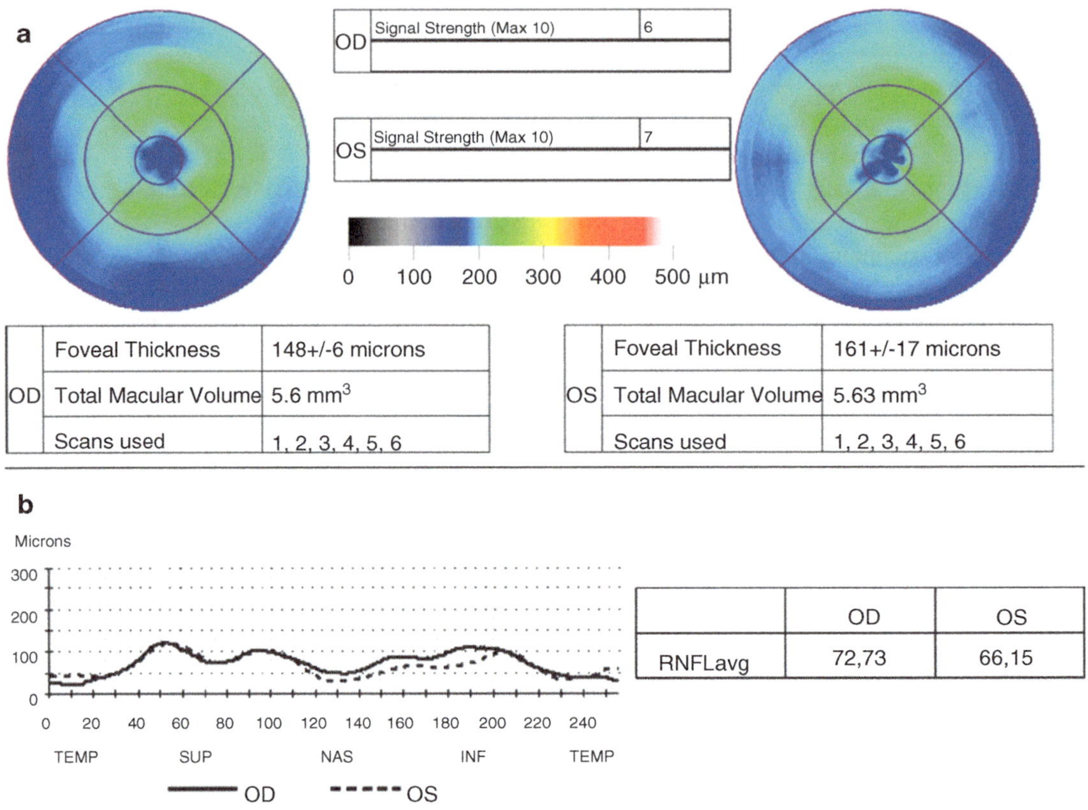

Fig. 20.8 The figure summarizes the OCT examination results of the macula and optic disc of a patient with secondary progressive multiple sclerosis. Previously, both eyes were affected by retrobulbar neuritis and, correspondingly, both macular volume (**a**) and mean peripapillary nerve fiber layer thickness (**b**) are considerably decreased in both eyes. It can be observed on the macular thickness map of the left eye that the scans are decentered, and the foveola is not in the center of the image, which is caused by improper fixation due to the poor visual acuity of the patient, explained by the loss of nerve fibers

head MRI findings are usually normal, or lesions not typical to MS are visible, and there is no oligoclonal gammopathy in the cerebrospinal fluid but pleocytosis can be observed. According to the currently accepted theory, the condition is a humoral autoimmune disease that affects the central nervous system and occurs in relapses. With the detection of the specific anti-aquaporin-4 (AQP4) antibody in the serum, which binds to the aquaporin receptors, a group of conditions collectively known as NMO spectrum disorders can be identified, which affect the optic nerve or the myelin in an isolated way, and are accompanied by demyelination. The relapse after the first symptom occurs within 1 year in 60 % and within 3 years in 90 % of the cases, but rarely decades may pass between the two episodes. The symptoms (both the decrease in visual acuity and the paresis) are more severe than usual in MS, and often residual symptoms may occur despite treatment. In addition to the imaging techniques and the detection of the serum antibody, OCT may provide further help in the future to make the diagnosis because, based on the first results, it may be suitable for the early differential diagnostics of optic neuritis.

The significant RNFL thinning and macular volume reduction measured during the OCT scan may help distinguish between NMO and MS. The nerve fiber layer thickness measured with OCT may be an objective indicator of disease severity, which currently can only be assessed by monitoring the clinical condition of the patient, and may also be a tool for the measurement of the efficacy of the immunosuppressant therapy.

In Devic's syndrome, as already mentioned, the inflammation is usually not followed by such a degree of complete resolution as it may happen in MS patients, which indicates a higher degree of axonal loss. Study results also support that RNFL thickness and macular volume are smaller in the eyes previously affected by ON of patients with Devic's syndrome than in the eyes previously affected by ON of MS patients. In the case of RNFL, a diffuse decrease in thickness can be observed, whereas in multiple sclerosis, mainly the temporal quadrant is affected. One might think that a history of several ON episodes in one eye may also be the reason for the higher-degree axonal loss observed in the eye affected by optic neuritis of NMO patients. It was calculated, however, that a single episode of ON leads to twice the decrease in RNFL thickness in NMO patients than in those with MS, the decrease being approximately 20 μm in the latter case. These data confirm that the optic neuritis that occurs in NMO is a much more severe condition, which is more likely to cause deterioration in vision than the one observed in MS patients. It is important to note that in patients who show myelitis alone, without neuritis, the RNFL thickness logically does not differ significantly from that measured in healthy subjects (Figs. 20.9 and 20.10).

The Role of OCT in Alzheimer's Disease

Alzheimer's disease is a chronic neurodegenerative condition of unknown origin, which is accompanied by impaired cognitive functions, changes in behavior and dementia. Its risk increases with age, whereas 1–5 % of the population aged 65 years are

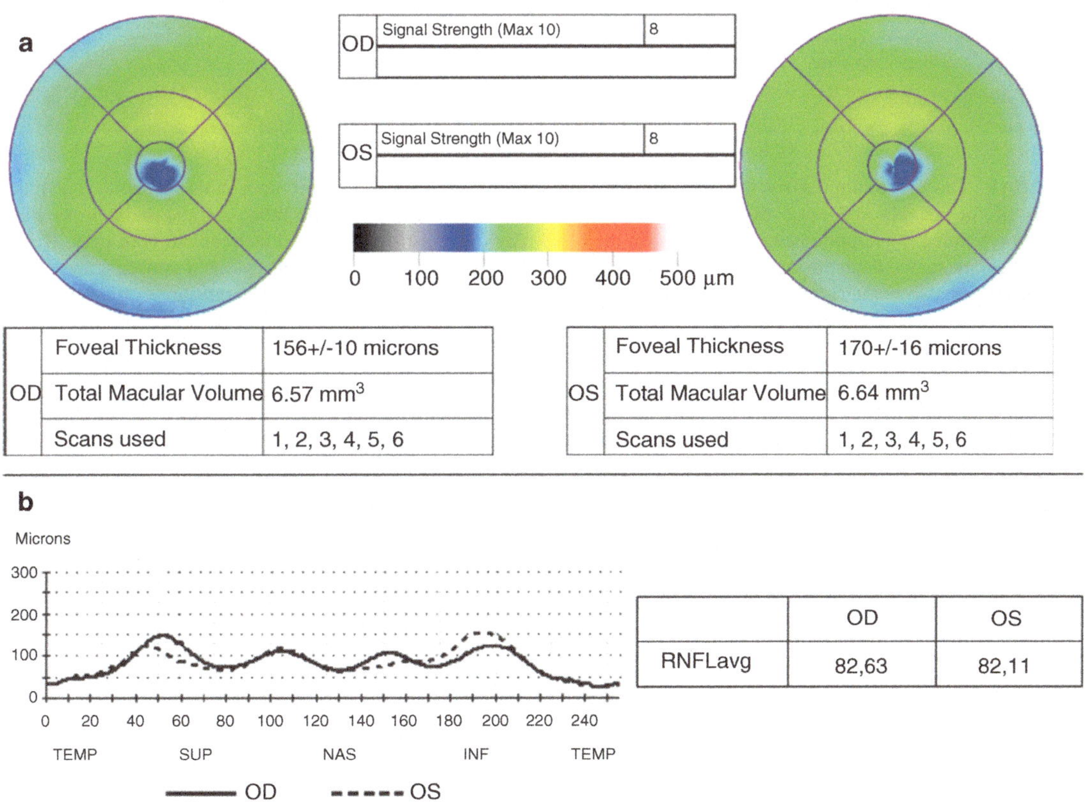

Fig. 20.9 The figure summarizes the OCT examination results of the macula and optic disc of a patient with primary progressive multiple sclerosis; there has been no previous optic neuritis in either eye. (**a**) The maculae are symmetric, and their thickness is on the lower limit of normal. (**b**) The peripapillary nerve fiber thickness curves run almost parallel to each other, and the mean nerve fiber layer thickness is decreased mildly and to approximately the same degree in both eyes. The above confirms that optic neuritis is rare in the primary progressive form, and there is continuous nerve fiber loss, the signs of which can be seen in both eyes

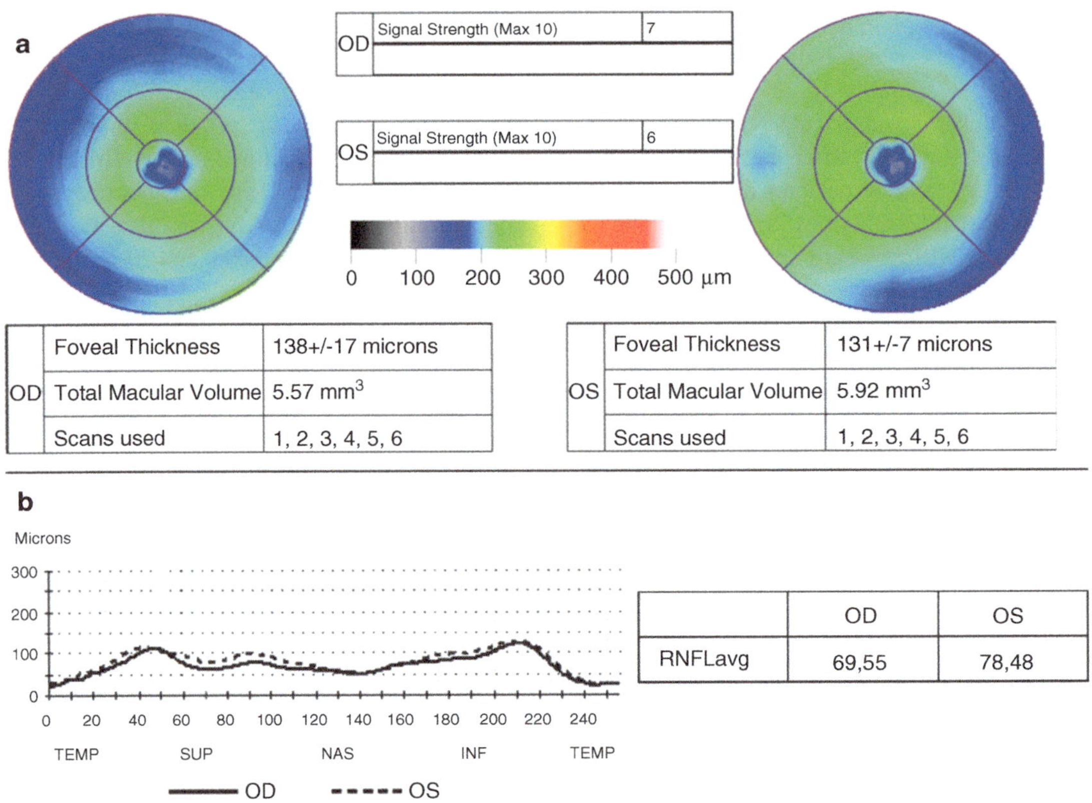

Fig. 20.10 The figure summarizes the OCT examination results of the macula and optic disc of a patient with Devic's syndrome. First, optic neuritis occurred in the left eye of the patient, and then, during the steroid therapy, ON was developed also in the right eye, which was accompanied by a considerable decrease in visual acuity. The macular volume (**a**) and the mean peripapillary nerve fiber thickness (**b**) shows a mild decrease in both eyes, with a higher decrease in the right eye as a consequence of the more severe prior optic nerve condition

affected, this ratio reaches 20 % above the age of 80 years, and therefore, it poses an ever-increasing epidemiological problem in the aging population of Western societies. The pathohistology of the disease is characterized by accumulation of amyloid beta and tau protein in the cerebral neurons, which leads to the death of these cells and, consequentially, a cerebral atrophy localized mainly to the frontal–temporal region. Patients with Alzheimer's disease often develop color vision defects and a decrease in contrast sensitivity. The reason for this may be the atrophy of the visual cortex or the involvement of the retina. Histological studies found the degeneration of retinal ganglion cells but there was no abnormal protein in the cells and, therefore, the death of the cells may be caused by another mechanism not yet known. The decrease in the number of ganglion cells was found to be the most pronounced in the temporal part of the macula. As a result of the loss of ganglion cells, the retinal nerve fiber layer that consists of their projections gets thinner and, correspondingly, several studies on OCT have confirmed that the mean thickness of the peripapillary nerve fiber layer is decreased in patients with Alzheimer's disease or mild cognitive dysfunction, when compared with healthy subjects. Pattern ERG examines the electrical function of the retinal ganglion cells, whereas pattern VEP assesses the electrical function of the optic nerve and the visual pathway, and both examinations show a prolonged latency and a decrease in the amplitude of the evoked potential in patients with Alzheimer's disease, which is related to the decrease in the peripapillary nerve fiber layer thickness. The loss of ganglion cells leads to a decrease in macular volume, the degree of which is proportional to the cognitive performance as measured with the Mini-Mental State Examination. Taking into account that OCT is a quick and non-invasive method, it has a possible role not only in the diagnosis and monitoring of the disease but even in understanding it better.

The Role of OCT in Parkinson's Disease

Similarly to Alzheimer's disease, Parkinson's disease is a slowly progressing, chronic neurodegenerative condition of unknown origin. It is also developed in older patients, with the first symptoms occurring at the age of 50 to 60 years, and the symptoms are caused by a decrease in dopamine production due to the degeneration of the substantia nigra. Dopamine is not only an important neurotransmitter of the brain but also an essential substance in the retinal stimulus transduction processes, and it is produced by the amacrine cells. On post-mortem examination of the eyes of patients with Parkinson's disease, a decreased level of dopamine was found in the retina. Similarly to the neurodegenerative diseases mentioned above, color vision and contrast sensitivity defects were also observed in patients with Parkinson's disease. When measuring the thickness of the inner (closer to the vitreous body) and the outer (farther from the vitreous body) part of the retina with OCT, thinning of the inner retina (consisting of the nerve fiber layer, the ganglion cell layer and the inner plexiform layer) was described, whereas there was no difference in the thickness of the outer retina compared to that of healthy subjects. The amacrine cells that contain the dopamine are located here, in the ganglion cell layer and the inner plexiform layer, and form synapses with the neurites of the ganglion cells. As a result of the loss of amacrine cells, the ganglion cells degenerate, which manifests in a decreased macular volume and a reduction in the peripapillary nerve fiber layer thickness. As of the writing of this chapter, no publications are available from longitudinal studies describing the time course of retinal degenerative changes, although knowing the time course of the changes would be indispensable for OCT to be a useful tool in the follow-up of patients and the assessment of drug effects. It is important to note that the OCT examination of patients with advanced Parkinson's disease is even more difficult due to their tremor, because the results are heavily affected by movement artifacts, which may be avoided, in a fortunate case, by the high scanning speed of fourth-generation devices.

Summary

We have reviewed the available diagnostic and monitoring possibilities of optical coherence tomography in neurodegenerative diseases. It is evident that OCT may be a useful help in the assessment of patients and, in certain cases, it may even be used as a 'surrogate marker.' It is expected that there will be considerable progress in this field in the future and that the OCT technology will become an important tool of cooperation with neurologists, which may be very useful not only in diagnostics but also in the assessment of progression. The study of neurodegeneration may lead to a deeper understanding of the morphological changes of the optic disc, which may provide ophthalmologists with a more accurate differential diagnostic method of the progressive optic neuropathy (i.e., glaucoma) accompanying the deterioration in visual function. The message of this chapter to be emphasized is that not only the classic measurement of peripapillary nerve fiber thickness but also the assessment of macular thickness and volume, and their symmetry, as well as the targeted assessment of the individual cell layers of the macula may serve as an important basis for the clarification of neurodegenerative conditions.

Further Readings

Altintas O, Iseri P, Ozkan B, Caglar Y. Correlation between retinal morphological and functional findings and clinical severity in Parkinson's disease. Doc Ophthalmol. 2008;116:137–46.

Balcer LJ, Baier ML, Cohen JA, et al. Contrast letter acuity as a visual component for the Multiple Sclerosis Functional Composite. Neurology. 2003;61:1367–73.

Berisha F, Feke GT, Trempe CL, McMeel JW, Schepens CL. Retinal abnormalities in early Alzheimer's disease. Invest Ophthalmol Vis Sci. 2007;48:2285–9.

Blanks JC, Hinton DR, Sadun AA, Miller CA. Retinal ganglion cell degeneration in Alzheimer's disease. Brain Res. 1989;501:364–72.

Blanks JC, Torigoe Y, Hinton DR, Blanks RH. Retinal pathology in Alzheimer's disease. I. Ganglion cell loss in foveal/parafoveal retina. Neurobiol Aging. 1996;17:377–84.

Bock M, Brandt AU, Dorr J, et al. Patterns of retinal nerve fiber layer loss in multiple sclerosis patients with or without optic neuritis and glaucoma patients. Clin Neurol Neurosurg. 2010;112(8):647–52.

Burkholder BM, Osborne B, Loguidice MJ, et al. Macular volume determined by optical coherence tomography as a measure of neuronal loss in multiple sclerosis. Arch Neurol. 2009;66:1366–72.

Costello F, Coupland S, Hodge W, et al. Quantifying axonal loss after optic neuritis with optical coherence tomography. Ann Neurol. 2006;59:963–9.

Costello F, Hodge W, Pan YI, Freedman M, DeMeulemeester C. Differences in retinal nerve fiber layer atrophy between multiple sclerosis subtypes. J Neurol Sci. 2009;281:74–9.

de Seze J, Blanc F, Jeanjean L, et al. Optical coherence tomography in neuromyelitis optica. Arch Neurol. 2008;65:920–3.

Fisher JB, Jacobs DA, Markowitz CE, et al. Relation of visual function to retinal nerve fiber layer thickness in multiple sclerosis. Ophthalmology. 2006;113:324–32.

Green AJ, Cree BA. Distinctive retinal nerve fibre layer and vascular changes in neuromyelitis optica following optic neuritis. J Neurol Neurosurg Psychiatry. 2009;80:1002–5.

Hajee ME, March WF, Lazzaro DR, et al. Inner retinal layer thinning in Parkinson disease. Arch Ophthalmol. 2009;127:737–41.

Harnois C, Di Paolo T. Decreased dopamine in the retinas of patients with Parkinson's disease. Invest Ophthalmol Vis Sci. 1990;31:2473–5.

Henderson AP, Trip SA, Schlottmann PG, et al. An investigation of the retinal nerve fibre layer in progressive multiple sclerosis using optical coherence tomography. Brain. 2008;131:277–87.

Henderson AP, Altmann DR, Trip AS, et al. A serial study of retinal changes following optic neuritis with sample size estimates for acute neuroprotection trials. Brain. 2010;133(9):2592–602.

Huang D, Swanson EA, Lin CP, et al. Optical coherence tomography. Science. 1991;254:1178–81.

Inzelberg R, Ramirez JA, Nisipeanu P, Ophir A. Retinal nerve fiber layer thinning in Parkinson disease. Vision Res. 2004;44:2793–7.

Kallenbach K, Simonsen H, Sander B, et al. Retinal nerve fiber layer thickness is associated with lesion length in acute optic neuritis. Neurology. 2010;74:252–8.

Katz B, Rimmer S. Ophthalmologic manifestations of Alzheimer's disease. Surv Ophthalmol. 1989;34:31–43.

Klistorner A, Arvind H, Nguyen T, et al. Axonal loss and myelin in early ON loss in postacute optic neuritis. Ann Neurol. 2008;64:325–31.

Krasodomska K, Lubinski W, Potemkowski A, Honczarenko K. Pattern electroretinogram (PERG) and pattern visual evoked potential (PVEP) in the early stages of Alzheimer's disease. Doc Ophthalmol. 2010;121(2):111–21.

Lu Y, Li Z, Zhang X, et al. Retinal nerve fiber layer structure abnormalities in early Alzheimer's disease: evidence in optical coherence tomography. Neurosci Lett. 2010;480:69–72.

Merle H, Olindo S, Donnio A, Richer R, Smadja D, Cabre P. Retinal peripapillary nerve fiber layer thickness in neuromyelitis optica. Invest Ophthalmol Vis Sci. 2008;49:4412–7.

Moschos MM, Tagaris G, Markopoulos I, et al. Morphologic changes and functional retinal impairment in patients with Parkinson disease without visual loss. Eur J Ophthalmol. 2011;21(1):24–9.

Naismith RT, Tutlam NT, Xu J, et al. Optical coherence tomography differs in neuromyelitis optica compared with multiple sclerosis. Neurology. 2009;72:1077–82.

Paquet C, Boissonnot M, Roger F, Dighiero P, Gil R, Hugon J. Abnormal retinal thickness in patients with mild cognitive impairment and Alzheimer's disease. Neurosci Lett. 2007;420:97–9.

Parisi V, Restuccia R, Fattapposta F, Mina C, Bucci MG, Pierelli F. Morphological and functional retinal impairment in Alzheimer's disease patients. Clin Neurophysiol. 2001;112:1860–7.

Pulicken M, Gordon-Lipkin E, Balcer LJ, Frohman E, Cutter G, Calabresi PA. Optical coherence tomography and disease subtype in multiple sclerosis. Neurology. 2007;69:2085–92.

Ratchford JN, Quigg ME, Conger A, et al. Optical coherence tomography helps differentiate neuromyelitis optica and MS optic neuropathies. Neurology. 2009;73:302–8.

Sepulcre J, Murie-Fernandez M, Salinas-Alaman A, Garcia-Layana A, Bejarano B, Villoslada P. Diagnostic accuracy of retinal abnormalities in predicting disease activity in MS. Neurology. 2007;68:1488–94.

Siger M, Dziegielewski K, Jasek L, et al. Optical coherence tomography in multiple sclerosis: thickness of the retinal nerve fiber layer as a potential measure of axonal loss and brain atrophy. J Neurol. 2008;255:1555–60.

Talman LS, Bisker ER, Sackel DJ, et al. Longitudinal study of vision and retinal nerve fiber layer thickness in multiple sclerosis. Ann Neurol. 2010;67:749–60.

Trapp BD, Peterson J, Ransohoff RM, Rudick R, Mork S, Bo L. Axonal transection in the lesions of multiple sclerosis. N Engl J Med. 1998;338:278–85.

Trip SA, Schlottmann PG, Jones SJ, et al. Retinal nerve fiber layer axonal loss and visual dysfunction in optic neuritis. Ann Neurol. 2005;58:383–91.

van Velthoven ME, Faber DJ, Verbraak FD, van Leeuwen TG, de Smet MD. Recent developments in optical coherence tomography for imaging the retina. Prog Retin Eye Res. 2007;26:57–77.

21 Diagnosis, Differential Diagnosis and Treatment of Congenital Ocular Motor Disorders

Anna Soproni and Patrícia Domsa

Contents

Introduction

Eye movement disorders diagnosed in adulthood do not necessarily mean that the specific problem is not of congenital origin. Sometimes it is not easy to prove that the paralysis of the ocular muscles is congenital. A skull MRI is required to confirm the trigger factor, and this intervention is not completely harmless in children as it has to be performed under general anesthesia. As a result, this chapter is going to focus on ocular motor disorders in childhood (including congenital ones), emphasizing certain elements of the differential diagnosis that can help avoid unnecessary and costly interventions.

The chapter is based on Brodsky (2010) (See the Acknowledgement at the end of the chapter). The paralysis of ocular muscles in children differs

A. Soproni, M.D. (✉)
Ophthalmologist, Pediatric Ophthalmologist, Private Medical Office, Budapest, Hungary
e-mail: sopronia@t-online.hu; http://sopronianna.hu

P. Domsa, M.D.
Ophthalmologist, Pediatric Ophthalmologist, Madarâsz Street Pediatric Hospital, Budapest, Hungary

Department of Ophthalmology, Semmelweis University, Budapest, Hungary

Rubrica Health Center, Budapest, Hungary
e-mail: patriciadomsa@gmail.com; http://rubrica.hu

J. Somlai, T. Kovács (eds.), *Neuro-Ophthalmology*, DOI 10.1007/978-3-319-28956-4_21

Table 21.1 Congenital ocular motor disorders

Congenital paralysis of ocular motor nerves
(cranial nerves III, IV, VI)
(for Duane retraction syndrome see section "Abducens nerve palsy")
Congenital infantile esotropia
Congenital cranial dysinnervation disorders: congenital ptosis
Marcus Gunn phenomenon
Congenital fibrosis syndrome
Congenital horizontal gaze palsy with scoliosis
Moebius's syndrome/sequence
Monocular elevation deficiency
Brown's syndrome
Latent nystagmus
Congenital motor nystagmus
Sensory nystagmus
Congenital oculomotor apraxia

from that of adults. Children suffering from *acute paralysis* of ocular muscles are provided medical help for diplopia, abnormal posture of the head, ptosis, strabismus or some systemic disease. Children with *chronic paralysis* of the ocular motor nerves are often referred to the specialist due to *amblyopia*. Their neurological diseases (e.g., brain tumor, congenital hydrocephalus, meningitis) are prone to develop *concomitant* and paralytic *(incomitant, synkinetic)* strabismus. It is also true the other way round: children with cranial nerve palsy have to be examined thoroughly to exclude other neurological diseases. When establishing the differential diagnosis of ocular motor nerve paralysis in children we have to remember that *congenital paralysis* is more frequent in this age group and they are also more susceptible to certain conditions (e.g. benign, recurrent abducens palsy, ophthalmoplegic migraine, bacterial meningitis) (Table 21.1).

Modern imaging techniques have become more readily available in the past 10 years, providing us with more information concerning the diagnostic assessment of ocular motor nerve paralysis. We can detect the occasional *lack or hypoplasia* of ocular motor nerves, follow their intracranial and orbital course, and we can also visualize blood vessels and extraocular *muscles* or their potential *hypoplasia*.

Before the formal assessment, we can get some initial impression by observing the posture of the child's head. With parallel alignment of the eyes, prolonged, marked *turning of the head* suggests acute abducens nerve palsy, while head tilt without visible strabismus raises the suspicion of trochlear nerve palsy. The sudden development of an asymmetrical, tilted neck associated with acquired cranial nerve palsy is rarely missed by parents; however, congenital paralysis accompanied by torticollis may go unnoticed. If cranial nerve palsy is suspected, we have to exclude neuromuscular conditions as well as restrictive disorders that mimic paralysis. This process should always start with thorough history taking.

History Taking

We Try to Get an Answer to the Questions Listed Below

1. *Is there head trauma in the history?*

   Recent head trauma is usually revealed fast, and the cause of the paralysis is less uncertain.

   In some cases, cranial nerve palsy associated with parasellar tumors is an accidental finding following a slight head injury. We also have to consider amniocentesis and perinatal skull injuries (forceps delivery and breech position, cephalhematoma and perinatal skull deformity). Old photos can be helpful as well.
2. *Is there any change during the day?*

   Diplopia or ptosis that is hardly noticeable in the morning but gets worse over the course of the day suggests myasthenia gravis.
3. *Does the patient complain of a headache?*

   Headaches can suggest increased intracranial pressure, meningitis or ophthalmoplegic migraine.
4. *Is the child otherwise neurologically normal (by history)?*
5. *Do the symptoms suggest a long or a short history?*

   Congenital paralysis of ocular motor nerves should always be considered in children presenting with prolonged symptoms and signs without diplopia. Patients often detect eye movement deficits associated with congenital paralysis of cranial nerve III or Duane syndrome. Visible strabismus is rare in the congenital paralysis of cranial nerve IV; old photos can confirm abnormal head posture and facial asymmetry (see Table 21.2).

6. *At what age did you first notice abnormal head posture? Does it disappear when the child lies down?*

   Head tilt associated with the congenital paralysis of nerve IV becomes detectable around the age of 6 months, while congenital torticollis of muscular origin can be observed in the first few months. This type of abnormal head position disappears when the child lies down, whereas the first one accompanying torticollis persists.

   If abnormal head posture disappears in a patient suffering from cyclovertical strabismus, it can indicate the cessation of paralysis, but it can also be the sign of suppression (risk of amblyopia!). Paradoxically, abnormal posture of the head is a good prognostic sign for binocular vision; therefore, we have to tell the parents to consult a specialist immediately if they cannot see it any more.

Examination Methods

The *physical examination* of children with paralytic (incomitant) strabismus includes inspection, sensory tests, examination of eye movements, visual acuity and field of vision, as well as additional tests. The *order* of these tests should be the following:

Table 21.2 Old versus recent paralysis?

	Old or congenital	Recent
Diplopia	Only in paretic gaze position	Prominent complaint
Image tilt	Absent	Diagnostic
Old photos	May show anomalous head posture	Normal head posture
Facial asymmetry	Common with fourth nerve palsy	Absent
Forced ductions	May show contracture	Negative
Amblyopia	May be present	Normal vision in both eyes
Comitance	Spread of comitance	Incomitant
Past-pointing	Absent	Common

von Noorden and Helveston (1994)

Sensory Test

Worth's four-dot test and especially polarization tests are used to assess binocular vision, while stereopsis is best examined with the help of *Lang, Titmus, Random dot* and polarization tests (See Polatest). Note the patient's current head posture as well.

Examination of Eye Movements

Smooth Pursuit Test

Examinations involving one eye only (duction) or both eyes (version). While paying attention to the upright posture of the child's head, we have to move an interesting object slowly in front of his/her eyes (at a distance of 40–50 cm) from side to side or from the nose to the appropriate direction. If we are uncertain whether a certain muscle has become weaker or not, we have to perform the *doll's head maneuvre.* During this maneuver, we try to establish eye contact with the patient, or show them an object straight in front of their eyes, and then we try to assess the function of the eye muscles while moving their head in a passive way. As a result of the *oculo-cephalic reflex,* the eyes will try to maintain the forward gaze while the head position is being changed (see Fig. 21.1).

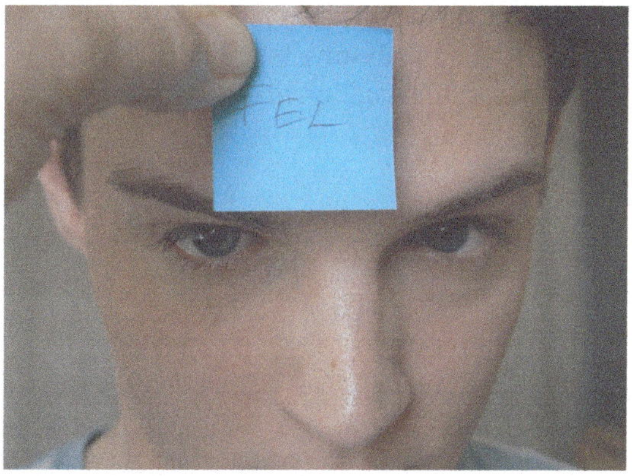

Fig. 21.1 Doll's head maneuver confirmed the bilateral restriction of upgaze: the examiners turned the patient's head down, but the eyeballs could not move upward even when forced to do so (From the photocollection of Anna Soproni)

Deviations

They serve to detect manifest (tropia) and latent (phoria) strabismus. The most significant examination when trying to detect manifest strabismus or differentiate between tropia and phoria is the monocular *cover-uncover test.* The precondition for the test is a relatively good vision and cooperation on the part of the patient. The best tool for covering is the translucent Spielmann occlude (Noorden and von Campos 2001). The *cover test* is used to detect *tropia.* The child sits with his/her head straight and fixates on a near or distant target (testing for near and distance deviation). While one eye is covered, the examiner watches the movements of the other, uncovered eye carefully. If any movement is detected, it suggests tropia. Obviously, if one eye is covered and the other one does not try to seek for a new position, the eye is not strabismic. The test has to be performed on the other eye as well.

The *uncover test* is used to detect *phoria.* We have to watch the eye in that moment when the cover is removed.

If the covered eye moves to one direction on covering (it can be seen with the help of the translucent occluder) and then performs an adjusting movement (fusion) when the occluder is removed, it indicates phoria. This motion is visible only when the alternating cover is fast enough to interrupt binocular vision (fusion). It can be elicited on both sides.

The angle of strabismus can be measured with the help of alternating cover test, prisms, near and distant objects, as well as near fixation in all 9 fields of gaze. The adjusting movement disappears when we reach the prism diopter (PD) appropriate for the angle of strabismus (see Table 21.3).

Differentiation of vertical strabismus and DVD (see below).

Table 21.3 Gaze matrix of left superior oblique muscle paralysis

LHT 35 PD	LHT 5 PD	X 2 PD
LHT 30 PD	LHT 10 PD	LHT 5 PD
LHT 33 PD	LHT 30 PD	LHT 12PD, E 4 PD

The higher position of the left eye can be detected in almost all directions, which suggests paralysis of longer duration. This phenomenon is called the spread of comitance, i.e. the initially paralytic strabismus gradually becomes comitant due to the formation of contractions
Abbreviations: *LHT* left hypertropia, *PD* prism diopter, *X* exophoria, *E* esophoria

We cover and uncover one eye while watching the other, uncovered eye. In vertical strabismus the uncovered eye drifts downward and the other eye drifts upward when uncovered. In DVD the uncovered eye drifts downward and the other eye may do the same when uncovered, but it never drifts upward.

Examination of Visual Acuity

The ophthalmological examination of children of all ages has to include a statement concerning vision. In infants and toddlers the accurate examination of vision is not feasible, but the vision-dependent behavior of the child (response to light, faces, toys, etc.) has to be assessed qualitatively. We can examine reaction to light, the blink reflex when objects are held close to the eyes, and we can also perform the *fixation preference test* with the help of alternating cover. At an early age, quantitative assessment is also possible by examining *optokinetic nystagmus,* and performing the preferential looking test and the visually evoked potential (VEP) test. Later the examination of visual acuity is performed with the help of age-appropriate optotypes. Ideally, we examine distance visual acuity, but if it is not successful, we assess near visual acuity. In *latent nystagmus,* we use a lens to cover the eye instead of an occluder. The refractive value of this lens has to be about 3.0D higher than the estimated one. Thus the vision of the 'covered' eye will be blurred enough so that we can examine the vision of the other eye. So, for example, if the estimated refraction is –2.0D, we have to use a lens of +1.0D.

Examination of the Field of Vision

The confrontational visual field examination is very effective at detecting neuro-ophthalmologically significant defects. The child sits in somebody's lap while another person moves an object in front of his/her face from behind. While the child is gazing strait ahead (keeping his/her attention with something), we monitor his/her reactions to objects that appear at surprising points of the visual field.

Additional tests *occlusion test, examination of torsion, three-step test, forced duction, Hess screen test*

Occlusion Test

Occlusion test helps to reveal the origin of abnormal head posture. During the test, we patch the eyes alternatively and watch for any change in the posture of the head. If the abnormal posture is not due to some ocular muscle disorder, it will stay the same when either eye is covered. (The only exception is when the null zone of a patient suffering from congenital nystagmus differs from his/her primary gaze.) If the head tilt disappears irrespective of which eye is covered, the patient has cyclovertical strabismus with fusion ability (see the section "Three-step test" below). If the disappearance of the head tilt is linked to the cover of one eye only (left or right), this eye has Brown syndrome (see below), or cyclovertical strabismus exists without fusion.

Examination of Torsion

The potential torsion of the eyeball (cyclodeviation, rotation) resulting from the paralysis of the vertical muscles can be measured subjectively by using two Maddox or Bagolini lenses of the same color. We hold the lenses with their axis vertical in front of the eyes. The patient is asked to set the horizontal lines produced by a spotlight parallel to each other. The extent of torsion (in degrees) can be read from the trial frame. If the patient has small vertical deviation, we might have to place vertically a weak prism in front of either eye, so that the lines of light could be differentiated more easily. The detection of objective torsion is of vital importance, especially in children. *Objective torsion* can be examined with a direct or indirect ophthalmoscope (see Fig. 21.2). Normally, the macula is at the level of the lower third of the optic disc.

Three-Step Test

The aim of this test is to find the muscle which is responsible for vertical deviation.

The diagnostic algorithm asks three questions:

1. Which eye is higher (hypertropic) in the primary position?
2. Does deviation increase when the patient gazes to the left or right?
3. Does deviation increase when the patient's head is tilted to the left or right? (Bielschowsky's head tilt test) (see Fig. 21.3).

In the majority of the cases, this test can reveal the paralysis of a cyclovertical eye muscle.

For example, if the patient is looking straight forward, and we can detect hypertropia of the right eye with *monocular cover test* (which means that the non-fixating eye adjusts from above to fixate), either the depressor muscles of the right eye (inferior rectus or superior oblique) or the elevators of the left eye (superior rectus or inferior oblique) are weak.

If the deviation is more significant when gazing to the left than to the right, the paralysed muscles are probably the right superior oblique or left superior rectus, as these muscles are responsible for depressing the right eye and elevating the left eye when gazing to the left.

During the head tilt test, if the deviation increases when the head is tilted to the right and decreases in the other direction, the paralysed muscle is the right superior oblique, as this muscle and the superior rectus turn the right eye inward (incycloduction) when the head is tilted to the right (see Figs. 21.3a, b).

Forced Duction Test

Its primary aim is to differentiate muscular paresis from *restrictive strabismus*. It is an important tool for differential diagnosis in the following cases: (1) prior trauma of the orbit, (2) prior eye surgery, (3) incomitant congenital strabismus with ptosis (congenital fibrosis syndrome), (4) inflammation or muscular hypertrophy in the orbit confirmed with imaging techniques, (5) prolonged paresis. In children it can only be performed in general anesthesia.

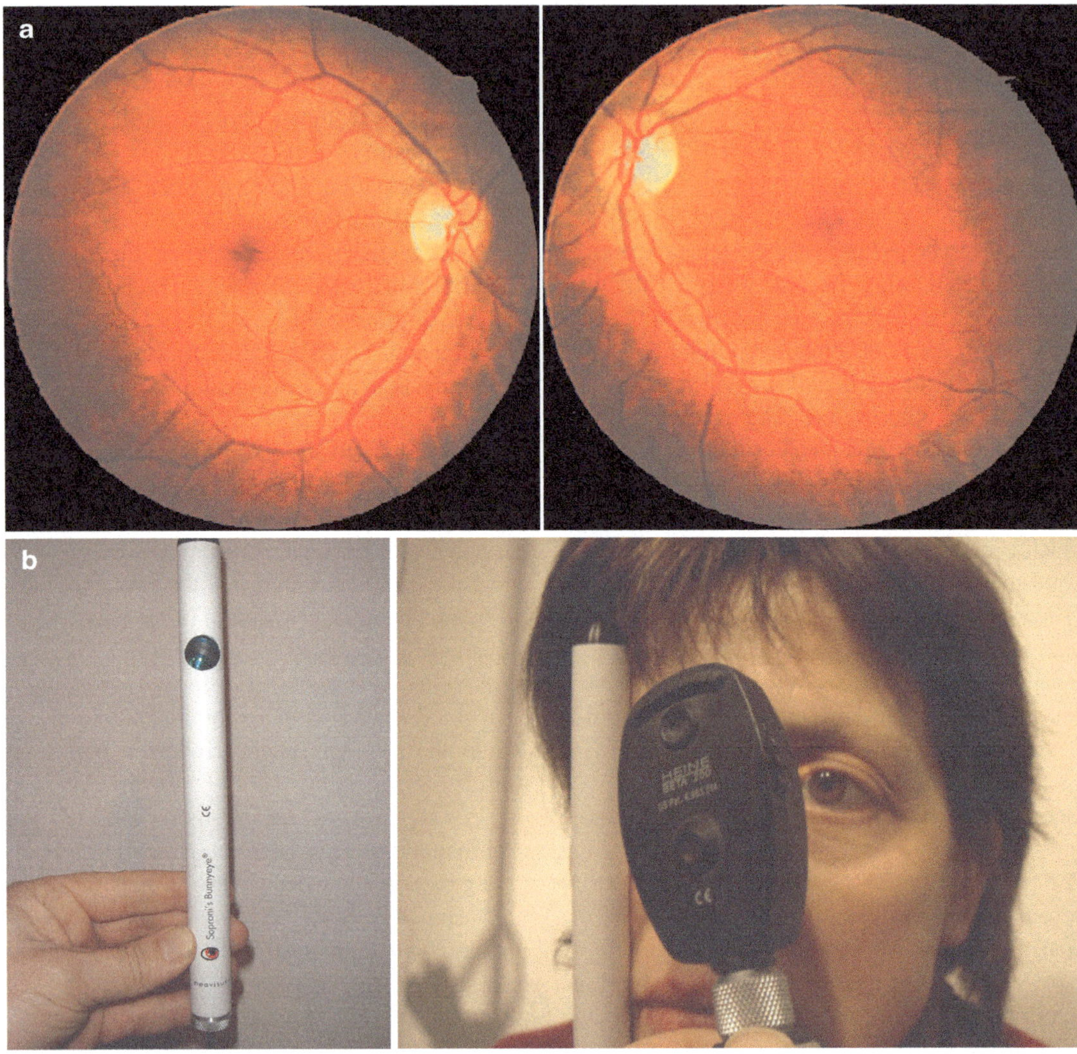

Fig. 21.2 (**a**) The objective measurement of torsion. In the left picture you can see the normal position of the optic disc and the macula. In the right picture the position of these fundal structures is different as a result of the extorsion of the eyeball. (**b**) A hand-held device that can be placed directly in front of the patient's eye to make him/her fixate at optical infinity (Soproni's Bunny Eye™). At the same time, objective torsion can be examined in the non-fixating eye with an ophthalmoscope. (The examination method and the device was presented by V. Paris at the 2009 conference of European Strabismological Association. The photos on the generous agreement of the lecturer) (Paris et al. 2009; Soproni 2003)

Hess Screen Test

This test is mostly used in patients whose diplopia is caused by incomitant strabismus, and it can only be performed in patients who have normal retinal correspondence, i.e., the objective angle measured with the cover test is the same as the subjective angle. So far, the youngest age it can be performed has been 6 years.

In these tests, the patients' two eyes fixate on two different targets, and we examine how they react to this situation. Deviation is measured in the eyes following fixation, e.g., on the Hess screen test, we use red–green glasses and a special screen with 8 fixation points. We also need a device that projects two spotlights; one green and one red. The test is performed from a distance of 50 cm. The patient's head is fixed, he/she is wear-

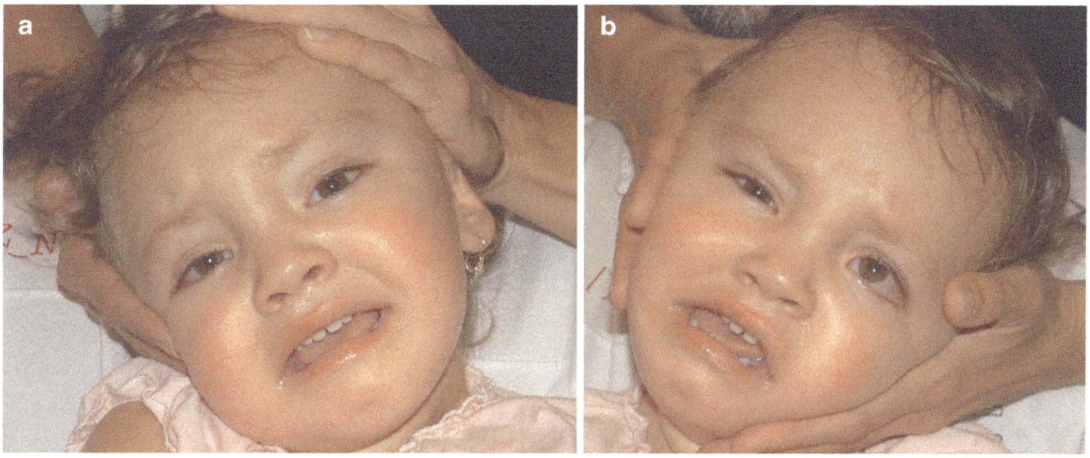

Fig. 21.3 Congenital paralysis of the superior oblique muscle in the left eye. Bielschowsky's head tilt test: The child is trying to prevent us (**b**) from changing the abnormal head posture she developed (**a**) as a result of left hypertropia (From the photocollection of Anna Soproni)

ing the red and green glasses and asked to use a hand-held device to project the green light on the red spots that are projected by the doctor on the fixation points. The points indicated by the patient are connected with straight lines. Then we turn the glasses around and have the patient perform the test once more, this time using the other eye for fixation. The registered data reveal which ocular muscles are responsible for the paralytic strabismus and to what extent (see Fig. 21.4).

A complete ophthalmological examination in childhood also includes *indirect fundoscopy,* measuring of the refractive value, detecting the *fixation and slit-lamp examination.*

Ocular Motor Nerve Palsies

Oculomotor Nerve Palsy

Incidence In a study of 30 children with isolated paralysis, 43 % of the cases was congenital, 20 % traumatic, 13 % caused by infection or inflammation, 10 % due to tumor, 7 % aneurysm and also 7 % ophthalmoplegic migraine (Brodsky 2010).

Clinical Anatomy

The nucleus of cranial nerve III is located in the tectum of the midbrain, anterior to the cerebral aqueduct. The superior rectus subnuclei are unique because they innervate the contralateral superior rectus muscle. On the contrary, cells innervating the levator palpebrae superioris muscle are located in the midline, posterior to the caudal part of the nucleus.

Clinical Symptoms

Lesions of the oculomotor nerve can cause complete or partial (lower or upper branch, or isolated) weakness in the affected muscles. In case of complete oculomotor nerve paralysis, the eyeball shows marked deviation downward and to the side (exohypotropia) with full ptosis and dilated pupil. Unilateral paralysis may result mild proptosis, imitating an orbital lesion.

Third nerve palsy rarely originates from the nucleus. However, damage to the nucleus is obvious if we detect

1. unilateral oculomotor paralysis with contralateral superior rectus paralysis and bilateral ptosis, or
2. bilateral oculomotor paralysis with normal levator function. Complete unilateral paralysis of oculomotor nerve cannot originate from the nucleus if the other eye is totally unaffected.

When the lesion primarily affects the *lower fasciculus* of the nerve, damage of the medialis rectus muscle causes exotropia, and the paresis of

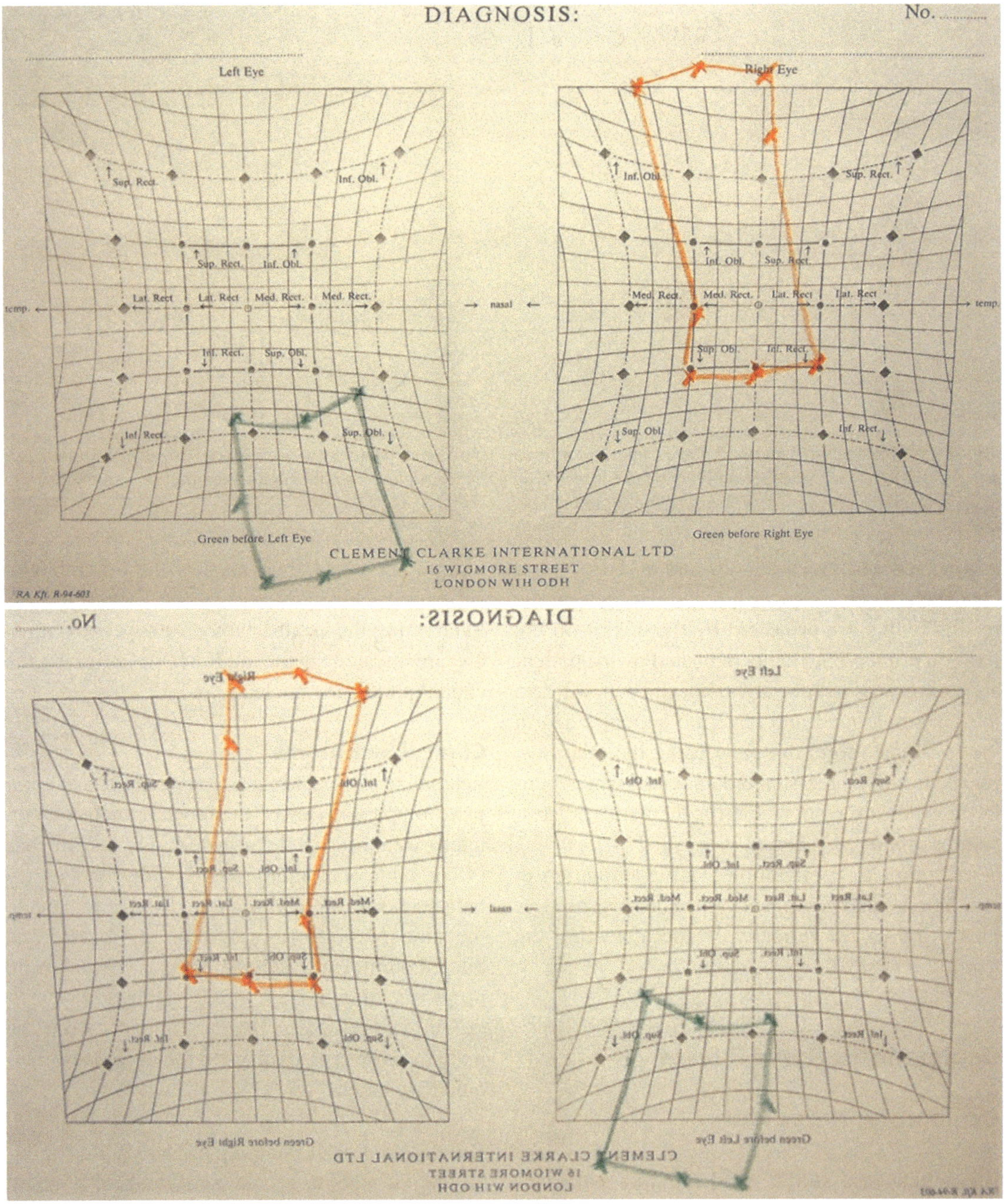

Fig. 21.4 Hess screen test image registered in congenital paralysis of the superior oblique muscle (cranial nerve IV) in the right eye. The upper image is the original that was registered, while the lower one is its mirror image along the vertical axis. It shows the pathological alignment from the specialist's aspect

the inferior rectus muscle leads to hypertropia. (see Fig. 21.5).

If the damage affects the *upper fasciculus,* the eye will be hypotropic in all gaze positions. Damage to the inferior oblique muscle makes the eyeball turn inward (incyclotorsion), causing torsion diplopia, which can interrupt fusion before the parallel alignment of the eyes is restored.

Partial Forms of Oculomotor Palsy

1. Isolated inferior rectus muscle palsy: MRI of the orbit can detect muscle aplasia as well.
2. Isolated inferior oblique muscle palsy: a rare condition; if adduction is limited, we have to consider Brown's syndrome. However, in the latter case (see page 197) the superior oblique muscle shows no overaction. Exotropia develops when the patient gazes upward, and forced duction is positive. The majority of patients suffering from paralysis of the inferior oblique muscle benefits from the weakening of the antagonist superior oblique muscle.
3. Isolated internal ophthalmoplegia: Unilateral, alternating mydriasis of the pupils can occur without other movement disorders in migraine. The initial symptom of compression damage to cranial nerve III is unilateral weakening of accommodation. The development of intermittent exotropia in children suffering from isolated internal ophthalmoplegia indicates incipient paralysis of cranial nerve III.

Oculomotor Synkinesis

The synkinesis (abnormal course) or aberrant regeneration of cranial nerve III develops over a period of some weeks to some months following damage to the oculomotor nerve (primarily disruption of the axon), but it can be associated with some congenital cases as well. The most widely accepted concept is still that of Bielschowsky, who suggested that the trigger factor is the abnormal regeneration of peripheral axons. The most characteristic features are the pseudo-von Graefe's sign (see Fig. 21.6), which gives a quite bizarre appearance to the patient, and the involuntary movements that can be reproduced when making a partly voluntary effort.

Congenital Third Nerve Palsy

In the congenital paralysis of cranial nerve III (associated with pathological regeneration) the pupil of the affected eye can be miotic compared to the unaffected one (see Fig. 21.5a). Approximately 40 % of oculomotor paralysis in childhood is congenital. Although frequently it is an isolated phenomenon, it may be accompanied by other neurological abnormalities. MRI scans show *hypoplasia* of the affected extraocular *muscles* and sometimes the *intracranial* portion of *cranial nerve III* may be absent as well.

Amblyopia is common. In some cases the paralyzed eye fixates (see Fig. 21.5), and this can lead to amblyopia in the unaffected eye. This symptom has been noted in patients with nystagmus, and it is probably related to the favorable decrease in nystagmus on the affected side. (This is exactly what we experienced in the case of the patient illustrated by Fig. 21.5.) Although binocular vision is not likely to be restored, surgical interventions aimed at correcting strabismus and ptosis can yield satisfactory cosmetic results.

Trauma-Induced Paralysis of Cranial Nerve III

Paralysis of cranial nerve III which is attributed to relatively mild trauma may actually be caused by a hidden intraocular tumor that compresses the nerve.

Treatment of Oculomotor Nerve Palsy

The primary objective of the therapy is to treat amblyopia, which is the combined result of strabismus and deprivation due to ptosis. Sometimes several surgical interventions are necessary to reach parallel alignment. Most commonly, patients have binocular vision when they keep their head in a normal position, but they experience diplopia at the sides. When planning to restore function, we have to put the most emphasis on the treatment of ptosis. Ptosis prevents the patient from experiencing diplopia. However, if we can reach some degree of binocular vision in such a patient, we have to perform surgical correction of the ptosis. This operation has to be postponed until we reach the most beneficial alignment (Table 21.4).

Myasthenia gravis
Blowout fracture
Congenital fibrosis syndrome
Internuclear ophthalmoplegia
Duane's syndrome type 2

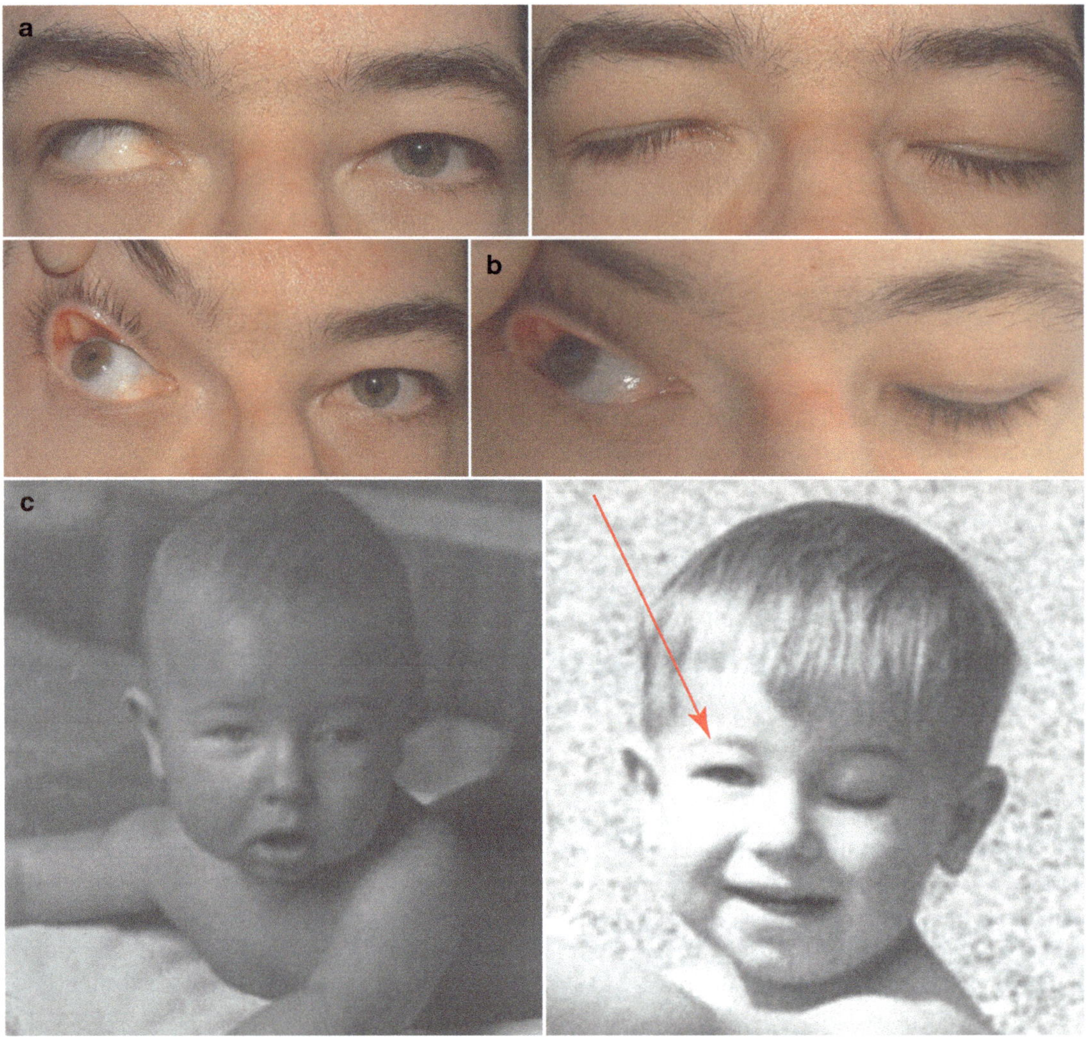

Fig. 21.5 Congenital, partial paralysis of cranial nerve III of the right eye. 43-year-old man. (**a**) Over the years, the right eye developed extreme outward-upward deviation due to the paralysis of the inferior and medialis rectus, as well as the inferior oblique muscles, combined with the contraction of the antagonist muscles (including the levator). As a result of eyelid pseudoretraction, palpebral fissure closure is not complete. The pupil is narrow due to pathological regeneration, and the unaffected eye shows mild nystagmus. Skull MRI did not reveal any pathological changes. (**b**) The right, paralytic eye is the dominant one (with smaller refractional value). The patient uses his finger to lift his eyelid when watching TV. When the right eye fixates, the left one deviates inward and downward with consequent pseudoptosis. (**c**) It is visible in both photos from childhood that the patient uses his right, paralytic eye for fixation (*red arrow*) (From the photocollection of Anna Soproni)

Trochlear Nerve Palsy

It is the most frequent isolated cyclovertical muscle paralysis that affects the superior oblique muscle. It can be congenital (a retrospective study of 92 children found that 56 cases were of congenital origin (Brodsky 2010), due to damage to the nucleus or the motor part of the nerve or *acquired*, due to closed skull trauma affecting the vertex.

The paralysis may be *uni- or bilateral;*

Unilateral paralysis can be caused by a direct injury to the tendon of the superior oblique muscle or the region of the trochlea. Congenital cases are usually unilateral, while acquired ones are mostly bilateral. Acquired paralysis which is certainly not related to injury raises the suspicion of a severe intracranial lesion; therefore, it requires a thorough neurological examination. To differentiate between congenital and acquired forms see Table 21.2.

Clinical Symptoms

Abnormal posture of the head is common: in more than 70 % of acute cases patients tilt their head in the direction of the contralateral shoulder. Patients suffering from unilateral paralysis may also feature hypertropia. Both the affected and the unaffected eyes may be dominant. Amblyopia is not common among acquired cases, but it may occur in congenital ones. Extorsion is common in patients suffering from acquired paralysis, and they often complain of the apparent tilt of objects. Sometimes, when they use their paretic eye for fixation, they report subjective excyclotropia (image tilt outward) in the unaffected eye.

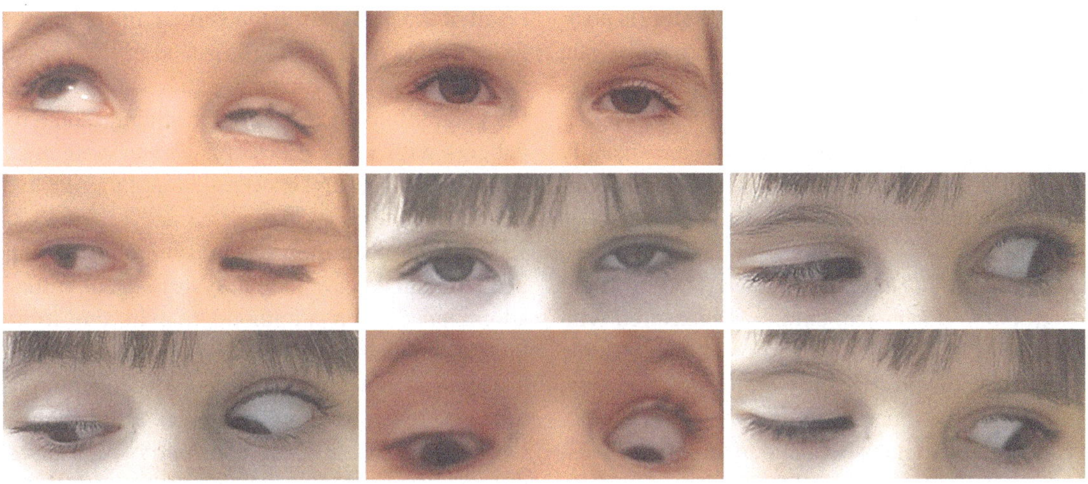

Fig. 21.6 Pathological, congenital synkinesis of the left eye (photos taken at the age of 5). When the eyeball is elevated, ptosis develops occasionally of the left eye (indicating pathological innervation), and eyelid retraction occurs when the patient gazes downward. The patient can control the occasional bizarre position of his eye relatively well (follow-up of 11 years) (From the photocollection of Anna Soproni)

Table 21.4 Clinical algorithm for the differential diagnosis of third nerve palsy in childhood Brodsky (2010)

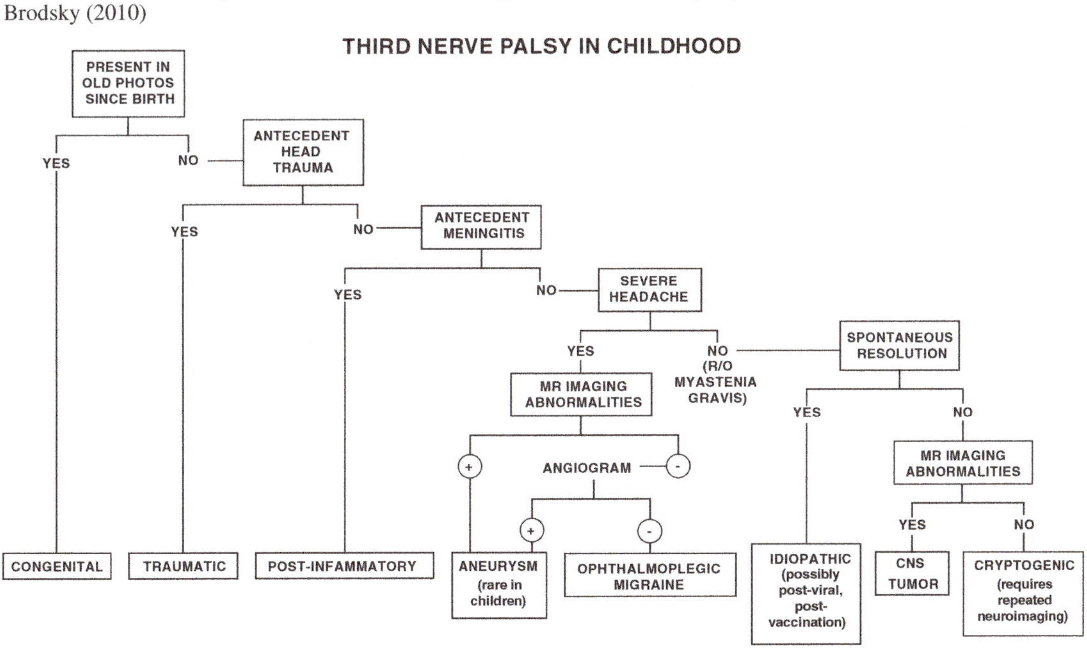

We always have to consider bilateral paresis.

Patients suffering from *bilateral paralysis* often feature a characteristic 'V' pattern esotropia in downgaze (i.e., esotropia increases when they look down), chin depression, and extorsion that is usually higher than 10°. Extorsion is visible in both fundi.

Another typical sign is right-sided hypertropia when gazing to the left and left-sided hypertropia when gazing to the right. The head tilt test is positive on both sides: hypertropia increases when the head is tilted in the direction of the hypertropic eye. The result is that ductions belonging to the superior oblique muscles are usually decreased and the overactions of the inferior oblique muscles suggests that the paralysis is bilateral.

Unilateral paralysis is characterized by slight esotropia in downgaze; extorsion measured with the double Maddox-rod test is lower than 10°; the head tilt test is positive only on the affected side; function of the superior oblique muscle is usually reduced. The diagnosis of superior oblique muscle paralysis can be helped by the *three step test* (the vertical deviation increases when the head is turned to the side of the paralysis and tilted to the opposite side), torsion measurement, careful analysis of duction and version. The three-step test can be misleading sometimes (DVD, presence of restrictive factors).

When establishing the diagnosis and planning the treatment, it is important to measure deviation in all 9 gaze positions and on tilting the head to both sides. When examining versions, we have to pay attention to the function of the affected superior oblique and antagonist inferior oblique muscles, as well as the depression of the affected eye (caused by the contracture of the ipsilateral superior rectus muscle). The change in deviation can be followed with the help of a Hess screen.

The *congenital paralysis* of cranial nerve IV often goes undiagnosed as a lot of children are asymptomatic, while others are thought to be suffering from torticollis of the neck muscles (see the case illustrated by Fig. 21.7: when the head is held upright, the cover test revealed mild right hypertropia. The slightly tilted posture of the head is apparent in old photos as well. The posture of the head was normalized by surgical weakening of the left inferior oblique muscle). There are children who turn their head away from the side of the paralyzed muscle to prevent incomitant hypertropia, while others combine head tilting and turning. In other cases the doctor notices *hypertropia* associated with vertical diplopia. Older children detect vertical *diplopia* as a result of the paralysis. High vertical fusion amplitudes are characteristic (16 instead of the normal value of 2–3 PD, which can reach as much as 30 PD in adulthood. Probably this is the reason why patients with vertical diplopia due to congenital cranial nerve paralysis do not complain of tilted images.)

It is not uncommon for the symptoms of congenital cranial nerve IV paralysis to occur around adolescence or in adulthood (maybe due to an increase in deviation caused by contractions or to a decrease in vertical fusional vergence amplitude as a result of aging). The face also becomes *asymmetric* (see Fig. 21.8) in almost all cases, possibly caused by the chronic tilting of the head (the cheek on the head tilt side will assume a more posterior position and the mouth will become lopsided as well. Facial asymmetry can be detected by drawing a line across the center of the two pupils and another one across the closed lips. If there is asymmetry, these lines converge and cross in the direction of the flatter, more retracted side of the face. This type of asymmetry has to be distinguished from the type seen in congenital muscular torticollis (synostotic plagiocephaly), which is not a specific form of asymmetry and it can occur normally in some people. In synostotic plagiocephaly asymmetry affects the forehead as well (see Fig. 21.9), while in the other two cases, it affects only the central part of the face.

Enophthalmus of the paralytic eye can be apparent as well. This phenomenon is caused by the lack of transmission force which would otherwise be exerted by the superior oblique tendon on the eyeball.

In patients suffering from congenital paralysis of the superior oblique muscle – as opposed to acquired cases – forced duction of this muscle

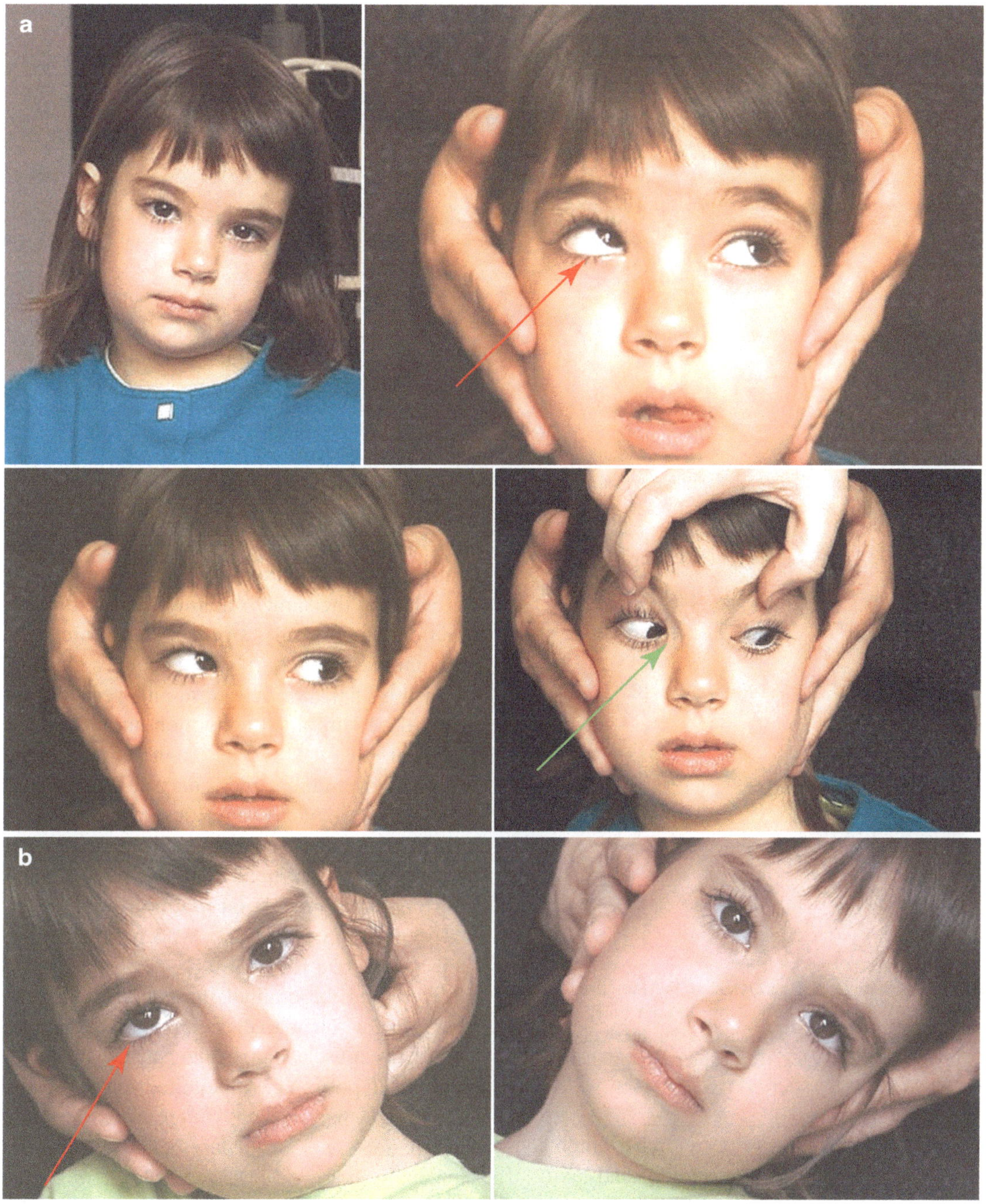

Fig. 21.7 (**a**) Congenital paralysis of cranial nerve IV in the right eye (Fodor et al. 2004). Compensatory head tilt towards the left shoulder. When the patient gazes downward to the left, the right superior oblique muscle lags behind (*red arrow*). When the patient gazes to the left or upward to the left, there is hypertropia of the right eye due to overaction of the inferior oblique muscle (*green arrow*). (**b**) Head tilt test: hypertropia of the right eye (*red arrow*) becomes visible when the head is tilted to the side opposite the habitual tilting (Fodor et al. 2004)

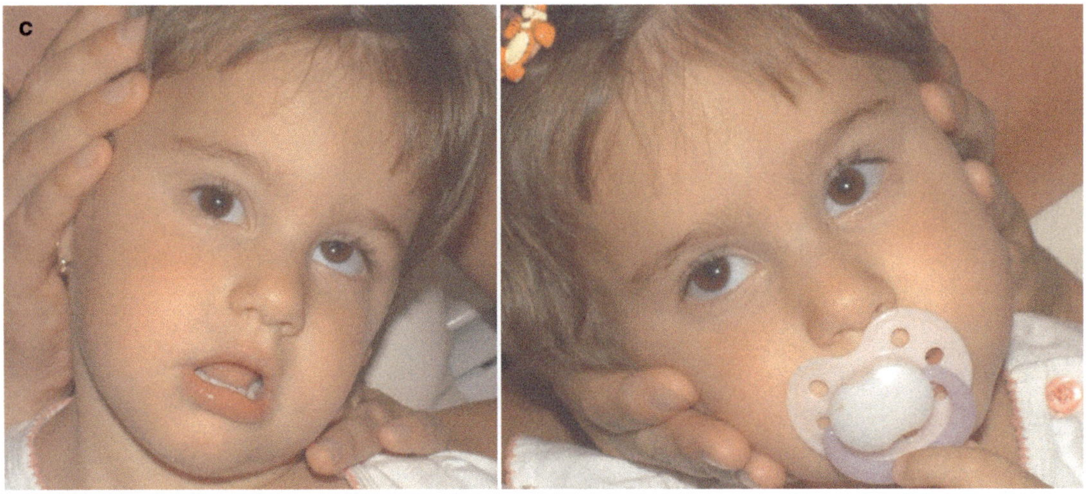

Fig. 21.7 (continued) (**c**) Head tilt test: congenital, bilateral paralysis of the superior oblique muscle (A.S.)

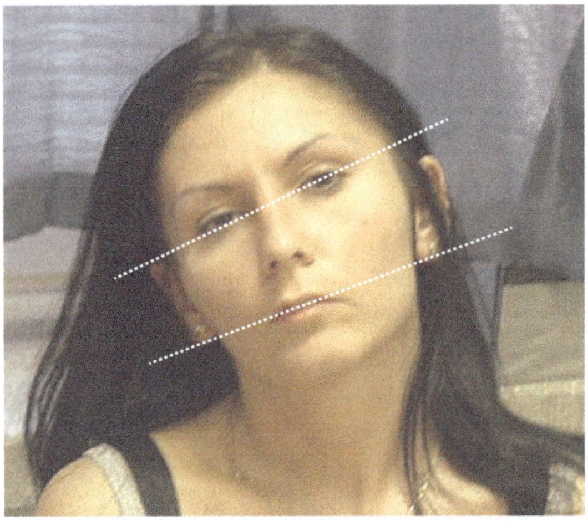

Fig. 21.8 Congenital paralysis of the superior oblique muscle of the left eye. The white dotted lines show the characteristic features of facial asymmetry associated with marked torticollis (for explanation see the text) (From the photocollection of A. S.)

requires excessive power (Guyton 5), which confirms the pathological size (length) and laxity of the tendon.

In 87 % of surgeries, the surgeon will find an abnormal (small or missing) superior oblique tendon, while the same figure is only 8 % in acquired cases (Helveston 5).

Even in acute cases of cranial nerve IV paralysis, where there has been no time for contractures to develop in the inferior oblique muscle, version assessment often detects overaction of the antagonist inferior oblique muscle, while at the same time the superior oblique function shows only slight or absolutely no weakening. Once paralysis becomes chronic, strabismus will become comitant: vertical values will be similar in abduction and adduction (see Table 21.3). This phenomenon is called the spread of comitance, and it may be the result of the contracture of the superior rectus muscle on the affected side (secondary to a chronic hyperdeviation) or contracture of the contralateral inferior rectus muscle (secondary to contralateral hypotropia in patients who habitually use their paretic eye for fixation).

Over time the compulsion to fixate with the paretic eye will lead to the contracture of the inferior rectus muscle of the other eye, which will result in hypotropia with limited elevation and sometimes enophthalmus *(fallen eye syndrome)*. Such patients are mistakenly believed to have a blowout fracture or paralyzed elevators in the other eye. However, MRI of the skull or the orbit reveals atrophy or hypoplasia of the paralyzed superior oblique muscle.

Prolonged paralysis of the trochlear nerve leads to decreased extorsion and increased hypertropia and head tilt, which probably reflects the superimposed contracture of the ipsilateral superior rectus muscle.

Synostotic Plagiocephaly

This unilateral deformity of the orbit imitates the paralysis of cranial nerve IV via the changed anatomical position of the trochlea (see Fig. 21.9) as it is accompanied by the overfunctioning of the inferior oblique muscle. On the contrary, in children suffering from congenital muscular torticollis and deformational plagiocephaly there is accompanying torticollis, which is not ocular in origin.

Idiopathic Cranial Nerve Palsy

The definition covers acute vertical diplopia and symptoms of isolated cranial nerve IV paralysis without recent head injury, congenital cranial nerve paralysis or accompanying neurological deficits. In adults, the condition usually needs 4 months to heal spontaneously. In older adults it is often attributed to a microvascular infarction affecting the cranial nerve. In children the natural (persistent of spontaneously healing) course of idiopathic cranial nerve IV paralysis is not known. In children the isolated paralysis of cranial nerve IV is rarely caused by a compressive lesion, therefore the clinical observation of the persistent paralysis may be sufficient. Imaging scans are not necessary unless other neurological signs develop.

Compressive Lesions

Routine MRI of the brain is not justified, as paralysis of the superior oblique muscle is rarely caused by compressive lesions in children. MRI of the orbit is performed to determine if the superior oblique muscle has become smaller. Recently high-resolution MRI has detected an increasing number of cranial nerve IV schwannomas (slow-growing benign tumors) in patients suffering from

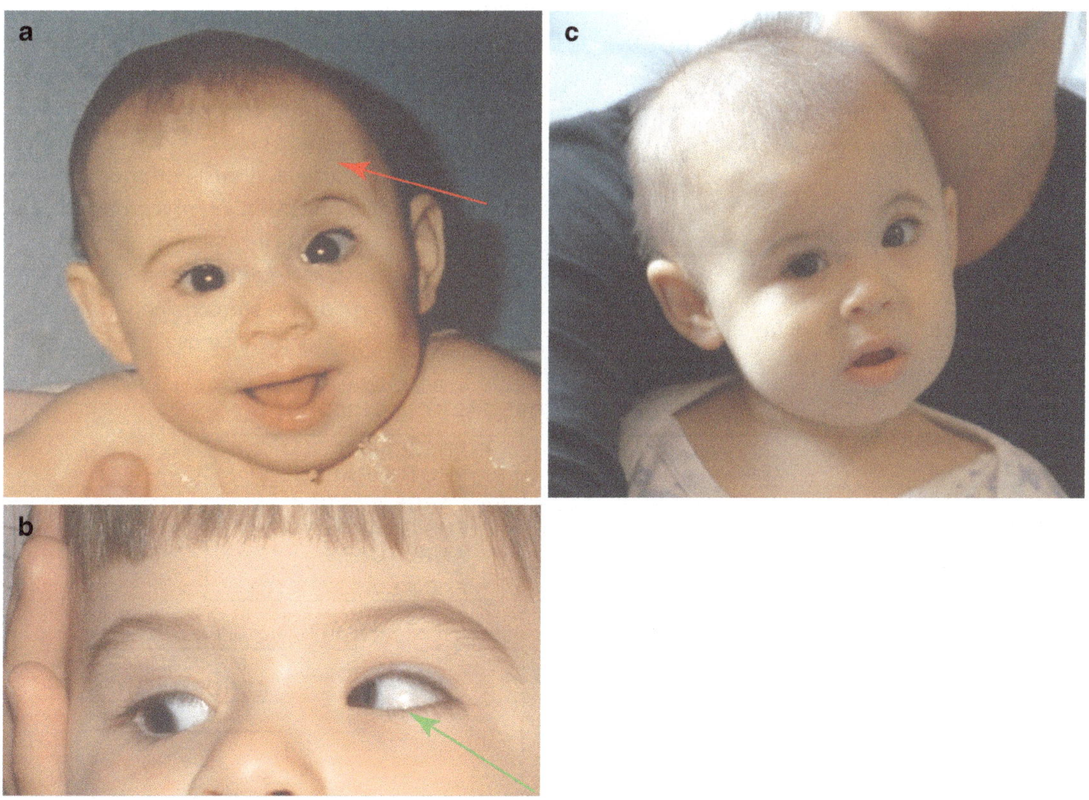

Fig. 21.9 Plagiocephaly. (**a**) The left frontal eminence is missing, the orbit is sunken (*red arrow*). (**b**) The higher position (hypertropia) of the left eye is more marked in adduction (*green arrow*). (**c**) Compensatory posture of the head (From the photocollection of Anna Soproni)

unilateral paralysis of cranial nerve IV. Tumor surgery is more frequently responsible for the isolated paresis of cranial nerve IV than the tumor itself.

Rare Causes of Cranial Nerve IV Paralysis

Differential Diagnosis

For considerations of the differential diagnosis of cranial nerve IV paralysis in children see Table 21.5. The isolated paralysis of the superior oblique muscle is generally more unequivocal in older children.

However, in children who sustained head injury we have to exclude skew deviation caused by functional impairment of the brainstem (Table 21.5).

Dissociated vertical deviation
Congenital muscular torticollis
Synostotic plagiocephaly
Double elevator palsy
Ocular tilt reaction
Incomitant oblique deviation

Treatment

In congenital cases the surgical correction of strabismus should not be delayed unnecessarily because of the pathological posture of the head and facial asymmetry. Patients with acquired paralysis have to be observed for 6 months before considering surgery. During this period, occlusion therapy is not recommended for unilateral cases as most children can reach fusion via some compensatory head tilting.

If amblyopia does develop in such conditions, we have to think about the presence of a coexistent motility disorder, which is responsible for the associated traumatic disruption of the fusion. The surgical treatment of unilateral paralysis needs individual solutions; the aim of the surgery is to create single binocular vision in the functional field of gaze and to normalize the head posture. Nevertheless, Bielschowsky head tilt test will still be positive following a successful surgical intervention, at least in congenital cases.

The Guiding Principle of Surgical Planning

In most cases, we will find isolated overaction of the ipsilateral inferior oblique muscle with little or no underaction of the superior oblique muscle. These cases can be treated with the surgical weakening of the antagonist inferior oblique muscle, i.e., via recession or myectomy. It can neutralize up to 15PD of hypertropia in primary gaze, and it is also self-adjusting.

In marked hypertropia (forced duction test: contracture of the superior rectus muscle!) recession of

Table 21.5 Clinical algorithm for the differential diagnosis of cranial nerve IV paralysis in childhood (Brodsky 2010)

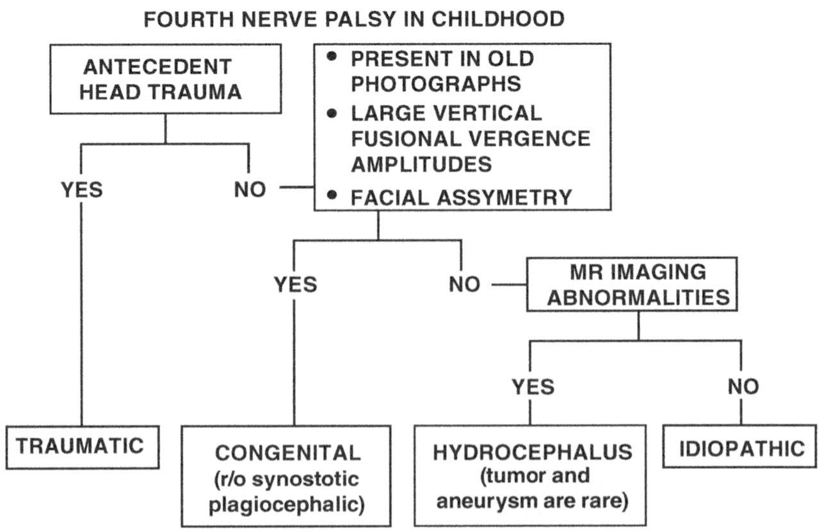

the ipsilateral superior rectus muscle may be necessary. In children who use their paretic eye for fixation, we can experience significant hypertropia in downgaze, and it should raise the suspicion of contralateral inferior rectus muscle contracture. In this case, a small recession of the contralateral inferior rectus muscle is recommended.

In congenital trochlear nerve palsy, if forced duction requires excessive strength, it means the absence of the superior oblique tendon or its laxity. If there is a tendon, *tendon tucking* is performed. However, we have to be careful with the size of the tuck, as a small tuck is not effective and a big one may cause *iatrogenic Brown's syndrome.*

Bilateral trochlear nerve palsy is more difficult to treat. In children who have alternating hyperdeviation when they gaze to the sides and they have marked esotropia in downgaze, bilateral tucking of the superior oblique tendon can often restore single binocular vision in primary gaze position; however, diplopia usually persists in downgaze and for near distance due to esotropia and the remaining torsion. The successful restoration of single binocular vision in downgaze was worked out by Kushner (Noorden and von Campos 2001).

The procedure was described by Forrest Ellis and Carlos Souza-Dias and it means the bilateral recession (5 mm OU) of the inferior rectus muscle. The procedure results a 'fixation duress', which leads to increased innervation in downgaze thereby increasing the function of the paretic superior oblique muscle, improving abduction and intorsion. However, it also needs some remaining function of the superior oblique muscle. According to Jampolsky (Noorden and von Campos 2001), the bilateral weakening of the superior rectus and inferior oblique muscles has to be performed so that the field of single binocular vision could be shifted from the upgaze to the primary position. The relative disadvantage of this procedure is the limitation of the upgaze.

Complaints of children suffering from bilateral superior oblique paralysis include torsion, alternating minimal hyperdeviation in sidegaze or V-pattern in downgaze. In such cases, instead of the superior oblique tuck, the anterior part of this tendon (which has a role in torsion) is dissected and moved anteriorly and inferiorly (*Harada–Ito procedure*). The procedure can reduce or eliminate excyclodeviation as well as increase abduction in downgaze, thereby decreasing V-pattern esotropia.

Abducens Nerve Palsy

Clinical Symptoms

As the only function of cranial nerve VI is abduction of the eye, the clinical signs and symptoms of its paralysis are easier to detect than those of oculomotor or trochlear nerve palsy. Paralysis of the lateral rectus muscle causes incomitant esodeviation. In acute paralysis (see Fig. 21.10) children turn their head to the affected side or incomitant esotropia develops, which increases when they gaze to the affected side, and decreases or disappears when they turn their gaze in the opposite direction. Older children complain of diplopia.

Esodeviation is usually more marked on distance fixation. The angle increases further when the child uses the affected eye to fixate. We can mistakenly diagnose gaze palsy in infants and children with abducens nerve palsy who try to avoid gaze in the field of diplopia. By turning the infant we can elicit the vestibulo-ocular reflex, and this way the noncomitant feature of the deviation becomes visible. Significant esotropia may persist during recovery, irrespective of the almost complete restoration of abduction. This phenomenon may be caused by the innervation imbalance following the paralysis of the rectus muscles, the secondary contraction of the internal rectus muscle or the decompensation of the previous esophoria (Table 21.6).

Causes of Abducens Nerve Palsy

More than one-third of acquired abducens nerve palsy cases in childhood are caused by brain tumors. When taking the history, we have to collect information concerning recent head trauma, infectious diseases or vaccinations, previous episodes and duration of abducens nerve paralysis, and symptoms of increased intracranial pressure.

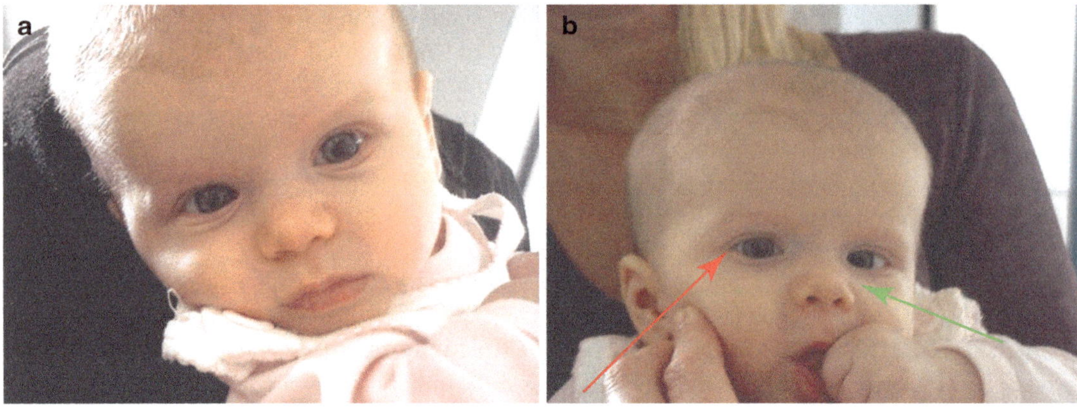

Fig. 21.10 Congenital paralysis of cranial nerve IV of the right (!) eye. (**a**) Compensatory posture of the head due to paralysis of the right lateral rectus muscle (**b**) when the head is turned to the left (doll's head maneuvre), the right eyeball is not able to move (*red arrow*). The contralateral pair of the right lateral rectus muscle, that is the left medial rectus muscle overfunctions (*green arrow*) (From the photocollection of Anna Soproni)

Table 21.6 Clinical algorithm for the differential diagnosis of abducens nerve palsy in childhood **Brodsky (2010)**

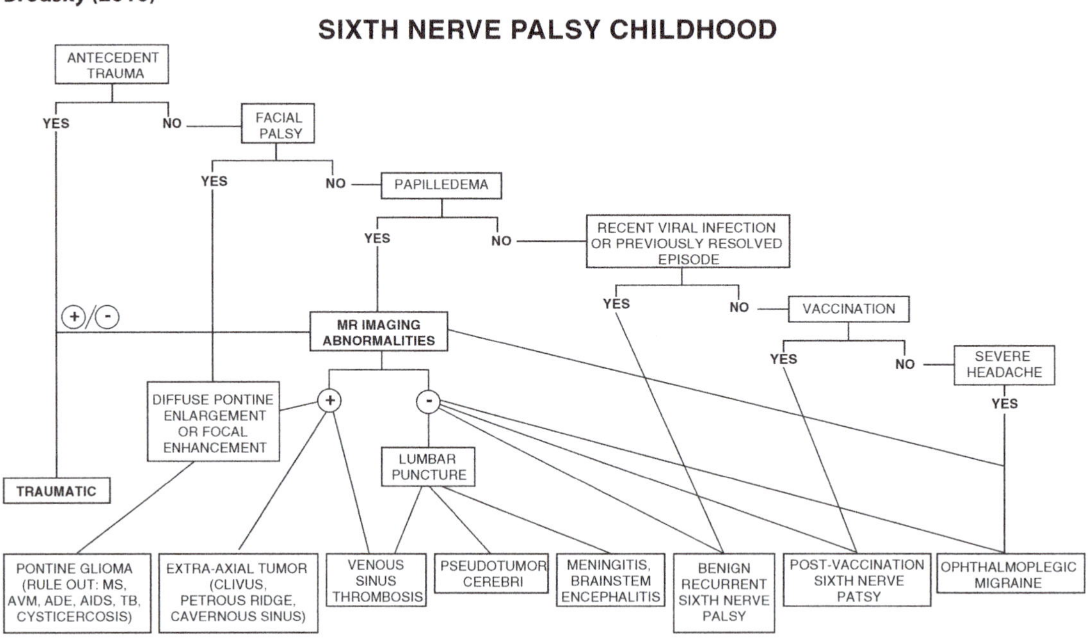

Complete neurological assessment and MRI are recommended in all children with cranial nerve VI palsy, even in cases where traumatic origin is obvious.

Congenital Abducens Nerve Palsy

This kind of paralysis is rare, but it often goes unnoticed as in neonates it is very difficult to rule out slight abduction deficits. Mostly there is no peripheral neural misdirection, and the condition is usually transient, attributable to some perinatal skull injury. Transient paralysis has two recognised forms. One of them presents as neonatal esotropia with unilateral abduction deficit and it usually disappears by the age of 1 month. These cases are likely to be the result of perinatal cranial injury. In the other type, neonatal esotropia is not accompanied by marked abduction deficit.

Trauma-Induced Abducens Nerve Palsy

Trauma-induced paralysis is frequent in patients who sustained a head injury. However, if it develops following a seemingly simple head injury, we have to consider a hidden intracranial tumor as well.

Benign, recurrent abducens paralysis of cranial nerve VI may be caused by a viral disease or vaccination. It is more frequent in women and on the left side. In contrast with paralysis caused by compression or increased intracranial pressure, benign and recurrent cases usually develop suddenly and they are associated with severe abduction weakness of the affected eye. These children feel well between the attacks and they have no other intracranial or metabolic disorders.

If the episodes are recurrent, they typically affect the same eye. In most cases complete recovery takes 8–12 weeks, but if relapses are frequent, esotropia will persist and it will have to be corrected surgically. As strabismus-induced amblyopia can develop before complete recovery, at ages when the risk of amblyopia is the highest, part-time occlusion has to be applied.

The diagnosis of recurrent, benign paralysis can be established based on the following signs: (1) acute onset, (2) complete lack of abduction, (3) recent febrile viral disease, (4) no other cranial nerve lesions and (5) no signs and symptoms of increased intracranial pressure. If a child is suffering from seemingly benign paralysis confirmed by normal imaging studies but he/she does not recover completely, the imaging scan has to be repeated as it might reveal pontine glioma.

The neurotoxicity of chemotherapeutic agents may also result in the paralysis of cranial nerve VI.

Although intracranial aneurysms are rare in childhood, aneurysms in the cavernous sinus may lead to isolated paralysis.

Pontine Glioma

Brainstem gliomas are especially common in children: more than 80 % originate from the pons. They mostly develop between the ages of 5 and 8 years. Facial weakness on the ipsilateral side detected during the initial neuro-ophthalmological examination suggests pontine glioma. Even intact sensory és motor fusion does not exclude the diagnosis of pontine glioma.

Increased Intracranial Pressure

Increased intracranial pressure may press on the brainstem stretching the sixth nerve, which is surrounded by Dorello's canal. When the intracranial pressure is normalized, the paralysis of sixth nerve almost always resolves.

As Chiari malformation may be associated with pseudotumor cerebri, the former condition has to be excluded, especially if the management of cranial nerve VI paralysis is not successful.

Management of Abducens Palsy

Children who are at risk of developing amblyopia due to their age may need occlusion therapy to preserve vision of the esotropic eye, especially if the child uses no compensatory head posture to maintain fusion. Diplopia that occurs in primary position can be corrected temporarily with the help of press-on Fresnel prisms. Spontaneous resolution is possible in more than half of the cases, especially if the paresis is unilateral. However, if there is no spontaneous recovery, we can inject *botulotoxin* into the antagonist (medial rectus) muscle thereby maintaining the primary position of the eyes.

Botulinum may help to prevent contraction of the medial rectus muscle while the patient is being observed before surgery. If there is no recovery in a period of 6 months or more, surgical intervention is recommended. Recession the antagonist medial rectus muscle combined with the resection of the lateral rectus muscle frequently proves to be a successful first-line surgical solution. Recession of the vertical muscles may also be necessary (Kestenbaum's precedure). In paralytic strabismus, if the patient is cooperative the application of adjustable sutures may be helpful.

Congenital Oculomotor Apraxia

It is a rare disorder that sometimes leads to strabismus. It is mostly detected together with developmental delay. Disorders of the central nervous system can also accompany the syndrome. It is important to use modern imaging technology when examining the skull, and the child has to undergo a thorough general investigation as well. One of the symptoms is inability to produce normal, voluntary horizontal saccades. Instead, changes in horizontal fixation are made by a head thrust that overshoots the target, followed by a rotation of the head back in the opposite direction once fixation is established. Joubert' syndrome and Gaucher's disease have to be considered and investigated.

Congenital Infantile Esotropia

Esotropia develops a few weeks or months following birth. Strabismus is frequently present in family history, but the etiology of the condition is not clear. Children suffering from early-onset esotropia are usually otherwise healthy; however, in those with neurological and developmental abnormalities this type of esotropia reaches 30 %. Due to the large angle of strabismus (>30 PD), cross fixation is common and it raises the suspicion of bilateral abducens palsy, but this latter condition can be excluded with the doll's head maneuvre. Following a few weeks' of alternating occlusion of the eyes, the abduction capacity of the eyes can be confirmed by checking if they can follow objects (see Fig. 21.11).

The condition is often accompanied by the overaction of the inferior oblique muscle, which causes an upward twitch in adduction. This phenomenon is the so-called dissociated vertical deviation (DVD). It is essential to distinguish it from vertical strabismus.

Latent nystagmus, which is often associated with infantile esotropia, requires a special solution during the examination (see section "Examination methods" at the beginning of this Chapter). The asymmetry of smooth horizontal pursuit (less developed when moving to the sides) in congenital esotropia persists beyond the age of 6 months. Amblyopia is relatively rare due to the mostly insignificant refractive error and alternating fixation. Treatment is basically surgical. It has been accepted in the profession to perform corrective surgery before the age of 2 in order to achieve good cosmetic results, as well as good fusion in a significant proportion of the cases. The most commonly used solutions are recession of both medial rectus muscles or recession one of the medial muscles and resection of the lateral rectus muscle.

Congenital Cranial Dysinnervation Syndromes

According to the most recent classification, the group includes the following conditions (see Table 21.1).

Marcus Gunn Phenomenon

The pathological synkinesis of the trigeminal and oculomotor nerves causes the development of this condition, which is associated with upward jerking of the upper eyelid during certain movements of the jaw (chewing, sucking, opening of the mouth) (see Fig. 21.12).

Monocular Elevation Deficiency

This descriptive diagnosis may cover the double elevator palsy (when the inferior oblique and the superior rectus muscles of the same eye become paralysed) or weakness of elevation (which is weakness of the inferior rectus muscle due to e.g., fibrosis) (see Fig. 21.13).

Monocular elevation deficiency means that elevation is limited in abduction, adduction, version and duction; however, this limitation is usually more marked in abduction than in primary position, and – contrary to Brown syndrome – it improves in adduction to some extent. True ptosis is present in 50 % of the cases. Treatment is justified if there is significant vertical deviation in primary position or if the patient presents with abnormal head posture (chin elevation). In case of underaction of the inferior rectus muscle, recession of this muscle is recommended. If there is no limitation, the transposition of the medial

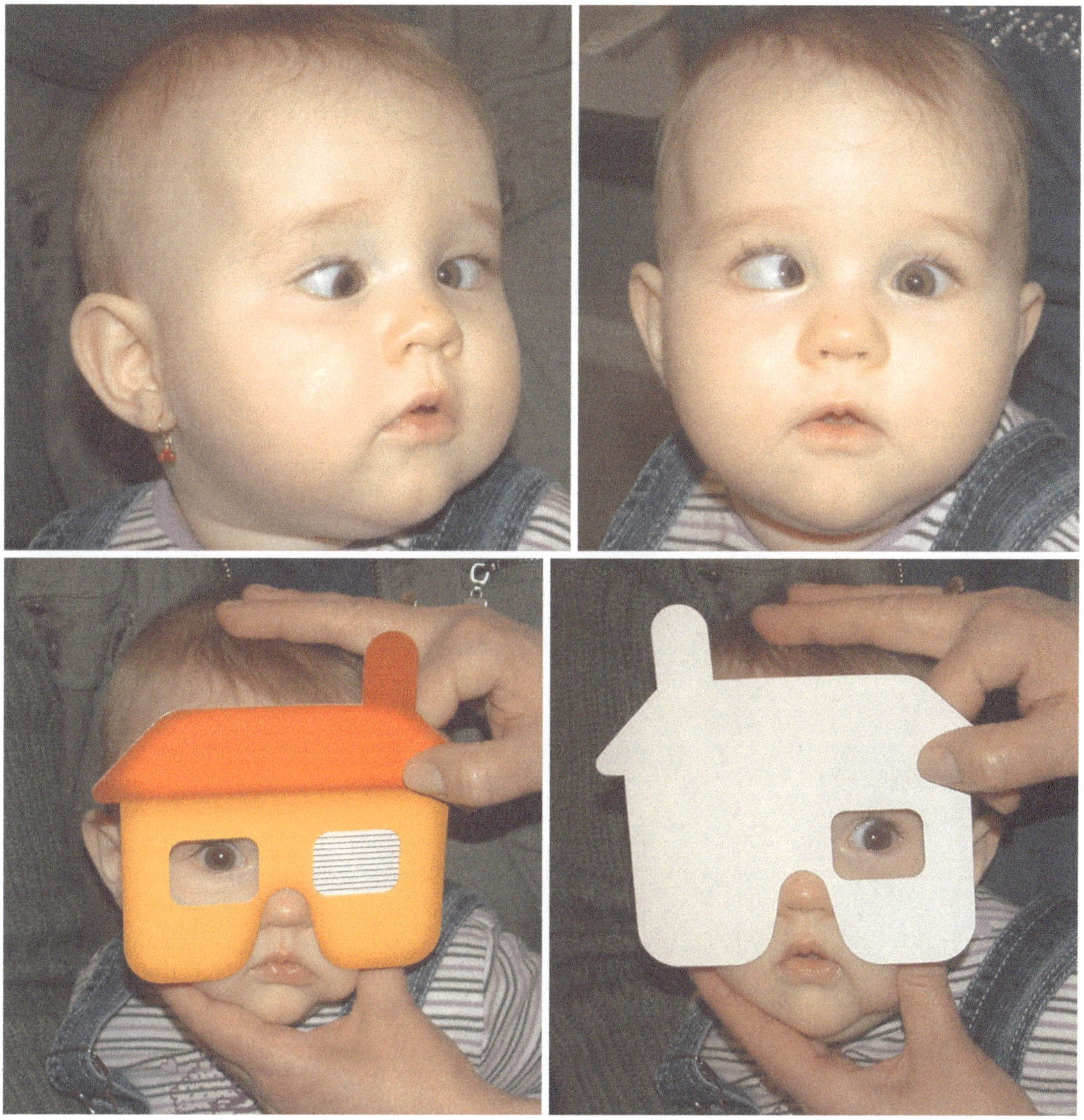

Fig. 21.11 Infantile esotropia, bilateral pseudoparesis of the abducens nerve. On monocular covering (with a disposable mask, <Soproni's Peep-n-See House ™>) the excursion of the lateral rectus muscles is almost normal (From the photocollection of A. S.)

and lateral rectus muscles is proposed in the direction of the superior rectus muscle (Knapp's procedure).

Moebius's Syndrome

There is simultaneous paralysis of cranial nerves VI and VII. Both abduction and adduction may be limited. The differential diagnosis is helped by the characteristic symptoms of cranial nerve VII paralysis (e.g., mask-like facial appearance).

Congenital Ptosis

Recently the presumption that this condition is caused by congenital muscular paresis has become outdated, as a significant proportion of

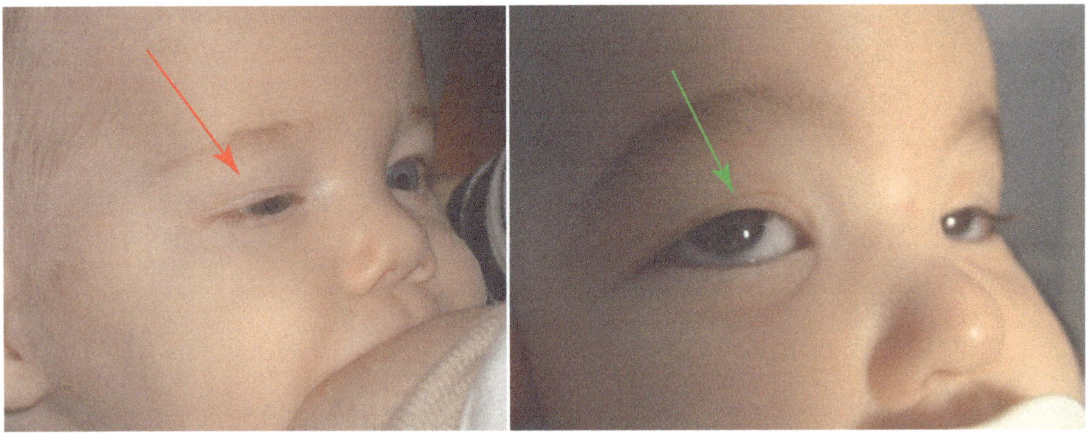

Fig. 21.12 Marcus Gunn phenomenon on the right eye. The right upper eyelid shows mild ptosis occasinally (*red arrow*), but during breast-feeding it retracts (*green arrow*) (From the photocollection of Anna Soproni)

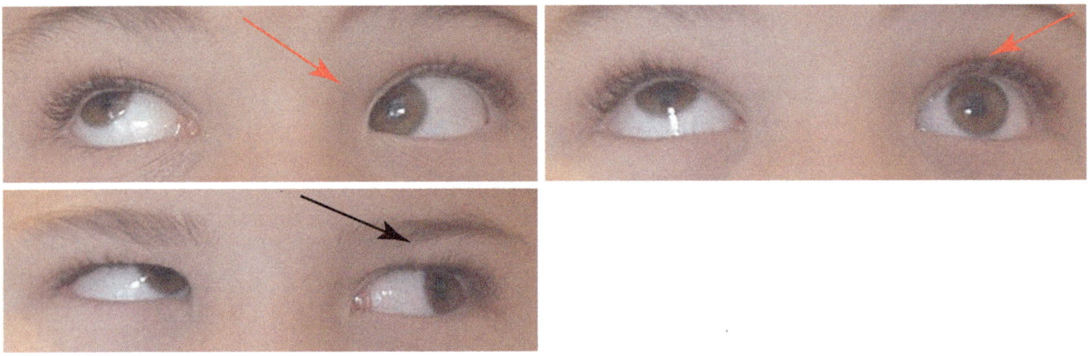

Fig. 21.13 Double elevator palsy in the left eye of a hemophiliac child. There is adducion on upward gaze. The limitation of abduction and upward gaze (*red arrows*) is also indicated by the simultaneous overfunctioning of the right eye (From the photocollection of Anna Soproni)

patients show symptoms of congenital cranial dysinnervation as well. Congenital ptosis can be considered an isolated form of congenital fibrosis syndrome, which affects the upper fasciculus of cranial nerve III only.

Congenital Fibrosis Syndrome (Congenital Fibrosis of Extraocular Muscles, CFEOM)

Restrictive ophthalmoplegia of autosomal dominant inheritance, which is associated with limited movement and fibrosis of the extraocular muscles. Its characteristic features are fixed downward gaze, ptosis, significant horizontal strabismus and compensatory posture of the head (elevated chin). The levator is the most frequently affected ocular muscle, followed by the inferior and lateral rectus muscles. Nowadays, the pathological regeneration is considered to be the most common symptom of congenital fibrosis syndrome. Forced duction is essential for the differential diagnosis, and genetic tests are becoming more readily available in major centers. Treatment: surgical correction is difficult. Even multiple, combined surgical interventions to treat ptosis and strabismus cannot ensure more than near-normal alignment in primary position.

Duane's Syndrome

Probably the most frequent eye movement disorder associated with isolated restriction of abduction.

It a frequent condition of unknown origin, in which the abducens innervation of the lateral rectus muscle is diminished or deficient, combined with the abnormal innervation of the lateral rectal muscle from a branch of third nerve. It means that the lateral and medial rectus muscles will contract at the same time. On attempted abduction the palpebral fissure gets wider, while in adduction it gets narrow and retraction of the eyeball is present. The latter phenomenon distinguishes the condition from the simple paralysis of the abducens nerve. Retraction may even cause visible enophthalmus when the patient gazes straight forward in some cases. Patients usually have good binocular vision, which is sometimes achieved via a compensatory head posture. It is a hereditary disorder in 10 % of the cases, and accompanying systemic conditions have to be considered as well.

Types

Type I (see Fig. 21.14): abduction is weak so esotropia is visible in the primary position.

Type II (see Fig. 21.15): adduction is weak so exotropia is visible in the primary position.

Type III (see Fig. 21.16): both adduction and abduction are weak. Differential diagnosis is easy, as there are no other syndromes that would cause a peculiar group of such symptoms. (Noorden and von Campos 2001)

Other clinical features: upbeat and/or downbeat nystagmus may occur on adduction

If the two horizontal muscles contract simultaneously in attempted adduction, the power of the lateral rectus muscle may be stronger than that of the medial one, therefore the affected eye will show paradoxical abduction (synergistic divergence). In view of the pathological innervation, the most important indication of surgery is a markedly abnormal head position. Careful planning of the surgery is a must.

Brown's Syndrome

In congenital Brown syndrome the cause of limited elevation in adduction (see Fig. 21.17) is the abnormal, congenital course of the superior oblique tendon. Acquired Brown syndrome may be caused by injuries or inflammation affecting the region of the trochlear nerve. The difference between Brown syndrome and isolated paralysis of the inferior oblique muscle is that in the latter condition the ipsilateral antagonist of the inferior oblique muscle, the superior oblique is overacted. Surgical treatment is not indicated unless the patient has strabismus in the primary position or markedly abnormal posture of the head. In this case the superior oblique muscle can be weakened (tenotomy, inserting a silicone tendon expander), with or without weakening the inferior oblique muscle.

Congenital/Infantile Nystagmus

The classification of congenital or infantile nystagmus is a difficult task. In 80 % of the cases the nystagmus can be attributed to a sensory defect (SDN or ocular nystagmus, can develop before the age of 6 months), and it is associated with the developmental abnormality of the retina/optic nerve. It is much more frequent than congenital idiopathic nystagmus (CIN), whose diagnosis can be established after everything else has been excluded. An accurate diagnostic classification enables us to provide a more precise prognosis and risk assessment for parents if they plan to have another child. In both cases there are characteristic features that can help us to rule out more extensive neurological diseases. If these characteristic features can be identified, we can differentiate the two diseases (sensory and idiopathic) as well. If the findings are atypical, we need complete neurological and neuroradiological investigations. It is also true when nystagmus is present together with other neurological diseases. In one third of the cases some form of albinism is revealed in the background.

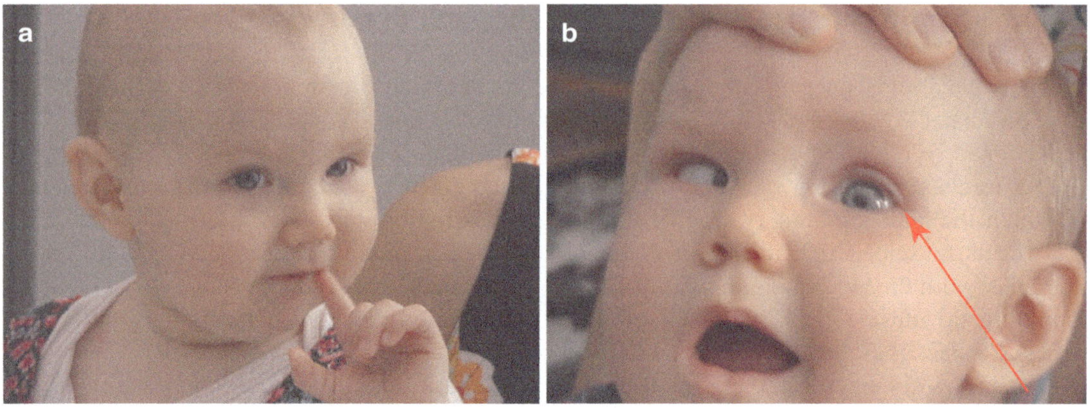

Fig. 21.14 Duane type I syndrome in the left eye. (**a**) Compensatory posture of the head; in dextroversion the left palpebral fissure gets narrow and the eyeball is drawn backward (**b**) When the head is turned to right, the left eye does not move (*red arrow*) and the palpebral fissure gets wider (From the photocollection of A. S.)

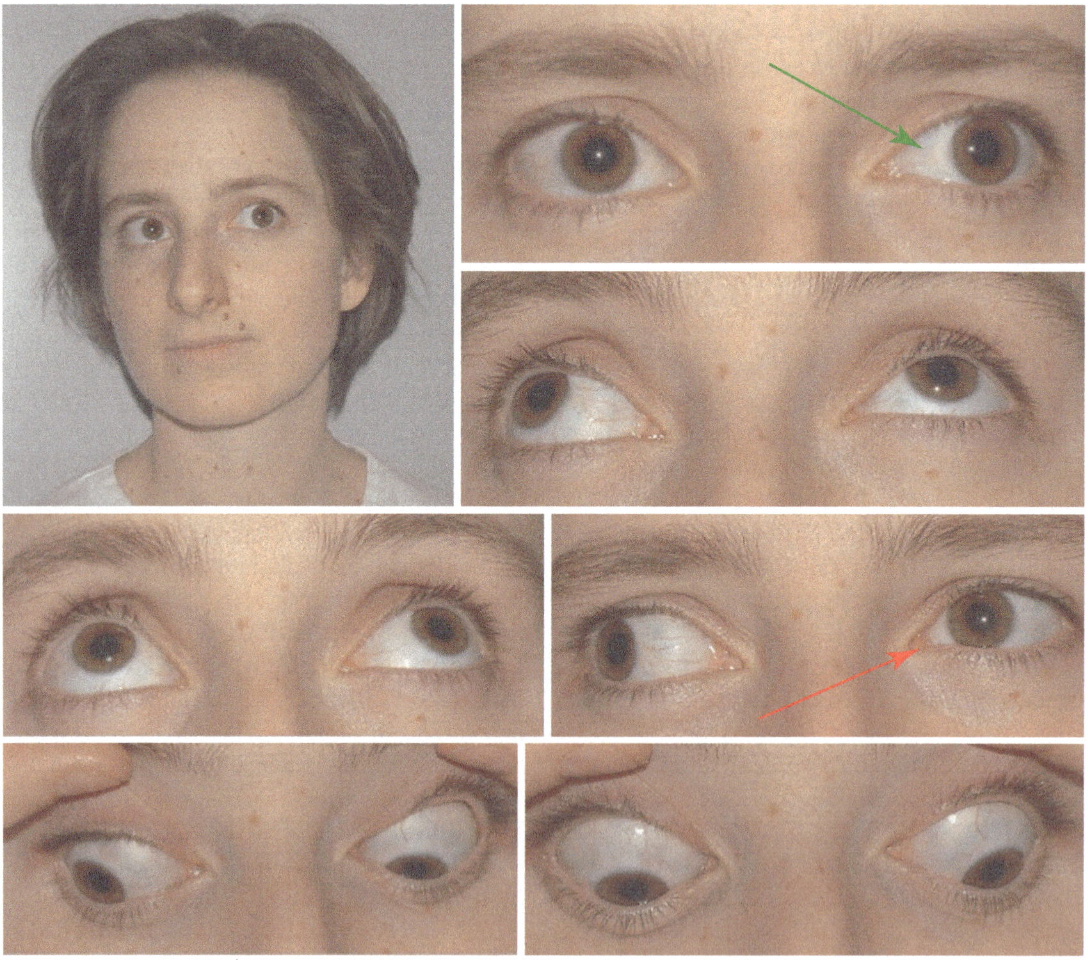

Fig. 21.15 Duane type II syndrome on the left eye. *First picture*: compensatory posture of the head due to the lack of the left medial rectus muscle function. *Pictures in the box*: When the patient gazes to the right, the left medial rectus muscle lags behind (*red arrow*) and retraction of the eyeball is visible. In primary position, the left eye diverges (*green arrow*). When the patient gazes to the right, upshot is visible on the left eye (*red arrow*) (From the photocollection of Anna Soproni)

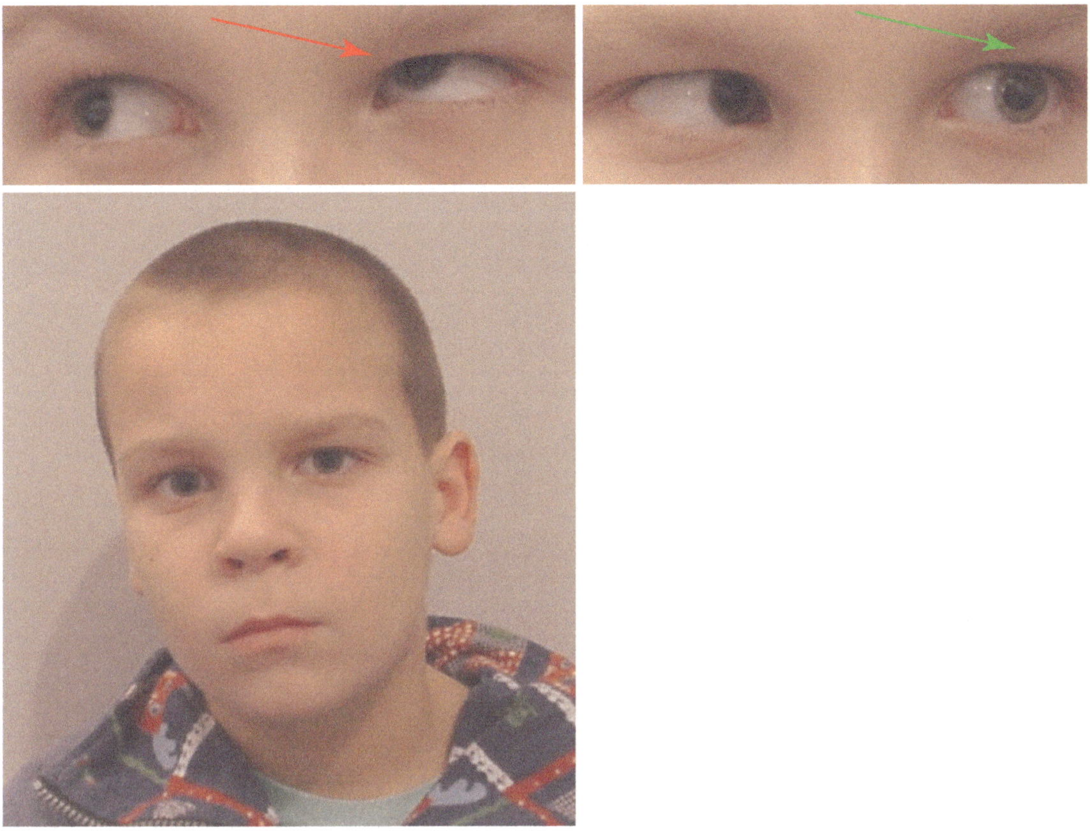

Fig. 21.16 Duane type III syndrome on the left eye. The left eye cannot move inward (*red arrow*) or outward (*green arrow*). In attempted adduction the palpebral fissure is markedly narrow, the eyeball shows upshot (*red arrow*) and retraction. In abduction the palpebral fissure gets wider (*green arrow*) (From the photocollection of Anna Soproni)

Manifest Congenital Motor Nystagmus

This type of nystagmus is mostly hereditary and binocular conjugated. It is generally horizontal, and it also remains horizontal when the patient gazes upward or downward. The form of the nystagmus can be pendular, jerk, circular or elliptical. Convergence frequently reduces congenital motor nystagmus, therefore it is often associated with esotropia (nystagmus blockage syndrome). Patients can have a null point or a neutral zone where the intensity of nystagmus is decreased and visual acuity is improved. If the neutral zone is outside the primary position, the abnormal head posture can be corrected with prisms or surgery. If we use prisms, the apexes of them show toward the deviation of the eyes. The treatment of motor nystagmus aims to improve eye stabilization.

Recession of all the horizontal rectus muscles to a position posterior to the equator is an alternative to the Kestenbaum-Amderson procedure for improving visual function when head position is not a problem, but newly generated deviation is possible (Pediatric Ophthalmology and Strabismus 2013).

Latent Nystagmus

It is congenital, conjugated, horizontal, jerk-like nystagmus, which develops on monocular fixation.

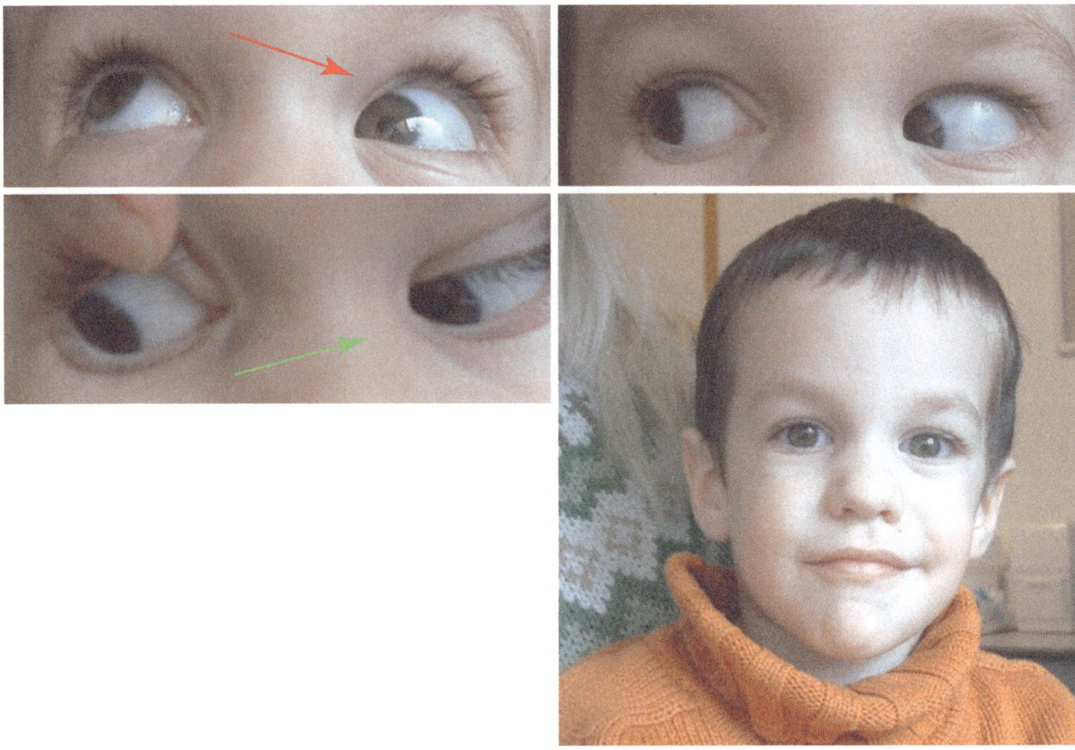

Fig. 21.17 Brown's syndrome on the left eye with normal head posture. There is limited elevation in adduction of the left eye (*red arrow*). The left superior oblique muscle does not overacted (*green arrow*) (From the photocollection of Anna Soproni)

Sensory Nystagmus

This form of nystagmus is secondary to damage to the afferent part of the visual pathway (hereditary retinal diseases, albinism, developmental abnormalities of the eyes). The amplitude of nystagmus usually depends on the severity of low vision (Lorenz and Borruat 2008).

Acknowledgement Special thanks to Professor Brodsky MC, who permitted me to modify Chapter 6 (Ocular Motor Nerve Palsies in Children) of his book's with some of my figures and text.

References

Brodsky MC. Pediatric Neuro-ophthalmology. 2nd ed. Springer. 2010.

Fodor M, Soproni A, Molnár K, Garai G. Congenital paralysis of the superior oblique muscle. Ophthalmologia Hungarica. 2004;141:102–8.

Lorenz B, Borruat F-X. Pediatric neuro-ophthalmology pediatric pphthalmology, neuro-ophthalmology, genetics. Springer. 2008.

Microdeviations and Macrosymptoms. What to do? V. Paris, Liege University, Private Center of Strabismology, Belgium. Presentation. Held at the 2009 conference of the European Strabismological Association (ESA).

Noorden GK, von Campos EC. Binocular vision and ocular motility. In: Theory and management of strabismus. 6th ed. Mosby. 2001.

Pediatric Ophthalmology and Strabismus. Basic and clinical science course. American Academy of Ophthalmology (2013–2014).

Soproni A. New handheld fixation device. Ophthalmologia Hungarica. 2003;140:271–2.

von Noorden GK, Helveston EM. A decision making approach. 1st ed. Mosby. 1994.

Polatest Procedure

22

Judit Pálfia and Ernő Pálfia✠

Contents

The various types of *heterophoria* (*latent strabismus*), the resting alignment errors of the eyes, may cause numerous complaints. The ones that should be highlighted for those involved in neuro-ophthalmology include headache that may turn into migraine, dizziness, deconcentration, occasionally diplopia, and spatial disorientation. If the neuro-ophthalmological examinations for these complaints find no abnormalities, a *proper* heterophoria test must be performed. Prism glasses made based on the result of this will eliminate the complaints due to heterophoria.

Physiological Background

Merely for didactic reasons, oculomotor and sensory components of binocular vision are distinguished. In natural vision, these two processes are merged together and can hardly be distinguished: the sensorium conducts and controls the oculomotor functions. The development of the ideal cooperation between the sensory functions of the two eyes is a result of a learning process that takes place in childhood. A motor prerequisite for this is the ability to direct both eyes precisely at the object to be viewed and maintain this state. This state may be ideal from the sensory aspect only, and as to the motor part, the work of the extraocular muscles is needed for bicentral image formation, and therefore the state is (now) not ideal from the motor aspect. Each pair of eyes has a rest and a work position. In an ideal case, the two positions are the same for both the far and the all-time near object distances, and the image of the fixated object point is formed simultaneously at the foveola in both eyes. This state is called *orthophoria*. In this case, the two images are fused quasi evidently into a single image in the visual cortex. Situations other than this can be classified into two major groups: if the binocular vision is lost, it is *strabismus* (monocular vision), whereas if the binocular vision

✠ Author was deceased at the time of publication

J. Pálfia, M.D. (✉)
Ophthalmologist, Pediatric Ophthalmologist, Pálfia Ltd., Budapest, Hungary
e-mail: palfia.judit@t-online.hu

E. Pálfia, M.D.
Ophthalmologist, Pediatric Ophthalmologist, Budapest, Hungary

J. Somlai, T. Kovács (eds.), *Neuro-Ophthalmology*, DOI 10.1007/978-3-319-28956-4_22

is maintained, although forced, we speak of *heterophoria*, which is the topic of this chapter.

Each point of the retina has its own sense of direction. They actually belong to the sensory cells of the center of vision and not to the retinal points. Retinal points that transmit the same sense of direction in the two eyes are called *corresponding retinal points*. The direction 'straight ahead' comes from the center of the retina (the foveola), which is the place of the highest visual acuity. These are called correspondence centers, since the other retinal points give a sense of direction in relation to this point in both eyes. Retinal points that give different senses of direction are called *disparate* retinal points. In theory, if the image of the outside world is projected onto such points, diplopia should occur. In case of normal binocular vision, however, there is no diplopia, owing to two different sensory mechanisms.

(a) The *Panum areas*, which ensure three-dimensional vision in an ideal case, are located around points that transmit the same sense of direction in the two eyes (naturally not in the retina but in the cortex). Their additional task is to prevent diplopia when one eye transmits the direction 'straight ahead' and the direction sensed by the other eye is slightly different (but within the boundary of the Panum area).
(b) The mechanism of inhibition is activated if the objects of the outside world are imaged in the binocular visual field by disparate retinal points that are too far away from each other (so far that the image is outside the Panum area in one eye). In this case, the visual impression of one eye is perceived, whereas that of the other eye is suppressed (inhibited).

Heterophoria

Heterophoria (latent strabismus) is a congenital disorder, a *resting alignment error*, where—with the help of the fusion stimuli continuously present under the conditions of natural vision—*normal, although not ideal, binocular single vision is maintained*. Therefore, there is no manifest strabismus, and the eye alignment appears to be parallel but the rest and work positions of the pair of eyes are different. The deviation between the resting lines of sight of the two eyes may have an outward, inward, upward or downward direction. In the literature, these are called *exo-*, *eso-*, *hyper-and hypophoria*, respectively. Horizontal and vertical heterophorias are often combined. A less common condition is *cyclophoria*, when the eye is rotated around its sagittal axis. This condition cannot be helped with prisms. In case of heterophoria, the line of sight of one eye is directed slightly beside the fixated object. In the resting position of the deviating eye, the image of the fixated object is formed beside the center. If it was not compensated, diplopia would occur, which would make work impossible.

Processes Compensating Heterophoria

Compensation may be achieved completely with motor functions, and sensory adaptation to the alignment error is also possible. In case of compensation completely achieved with motor functions, fusion of the images is initially (in childhood) achieved purely in a motor way: the pair of eyes assumes its work position using the extraocular muscles in a direction opposite to that of the heterophoria (vergence).

The result is that the image of the fixated object is formed, in both eyes, at the site of highest resolution, the foveola, which is at the center of the retina. Maintaining this state involves keeping a continuous tone in the oculomotor muscles. The nature of the tone is subject to changes; over time, the initially completely mobile tone, owing to the continuous practice, turns in an ever-growing part into *contractile* tone. In certain cases, especially in some moderate to severe esophorias *plastic tone* may appear with a higher and higher degree over time. (The term 'eye muscle tone' always means the complete, joint compensatory tone.)

The change in tones does not mean an increase in the original, mobile tone but the change in its rigid part due to permanent tension, whereas the development of a plastic tone means the (partial) transformation of the muscles. (It is supposedly about the ratio of fast and slow twitch muscle fibers, which can be found mixed in the extraocular muscles.) With the use of proper prisms, first the contractile, and then the plastic tones become 'spasm-free' and mobilized. This process is called *tone reduction*. Reduction of the plastic tones is never achieved with the first prism glasses0; they can be mobilized only slowly and gradually. Often several post-corrections are required, with intervals that last for weeks or even months, but finally, the total value of (the until then, latent components of) heterophoria/angle-deviation binocular vision can be measured even in 'obstinate' cases. *The need for vergence and the tone may never exceed the actual value of uncorrected heterophoria.* If the final resting position of the pair of eyes is achieved, and the prisms ensuring this are removed, the entire mobile reserve is activated. The blurred vision and/or diplopia lasting for a fraction of a second trigger the fusion stimulus. In response to this, the eyes immediately assume with the help of the oculomotor muscles a parallel alignment. The patient utilizes their entire fusion width, since no part of it is engaged in maintaining the tone. Those that oppose treatment with prisms say in such cases that prism glasses are completely unnecessary since the eyes already have a parallel alignment without them. *Sensory adaptation* is required if the purely motor compensation for the misalignment begins to decompensate, and the fixation point is no longer imaged at corresponding retinal points but in a disparate position in the deviating eye, although within the central Panum area. At this stage of heterophoria, extraocular muscles now need to pull the deviating eye only until the boundary of the Panum area. The remaining portion of heterophoria is compensated by the cortex with sensory adaptation, taking advantage of the Panum areas. The sense of direction at the given point is altered under the conditions of binocular vision. (In case of monocular vision, the original sense of direction still applies.) This state is called *fixation disparity* (FD). This is considered a normal although not ideal state of binocular single vision.

The *Panum areas may enlarge* due to the continuous practice during binocular vision (especially in case of esophoria). (This is not an anatomical enlargement but merely a change in the sense of direction of the affected cortical cells.) Because of this, the extraocular muscles have to do less work, and sensory adaptation compensates for a larger portion of the heterophoria. Fusion, therefore, is the result of a partly motor, partly sensory work in this case. Both stages put an unnecessary load on the sensorymotor system, which may lead to symptoms under certain circumstances.

The Symptoms

The majority of the stimuli from the outside world are perceived visually, with the eyes. If accurate perception can be achieved only with exhausting work, symptoms can be considered just natural.

Eye-related symptoms that cannot be eliminated with conventional glasses include a vision that feels uncertain or forced, difficulty estimating distance, burning eyes, tearing when watching television or reading, light sensitivity, and chronic inflammations. Transient, or rarely more persistent, diplopia and spatial disorientation may also occur. A detailed neuro-ophthalmological examination is indispensable in these cases.

Since the innervation of the oculomotor muscles is closely connected to the autonomic nervous system, heterophoria often causes *autonomic symptoms* as well. It should be noted that patients visit the ophthalmologist only with symptoms specifically related to vision, and do not even suspect an ophthalmological cause in case of other problems. The evaluation of the symptoms is determined by the degree of the defect, the individual sensitivity, the physical-mental status, and other circumstances. Autonomic symptoms most often present as *headache*. These may often worsen to a migraine episode (sometimes accompanied by vomiting). At other times, the main symptom is dizziness, a feeling of uncertainty, undue tiredness or, sometimes, a transient visual field defect. Symptoms are often triggered by a physical or mental trauma or stress situation. There is often a history of a viral or other disease (especially one that is accompanied by high fever), which causes a deterioration in general condition. If the heterophoria decompensates following a trauma (such as commotion or cerebral contusion), health care professionals usually consider it as a transient consequence of that. They prescribe restricted physical activity and strengthening for the patient. In case of persistent symptoms, experience shows that they advise a change in work or a request for (disability) pension. If the above symptoms occur, detailed neurological and medical investigations have the priority but if they do not find abnormalities, examinations for heterophoria must be performed.

Examination of Heterophoria, Diagnostic Problems

Ophthalmologists already knew in the nineteenth century that if the image of the fixated object was projected onto the center of the retina in the resting position of the deviating eye, the symptoms related to heterophoria would be gone. Prism glasses that suit the angle of deviation are designed exactly for this purpose. (Prism glasses change the direction of the light ray in accordance with their strength.)

The only objective examination method is the *cover test*, which is actually suitable for ruling out strabismus only. In case of strabismus, the uncovered eye shows movement when the leading eye is covered but returns to its original position when the cover is removed. There is no fusion stimulus while the cover is in place. The alternate cover test involves covering and uncovering the eyes in alternation. If the result of the cover test is normal but during the alternate cover test, a movement to take up a parallel position is observed on the uncovered eye, the diagnosis is heterophoria. Observation of the movement to take up fixation may therefore provide a clue but it does not provide a usable prism diopter value.

All other options for detecting heterophoria are based on subjective reports from the patient. Since the previous century, numerous procedures have been designed to separate the images of the two eyes in the cortex, to be able to determine the direction and degree of the deviation in the line of sight/direction of one eye compared with the leading eye. All older procedures differ from the circumstances of everyday life, which leads to inaccurate measurements.

An example for this is a procedure that is still used in many places: the *Maddox rod test* (see Chap. 24 on page 217 for more information, and see Fig. 24.2a, b for a photograph of the device). A disadvantage of this procedure is that in everyday life, we see in possession of our fusion abilities, and therefore their complete elimination cannot provide information about the strength of the prism diopter to be prescribed and worn. Further disadvantages are that it determines the resting position of the eye in darkness (which differs from that under daytime circumstances) and that it does not provide the two eyes with the same visual stimulus.

Prisms prescribed based on conventional examination methods do not (or only in rare cases) eliminate the symptoms of the patient. Some textbooks still oppose the prescription of prism glasses and mention it as a last resort only. One of their arguments is that if someone starts to wear the prism glasses, the value of the prisms must be increased more and more, while the fusion ability of the patient is weakened further. This is a wrong supposition because, as already mentioned, the prism value that compensates for the heterophoria cannot exceed the deviation angle of the eye. The reason for the difference in opinions is that the exact degree of this deviation cannot be determined with traditional examination methods.

Three different tests are required for diagnosing and compensating for the stages of heterophoria. The Polatest device contains all three. Prior to the examination, the possibly required optimal monocular correction must be determined.

Test Figures of the Polatest Device and the Examination Procedure of H.- J. Haase

The problem was solved with the Polatest procedure of *H.J. Haase*. It involves dissociating the image of the two eyes with positive polarization. To this end, filters with opposing polarization (analyzers) are placed in the test frame, in front of the right and the left eye.

The device, located 5–6 m from the subject, displays test figures—also with opposing polarization for the right and the left eye – in front of a bright background. When the test field is viewed without analyzers, the zero or baseline position of the entire figure appears gray. If this is presented to the subject, it will be easier for them to notice and assess any differences. Through the analyzers, only one half of each test figure appears black when viewed with one eye, whereas the part for the other eye cannot be distinguished from the background. This solution is called *positive polarization*, where the image of the test figures is seen dissociated by the subject because of the two, separately functioning foveas. Meanwhile, peripheral stimuli have the same effect as in everyday life. The patient sees the entire environment undistorted through the analyzers, just like a car driver sees it through their polarized glasses. (The device also contains stereo figures but, unfortunately, these cannot be demonstrated.)

Interpretation of the Polatest Figures

In *Figures 1, 2, and 3*, the first pictures show the image as seen without analyzers, whereas the second and third pictures show the image as seen through the analyzer with the right eye and the left eye, respectively. Picture 4 of each figure demonstrates how a person with orthophoria (or with a heterophoria completely compensated with proper prisms) sees the image through the analyzers, binocularly. (That is, in black and in zero/baseline position.) Picture 5 of each figure shows a characteristic deviation with explanation below.

When the patient is looking through the analyzers, there is a defect in binocular vision if the patient sees one half of each test figure shifted in the lateral direction or upwards/downwards. The defect may manifest as one half of each test figure being gray or completely absent. The first figure is a cross. Since it has no part that would serve as a fusion stimulus, the (fusion-free) sensory state can be assessed with this figure. In the stage of purely motor compensation, the defect can only be diagnosed with this figure because when the patient is looking at figures that contain a fusion stimulus, the eyes involuntarily and immediately assume a parallel alignment. At the center of the other test figures (2–3, and the stereoscopic images), there is a detail that is black in itself, which can be seen with both eyes and, therefore, serves as a fusion stimulus. With these fixation disparity (FD) figures, the direction and degree of both horizontal and vertical deviations can be diagnosed well

Observing the rules of the examination, prisms of proper direction and strength are placed in the test frame until all test figures appear black and in zero position to the subject, and spatial vision becomes perfect both proximal and distal to the fixated object point.

The figures and the examination technique developed in relation to the procedure provide a

1. Cross test

1.1 *1.2* *1.3*

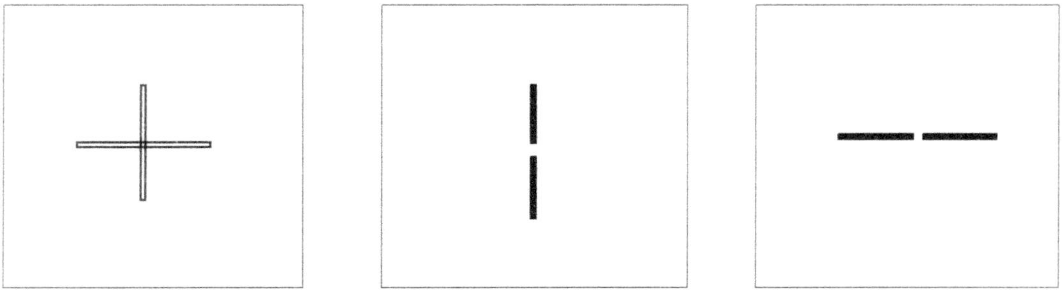

As seen without analyzer — *As seen with the right eye through analyzer* — *As seen with the left eye through analyzer*

On the subsequent figures, there is an analyzer in front of each eye

1.4

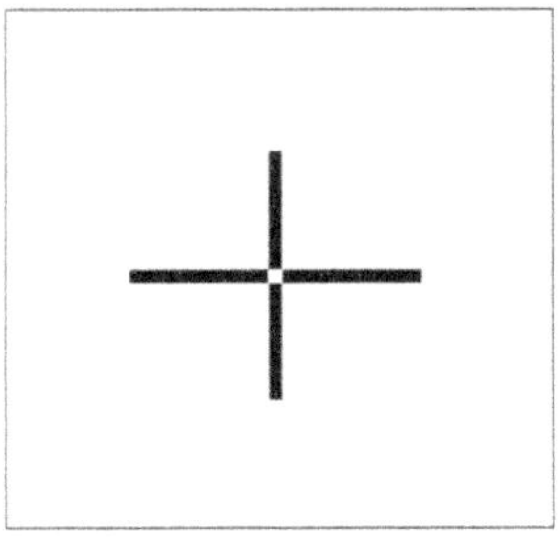

Normal alignment

1.5

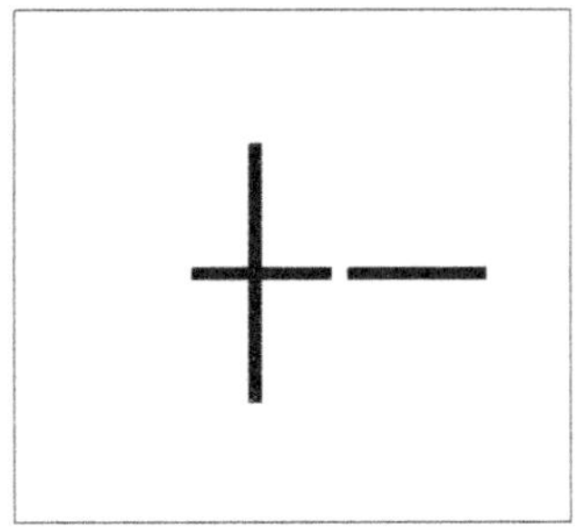

Exophoria

1.6

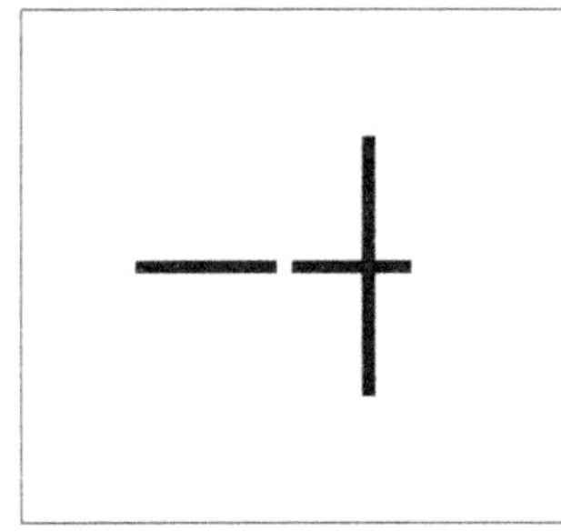

Esophoria

1.7

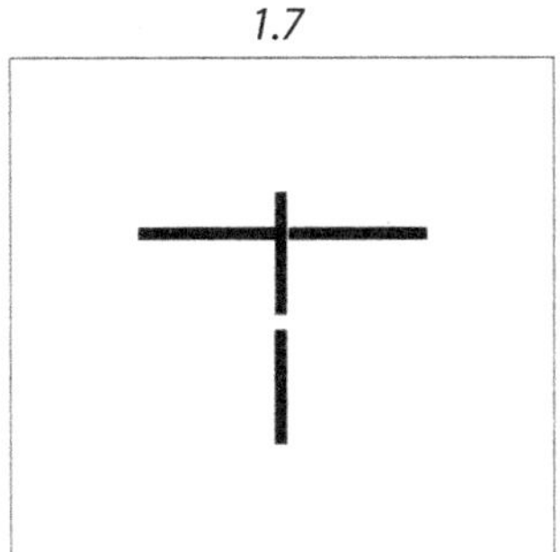

Hyperphoria, right side

1.8

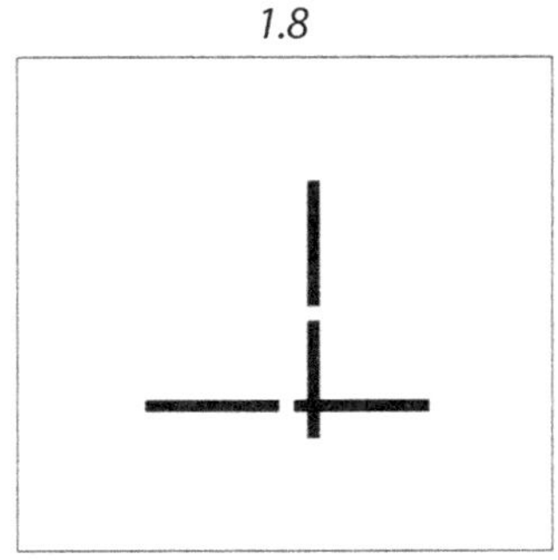

Eso- and hyperphoria, left side

firm ground for detecting all types and stages of heterophoria/angle-deviation binocular vision and, by correcting the defect (except in the case of cyclophoria), for determining the prism correction accurately. An important advantage of the procedure is that there is no harm in it whatsoever because the only thing that happens is that the patient, despite their resting alignment deviating from parallel, sees the details of the test figures, with the help of the prisms, at the same place and in the same way (in the zero/baseline position and in black) where and how they actually appear. The advantage of the procedure is that it perfectly corresponds to the circumstances of everyday life. The procedure is performed under daytime light conditions, the movement of the patient's head does not have an effect on the perception of the figures, and both eyes are provided with the same illumination, and stimuli of the same strength. The procedure detects the fixation disparity conditions that occur during binocular vision, and what is more, also the different stages of FD, which cannot be demonstrated with the conventional procedures.

According to *H.J. Haase*, who developed the procedure and its rules, the prism diopter values determined can be and should be prescribed in their completeness. Glasses with adequate correction and combined with prisms, after the potential temporary difficulties in getting used to them, are well tolerated and eliminate the symptoms caused by the heterophoria. A larger and

2. Clock test

2.1

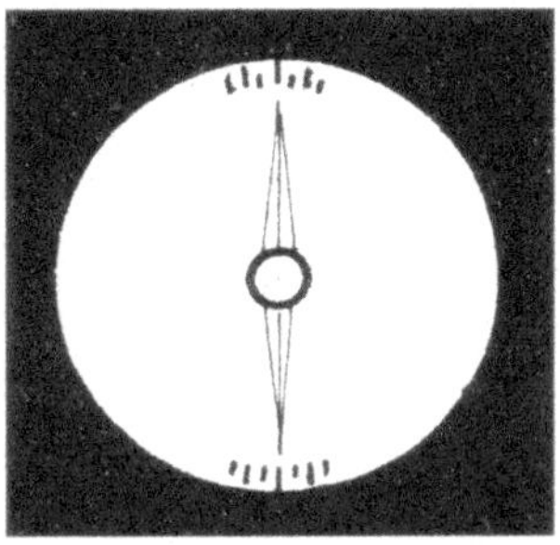

As seen without analyzer (the scales and the hands are gray)

2.2

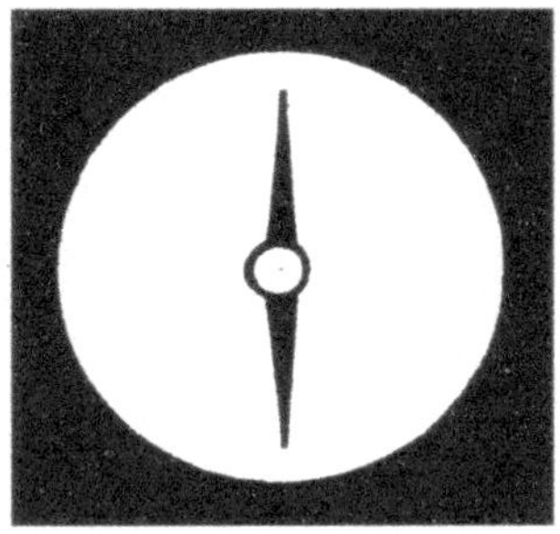

As seen with the right eye through analyzer

2.3

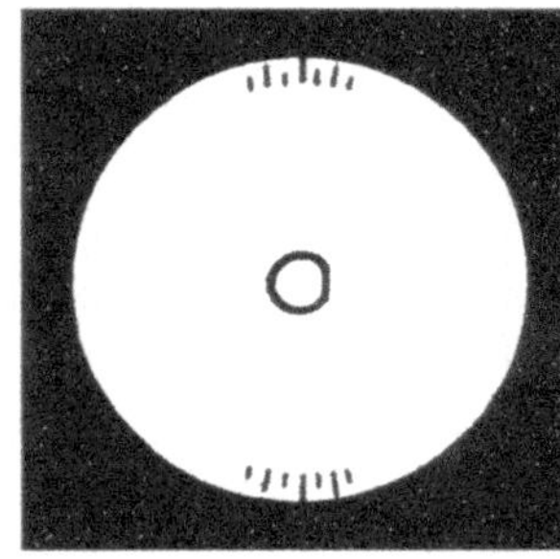

As seen with the left eye through analyzer

On the subsequent figures, there is an analyzer in front of each eye

2.4

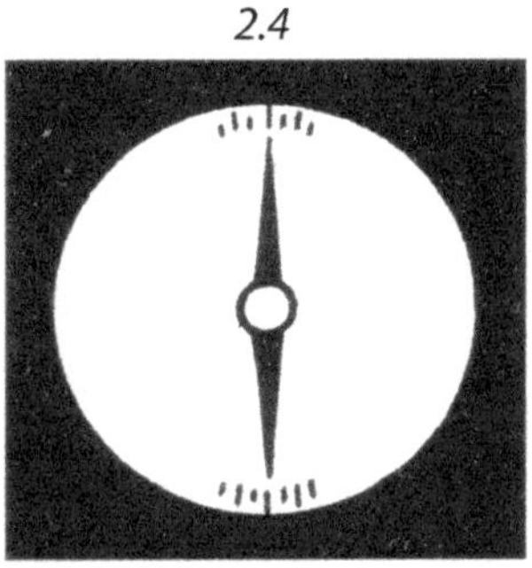

Normal alignment

2.5

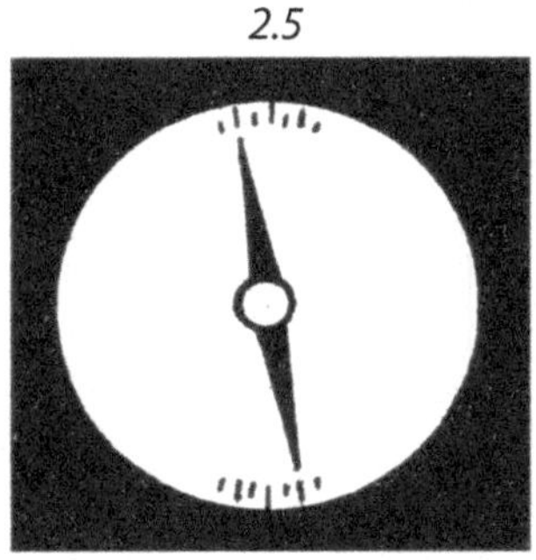

Excyclophoria

2.6

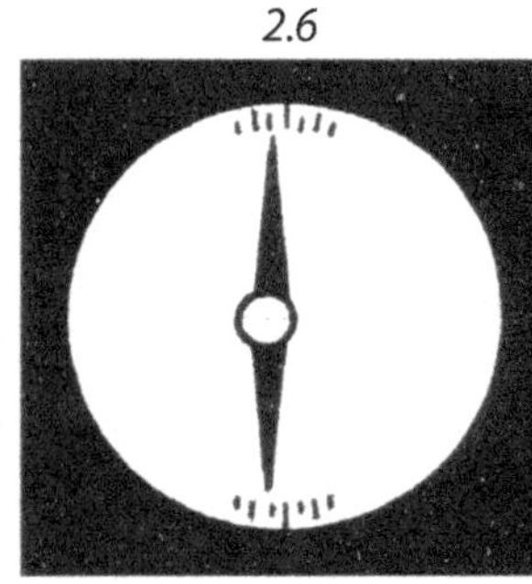

Exophoria

2.7

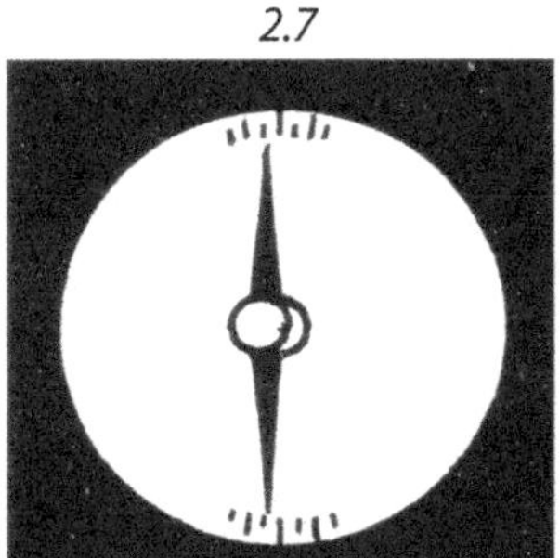

Exophoria with microdiplopia

2.8

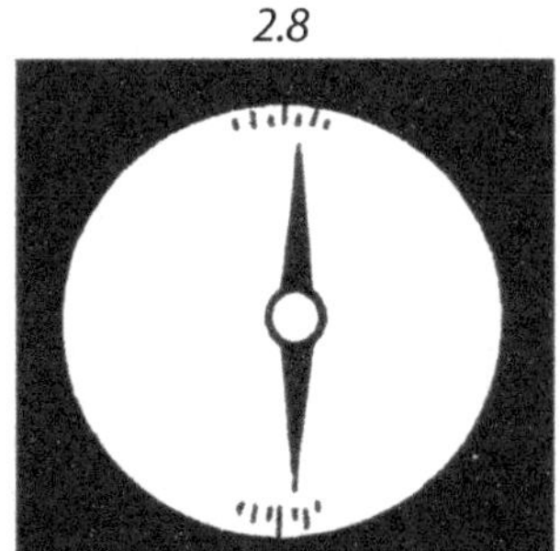

Esophoria

3. Bracket test

3.1

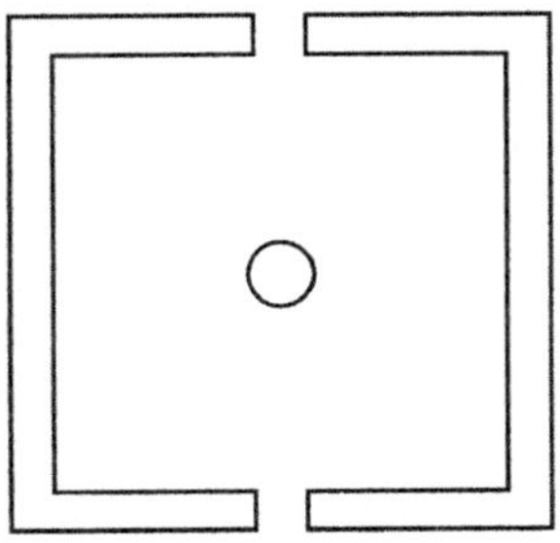

As seen without analyzer

3.2

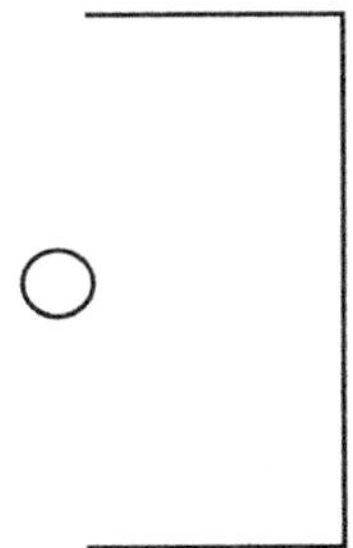

As seen with the right eye through analyzer

3.3

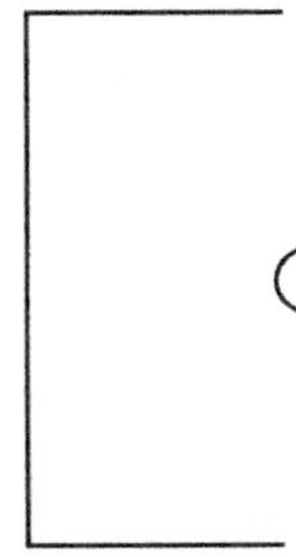

As seen with the left eye through analyzer

On the subsequent figures, there is an analyzer in front of each eye

3.4

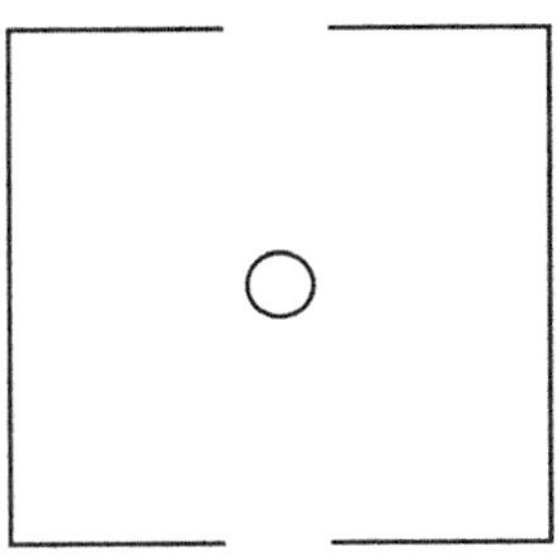

Normal alignment

3.5

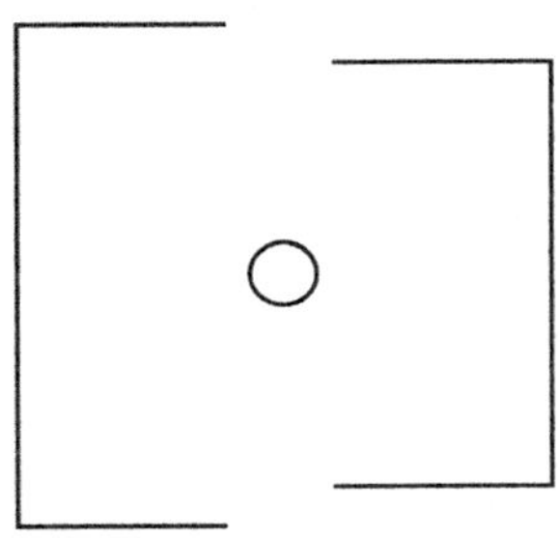

Aniseikonia (left image is greater than the right one)

3.6

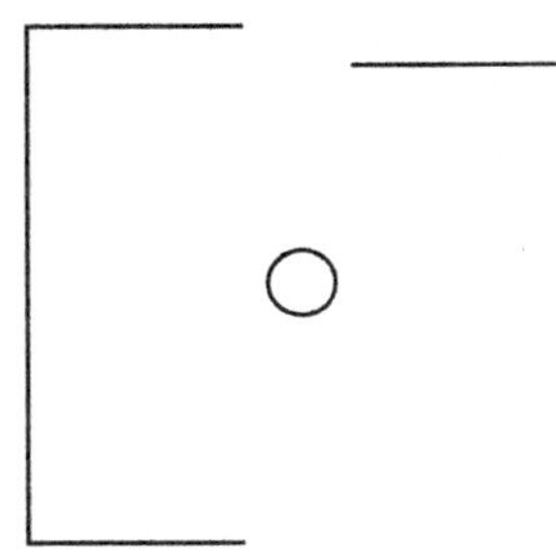

Hyperphoria

3.7

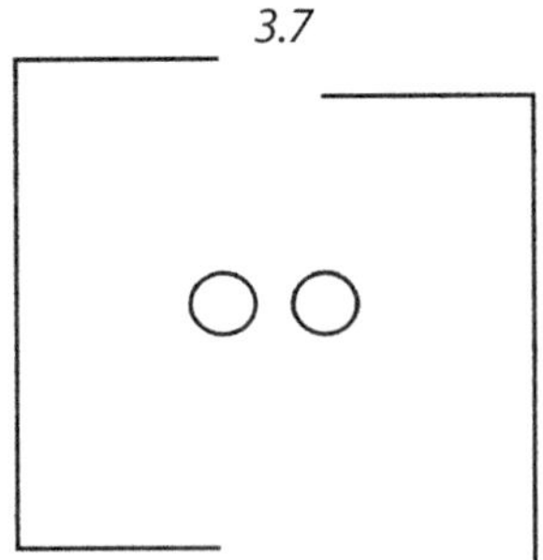

Esophoria with microdiplopia

larger portion of fusion (burdened until then) is released and the oculomotor muscles assume their resting position because the difference between their resting and work positions is compensated by the prisms.

The English and, recently, the German language literature makes a distinction between the traditional state of deviation of one eye called heterophoria and the deviation found during the examination performed under circumstances of everyday life. This is distinguished with the term 'angle-deviation binocular vision.'

The vergence system, depending on the external conditions, has different resting alignments. For example, if there is no fusion stimulus whatsoever (such as when binocular vision is deliberately interrupted), we speak of resting vergence position without fusion stimulus. The term heterophoria has always, since its first use, referred to the deviation of vergence from the ortho-alignment when the fusion is obstructed on purpose during examination. The conventional concept of heterophoria, therefore, is clearly related to the fusionfree resting vergence position. (This fusion stimulus-free resting vergence position has no importance from the optometric aspect.) The optometric resting position of vergence is the state that the vergence system intends to assume under the circumstances of natural vision, when looking at a distant fixation point. Angle-deviation binocular vision is a state of binocular vision where the optometric resting position of vergence does not matches the ortho-alignment. This is to be determined with the examination of angle-deviation binocular vision.

The purpose of optometric correction is to find the optimal glasses correction that is in accordance with the conditions of natural vision. To this end, the resting position of the vergence system with fusion stimuli (the optometric resting position of vergence) must be determined. This is achieved by using the figures with central parts that provide a fusion stimulus during the fixation disparity tests of the Polatest procedure.

Based on the above, the concept of angle-deviation binocular vision differs considerably from that of heterophoria, and they should not be confused with each other in the future.

Further Readings

Haase H-J. Über binokulare Prüfverfahren. Der Augenoptiker 10 (1957) bis1 (1961).

Haase H-J. Binokulare Korrktion. "Optometrie." Heft 2, 3, 4. Berlin: Verlag Deutsche Gesellschaft für Optometrie; 1959.

Haase H-J. Grenzfälle der heterophorie-Korrektion "Optometrie." Heft 1, 2. Berlin: Verlag Deutsche Gesselschaft für Optometrie; 1960.

Goersch H. Die drei Notwendigen Testarten dzur vollständigen Heterophoriebestimmung. Heidelberg: Dtsh Opticerz.; 1978/11.

Goersch H. Einführung in das Binokularsehem. Der Augenoptiker: 1980/12; 1981; 1982; 1982; 1984; 1988.

Goersch H. Dekompensierte Heterophorien und ihre Auswirkungen auf das Sehen. Der Augenoptiker. 1978;5:13–23.

Goersch H. Sensorische Abweichungen vom idealen Binukularsehen. NOJ 1979/2: 8, NOJ 1987/11.

Haase H-J. Zur Fixationsdisparation. Der Augenoptiker Heft. 1980;6:17–21.

Goersch H. Fixationdisparation erster und zweiter Art. NOJ. 1987/11.

Goersch H. Stereopsis unter phorischer Belastung. Deutsche Optikerzeitung. Heidelberg. 1982/9.

Pestalozzi D. Resultate binokularer Vollkorrektion versus konventionelle Methoden. Klin Monatsbl Für Augenheilkunde. 1991;198:464–9.

Pintér K. Miozin izoformák a harántcsíkolt izmok rostjaiban [Myosin isoforms in skeletal muscle fibers]. Kandidátusi értekezés. 1983.

Physiology and Examination Methods of the Pupillomotor Pathway

23

Bernadett Salomváry

Contents

For ophthalmologists, examination of the pupillomotor pathway starts with screening for the conditions of the intraocular segment. Neurologists, during the routine examination of the cranial nerves, regularly use the examination methods of the pupillomotor pathway. In topographical diagnostics, knowing the physiological phenomena and the examination methods is important for both ophthalmologists and neurologists.

Anatomy

The pupil is the aperture of the iris and a kinetic indicator of the functional status of the adjacent tissues and of a special sensory apparatus, the retina. The neural mechanisms which control pupil size and reactivity are highly complex but the examination of the pupil with simple clinical methods may provide important information.

The dynamics of the pupil are influenced by the amount of light that reaches the retina, the integrity of the retinal receptors and afferent axons in the optic nerve, the mesencephalic nuclei and the interconnecting neurons, and the efferent parasympathetic pathway. In addition, supranuclear influences from the frontal and occipital cortices, the sympathetic nervous system and the brainstem reticular formation also have an important role in controlling the pupil. The importance of pupil symptoms is that a lesion in any of the above structures usually causes a pupil defect as well.

The iris, among the optical elements of the eyes, serves as a diaphragm. Its main task is to control the amount of light that reaches the retina by changing the diameter of the pupil. This function is enabled by its muscles, the circular part of which is the sphincter, whereas the radial part is the dilator of the pupil. Contrary to the classic view, recent studies suggest that both the sphincter and the dilator muscles receive sympathetic and parasympathetic fibers. The innervation of the sphincter muscle is mainly parasympathetic, whereas that of the dilator muscle is predominantly sympathetic. The primary factor during the dilation of the pupil is not a sympathetic stimulation but the supranuclear inhibition of the parasympathetic innervation.

The afferent pupillomotor pathway starts at the retinal photoreceptors, since the photoreceptors of

B. Salomváry, M.D.
Head of Department, Head Physician Ophthalmologist, Neuro-ophthalmologist, Orbital Surgeon, National Institute of Neurology, Budapest, Hungary

Neuro-Ophthalmology Section, Hungarian Ophthalmological Association, Budapest, Hungary
e-mail: salom.betty@gmail.com

J. Somlai, T. Kovács (eds.), *Neuro-Ophthalmology*, DOI 10.1007/978-3-319-28956-4_23

the retina likely have a pupillomotor activity. In the chiasm, the pupillomotor fibers, similarly to the optic tract, partially cross, and then their course until the lateral geniculate body is the same as that of the optic tract. In the posterior third of the optic tract, before the lateral geniculate body, the pupillomotor fibers detach from the optic fibers, and are relayed to an interconnecting neuron in the pretectal region that corresponds to the superior colliculus. The axons that start from here make a turn in the medial direction and, after mostly crossing in the posterior commissure, run in part to the contralateral pretectal nucleus, and in part to the ipsilateral and in small part to the contralateral Edinger–Westphal (EW) nucleus. The afferent limb of the light reflex arc of the pupil, therefore, reaches the EW nucleus after three partial crossings. Based on this, it is clear that the light reflex of either pupil can be evoked from any of the retinal halves. The preganglionic fibers from the EW nucleus join the fibers from the somatomotor nuclei of the 3rd cranial nerve, and leave the mesencephalon ventrally, at the inferior-lateral wall of the interpeduncular fossa. The oculomotor nerve runs between the posterior cerebral artery and the superior cerebellar artery, parallel to the posterior communicating artery. The nerve runs between the free edge of the tentorium and the lateral side of the posterior clinoid process, and then, before perforating the dura, crosses the sphenopetrosal ligament and enters the cavernous sinus. It is located in the upper part of the cavernous sinus, directly above the trochlear nerve. Later on, the trochlear nerve and the ophthalmic nerve get to the top. The pupillomotor fibers are located superficially in the oculomotor nerve, directly beneath the epineurium. This explains the high sensitivity of the pupillomotor fibers to compression.

The oculomotor nerve passes through the superior orbital fissure, and then divides into two branches before entering the orbita. The superior branch runs laterally to the optic nerve and supplies the superior rectus and the levator palpebrae superioris. The inferior branch supplies the inferior rectus, the medial rectus and the inferior oblique. The parasympathetic preganglionic fibers form the oculomotor root of the ciliary ganglion, and they are relayed in the ganglion. The parasympathetic postganglionic fibers enter the eyeball as 6–10 short ciliary nerves, near the exit of the optic nerve. The nerve fibers run between the sclera and the choroidea, in the suprachoroidal space, and after further divisions, they end in the iris and the ciliary body. By innervating the sphincter muscle, they have a partial pupillomotor function, and by supplying the ciliary muscle, they also have a role in the control of accommodation (Fig. 23.1).

The dilator muscle is supplied by three neurons. The sympathetic nucleus system, the ciliospinal center, is located in the lateral grey column of the spinal cord between C8 and T2. From here, the axons leave the spinal cord through the anterior root. The preganglionic fibers, through the communicating branches, run upwards in the cervical segment of the sympathetic chain, and are relayed in the superior cervical ganglion. The sympathetic chain is in close contact with the pleura of the apex of lung, and the fibers go around the subclavian artery. The postganglionic fibers enter the skull accompanying the internal carotid artery and, through the cavernous sinus, reach the orbita along the artery, where they form the sympathetic root of the ciliary ganglion. Passing through the ganglion without being relayed, they reach the uveal structures as short and long ciliary nerves (Fig. 23.2).

The afferent pathway to the ciliospinal center is not completely clarified. The central sympathetic pathway starts from the posterior lateral hypothalamus. The fibers reach the ciliospinal center of the spinal cord via the mesencephalic reticular formation, without crossing. The sympathetic nerves in part have a vasomotor and sudomotor function (innervating the lacrimal glands), and in part provide sympathetic innervation to certain muscles, such as the dilator pupillae, the superior and inferior tarsal and the orbitalis muscles. The fibers that run towards the sweat glands of the face follow the ipsilateral common carotid artery but detach from it before it enters the skull, and continue along the external carotid artery.

Supranuclear pathway of the accommodation reflex: when focusing on a near object, the accommodation of the lens and the convergence is accompanied by miosis. This is not a reflex but rather a synkinesis. When focusing on a near object, the medial rectus muscles, the ciliary

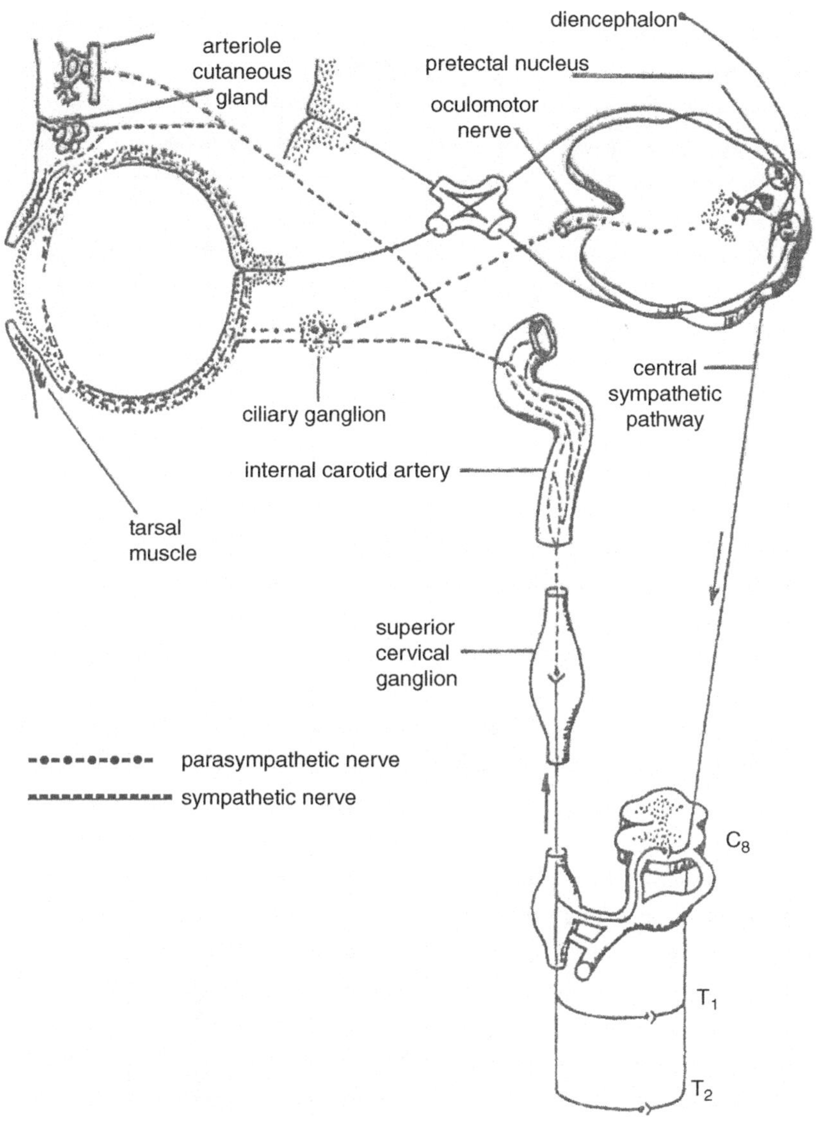

Fig. 23.1 Sympathetic and parasympathetic innervation of the intraocular muscles (Redrawn after Peter Duus: *Topical Diagnosis in Neurology*. 1989. p. 100 Fig. 3.26, Springer)

muscles and the sphincter pupillae muscles become innervated simultaneously on both sides. These three movements can be triggered by voluntary on a nearby object. The afferent pathway likely starts in the retina, and runs with the optic tract into the area striata. From here the efferent impulses, proceed over the pretectal area (although the nuclei are not involved in the synkinesis), to a group of parasympathetic nuclei, called Perlia's nuclei located at the midline ventral to the EW nuclei. This nucleus sends impulses to the neurons that supply the medial rectus on both sides and to the EW nuclei, which supplies the sphincter pupillae and the ciliaris through the ciliary ganglion. The central connections to the ciliary muscle and to the sphincter muscle of the pupils are probably not the same, since the pupillary reflex for accommodation and that to light may be impaired separately. This can be observed for example in the case of Argyll Robertson pupils.

Normal Pupil – Physiological Variations

The diameter of the pupil is 7.5–8 mm in full mydriasis and 1.5–2 mm in full miosis. The resting pupil

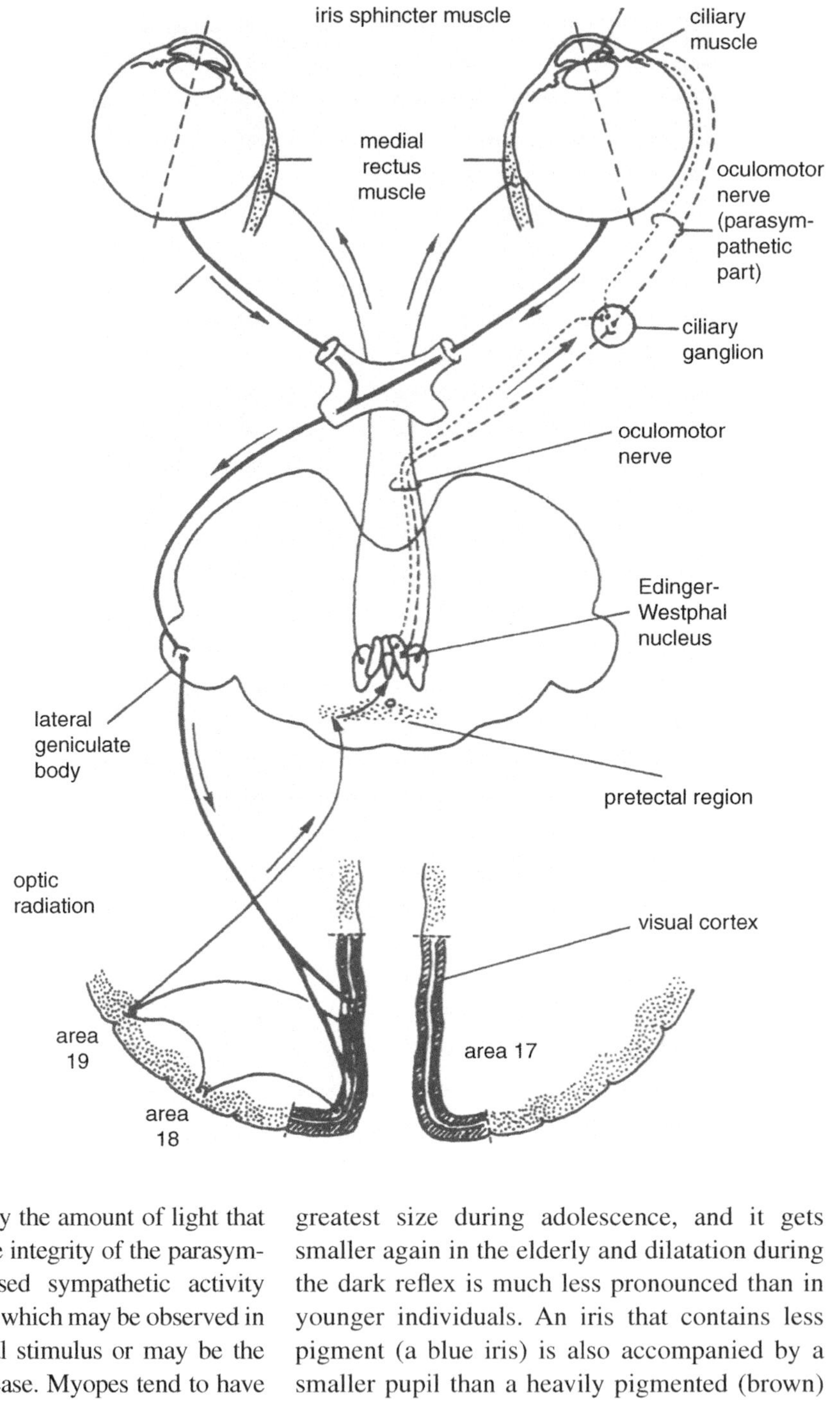

Fig. 23.2 The central pathways of convergence and accommodation (Redrawn after Peter Duus: *Topical Diagnosis in Neurology*. 1989. p. 97. Fig. 3.23, Springer)

diameter is determined by the amount of light that reaches the retina and the integrity of the parasympathetic system. Increased sympathetic activity results in mild mydriasis, which may be observed in response to an emotional stimulus or may be the symptom of Graves' disease. Myopes tend to have larger pupils than emmetropes and hyperopes.

The diameter of the pupil also depends on age. In the first year of life, the pupil is small because the dilator pupillae is poorly developed in the newborn and even adrenergic drugs produce very little mydriasis at that age. The pupil attains its greatest size during adolescence, and it gets smaller again in the elderly and dilatation during the dark reflex is much less pronounced than in younger individuals. An iris that contains less pigment (a blue iris) is also accompanied by a smaller pupil than a heavily pigmented (brown) iris. The diameter of the pupil of an emmetropic eye does not have an effect on visual acuity. In case of uncorrected ametropia, however, visual acuity shows a pronaunced dependence on pupil size, the degree of this dependence increasing with the degree of the refractive error.

Essential (Physiological, Simple) Anisocoria

Almost everyone has a certain degree of anisocoria, and it can be demonstrated clinically in 17 % of the population but the difference is pronounced in only about 4 %. The diagnosis of essential anisocoria can be made only after ruling out other causes and abnormal conditions. Pupil reactions are always normal, and no abnormal reactions can be observed during pharmacological tests either. The difference in diameter between the two pupils is quite constant and independent of illumination. It is not unusual that someone suddenly discovers their pupil asymmetry that has been present for a long time. In this case, the examination of old photographs may help.

Examination of the Pupillary Diameter

The simplest device is the Haab scale, which has black circles of gradually increasing size painted on it. These are compared with the pupil of the subject. Pupillography is a more modern examination, which involves the registration of the diameter or the area of the pupil under specified illumination conditions. The examination is performed using infrared photography or a photoelectric method. If a pupillary defect is observed, *local ophthalmological lesions* must be ruled out first: congenital disorders, e.g., corectopia when the pupil is not in the central position and not round; microcoria, which is due to the absence of the dilator pupillae, and causes extreme miosis; and colobomas and aniridia.

The inflammatory processes of the iris are accompanied by a small pupil. An irregular pupil developed during iritis is due to the presence of posterior synechiae. The pupil is large and irregular during an acute angle-closure glaucoma. The tumors of the iris may also lead to an irregular pupil. Contusion injuries of the eyeball, may cause cracks in the sphincter of the iris, which may lead to zig-zagged pupils. The iris may be torn away from its attachment at a circumscribed site (iridodialysis) or a circumferencial iris root avulsion may result in complete absence of the iris (aniridia). A trauma may cause either mydriasis or miosis. Mydriasis is more common and is due to the injury of the short ciliary nerve fibers in the choroidea (post-traumatic iridoplegia).

Physiological Pupillary Reactions

When the eye is illuminated, the pupil shows constriction, this is the *direct light reaction*. The degree and the speed of the constriction depend on the brightness and wavelength of the light, its duration and the adaptation state of the retina. It is examined with a point-like source of light, under dim light conditions, while the patient is fixating at a far distance. The speed and degree of the constriction, and its duration must be observed.

Together with the pupillary reaction of the illuminated eye, the same reaction is evoked in the other eye, this is the *indirect or consensual light reaction*. The reflex is bilateral because both retinas are connected to both optic tracts, and both optic tracts are connected to both oculomotor nuclei.

When the two eyes are illuminated simultaneously, the direct and indirect reactions add up, i.e. the miosis is greater than in the case of monocular illumination. If, after illuminating one eye, the other one is illuminated, the pupil of the first eye shows further constriction, which is called Weiler's secondary light reaction. In response to long-term illumination, the diameter of the pupil gradually becomes stable after large initial oscillations. This is the tonic pupillary reaction. A short illumination induces a short pupillomotor reaction. Constriction is followed by pupil dilation, which is the transient or phasic light reflex. Similarly to the tonic pupillary reaction, this reflex is also consensual.

A quick examination of the afferent pupillomotor pathway, which can be performed even at the bedside, is the *swinging-flashlight test*, which indicates even a mild disorder. The examination compares the direct and consensual light reactions of the given pupil. In case of unilateral optic nerve lesion, the direct reaction results in a lower degree of miosis than the consensual reaction from the unaffected side. In a dimly lit room, the pupils of the patient are illumined with a strong light in alternation. If the light is directed on the unaffected eye, both pupils show constriction. If the light is returned to the affected eye, both pupils show dilation. The *convergence and accommodation reactions* of the pupil are physiological pupil reactions. Fixation at a near object results in convergence, accommodation and pupil constriction, i.e., the three-component physiological synkinesis. It is examined by instructing the patient to fixate at a near object and observing whether the eyeballs are converging, the pupils are showing miosis and the patient has sharp near vision. Convergence and accommodation are reduced in the elderly. The light and accommodation reaction of the pupil are usually impaired simultaneously, isolated impairment is rare. This latter is seen in case of Argyll Robertson pupils.

The lid closure *pupil reaction* is also a synkinesis. Pupillary contraction occur whenever the eyelids are suddenly and temporarily closed, whether voluntarily or involuntarily.

Pharmacology of the Pupils

Agents acting on the pupils have an effect on either the dilator pupillae through the sympathetic nervous system, or the sphincter pupillae through the parasympathetic innervation. Of the *adrenergic agents*, epinephrine and phenylephrine act by binding directly to the sympathetic receptors. Cocaine increases the effect of endogenous norepinephrine by inhibiting its re-uptake into the sympathetic end-plate. Tyramine, ephedrine and hydroxyamphetamine mobilize the stored endogenous norepinephrine.

- *Antiadrenergic agents* cause miosis by inhibiting the sympathetic nerve–dilator muscle system, blocking the sympathetic transmission. These include guanethidine, which is an adrenergic neuron blocker. It accumulates in the end-plates of adrenergic neurons, and reduces the release of norepinephrine, thus inhibiting these neurons.
- Cholinergic agents may stimulate the oculomotor nerve–sphincter pupillae system with two different mechanisms: directly, acting similarly to the natural mediator (acetylcholine, pilocarpine, carbachol, mecholyl), or indirectly, by inhibiting cholinesterase (physostigmine, prostigmin, tosmilen, mintachol, phospholine iodide).

Anticholinergic agents specifically inhibit the effect of acetylcholine that is released from the parasympathetic end-plate. Tropane alka-

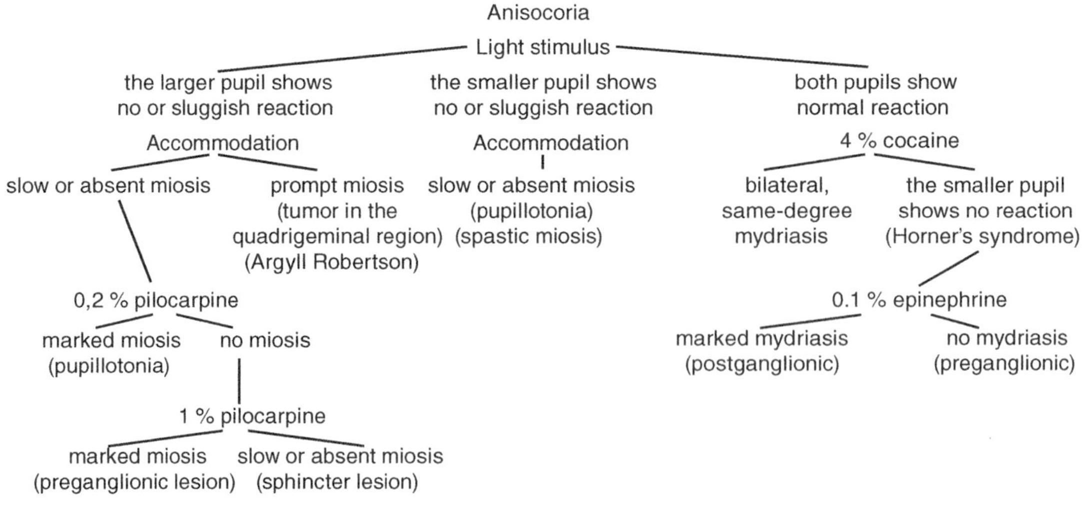

Fig. 23.3 Differential diagnostics of anisocoria (Redrawn after Alexandridis: *The Pupil* p. 69 Fig. 33, Springer 1988)

loids, such as atropine, scopolamine and homatropine, bind to the acetylcholine-sensitive receptors of the effector cell, and competitively inhibit the effect of acetylcholine. They cause not only pupil dilation but also a smaller or larger degree of cycloplegia.

In case of *anisocoria* (Fig. 23.3), usually the lesion of the efferent pupillomotor pathway is supposed. The first step during the examination is to determine if the difference between the two pupils increases in darkness by a further dilation of the wide pupil, or if it decreases due to the dilation of the narrow pupil. In the first case, the narrow pupil is abnormal, whereas in the second case, it is the wide pupil that is impaired. If the wide pupil is abnormal, the disorder should be looked for in the parasympathetic nervous system or the muscles of the iris. If the pupil shows no (or only decreased) reaction to light and accommodation, the lesion may be localized with a pharmacological test.

- The *pilocarpine test* is based on the fact that a 0.2 % solution of pilocarpine normally does not cause notable miosis. A marked pupil constriction indicates the denervation hypersensitivity of the muscle receptor. The lesion in such cases is postganglionic, and pupillotonia can be diagnosed. If the pupil shows no reaction to the diluted pilocarpine, the lesion must be located in the 1st neuron of the oculomotor nerve or in the iris musculature. The question is resolved by instilling 1 % pilocarpine drops into both eyes. If miosis occurs on both sides, the lesion affects the 1st neuron of the oculomotor nerve, and if the pupil shows little or no reaction compared with the unaffected eye, the lesion is located in the iris muscle. In case of pupillotonia, the increased sensitivity to pilocarpine is demonstrated with the *cocaine–pilocarpine test*. Thirty minutes after the administration of 2 % cocaine drops into both eyes, 0.5 % pilocarpine (or 0.75 % carbachol) drops are administered. In case of pupillotonia, both mydriasis and miosis will be of higher degree than in the unaffected eye (Fig. 23.4; Table 23.1).

If both pupils react briskly to light, two possibilities exist: simple anisocoria (without pathological significance) or Horner's syndrome. To find out, 4 % *cocaine drops* are administered into both eyes. If both pupils respond with mydriasis, the anisocoria does not indicate pathologic significance. If the originally small pupil shows no or only slight dilation, the

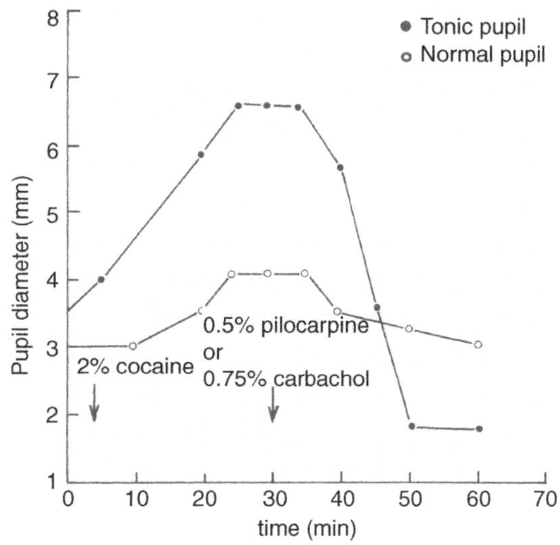

Fig. 23.4 Cocaine–pilocarpine test in pupillotonia (Redrawn after Alexandridis: *The Pupil* p. 70. Fig. 34. Springer 1988)

Table 23.1 Pharmacological tests in Horner's syndrome

	Intact sympathetic pathway	Impaired sympathetic pathway		
		Preganglionic		Postganglionic
		1st neuron	2nd neuron	3rd neuron
4 % cocaine	Mydriasis	Slight mydriasis	No change	No change
0.1 % epinephrine	Mild mydriasis or no change	No change	Very mild mydriasis or no change	Mydriasis
1 % hydroxyamphetamine	Mydriasis	Mydriasis	Mydriasis	No change

Table 23.2 Pupil disorders in neuro-ophthalmological conditions

	General properties	Light and accommodation (convergence) reaction	More pronounced anisocoria	Effect of mydriatic agents	Effect of miotic agents	Effect of mydriatic agents
Essential anisocoria	Round, regular	Good reaction to both	No change	Dilation	Constriction	
Horner's syndrome	Round, unilateral	Good reaction to both	In darkness	Dilation	Constriction	4 % cocaine, 0.1 % epinephrine, Paredrin
Pupillotonia (Holmes-Adie)	Usually more dilated in daylight, unilateral in 90 %	No reaction to light, prolonged reaction to convergence, tonic redilation	In daylight	Dilation	Constriction	0.2 % pilocarpin-test
Argyil-Robertson	Small, irregular, bilateral	No reaction to light, intact convergence reaction	No change	No dilation	Constriction	
Mesencephalic lesions	Submaximally dilated, bilateral	No or sluggish reaction to light and convergence	No change	Dilation	Constriction	
Effect of atropin	Maximally dilated, round	Fixed pupil	In daylight		No constriction	No constriction to 1 % pilocarpine
Oculomotor nerve palsy (non-diabetic)	Submaximally dilated, unilateral, rarely bilateral	Fixed pupil	In daylight	Dilation	Constriction	

diagnosis is Horner's syndrome. The next step is to locate the lesion (Fig. 23.1): *0.1 % epinephrine (adrenaline)* has no effect on an intact pupil but in case of Horner's syndrome, it causes marked mydriasis on the affected side if the lesion is located at the level of the 3rd neuron (postganglionic), indicating denervation hypersensitivity. When *1 % hydroxyamphetamine (Paredrin) drops* are administered, both pupils show dilation in case of a preganglionic lesion. In case of a not-too-recent lesion of the postganglionic sympathetic segment, the norepinephrine storages are depleted, hydroxyamphetamine is unable to release norepinephrine, and the pupil remains small on the affected side (Table 23.2).

Further Readings

Alexandridis E. The pupil. New York: Springer; 1988.

Collins JF. Handbook of clinical ophthalmology. New York: Masson Pub; 1982.

Duus P. Topical diagnosis in neurology. Stuttgart: Georg Thieme Verlag; 1983.

Glaser JS. Neuroophthalmology. Hagerstown: Harper and Row; 1978.

Huber A. Eye symptoms in brain tumors. Saint Luis: CV. Mosby; 1971.

Mumenthaler M. Neurológia [Neurology]. Budapest: Medicina Kiadó; 1989.

Patten J. Neurological differential diagnosis. London: Harold Starke; 1977.

Somlai J. Neuroophthalmologia [Neuro-ophthalmology]. Budapest: Literatura Medica Kiadó; 1996.

Somlai J. Neuroophthalmologia [Neuro-ophthalmology]. Budapest: PressCon Kiadó; 2007.

Neuro-ophthalmological Methods for the Clinical Analysis of Double Vision

24

Judit Somlai

Contents

Bedside Eye Movement Examinations

The first task at the bedside, regardless of whether that patient is unconscious or of intact consciousness, is to establish whether the ***palpebral fissures are identical***. It is assessed if there is incomplete or complete ptosis, if eye opening is unilateral or bilateral, and if there is abnormal contraction of the eyelid (blepharospasm). The second step is to observe the ***primary position***, i.e., if the two eyes looking straight ahead are parallel or they are misaligned in the horizontal or vertical plane. Is any type of nystagmus visible already when looking straight ahead? ***State of the pupils*** before the reflex tests: whether they are identical in size (isocoria), and whether one or both are constricted–dilated are important information, and eye drops that affect pupillary function must never be used, especially in case of an altered level of consciousness. Evoking and accurately recording the ***pupillomotor functions***, i.e., the direct and indirect pupillary reflexes are among the most important parts of neurointensive care and the first neurological examination. Unilateral pupil dilation with decreased indirect reaction (anisocoria) can be decisive already at the bedside, since it may be the leading and first symptom of higher intracranial pressure (HIP), even without papilledema or other symptoms. In conscious patients: the examination of *smooth pursuit* and *saccadic eye movements*, and the *optokinetic reflex test (OKN)* are of differential diagnostic value in the distinction between the dysfunctions of the *slow* pursuit supranuclear oculomotor system.

Outpatient Neuro-ophthalmological Examinations of Eye Movement Disorders

The sudden-onset symptoms of the patients that start with intolerable double vision make them to visit either an ophthalmologist or a neurologist for an outpatient examination. Taking a detailed ***history*** is therefore extremely important. A marked or

J. Somlai, M.D.
Unit of Neuro-Ophthalmology, Department of Neurology & Stroke, Military Hospital, Budapest, Hungary

Neuro-Ophthalmology Section, Hungarian Ophthalmological Association, Budapest, Hungary

Trustee, NOSZA Foundation (for the Prevention and Screening of Ocular Storke), Budapest, Hungary
e-mail: dr@somlaijudit.hu; http://somlaijudit.hu

J. Somlai, T. Kovács (eds.), *Neuro-Ophthalmology*, DOI 10.1007/978-3-319-28956-4_24

symmetric image displacement is the first sign of neurogenic paresis. An incomplete gaze paresis rather causes a spatial perception or fixation disorder, reading disability and dizziness. A diurnal variation of image displacement, or difficulty swallowing or breathing may indicate a neuro – muscular or myogenic origin. In addition to the bedside examinations listed above (such as the establishment of whether the palpebral fissures are identical, their measurement, primary position, pupil status, pupil reactions), more detailed and, principally, instrumental examinations and measurements are performed at the outpatient clinic.

Examination Algorithm of the Pupillomotor Functions

- Examination of direct and indirect pupil reactions
- Assessment of pupil constriction during induced convergence; it is the consensual pupillary reflex
- Topographical diagnostics of the lesions in the parasympathetic afferent and efferent pupillomotor pathways with conventional reflex tests and pharmacological tests
- Topographical diagnostics of the three-neuron sympathetic pupillomotor pathways with conventional and drop tests

Examination of the Eye Movements

First, the *conjugate, Slow Eye Movement (SEM) system* is assessed by instructing the patient to look in the nine gaze directions and fixate at an object 30–35 cm away, and observing:

- whether eye movements are conjugate when looking in a given gaze direction
- if there is movement to take up fixation during the alternating cover test (when fusion is suspended)
- which gaze direction(s) is (are) characterized by lagging behind – paresis
- the near triad (instructing the patient to fixate at a near object):
  - bilateral decrease in adduction
  - pupil constriction during induced convergence (consensual pupil reaction)
  - lens adduction (can only be assessed by diopter measurement)

Fast – saccadic – eye movements *(Fast Eye Movement system, FEM)* are assessed by instructing the patient to fixate in alternation at an object point 30 cm away, both in the horizontal and the vertical planes.

Optokinetic nystagmus (OKN) test With a revolving cylinder that has even stripes on it, the smooth pursuit and fast refixation movements are observed. This examination enables the examination of both the FEM and the SEM systems.

Double vision tests enable the measurement of the degree of the image displacement due to the eye movement disorder and, indirectly, the assessment of the type of the eye movement disorder.

Cover test The eyes of the patient are covered separately and then in alternation, and the fixation or (after the suspension of binocular vision, i.e., the fusion ability) the movement to take up fixation helps detect the direction of the movement disorder of the paretic ocular muscle(s). The direction in which the gaze of the eye that takes up fixation moves is the direction in which the patient has difficulty pulling the eyeball, i.e., it '*points at the direction of the paresis*.' For example, in case of abducens nerve palsy, the eyeball moves outwards, i.e., in the direction of the decreased abduction when the cover is removed. At the same time, this simple test helps distinguish between peripheral and central palsies. This is because a disorder indicated by the monocular cover test is rather typical of peripheral palsy, whereas if an abnormality is found during the alternating cover test, a central eye movement disorder should be considered first.

Prism bar set combined with cover test While the changing diopter of the prism bar is moved in front of the patient, the disappearance of the movement to take up fixation during the cover test indicates the diopter which can eliminate paretic strabismus. This way, paretic strabismus (that is, heterotropia) can not only be measured but also improved with the proper correction (see Table 11.3 on page 75).

Maddox lens and rotary prism Disconjugate eye movement disorders or gazing palsies due to brainstem dysfunction can be quantified in the horizontal, the vertical and even an oblique plane. It requires a higher level of cooperation from the patient, and it is not a widespread method in the assessment of neurological patients in Hungary.

Hess screen test This is an examination tool for the double vision and eye movement disorder that occurs when the patient is fixating at distant points. Through red-green glasses, the patient is looking at specified points of the Hess screen that is 80–90 cm away. These test points are illuminated with a red light, and the patient projects a green light source given to them onto the test points. In the straight ahead gaze direction, the patient marks for at least nine points where they think the red and green lights meet. The points marked by the patient are copied by the examiner onto the paper copy of the Hess screen, plotting a diagram by the end of the examination, which shows whether the patient directs their gaze at the same or different points compared with the normal positions. (See Fig. 24.1 of this chapter and Chap. 21 on page 171).

The solid black-printed line is the normal, orthophoric position, and the displaced points of the left and right eyes of the patient are marked with a red line. This procedure is suitable not only for making the diagnosis but also for measuring the efficacy of the prism correction used for the elimination of double vision.

Handheld Maddox wing (near diplopia test) The patient is fixating at near object points in the horizontal, and then the vertical plane, and if they are unable to maintain the images of the two eyes in fusion, it indicates an ocular muscle dysfunction that occurs during convergence (Fig. 24.2).

If this phenomenon occurs in the horizontal plane, it indicates abduction paresis or convergent (inward) squinting, or adduction paresis or divergent (outward) squinting of the two eyes. (These are esophoria and exophoria, respectively.) When the same happens in the vertical plane, the position of the more elevated eye can be measured in relation to the lower position of the other eye due to the gaze elevation disorder (hyperphoria and hypophoria). The double vision due to the asymmetric movement of the two eyes can be measured numerically and followed with this device, and it also helps measure the correction effect of the prism prescribed to eliminate the diplopia due to the eye movement disorder. For example, in case of a weak convergence, a white arrow shifted to the left indicates that one eye shows central fixation, whereas the other eye is in a divergent position due to its weak fusion. This is used to detect latent strabismus (heterophoria). This device is suitable for the measurement of adduction and abduction weaknesses in the horizontal plane, as well as gaze elevation and depression disorders in the vertical plane. With a third function, the abnormal cyclorotational movement and its degree can also be determined. For details of the clinical importance of these examination procedures, see Chap. 55 on page 493.

Supplementary Tests

These help in the detection of neurogenic and myogenic, as well as neuromuscular conditions, and in their differential diagnostics.

- *Looking upwards test:* the procedure to clinically confirm ocular myasthenia gravis (OMG)
- *Edrophonium and/or looking upwards test:* it also confirms the conduction disorder due to OMG when combined with a double vision test. (See Chap. 60 on page 545).
- *Forced duction test:* a procedure for the detection of incipient scarring due to endocrine myopathy, which also helps its physical release

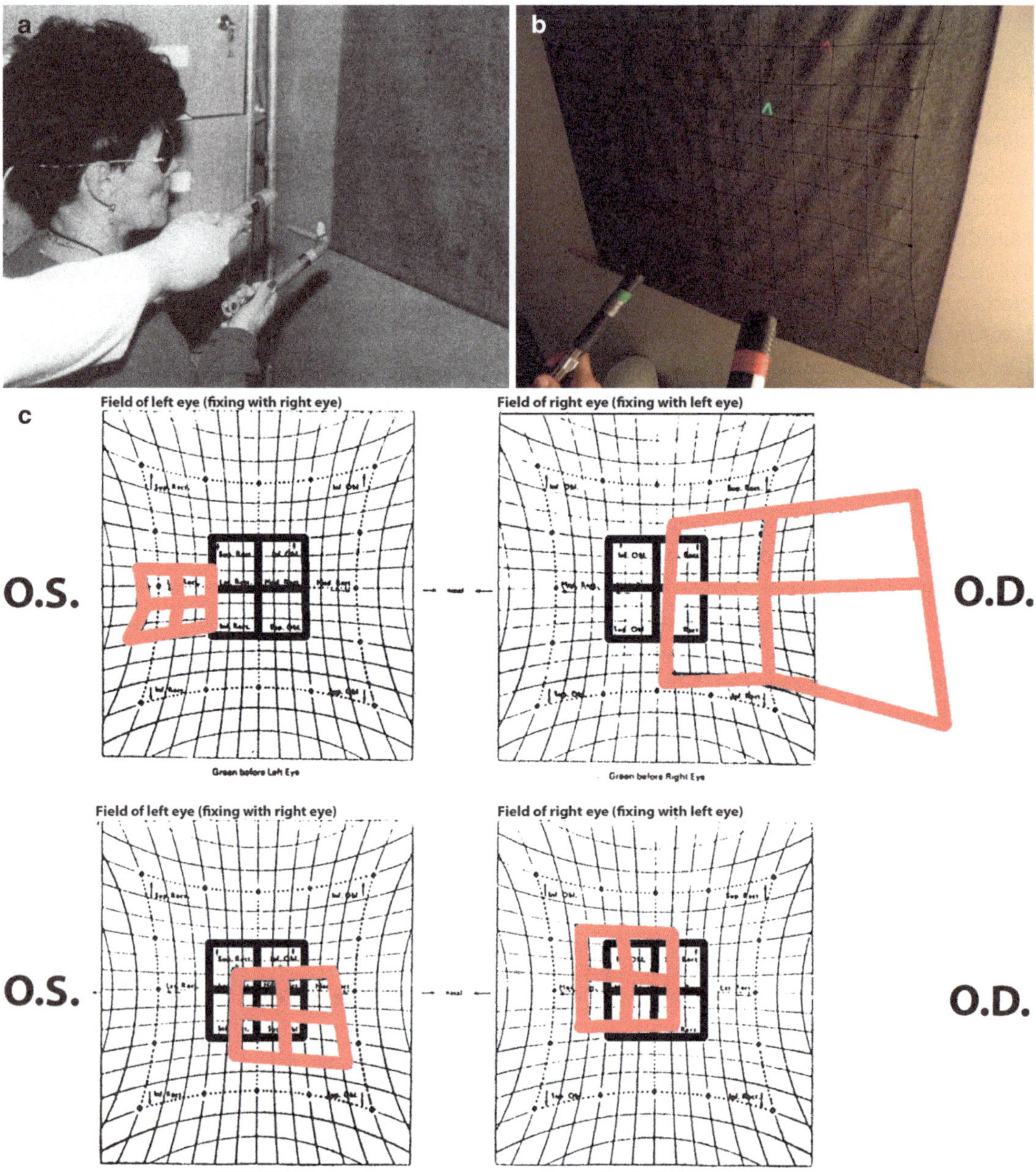

Fig. 24.1 (**a**, **b**) Double vision test with red-green glasses and a Hess screen, (**c**) The image displacement indicated by the patient are marked on the diagram of the Hess screen (the image displacement is marked with a color line against the normal image position marked with a *black line*)

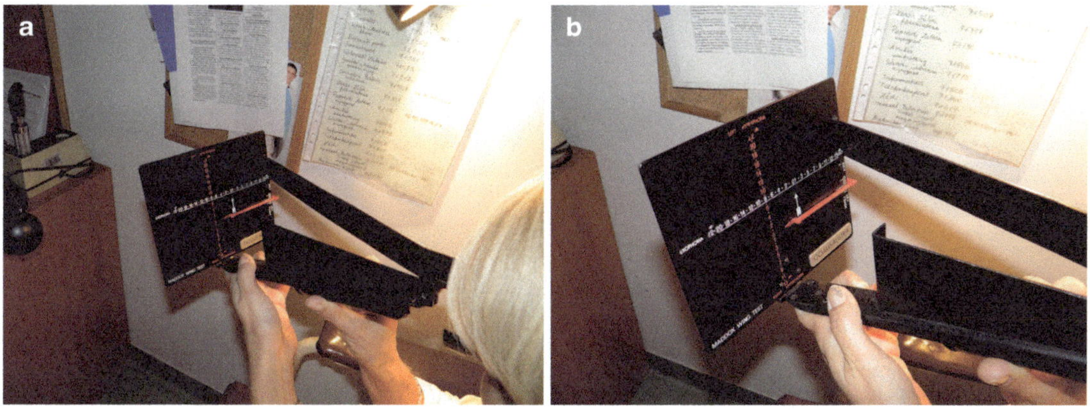

Fig. 24.2 (**a**, **b**) Near diplopia test with a Maddox wing-near diplopia test

- *Video recording:* it documents the type and degree of the eye movement disorder, primarily for teaching purposes.
- *Fundus photography series:* it is used to detect and measure the change in the angle of the papillomacular axis, the cyclorotational eye movement disorder.
- Electrophysiological tests:

  The brainstem auditory evoked potential (BAEP) test attempts to test the change in the vestibulo-ocular reflex by stimulating the auditory pathway.

  Electrooculography (EOG): a recording of the eye movement disorder, which measures its change.

The practical importance of the examination procedures is detailed at the description of the clinical conditions. The references can also be found at the end of that chapter.

Duplex Ultrasound Examination of the Carotid and Vertebral Arteries

25

Péter Barsi

Contents

The whole neuro-anatomical background of the vision from the retina to the visual cortex is supplied by the branch system of the internal carotid artery and the vertebral artery bilaterally. A non-invasive, easily performed test method detecting various abnormalities of the large arteries supplying the area plays an important role in neuro-ophthalmological diagnostics, which is explained partly by the above fact, partly by the incidence of degenerative vascular diseases.

P. Barsi, M.D., PhD Habil
Szentâgothai Knowledge Center – MR Research Center, Semmelweis University, Budapest, Hungary

Unit of Neuroradiology, Department of Neurosurgery, University of Pécs, Pécs, Hungary
e-mail: barsipeterdr@gmail.com

The Main Point of the Method

The test combines two ultrasound methods, as described by its name: the large frequency, high resolution, two dimensional imaging and Doppler technique. The first one usually uses a 7.5 or 10 MHz frequency ultrasound beam resulting in a high resolution image with poor penetration. However, the carotid arteries are found near the surface, and the vertebral arteries can usually be visualized as well.

The main point of the Doppler technique is that frequency of the ultrasound reflected from the red blood cells moving in the blood changes proportionally to the velocity of the red blood cells in accordance with the Doppler formula. From the changes in the frequency, the computer calculates the flow velocity and prepares a velocity to time curve which is similar to the pulse wave (Figs. 25.1, 25.2, 25.3, and 25.4).

The shape of the curve and the filling of the area under the curve at the maximum value of systole show the type of the flow and the presence of turbulence, while the systolic peak velocity and the diastolic end velocity show the extent of hemodinamically significant stenoses with 10–20 % accuracy. However, the duplex technique does not use the two methods independently: the pulse wave Doppler curves are obtained from a selected region of the vessel segment on the good quality two-dimensional images. Therefore, the method can be standardized, the environment of the mural lesions can be

J. Somlai, T. Kovács (eds.), *Neuro-Ophthalmology*, DOI 10.1007/978-3-319-28956-4_25

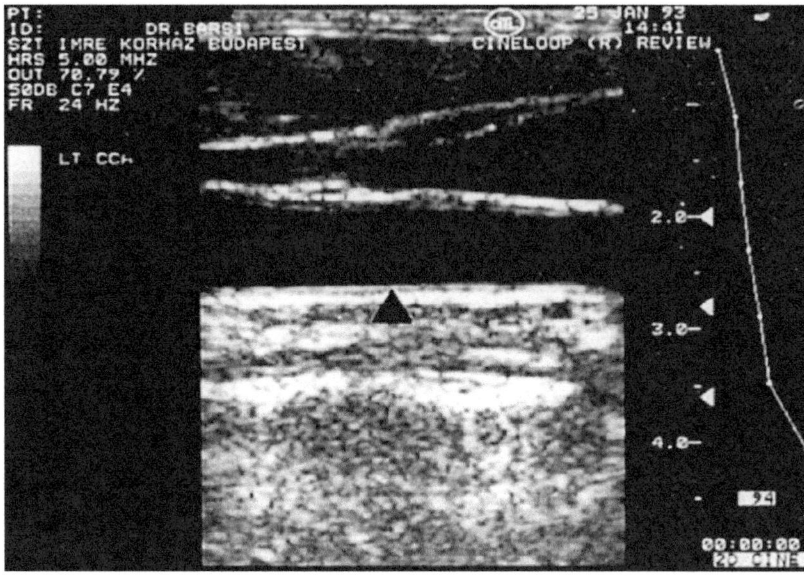

Fig. 25.1 A healthy common carotid artery with an intimal layer of normal width

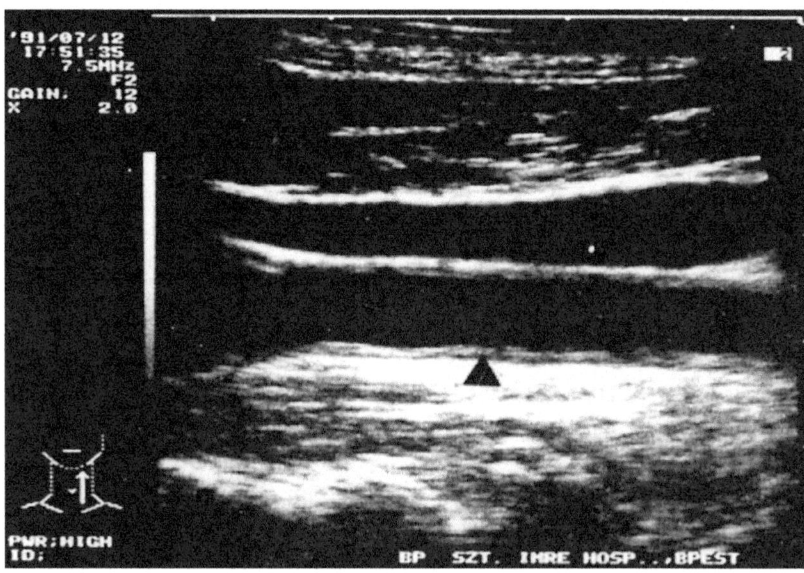

Fig. 25.2 Partially plaque-like widening of the intimal layer is observed in the region at the bifurcation of the common carotid artery

examined in detail, and significant luminal stenoses can be located. Conversely, the Doppler examination indicates stenosis where no lesion is seen with regular image quality, and the presence of a thrombus with density similar to that of blood can be detected only in images using increased gain. The method is complemented by a useful sound phenomenon accompanying the Doppler measurement. A more important thing is that the majority of the modern devices use the colour Doppler technique to help the diagnostic work. The computer technique assigns color codes to the velocities measured at each image point indicating the direction and the intensity of the flow, and these color codes are placed on the two-dimensional black and white images. The technique increases the speed of the examination and makes it easier; it is especially important in differentiating between subtotal stenoses and occlusions.

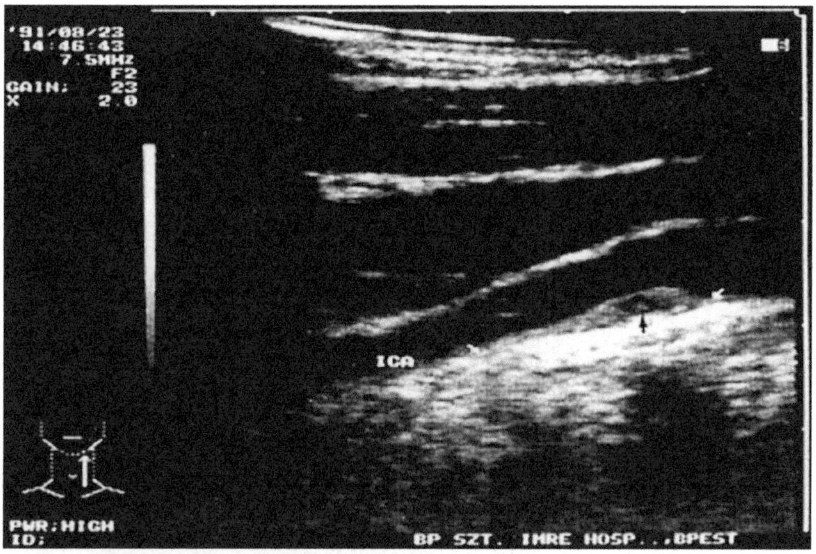

Fig. 25.3 Inhomogeneous plaque (*white arrow*) with smooth surface and moderately poor central echogenicity (*black arrow*) at the origin of the internal carotid artery

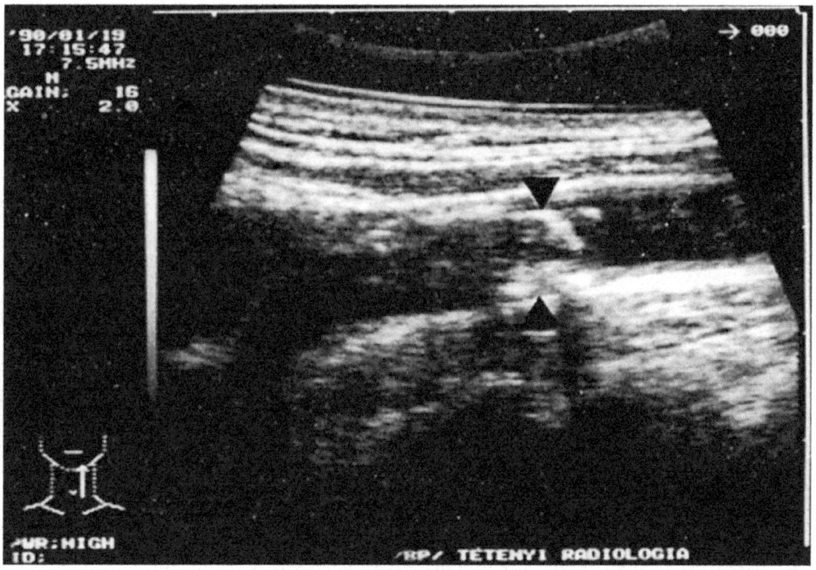

Fig. 25.4 Significantly calcified, inhomogeneous plaques with uneven surface at the origin of the internal carotid artery

Course of the Examination

During the examination, the structure of the wall is reviewed from the origin of the common carotid artery to the highest level of the internal carotid artery that can be visualized. The thickness of the intimal layer, normally a linear echo between the intima of the vessel and the layer of media, is analyzed in the common carotid artery; the thickness reflects the condition of the whole arterial system. Mural lesions, plaques, are examined; the homogeneity, calcification and surface of the lesions, echo poor regions indicating bleeding in the plaque, and mural thrombi are investigated. Inhomogeneous areas, calcified regions, uneven, or ulcerated surfaces, mural thrombi, and plaque bleeding increase the chance that an embolus develops at the affected region. If color Doppler is available as well, the whole vascular system can be examined for turbulence, stenosis, and occlusion (Figs. 25.5, 25.6, 25.7, and 25.8).

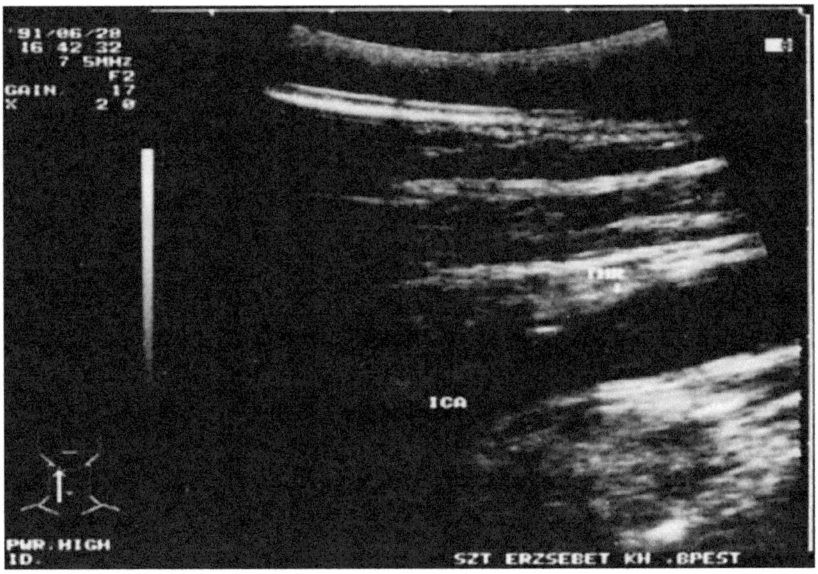

Fig. 25.5 Thrombus (THR) with echodensity similar to that of blood at the origin of the internal carotid artery

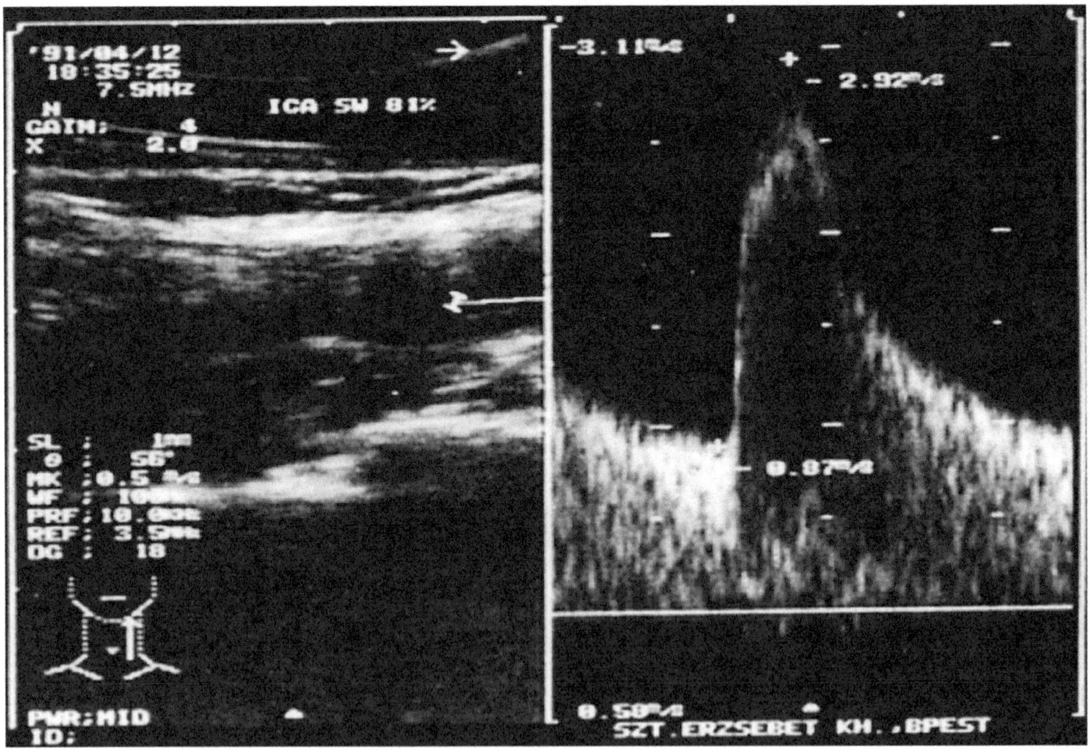

Fig. 25.6 Mural lesions causing 80–90 % stenoses at the origin of the internal carotid artery (systolic peak velocity is normal up to 1 m/s, and diastolic end velocity is normal up to 0.4 m/s)

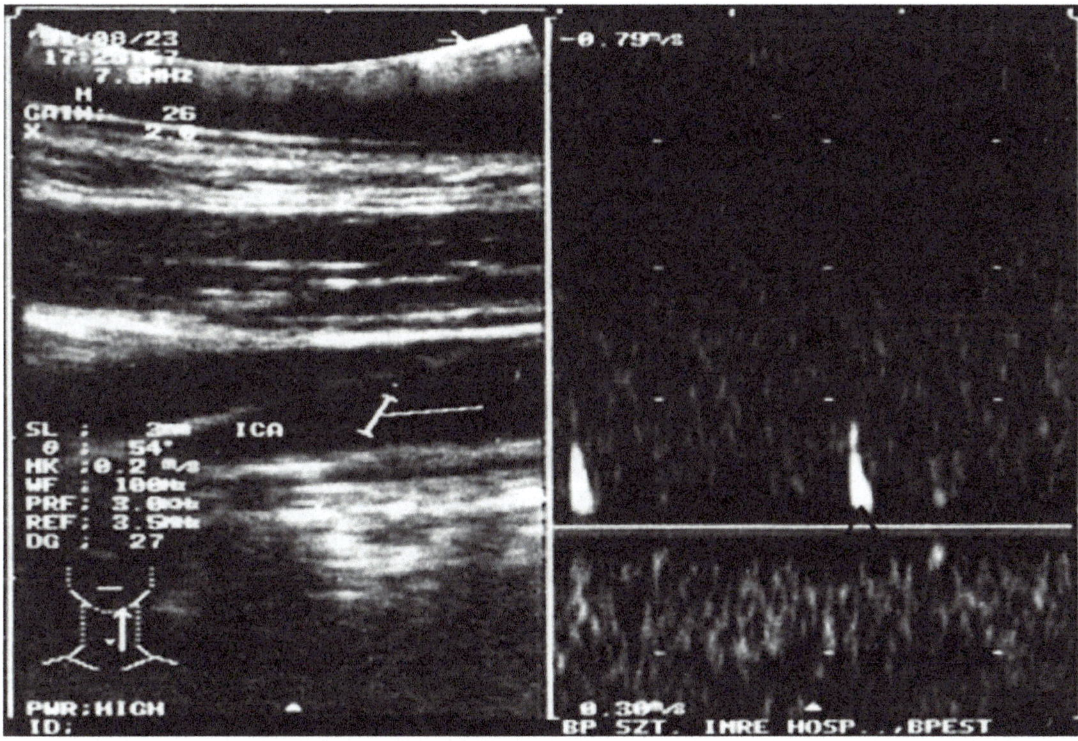

Fig. 25.7 Only spikes (*empty arrow head*) can be measured at the origin of the internal carotid artery with Doppler technique; it is characteristic of the occlusion of the distal segment

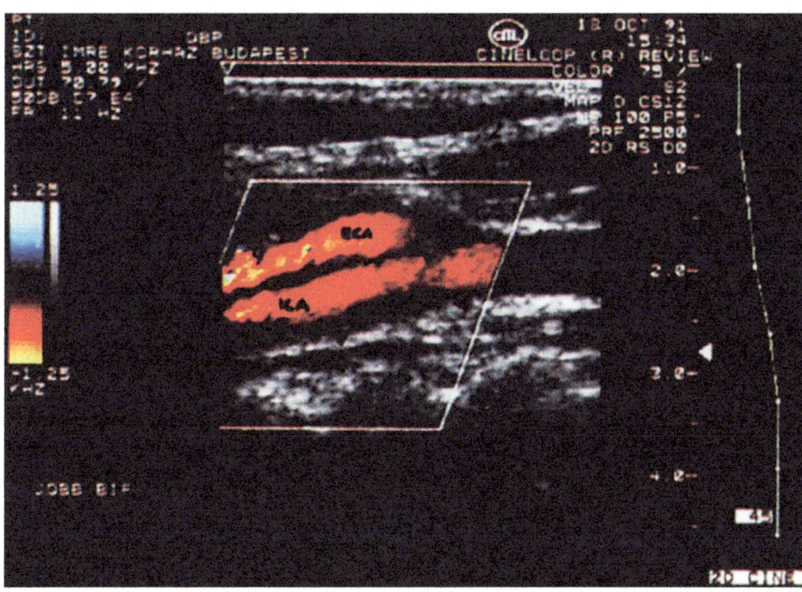

Fig. 25.8 The bifurcation and the origin of the internal and external carotid arteries are seen in the color Doppler image. The flow is diverted due to a small mural lesion (*arrowhead*) at the origin of the internal carotid artery

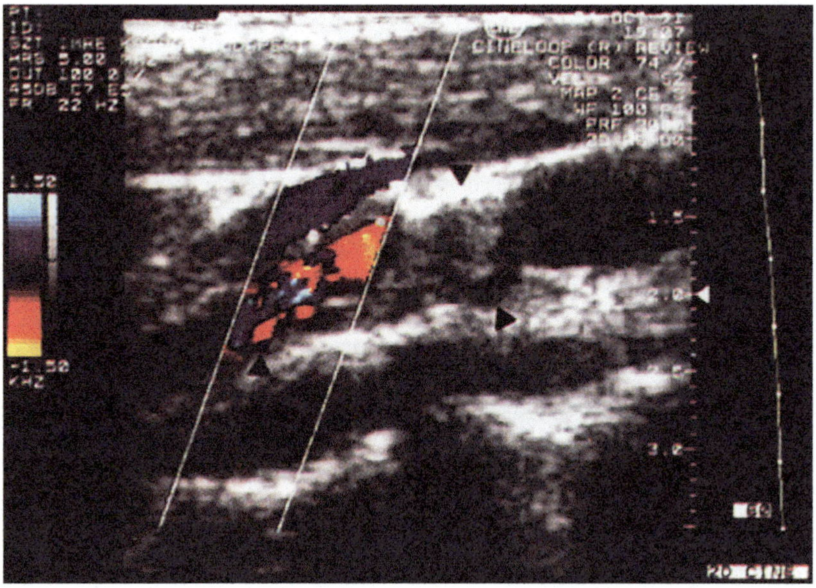

Fig. 25.9 The color Doppler image is inhomogeneous at the origin of the internal carotid artery, the surface of the artery is uneven, and significant turbulence is seen caused by calcified plaques (mixed color band). The blue band is the internal jugular vein

After that, a Doppler measurement is performed at defined locations even if the structure of the wall is regular, and the flow is examined in more details near mural lesions. The external carotid artery and then the vertebral artery are then examined. The latter artery is usually covered by bony structures (clavicle, transverse processes of the vertebrae), the origin cannot be visualized in all cases, but the presence and direction of the flow can be established in 90 % of the cases, even in case of patients with disadvantageous physique. The examination of the branches of the four large vessels can be performed by an experienced professional in about 20–30 min.

What Lesions Can Be Detected with the Method?

In the Carotid System

- Congenital abnormalities and abnormalities in the course of the arteries (aplasia, hypoplasia, kinking, and coiling),
- Alterations in the intima of the common carotid artery reflecting the condition of the whole arterial system,
- Less dangerous mural lesions can be differentiated from specifically high-risk plaques and thrombi that may be the source of emboli, hemodinamically significant stenoses or complete occlusions,
- The condition of the operated segment can be continuously monitored after endarterectomy, patch plastic surgery, or prosthesis surgery,
- Arrhythmia, hyperkinesis, or slow flow may be found as an additional finding.

In the Vertebral Artery

- Based on the above facts, no analysis of the structure of the wall can be performed in many cases, but the presence and the direction of the flow (subclavian steal syndrome) can be determined in 90 % of the cases if the examiner has enough experience. In fortunate cases, the origin of the artery can be visualized; it is the region where 50–60 % of the atherosclerotic lesions occur (Figs. 25.9, 25.10, 25.11, and 25.12).

Summary

The described examination method provides a diagnostic device for neuro-ophthalmology that can gather data on the mural structure and flow characteristics of every artery supplying the whole

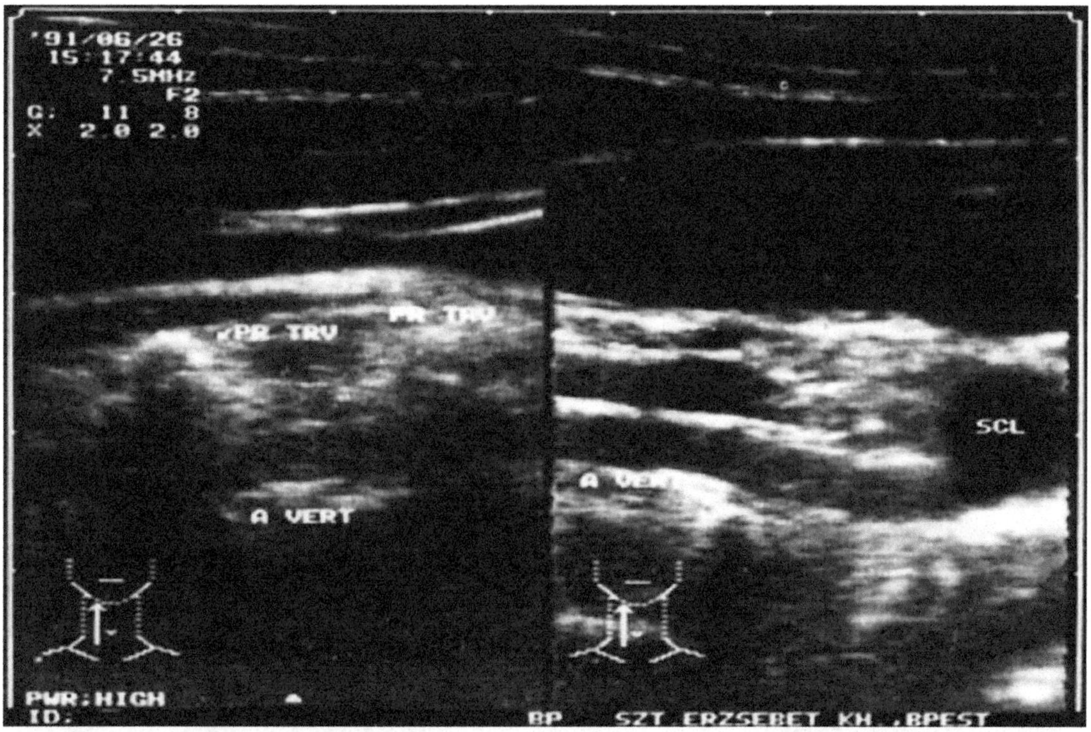

Fig. 25.10 The origin of the vertebral artery (A VERT) from the subclavian artery (SCL) can rarely be visualized such clearly due to the design of the transducer and the physique of the patient. The vertebral vein is seen along the artery as well (PR TRV: transverse processes of the vertebra)

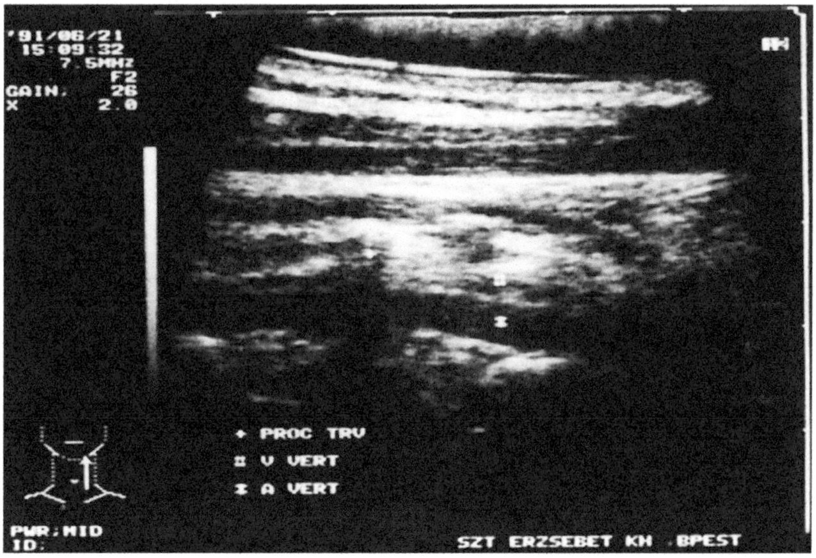

Fig. 25.11 Usually, a small segment covered partly by the transverse processes (PROC TRV) is visualized from the vertebral artery and vein

visual pathway and visual cortex, and areas of the brainstem containing the eye movement regions; in addition, data can be collected on the postoperative condition of the arteries, condition of the whole arterial system, and heart function. The method is non-invasive, reproducible, easy to

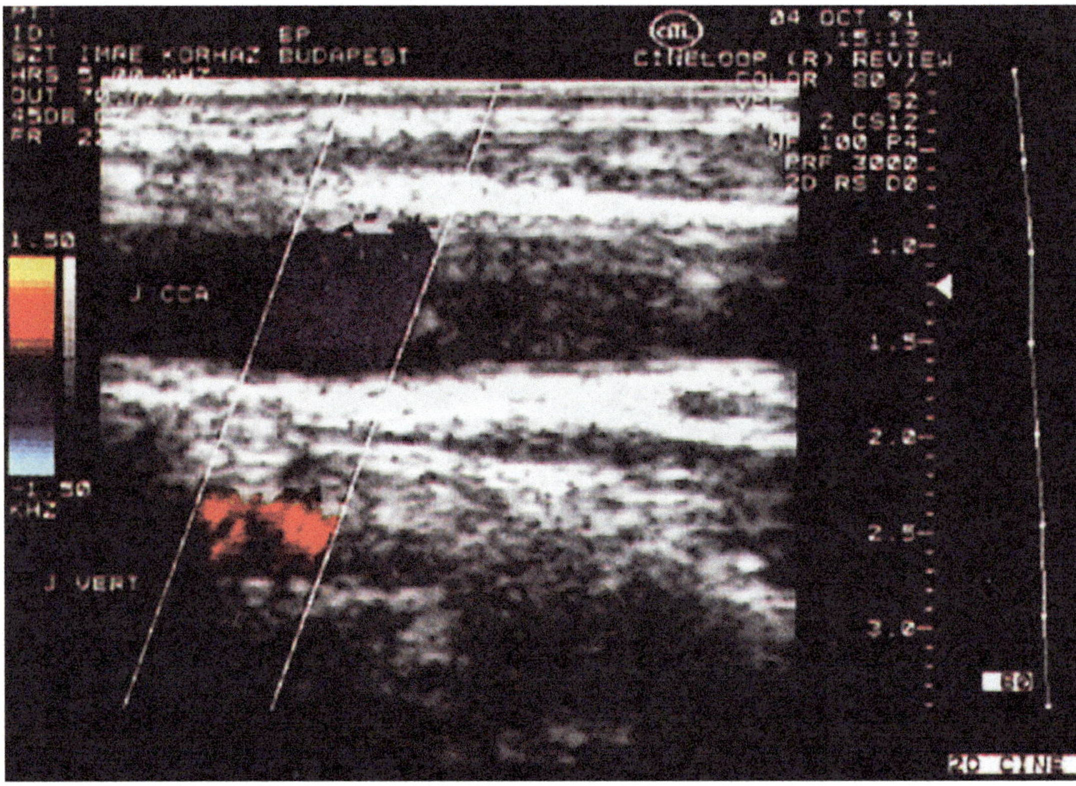

Fig. 25.12 The color Doppler technique shows that the flow in the right vertebral artery (R VERT) is in the opposite direction to the flow in the common carotid artery (R CCA) characteristic of subclavian steal syndrome

learn, relatively short to perform and cheap. It can be considered a very effective method combined with transcranial Doppler examination. Performed parallel with the cranial CT scan, it may substitute angiography that represents a risk unnecessary.

References

Bluth EI, Wetzner SM, Stavros AT, Aufrichtig D, Marlch KW, Baker JD. Carotid dulplex sonography: a multicenter recommendation for standardized imaging and Doppler criteria. Radiographics. 1988;8(3): 487–506.

Caroll BA. Carotid sonography. State of the art. Radiology. 1991;178:303–13.

Davis PC, et al. A prospective comparison of duplex sonography vs angiography of the vertebral arteries. AJNR. 1986;7:1059–64.

Grant EG, Wong W, Tessler F, Perella R. Cerebrovascular ultrasound imaging. Radiol Clin North Am. 1988;26(5): 1111–30.

Harkányi Z. Duplex ultrahang [Duplex ultrasound]. Budapest: Springer Hungaria; 1991.

Jack JG, Hoenveld H, van der Windt JM, van Doorn JJ, Ackerstaff RGA. A six year evaluation of duplex scanning of the vertebral artery. A non- invasive technique compared with angiography. J Vasc Technol. 1989;13:26–30.

Reilly LM, Lusby RJ, Hughes L, Ferrel LD, Stoney RJ, Ebrenfeld WK. Carotid plaque histology using real-time ultasonography. Clinical and therapeutic implications. Am J Surg. 1983;146:188–93.

26 Transcranial Doppler Examination

Gyula Pánczél

Contents

G. Pánczél, M.D., PhD
Department of Neurology,
Pest County, Flór Ferenc Hospital, Kistarcsa,
Budapest, Hungary
e-mail: panczel@t-online.hu

Abbreviations

RBC	Red blood cell
US	Ultrasound
TCD	Transcranial Doppler
MCA	Median cerebral artery
ACA	Anterior cerebral artery
PCA	Posterior cerebral artery
VA	Vertebral artery
BA	Basilar artery
OA	Ophthalmic artery
ACoA	Anterior communicating artery
PCoA	Posterior communicating artery
AVM	Anteriovenous malformation
PM D	Power motion Doppler
CCC	Common carotid compression (compression test of the common carotid artery
AVM	Arteriovenous malformation

Flow in the intracranial vessels, especially in the arteries, can be examined with TCD. The ultrasound can hardly penetrate the skull, but in certain regions, the ultrasound windows, the bone is missing (such as the orbit, foramen magnum) or thin, the trabecular layer is missing (such as the temporal window), so the examination can be performed via these windows.

J. Somlai, T. Kovács (eds.), *Neuro-Ophthalmology*, DOI 10.1007/978-3-319-28956-4_26

The Theory of Operation of TCD

The operation of TCD is based on the Doppler principle. The transducer omits a short ultrasound vibration package, which penetrates the ultrasound window, reaches the examined artery and is reflected from the red blood cells in the circulation, and then gets back into the transducer. The omitted ultrasound frequency changes during reflection; this change is proportional to the velocity of the red blood cells, so the velocity can be calculated from the frequency shift.

Frequency shift based on the Doppler formula:

df = (2f0 v cos Φ)/c

Where df is: the Doppler shift (frequency shift)

f0: the frequency of the emitted ultrasound beam

v: the velocity of the examined object (in this example: velocity of the RBCs)

cos Φ: cosine of the angle between the direction of the flow of the RBCs and the ultrasound beam

c: speed of the ultrasound in a certain environment

It calculates the difference between the frequency of the emitted ultrasound beam and the reflected ultrasound beam, which is the frequency shift. The TCD examination usually examines in 30–90 mm depth, the optimal frequency of the transducer (f0) is 2 MHz. In case of examinations performed from the temporal window, the ultrasound beam and the course of the MCA and/or the anterior cerebral artery (ACA) are almost parallel (the difference is usually within 30°), so it means only a small error if Φ is considered to be zero. The c constant: ≈ 1540 m/s. As f0, Φ and c are constant variables, v depends only on the frequency shift, and therefore, the device calculates the result directly in velocity (cm/s). If the direction of the flow is towards the transducer (v is positive), the frequency increases, df will be positive, so the resulting flow spectrum will be positive as well (it is above the zero line), while if the direction of the flow is away from the transducer, the spectrum will be negative (below the zero line) (Fig. 26.1; Table 26.1).

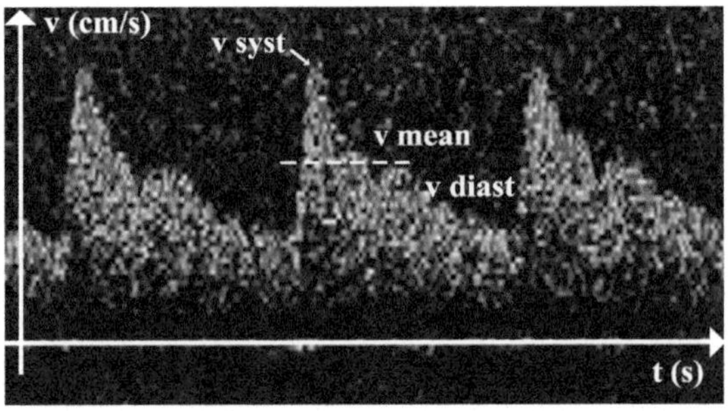

Fig. 26.1 The Doppler spectrum and its characteristics: *v syst*: systolic peak velocity; *v mean*: mean velocity; *v diast*: end diastolic velocity

The Doppler spectrum is the time–velocity curve of the blood flow, and it contains the following information:

The US Windows

TCD examination can be performed through the following windows:

- The MCA, the ACA, the posterior cerebral artery (PCA) and the distal segment of the ICA before the bifurcation can be best examined through the temporal window (via the squamous part of the temporal bone).
- The ophthalmic artery (OA) and the carotid siphon can be examined through the orbital window (via the optic canal and the superior orbital fissure). The performance of the emitted ultrasound has to be decreased (maximum 10 mW/cm^2) in this case due to the risk of developing a cataract.
- The two vertebral arteries (VAs) and the basilar arteries (BAs) can be visualized suboccipitally, via the foramen magnum window. In some cases, flow of smaller arteries (such as the superior cerebellar artery, the posterior inferior cerebellar artery, and the communicating arteries in case of collateral circulation) can be detected as well (Fig. 26.2).

Table 26.1 Characteristics of the Doppler spectrum

Amplitude of the curve	Represents the velocity of blood flow at a certain time.
Polarity (curve below or above the zero line)	Represents the direction of flow (in case of standard settings, flow towards the transducer results in a positive curve, flow away from the transducer results in a negative curve).
Filling of the area under the curve (systolic window)	Refers to turbulent flow (if the area is filled, especially if there is a component with opposite polarity as well, the flow is turbulent, if the spectrum is narrow, linear, the flow is laminar). Its importance in case of a TCD examination is inferior as the spectrum is usually filled in case of laminar flow as well (opposed to the carotid duplex ultrasound scan where normal spectrum is seen which is usually linear)
Pulsatility (Gosling pulsatility index: $PI = (v_{systolic} - v_{diastolic})/v_{mean}$)	Indicates the distal vascular resistance (High PI: indicates increased resistance [for example distal stenosis, old age, increased intracranial pressure], in this case spikes are seen on the curve, and the curve suddenly starts to decrease after reaching the peak systolic velocity, the diastolic velocity is significantly low. Low PI: indicates decreased resistance [for example AVM feeder, hypercapnia], the end diastolic velocity increases to a larger extent compared with the systolic velocity, the curve becomes wider).
Resistance index $RI = (v_{systolic} - V_{diastolic})/V_{systolic}$)	Indicates the distal vascular resistance as well. (Pourcelot, 1976.) Clinically, it is important mainly for monitoring intracranial pressure; its value is abnormally high in this case.
Systolic upward slope (systolic acceleration)	It represents the pressure gradient maintaining flow (post-stenotic flow is characterized by decreased systolic acceleration, the curve is flattened in this case [delta sign], as distally, the perfusion pressure significantly decreases due to decreased pressure through the stenosis).
The heart rate	Can be characterized by the number of heart cycles in a minute.
Hemispheral index Lindegaard (vMCA/vICA)	It differentiates between vasospasm and systemic flow hyperkinesis. Flow velocity of the ICA should be determined by submandibular measurement in 40–50 mm depth: A value above 3 refers to vasospasm.

The TCD Examination

The examination of the arteries of the circle of Willis should be started with the MCA. A little US gel is placed on the transducer, and it is placed to the temporal window directed towards the contralateral temporal window (the head of the US transducer is almost perpendicular to the temporal bone). The depth of the examination is set to 50–55 cm, and fine scanning movements are used to find the ipsilateral MCA. The TCD is not an imaging study, the artery has to be defined from the characteristics of the resulting spectrum (Table 26.2). Thus, for example the spectrum of the MCA can be measured in about 40–65 mm depth via the temporal window, it is positive, so it is located above the zero line, and the highest velocity can be measured here in most cases (v mean: usually between 50 and 65 cm/s). By increasing the depth but leaving the transducer's position unchanged or by hardly changing the transducer's position, more proximal segments of the MCA are visualized, and then the bifurcation of the internal carotid artery is examined (origin of the MCA–ACA; in 60–64 mm depth). This is an important reference point, as the positive spectrum of the MCA and the negative spectrum of the ACA are seen simultaneously in the bifurcation of the internal carotid artery. By further increasing the depth, the A1 segment of the ipsilateral ACA (65–75 mm; negative spectrum), and then the A1 segment of the contralateral ACA (75–85 mm; positive spectrum), and finally the contralateral MCA (85–100 mm; negative spectrum) can be examined (Fig. 26.3).

In order to find the PCA, the ipsilateral bifurcation of the internal carotid artery (approximately

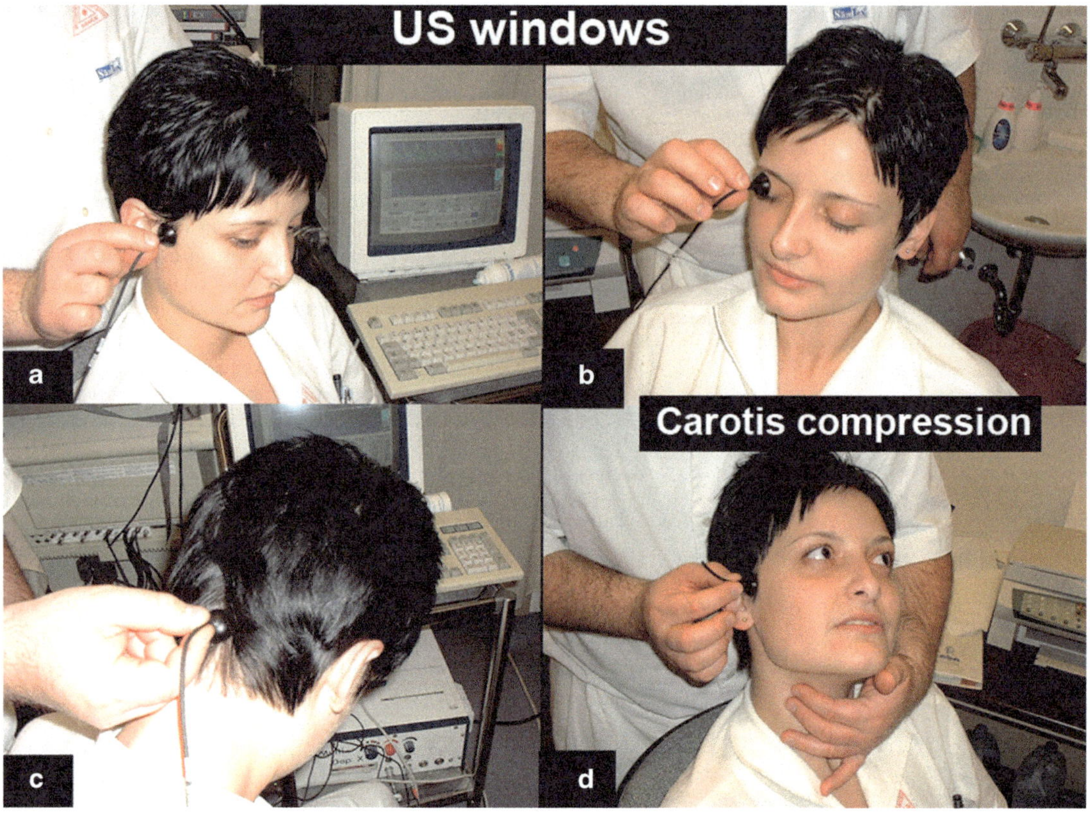

Fig. 26.2 The US windows: (**a**) temporal window; (**b**) orbital window; (**c**) foramen magnum window; (**d**) compression test of the common carotid artery

Table 26.2 Characteristic values of certain arteries

Artery	Depth (mm)	v (cm/s)	Direction	Window
Ipsilateral MCA	40–65	62 ± 12	Positive	Temporal
Ipsilateral ACA	65–75	50 ± 12	Negative	Temporal
Contralateral ACA	75–85.5	0 ± 12	Positive	Temporal
Contralateral MCA	85–100	62 ± 12	Negative	Temporal
Ipsilateral PCA (P1 segment)	55–75	42 ± 10	Positive	Temporal
Ipsilateral PCA (P2 segment)	55–65	42 ± 10	Negative	Temporal
Contralateral PCA (P1)	75–85	42 ± 10	Negative	Temporal
OA	38–60	35 ± 10	Positive	Orbital
Carotid siphon	60–75	54 ± 13	Positive/negative	Orbital
VA	50–80	36 ± 10	Negative	Foramen magnum
BA	80–100	40 ± 10	Negative	Foramen magnum

60–64 mm depth) is usually a reliable reference point. P1 segment of the PCA can usually be visualized by tilting the US beam a little backwards in posterior direction from the bifurcation of the internal carotid artery (so that the US beam gets about 1 cm backwards in the depth of the bifurcation of the internal carotid artery [60–64 mm]).

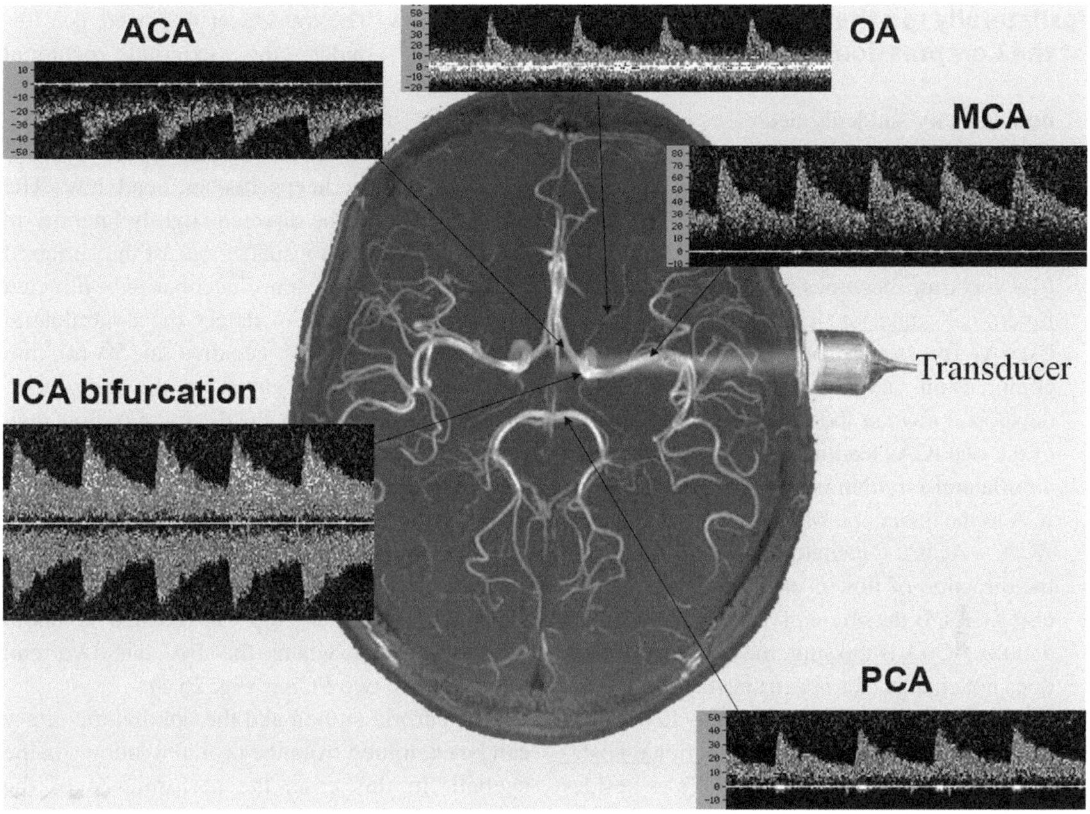

Fig. 26.3 Spectrums of the intracranial arteries examined through the right temporal window. *MCA* median cerebral artery, *OA* ophthalmic artery, *ACA* anterior cerebral artery, *ICA bifurcation* bifurcation of the internal carotid artery, *PCA* posterior cerebral artery

The spectrum is positive as the blood flow is towards the transducer; velocity is significantly lower in case of the MCA (v mean: 32–52 cm/s). By increasing the depth, more proximal segments of the ipsilateral PCA, and then the bifurcation (in this region, the positive spectrum of the ipsilateral PCA and the negative spectrum of the contralateral PCA can be seen simultaneously), and then finally the contralateral PCA can be examined. When examining the P2 segment of the ipsilateral PCA, the transducer in 55–60 mm depth has to be tiled a little backwards compared to the position described when examining the P1 segment; the negative spectrum of the P2 segment appears in case of a good window (as the P2 segment of the PCA is directed backwards, bypasses the mesencephalon and continues in occipital direction; the blood flow is away from the transducer in this segment). The amplitude of the PCA decreases when the eyes are closed and increases when the eyes are open (approximately 10 % change), this helps identifying the vessel.

The MCA is the easiest to examine, the second one is the ACA, and the PCA cannot be identified safely in about 20 % of the cases. If it cannot be determined which artery the spectrum originates from, the compression test of the common carotid artery (CCA) should be performed. The CCA has to be palpated on the examined side, and then it has to be compressed with a finger (Fig. 26.2d). Flow of the intracranial artery changes characteristically as described below after the compression:

Ipsilaterally (on the Side of the Compression)

- flow velocity suddenly decreases in the MCA (flow does not stop completely, as the vessel still receives blood supply via collateral arteries)
- the direction of the flow in the ACA changes (the spectrum becomes positive) if there is a functional anterior communicating artery (AcoA) (pressure drops on the side of the compression, significant pressure gradient develops between the intracranial bifurcation of the two ICAs leading to the development of a collateral circulation from the contralateral ICA to the ipsilateral MCA in the contralateral ACA – ACoA – ipsilateral ACA pathway, so the direction of flow is changed in the ipsilateral ACA). If the circle of Willis is incomplete and the ACoA is missing, the direction of flow does not change (the spectrum stays negative), but the velocity decreases, velocity in the PCA slightly increases if there is a functional posterior communicating artery (PCoA), as besides the normal region the posterior artery supplies, collateral flow commences towards the region of the MCA via the PCoA. The flow does not change if there is no PCoA.

Contralaterally

- flow of the MCA and that of the PCA do not change
- flow velocity of the ACA increases if there is a functional ACoA (as the amount of blood volume flowing through a certain region in a unit of time increases, the size of the supplied area is increased [the region of the compressed ICA/accordingly], or the flow velocity does not change if there is no ACoA.

It is important to examine the wall structure of the CCA before the carotid compression with duplex ultrasound examination to avoid embolism from potential unstable plaques as a consequence of the compression. The vertebrobasilar system can be examined via the foramen magnum window. The transducer is placed 1–2 fingerbreadths under the external occipital protuberance in the midline or slightly laterally. The ultrasound beam is directed towards the nasal bridge, while the examined person is sitting, and he/she keeps his/her head low. The transducer has to be directed slightly laterally in 50–80 mm depth to visualize one of the vertebral arteries, and then the transducer has to be directed to the opposite side to detect the contralateral VA. The spectrum is negative in 50–60 mm depth, thus flow is away from the transducer; between 60 and 80 mm, the direction of flow may change reflecting the bends of the VA. Increasing the depth to about 80 mm, flow velocity slightly increases, the spectrum is negative (flow is away from the transducer) indicating the origin of the basilar artery (BA). Moving the transducer along the BA, the basilar "top" is reached at about 100 mm depth where the BA has two end branches, the two PCAs (Fig. 26.4).

The carotid siphon and the ophthalmic artery can be examined from the orbital window via the eyeball. In this case, the performance of the omitted ultrasound has to be decreased to 10 % of the maximal value (to avoid the development of cataract). Abundant amount of gel has to be placed on the transducer and the eyeball should not be pressed. The OA can be visualized in most cases at about 50 mm depth. Distal segments of the OA can be examined by decreasing the depth (till about 38 mm) without changing the position of the transducer. The carotid siphon is reached by increasing the depth to about 60–70 mm. At this depth, the slow flow with large pulsatility of the OA (25–45 cm/s), which is an external type flow, is exchanged by the flow of the carotid siphon, which has smaller pulsatility and larger velocity (41–67 cm/s), it is an internal type flow which may have positive or negative polarity depending on whether the inferior or superior segment of the siphon is visualized. The carotid siphon can be examined at approximately 65–75 mm depth.

The flow in the OA is normally anterograde, the Doppler wave is positive. In case of severe ICA stenosis or occlusion, usually retrograde flow is present in the OA with good ECA collat-

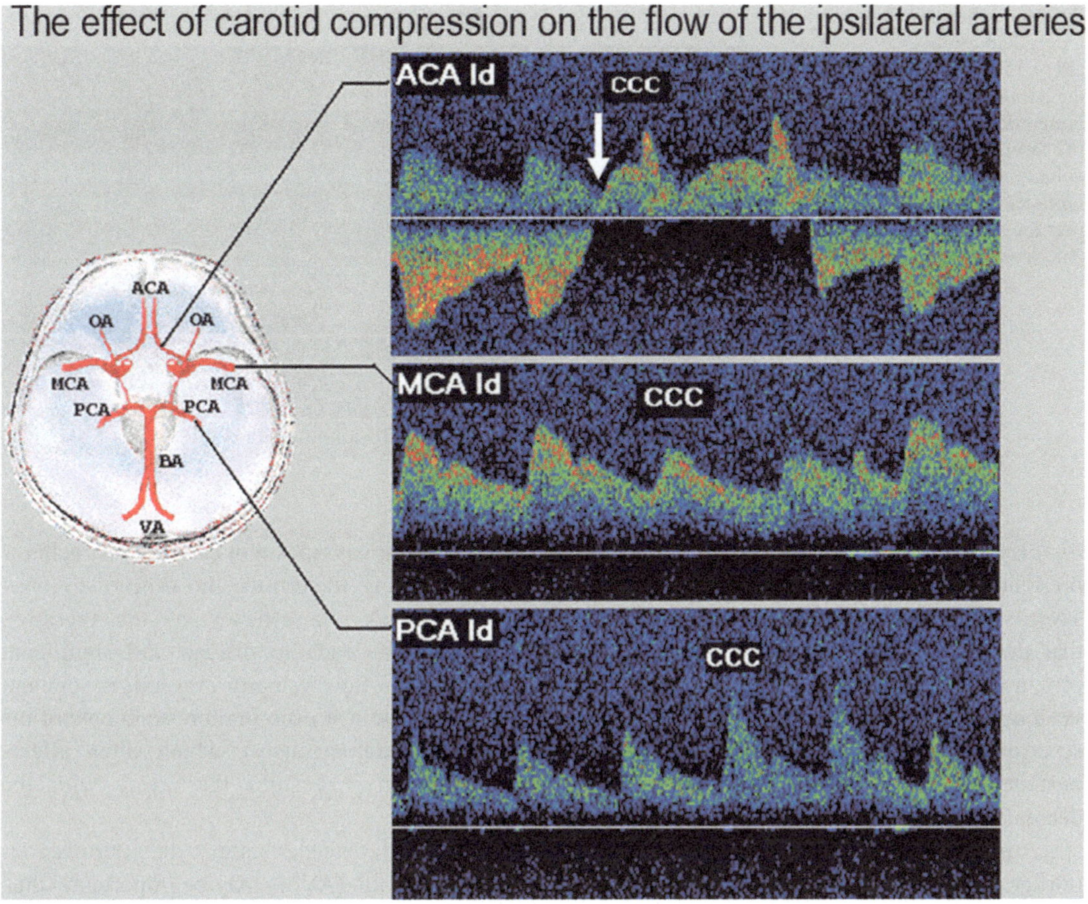

Fig. 26.4 The effect of the common carotid artery compression (*CCC*): As a consequence of the CCC, flow in the ipsilateral (in this case the right) anterior cerebral artery changes (*upper spectrum*); flow in the median cerebral artery decreases (*middle spectrum*); flow in the posterior cerebral artery slightly increases. *ACA* anterior cerebral artery, *MCA* median cerebral artery, *PCA* posterior cerebral artery

eral arteries, the Doppler wave is negative (flow is away from the transducer).

If severe stenosis or occlusion is present in the ICA, but flow from the intracranial collateral arteries (ACoA, PCoA) maintains larger pressure in the siphon (at the origin of the OA) than the pressure the ECA generates at the distal end of the OA (via the angular artery), then the flow will not turn and will remain to be anterograde, but the spectrum will be abnormal: low pulsatility (internalized), flattened, collateral type flow will be seen. If the perfusion pressure is similar in the intracranial collateral arteries and in the ECA–periorbital arterial system, flow cannot be measured in the OA (Table 26.2).

Indications of the TCD Examinations, Alterations of the Spectrum in Certain Diseases

TCD is indicated in the following cases:

- If the clinical symptoms or the CT/MRI lesions (territorial infarction, borderline zone infarction) indicate arterial stenosis or occlusion in the background of the ischemic stroke, but it is not found with duplex ultrasound examination. In this case, TCD will be used to find intracranial stenosis or occlusion.

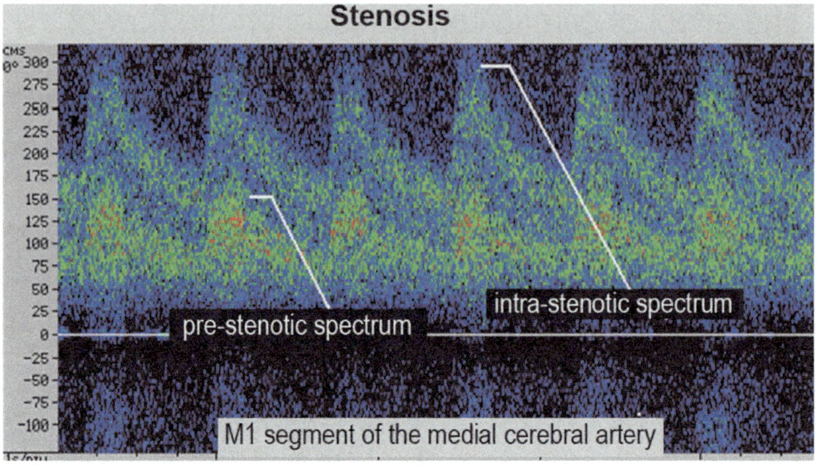

Fig. 26.5 Stenosis of the median cerebral artery. Flow velocity in the intra-stenotic artery is significantly increased. The sample volume contains the post-stenotic segment near the stenosis (spectrum with decreased velocity)

Abnormalities found in case of stenosis In the prestenotic region, flow is usually normal. As the severity of the stenosis increases, it is more likely that the flow is more pulsatile and depressed proximally. In the intrastenotic region, flow velocity is increased; velocities correlate with the severity of the stenosis well (Fig. 26.5). In the post-stenotic region, flow velocity is significantly decreased, significant turbulence is seen, the spectrum contains spikes, split segments, and a retrograde component is seen as well. The systolic velocity is decreased, the curve is flattened (delta sign). The larger the stenosis, the more distally the regeneration of the spectrum starts.

Abnormalities characteristic to occlusion In case of an occlusion of the intracranial arteries, the flow cannot be measured in the occluded vessel. If the occlusion does not affect the main branch of the MCA (M1 segment) but only a distal branch, decreased flow with low velocity and spectrum with increased pulsatility can be measured in the M1 segment. The flow of some arteries cannot be measured due to technical reasons (poor bone window), this has to be considered when diagnosing an occlusion (Fig. 26.6).

- If we wish to clarify the abnormalities of the intracranial flow in case of the stenosis of the internal carotid artery (extent of residual flow, presence of collateral flow), primarily before a vascular surgical intervention, or rarely for intraoperative monitoring (to determine the vascular reserve or detect embolisation).
- To monitor vasospasm in case of subarachnoidal bleeding (determine the time of the surgery, check the efficacy of the therapy). Vasospasm leads to diffuse and significant increase in flow velocity in a longer segment of the vessel (or even in more segments of the vessel simultaneously), which often affects other arteries besides the artery with the aneurysm.
- Defining the "feeder" artery, the arteriovenous malformation (AVM) may be important, when examining AVM, for example before embolization. The Doppler spectrum of the feeder artery is characteristic: flow velocity is increased, diastolic velocity is relatively more increased compared with the increase in systolic velocity; therefore, pulsatility is very low ($PI<0.5$). As a consequence, the main vascular resistance segment, the arteriolo-capillary system is missing in the angioma. Vasoreactivity is significantly reduced as well.
- If cerebral embolism is suspected, for example cardiac (artificial valve, AF) or the arterial (soft or ulcerated plaque) source of the embolus is known, or in case of a CT/MRI suggestive of a source of the embolus, an embolus detection is performed.
- During the examination, a transducer holding head band is placed on the patient and a transducer is fixed over the right temporal lobe, and another one is stabilized over the left temporal lobe. Two MCA flows are found by slightly moving these transducers, and flow is moni-

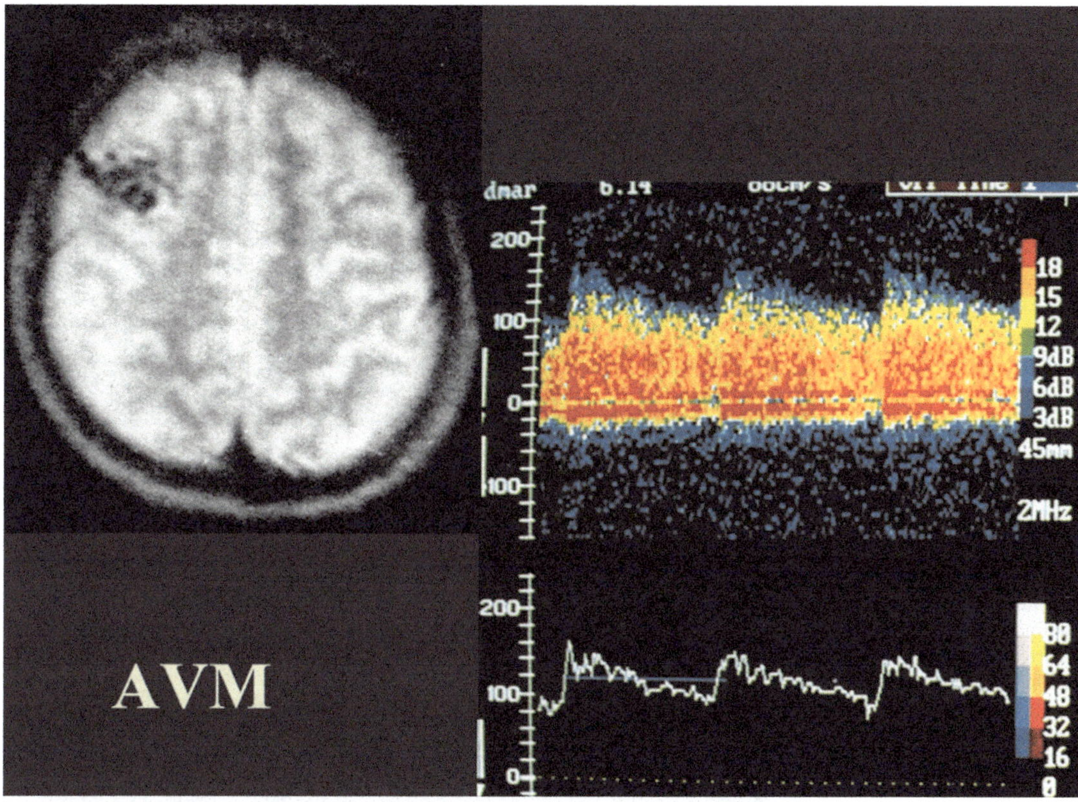

Fig. 26.6 Spectrum of a so called feeder artery feeding an arteriovenous malformation (*AVM*), and the MRI of the AVM. It is well seen that the increase in velocity during diastole is larger than the increase seen in the systolic velocity, so the curve is flattened, pulsatility decreases

tored continuously for 40–60 min. If an embolus is detected in the examined vessel segment, it is detected by TCD: a high intensity transient signal (HITS) appears in the flow spectrum. The device saves every embolus signal into the memory and the signals are counted.

- If paradox embolism is suspected, a "bubble study" has to be performed to detect permanent foramen ovale (PFO): after the administration of an intravenous contrast agent (for example physiological saline mixed with air); the patient is asked to perform a Valsalva maneuver, and TCD is performed to see whether the contrast medium appears in the contralateral median cerebral artery.
- Lesions characteristic to increased distal resistance are seen in case of increased intracranial pressure (for example cerebral sinus thrombosis, cerebral edema, apoplexy): velocity is decreased, diastolic decrease is somewhat larger, therefore, pulsatility increases, and the area under the curve decreases (externalized type curve). If the intracranial pressure is higher than the diastolic pressure measured in the intracranial large arteries, diastolic flow will be blocked while systolic flow will be maintained. Further increase in the pressure leads to shortened flow during systole, and finally, systolic flow stops.
- TCD may be a useful ancillary examination to determine brain death. If organ donation is considered, compulsory waiting time may be shortened with TCD. (In case of brain death, extremely high pulsatility, an oscillating spectrum may be seen with back and forth flow, practically it is a series of positive and negative spikes.) (Figs. 26.7 and 26.8)

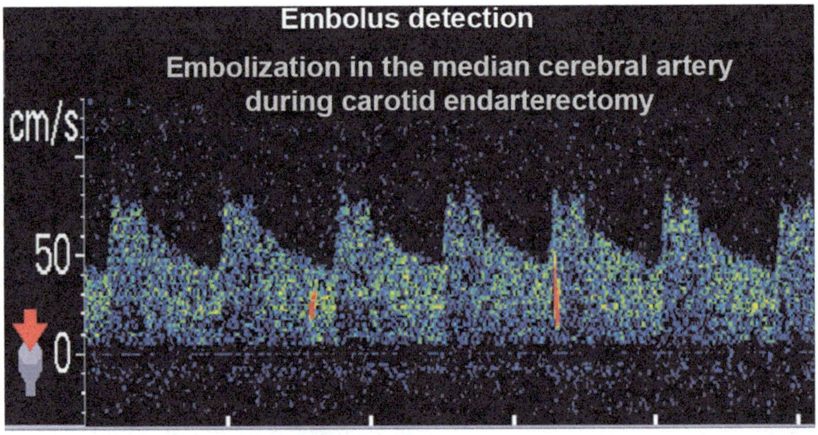

Fig. 26.7 Embolus detection. Short-term increases in signal intensity inside the spectrum (High-Intensity Transient Signal, HITS) indicate the transition of the embolus through the examined vessel segment. Emboli registered during carotid endarterectomy)

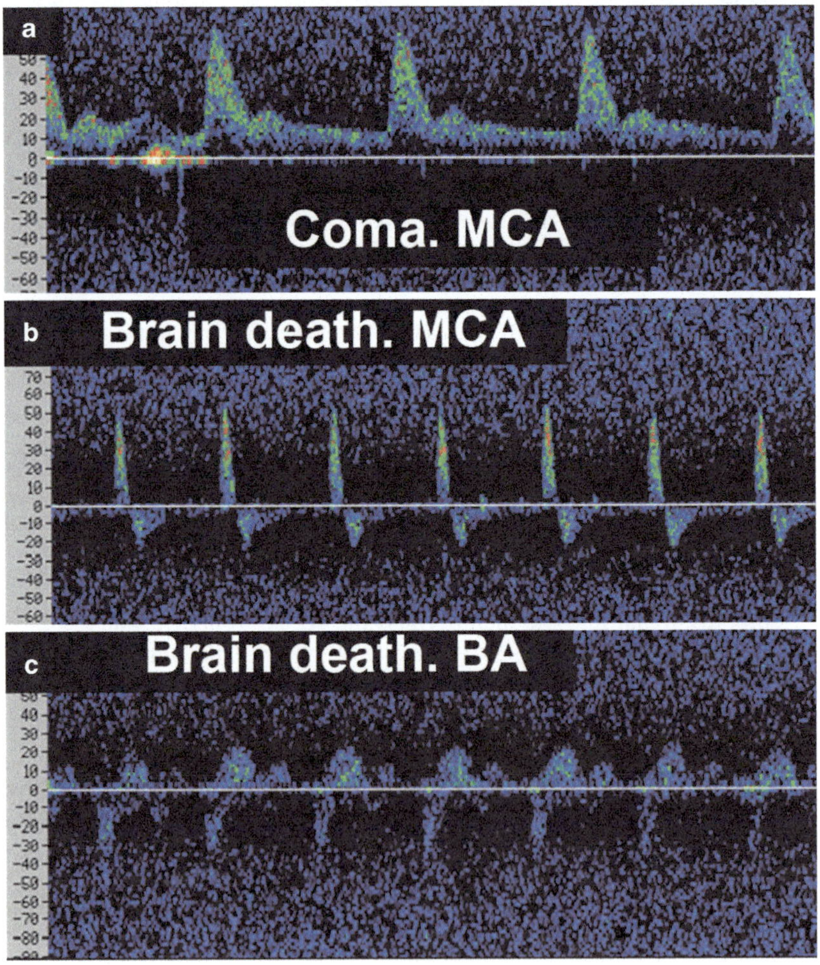

Fig. 26.8 Respiratory arrest, permanent cerebral anoxia, coma, and finally, brain death occurred in a young patient with drug overdose. (**a**) the spectrum of MCA on the day of the respiratory arrest. As a consequence of diffuse cerebral edema, the diastolic velocity is low, and the pulsatility is high. Brain death occurred in 2 days. (**b**) shows the spectrum of the MCA and (**c**) represents the spectrum of the BA; spikes, back and forth flow are seen, no effective blood flow is present. *MCA* median cerebral artery, *BA* basilar artery

Special Uses

Vasoreactivity

Cerebral vasoreactivity may be examined by various functional tests, such as hyper- and hypocapnia, tilting tests, or transient pharmacological vasodilatation (acetazolamide).

In case of altered vasoreactivity, arteriole constriction/dilatation expected in the test will be missing or decreased. Vasoreactivity may be altered in case of severe stenosis/occlusion of the large arteries (for example internal carotid artery) or in case of a small vessel disease (hypertension, diabetes).

In case of occlusion of the large vessels, chronic, compensatory vasodilatation develops in the arterioles above the occlusion, further vasodilatation is hardly or not possible, and therefore, the autoregulatory capacity decreases or is lost. Generally, vasoreactivity of patients is impaired if the function of the intracranial collateral arteries is not satisfactory in addition to occlusion in the internal carotid artery. Degenerative lesions of the arterioles (for example lipohyalinosis) limit the vasodilator capacity in case of disease of the small vessels. In case of limited vasoreactivity, additional compensatory vasodilatation is not possible, ischemic symptoms may develop if the blood pressure further decreases for any reason (cardiac, orthostatic, etc.) or in case the CO_2 level increases (for example in case of sleep apnea) (Fig. 26.9).

In case of the examination of vasoreactivity, changes in flow velocity as a response to certain provocation methods (for example hypercapnia, acetazolamide) are measured. Change in velocity per unit change in pCO_2 is the CO_2 reactivity and maximal change in velocity to (usually 1 g) intravenous acetazolamide (Diamox) is the acetazolamide reactivity. These parameters may be more precise indicators of the disorder of the cerebral circulation compared to flow velocity values.

Ultrasound Contrast Agent

The sensitivity of the transcranial Doppler examination may be significantly increased by the administration of an intravenous contrast agent. The contrast agent (such as Levovist) administered in bolus may lead to significant increase in the intensity of the flow spectrum monitored by TCD (blooming effect). This method should be used in case of poor bone window if an intracranial vascular lesion is significantly suspected. The administration of contrast agent enables harmonic imaging. The essence of the method is that the administered contrast agent resonates in the

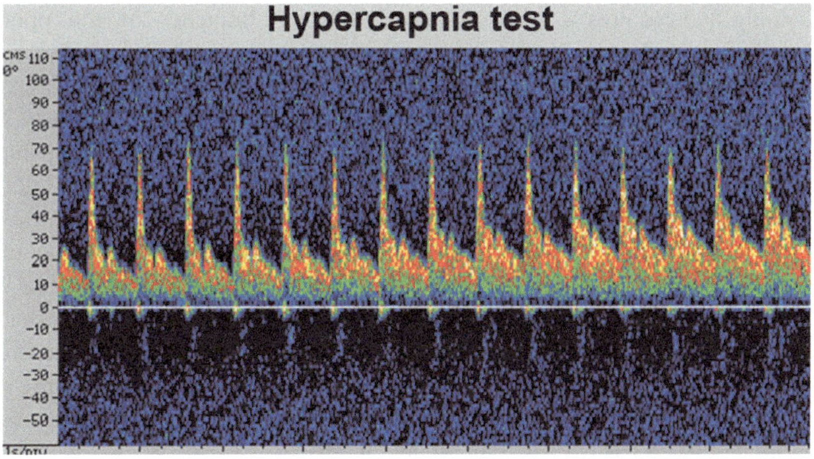

Fig. 26.9 Hypercapnia test. Flow velocity of the median cerebral artery gradually increases with inhaling air rich in CO_2 as a consequence of the dilatation of the arteriolar system

ultrasound field, and in addition to the basal frequency, it resonates its whole-number multiples (so called harmonics) as well. By detecting the second harmonic (double of the basal frequency) and filtering the other frequencies, the vascular system will be visualized selectively (including arterioles with 30–40 μm diameter too) as the contrast agent is located intravasally; the surrounding tissues will not be visualized.

Transcranial Power Motion (M mode) Doppler (PMD)

PMD enables that information be collected from the whole length of the US beam at the same time from the flow of the vessel in the direction of the beam, therefore, it may give data from the flow of the median cerebral artery and the flow of the anterior cerebral artery simultaneously. The method was described by Mark Moehring in 2002.

The essence of PMD is that 33 partly overlapping sample volumes are placed along an approximately 6-cm segment of the intracranial region of the US beam. All sample volumes indicate the intensity and direction of flow simultaneously, at the same time. Flow towards the transducer is coded by red, flow away from the transducer is blue, and increasing signal intensities are indicated by lighter tones.

While finding the intracranial flow is time consuming and requires a lot of practice, with the standard one-channel device, it can be easily found even by an inexperienced operator with the 33 simultaneous channels of the PMD (Fig. 26.10).

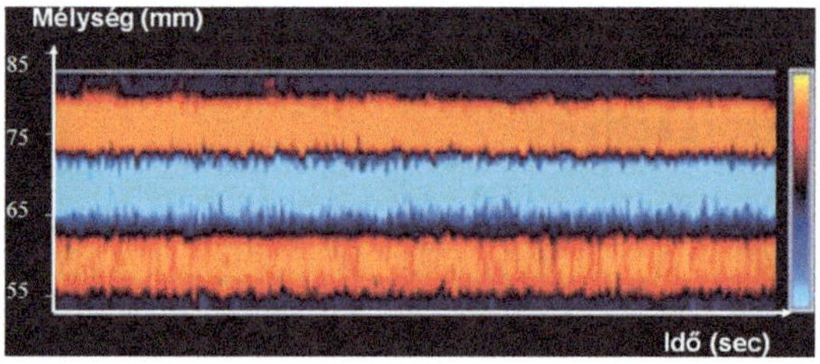

Fig. 26.10 Transcranial Power Motion Doppler (PMD). Three spectrums are seen in the figure at the same time. The lower red band indicates the flow towards the transducer in the ipsilateral median cerebral artery in 55–60 mm depth. The middle blue band indicates the flow in the ipsilateral anterior cerebral artery directed away from the transducer in approximately 65–70 mm depth, while the upper red band represents the flow towards the transducer in the contralateral anterior cerebral artery in about 70–80 mm depth

Neuro-ophthalmologic Indications

The symptoms of ischemic stroke are often accompanied by ophthalmologic symptoms. The anterior ischemic optic neuropathy (AION) develops based on the occlusion of the short posterior ciliary artery, posterior ischemic optic neuropathy (PION) is less common, and it develops as a consequence of occlusion of the more posterior branches of the ophthalmic artery.

Characteristic symptoms include sudden onset deterioration in vision without pain, disorder of color vision and visual field deficits (for example inferior nasal or inferior horizontal). Amaurosis fugax is temporary visual loss which lasts for a few seconds or minutes, is usually unilateral, and affects the whole visual field or only a part of the visual field. Temporary occlusion of the ophthalmic artery or the central retinal artery is in the background in most cases (most commonly caused by embolism). Common characteristic of the mentioned ophthalmologic symptoms is that circulatory disorder of the ophthalmic artery originating from the internal carotid artery or branches of the ophthalmic artery is in the background.

It is understandable that the above ophthalmologic symptoms may be accompanied by other cerebral ischemic symptoms from the region of the internal carotid artery. In most cases, accompanying symptoms include contralateral hemiparesis, hemiparesthesia or if the dominant side is affected, aphasia. However, it is more important that isolated temporary ophthalmic symptoms may indicate imminent ischemic stroke. Permanent blindness or ischemic stroke develops in 16 % of patients having amaurosis fugax (within 4 years).

Case Report An ophthalmologist colleague refers a young female patient having amaurosis

fugax to carotid US examination. 70 % stenosis of the ipsilateral internal carotid artery was confirmed, which was caused by a significantly embologenic plaque (soft, uneven plaque which was moving in case of every systole). The neurologists examining the patient recommended emergency carotid endarterectomy, however, the patient had hemiparesis before the end of the late vascular surgical intervention, and the severe symptoms did not improve.

Homonymous hemianopsia, quadrant anopsia in the region of the posterior cerebral artery, and anopsia in the lower quadrant may refer to circulatory disorders in the region of the medial cerebral artery. In this case, examination of the carotid and vertebral systems is recommended with duplex US.

Circulatory disorder of the vertebrobasilar system may lead to eye movement disorders, the patient may complain about diplopia. Infarction in the pons (such as lacuna) may lead to abducens nerve palsy; mesencephalic infarction may cause oculomotor paresis (for example oculomotor paresis and contralateral hemiparesis in case of Weber syndrome). Medial thalamus infarction may lead to disorder of the vertical eye movements. In the above listed cases, duplex US of the vertebral arteries may clarify the diagnosis.

If the cause of the ophthalmologic symptoms with vascular origin is not found with duplex US (mainly significant stenosis causing embologenic plaque or hemodynamic disorder), TCD may be performed. In case of symptoms in the carotid region, flow of the carotid siphon and that of the ophthalmic artery may be examined, and flow of the vertebral, basilar and posterior cerebral arteries may be examined in case of vertebrobasilar symptoms. If the patient has small vessel disease and the symptoms are caused by lacunar infarction, no abnormal lesion is usually found with TCD, pulsatility may be slightly increased or be at the upper limit of the normal level at most. In such cases, examination of vasoreactivity (for example CO_2 inhalation test, hypercapnia test) may indicate significantly decreased reactivity reflecting the severity of the small vessel disease.

If an embolism is suspected, emboli may be detected by monitoring the medial cerebral artery and the posterior cerebral artery in addition to cardiac examination (Holter).

References

Aaslid R, Markwalder T-M, Nornes H. Noninvasive transcranial Doppler ultrasound recording of flow velocity in basal cerebral arteries. J Neurosurg. 1982;57:769–74.

Aaslid R, Huber P, Nornes H. Evaluation of cerebrovascular spasm with TCD. J Neurosurg. 1984;60:37–41.

Ackerstaff RG, Moons KG, van de Vlasakker CJ, Moll FL, Vermeulen FE, Algra A, Spencer MP. Association of intraoperative transcranial doppler monitoring variables with stroke from carotid endarterectomy. Stroke. 2000;31(8):1817–23.

Alexandrov AV, Demchuk AM, Burgin WS. Insonation method and diagnostic flow signatures for transcranial power motion (M-mode) Doppler. J Neuroimaging. 2002;12(3):236–44.

Arenillas JF, Molina CA, Montaner J, Abilleira S, González-Sánchez MA, Alvarez-Sabín J. Progression and clinical recurrence of symptomatic middle cerebral artery stenosis: a long-term follow-up transcranial Doppler ultrasound study. Stroke. 2001;32(12):2898–904.

Arnold M, Sturzenegger M, Schäffler L, Seiler RW. Continuous intraoperative monitoring of middle cerebral artery blood flow velocities and electroencephalography during carotid endarterectomy. A comparison of the two methods to detect cerebral ischemia. Stroke. 1997;28(7):1345–50.

Barzo P, Pavics L, Borda L, Bodosi M, Doczi T, Katona E. Az agyi rezisztenciaerek rezervkapacitasanak meghatarozasa acetazolamid teszt soran vegzett transcranialis Doppler es SPECT vizsgalattal [Assessment of reserve capacity of cerebral resistance vessels by transcranial Doppler and SPECT scans during acetazolamide test]. Orv Hetil. 1992;133(37):2347. -50, 2355.

Baumgartner RW, Regard M. Role of impaired CO2 reactivity in the diagnosis of cerebral low flow infarcts. J Neurol Neurosurg Psychiatry. 1994;57(7):814–7.

Cartier R, Cartier P, Fontaine A. Carotid endarterectomy without angiography. The reliability of Doppler ultrasonography and duplex scanning in preoperative assessment. Can J Surg (Canada). 1993;36(5): 411–6.

De Bray JM, Le Jeune JJ, Pourcelot L, Saumet JL, Jallet P. 99Tcm-HMPAO cerebral scintigraphy and transcranial pulsed Doppler in acute intracranial hypertension in rabbits. Br J Radiol. 1994;67(798):540–5.

Diehl RR. Cerebral autoregulation studies in clinical practice. Eur J Ultrasound. 2002;16(1-2):31–6. Review.

Diehl RR, Henkes H, Nahser HC, Kuhne D, Berlit P. Blood flow velocity and vasomotor reactivity in patients with arteriovenous malformations. A transcranial Doppler study. Stroke. 1994;25(8):1574–80.

Doppler C. Über das farbige Licht der Doppelsterne und einiger anderer Gestirne des Himmels.Abhandl Kőnigl Bőhm Ges. 1843;2:465–82.

Feri M, Ralli L, Felici M, Vanni D, Capria V. Transcranial Doppler and brain death diagnosis. Crit Care Med. 1994;22(7):1120–6.

Garami ZF, Bismuth J, Charlton-Ouw KM, Davies MG, Peden EK, Lumsden AB. Feasibility of simultaneous pre- and postfilter transcranial Doppler monitoring during carotid artery stenting. J Vasc Surg. 2009; 49(2):340–4.

Gattuso R, Martinelli O, Alunno A, D'Angeli I, Felli mm, Castiglione A, Izzo L, Gossetti B. Carotid Stenting and Transcranial Doppler Monitoring: Indications for Carotid Stenosis Treatment. Vasc Endovasc Surg. 2010.

Giller CA, Mathews D, Purdy P, Kopitnik TA, Batjer HH, Samson DS. The transcranial Doppler appearance of acute carotid artery occlusion. Ann Neurol. 1992; 31(1):101–3.

Goode SD, Altaf N, Auer DP, MacSweeney ST. Carotid endarterectomy improves cerebrovascular reserve capacity preferentially in patients with preoperative impairment as indicated by asymmetric BOLD response to hypercapnia. Eur J Vasc Endovasc Surg. 2009;38(5):546–51.

Harper C, Cardullo PA, Weyman AK, Patterson RB. Transcranial Doppler ultrasonography of the basilar artery in patients with retrograde vertebral artery flow. J Vasc Surg. 2008;48(4):859

Hartl WH, Janssen I, Furst H. Effect of carotid endarterectomy on patterns of cerebrovascular reactivity in patients with unilateral carotid artery stenosis. Stroke. 1994;25(10):1952–7.

Hartmann A, Mast H, Thompson JL, Sia RM, Mohr JP. Transcranial Doppler waveform blunting in severe extracranial carotid artery stenosis. Cerebrovasc Dis. 2000;10(1):33–8.

Hilgertner L, Szostek M, Malek AK, Staszkiewicz W. Collateral role of the external carotid artery and its branches in occlusion of the internal carotid artery. Int Angiol. 1994;13(1):5–9.

Jeon HW, Cha JK. Factors related to progression of middle cerebral artery stenosis determined using transcranial Doppler ultrasonography. J Thromb Thrombolysis. 2008;25(3):265–9.

Kelley RE, Namon RA, Mantelle LL, Chang JY. Sensitivity and specificity of transcranial Doppler ultrasonography in the detection of highgrade carotid stenosis. Neurology. 1993;43(6):1187–91.

Kessler C, von Maravic M, Albrecht DM, von Maravic C, Muller M, Schmidt P, Kompf D. Doppler CO2-test in patients with vertebrobasilar ischemia. Acta Neurol Scand (Denmark). 1991;84(6):519–22.

Kim DW, Min JH, Lee YS. Transcranial Doppler in asymptomatic carotid stenosis representing hemodynamic impairment: correlation study with magnetic resonance imaging. J Neuroimaging. 2004;14(4): 331–5.

Maeda H, Matsumoto M, Handa N, Hougaku H, Ogawa S, Itoh T, Tsukamoto Y, Kamada T. Reactivity of cerebral blood flow to carbon dioxide in hypertensive patients: evaluation by the transcranial Doppler method. J Hypertens. 1994;12(2):191–7.

Manchola IF, De Salles AA, Foo TK, Ackerman RH, Candia GT, Kjellberg RN. Arteriovenous malformation hemodynamics: a transcranial Doppler study. Neurosurgery. 1993;33(4):556–62; discussion 562.

Marshall J, Meadows S. The natural history of amaurosis fugax. Brain. 1968;91:419.

Massaro AR, Young WL, Kader A, Ostapkovich N, Tatemichi TI, Stein BM, Mohr JP. Characterization of arteriovenous malformation feeding vessels by carbon dioxide reactivity. AJNR Am J Neuroradiol. 1994; 15(1):55–61.

Miller JD, Smith RR. Transcranial Doppler sonography in aneurysmal subarachnoid hemorrhage. Cerebrovasc Brain Metab Rev. 1994;6(1):31–46.

Moustafa RR, Izquierdo-Garcia D, Fryer TD, Graves MJ, Rudd JH, Gillard JH, Weissberg PL, Baron JC, Warburton EA. Carotid plaque inflammation is associated with cerebral microembolism in patients with recent TIA or stroke: a pilot study. Circ Cardiovasc Imaging. 2010;16.

Navarro JC, Lao AY, Sharma VK, Tsivgoulis G, Alexandrov AV. The accuracy of transcranial Doppler in the diagnosis of middle cerebral artery stenosis. Cerebrovasc Dis. 2007;23(5-6):325–30.

Palombo D, Porta C, Peinetti F, Brustia P, Udini M, Antico A, Cantalupi D, Varetto T. Cerebral reserve and indications for shunting in carotid surgery. Cardiovasc Surg. 1994;2(1):32–6.

Rorick MB, Nichols FT, Adams RJ. Transcranial Doppler correlation with angiography in detection of intracranial stenosis. Stroke. 1994;25(10):1931–4.

Rozsa L, Szabo S, Gombi R, Miko L, Balazs E. Koponyauri nyomasfokozodast es agyhalalt kisero agyi veraramlas valtozasok vizsgalata transcranialis Doppler szonografiaval [Examination of changes in cerebral flow accompanying increased intracranial pressure and brain death by transcranial Doppler sonography]. Orv Hetil (Hungary). 1991;132(50): 2785–8.

Russell SM, Woo HH, Siller K, Panasci D, Leroux PD. Evaluating middle cerebral artery collateral blood flow reserve using acetazolamide transcranial Doppler ultrasound in patients with carotid occlusive disease. Surg Neurol. 2008;70(5):466–70.

Saqqur M, Demchuk AM, Hill MD, Dean N, Schebel M, Kennedy J, Barber PA, Shuaib A. Bedside emergency transcranial Doppler diagnosis of severe carotid disease using orbital window examination. J Neuroimaging. 2005;15(2):138–43.

Saqqur M, Hill MD, Alexandrov AV, Roy J, Schebel M, Krol A, Garami Z, Shuaib A, Demchuk AM. Derivation of power M-mode transcranial Doppler criteria for angiographic proven MCA occlusion. J Neuroimaging. 2006;16(4):323–8.

Siebler M, Rose G, Sitzer M, Bender A, Steinmetz H. Real-time identification of cerebral microemboli with US feature detection by a neural network. Radiology. 1994;192(3):739–42.

Tatemichi TK, et al. Hemodynamic role of ophthalmic artery collateral in internal carotid artery occlusion. Neurology. 1990;40:461–4.

Telman G, Kouperberg E, Sprecher E, Hoffman A, Yarnitsky D. Assessment of ophthalmic artery collateral pathway in the hemispheric cerebral hemodynamics in patients with severe unilateral carotid stenosis. Neurol Res. 2003;25(3):309–11.

Telman G, Kouperberg E, Hlebtovsky A, Sprecher E, Hoffman A, Beyar R. Determinants of micro-embolic signals in patients with atherosclerotic plaques of the internal carotid artery. Eur J Vasc Endovasc Surg. 2009;38(2):143–7.

Velkey I, Lombay B, Panczel G. Obstruction of cerebral arteries in childhood stroke. Pediatr Radiol. 1992; 22(5):386–7.

Visser GH, van der Grond J, van Huffelen AC, Wieneke GH, Eikelboom BC. Decreased transcranial Doppler carbon dioxide reactivity is associated with disordered cerebral metabolism in patients with internal carotid artery stenosis. J Vasc Surg. 1999;30(2):252–60.

Wardlaw JM, Vaughan GT, Steers AJ, Sellar RJ. Transcranial Doppler ultrasound findings in cerebral venous sinus thrombosis. Case report. J-Neurosurg. 1994;80(2):332–5.

You Y, Hao Q, Leung T, Mok V, Chen X, Lau A, Leung H, Wong KS. Detection of the siphon internal carotid artery stenosis: transcranial Doppler versus digital subtraction angiography. J Neuroimaging. 2010;20(3):234–9.

Color Doppler Ultrasound Examination in Orbital Diseases

27

János Németh, Zoltan Harkányi, and Zita Morvay

Contents

The diameter of the vessels in the eyeball is small, less than 1 mm in healthy people; therefore, these vessels are not seen in the ophthalmologic ultrasound. The diameter of the large veins is about 1 mm, but these veins collapse or their lumen decreases as a consequence of slightly increased intraocular pressure due to positioning the transducer. In abnormal cases, the diameter of the vessels may be more than 1 mm and the vessels are visualized as an echopoor band. The ophthalmic vein may be seen in healthy crying newborns.

J. Németh, M.D.
Department of Ophthalmology, Faculty of Medicine, Semmelweis University, Budapest, Hungary
e-mail: nemeth.janos@med.semmelweis-univ.hu

Z. Harkányi, M.D., PhD (✉)
Department of Radiology, CT Laboratory, Heim Pál Pediatric Hospital, Budapest, Hungary
e-mail: harkanyi@heimpalkorhaz.hu

Z. Morvay, M.D., PhD
Diagnoscan, Szeged, Hungary
e-mail: info@diagnoscan.hu

Currently, there are two ultrasound methods the vessels of the eyeball can be visualized with: the color Doppler ultrasound examination (color Doppler imaging, CDI) and the ultrasound angiography (power Doppler). Both methods register the movement of the blood, and therefore, visualize the vessels. In addition to examining the topography, flow velocity of the blood can be measured accurately. Usually the orbital vessels listed in Table 27.1 are examined with ultrasound flow examination. Transcranial and duplex Doppler ultrasound examinations do not show the orbital vessels (Table 27.2), only the flow velocity can be measured with these methods in the ophthalmic artery and in the central retinal artery and vein. As no angle correction can be performed with these methods, accuracy of these measurements is disputable.

The advantage of vascular ultrasound examinations is that they are non-invasive, fast, and give an immediate result. Administration of the contrast agent is not necessary, it is harmless for

Table 27.1 Color Doppler, ultrasound angiography – orbital vessels that can be examined with ultrasound methods

Ophthalmic artery and vein
Short and long ciliary arteries
Central retinal artery and vein and their branches
Choroidal vascular network
Pathologically appearing larger vessels
Vessels in neoplasms

J. Somlai, T. Kovács (eds.), *Neuro-Ophthalmology*, DOI 10.1007/978-3-319-28956-4_27

Table 27.2 Services of ultrasound vascular examinations when examining orbital vessels

	B scan image	Velocity measurement	Direction of flow	Vessel position
Transcranial Doppler	–	++	+	–
Duplex Doppler	+++	+++	+	–
Color Doppler	+++	+	+++	+++
Power Doppler	+++	–	–	+++

the patient, so it can be repeated as necessary. An additional advantage is that both the arterial and the venous circulations can be examined from the apex of the orbit to the retina, and topographic and hemodynamic information is available at the same time. Accurate measurement of velocity makes quantitative description of the circulation and follow-up of timely changes possible. Ultrasound vascular examinations have no contraindications, but it should be noted that the Doppler examination poses larger ultrasound energy exposure than the B scan ultrasound examination. During an ophthalmologic vascular examination, the amount of maximal energy exposure (Spatial Peak Time Average Intensity) is below 100 mW/cm^2. It is significantly lower than the energy causing a choroidal lesion or cataract in experimental conditions. Despite it, our aim should be to minimize the energy exposure of the patient during the examination. In order to ensure minimal exposure, low energy ultrasound should be used, and the examination should be short.

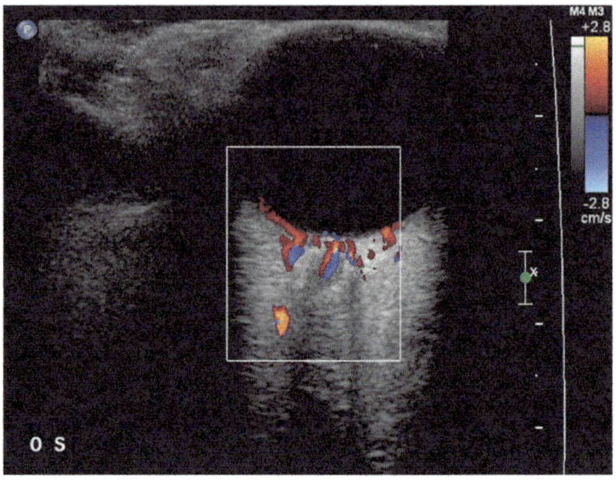

Fig. 27.1 Color Doppler image of the eye and orbit in a healthy person. The normal blood circulation is well seen in the central retinal artery and vein and in the short ciliary arteries and in the choroid-retina

Color and Duplex Doppler Ultrasound Examination

The aforementioned vascular examinations, are based on the Doppler effect. The essence of the phenomenon is that the frequency of the transducer is known, and this ultrasound is reflected by the red blood cells circulating in the vessels, the transducer receives the reflected ultrasound. The difference between the emitted and reflected ultrasound frequency is the Doppler frequency shift, which depends on the direction of the flow and the velocity. Color Doppler examination is the combination of the black and white ultrasound B scan and the color image indicating blood flow (Fig. 27.1.). During the examination, steady structures are seen in two-dimensional black and white B images, while moving areas are represented by colors. Standard coding indicates flow towards the transducer with red color and flow away from the transducer with blue color. Lighter colors represent increased velocity, darker colors indicate slow flow, therefore indicating the extent of the frequency shift. In order to accurately measure the flow velocity, the device has to be switched to pulse Doppler mode, when the Doppler spectrum from the selected area becomes visible, and flow velocity can be measured after an angle correction (Fig. 27.2.).

The following parameters are usually defined to characterize blood flow: systolic peak velocity, end diastolic velocity, mean velocity, acceleration, acceleration time, and various flow indices. Normal values detected in the orbital vessels are seen in Table 27.3.

Based on our observations, flow velocity is highly dependent on the depth of the Doppler measurement performed in the eyeball in case of the ophthalmic artery (Table 27.4). The reason

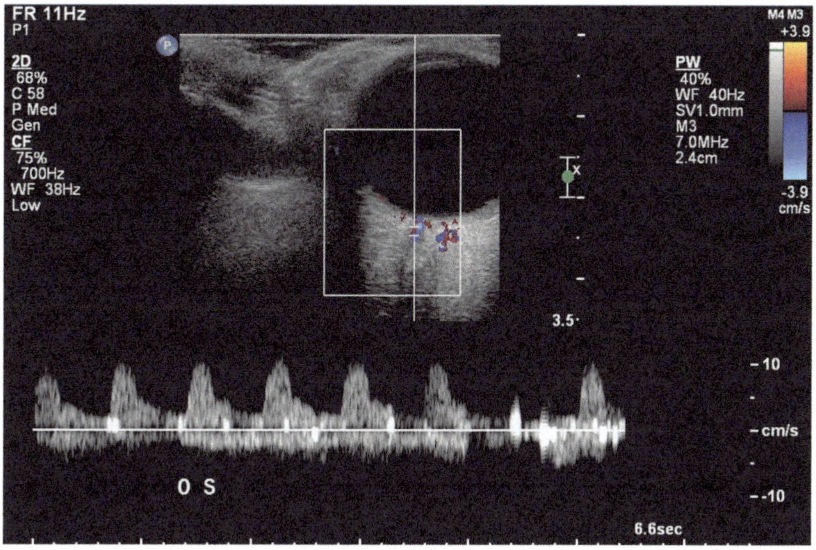

Fig. 27.2 Color Doppler and Duplex Doppler image of the eye and orbit. The Doppler spectrum is showing normal circulation in the central retinal artery and vein

Table 27.3 Flow velocity values in healthy orbital vessels (mean ± SD, cm/s)

	Lieb (1991)	Guthoff (1991)	Ho (1992)	Németh (1996)
Case number	40	72	27	48
Ophthalmic artery systolic peak velocity, end diastolic velocity, mean velocity	31.4 ± 4.2	31.6 ± 9.0 8.2 ± 3.7 15.9 ± 5.3	30.6 ± 8.9	34.2 ± 9.9 9.0 ± 2.9 17.2 ± 5.6
Central retinal artery systolic peak velocity, end diastolic velocity, mean velocity	10.3 ± 2.1	9.5 ± 3.1 3.1 ± 1.6 5.7 ± 2.0	10.5 ± 2.4	9.3 ± 2.1 3.0 ± 0.9 5.2 ± 1.4
Posterior ciliary artery systolic peak velocity, end diastolic velocity, mean velocity	12.4 ± 4.8		9.1 ± 2.6	11.9 ± 3.0 3.6 ± 1.3 6.7 ± 2.1
Max. velocity, min. velocity of ophthalmic vein				10.1 ± 3.1 7.9 ± 2.7
Max. velocity, min. velocity of retinal central vein	2.9 ± 0.73	5.7 ± 1.5 4.0 ± 1.0		5.1 ± 0.9 3.7 ± 0.8

Table 27.4 Flow velocity measured in the ophthalmic arteries of healthy volunteers in various depths (mean ± SD, cm/s)

Depth of the measurement	Case number	Systolic peak velocity	End diastolic velocity	Mean velocity
3.0–3.9 mm	22	28.0 ± 7.4	7.1 ± 1.8	13.3 ± 3.0
4.0–5.0 mm	23	40.1 ± 8.5	10.8 ± 2.7	20.8 ± 5.0
p value		<0.001	<0.001	<0.001

for this is that the ophthalmic artery has end branches shortly after it enters the orbit. The deeper the measurement is performed, the more likely it is that the main branch of the ophthalmic artery is examined in which flow velocity is increased, and not a branch is examined with slower velocity.

Flow indices are parameters suitable to characterize peripheral resistance. The resistance index (RI) (or Pourcelot Index) is the difference of systolic and diastolic frequency shifts divided by the systolic frequency shift. The pulsatility index (PI) is the difference of systolic and diastolic frequency shifts divided by the mean velocity. The A/B ratio (or S/D ratio) is the quotient of the systolic and diastolic frequency shifts. Table 27.5 contains normal values of flow indices based on our own measurements.

Clinical Use of Color Doppler Ultrasound Examination

In case of occlusive arterial and venous diseases, color Doppler ultrasound examination may be used to prove changes in orbital blood supply (Table 27.6). If the flow velocity decreases, stenosis may be suspected in the vessel segments proximal to the examined vessel. If no sign of circulation is detected in the affected vessel in the acute phase of the disease, a complete vascular occlusion is suspected. Usually reperfusion is seen in 1 week.

Detection of orbital vascular malformations is easy in case of arterial lesions; however, venous anomalies (varices) are significantly more difficult to diagnose as blood flow is often very slow.

Color Doppler ultrasound is diagnostic in detecting carotid–cavernous fistulas: it confirms retrograde and arterialized flow in the dilated ophthalmic vein branch(es) (Fig. 27.3.). In addition to diagnosis, color Doppler ultrasound can be well used in measuring the efficacy of embolization or balloon surgeries, and in pre- and post-operative follow-up.

In case of intraocular and orbital tumors, color Doppler ultrasound can be used as a differential diagnostic tool by detecting the internal blood flow inside the tumor (Fig. 27.4.). It helps differentiating between tumors and non-vascularized disorders (hemorrhages) masking tumors. Precaution should be taken when evaluating the finding as there are certain non-tumor lesions with an echographic image characteristic of a tumor (such as scleritis, PVR) having an internal circulation.

Having information on the blood supply of the tumors is important in the treatment of the tumor as well, as it influences the response to conservative treatment. Examination of the circulation may help in following the fibrosis of conservatively treated tumors and in recognizing potential recurrence of the tumor.

Table 27.5 Flow indices in healthy volunteers (mean ± SD)

	Ophthalmic artery	Central retinal artery
Resistance index	0.74 ± 0.07	0.67 ± 0.08
Pulsatility index	1.57 ± 0.58	1.21 ± 0.26
S/D ratio	4.52 ± 3.86	3.28 ± 0.91

Case number: 48

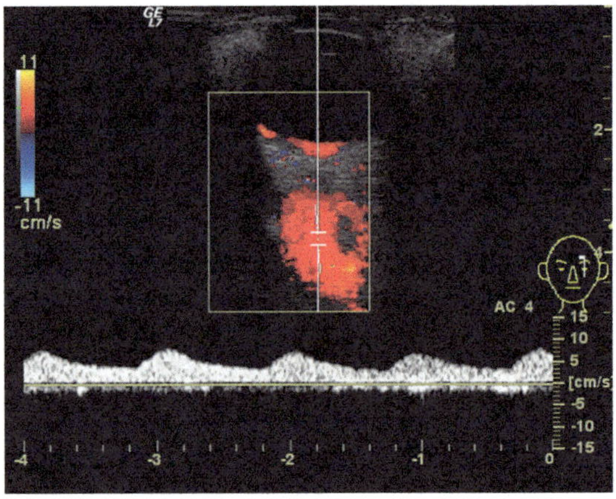

Fig. 27.3 Color Doppler image of a carotid-cavernous fistula. The circulation in the dilated superior ophthalmic vein is reversed and the spectrum is arterialized

Table 27.6 Flow velocity in various diseases and in healthy controls, based on our own measurements (systolic peak/end diastolic velocity values in cm/s)

Patient groups (n)	Ophthalmic artery	Central retinal artery	Central retinal vein	Ophthalmic vein
Healthy controls (17)	35.5/8.3	13.1/4.2	4.7	13.9
Optic ischemia (AION) (15)	32.3/12.0	12.1/4.2	4.3	9.4
Glaucoma (6)	21.6/7.2	15.8/2.2	5.1	7.0
Intraocular tumors (10)	44.3/15.0	13.0/4.5	5.8	13.6
Tumors of the orbit (4)	44.7/11.3	15.7/4.7	6.2	11.5

Németh and Forster (1993)

Our own experience and results of previous studies show that the lack of signs of circulation does not exclude the presence of a tumor. Based on the literature, no Doppler sign suggestive of circulation was detected in 2–17 % of choroidal melanomas and metastatic carcinomas. Detecting signs of circulation is strongly related to the technique of the vascular examination and the experience of the examiner. Several various technical and biological factors influence the detectability of tissue circulation. Technical factors: spatial and time resolution of the device and the transducer, Doppler sensitivity, angular dependence and spontaneous movements of the examiner. In case of orbital vessels with a small lumen, low velocity range and low wall filter settings are recommended. Biological factors influencing the detectability of signs of circulation are the following: the size of the vessels, the direction of the vessels, blood flow velocity, eye movements of the examined person, and spontaneous tissue movements occurring simultaneously with the heart rate and breathing. As the size of the color sign is generally larger than the actual size of the vessel, determining the presence or lack of internal circulation of small tumors or structures which are considered to be tumors and differentiating them from the circulation of the surrounding structures (retina, choroid) is impossible.

Color Doppler ultrasound in case of patients with glaucoma showed decreased flow velocity in the ophthalmic artery and in the central retinal artery, and increased peripheral resistance was found in the posterior short ciliary vessels. Flow velocity was increased and peripheral resistance was decreased in the central retinal artery and in the posterior short ciliary arteries after trabeculectomy, suggesting improved circulation. In case of other diseases (inflammations, hypertension, diabetes mellitus), vascular disorders are examined for research purposes only, but may have diagnostic and differential diagnostic importance in the future. Wong et al (1994) and Hilborn et al (1993) have differentiated the detached retina and the limiting membrane of the vitreous body as well as diabetic proliferative membranes with color Doppler ultrasound. The method was found to be useful in differentiating between the retina and the chorioidea after severe injuries as well.

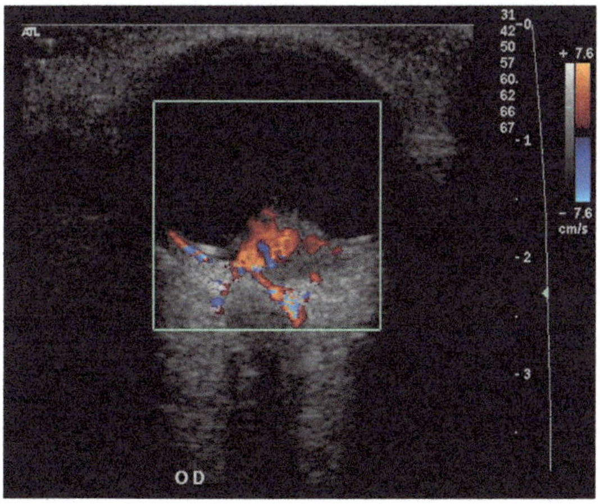

Fig. 27.4 Color Doppler image of an intraocular tumor

References

Balázs E, Rózsa L. Diagnosztikus lehetőségek a szemészetben transcraniális Doppler-szonográfiával. I. Vasculáris betegségek [Diagnostic possibilities in ophthalmology with transcranial Doppler sonography. 1. Vascular diseases]. Szemeszet. 1988;125:168.

Balázs E, Rózsa L, Szabó S. A carotideo-cavernosus fistulákat követô véráramlás-változások [Changes in blood flow after carotideo–cavernous fistulas]. Szemeszet. 1992;129:159–62.

Balázs E, Rózsa L, Szabó S. A véráramlás sebessége az artéria ophthalmicában. Transcranialis Doppler-tanulmány [Blood flow velocity in the ophthalmic artery. A transcranial Doppler study]. Szemeszet. 1993a;130:153–5.

Balázs E, Rózsa L, Szabó S. Véráramlási viszonyok a vena ophthalmica superiorban [Blood flow in the superior ophthalmic vein]. Szemeszet. 1993b;130:221–4.

Balázs E, Rózsa L, Fülesdi B, Szabó S. Transcranialis Doppler-vizsgálatok ischaemiás szembetegségekben [Transcranial Doppler tests in ischemic eye diseases]. Szemeszet. 1994a;131:169–75.

Balázs E, Fülesdi B, Rózsa L. Transcranialis Doppler- és duplex ultrahangos vizsgálatok normális tenziójú glaukómás betegekben [Transcranial Doppler and duplex ultrasound scans in glaucoma patients with normal pressure]. Szemeszet. 1994b; 131:233–6.

Barta M, Sandy RM, Merton DA, Goldberg B. A szem és az orbita színes Doppler vizsgálata [Color Doppler test of the eye and the orbit]. Lege Artis Med. 1993;3:630–5.

Berges O. Colour Doppler flow imaging of the orbital veins. Acta Ophthalmol. 1992;70 Suppl 204:55–8.

Flaharty PM, Lieb WE, Sergott RC, Bosley TM, Savino PJ. Color Doppler imaging. A new non-invasive technique to diagnose and monitor carotid cavernous sinus fistulas. Arch Ophthalmol. 1991;109:522–6.

Guthoff RF, Berger RW, Winkler P, Helmke K, Chumbley LC. Doppler ultrasonography of the ophthalmic and central retinal vessels. Arch Ophthalmol. 1991a;109:532–6.

Guthoff RF, Berger RW, Winkler P, Helmke K, Chumbley LC. Doppler ultrasonography of malignant melanomas. Arch Ophthalmol. 1991b;109:537–41.

Guthoff R. Ultrasound in ophthalmologic diagnosis. A Practical Guide. Stuttgart/New York: Thieme; 1991.

Harkányi Z. Duplex ultrahang. Gyakorlati útmutató duplex és color Doppler-ultrahang-vizsgálatokhoz [Duplex ultrasound. A practical guide to duplex and color Doppler ultrasound scans]. Budapest/Berlin: Springer; 1991.

Harkányi Z, Merton D, Lui JB, Goldberg BB. Új ultrahangmódszer a vérkeringés vizsgálatában: color velocity imaging [A new ultrasonography method in detecting the blood flow: color velocity imaging]. Lege Artis Med. 1992;2:964–51.

Harkányi Z, Morvay Z, editors. UltraSzonográfia. 2. bővitett kiadás [Ultrasonography 2. An extended version]. Budapest: Minerva; 2006.

Horóczi Z, Morvay Z, Szabó Á. Color Doppler ultrahangos vizsgálatok endocrin orbitopathiában [Color Doppler ultrasound scans in endocrine orbitopathy]. Szemeszet. 1995;132:33–4.

Lieb WE, Shields JA, Cohen SM, Merton DA, Mitchell DG, Shields CL, Goldberg BB. Color Doppler imaging in the management of intraocular tumors. Ophthalmology. 1990;97:1660–4.

Lieb WE, Flaharty PM, Ho A, Sergott RC. Color Doppler imaging of the eye and orbit. A synopsis of a 400 case experience. Acta Ophthalmol. 1992;70 Suppl 204:50–4.

Morvay Z, Németh J, Horóczi Z, Nagy E. Az orbita ereinek vizsgálata színkódolt Doppler-ultrahang eljárással [Examination of the vessels in the orbit by color Doppler ultrasound]. Magy Radiol. 1993;67: 133–6.

Nagy ZZs, Barzó P, Pelle Zs, Az a. ophthalmica és az agyi erek keringésviszonyainak meghatározása EME TC-2-64B transcraniális Doppler készülékkel kora- és egészséges újszülöttekben, valamint inaktív stádiumú ROP-os és egészséges kontrollszemeken [Assessing the flow in the ophthalmic artery and the cerebral arteries by EME TC-2-64B transcranial Doppler in premature and healthy newborns and in ROPs in inactive stage and healthy controls]. Szemészet. 1992;129: 111–4.

Nagy ZZs, Németh J, Süveges I, Lányi F, Bodosi M, Facskó A. Panretinalis fotokoaguláció a paradox módon rosszabbodó duralis-sinus cavernosus arteriovenosus malformatio egy esetében [Panretinal photocoagulation ina case of paradox exacerbation of dural–sinus cavernous arteriovenózus malformation]. Szemészet. 1994;131:43–7.

Németh J, Morvay Z, Horóczi Z, Nagy E. A színkódolt Doppler ultrahangvizsgálat szemészeti alkalmazása [Use of color Doppler ultrasound scan in ophthalmology]. Szemeszet. 1992a;129:34–7.

Németh J, Végh M, Horóczi Z, Süveges I. A szemgolyó és az orbita vizsgálata nem-szemészeti ultrahang készülékekkel [Examining the eye-ball and the orbit with non-ophthalmologic ultrasound scan]. Orv Hetil. 1992b;133:2563–5.

Németh J, Forster T. Carotideo-cavernous fistula diagnózisa ultrahanggal [Diagnosing carotieo-cavernous fistula with ultrasound scan]. Szemeszet. 1993;130:25–7.

Németh J, Tapasztó B, Morvay Z, Nagy E. Orbitális keringésváltozások glaucomás betegekben. Előzetes közlemény [Changes in orbital circulation in patients with glaucoma. A preliminary study]. Szemeszet. 1994;131:31–4.

Németh J, Sényi K, Harkányi Z, Kovács R, Morvay Z, Kovács E, Tóth J. A color Doppler-ultrahang szerepe a szemgolyó és az orbita daganatainak diagnosztikájában [The role of color Doppler ultrasound scan in diagnosing tumors of the eye-ball and the orbit]. Szemeszet. 1995;132:239–42.

Németh J, Harkányi Z, Kovács R, Sényi K, Tapasztó B, Marsovszky I, Barta M. Normális áramlási értékek meghatározása egészséges személyek orbitaereiben color Doppler-ultrahang módszerrel [Assessment of normal flow values with color Doppler ultrasonography in the vessels of the orbit of healthy subjects]. Szemeszet. 1996;133:221–4.

Németh J. Szemészeti ultrahang-diagnosztika és biometria [Ophthalmology utrasound diagnostics and bimetry]. Nyctalus Orvosi Kiadó, Bp. 1996.

Németh J. Szemtumor vagy vérzés? In: Harkányi Z, Morvay Z, editors. UltraSzonográfia. Általános és vaszkuláris ultrahang-diagnosztika orvosok és szonográfusok részére [Tumor of the eye or bleeding? In: Harkányi Z, Morvay Z, editors. Ultrsonography. General and vascular ultrasound diagnostics for doctors and sonographists]. Minerva: Budapest; 2001. p. 351–7, 4.

Németh J, Kovács R, Harkányi Z, Knézy K, Sényi K, Marsovszky I. Observer experience improves reproducibility of color Doppler sonography of orbital blood vessels. J Clin Ultrasound. 2002;30:332–5.

Németh J, Harkányi Z, Humml F. Non-invasive volumetric blood flow measurement in the orbit. Br J Ophthalmol. 2003;87:927–8.

Németh J, Tapasztó B, Harkányi Z, Tóth J. Colour Doppler imaging of intraocular and orbital tumors and comparison with pathological findings. South-East Eur J Ophthalmol. 2006;1:60–3.

Trible JR, Sergott RC, Spaeth GL, et al. Trabeculectomy is associated with retrobulbar hemodynamic changes. A color Doppler analysis. Ophthalmology. 1994;101: 340–51.

The Role of the Ophthalmologic Ultrasound in Neuro-ophthalmology

28

Béla Csákány and János Németh

Contents

The ophthalmologic ultrasonography includes several examination methods with various techniques that are performed for different purposes. The most important examinations are the following:

1. Biomety with A-scan method – most commonly used to measure the axial length (AL).
2. Ultrasound biomicroscopic (UBM) examination of the anterior segment of the eyeball.
3. Diagnostic B-scan examination of the posterior segment of the eyeball and the parabulbar and retrobulbar orbital tissues.

B. Csákány, M.D., PhD (✉)
Department of Ophthalmology,
Semmelweis University, Budapest, Hungary
e-mail: csakanybela@gmail.com

J. Németh, M.D.
Department of Ophthalmology, Faculty of Medicine,
Semmelweis University, Budapest, Hungary
e-mail: nemeth.janos@med.semmelweis-univ.hu

A-Scan Examination for Biometric Purposes

The examination is performed with a 10 MHz A-scan ultrasound probe; currently other biometric devices that are not based on the reflection of ultrasound are available as well. The method can be used to determine the axial length of the eyeball. This examination method can help differentiate between real exophthalmus and pseudoexophthalmus seen in patients with extreme short-sightedness who have significantly elongated eyeball. As lesions in the orbit rarely change the length of the eyeball, and other examination methods are more informative in these disorders, this examination has no other neuro-ophthalmologic aspect.

Ultrasound Biomicroscopy (UBM)

The size of the pupil and dynamic changes in the size of the pupil can be documented with UBM. However, the slit lamp examination or macrovideo recording and pupillometry are more suitable for this purpose, so UBM is necessary only in rare cases when functional alteration of the pupil can be assumed (not as a consequence of a topical reason), and the patient has corneal opacity or the anterior chamber is cloudy. In case of accommodative spasm caused by the lesion of the brainstem, UBM may be used to examine the ciliary body and the thickness of the lens, but it is not necessary for the diagnosis.

J. Somlai, T. Kovács (eds.), *Neuro-Ophthalmology*, DOI 10.1007/978-3-319-28956-4_28

Diagnostic B-Scan Examination

This examination is performed with a 10 MHz or 20 MHz ophthalmologic ultrasound transducer; but if necessary, it may be performed with a non-ophthalmologic ultrasound device.[1] Neuro-ophthalmological intraocular lesions may be examined with this device; in addition, parabulbar tissues of the orbit and the retrobulbar space may be examined to 40 mm depth from the transducer. The posterior 1/3 of the orbit and the apex of the orbit cannot be examined with this method.

Intraocular Lesions

They may affect the vitreous space, the wall of the eyeball or the optic disc. B-scan examination is necessary in any disorder that is accompanied by visual loss, if the examination of the fundus is not possible due to the not clear media. In these cases, the purpose of the ultrasound is to exclude or confirm potential local origin of the loss in the visual field.

Vitreous Space

Terson's syndrome: intraocular bleeding accompanied by subarachnoidal bleeding. If the bleeding affects the vitreous gel or is retrohyaloid, it can be seen easily with B-scan images. Intragel vitreous hemorrhage in the vitreous space is usually seen next to the optic disc, and it is less likely to sediment compared to bleeding in proliferative diabetic retinopathy.

Posterior Wall of the Eyeball

Tuberous sclerosis: astrocytic hamartoma of the retina has an extremely high reflectivity; it has a strong acoustic shadow, and is usually protruding into the eyeball in the images. It cannot be differentiated from a calcified retinoblastoma focus with ultrasound, but other diagnostic signs of tuberous sclerosis and the fact that the retinal lesion is not progressive are usually helpful.

Posterior pole and optic nerve coloboma: imaging these abnormalities is relatively easy with ultrasound: circumscribed posterior staphyloma bulging of the wall (more common) and low reflectivity area located to the optic nerve (rare) are the typical signs of this developmental disease. The location of the retina in the area of the coloboma can be better evaluated with echography than with other imaging studies.

Disorders of the Optic Disc

Optic disc drusen is a common, relatively harmless disorder. In young patients, hyaline nodules in the area of the optic disc are still under the surface, and a bilateral, protruding optic disc with a blurred edge may refer to increased intracranial pressure.

A round structure with very high reflectivity is seen in the region of the optic nerve head (Fig. 28.1) with ultrasonography. This structure can easily be differentiated from the true optic disc edema which is protruding as well but has decreased reflectivity compared to its surrounding.

Anterior ischemic optic neuropathy (*AION*): according to the literature, the optic nerve is wider and has a dual contour, but it is often questionable whether it can be judged or not. Therefore, B scan examination is considered to be unnecessary to perform in this disease.

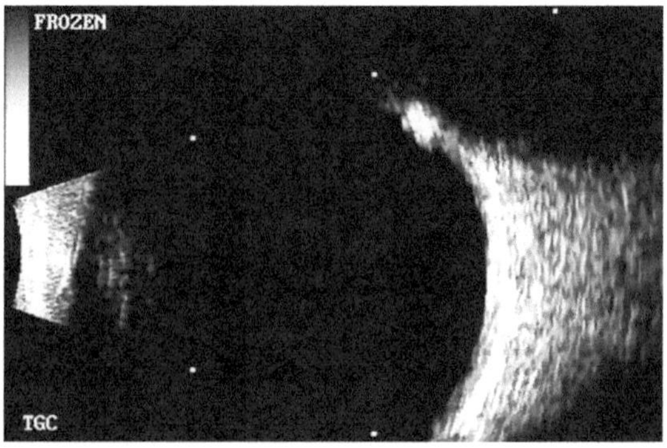

Fig. 28.1 Optic disk

[1] Note: in addition to diagnostic B-scan examination, standardized echography described by Karl C. Ossoinig is often recommended in the literature. The most important tool of this examination is the diagnostic A-scan head with 8 MHz frequency. There is no clear agreement regarding the benefits of this method; as it is not widely used in Hungary, this examination is not described in details here

Disorders of the Orbit

May affect the optic nerve, the muscles, the orbital fat tissue, or the vessels of the orbit. The tumors may be intraconal or extraconal.

Optic Nerve

The optic nerve thickness and its reflectivity can be evaluated with ultrasonography. In order to measure the thickness in B scan cross sectional images, the transducer has to be placed to the eyelid from lateral direction in vertical examination plane, and the patient should be asked to look strictly in the direction of the transducer. In this case, the cross section of the optic nerve can be visualized behind the eyeball (Fig. 28.2).

Increased intracranial pressure: the diameter of the optic nerve may be even 5.5–6.0 mm large, (the average diameter of the optic nerve in normal condition is around 3.8 mm); the optic nerve sheath can be differentiated in the images (Fig. 28.3). Similarly, the optic nerve may be thicker in case of advanced *thyroid associated orbitopathy* as well (TAO, see below).

Acute phase optic neuritis may be detected as a defined thickening in some cases. The optic nerve thickness does not change detectably in *optic atrophy*, even in cases without light sensation either. The thinner than normal optic nerve is rather characteristic of *optic nerve hypoplasia*.

Traumatic damage of the optic nerve is rare; in this case, B scan examination may help deciding whether functional impairment is caused by a treatable condition (orbital bleeding with the compression of the optic nerve) or by direct injury of the optic nerve.

For the same reasons, emergency ultrasound is recommended in case of visual loss after a retrobulbar injection. Retrobulbar bleeding is an area with low reflectivity.

Muscles of the Eye, Orbital Fat Tissue

In case of thyroid associated orbitopathy, increased muscle thickness is seen (Fig. 28.4), reflectivity of the muscles is low at the beginning, and then as the process worsens, and fibrosis of the muscles develop, an uneven increase is seen in the reflectivity.

Reflectivity of the orbital fat tissue may be uneven as well. A thicker than normal optic nerve is seen only in case of advanced TAO, when enlarged muscles compresses the optic nerve.

Orbital Vessels

The reflectivity of the intraorbital varix is low, it is a system of vascular spaces communicating with each other behind and next to the eyeball. Reflectivity of the *orbital hemangioma* is low

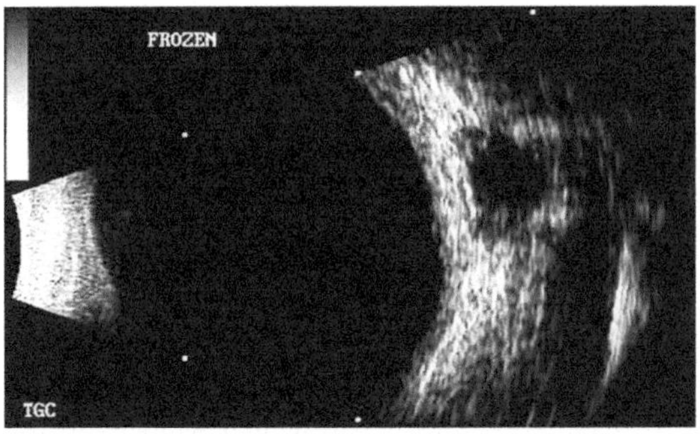

Fig. 28.2 Cross sectional image of the optic nerve

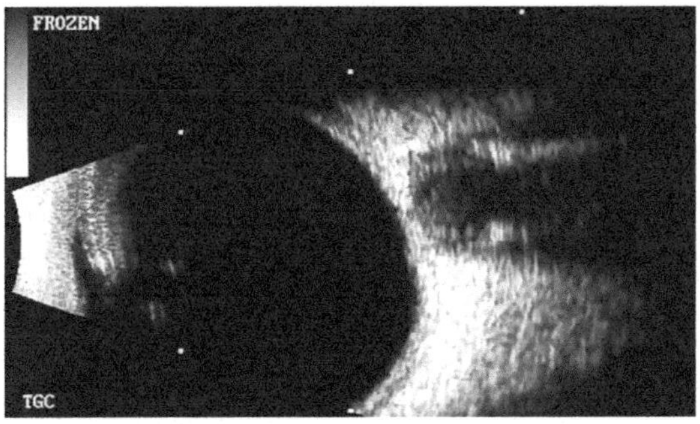

Fig. 28.3 Longitudinal section of the optic nerve. The optic sheath is easily visible

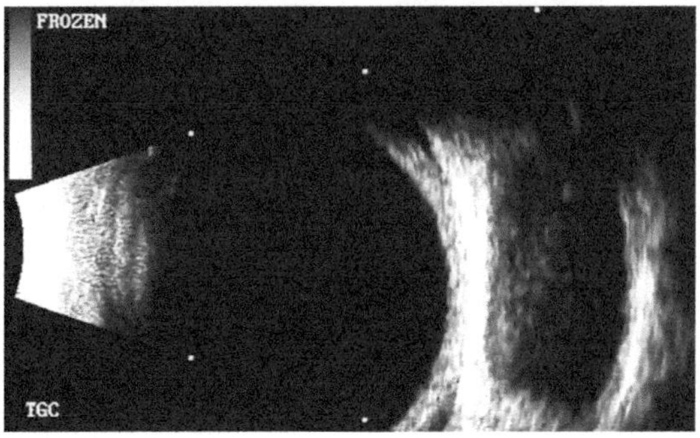

Fig. 28.4 Significantly thicker medial rectus eye muscle with low internal reflectivity

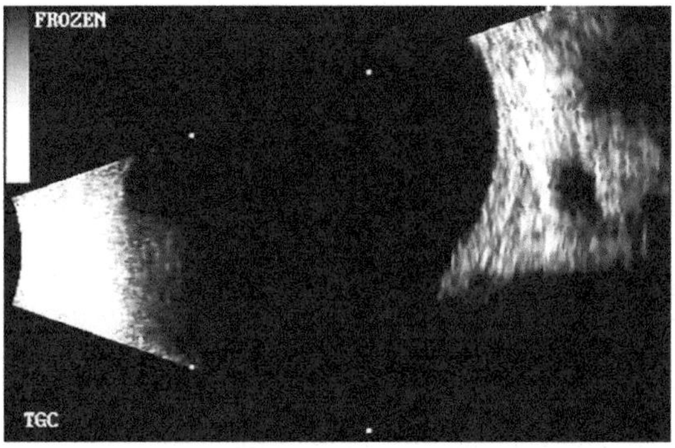

Fig. 28.5 Dilated superior ophthalmic vein behind the eyeball

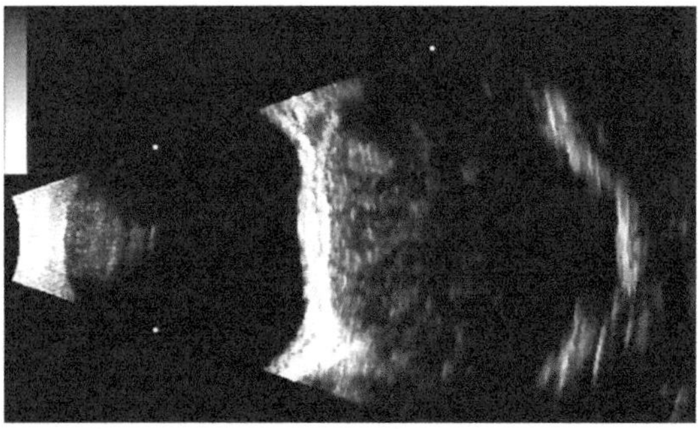

Fig. 28.6 Soft tissue tumor in the orbit leading to a protrusion in the posterior wall of the eyeball

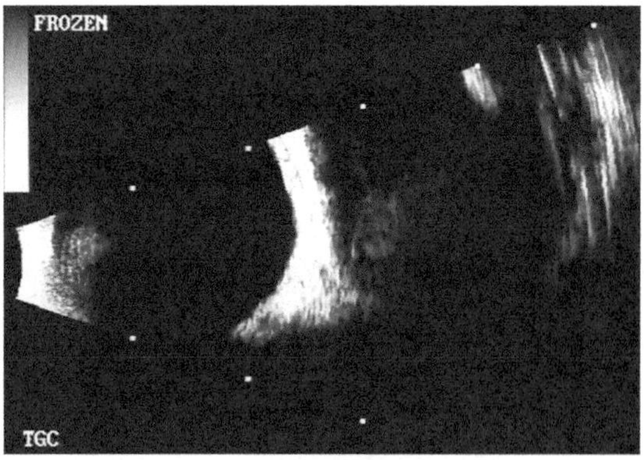

Fig. 28.7 Large orbital mucocele

and inhomogen; the lumen of the vessels is often just susceptible. The dilated orbital veins are easily differentiated from both disorders based on their course; their lumen may be 4–5 mm instead of the physiological 1 mm in case of *carotid-cavernous fistule* (Fig. 28.5).

Tumors of the Orbit

Glioma of the optic nerve (pilocytic astrocytoma) and meningeoma of the optic sheath are usually detectable by ultrasound: the anterior surface and the intraconal localization of the tumor are seen. However, the method is not suitable in determining the exact size and extent of the tumor, and it cannot be clearly differentiated from each other or from other soft tissue tumors (rhabdomyosarcoma, neuroblastoma) (Fig. 28.6) or from non-neoplastic space occupying lesions (Fig. 28.7) based on the examination of the inner reflectivity of the tumors. Tumors of the orbit usually require further imaging studies, the final diagnosis can only be set up after histological sampling in some cases.

Further Readings

Byrne SF, Green RL. Examination techniques for the orbit; orbital tumors; vascular lesions. In: Byrne SF, Green RL, editors. Ultrasound of the eye and orbit. St. Louis: Mosby; 2002. p. 275–366.

Hidasi V, Kolozsvári L. A szem tengelyhosszának és konfigurációjának korral összefüggő változása progresszív myopiában [Changes of the axial length and configuration of the eye related to aging in progressive myopathy]. Szemészet. 1995;132:119–21.

Németh J. Orbita betegségek echográfiája. In: Németh J. Szemészeti ultrahangdiagnosztika és biometria [Echography of diseases of the orbit. In: Németh J. Ophthalmology ultrasound diagnostics and bimetry]. Budapest: Nyctalus; 1996. p. 107–118.

Szabó Á, Valkusz Z, Németh J, Horváth E. A nervus opticus méretváltozásainak echográfiai követése endocrin orbitopathia kezelése során [Following changes in the size of the optic nerve in the treatment of endocrine orbitopathy with echocardiography]. Szemészet. 1995;132:41–4.

The Role of the EMG-ENG in Diagnosing Neuro-ophthalmologic Diseases

29

Mária Judit Molnár

Contents

From the electrophysiological examinations, electromyography (EMG) and electroneurography (ENG) help neurologists and neuro-ophthalmologists in diagnosing diseases affecting the skeletal muscle, the neuromuscular junction, or the peripheral nerves, or if the neuro-ophthalmological symptom is part of a multisystemic disease affecting one of the above organs. This chapter briefly describes the role of EMG–ENG examinations in neuro-ophtalmologic diseases and then describes the most characteristic differences that help the clinician in recognizing neuro-ophthalmological diseases.

Electromyography

EMG registers bioelectric voltage changes developing as a consequence of the function of the striated muscle. In the clinical practice, the most important examination is the concentric needle electrode test. The EMG examination is performed in 4 steps: (1) registering the insertional activity, (2) observing spontaneous activity at rest, (3) analyzing motor unit potentials with slight innervation, (4) registering the interference pattern with maximal voluntary innervation. In addition, response to repetitive stimulation of the peripheral nerve can be examined as well as the degree of the jitters with single fiber EMG.

Insertional Activity

Normally, inserting or suddenly moving the needle leads to a burst consisting of high frequency potentials lasting a few milliseconds. Inserting the needle may lead to abnormally long spontaneous activity in abnormal cases. The insertion potential is different in each muscle and is different near the end plate and far from the

M.J. Molnár, M.D., PhD, med. habil
Department of Molecular Neurology and Research Center, Center for Rare Neurological Diseases, Semmelweis University, Budapest, Hungary
e-mail: molnarmj@neur.sote.hu;
http://molneur.eoldal.hu

J. Somlai, T. Kovács (eds.), *Neuro-Ophthalmology*, DOI 10.1007/978-3-319-28956-4_29

end plate. Insertion activity is increased if the muscle is abnormally excitable. This can be detected primarily in denervation procedures, but increased excitability is often detected in myotonia, inflammatory myopathy as well.

Spontaneous Activity

Normally, action potential cannot be registered in the muscle at rest. In certain diseases, fibrillation potentials and monophasic positive sharp waves may appear. Fibrillation potentials are 1–5 msec long bi- or triphasic spontaneous bursts with 100–200 μV amplitude. Positive sharp waves are 5–10 msec long monophasic potentials with amplitude of over 100 μV. Both findings are seen primarily in denervation procedures, but may occur in inflammatory, metabolic, or endocrine myopathies as well.

The complex repetitive discharge (pseudomyotonic burst) is the elongated burst of small and large frequency potentials developing as a consequence of synchronous repetitive discharge of a group of muscle fibers and sound similar to the crackling sound of a machine gun. The series of discharges start and end suddenly, and the shape of each potential may be bizarre sometimes. This may be present in motor neuron diseases, myopathies, muscular dystrophies, polymyositis, myxedema, and chronic polyneuropathy. The myotonic discharges are high frequency repetitive discharges with frequency and amplitude values increasing gradually reaching the maximum value, and then the amplitude and the frequency start decreasing gradually. It occurs usually when the needle is inserted, it can be provoked by moving the needle, but sometimes it may be registered spontaneously. In the speaker, a crescendo-decrescendo sound effect, the sound of a dive bomber is heard. In addition to myotonic diseases, myotonic discharges are seen in periodic paralysis, rarely in chronic myositis and hypothyroidism. It may appear when the needle electrode is inserted, when the electrode is moved, or when percussion is applied on the muscle.

Motor Unit Potentials (MUP)

Isolated discharges of single motor axons give rise to motor unit potentials. Characteristics of motor unit potentials: the duration, amplitude, wave form, phases, stability and discharge frequency of the potential. The size of the MUP increases lowering temperature or advanced age. In case of a concentric needle electrode examination, the registered amplitude may vary between 100 μV and 2000–3000 μV. The shape of the wave is normally biphasic or triphasic. A potential is polyphasic if it has four or more phases. The polyphasic potential is the consequence of the temporal dispersion of each fiber potential discharging within a motor unit. Normally, the incidence of polyphasic potentials is 3–5 %. Incidence above 10 % is considered to be abnormal. The shape of the wave may be influenced by the spatial position of the needle electrode related to muscle fibers, and the temperature of the muscle tissue. Decreasing the temperature increases the number of poplyphasic potentials.

The amplitude and duration of the MUP decrease in myopathic diseases, few polyphasic potentials are seen, the waveform is stable. In case of maximal innervation, low amplitude interference pattern is seen in weak and atrophic muscles as well. The duration of MUP increases in neurogenic diseases. The amplitude may increase, but this is not generally applicable. Several complex, polyphasic potentials and large unit potentials are seen with increased duration in lesions of the frontal horn. Collateral reinnervation is in the background during which muscle fibers innervated by destroyed motor units are innervated by the surrounding, still functional motor units with new collaterals. Denervation activity such as fibrillation potentials, positive sharp waves, sometimes fasciculation potentials may be seen at rest. The duration and the amplitude of the MUP increase in case of peripheral nerve damage as well, but the extent of this increase is less compared with that seen in motor neuron lesion. Polyphasic potentials with low amplitude are seen even before the clinical improvement as a sign of regeneration.

Interference Pattern

In case of slight voluntary innervation of the skeletal muscle, only a few motor units are discharging, increasing the intensity of innervation activates further motor units. This process is called recruitment. Interference pattern is defined as a condition when individual motor unit potentials are not recognized, only the summarized potentials are seen in the screen of the EMG device. In neurogenic diseases, motor nerve cells not involved have to discharge faster in order to develop the desired force, so the recruitment is limited or decreased, the interference pattern is incomplete, and individual MUP can be recognized in case of maximal force production as well. While in myopathies, in order to develop the same force, more motor units have to activate as the number of muscle fibers decreased, so complex interference pattern develops even in case of small effort. This is the phenomenon of early recruitment. As in case of myopathies, early recruitment is seen in case of neuromuscular junction disorders.

Repetitive Stimulation

Depolarization of the motor end plate leads to the release of a certain amount of acetylcholine molecules from the synapses The acetylcholine molecules bind to the ACh receptors of the end plates of the muscles and induce depolarization, the so called end plate potential, by opening the ion channels. If the end plate potential is large enough, running action potential develops in the surrounding muscle cell membrane. In Lambert–Eaton syndrome, in certain congenital forms myasthenia and botulism, complaints occur due to the presynaptic damage of the neuromuscular junction, the amount of ACh molecules released is insufficient, therefore proper end plate potential does not develop. On the other hand postsynaptic part is damaged in myasthenia gravis for example. The simplest way to examine the transmission disorder of the neuromuscular junction is repetitive stimulation. The repetitive supramaximal peripheral nerve stimulation and the analysis of the resulting muscle action potentials can be performed easily; it is a relatively simple technique. Most commonly used methods: stimulation of the ulnar nerve at the wrist, registration with a superficial electrode in the abductor digiti minimi muscle, or stimulation of the brachial plexus at the Erb point and registrating electrode placed above the deltoid muscle. First, the amplitude of the CAMP (compound action muscle potential) is determined with 3c/s supramaximal series of triggers, the 4–9th amplitudes are compared to the first one. If the CAMP decreases rapidly (with at least 8 % after the 7–8th stimulation), so decrement is seen, neuromuscular transmission disorder is likely to be present. After this, tetanic stimulation is applied (31 c/s), or the patient is asked to perform maximal innervation for one minute. Tetanic stimulation may be more painful for the patient than the maximal voluntary innervations. Slight facilitation (CAMP amplitude increases due to the increased number of the activated muscle fibers) or pseudofacilitation (CAMP amplitude increases as the duration of the potential decreases, but the area under the negative peak does not change) may develop in case of healthy individuals… Both the tetanic and the 30–60 s long maximal voluntary innervation methods lead to calcium accumulation in the nerve ending, therefore increased CAMP amplitude. This is called postactivation facilitation (PAF). The PAF may be very significant in Lambert–Eaton syndrome (more than 100 %), while in case of myasthenia gravis, temporary improvement can be seen in the decrement detected after stimulation with lower frequency. If the maximal innervation lasts longer, the decrement increases, and this is called post-tetanic exhaustion. After tetanic stimulation or maximal voluntary innervation, 3 c/s stimulation is used again 40, 60 and 120 s later, and the parameters of CAMP are monitored. The diagnostic value of repetitive stimulation is largely dependent on the optimal selection of the muscle. A clinically affected muscle should be used all the time, but this cannot be performed in all cases in the clinical practice. For example, the examination of the facial muscles is very painful, and in many times it is difficult to stabilize the electrodes on the muscles of the proximal extremities for the complete duration of the examination. In myasthenia gravis, in case of repetitive stimulation, decrement is seen in about 66 % of the cases in the distal muscles and in about 83 % of the cases in the proximal muscles. Repetitive stimulation is often normal in case of ocular myasthenia gravis. The most common disorders in myasthenia gravis: in case of single stimulation, the amplitude of the action potential of the muscle is normal, decremental response is seen after low frequency stimulation, and no significant decrement is detected in case of large frequency stimulation. Repetitive stimulation is the only diagnostic methods that can be used to confirm Eaton–Lambert syndrome. The result of classic repetitive stimulation is the following: action potential of muscles in response to single stimulation is low, decremental response is seen in case of low frequency stimulation, and incremental response can be recorded in case of high frequency stimulation. The results of repetitive stimulation are similar in case of drug induced myasthenia and botulism as those described in case of Eaton–Lambert syndrome.

Single Fiber EMG (SFEMG)

Single fiber EMG is the most sensitive method to examine the neuromuscular transmission. SFEMG detects the action potential of a single muscle fiber with a fine needle electrode the diameter of which is 25 μm. This is smaller than the diameter of an average muscle fiber. If this fine electrode is inserted between two muscle fibers in the same motor unit, the action potential of both muscle fibers can be recorded simultaneously. SFEMG is triggered by voluntary innervation or electric stimulation. 20 single fiber potentials have to be collected in both cases and the average jitter has to be measured. The extensor digitorum muscle, the frontal muscle, and the orbicular ocular muscle are the most commonly used muscles for the examination. Normally, the action potentials of the muscle fiber develop at about the same time within a motor unit. There may be a short time shift between the two action potentials, this timely latency is the jitter which means variability. Normally, the maximal jitter is 21 μsec. The phenomenon can be explained by the fact that the distance of the two motor end plates from the stimulation is different. If the neuromuscular transmission is damaged, the jitter is elongated. If the damage is very severe, no action potential is seen after the impulse of the nerve, and *so called conduction block develops*.

In 77–100 % of the cases, SFEMG disorder is seen in myasthenia gravis. Based on the studies of Stalberg and Trontelj, if the jitter is normal, the diagnosis of myasthenia gravis can be excluded. Jitter may be abnormal is several neuromuscular diseases where the motor neurons, peripheral nerves or muscle fibers are damaged. Therefore, thorough neurological examination, ENG and standard EMG have to be performed before each SFEMG. Cholinesterase inhibitors may influence the result of the SFEMG; therefore, the drug should not be taken for at least 24 h before the examination.

Electroneurography

The conduction time of electric impulse running on motor and sensory nerves can be measured with great accuracy. The conduction time of the nerve characterizes the physiological and pathophysiological condition of the nerves. There are three types of nerve conduction velocity tests: 1. motor conduction velocity, 2. sensory conduction velocity, 3. mixed conduction velocity.

Motor Conduction Velocity (MCV)

Measurement of the motor conduction velocity is performed by supramaximal stimulation of the nerve in two proximal points of the peripheral nerve, while the summarized action potential of the muscle is registered with a superficial electrode in the muscle innervated by the examined nerve. For example the median nerve is stimulated in the elbow and wrist, and the recording electrode is fixed above the abductor pollicis muscle. In case of distal stimulation, the so called distal motor latency is determined by the beginning of the potential. In order to calculate the conduction velocity, the distal latency has to be extracted from the latency measured in case of proximal stimulation, and the distance between the two points of stimulation has to be divided by the difference of the latencies. The amplitude and shape of the CAMP are also informative.

Sensory Conduction Velocity (SCV)

The sensory conduction velocity may be measured with orthodromic and antidromic methods. In case of the orthodromic method, the sensory nerve is stimulated at the distal end of the nerve, and the sensory action potential of the nerve is recorded above the proximal segment. For example in case of the examination of the sensory fibers of the ulnar nerve, ring electrodes are used to perform stimulation in the 5th finger, the action potential is then recorded above the wrist. In case of proximal stimulation and distal recording, antidromic stimulation is performed. The amplitude of the SANP is measured from negative peak to positive peak. Theoretically, the motor, sensory, and mixed NCV means the conduction velocity of the motor, sensory, and mixed type fibers conducting with the largest velocity. The conduction velocity is influenced by: the age (very slow below 3 years of age), skin temperature (1 °C decreases conduction with 2 m/s), and the characteristics of the peripheral nerve (for example conduction of the fibers of the median nerve is larger than that of the peroneal nerve). Every EMG laboratory has to determine the normal values in case of each age group with the technique used by the laboratory. Conduction velocity is considered to be abnormal in case of velocity below about 50 m/s in case of the upper extremity and below about 40 m/s in case of the lower extremity. Decreased NCV refers to peripheral nerve damage or injury. The sensory fibers are more sensitive, injury may develop more easily, and therefore the SCV is a more sensitive parameter compared with the MCV in diagnosing peripheral neuropathy.

Abnormalities of Nerve Conduction Velocity

Abnormalities of conduction velocity are not specific to a single disease. These electrophysiological data can only be evaluated together with the clinical data and other laboratory findings. Nerve conduction tests are very useful in the diagnosis of peripheral neuropathy, tunnel syndromes, and peripheral nerve injuries. In case of peripheral neuropathy, motor and sensory conduction velocities of at least one upper extremity and both lower extremities have to be measured as peripheral neuropathy does not affect the certain fibers similarly. The more nerves are selected, the more accurate the result will be. In a few cases, only slight abnormality can be detected in a number of nerves. The amplitude of the CAMP and the SANP, temporal dispersion, and conduction blocks are informative in addition to NCV. The NCV may be normal in case of axonal damage. In this case, the amplitude of CAMP and SANP is low which suggests axon lesion. The extent of the decrease in NCV helps determining the type of the peripheral neuropathy. Axonal degeneration results in minimally decreased NCV, as the axon is less effective in conducting the action potential. As a contrary, segmental demyelination significantly decreases NCV. Slow NCV is often accompanied by low CAMP and CANP, although action potentials with low amplitude may be measured with normal NCV in case of axonal lesions as mentioned above. Conduction blockage and abnormal temporal dispersion indicate segmental demyelination. This is most likely to be detected with low NCV. Multiple motor blockages may be detected in motor conduction blockage syndrome in the nerves of the upper extremity.

The following electrophysiological abnormalities are seen in the most common neuro-ophthalmologic diseases:

Muscular Diseases

The following muscular diseases have neuro-ophthalmological importance: muscular dystrophies (congenital muscle dystrophies, myotonic dystrophy, and oculopharyngeal muscle dystrophy), mitochondrial myopathies from the metabolic myopathies, and myositis from autoimmune muscle diseases. In muscular dystrophies, the EMG registers early recruitment, and motor unit potentials with low amplitude and short duration indicating myogenic lesion. Few polyphasic potentials and stable waveforms are seen. In mitochondrial diseases, usually mixed type changes are seen, which means that spontaneous activity and MUP with larger than average amplitude and duration are seen suggesting the presence of the neurogenic lesion in some muscle groups while MUP with shorter duration and decreased amplitudes suggestive of myogenic lesion are seen in other muscle groups. In this case the number of polyphasic potentials are usually larger than the average.. In inflammatory myopathies, the insertional activity is increased, and spontaneous activity could be seen as well, and several polyphasic potentials are seen. In myotonic dystrophy, myotonic discharges detected in the resting muscle helps the electrophysiologist in making a decision.

Disorders of Neuromuscular Transmission

The most common disorder of neuromuscular transmission a neuro-ophthalmologist sees is myasthenia gravis, as the main symptoms in the ocular forms are ptosis and diplopia, so these patients often visit an ophthalmologist. In this disease, malfunction of the neuromuscular junction can be confirmed by identifying a decrement with repetitive stimulation. It is important to know that a negative repetitive stimulation does not exclude ocular myasthenia gravis. If the other causes are excluded, SFEMG should be performed as a following examination. Repetitive stimulation is highly dependent on the applied technique, the experience of the examiner, and the co-operation of the patient. Repetitive stimulation is the most important electrophysiological diagnostic method in congenital myasthenia syndromes as well. Although, in some cases, ENG examination may be useful, as in certain forms of the disease, dual action triggered response develops when measuring conduction speed of motor nerves, and this finding may be an important clue for the observant examiner. In Eaton–Lambert syndrome, action potential of muscles in response to stimulation is low, decremental response is seen in case of low frequency stimulation, and incremental response can be recorded in case of high frequency stimulation.

Peripheral Neuropathies

In some cases, peripheral neuropathies may be accompanied to neuro-ophthalmologic diseases, such as type 2 Charcot–Marie– Tooth disease developing as a consequence of mitofusin gene lesion. It is a classic form of congenital axonal type neuropathy. In such cases, characteristic symptoms of the peripheral nervous system are detected in addition to ophthalmologic symptoms, and an ENG finding supporting the peripheral neuropathy is received from the electrophysiologist. The most common cause of external progressive ophthalmoplegia (EPO) occurring from young adulthood is the mitochondrial disease in which axonal or mixed type lesions are seen in the peripheral nerves in addition to mixed type EMG changes seen in the muscles. The involvement of the peripheral nerves is not uncommon in autoimmune diseases as well. This may develop as a direct damage of the nerve due to immunological reasons, or due to the inflammation of the small vessels of the vasa nervorum in many cases.

Further Readings

Karpati G, Hilton Jones D, Bushby K, Griggs R. Disorders of voluntary muscle. Cambridge/London: Cambridge University Press; 2010.

Kimura J. Electrodiagnosis in diseases of nerve and muscle: principles and practice. 3rd ed. New York: Oxford University Press, USA; 2001.

Molnar MJ. Neuromuscularis betegségek [Neuromuscular diseases]. In: Oláh É, editor. Gyermekgyógyászati Kézikönyv. 2nd ed. Budapest: Medicina; 2009. p. 993–1035.

Molnár MJ, Karpati G. Az izombetegségek alapjai és modern szemlélete [Basics of myopathies and their modern assessment]. Budapest: Springer; 2001.

Preston CD, Shapiro B. Electromyography and neuromuscular disorders. 2nd ed. Butterworth-Heinemann; 2005.

Computed Tomography Examinations

30

József Kenéz

Contents

J. Kenéz, M.D., PhD
MR Laboratory, Székesfehérvár, County Hospital, Székesfehérvár, Hungary

Department of Radiology, Semmelweis University, Budapest, Hungary

Department of Radiology, National Traumatology Institute, Budapest, Hungary

Department of Neurology, Semmelweis University, Budapest, Hungary

Department of Neuroradiology, Haynal Imre Postgraduate University of Health Sciences, Budapest, Hungary
e-mail: j.kenez@chello.hu

The rapid development seen in the last 20–25 years in neuroimaging had the largest effect perhaps on neuro-ophthalmologic diagnostics. The main purpose of this chapter is to select the methods that give reliable answers from the various available examinations in neuroimaging in the field of neuro-ophthalmology to questions rising during a thorough preliminary clinical examination. Primarily, data collected with CT examination will be discussed, but other examinations will be mentioned regarding indications. Examination of the following anatomical areas may be performed regarding visual disorders in a broader sense:

- the orbit and its content with the optic nerve,
- the sinus cavernous and the sellar region,
- the optic chiasm,
- the retrochiasmal optic path and the visual cortex,
- the brainstem and the posterior fossa./scala./

It should be mentioned in the introduction that the orbit and its content are usually better examined with CT examinations, while the other anatomic regions should be examined with MRI, but analogous X-ray examinations and, in case of some special questions, invasive examinations (angiography) may become necessary as well in the era of modern digital imaging.

J. Somlai, T. Kovács (eds.), *Neuro-Ophthalmology*, DOI 10.1007/978-3-319-28956-4_30

Methodology of the CT Examination of the Orbit

The orbit is ideal to be examined with CT regarding the fact that the large amount of orbital tissue is fat tissue which is in the negative Hounsfield unit; its density gives proper contrast to visualize orbital structures and bony structures can be visualized excellently as well. In case of the standard CT examinations performed in the transverse plane, using planes parallel to the optic nerve is obvious (this plane may be performed by tilting the gantry forward with 20° if the Reid baseline is perpendicular to the table, and by tilting the gentry forward with 30° if the orbitomeatal line is perpendicular to the table [its plane]). The finest potential layer has to be selected for the CT examination of the orbit; this is usually 1.5 mm in case of the currently used devices. Coronal acquisition is very important in CT diagnostics of the orbit; this may be performed with direct coronal scanning or reconstruction methods. Resolution is somewhat better in case of direct coronal imaging, but the examination is time consuming, often uncomfortable for the patients, and dental fillings may disturb the examination in many cases. The quality of coronal reconstructions may be improved by the overlap technique, 1.5 mm slice thickness should be used in this case with 1-mm table movements. An additional advantage of the reconstruction method is that in addition to the coronal plane, examinations may be performed in oblique planes parallel to the optic nerve as well. The bulb, the optic nerve, muscles, vessels, the lacrimal gland, and the bony wall are well visible in the CT images of the eyeball. Smaller nerves (oculomotor nerve) may be examined with very thorough technique. Patient co-operation is very important in examining the anatomical characteristics of the orbit in detail, as it is a moving object, and accurate CT cannot be performed of a moving object. Rapid availability of the advanced spiral CT devices significantly increased the information content of the examination, the examinations became faster, reconstruction options, including 3D images may be performed almost every time, but radiation hygienic considerations should be remembered. The eye is particularly sensitive to radiation.

Clinical Practice of the CT Examination

Congenital Abnormalities

Coloboma of the optic nerve developing as a disorder of the closing of the choroidal fissure of the primitive optic nerve is easily detectable with CT. The vitreous body significantly protrudes in the optic nerve in the projection of the optic disc in the CT image. This condition may lead to the development of a cyst within the optic nerve which is often accompanied by congenital microphthalmus. *Septo-optic dysplasia* is a significant congenital abnormality. This is characterized by hypoplasia of the optic nerve and decreased vision, hypophysic hormonal insufficiency, and midline defect of the cerebral structures. The septum pellucidum is missing in most cases. Cleft palate is often seen in this condition. In the CT image, the optic canal is narrow, hypoplasia of the intraorbital and intracranial segment of the optic nerve is present, and dysraphic cerebral congenital abnormality is detected as well. MRI is more suitable to detect intracranial lesions than the CT. For other rare congenital abnormalities that can be detected with neuroimaging (congenital cystic eye, anophthalmus, morning glory defect, etc), see the referred manuals.

Space Occupying Processes

Meningeomas may be primarily intraorbital originating from the sheath of the optic nerve, and may spread to the orbit secondarily from the surrounding intracranial regions (Fig. 30.1a, b). The appearance of *optic sheath meningeoma* is very characteristic: it is hyperdense in plain CT scans, and an intense contrast enhancement is seen after the administration of intravenous contrast medium. The optic nerve located inside the sheath is less dense, it is usually easy to differentiate, and the optic nerve inside the meningeoma often has a *tram track* sign. The symptoms are seen in case of the other disorders affecting the optic sheath as well (Fig. 30.2a–c).

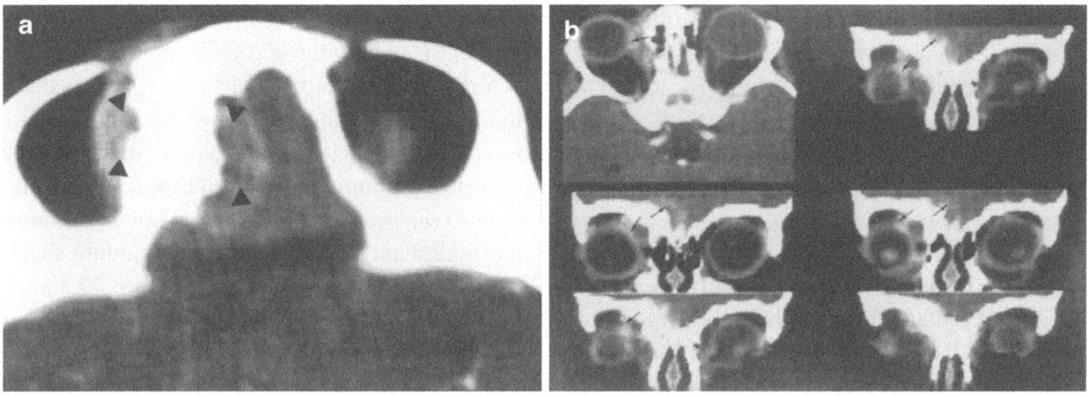

Fig. 30.1 Contrast enhanced image of fronto-basal meningeoma, primary (**a**) and coronal reconstruction images (**b**) Intraorbital spreading and intracranial segments of the tumor are shown by the *arrows* and *head of arrows*

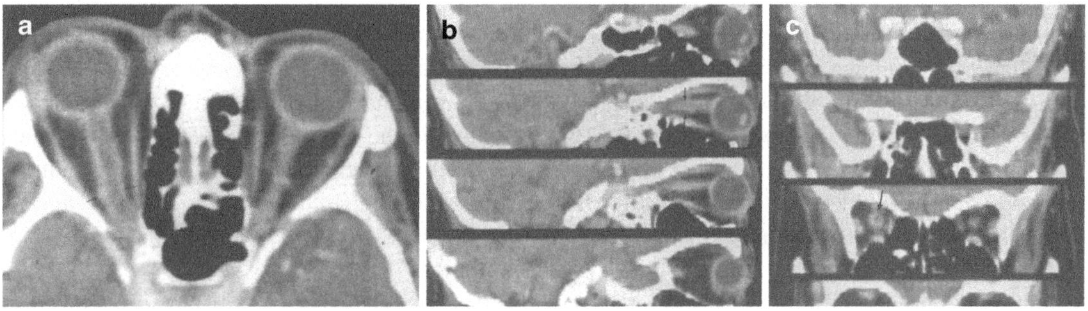

Fig. 30.2 The sheath of the right optic nerve is wider due to leukemic infiltration (tram track sign). Primary axial contrast enhanced image (**a**), parasagittal reconstructions parallel with the optic nerve (**b**) and coronal reconstruction images (**c**). It is characteristic, that the optic nerve stays hypodense

When the meningeoma of intraorbital origin reaches a large size, it may deform the orbital wall. Every form of the meningeoma is often accompanied by calcification. The appearance of the *optic glioma* is similar to that of the meningeoma on plain images, but the enhancement seen after the administration of the contrast medium is smaller, and the optic nerve cannot be differentiated inside it. It often spreads along the visual pathway. MRI is more suitable to detect its intracranial segments than the CT. It is a common childhood tumor. *Neurinomas and schwannomas* originate from the region of the superior orbital fissure in most cases. It is considered to be characteristic feature of the schwannomas to have a longitudinal form, the affected nerve is wider, while the neurinomas are usually round or oval. Neurinomas are often multiple, their contrast enhancement is rather homogeneous. Schwannomas are often part of neurofibromatosis. Their contrast enhancement is often inhomogeneous. Sarcomatous degeneration may be seen as well. *Dermoids and epidermoids* are congenital tumors mainly occurring in childhood, they often destroy the surrounding bones, they grow slowly, and lead to slight visual disturbance in most cases. Adipose tissue and calcification is often seen in these tumors, their contrast enhancement is inhomogeneous and often very weak. From the muscular tumors, *rhabdomyosarcoma* is a common malignant tumor in childhood leading to bone destruction. This tumor grows rapidly, and leads to significant exophthalmus. It is a hyperdense tumor with very intense enhancement. Myoblastomas of other origin may also occur in adults, their embolic origin is not clear, and they are often considered to be neurogenic. They have well defined, moderate contrast enhancement. If they are located centrally in the muscle, they cannot be differentiated from muscular enlargements of other origin. *Tumors of the lacrimal gland* may be benign or malignant as well. Benign tumors are usually mixed type, they grow slowly, while the malignant tumors grow rapidly.

Both types of the tumor often affect the surrounding bone structures. *Orbital lymphomas* have localized and diffuse forms, they often originate from the region of the lacrimal fossa, have moderate contrast enhancement, and their lateral regions are not welldefined. The diffuse forms cannot be differentiated from other diffuse diseases, such as pseudotumors or aggressive inflammatory reactions. *Pseudotumors* are all space occupying lesions in the orbit the etiology of which is unknown and they lead to the expansion of the retro-orbital tissue. The pseudotumor may be unilateral or bilateral, defined or diffuse. On plain CT images, the tumor is characterized by the lack of normal structures, opacity, and intense contrast enhancement. Several authors consider it to be an early sign of lymphoma, but others consider it to be an autoimmune disease. The most important clinical task is to identify the etiology. *Metastatic tumors* are most commonly intraorbital metastases of lung, breast, kidney, or colon tumors. Metastases are often localized in the apex of the orbit, and are characterized by intense contrast enhancement. It is important to note that in case of metastatic tumors, the CT scan usually provides more information than the MRI. For example, metastasis of prostate carcinoma in the orbital wall is very difficult to diagnose with MRI. It is not uncommon that malignant lesions in the surrounding facial skull spread to the orbit directly (Fig. 30.3a, b). *Vascular space occupying lesions* are interesting and diverse disorders in the orbit. *Orbital varices*, similarly to varices in the other parts of the body result from the extreme dilatation of a venous channel. A very characteristic feature of varices is that if a Valsalva maneuver is performed during the CT, the size of the varices increase significantly, and their contrast enhancement is significant. *Capillary hemangiomas* usually occur in infantcy or childhood as a pathological structure in the orbit. Intense but inhomogeneous contrast enhancement is seen, and these tumors are often accompanied with skin lesions (*encephalotrigeminal angiomatosis*) (see phakomatoses). *Cavernous hemangiomas* are the most common lesions in adults, and these lesions often occur in the muscle conus of the orbit, form a well-defined structure and dislocate the surrounding structures but are not invasive. Their contrast enhancement is always very intense (Fig. 30.4a, b). The MRI

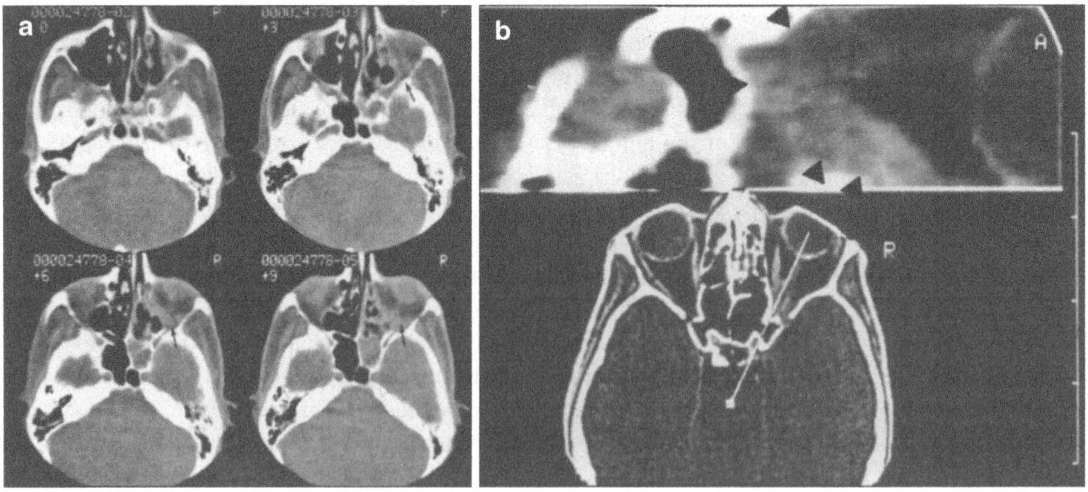

Fig. 30.3 Malignant maxillary tumor spreading into the orbit via the inferior orbital fissure. This is seen in the primary axial contrast enhanced image (**a**) and in the parasagittal reconstructions (**b**)

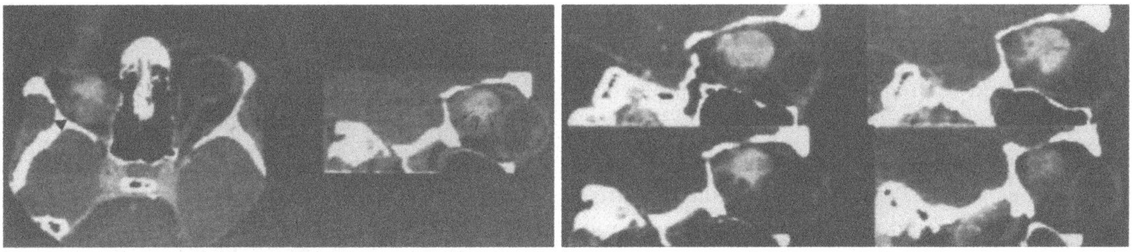

Fig. 30.4 Tumor of intraconal origin with intense contrast accumulation in axial and parasagittal reconstructions parallel to the optic nerve. Only slight visual impairment, large exophthalamus and optic dislocation are present. The slowly growing benign tumor is well-defined from the dislocated optic nerve, the optic disc is intact

results may be misleading due to the slow velocity. A bleeding cyst may occur in the apex of the orbit that may be of traumatic or inflammatory origin. It is seen as a round structure in plain images, slight contrast enhancement is seen only long after the administration of an intravenous contrast medium. The *arteriovenous fistula* is an important vascular lesion which usually occurs as a carotid-cavernous fistula and is mainly of traumatic origin.

The fistula may develop spontaneously as well due to the rupture of an aneurysm or vascular disease, and may occur between the system of the external carotid artery and the venous system of the orbit. Spontaneous fistulas are usually less space occupying than the traumatic ones. *Intense dilation of the intraorbital veins* is characteristic, in addition, significant enlargement is seen in the extraocular muscles. Vascular pathological lesions are *hemangiopericytomas and glomus tumors* as well, they may occur in the orbital region, too. They are usually invasive, spread to the bony wall of the orbit, and intense contrast enhancement is seen in these tumors. *From the tumors of the eyeball, retinoblastoma* is a childhood tumor originating from the retinal surface of the eyeball. It usually contains fine calcified regions and often leads to bleeding. CT detects the posterior extent of the tumor and the potential involvement of the central nervous system. The MRI needs special acquisitions to detect calcification. *Melanomas* are tumors affecting all age groups and may appear as tumors protruding in the vitreous body, spreading thorough the wall of the eyeball, and leading to metastases in almost all cases. These tumors have high density even in plain images, and have intense contrast enhancement. As in case of the tumors of the eyeball, primarily a CT scan should be performed in case of a melanoma if the ophthalmologic examination does not provide proper information due to bleeding or if the posterior extent of the tumor is intended to be determined.

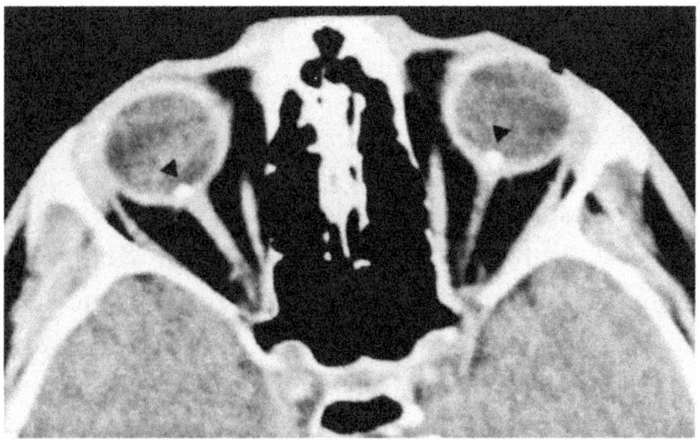

Fig. 30.5 Drusen bodies in both optic discs

Drusen

A rare anomaly, pathologically hyaline accumulation develops in the optic disc due to degenerative processes. A point-like calcification is detected in the central region of the optic disc with CT (Fig. 30.5). The disease has differential diagnostic importance, it has to be differentiated from other calcifications of tumor origin.

Endocrine Ophthalmopathy

Endocrine myo- and orbitopathies (Graves disease) are the most common causes of exophthalmus that may be unilateral or may occur in completely euthyroid condition. Pathologically, in case of this disease, myositis is present, and it affects the extraocular muscles, leads to the enlargement of these muscles. Sometimes it affects one muscle, usually the rectus medial and/or the inferior. In orbitopathy, increased intraorbital pressure, the compression of the optic nerve and its tension is responsible for the visual disturbance. Enlarged muscle tissue can be well-visualized with CT scan. Coronal scans are especially important to determine the relation to the other structures. Increased contrast enhancement is seen in the enlarged muscles.

Foreign Body

The CT scan is ideal to localized intraorbital or intraocular foreign bodies (Fig. 30.6). Metal foreign bodies can ideally be detected from the size of 0.1–0.2 mm, glass foreign bodies are well visible, wooden foreign bodies are difficult to detect depending on their size and nature. Fine slice thickness has to be selected to detect foreign bodies. Multiplanar reconstruction may help in the exact localization.

Orbital Trauma

Fractures of the orbit may affect any wall of the orbit or the inlet. CT plays a crucial role in diagnosing fractures of the orbit as it provides very important information regarding soft tissue injuries. The CT scan is very informative in perforating eye injuries, collapse of the eyeball, vitreous bleeding, lens luxations (Fig. 30.7), dislocations, and retinal detachment. *Blow out fractures* important in posttraumatic eye movement disorders have to be mentioned as well. Suddenly increasing intraorbital pressure during the trauma breaks the inferior wall of the orbit into the Highmore cavity.

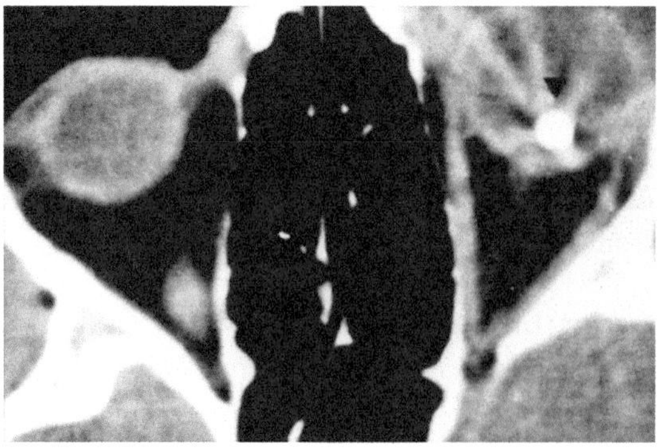

Fig. 30.6 Air rifle bullet in the left eye

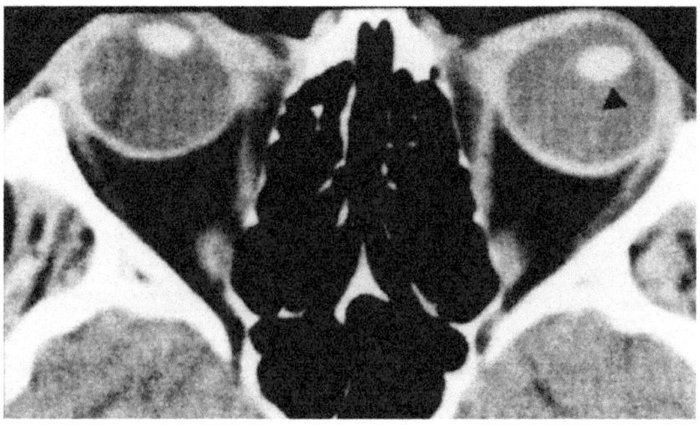

Fig. 30.7 Lens luxation on the left side

Injury of the eye moving musculature is often seen in connection to the fracture; primarily the inferior muscle and the superior rectus muscle are damaged. During the healing, these muscles may become deformed, adhesions may occur, and consequential severe posttraumatic eye movement disorders, dual images, enophthalmus may occur. The CT scan may be suitable to accurately analyze these important accompanying symptoms and complications, for proper planning of the correction surgery, and to analyze the result of the surgery.

Changes in the Size of the Eyeball

In severe myopathy, the eyeball may be significantly enlarged, in hypermetropy, the eyeball may be smaller, but these changes in size are usually accidental findings in the CT. In severe myopathy, the optic disc may become excavated, an extreme case is called *staphyloma*. Permanent and malignant *glaucoma* may lead to the enlargement of the eyeball as well. Congenital maxillary sinus hypoplasia may lead to significant enophthalmus. It is important to note that inflammatory or tumorous processes of the nearby sinuses often affect the orbit, like the intracranial abnormalities, vascular disorders, venous occlusion, leading to secondary orbital symptoms. In such cases like in other cases as well, knowledge of clinical

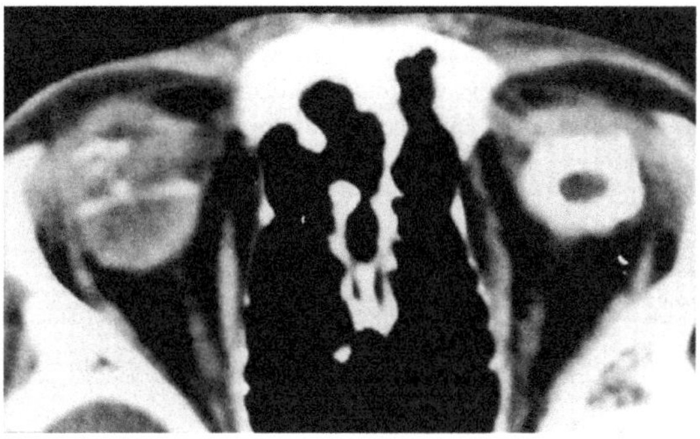

Fig. 30.8 Deforming, calcified scars with shrinkage and complete blindness after suppuration following childhood bilateral perforating eye injury and infection

data is essential for the proper analysis of the CT results. Deforming, fibrous, calcified shrinkage may also occur after old purulent inflammations (Fig. 30.8).

Incidence of Lesions Based on Localization

The most common disease affecting the *extraocular muscles* is *endocrine exophthalamus*. Metastases, vascular malformations, or a pseudotumor and myositis may occur in the muscles. Primarily, the abnormal lesions of the optic nerve are visualized inside the muscle conus. Vascular pathologies may occur in this region as well. *Dermoids*, abnormal lesions of the lacrimal gland, granulomas, lymphomas, histiocytosis, neurofibromas, schwannomas, or metastases may occur in the extraconal region, or inside the bony wall of the orbit. A CT examination is important in determining the abnormal lesion of the eyeball if the ophthalmologic examination is not informative due to bleeding, cataract or other reason. Similarly, the exact size of the tumors extending beyond the eyeball can be determined with CT, such as in case of retinoblastomas, melanomas or rare metastatic tumors of the eyeball. In the majority of patients presenting with eye complaints, the reason for the complaint is found outside the orbit. Inflammatory or tumor diseases of the paranasal sinuses most commonly cause visual disorders or eye complaints. Abnormal intracranial lesions may lead to visual disorders or eye complaints similarly: aneurysms, meningeomas, increased intraocular pressure or intracranial gliomas. The reason for the visual disorder is often found near the sella or in the parasellar region. Rarely the diseases of the nasal cavity or the epipharynx cause orbital complications. Malignant tumors of the nasal cavity, the epipharynx, or the parapharyngeal space may lead to the orbit through neighboring tissues.

Abnormal Lesions Based on the Age of the Patients

The most common malignant lesions in infants and children are retinoblastomas, neuroblastomas, leukemic infiltrations, or lymphomas. Colombomas, cysts, and dermoids are benign lesions. In early childhood, rhabdomyosarcomas, optic gliomas, lymphangiomas, and hemangiomas may occur. Metastatic tumors or intraorbital spreading of the malignant tumor of the epipharynx or the sinuses are common above the age of sixty. No significant correlation with age is seen in the other disorders. As a consequence, CT as a diagnostic tool gives new dimensions in the diagnosis of abnormal lesions in the orbit. Conventional X-ray diagnostics may help a lot in reviewing the whole skull, estimating the proportions, and evaluating abnormal lesions affecting primarily the structure of the bones. Although MRI diagnostics were not mentioned in this chapter, it has to be noted that it is still intensely developing. More and more novel data acquisitions and continuous development of the computer background, as well as the modern devices are so promising that the role of the MRI will surely increase in the imaging of the orbit, too. *Fat suppression* technique may especially be important in intraorbital imaging. As it was mentioned in the introduction, MRI already plays a larger role in the diagnosis of retro-orbital neuroophthalmologic disorders than the CT scan. Depending on the capacity of the MRI devices to be set up in the future in Hungary, MRI examinations will be in the focus. It does not mean that CT does not provide important information regarding these regions of course.

Further Readings

Atlas SW. Magnetic resonance imaging of the brain and spine. New York: Raven; 1994.

Mafee MM. Imaging in ophthalmology part I-II, The radiologic clinics of North America, vol. 25. Philadelphia: Saunders; 1987. p. 3–4.

Mancuso AA, Hanafee WN. Computed tomography and magnetic resonance imaging of the head and neck. Baltimore: Williams and Wilkins; 1985.

Osborn AG. Diagnostic neuroradiology. Mosby-Yearbook; 1994.

Zonneveld FW. Computed tomography of the temporal bone and orbit. Urban-Schwarzenberg; 1987.

Neuroradiology, Functional MRI 31

György Várallyay and Lajos Rudolf Kozák

Contents

G. Várallyay, M.D. (✉)
Radiologist, Neuroradiologist, Szentágothai Knowledge Center – MR Research Center, Semmelweis University, Budapest, Hungary
e-mail: varally@gmail.com

L.R. Kozák, M.D., PhD
Bolyai Research Fellow, MR Research Center, Semmelweis University, Budapest, Hungary
e-mail: lkozak@mrkk.sote.hu

Introduction

Since the publication of the book titled "Neuroophtalmology" in 1996, the development of CT and MRI and PET techniques are the most relevant to follow up in neuroradiology. The reason is that these modalities, as well as their advanced imaging methods are widely available. Therefore the structure of this chapter will follow technical considerations. Radiologists often use new terms, and getting familiar with those is essential to fully understand the reports.

Computed Tomography (CT)

The multidetector CT (Multi Slice CT, MSCT) brought quality improvements compared to earlier CT techniques. Due to submillimeter slice thickness it is also called "volume CT": imaging data can be reconstructed in any imaging planes. As the speed of the examination increased significantly (a few seconds are enough to examine a whole region), good quality angiography can be performed after the administration of contrast agent, and useful data can be obtained about the perfusion of certain cerebral areas. Immediately after arterial occlusion, the non-perfused area can be depicted. In tumors, dynamic perfusion measurement and the derived parametric maps may indicate differential diagnosis of various histologies. Using MSCT, radiation exposure has to be taken into account, which is not negligible

J. Somlai, T. Kovács (eds.), *Neuro-Ophthalmology*, DOI 10.1007/978-3-319-28956-4_31

especially in head CTs due to the risk of developing cataracts. For more information on radiation exposure see chapter 3.3.6 on page 153.

Magnetic Resonance Imaging (MRI)

The development of MR scanners involves both software development as well as utilizing higher magnetic field strengths. Whereas 7 Tesla human scanners are mostly used for research, magnets with 3 Tesla field strengths are increasingly used clinically. The advantage of higher field strength is obvious in brain imaging, especially for recent applications, such as diffusion, tractography, perfusion, functional MRI and spectroscopy.

Water- and Fat-Suppressed MRI Sequences

Among the large number of new MRI sequences (with often confusing physics and nomenclature) the suppression techniques are important in the everyday practice. The FLAIR (Fluid Attenuated Inversion Recovery) is a T2 weighted sequence in which the water signal is suppressed, therefore water gives low instead of high signal. Most of the MRI detectable lesions are visualized on FLAIR (Fig. 31.1). Fat suppressed (FS) images play an important role in orbital imaging. The FS T2 weighted images show diseases of the optic nerve with high signal intensity within the dark orbital fat tissue. The post contrast (+C) FS T1 weighted images show enhancing lesions in the dark surrounding fat.

Clinical findings: Sudden onset of right homonym hemianopia in a pregnant woman at 35th week of gestation. There is high signal on FLAIR and diffusion weighted images. Restricted diffusion refers to a cytotoxic edema. MRI angiography indicated significant stenosis of the left posterior cerebral artery. A: FLAIR B: DWI C: MRI angiography (Fig. 31.2a-c).

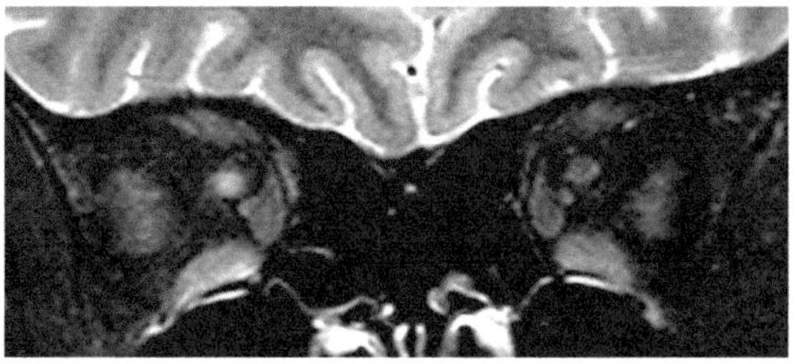

Fig. 31.1 Retrobulbar neuritis on the right side. Clinical findings: right sided loss of vision. Coronal plane, T2 weighted fat supressed image. There is high signal of the right optic nerve. Slightly increased signal is seen adjacent to this structure inside the dark fat tissue indicating edema

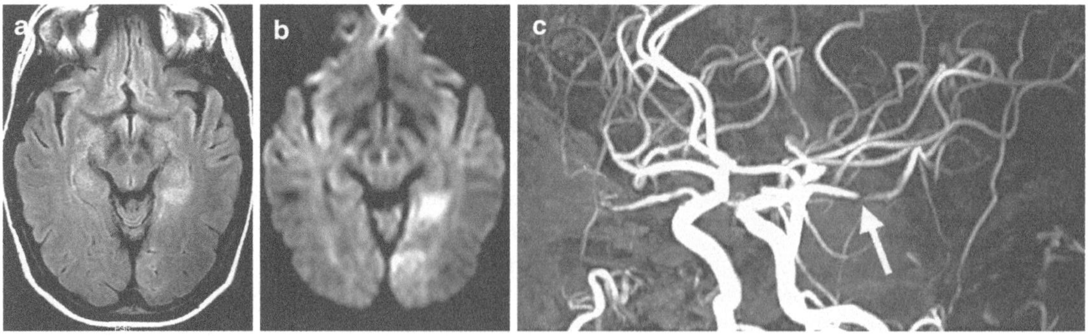

Fig. 31.2 Acute infarct in the distribution of the left posterior cerebral artery. Clinical findings: Sudden onset of right homonym hemianopia in a pregnant woman at 35th week of gestation. There is high signal on FLAIR and diffusion weighted images. Restricted diffusion refers to a cytotoxic edema. MRI angiography indicated significant stenosis of the left posterior cerebral artery. (**a**) FLAIR (**b**) DWI (**c**) MRI angiography

Imaging Based on the Diffusion of Water Molecules

Diffusion Weighted Imaging (DWI) is nowadays part of routine cerebral MR protocols. The diffusion of water molecules largely depend on the structure of the environment. In geometrically homogeneous fluids, diffusion of molecules is free in every direction. However, if there are structures in the fluid space that inhibit diffusion, the molecules collide with each other, and their straight paths shorten. In case of free diffusion, DWI shows decreased signal, (similarly to flow related signal loss) whereas restricted diffusion gives high signal. Barriers restricting diffusion can be irregular, such as in cytotoxic edema, when the extracellular space (primarily providing free diffusion) decreases due to cell swelling. The diffusion movement of the molecules significantly decreases due to the increased size of the cells, therefore DWI shows diffusion restriction. This way, a new infarction can be differentiated from several other lesions (Fig. 31.3).

In case of vasogenic edema occurring in various pathologies, the extracellular fluid space increases at the expense of the cells. So an increased diffusion can be detected in the images. With this method, a newly developed infarction in the occipital lobe (Fig. 31.2b), cytotoxic edema – restricted diffusion can be safely differntiated from the PRES (Fig. 31.4) as the cause of homonymous hemianopsia.

Vasogenic edema (which has increased diffusion) may be due to hypertensive crisis, eclampsia, or overdose of some medications.

DWI shows the restricted diffusion in highly cellular tumors, and in early stages of cerebral abscesses.

If water diffusion is limited by barriers with regular morphological structures, diffusion may be free in certain directions but restricted in other directions. The best example of this is the fibers of the white matter in the brain. Molecules move freely along the fibers, but the diffusion pathway of the molecules perpendicular to the fibers is shorter. Based on diffusion measurements performed in several (32 or more) directions, the most free diffusion direction can be determined in each volume (Diffusion Tensor Imaging, DTI). The neighboring voxels in the direction of the boxes can be linked: the resulting line represents a free "water pathway" between the voxels along the line. The direction of the line is the same as the direction of the

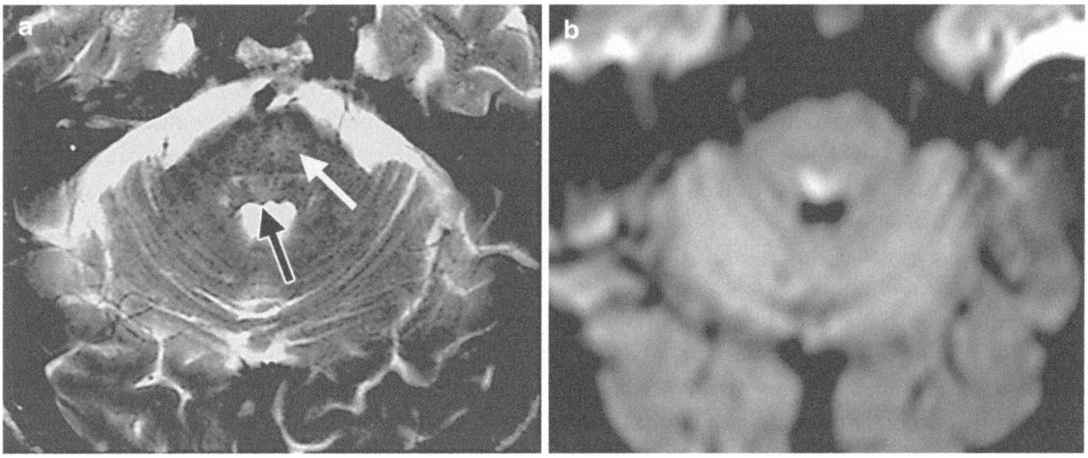

Fig. 31.3 An acute infarction in the tegmentum of the pons. Clinical: One-and-a-half syndrome. Increased signal intensity is seen in the tegmentum (*black arrow*) and ventrally (*white arrow*) in T2 weighted images. The DWI shows increased signal intensity only in the tegmentum: the restricted diffusion is consistent with acute infarction. The ventral lesion is older. (**a**) T2 weighted (**b**) DWI

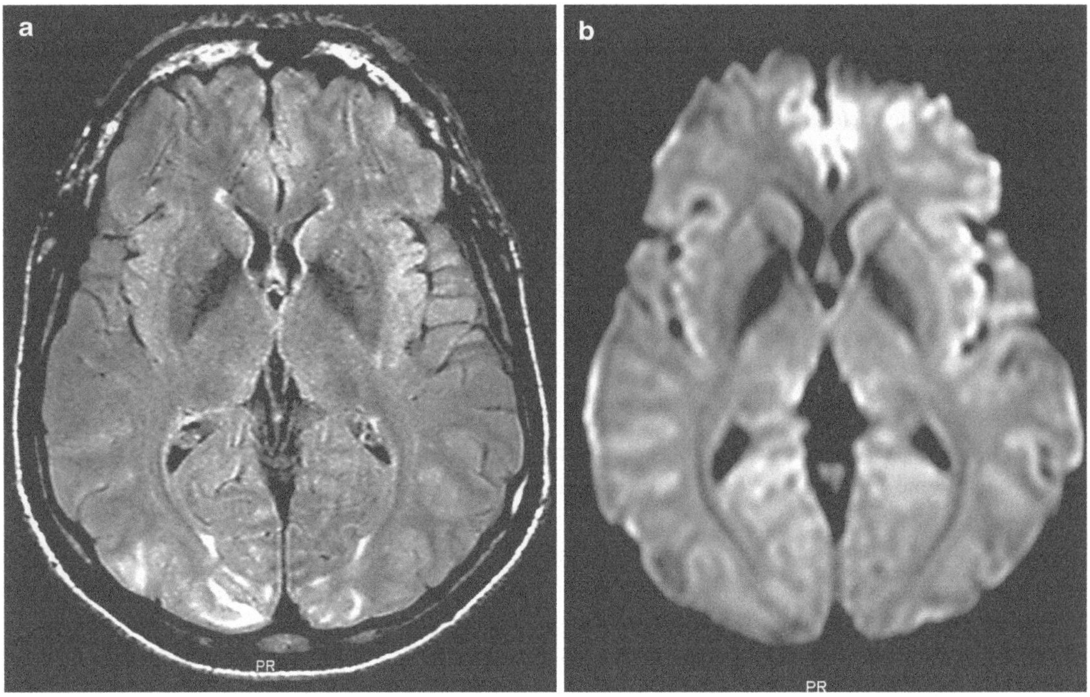

Fig. 31.4 Posterior reversible encephalopathy syndrome. Clinical: Cortical blindness developing after hypertensive crisis. The occipital FLAIR images show increased signal intensity on both sides, signal intensity is decreased in diffusion weighted images. The increased diffusion refers to vasogenic edema. (**a**) FLAIR (**b**) DWI

fibers. With special software, three dimensional bands can be displayed on the screen with their direction refering to the fibers of the white matter (diffusion tractography). These images can be considered as in vivo depiction of white matter tract anatomy. The optic radiation is particularly well-visualized. In abnormal cases, lesions dislocating the fibers can be differentiated from lesions infiltrating the fibers with this method. The first lesions alter the course of the fibers while the latter involves the fibers, more precisely: the regular interstitial fluid space disappears around the fibers. Despite of the spectacular color images of tractography, being aware of its limitations is important. The technique is not visualizing fibers directly, what we see are lines generated based on the fluid spaces between the fibers. The problem of the crossing fibers cannot be completely resolved by increasing the spatial resolution of the acquisition. For example, a portion of the fibers representing the right optic nerve seems to be turning into the left optic nerve from the chiasm.

MR Perfusion

MR perfusion imaging (similarly to CT perfusion), is based on the temporal distribution of the contrast agent. Images are repeatedly acquired at the examined cerebral region after the administration of the contrast agent. Based on signal intensity changes in pixels, contrast agent concentration in corresponding voxels can be determined. The time course of these values represents the blood supply of the area. Similar to certain phases in catheter angiography, perfusion parametric maps and the derived numerical values may refer to the histology of the tumors.

The perfusion and diffusion MRI have a special role in diagnosing stroke. Perfusion images indicate the area that has no blood supply, and areas with restricted diffusion indicte ischemic damage (cytotoxic edema). The difference between these two (mismatch) represents areas without blood supply but still viable, and where there is a chance of recovery after restoring the blood supply.

MR Angiography

MR angiography images of the last few years are of such a good quality that they make diagnostic catheter angiography unnecessary in the majority of the cases. Primarily, time of flight (TOF) angiography based on detecting the rapid flow is used to visualize the intracranial arteries without the administration of the contrast agent (Fig. 31.2c). Occlusions, stenoses, vascular malformations, and aneurysms are well-visualized. The latter ones may lead to visual symptoms and eye movement disorders but may also be incidental findings in many cases.

In the so-called angiographic source images, high signal intensity arteries are visualized together with intermediate signal of the cerebral parenchyma and the cranial nerves. Neurovascular compressions can be detected this way. Mostly the lesion of cranial nerves V, VII, and VIII may be explained by the compression effect of an artery (rarely a vein) crossing the nerve, but the phenomenon should be noted in Neuro-Ophthalmology as well: the elongated and torturous internal carotid artery may compress the optic nerve, and the elongated basilar artery with a bifurcation at a high level or the posterior cerebral artery may compress the the optic tract. In both cases, the result is visual field loss, corresponding to the lesion location. Venous angiography is mainly performed if venous sinus thrombosis is suspected. However venous angiography alone is usually not sufficient to make the diagnosis. Significant hypoplasia or the lack of the transverse sinus on one side is very common.

MR Spectroscopy

Long before MR imaging spectroscopy was used for in vitro chemical analysis of the material. It is based on the fact that hydrogen atoms resonate with different frequency in different chemical environment. Excitation is performed using a continuous broad frequency spectrum of radio waves, so every hydrogen atom resonates and absorbs energy. However, when the radio wave is stopped, the spectrum of the energy emitted by the excited atoms will not be continuous, only frequency proper for the chemical binding of the hydrogen atoms will be seen. The height of each peak seen in the spectroscopic curve (and rather the size of the area under the curve) represents the concentration of a compound in the examined volume.

Main Metabolites That Can Be Detected in the Normal Cerebral Tissue

- N-acetyl aspartate (NAA): indicating the integrity of normal cells. It is decreased in case of cell damage, such as in tumors and inflammation, but in post-irradiation necrosis as well. In non-glial tumors (for example meningeoma), no NAA is present.
- Creatine (Cr): representing the energy reserve of the cells. It is decreased in malignancies.
- Choline (Cho): indicator of cell dividing activity. Its level is increased in tumors and inflammation (Fig. 31.6), it can detect tumor recurrence. Normal or decreased choline level indicates that malignancy is unlikely (Fig. 31.5).
- Lactate, lipid: can be detected in necrosis.
- Myoinisitol: characteristic of gliosis.

Decreased and increased amount of the above metabolites and the appearance of other special metabolites may result in many types of curves. Based on this information, malignancies, inflammation, ischemic disease, and special metabolic disorders may be diagnosed. The normal cerebral spectrum changes with age and various curves are seen in various cerebral areas (Fig. 31.5a–d). Unfortunately uncertain findings on spectroscopy are not rare. This is partly due to technical reasons; on the other hand, our knowledge is still incomplete in several questions, despite the currently available large amount of literature data.

Choosing the Imaging Modality

In Neuro-Ophthalmology, CT alone may have a role mainly in diagnosing intraorbital lesions. CT may be a complementary modality in evaluating

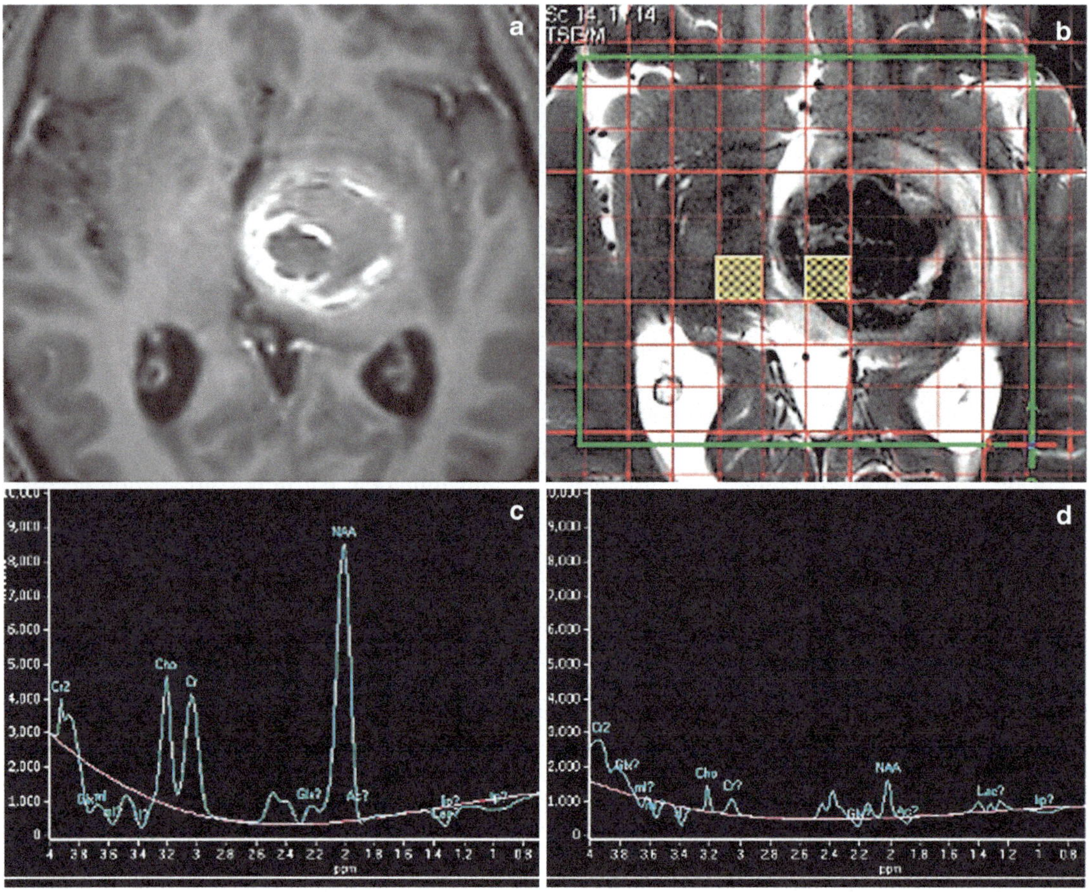

Fig. 31.5 Hemorrhagic cavernoma in the left thalamus. Clinical: Right hemiplegia and right homonym hemianopia, mixed type aphasia developing in a few days. (**a**) Post-contrast T1 weighted image: there is a fluid containing, space occupying structure with peripheral enhancement. (**b**) MR spectroscopic measurement in the normal and abnormal regions. (**c**) Normal side, normal curve. (**d**) In the abnormal area, the peaks of each metabolite are very low. The low choline value makes the presence of a tumor very unlikely

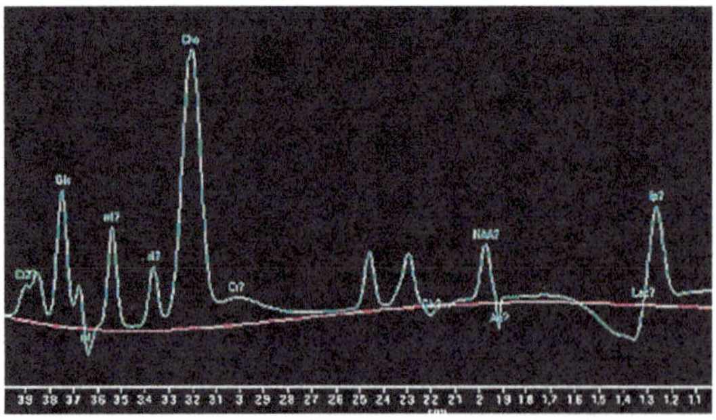

Fig. 31.6 MR spectroscopy of a malignant tumor: The N-acetyl aspartate and creatine levels are significantly decreased, the choline level is very high

bones and detecting calcifications. CT has to be performed if the MRI is contraindicated or as the MRI images cannot be evaluated due to dental artifacts. Otherwise, MRI is the most suitable to answer questions in the majority of the cases using the standard sequences and the above described new methods as well.

For a good quality imaging study, modern hardware and software are necessary in the MRI device, as well as well-trained MRI technicians and proper scan time are also important. In more complicated cases, the good co-operation between the ophthalmologist, neurologist, neurosurgeon, and radiologist has to be highlighted. In order to be able to choose the appropriate MRI technique and to evaluate results, detailed clinical information as well as prior images/imaging findings have to be available for the neuroradiologist.

Functional Magnetic Resonance Imaging (fMRI)

The main purpose of functional magnetic resonance imaging is the mapping of neural activity patterns; for this reason, usually the BOLD (blood-oxygenation-level dependent) contrast is used, which gives information on the complex interaction of local blood supply, blood volume, and hemoglobin concentration. Changes in cerebral blood flow (CBF) in response to fluctuations in energy requirement depending on the neural activity provides the physiological basis of the method (Roy and Sherrington 1890); these changes can represent activation and inhibiton, as well. The physical basis of the method lies in the different magnetic properties of oxy- and deoxyhemoglobin: the paramagnetic deoxyhemoglobin causes slight distortions (susceptibilities) in the magnetic field which decrease signal intensity in T2* weighted gradient echo sequences (Ogawa et al. 1993). The exact mechanism of the neurovascular coupling, i.e. the connection between neural activity and changes in blood flow, is still not completely known. Yet, the course of the BOLD response is fairly consequent. Neuronal activation is followed by a rapid decrease in signal intensity, which may be the consequence of increased oxygen extraction. This is followed 0.5–1.5 s later by a signal intensity increase as a result of increasing oxy- and deoxyhemoglobin ratio due to the increased blood flow. The highest signal intensity is seen 4–8 s later, and then the BOLD response returns to the baseline after 15–20 s from onset.

The BOLD signal shows close correlation with the local field potentials that provide the basis of EEG, but not with the excitation pattern of certain cell groups (Logothetis et al. 2001). Maximal amplitude of the BOLD signal has almost linear correlation with the level of local neuronal activity (Heeger and Ress 2002).

There is an inverse relation between the achievable spatial resolution and the temporal sampling, so the spatial resolution of fMRI is significantly lower than the theoretical maximal resolution of MRI. The whole brain volume has to be scanned in 1000–3000 ms to achieve acceptable temporal resolution, therefore the minimal slice thickness is limited to 2–3 mm in this case. This, however, does not lead to significant loss of spatial information as the spatial resolution of the hemodynamic response is on similar magnitude. Increasing the magnetic field strength can lead to better image quality in shorter acquisition time, moreover functional accuracy can be increased simultaneously as the contribution of microvasculature to BOLD signal is more pronounced at higher field strength than that of the macrovasculature.

In comparison with other functional mapping methods: the time resolution of the fMRI is worse than that of electrophysiological examinations, but its spatial localization is magnitudes more accurate due to direct volumetric data recording. Compared with PET – a technique used in functional mapping, as well – the most important advantage of fMRI is that there is no need for the administration of radioactive tracers, moreover fMRI's spatial resolution is better and the examination protocols may be more flexible. Nevertheless, fMRI provides information only about the blood-oxygenation, while the PET can quantify other metabolic effects, as well, depending on the tracer used.

As neuronal activation patterns can be followed non-invasively, with good spatial resolution and almost in real-time, functional magnetic resonance imaging has been increasingly utilized in the clinical practice, lately. Its main use is for preoperative planning of brain surgeries in cases of cerebral tumors and/or pharmacoresistant epilepsies where mapping the language, memory and sensory-motor networks (Auer et al. 2008; Kozák et al. 2009) helps providing better post-operative quality of life, but neuro-ophthalmological indications are gaining importance lately, as well (Beauchamp et al. 2000; Szatmáry et al. 2007).

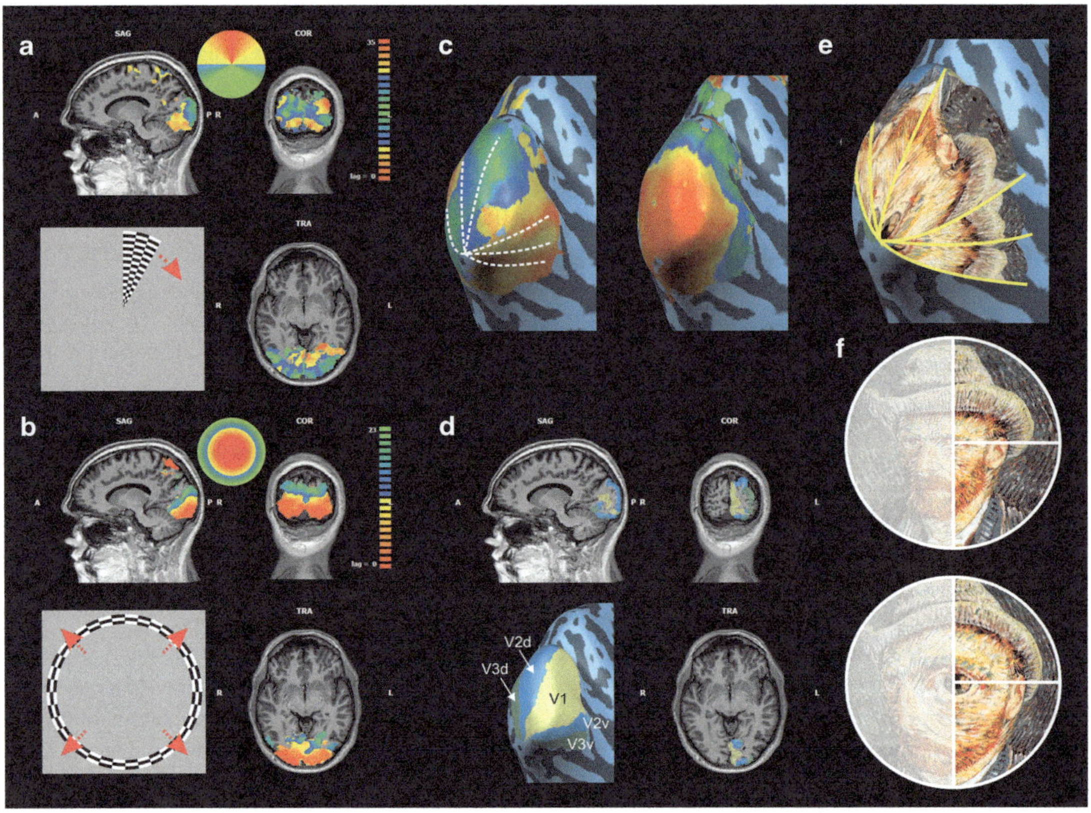

Fig. 31.7 Retinotopic mapping (**a**, **b**) The evoked cortical maps representing polar angle and distance from the fovea with the stimuli used for mapping. In case of polar angle mapping a rotating wedge is presented, while in the other case an expanding ring is shown. Both stimuli are presented in cycles during the examination, and they are overlaid with a checkerboard pattern changing its polarity with 8 Hz frequency. Coloring of the activation maps is according to colored circles representing the visual field. (**c**) Activation maps shown on the inflated and flattened gray and white matter boundary. The light blue regions represent the gyri, the darker, grayish-blue regions represent the sulci. In the polar angle map, the edge of the primary, secondary, and tertiary visual cortical areas are indicated by a white dashed line. (**d**) The location of the primary (V1), secondary (V2), and tertiary (V3) visual cortical areas in the left hemisphere. In the name of the areas, "d" means dorsal, and "v" refers to ventral. (**e**) Schematic representation of the visual field on the cortex using the self-portrait of van Gogh in panel (**f**). The yellow lines represent the edges of the visual areas seen in Panel (**c**, **d**). A complete but upside-down representation of the contralateral visual field is projected onto the primary visual cortex, while the representation of the lower and upper quadrant of the visual field are processed separately in the secondary and tertiary visual cortical areas. Cortical representation of the fovea and its surrounding is more extensive then that of the peripheral retinal areas, this is the so called cortical magnification effect which is shown schematically in Panel (**f**) where an image of van Gogh's self-portrait is seen with normal proportions above, and a distorted image representing cortical magnification is seen in the *bottom*

Special equipment is necessary for the fMRI examination of the visual system to perform visual stimulation and to record the patient's response with a push button if necessary. There are two widely used methods for visual stimulation: (a) projecting the image on a screen set up at the MRI machine, in this case the patient sees the screen via a mirror fixed to head coil, this method is used by the Szentágothai Knowledge Center, Semmelweis University, MR Research Center, Budapest; (b) another possibility is to use a special MRI compatible video goggle mounted to the head coil or to the patient, the image is then seen at the lenses.

Retinotopic mapping is used to identify and describe the cortical representation of the visual field with functional MRI (Warnking et al. 2002) (Fig. 31.7). With this procedure, a polar coordinate system is projected onto the cortex with the center on the fovea. It is performed in

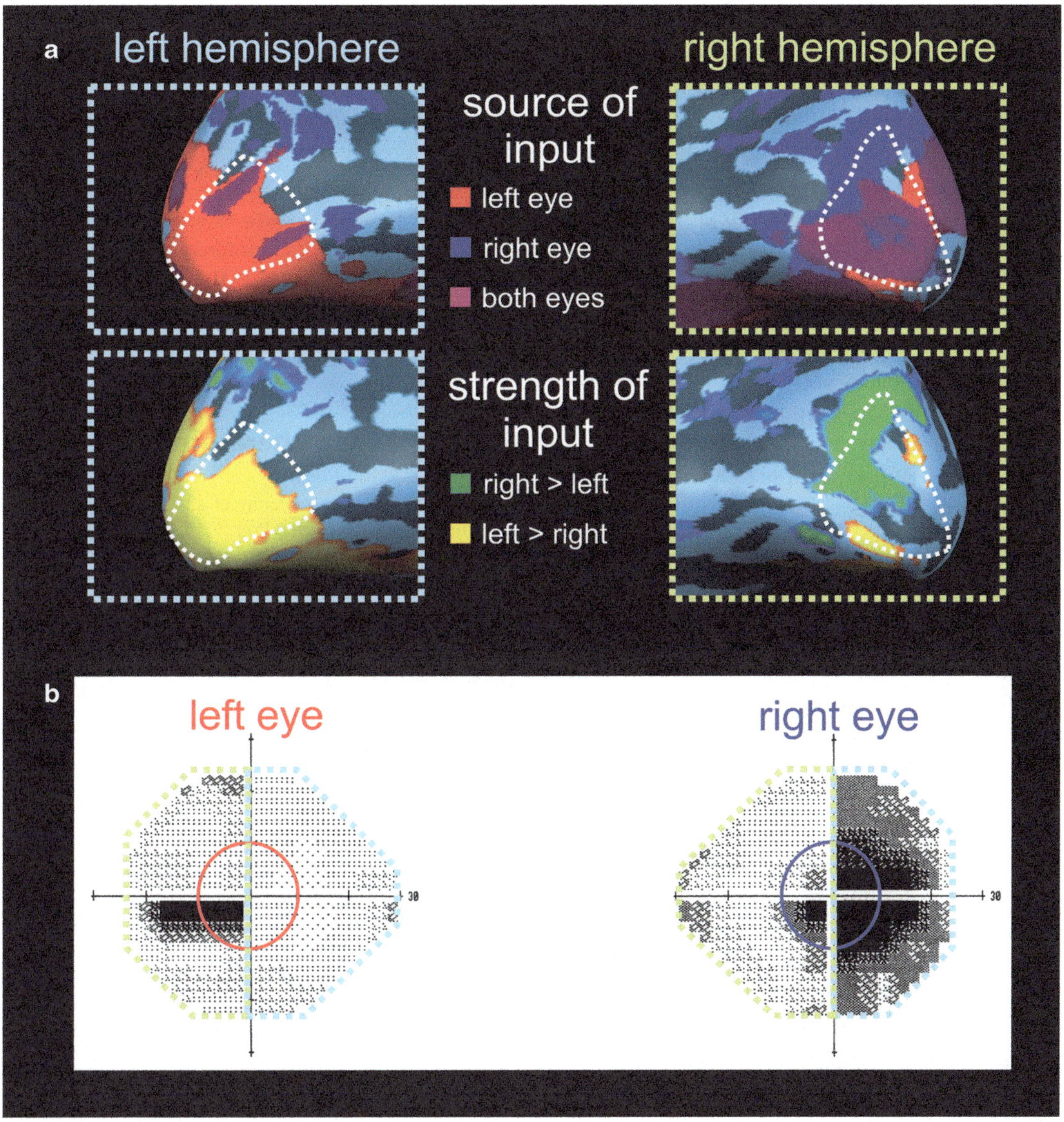

Fig. 31.8 Cortical representation of visual field defects caused by compression of the optic chiasm after suprasellar cyst removal surgery. (**a**) The *top panels* represent the input to the hemispheres; *red areas* represent the left eye, while the *blue* ones represent the right eye, the purple regions get input from both eyes. The *lower panels* show the relative strength of the signal coming from the eyes; *green* parts represent dominant activation originating from the right eye, *yellow areas* represent dominant information originating from the left eye, areas not shown receive about equal input from both eyes, or none. (**b**) Results of perimetry; the *red* and *dark blue circles* indicate the border of the 10° central visual field stimulated during retinotopic mapping. The *colored dashed lines* around the visual fields indicate the cortical regions in panel (**a**). The left sides of the visual fields (represented by *blue dashed lines*) project to the right occipital lobe, while the right sides of the visual fields (represented by *green dashed lines*) project to the left occipital lobe

two steps: first, the polar angle is defined using a slowly rotating wedge, and then the distance from the foveal center is determined using a slowly dilating ring; full movement cycles are repeated several times in both cases. The presented moving stimuli are overlaid with a dartstable like checkerboard pattern, with black and white polarity changing at 8 Hz frequency optimal for the stimulation of the primary visual cortex. During the analysis, the cortical activity pattern is correlated to the known spatial and temporal parameters of the stimuli; the retinotopic map is based on these correlations. As retinotopic organization is not only present in the primary visual cortex, the map represents a series of lower level visual areas.

In case of visual field deficiencies, the retinotopic maps change as well, for example in case of a lesion compressing the optic chiasm (Fig. 31.8) it can be well seen that the activity detected in the cortex depends clearly on the input to the cortex and that the distribution of the maximal BOLD response in the visual cortex is a good representation of the pattern seen with perimetry. Similar changes in the cortical representation of the visual field were detected in primary open angle glaucoma (POAG) as well, where the maps of the affected and less affected eyes were compared, and correlation was found between the maximal BOLD response measured at certain points and the retinal sensitivity threshold values of certain cortical areas (Duncan et al. 2007).

The development of methods suitable for mapping the lateral geniculate nucleus (Schneider et al. 2004) was a great leap forward in the functional examination of the optic pathway and in the localization of lesions of the pathways. The introduction of multifocal MRI (mfMRI) method analogous to the clinically widely used multifocal visual evoked potential (mfVEP) and the multifocal electroretinography (mfERG), and suitable to directly compare data collected from retinal electrophysiology and fMRI was of similar importace (Vanni et al. 2005).

Additional to the previously mentioned uses, fMRI can help in the differential diagnosis of visual-cognitive functional disturbances developing as a consequence of brain damage (Castelo-Branco et al. 2006; Kozák et al. 2009; Sorger et al. 2007), and can further our knowledge about the plasticity seen after functional loss, and about the potential cortical effects of rehabilitation (Henriksson et al. 2007). New results in the investigation of eye movement related functional activations (Brown et al. 2006) may in the future help the accurate differential diagnosis of eye movement disorders.

Functional MRI is already a versatile tool for neuro-ophthalmologists. Although the majority of procedures mentioned above are not as well established clinically as fMRI mapping for neurosurgical planning, there is a wide-spread serious research and clinical interest in the visual and ophthalmology-oriented fMRI, so these examinations may indeed be part of the routine neuroophthalmological practice in the near future.

Recommended Literature

Frackowiak, Ashburner, Penny et al. Human brain function, 2nd ed. Academic Press; 2003.

Huettel SA, Song AW, McCarthy G. Functional magnetic resonance imaging. Sinauer; 2004

References

Auer T, et al. Functional magnetic resonance imaging in neurology. Ideggyogy Sz. 2008;61(1–2):16–23.

Beauchamp MS, et al. A functional MRI case study of acquired cerebral dyschromatopsia. Neuropsychologia. 2000;38(8):1170–9.

Brown MR, et al. Inhibition and generation of saccades: rapid event-related fMRI of prosaccades, antisaccades, and nogo trials. Neuroimage. 2006;33(2): 644–59.

Castelo-Branco M, et al. Specific retinotopically based magnocellular impairment in a patient with medial visual dorsal stream damage. Neuropsychologia. 2006; 44(2):238–53.

Duncan RO, et al. Retinotopic organization of primary visual cortex in glaucoma: comparing fMRI measurements of cortical function with visual field loss. Prog Retin Eye Res. 2007;26(1):38–56.

Heeger DJ, Ress D. What does fMRI tell us about neuronal activity? Nat Rev Neurosci. 2002;3(2):142–51.

Henriksson L, et al. Training-induced cortical representation of a hemianopic hemifield. J Neurol Neurosurg Psychiatry. 2007;78(1):74–81.

Kozák LR, et al. A clonazepam elősegítheti a szenzomotoros funkcionális MR lebonyolítását alvás közbeni elektromos status epilepticusban [Clonazepam my promote the performance of sensomotor functional MRI in electrical epileptic state during sleep]. Ideggyogy Sz. 2009;62(3–4):130–5.

Kozák LR, et al. Az arcfeldolgozás hálózaton-belüli reorganizációja a gyrus fusiformist érintő dysembrioplasticus neuroepithelialis tumor esetében, in MNRT Kongresszusa. 2009.

Logothetis NK, et al. Neurophysiological investigation of the basis of the fMRI signal. Nature. 2001;412(6843):150–7.
Ogawa S, et al. Functional brain mapping by blood oxygenation level-dependent contrast magnetic resonance imaging. A comparison of signal characteristics with a biophysical model. Biophys J. 1993;64(3):803–12.
Roy CS, Sherrington CS. On the regulation of the blood-supply of the brain. J Physiol. 1890;11(1–2):85–158. 17.
Schneider KA, Richter MC, Kastner S. Retinotopic organization and functional subdivisions of the human lateral geniculate nucleus: a high-resolution functional magnetic resonance imaging study. J Neurosci. 2004;24(41):8975–85.
Sorger B, et al. Understanding the functional neuroanatomy of acquired prosopagnosia. Neuroimage. 2007;35(2):836–52.
Szatmáry G, Kozák LR, Vidnyánszky Z. Functional MRI-perimetry: a novel technique for simultaneous neural and behavioral mapping of the visual field, in EUNOS. Istambul; 2007.
Vanni S, Henriksson L, James AC. Multifocal fMRI mapping of visual cortical areas. Neuroimage. 2005;27(1):95–105.
Warnking J, et al. fMRI retinotopic mapping – step by step. Neuroimage. 2002;17(4):1665–83.

Novel Information Regarding the Visual and Eye Movement Systems in Otoneurology

32

Ágnes Szirmai

Contents

Examination of Vestibular Nystagmus

Contact point of Neuro-ophthalmology (borderline area of Ophthalmology and Neurology) and Otoneurology (borderline area of Otology and Neurology) can be defined with one word: nystagmus. The cause of this eye movement disorder can be partly in the inner ear or in the central nervous pathway originating from the inner ear. This diagnostic procedure makes it possible that examination of a patient having vertigo is described in this Neuro-Ophthalmology book. When a patient with vertigo has an episode of vertigo, he/she is so sick that a detailed examination may be very burdensome for him/her. During an episode of vertigo, the patient seems to be in a very severe condition, the patient is unable to move and have autonomic symptoms. Standard statokinetic examinations cannot be performed, as the patient is unable to move and the slightest movement may trigger vomiting. However, the most important diagnostic sign is spontaneous nystagmus. If the acute episode of the patient is of vestibular origin, spontaneous nystagmus is always present. If the patient sees a doctor when the patient does not have an episode, taking a thorough, detailed past medical history is very important: if the patient has any disease that makes him/her susceptible to vertigo, what the characteristics of vertigo are, how long an episode lasts, and how it develops and stops. Symptoms accompanying

Á. Szirmai, M.D., PhD
Department of Otorhinolaryngology, Head and Neck Surgery, Faculty of Medicine, Semmelweis University, Budapest, Hungary
e-mail: szirmai.agnes@med.semmelweis-univ.hu; http://drszirmaiagnes.hazipatika.net

J. Somlai, T. Kovács (eds.), *Neuro-Ophthalmology*, DOI 10.1007/978-3-319-28956-4_32

vertigo are very important. Examination of the patient starts with an explorative neurological and ophthalmologic examination. If the patient has spontaneous nystagmus, it is already known that he/she has vestibular disease.

Examination of Spontaneous Nystagmus

Examination of spontaneous nystagmus is very important. Nystagmus can be classified from several points of view. Its direction may be horizontal, rotatory, horizontorotatory, vertico-rotatory or retractional. Nystagmus may be examined visually, but may be better seen with a +20 diopter eyeglass, Bartels' spectacles or Frenzel goggles with electric illumination system. Regarding the type and intensity, peripheral vestibular nystagmus usually follows the Alexander's law:

1st degree: eyes move only into the direction of gazing.
2nd degree: nystagmus is present in primary gaze as well.
3rd degree: nystagmus is present in the direction opposite to the direction of gaze as well, it is present in case of the most severe and acute forms (Fig. 32.1).

Nystagmus in the direction of gaze may be:

- ophthalmologic (tiredness of the eye muscles, or fixation; fixation nystagmus cannot be detected with the 20 diopter Frenzel goggles),
- central nystagmus can be seen in case of a functional disorder of the brainstem.

Abnormalities seen with statokinetic tests can be evaluated together with spontaneous nystagmus. The statokinetic tests give information on the function of the vestibulospinal pathways.

Examination of Positional Nystagmus

Changing the position of the head and the body often causes vertigo and nystagmus. Based on how the nystagmus is developed, the following types are differentiated: positional nystagmus, which is persistent and positioning nystagmus, which is temporary. Positional nystagmus is triggered by a static stimulus, the certain supine position should be considered. Positioning nystagmus is a dynamic stimulus, movement when changing a body position triggers the nystagmus. Both positional and positioning nystagmus may be direction-fixed or direction-changing. Direction-fixed nystagmus is usually present in peripheral vestibular lesions, direction-changing nystagmus is characteristic in central lesions. When triggering positional or positioning nystagmus, it is important to observe whether nystagmus can be exhausted, extinguished or increased in intensity.

Examination of the Eye Movement System

Examining Pursuit Eye Movements

Usually it is the examination of the optokinetic nystagmus, but examination of saccadic eye movements and smooth pursuit eye movements are included as well. Examination using nystagmographic registration is the most practical, but significant changes may be seen with the naked eye as well. During the examination, the eye follows a continuously moving visual target. Movement of the visual field plays a role in the development of nystagmus. Optokinetic nystagmus is normal.

Impulse Test

Physiological background of the examination is that in case of normal labyrinth function, after a sudden movement of the head, the examined person is still able to fixate on a certain point as the eye movement system makes a correction. In case of decreased labyrinthine function, if the patient's head moves to the affected side, temporary saccadic nystagmus develops to the opposite

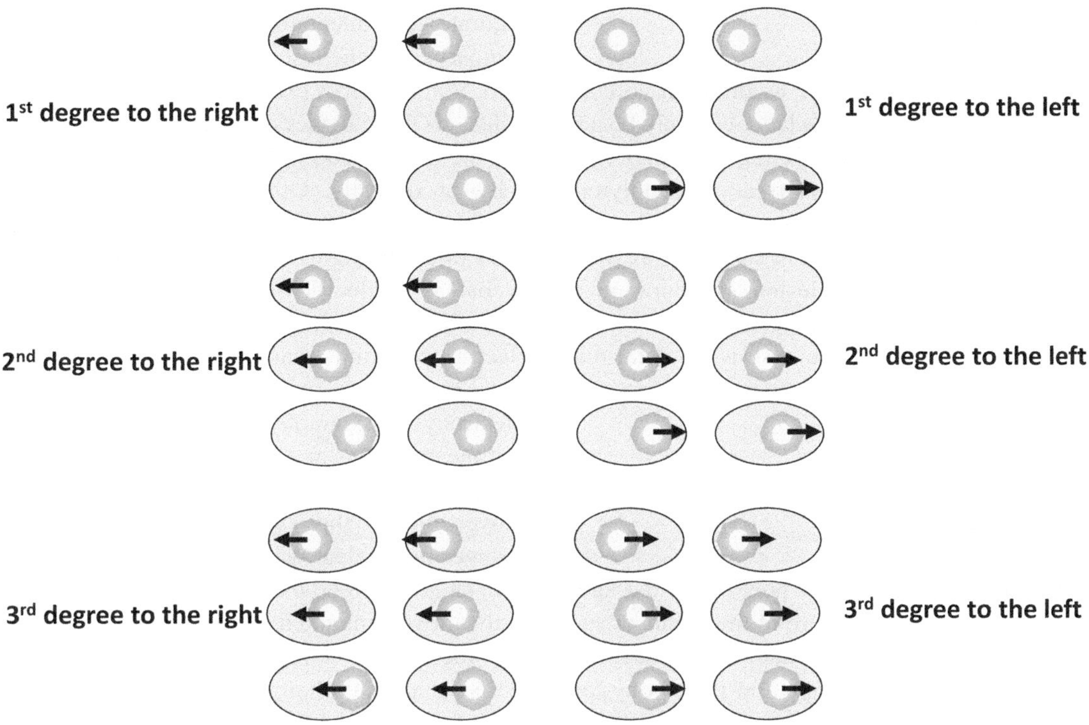

Fig. 32.1 Nystagmus following the Alexander's law

direction. As the examination is based on fixation, the nystagmus cannot be seen under Frenzel goggles.

Labyrinth Stimulation Tests

Provocation tests may provide information about the function of the labyrinth. The two labyrinths can be stimulated separately with thermal or caloric stimulation, while the rotatory test stimulates both labyrinths at the same time. The response to the stimulation develops via three reflex arcs:

- Vestibulospinal reflex arc
- Vestibulo-vegetative reflex arc
- Vestibulo-ocular reflex arc: nystagmus develops via the connection between the labyrinth and the eye movement muscles. The purpose of the stimulation is to examine the nystagmus as the triggered nystagmus may reflect the function of the labyrinth.

Caloric Stimulation

Caloric stimulation is one of the most useful examination methods in the hands of an otoneurologist. If the external auditory tube is heated or cooled with water or air at least 7 degrees of Celsius different from the body temperature, caloric nystagmus develops. In case of a warm stimulus, the direction of nystagmus is towards the stimulated ear, the direction is the opposite in case of cold stimulus. From the four caloric reactions performed on the two sides, two caloric tests examine one ear. Normally, the amplitude, frequency, and duration of the resulting nystagmus seen after the two cold and two warm stimulations are the same. Semicircular canal paresis is present if excitability of one or both labyrinths is decreased to cold and warm temperature. It is characteristic of peripheral lesions. The directional preponderance is seen in central lesions. In this case, nystagmus reactions are more pronounced to one direction (nystagmus after a cold stimulus on one side and nystagmus after warm stimulus on the other side are more intense).

Rotating Stimulation

The rotating stimulus may be different, circular or sinus wave-like, and the latter can only be performed with an electric rotating chair and computed analysis. In case of rotation, endolymph flow is present in both labyrinths. In case of an intact vestibular system or in case of a previous, compensated vestibular lesion, the duration of nystagmus seen after bilateral rotation is the same. A purpose of the test is to determine whether central compensation is present or not.

Mechanical Stimulation (Fistula Symptom)

Increased or decreased air pressure in the auditory canal (such as pressure of the tragus or suction discharge from the auditory canal) may cause temporary endolymph flow if the bony capsule of the labyrinth gets injured, and consequential nystagmus develops. This is called a fistula sign. If we are changing the pressure in the auditory canal (such as using a Politzer balloon), the fistula symptom can be well examined. Most commonly otitis media with cholesteatoma leads to fistula symptom as a consequence of destroying the labyrinth.

Instrumental Examination of Vertigo

Diseases accompanied by vertigo are usually easy to diagnose without special devices; however, requirements of modern medicine is to make test results objective, and to prepare accurate documentation, reproducibility and comparison of the test findings are important as well. Some devices examine the vestibulospinal reflex, so these devices are capable of visualizing the statokinetic reflex in an image, graphically or digitally. Other devices register the vestibulo-ocular reflex, the nystagmus. The basis of recording nystagmus is the fact that the eyeball is an electric dipolar object (the cornea is positive, the retina is negative); therefore, electric potential changes may be measured and recorded after proper amplification. Electronystagmography (ENG) is based on the fact the eyeball is an electric dipolar object (the cornea is positive, the retina is negative). Movement of the eyeball induces potential changes in the electrodes placed around the eyeball, and the potential changes are proportionate to the movement and direction of the movement of the eye. Photo-electronystagmography (PENG): a small photocell detects and registers the infrared light beam reflected from the corneo-scleral border. Video nystagmography (VNG): the most recent registering option is video recording. The most important thing is an eyeglass which has two built-in digital cameras. If the eyeglass is connected to a computer, nystagmus can be analyzed.

Further Readings

Szirmai Á. Instrumental examination of dizziness. International Békésy Conference, Budapest, 1999. június 24–26. Abstract 241–245. o.

Szirmai Á. Az egyensúlyzavarok differenciáldiagnosztikája és terápiája [Differential diagnostics and therapy in balance diseases]. Budapest: Semmelweis Kiadó; 2006.

Electro-Oculography (EOG) Examination of Eye Movements

33

Szilvia Gulyás

Content

Measurement of the characteristics of eye movements may provide important information in several neurological disorders. Timely course, progression of the disease, and the efficacy of the therapy can be followed up with the objective methods. The essence of electrophysiological methods is that in addition to the morphological evaluation of eye movements, it makes certain characteristics of the eye movements, their latency, speed, and amplitude measurable. Evaluation of conjugated eye movements becomes possible as well if these parameters are compared when the two eyes are moving in the same direction.

Electro-oculography (EOG) is a very commonly used test procedure, neuro-ophthalmological workshops, mainly in the USA, Germany, Italy, and France use them in the clinical practice for about 25 years and for more than 85 years in scientific research. In Hungary, it is less commonly used as a complementary diagnostic tool. Its simple form recording by two electrodes is used e.g. to monitor REM phases in sleep laboratories. International organizations have standardized the routine method of examinations, so data of laboratories all over the world can be compared. The International Society for Clinical Electrophysiology of Vision (ISCEV, www.iscev.org) created a recommendation first in 1993. The latest protocol was published in 2006; it can be downloaded from the website of the Society free.

The registration is based on the difference in potentials between cornea and retina (corneo-retinal or corneo-fundal potential) discovered by *du Bois Reymond* in 1849. This difference in potentials is present due to the ion permeability of the pigment epithelium of the retina in case of normal structures. The cornea is positively discharged compared to the retina due to the difference in corneo-retinal potential; the resting potential is about 1 mV. The difference in potential changes in time; its value depends on the amount of light getting to the retina, the blood supply, and how tired the person is. If the bulb is placed between two electrodes as a dipole object, its movement generates voltage difference between the two electrodes. If the cornea moves towards the active electrode, a positive change occurs (upward deflection), if it moves towards the reference electrode, the change is negative (downward deflection). If the signals are recorded in DC mode, linear correlation is seen between the generating voltage and the movements of the bulb. The movement can be measured in degrees as the bulb has a nearly spherical sur-

S. Gulyás, M.D., PhD
Electrophysiology Unit, Department of Neurology, Faculty of Medicine, Semmelweis University, Budapest, Hungary
e-mail: gulyszi@yahoo.co.uk

J. Somlai, T. Kovács (eds.), *Neuro-Ophthalmology*, DOI 10.1007/978-3-319-28956-4_33

face, and the speed of the movement is angular velocity, therefore °/sec is used. An advantage of the method is that it is non-invasive; it can register eye movements in a wide range, horizontally in both directions approx. in 40–40°, while vertically in almost 30–30°. Deflection of eye movements can be evaluated with 1° accuracy. With this device, less cooperating patients and children can be examined as well. A disadvantage of the examination is that the baseline is fluctuating due to the dynamic characteristic of the corneo-retinal difference. The recording is often disturbed by the electromyography (EMG) artifacts of the mimic muscles and blinking, it makes evaluation of especially the vertical eye movements difficult. After cleaning and degreasing the skin around the eyes, four Ag/AgCl electrodes are placed on each side on the horizontal and vertical axes crossing the pupil under and below the eye, and in the nasal and temporal regions (Fig. 33.1). The active electrodes are the ones above the eyebrow and on the right side, that is the temporal electrode in case of the right eye and the nasal electrode in case of the left eye, so positive movement is seen in the electrooculogram in case of looking upwards and to the right. The ground electrode is placed on the forehead. The twice four electrodes make horizontal and vertical eye movements to be evaluated separately and simultaneously in case of both eyes. The computer registers the DC signs in four channels; the channels are recording the horizontal movement of the right and then the left eye, and the vertical movement of the right and then the left eye respectively. During the EOG examination, the patient sits in a dark room in a comfortable chair with a headrest 130 cm from a 150 × 100 cm large screen. Horizontally, the screen is seen at 30–30°, this value is 21–21° vertically (Fig. 33.2). A white

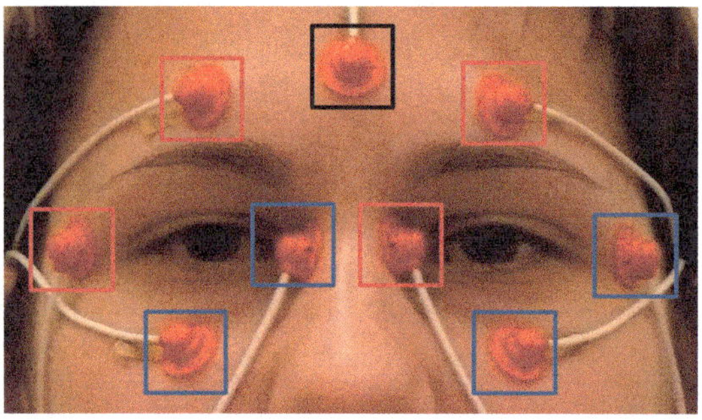

Fig. 33.1 The position of the electrodes around the eyes (the *red* ones are the active electrodes, the *blue ones* are reference electrodes, and the ground electrode is *black*)

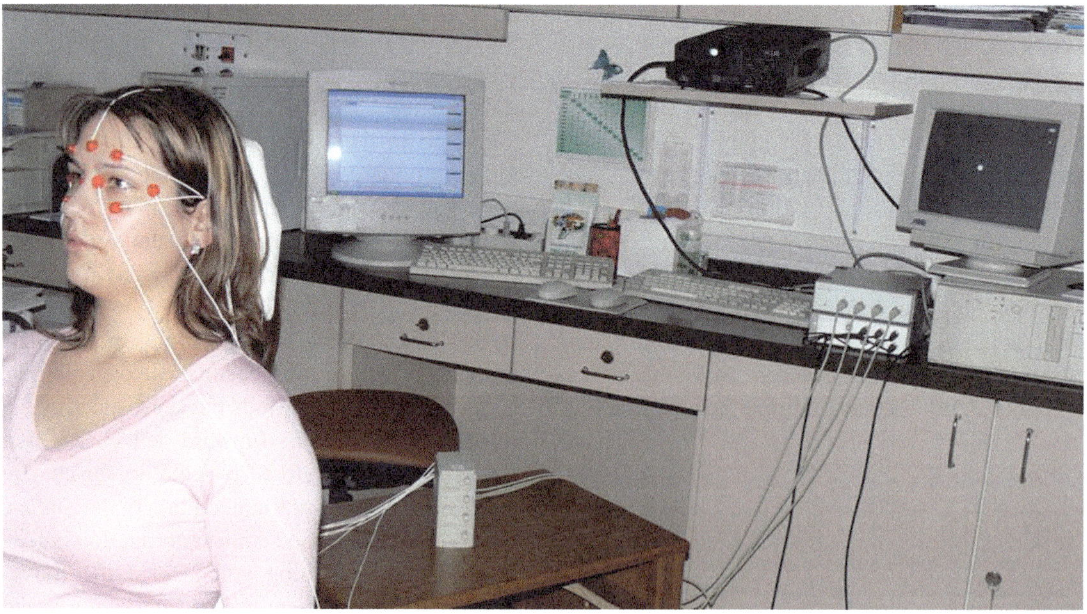

Fig. 33.2 The DC recorder, the collector head connecting to the amplifier device and the computer are behind the examined subject

disc with 2° radius and 4° wide white bands are projected on the screen with a projector, and these objects move on the screen depending on the type of the test.

During the examination, the role of the patient is to follow the moving object on the screen without moving his/her head.

After approximately 10 min of dark adaptation, **eye movements during fixation** are recorded with a white disc located on the center of the screen. In case of a normal recording, no abnormal oscillation (square-wave jerks, macrosquare-wave jerks, ocular flutter, opsoclonus, etc. See Fig. 33.3) or resting nystagmus is seen during the fixation.

Voluntary, **commanded rapid eye movements** (**saccades**) are triggered with rapid commands, "Look to the right, left, look up and down." Latency of the triggered movement cannot be examined, as the time of the auditory information processing has to be added to the latency of the saccade. However, the velocity, amplitude of the saccade, or extent of conjugation of the eye movements can be measured. It can be observed whether voluntary saccades are dysmetric, and whether nystagmus is present or not, if yes, in what directions.

During the examination of **reflexive**, **visually guided saccades**, the disc projected on the center of the screen randomly moves to the right or left side of the screen, back to the center, upper or lower border, time between each movement changes randomly as well. The time the disc changes its position is indicated by a marker given by the computer projecting the task; therefore, the latency of the saccade can be calculated properly in the various directions. This value in case of healthy is 200–250 msec (Fig. 33.4), in frontal or parietal lesions, the latency of the saccade in the opposite direction is increased; this can be seen in the early stage of corticobasal degeneration (CBD) as well. The average speed of the saccade regarding the whole saccade is 360°/s (Fig. 33.4), a value below this number is abnormal. The average speed of the saccade of young, healthy persons is about 450°/s, but it may be decreased in case of frontal or parietal cortical lesions. The latter is seen in progressive supranuclear paresis (PSP) (in a parkinsonian syndrome). The velocity of the horizontal and vertical saccades decreases without vertical gaze palsy, even in a very early stage of the disease.

Examining the amplitude of the saccades may lead to the discovery of impaired horizontal or vertical movement for example in PSP. In case of dysmetric saccades (Fig. 33.5), the eye reaches the target in several steps, the eye movement may be hypometric and hypermetric, with or without corrective saccades. Dysmetry may be caused by the lesion of the dorsal vermis of the cerebellum; certain publications mention hyper-, others mention hypometry, in our experience, it is hypometry. Hypometry may be caused by, for example, the lesion of the frontal eye field also (Fig. 33.5). Saccades of healthy subjects are conjugated; however, for example, in rare pseudo-abducent palsy, the abducting eye moves more slowly than the adducting eye leading to diplopia. Eye movements are disconjugate in peripheral palsy of nerves III, IV, and VI, in skew deviation, one-and-a-half syndrome, etc.

Smooth pursuit eye movement (**SPEM**) may be stimulated by moving a disc with constant velocity in right, left, upward, and downward directions. The speed of the disc is most commonly 30°/s. It leads to a healthy sinusoidal SPEM curve, and no saccadic movement or nystagmus is seen in the EOG acquisition. Movements of the eyes are conjugated, the extent of pursuit (gain), that is the ratio of the velocity of SPEM and that of the object, around 1 (Fig. 33.6). Saccadic SPEM may be caused by several diseases, such as lesion of the cerebrocerebellum (Fig. 33.7), the frontal eye field (FEF) or the paramedial region of the thalamus.

At the end of the examination, **optokinetic nystagmus** (**OKN**) may be stimulated with a computerized rotating drum. The black and white stripes move with 30°/s velocity in the right, left, upward, and then downward directions, which may stimulate typical train nystagmus (Fig. 33.8). The speed of the slow phase of the OKN divided by the speed of stimulation is the gain, which is around 1 in healthy. Temporo-parietal lesions alter the contralateral, while lesions of the brainstem alter the ipsilateral OKN.

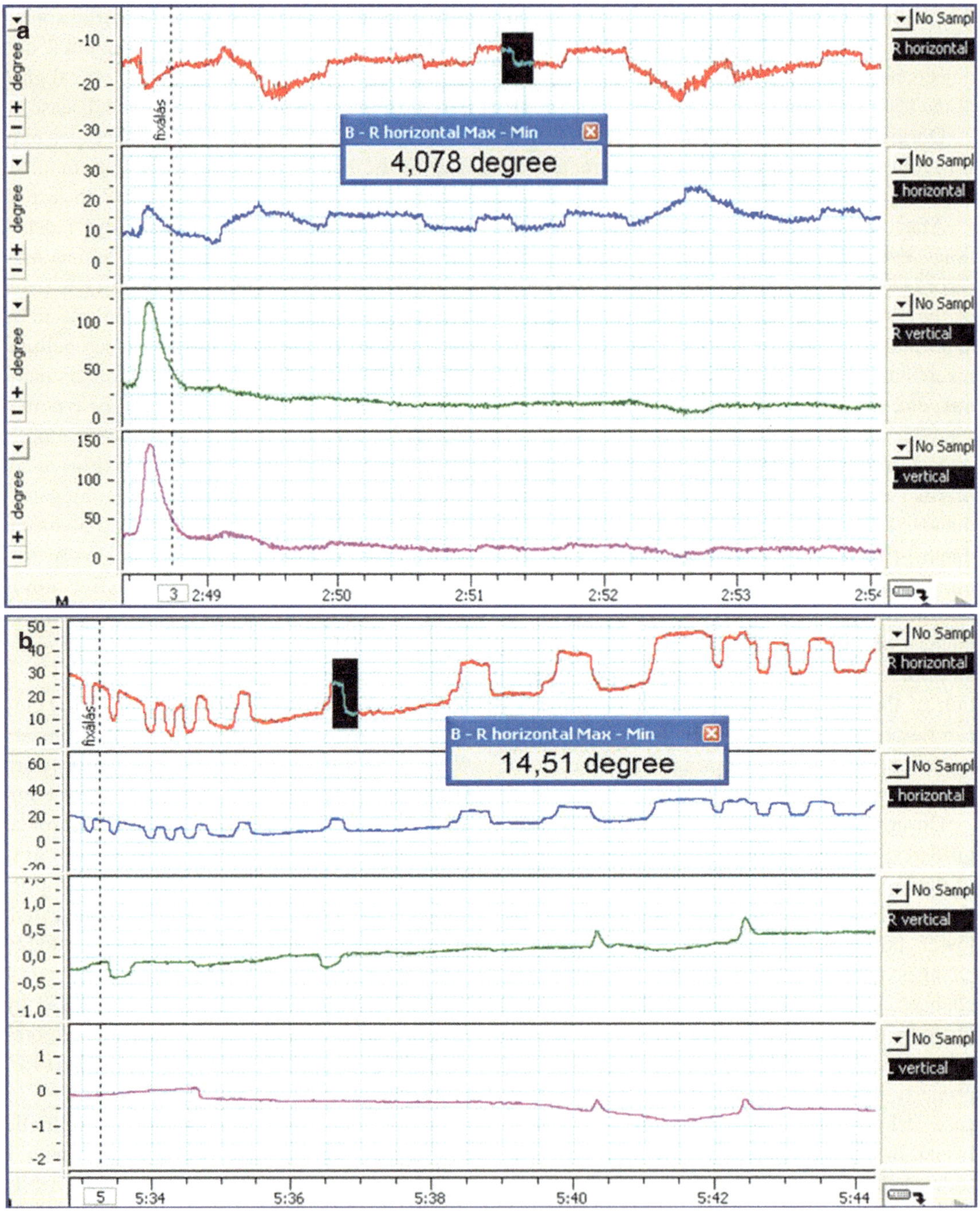

Fig. 33.3 EOG recording of abnormal horizontal oscillation in Parkinson's syndrome. (**a**) Square-wave jerks in progressive supranuclear paresis (PSP), abnormal saccades, lasting for 250–350 msec with an amplitude of around 4°. Blinking is seen at the beginning of the recording which leads to artifacts on the horizontal channels (Channel 1–2) as well. (**b**) Macrosquare-wave jerks in multisystemic atrophy (MSA), the extent of oscillation is around 15° which can be seen with the naked eye as well

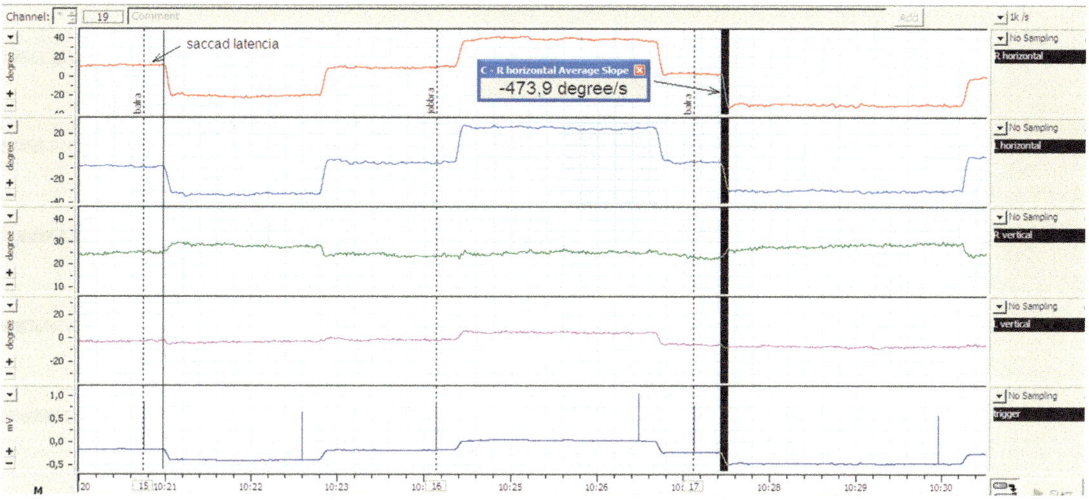

Fig. 33.4 EOG record of reflexive, visually guided horizontal saccades in healthy. The latency of the saccades is between 210 and 250 msec, deflection to the right and left is 30° similarly. The average speed of the saccade highlighted with a black band is around 470°/s

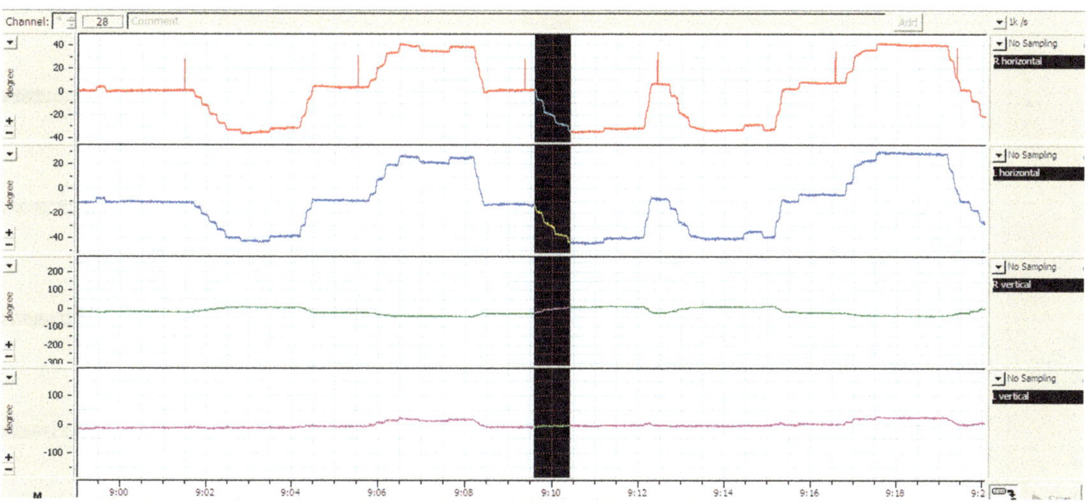

Fig. 33.5 Hypometric horizontal saccades in the early stage of PSP. The eyes reach the target in several (4–5) steps. Some abnormal horizontal oscillation below 5° (square-wave jerks) are seen during fixation at the saccade's end position

In summary, EOG examination of the eye movements is a complementary diagnostic procedure, it gives little additional information in case of the lesion of nerves III, IV, and VI, but it is rather useful in the diagnosis of dysfunction of central structures. As different cerebral structures may lead to the same alterations in eye movement, the results of the electro-oculography are valuable only with the complex clinical picture.

It largely helps the differential diagnosis of parkinsonian syndromes at very early stage, and

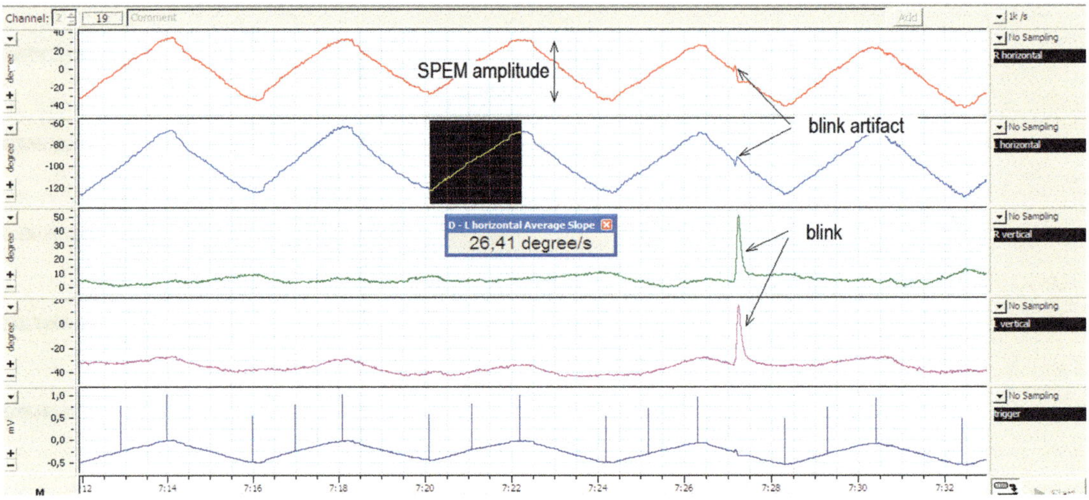

Fig. 33.6 EOG recording of smooth pursuit stimulated by an object moving horizontally with 30°/s. The healthy SPEM curve is a sinusoid curve, the extent of pursuit is between 0.8 and 1. In the figure, it is 26.4/30=0.88. Blinking is seen in the vertical movement of the *right* (Channel 3) and *left* (Channel 4) eye, it leads to artifacts on the horizontal channels also (Channels 1–2)

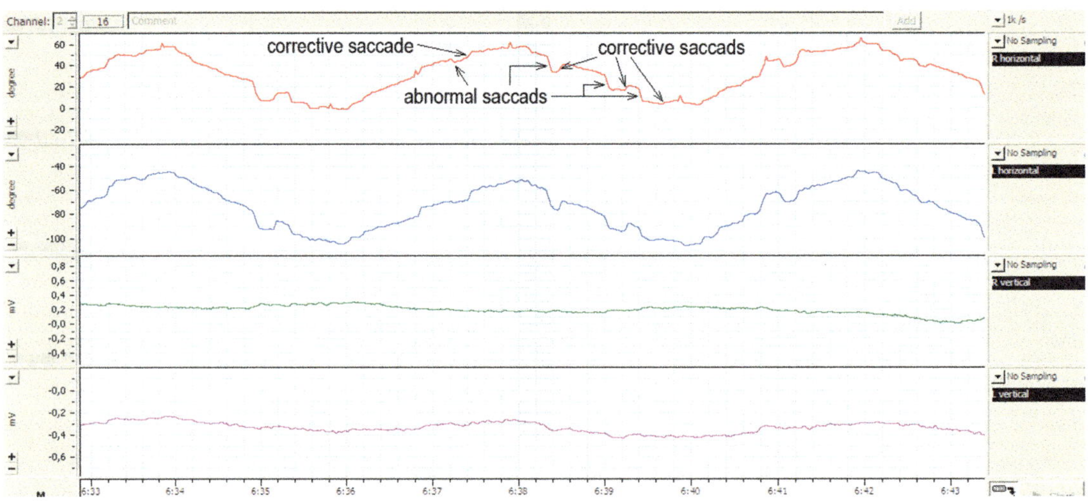

Fig. 33.7 Saccadic horizontal SPEM. The object is moving with 30°/s speed on the screen. In the curve of a female patient with celiac disease there are abnormal saccades due to the cerebellar dysfunction corrected with new saccades in the opposite direction trying to bring the image of the object to the fovea again

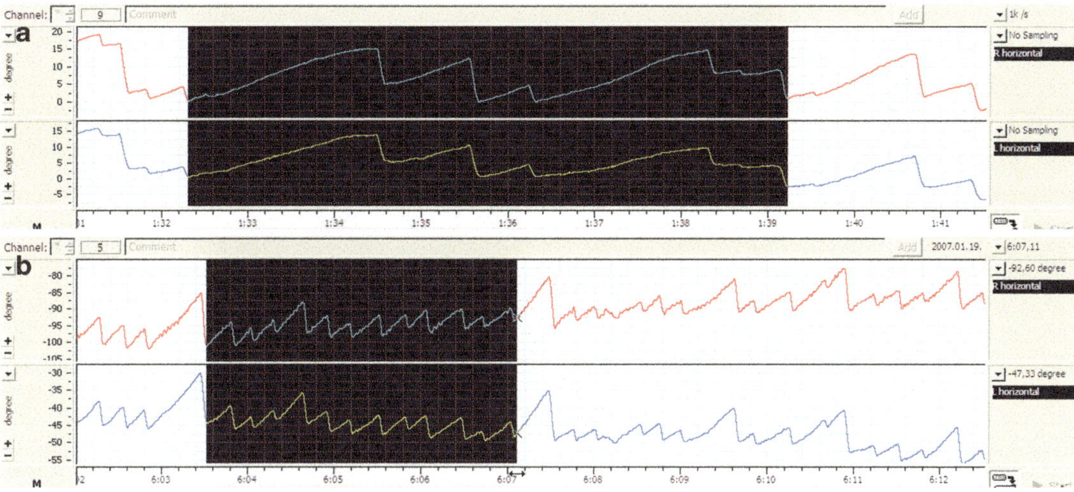

Fig. 33.8 EOG curve of a horizontal optokinetic nystagmus stimulated by a rotating drum moving to the right with 30°/s velocity. (**a**) Cortical, attentive or "look" nystagmus. Lower frequency movement. (**b**) Subcortical, inattentive or "stare" optokinetic nystagmus. High frequency movement

in case of cortical, cerebellar or brainstem dysfunctions, it contributes to the diagnosis of the disease, for example, in fronto-temporal dementia or spinocerebellar atrophy.

Further Readings

Barry W, Jones GM. Influence of eye lid movement upon electro-oculographic recording of vertical eye movements. Aerosp Med. 1965;36:855–8.

Brown M, Marmor M, Vaegan ZE, Brigell M, Bach M. ISCEV standard for clinical electro-oculography (EOG) 2006. Doc Ophthalmol. 2006;113:205–12.

Carpenter RHS. Movements of the eyes, second. London: Pion; 1988.

Homer LD, Kolder H. Mathematical model of oscillations in the human corneo-retinal potential. Pflugers Arch. 1966;287:197–202.

Marmor MF. Standardization notice: EOG standard reapproved. Doc Ophthalmol. 1998;95:91–2.

Marmor MF, Zrenner E. Standard for clinical electro-oculography. Doc Ophthalmol. 1993;85:115–24.

Miles W. Modification of the human-eye potential by dark and light adaptation. Science. 1940;91:456.

Mowrer OH, Ruch TC, Miller NE. The corneo-retinal potential difference as the basis of the galvanometric method of recording eye movements. Am J Physiol. 1935;114:423–8.

North AW. Accuracy and precision of electro-oculographic recording. Invest Ophthalmol. 1965;4:343–8.

Schott E. Über die Registrierung des Nystagmus und anderer Augenbewegungen vermittels des Saitengalvanometers. Deutsch Arch Klin Med. 1922;140:79–90.

van der Stappen A, Wuyts FL, van de Heyning PH. Computerized electronystagmography: normative data revisited. Acta Otolaryngol. 2000;120:724–30.

The Importance of Familiar Thrombophilias in the Clinical Practice. Novel Ways in Anticoagulant Therapy

34

László Nemes

Contents

Importance

Thrombophilic diseases are among the most common causes of death; its mortality is three-four times as high as all cancer mortality in the developed countries. With the currently available laboratory methods, about 50% of the cases, acquired or congenital coagulation disorder or platelet defect can be found in the background of thromboses. These are the hypercoagulability conditions with a varying diagnosis rate depending on the localization of the thromboembolic process: approximately 80% in patients with venous diseases, 50% in early myocardial infarction and 33% in juvenile stroke. Thrombophilic conditions clearly play a role in arterial thromboses as well with the other well-known risk factors; however, they are essentially important in the pathogenesis of venous diseases. Venous thromboembolism is very common as well, and its mortality is surprisingly high: the incidence is about 1–1.5 % oper year based on large international surveys, and the mortality of the disease is 20/100,000 according to national data. Mortality has doubled in the past two decades. Previous or new pulmonary embolism can be detected in 10–60% of the cadavers undergoing autopsy. Diagnosing genetic susceptibility to thrombosis may be essential, as it enables adequate antithrombotic therapy in the patients, it clearly influences the method and time of secondary prevention (anticoagulant therapy), and the risk of the direct family members can be determined with this diagnosis.

Definition and History of Thrombophilia

The classic triad of susceptibility to thrombosis has been known since Virchow's description: venous stasis, injury of the vascular wall, and coagulation

L. Nemes, M.D., PhD
National Hemophilia Center and Hemostasis Outpatient Unit, Military Hospital, Budapest, Hungary
e-mail: lnemes@hm.goc.hu

J. Somlai, T. Kovács (eds.), *Neuro-Ophthalmology*, DOI 10.1007/978-3-319-28956-4_34

disorder (Table 34.1). It has been observed for a long time that thrombosis may often develop in young patients having no known acquired risk factors. These "idiopathic" cases where thrombosis occurs without any clear cause, and thromboembolic episodes occur in several family members lead to intense research focusing on finding congenital thrombophilias. The expression thrombophilia was first used by Egeberg as an analogue of hemophilia, and the first congenital thrombophilia, antithrombin III defect was found in 1965 in a Norwegian family. Every acquired or inherited coagulation disorder that makes a person susceptible to thrombosis is thrombophilia in a broader sense. It means a thrombophilic predisposition, the disorder of the natural anticoagulant and fibrinolytic mechanisms can be found in the background.

Table 34.1 Acquired susceptibility to thrombosis

1. Venous stasis
Immobilization: trauma, postoperative conditions
Pregnancy
Decompensation
Obesity
Previous deep venous thrombosis
Varicosity
Old age
2. Injury of the vascular wall
Trauma
Veno-occlusive disease (VOD) in bone marrow transplantation
Smoking
Diabetes
TTP (Moschcowitz syndrome)
Atherosclerosis
Hyperhomocysteinemia
Vascular and valvular prostheses
3. Coagulation disorder
Malignancy: Trousseau syndrome, chronic DIC
Antiphospholipid antibody syndrome: lupus anticoagulant, anticardiolipin antibody, B-2GPI
Excess estrogen: oral contraceptive, hormone supplementation, hormone therapy of prostate cancer, pregnancy
Hyperlipidemia
Hyperviscosity
Myeloproliferative diseases

In a narrower sense, thrombophilia means only congenital (primary) hypercoagulability conditions leading to thrombosis without known (acquired) risk factors, and that is characterized by increased risk for recurring thrombosis. Naturally, any risk factors listed in Table 34.1 may trigger a thromboembolic episode in a patient with thrombophilia (inherited susceptibility to thrombosis).

In another approach, a patient has thrombophilia if hypercoagulability is confirmed with currently available laboratory methods. "Clinically", a patient has thrombophilia if he/she has juvenile, "idiopathic" thrombosis in case of which no evident underlying cause is found according to our current knowledge. As clinical manifestations may be variable depending on the severity of hemophilia (bleeding occurs after a large trauma or surgery in case of slight to moderate hemophilia, but spontaneous articular or intramuscular bleeding is common in patients with severe hemophilia, and these conditions lead to deformity later), the clinical spectrum of thrombophilia is significantly varying as well.

There are forms that are incompatible with life in the long term (such as homozygous antithrombin and protein C deficiency), and there are slight mutations that do not lead to thrombosis without accompanying risk factors (such as Factor V Leiden, Factor II 20210). It is understandable that first, the less common, but more severe forms of thrombophilia with significant susceptibility to thrombosis are discovered, in order: antithrombin III defect, protein C deficiency, protein S deficiency (Comp and Esmon, and Griffin, 1984). In these forms, the genetic abnormality is localized to the gene of the natural anticoagulants (inhibitors), the mutations are significantly heterogeneous: approximately 80 mutations were identified in antithrombin III defect, more than 300 mutations were found in protein C deficiency, and at least 60 mutations are known in protein S deficiency. However, thrombophilias described in the past 5 years with less severe susceptibility to thrombosis are caused by a single mutation, Leiden mutation of factor V may be an example, or the mutation of the methylenetetrahydrofolate reductase gene, or the prothrombin 20210 A polymorphism. Newly discovered mutations do not affect the inhibitors but the substrates of the coagulation pathways (such as factors Va, IIa). The mutant coagulation factor is produced in lager amount (such as prothrombin polymorphism) or breakdown of the activated form is more difficult (such as factor V Leiden mutation). Besides the slight thrombogenicity, these conditions may have great importance regarding public health as they are very common.

Clinical Picture

Even the simple data of the past medical history may raise the suspicion of congenital susceptibility to thrombosis in a careful examiner. Clinical characteristics of familiar thrombophilia are described in the following points. (Certain clinical manifestations may be characteristic to a certain thrombophilia, in this case, the defect is indicated in brackets).

1. Thromboembolic disease at a young age in the family history.
2. Thrombophilia confirmed with laboratory methods in a close relative.
3. Thromboembolic disease at a young age in the past medical history (arterial thrombosis below the age of 35, or venous thrombosis below the age of 40, spontaneous thrombosis in the newborn).
4. Recurrent thromboembolic episodes.
5. "Idiopathic" deep venous thrombosis (cause cannot be identified).
6. Venous thromboembolism with minimal provoking factors (such as pregnancy, oral anticoagulant therapy, hormone supplementation, short immobilization, such as "economy class syndrome" of passengers of transcontinental flights).
7. Combined venous and arterial thrombosis (protein S deficiency).
8. Venous thrombosis in multiple locations (such as upper and lower extremity + mesenterial).
9. Thrombosis in uncommon localizations:
   - inferior vena cava,
   - mesenteric vein,
   - cerebral sinus thrombosis,
   - renal vein,
   - deep venous thrombosis in the upper extremity,
   - thrombosis in the splenic, hepatic, or portal vein.
10. Progressive thrombosis besides anticoagulant treatment (antithrombinopathy, but malignant diseases as well).
11. Thrombosis from adolescence (such as type 1, severe antithrombin III deficiency, combined defects).
12. Fulminant purpura in newborns (homozygous protein C and protein S deficiency).
13. Skin necrosis caused by coumarin (protein C and S deficiency, antiphospholipid syndrome).
14. Clinical and laboratory heparin resistance (antithrombin III deficiency)
15. Migrating thrombophlebitis (protein C deficiency, but it may be characteristic in case of malignant tumors as well).
16. Increased thromboembolic risk during pregnancy and after giving birth.
17. Increased risk of fetal death.

As the hemostatic balance is essential in maintaining the uteroplacental circulation, it is not surprising that international, multicenter studies confirmed that the ratio of fetal death was increased in pregnant women with thrombophilia compared to the average ratio. There was an about four-fold increase in preterm births, and the risk of spontaneous miscarriage was one and a half times increased compared to the control group, but the risk was ten-fold in some severe or combined thrombophilias.

Basics of the Pathomechanism

Physiologically, the hemostatic balance ensures that we do not bleed out in case of a vascular injury, and that blood clots do not develop in the vessels if not necessary. This finely controlled process may become thrombogenic if

1. The production of procoagulants (classic coagulation factors) increases or the breakdown of activated coagulation factors is impaired.
2. Efficacy of the natural anticoagulant inhibitor systems (antithrombin, thrombomodulin – protein C – protein S, and Tissue Factor Pathway Inhibitor) decreases.
3. The developed blood clot dissolves abnormally due to the imbalance of the profibrinolytic – fibrinolytic proteins.

A key component of coagulation is the prothrombin (factor II) – thrombin conversion, as the resulting active serine protease IIa has a diverse role in the coagulation process (Table 34.2).

If produced in a proper amount, it induces and multiplies the speed of the coagulation processes with positive feed back cycles. Therefore, it is understandable that the deficiency of natural anticoagulants inhibiting the function and regulating the production of thrombin increases the risk of thrombosis. Characteristics of the most important inhibitors of the coagulation system are summarized in Table 34.3.

Table 34.2 Diverse role of thrombin in coagulation

Releasing factor VIII from the carrier von Willebrand factor
Activation of coagulation cofactors V and VIII
Activation of factors IX and XI (acceleration of coagulation)
Release of prothrombin fragment 1 (autoactivation)
Creating the fibrin net
Activation of factor XIII (stabilizing the fibrin net)
Activation of platelets (phospholipase A2-TXA2-aggregation)
Activation of protein C (TM/PC/PS-APC system)
Inactivation of factor Va and VIIIa Stimulation of the endothelium (prostacyclin and TPA release)
Activation of the complement system (cleavage of C3 and C5)
Mitogenic stimulation of fibroblasts

Several inhibitor type proteins play a role in the inactivation of the developed thrombin (alpha 2 macroglobulin, trypsin inhibitor, heparin cofactor II), but the majority of the thrombin inhibiting capacity of the plasma (approximately 80 %) originates from antithrombin III.

Another clinically important anticoagulant mechanism is the activated protein C system. Members of this system are the thrombin, the vitamin K dependent coagulation inhibitor proteins C and S, and thrombomodulin, a membrane protein that can be found everywhere on the surface of the intact vascular endothelium. As thrombin produced in the coagulation processes binds to thrombomodulin, its procoagulant effect disappears, and it becomes able to activate protein C. Protein S is a cofactor increasing the speed of the reaction. The produced activated protein C (APC) has an important role in the coagulation cascade as a cofactor inactivating activated V and VIII factors (Va, VIIIa), thus, it "decreases the speed" of coagulation and leads to decreased thrombin production. Therefore, thrombin, via the protein C system, has a paradox anticoagulant role preventing its own "overproduction".

Inherited Defects Causing Thrombophilia

Several procoagulant and inhibitor factors known to play a role in coagulation were found to increase the risk of thrombosis if produced in a

Table 34.3 Characteristics of coagulation inhibitors

	Molecular weight	Production site	Function	Plasma concentration in μg/mL	Chromosome
Antithrombin	60,000	Liver	Serpin	150	1
Protein C	62,000	Liver	Va, VIIIa inactivation	5	2
Protein S	80,000	Liver	Cofactor of PC	25	3
TFPI	33,000	Endothelium	VIIa-TF inactivatio n	115	2

Table 34.4 Indicence of inherited defects leading to throbophilia

	General population	Patients with thrombosis
APC-R (FV Leiden mutation)	5–10 %	30–65 %
Protein C deficiency	0.2 %	3–5 %
Protein S deficiency	0.1	2–5 %
Antithrombin III defect	0.02 %	1–4 %
Heparin cofactor II deficiency	?	1
F XII (Hageman) deficiency	?	5–10 %(?)
Plasminogen defect	<0.01 %	1–2 %
Dysfibrinogenemia	<0.01 %	0.1–1 %
Abnormal fibrinolysis	?	10–15 %
Thrombomodulin defect	<0.01 %	<0.1 %
Prothrombin allele 20 210A	1–2 %	6 %

smaller amount or in case of abnormal function. Clinical significance of each defect is different of course, as the incidence and thrombogenic effect of these abnormalities vary. The incidence of familiar thrombophilias in the "healthy" population and in patients with previous venous thromboembolism is summarized in Table 34.4.

Data refer to the "Caucasian" (European and North-American white) population, and for example data regarding APC resistance and prothrombin mutation are similar to data found in Hungary. Hereditary thrombophilic conditions with increased incidence or significant thrombogenicity are described below.

Antithrombinopathy

It is an autosomal dominant disease, antithrombin III (AT III) activity of the heterozygotes is usually 50–60 %. The protein was described by Morawitz in 1905, and its role in human pathology is known since 1965 when Egeberg described a case. AT III deficiency/dysfunction can occur not only as a consequence of mutation, it may be seen in several acquired conditions (such as cirrhosis, protein-losing enteropathy, nephrosis syndrome, DIC, sepsis, heparin-, estrogen-, L-asparaginase therapy), where thrombotic risk is increased just like in case of the congenital forms.

The AT III gene is localized in region 23–25 of the long arm of chromosome 1. The protein is a member of the serine protease inhibitors (SERPIN), it is able to irreversibly bind activated coagulation factors (IIa, IXa, Xa XIa, XIIa, VIIa-tissue factor complex); these reactions are enhanced by heparin as a cofactor. AT III is a single chain peptid with 425 amino acids and a biological half life of 48–60 h. This value may be significantly lower in case of consumption disorders, extensive thromboembolic processes or during intense heparin treatment.

AT III deficiency is characterized by relative heparin resistance and thromboembolic episodes in unusual localization from adolescence or early adulthood. Two thirds of the patients are between the ages of 15 and 30 when they have the first thromboembolic disease. It is important to note that it is not a uniform disease; the clinical spectrum varies from mild (heterozygous) heparin binding site defect, which does not lead to thrombosis alone, to the severe reactive binding site defect or quantitative defect accompanied by significant susceptibility to thrombosis.

Protein C Deficiency

Protein C is a vitamin K dependent glycoprotein, which is produced in the liver in the form of a single chain polypeptide and undergoes post-translational gamma carboxylation. In addition to the acquired deficiency (such as vitamin K deficiency, liver disease, DIC, sepsis, postoperative conditions, ARDS, extensive thromboembolic diseases), the inherited form has been known since 1981. Heterozygous protein C deficiency is accompanied with eight to ten-fold increased thrombosis risk independent from the type of the defect (type 1: quantitative, 2: functional).

At least 50 % of the patients with the deficiency have the first thromboembolic disease before the age of 40.

Protein S Deficiency

Protein S is a vitamin K dependent coagulation factor as well; it is the cofactor of the activation of protein C. In addition to liver cells, this protein is produced by the endothelium and the megakaryocytes. A unique feature of this protein is that 60 % of the circulating protein S forms a complex with the C4b-binding protein. It explains the close pathophysiological relationship between the protein C/protein S/ thrombomodulin system and the complement system, inflammatory processes. The incidence and thrombogenicity of hereditary protein S deficiency is similar to those of protein C deficiency. Like in case of protein C, acquired protein S deficiency may occur as well, and its activity is decreased during pregnancy and estrogen therapy (oral anticoagulant therapy and hormone supplementation) as well.

APC Resistance

The importance of APC resistance was recognized by Dahlback in 1993. Dahlback examined patients with idiopathic thrombosis and found that the known amount of activated protein C (APC) did not increase coagulation time in some patients as seen usually in an in vitro APTT-based system. It is an insufficiency of the anticoagulant response to APC, APC resistance. In 95 % of the cases, Leiden mutation of the gene of coagulation factor V is in the background (G 1691 A) as it was described by Bertina in 1994. Based on population genetic studies performed later, this mutation potentially occurred 25–30 thousand years before, and first it may have posed certain selection advantage in the heterozygous population. For example, in case of important factors of morbidity at that time, puerperal bleeding or injuries in the battlefield. Ethnicity of the mutation is interesting: FV Leiden mutation cannot be found in people originally living in Europe (for example Basques) and in Asian people (such as Japanese, Chinese), while a considerable ratio (5–10 %) of the current European and North-American population is heterozygous to this disease. APC resistance is not the most important disease regarding thrombogenicity, but it is the most common thromboembolic condition. Heterozygous individuals have venous thromboembolism before the age of 50. The calculated thrombosis risk is seven-fold in heterozygous individuals, and 50 to 100-fold in case of the homozygous forms. APC resistance combined with other acquired or hereditary risk factors is especially important as well. A good example is the oral contraceptives: the risk of venous thrombosis is 3–4 times increased in healthy women taking the tablet, and is about 7 times increased in people with heterozygous Leiden mutation as mentioned above. However, if a Leiden mutation positive individual is taking a contraceptive, the risk is 35 to 50-fold, it is a classic form of "super additive" potentiation of risk factors.

Prothrombin 20 210 GA

Poort et al. published factor II polymorphism with moderate susceptibility to thrombosis in November 1996. The single-point mutation was identified in the 3′ terminal region of the untranslated region of chromosome 11. It leads to higher translational rate or more stable mRNA formation, the amount of prothrombin produced increases leading to a procoagulant effect in hemostasis. 2 % of the healthy population, 6 % of patients having a thrombosis, and 18 % of patients examined for having idiopathic thrombosis were found to be heterozygous. Based on previous studies, it can be considered to be a moderate but very common, independent risk factor of thrombosis, the risk of venous thrombosis is about three-fold in heterozygous persons, it may be important especially in combination with other thrombophilias.

Significance of Combinations

Hungarian researchers were the first to find the importance of the combination of mild defects not causing thrombosis alone. Based on current modern approach, venous thrombosis at a young age is more or less considered to be a multiple genetic disease.

Practical Considerations

Summarizing the above data from the point of view of daily medical practice,it is an important question to determine when to perform hemostasis examinations on familial thrombophilia. Laboratory screening is obviously indicated in case of thromboembolism detected with objective methods and developing under the age of 40, and in case of recurrent thromboembolism or thromboembolism in an unusual location. Targeted screening of family members in case of a positive result is understandable, too. Unlimited screening of healthy individuals with another serious risk factor is confined mainly by economical, financial/beneficial considerations. The screening and verifying complementary tests that should be performed are listed in Table 34.5.

Another important practical consideration is that blood draw has to be performed after at least 3 months of the episode, when the inhibitors and acute phase reaction is over, and the patient should stop taking the oral anticoagulant before the test. In case of acenocoumarol, the patient should stop taking the drug 1 week before the test, this period should be 2 weeks in case of warfarin derivatives. During this period, increased dose of low molecular weight heparin prophylaxis may be administered once daily, and then the oral anticoagulant therapy may be continued with an overlapping period.

Table 34.5 Diagnostics of thrombophilia

Screening tests
Antithrombin III activity
Protein C activity
Free Protein S antigen or functional measurement of Protein C activity
APC resistance (with FV deficient plasma)
Plasma homocystein level
Prothrombin 20 210 A mutation PCR
Verifying – complementary tests
Antithrombin III crossed immun ELFO (CIE)
Antithrombin III crossed immune electrophoresis (CIE)
Protein C antigen
Whole Protein S antigen + free antigen or activity
F V Leiden mutation PCR
Antiphospholipid antibody tests:
Lupus anticoagulant, anticardiolipin antibody, Beta 2 glycoprotein I

Novel Ways in Anticoagulant Treatment

Currently available heparin and coumarin products used to prevent and treat venous thromboembolic diseases have been a great success in medicine. Heparins have been used for seven years and coumarins for five years in the treatment. It can be stated that the prevention and therapy of deep venous thrombosis and pulmonary embolism are performed with effective drugs. However, the currently used anticoagulants have limitations as well.

Vitamin K antagonist coumarin derivatives are indirect anticoagulants, they take effect by influencing the synthesis of vitamin K dependent coagulation factors (II, VII, IX, X). Therefore, there is a significant latency in the development and elimination of the anticoagulant effect: the therapeutic effect develops relatively slowly, and in case of overdose, if the patient has a serious bleeding complication, it is not enough to stop the administration of the drug. The development or expansion of the thrombus is inhibited by these drugs, they have no thrombolytic effect, and therefore, they are suitable for the prophylaxis of the spreading, extension of the thromboembolic process. In the arterial system, the effect of the administration of these products is questionable, rather adjuvant. There is great individual difference in the effective dose of coumarins, which is primarily the result of the different biodegradation of the active agent. The vitamin K content of the diet largely influences the dose of the drug necessary to maintain therapeutic level. A large number of clinically significant coumarin – drug interaction is known. Coumarin derivatives have a narrow therapeutic window: there is a small difference between the effective preventive dose and the dose leading to hemorrhagic side effect. Therefore, relatively frequent laboratory (prothrombin, INR) check-ups are necessary, which is unfavorable regarding compliance. Frequent dose adjustment is necessary, and the administration of coumarins requires a certain intelligence level of the patient.

Prothrombin time, APTT, and coagulation time increase in case of the administration of vitamin K antagonists. Decreased activity of coagulation factors II, VII, and X can be characterized by the prothrombin time, or by comparing prothrombin ratio (%) based on the normal plasma; however, the sensitivity of the applied reagents are different, and certain laboratories use different methods and different coagulometers. These variables can be eliminated by consequently using the International Normalized Ratio (INR). The INR value can be calculated from the ISI (International Sensitivity Index) value of the reagent. INR should be measured in every 4–6 weeks even in case of well tailored, stable coumarin treatment. A significant ratio of patients requires long-term or permanent oral anticoagulant prophylaxis (for example for having atrial fibrillation, mechanical valve, familial thrombophilia, recurrent thromboembolic diseases). In these cases, compliance may be significantly improved by self-checking at home. The CoaguCheck system is a widely used example applied in several countries. The portable device can be used at home or bedside, it gives an immediate result, and can be used to determine prothrombin level or APTT as well. Capillary (fingertip) or venous blood may also be used to measure the prothrombin level. In the therapeutic INR range, the specificity and sensitivity of this method is the same as those of standard coagulometers based on studies. Financial consideration limits the wide-spread use of this device.

Vitamin K antagonists may cross the placenta and have a teratogenic effect. Coumarin embriopathy may occur for example as nasal hypoplasia, bleeding in the central nervous system, or deformities of the extremities. Therefore, coumarins are contraindicated in case of pregnancy. Certain coumarin derivatives can be detected in the breast milk, but in therapeutic doses, these derivatives have no anticoagulant effect in the newborn. Osteoporotic side effects have to be considered in case of long-term use as well. Standard oral anticoagulant therapy may be impossible in case of rare coumarin resistance or coumarin necrosis. Alopecia, "purple toes" syndrome, liver function disorders, or gastrointestinal complaints are rare side effects of the drug. The most common and severe side effect is bleeding. The incidence of fatal hemorrhage is <0.5 %/year; major, life- or limb-threatening bleeding occurs in 2–5 %/year. In such cases, it is not enough to suspend the administration of the drug and the administration of vitamin K, but a blood product (FFP, Prothrombin Complex Concentrate, PCC or recombinant, activated factor VII – NovoSeven) transfusion is necessary as well. Vitamin K antagonists are usually not used in the perioperative period due to the risk of bleeding, and low molecular weight heparin bridging therapy is required.

Therefore, it is not a coincidence that intense research is focused on the development of new oral anticoagulants. Advanced clinical studies were performed with the direct, reversible thrombin inhibitor, melagatran (AstraZeneca). The theoretical advantage of this low molecular weight anticoagulant product is that it is able to inhibit the last step of the anticoagulant cascade and its "key participant", thrombin. This drug does not require a cofactor as opposed to heparins (such as antithrombin III, heparin cofactor II), and it is selective unlike coumarin derivatives. It reversibly inhibits thrombin compared with tested direct thrombin inhibitors (such as hirudin or hirulog); researchers expect this drug to have wider therapeutic window and fewer hemorrhagic side effects. Another advantage of this drug compared to standard anticoagulants is that it is able to inhibit thrombin that is already bound to the fibrin net and is important in local propagation to a significantly larger extent. Melagatran had comparable effect with low molecular weight heparin (1x5000 U dalteparin – Fragmin subcutaneously) in the prevention of venous thromboembolism in patients with hip and knee endoprosthetic surgeries in the Metro II study. The introduction of melagatran was not approved by the FDA due to side effects affecting liver function that were clinically significant in a large percentage of patients, but it is an example for the direction of the development of new oral anticoagulants. When this chapter was written, two new oral anticoagulant drugs had been registered: the direct thrombin inhibitor dabigatran and rivaroxaban having an anti-Xa effect. Currently, these drugs are used in the prophylaxis of thromboembolism in case of large, elective orthopedic surgeries in the everyday clinical practice, but there are advanced clinical studies with these compounds in the treatment of venous thromboembolism (deep venous thrombosis and pulmonary embolism) and in the prophylaxis of thromboembolism in atrial fibrillation.

Low Molecular Weight Heparin (LMWH) has taken the leading role in the prophylaxis and treatment of venous thromboembolic disease from standard Unfractionated Heparin (UFH) in the last decade. The reason for this is primarily the fact that if only the low molecular heparin chains important for the effect are administered, the side effect profile will be better. Biological availability improves, individual differences in plasma level decrease, dose effect connection can be better estimated, and half life increases making a single daily administration possible, fewer Heparin-Induced Thrombocytopenia (HIT) cases occur, and the risk of osteoporosis decreases in case of long-term prophylaxis, and usually there is no need to monitor coagulation. This is achieved with the same prophylactic and therapeutic efficacy, and the incidence of hemorrhagic side effects is at least the same or LMWH products are rather beneficial from this point of view as well based on the majority of large multicenter, comparative studies. It seems that decreasing the molecular weight has not stopped: the smallest but still effective pentasaccharide with anti-Xa activity has appeared in the clinical practice, it can be produced synthetically as well. The maximal plasma concentration of the selective and synthetic Xa inhibitor pentasaccharide (fonparinux) develops two hours after the subcutaneous injection. Idraparinux having a long half life and indraparinux combined with biotin are under clinical development; the effect of these forms can be suspended in case of an overdose. Developers expect selective Xa antagonists to lack some of the side effects of heparin derivatives (such as heparin induced thrombocytopenia, alopecia, or osteoporosis).

Further Readings

Baglin T. What happens after venous thromboembolism. J Thromb Haemost. 2009;7 Suppl 1:287–90.

Baglin T. Unraveling the thrombophilia paradox: from hypercoagulability to the prothrombotic state. J Thromb Haemost. 2010;8:228–33.

Bounameaux H, Reber G. New oral antithrombotics: a need for laboratory monitoring. Against. J Thromb Haemost. 2010;8:627–30.

Castoldi E, Rosing J. APC resistance: biological basis and acquired influences. J Thromb Haemost. 2010;8: 445–53.

Ehrenforth S, Nemes L, et al. Impact of environmental and hereditary risk factors on the clinical manifestation of thrombophilia in homozygous carriers of factor V:G1691A. J Thromb Haemost. 2004;2:430–6.

Eichinger S, Kyrle PA. Duration of anticoagulation after initial idiopathic venous thrombosis – the swinging pendulum: Risk assessment to predict recurrence. J Thromb Haemost. 2009;7 Suppl 1:291–5.

Kearon C. Balancing risks and benefits of extended anticoagulant therapy for idiopathic venous thrombosis. J Thromb Haemost. 2009;7 Suppl 1:296–300.

Mismetti P, Laporte S. New oral antithrombotics: a need for laboratory monitoring. For. J Thromb Haemost. 2010;8:621–6.

Pabinger I, Nemes L, et al. Pregnancy-associated risk for venous thromboembolism and pregnancy outcome in women homozygous for factor V Leiden. Hematol J. 2000;1:37–41.

Rangarajan S. Commentary. Inhibitors of coagulation. Haemophilia. 2010. doi:10.1111/j1365-2516.2010.02335.x.

35 Novel Consideration Regarding the Role of Evoked Potential in Confirming the Diagnosis of Eye Movement Disorders of Brainstem Origin

Szabolcs Tóth✠

Currently, it is generally accepted that Brainstem Acoustic Evoked Potential (BAEP) may be used to diagnose functional disorders of brainstem origin. However, it is clear that the acoustic evoked potential gives proper information of the function of only a part of the brainstem. Therefore, it seems necessary to involve the examination of the **functional disorder** of the sensory and motor segments of the brainstem and the **functional disorder of the border zone of the diencephalon** having direct connection to the brainstem to the examination. The acoustic evoked potential examination of the first, 10 msec long section and the second 10 msec (10–20 msec) long section can be well used to determine the functional disorder of the latter area, as seen in case of severe, traumatic conditions of the brainstem. Severe disorders may be present in the second 10 msec long segment even if the first 10 msec long segment is intact. Lesions of the sensory and motor pathways in the brainstem lead to increased conduction time, and impaired sensory and motor functions, often on the opposite side.

Studies show that evaluation of the functional disorder of the brainstem is easier and more unequivocal when examined with multimodal evoked potential compared with the examination of only the first 10 msec of the evoked potential of the brainstem. Changes in the multimodal evoked potentials are better and more reliable methods to determine the potential changes in brainstem conditions which are often severe.

✠ Author was deceased at the time of publication

S. Tóth, M.D.
University Professor, DMSC Neurosurgeon, Electrophysiologist, Budapest, Hungary

J. Somlai, T. Kovács (eds.), *Neuro-Ophthalmology*, DOI 10.1007/978-3-319-28956-4_35

Part IV

Diseases of Retina and the Optic Nerve (Visual and Sensory System)

Acquired Diseases of the Optic Nerve: Toxic and Deficiency Optic Neuropathy

Acquired Diseases of the Optic Nerve: Eye-related Symptoms and Signs of Intracranial Hypertension

Hereditary Diseases of the Retina 36

Ágnes Farkas

Contents

The clinical presentation and the genetic background of hereditary retinal disorders are heterogeneous (at present the pathogenic roles of more than 100 genes are known). Below we discuss the diseases in an order based on the anatomical localization of the pathology (the primarily affected retinal layers), without being exhaustive.

In addition to psychophysical examinations (such as examination of visual acuity, visual field, dark adaptation, color vision and contrast sensitivity) the application of objective electrophysiological methods is essential in the clinical diagnosis of the diseases, i.e., the characterization of the phenotype. In a proportion of the diseases molecular genetic examinations can be performed for the unequivocal confirmation of the genotype. Despite the ongoing promising research worldwide, there is no effective therapeutic possibility to treat hereditary retinal diseases (retinal dystrophies) at present.

Retinal diseases originating from the pigment epithelium
- 1.1 Gyrate atrophy of the choroid and retina
- 1.2 Stargardt disease
- 1.3 Leber congenital amaurosis
- 1.4 Best vitelliform macular dystrophy

Diseases of the outer retinal layers
- 2.1 Retinitis pigmentosa
- 2.2 Cone dystrophies

Diseases of the inner retinal layers
- 3.1 X-linked juvenile retinoschisis
- 3.2 Congenital stationary night blindness

Retinal Diseases Originating from the Pigment Epithelium

Gyrate Atrophy of the Choroid and Retina

Gyrate atrophy is a rare autosomal recessively inherited, progressive chorioretinal dystrophy.

Á. Farkas, M.D., PhD
Department of Ophthalmology, Semmelweis University, Budapest, Hungary
e-mail: faragnes@gmail.com

J. Somlai, T. Kovács (eds.), *Neuro-Ophthalmology*, DOI 10.1007/978-3-319-28956-4_36

The clinical presentation of the disease was described by Cutler and Fuchs in 1895–96 (Cutler 1895), whereas its pathomechanism (i.e. hyperornithinemia) was clarified by Simell and Takki (Simell et al. 1973; Takki 1974).

Clinical symptoms and signs: night blindness in young adulthood followed by severe deterioration of peripheral and central vision. Most of the affected individuals are short-sighted. Posterior cortical cataract is frequent. The appearance on fundoscopy is characteristic presenting in atrophic tortuous confluent patches of the pigment epithelium and the choriocapillary layer with apparent large choroidal vessels within them.

Preserved retinal structure can be observed only in form of small islands (Fig. 36.1). *ERG examination:* The response of both the cones and rods is diminished or extinguished.

This disease is one of the few retinal dystrophies in which the background of the metabolic disturbance is rather well known, and the ornithine level can be theoretically reduced by the restriction of arginine intake and the administration of pyridoxine (vitamin B6). Diet restriction (arginine-free diet) can temporarily improve the patient's condition (visual acuity) (Kaiser-Kupfer et al. 1985). The heterogeneity of the disease at the molecular level is reflected by the observation that only a small proportion of patients show a positive response to pyridoxine therapy (Kennaway et al. 1989); the responsivity to pyridoxine has to be clarified before beginning the therapy. The vision of 'responsive' patients slightly improved with a daily intake of 100–200 mg vitamin B6 (Weleber et al. 1981). Therapeutic benefit can only be expected in cases with early diagnosis.

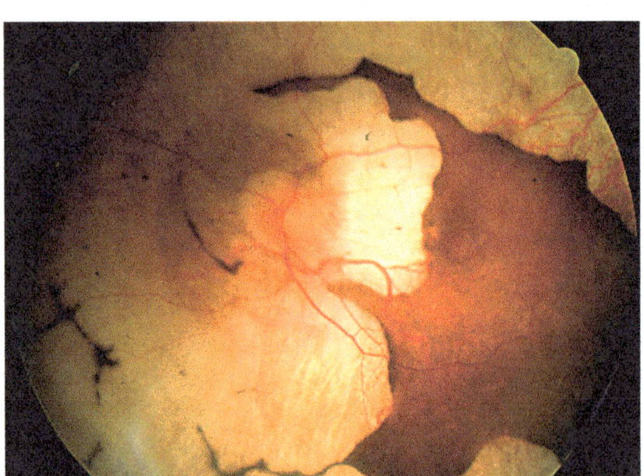

Fig. 36.1 The characteristic fundoscopic appearance of gyrate atrophy in the left eye. Biochemical background: The plasma and urine ornithine levels are 10–20 times elevated compared to normal levels, which is caused by the dysfunction of the ornithine aminotransferase (OAT, a pyridoxal phosphate-dependent enzyme, the gene of which is localized in chromosome 10) (Sengers et al. 1976)

Stargardt Macular Dystrophy

The most frequent and mostly autosomal recessively inherited juvenile macular 'degeneration' was described by Karl Stargardt in 1909 (Stargardt 1909). A variant of the disease called fundus flavimaculatus was described in 1965 by Franceschetti and Francois (Franceschetti et al. 1965), in which diffuse yellow patches of variable shape and preserved posterior pole are apparent on the fundi of affected individuals, and the visual acuity does not deteriorate remarkably with aging. The typical age of onset in Stargardt disease (STGD) is within the first two decades of life. The most characteristic sign is the non-correctable, reduced vision, which deteriorates to 0.1–0.05 by reaching adulthood (Fishman et al. 1987). In the early stages, the characteristic fundoscopic findings include subtle pigment irregularity and yellowish deposits in the posterior pole, which become more pronounced over time, showing bronze-like flare, and subsequently an atrophic scar develops. In 1980, Eagle et al. described deposits of lipofuscin-like substance in retinal pigment epithelial cells and cellular hypertrophy (Eagle et al. 1980). This abnormality may be responsible (at least in part) for the phenomenon of 'dark choroid', which is of a differential diagnostic value during fluorescein angiography in STGD.

Further Diagnostic Approaches

Ganzfeld ERG: useful in the differentiation of the disease from diffuse retinal dystrophies, showing pathological changes already in the early stages (e.g., rod–cone dystrophies) (Berson 1993). At the early stage of STGD both rod and cone functions are intact or close to normal (Lachapelle et al. 1990), and remain preserved even at an advanced stage. On the examination of rod functions the prolonged time of dark adaptation (at least 45 min) has to be taken into account.

Multifocal ERG: sensitively detects degree and localization of macular damage, by recording waves with pathological shape and amplitude, and represent a useful objective method for patient follow-up. (Considering the patient's difficulties in fixating, which is inherent in this disease, a special attention is to be paid to monitor the direction of the patient's gaze (if possible, the fixation should be monitored by a video camera). More recent (1997) research at the molecular level has suggested that autosomal recessive forms of fundus flavimaculatus and STGD as well as certain forms of cone-rod dystrophies (CRD) and retinitis pigmentosa (RP) are caused by mutations in the ABCA4 (previously ABCR) gene.

Examination of patients with Stargardt disease and cone–rod dystrophy and experiments with animal models may shed light on the mechanisms of age-related macular degeneration (AMD). Analysis of data obtained from 1700 patients with AMD suggested that certain alleles of ABCA4 increase the risk of AMD (Allikmets 2000). Mata et al. (2001) have revealed a pathological transport (and light-inducible accumulation) of toxic (all-trans) retinaldehydes in the outer segment of rods and in the pigment epithelium in ABCA4 mutation (Mata et al. 2001). It is presumed that this may be responsible for the characteristic prolonged dark adaptation in the affected patients. The eyes are to be protected from intense light. The inhibition of A2E accumulation in the pigment epithelium may represent a therapeutic possibility. (A beneficial effect of isotretinoin has been reported in mice.) Gene therapy may also become a therapeutic option in the foreseeable future.

Leber Congenital Amaurosis

It was Leber who first described the disease in 1869, as a congenital form of retinitis pigmentosa. Leber highlighted the extremely severe visual impairment present as early as (or soon after) birth, as well as nystagmus, amaurotic pupil, pigmentary retinopathy and an autosomal recessive inheritance as characteristic signs of the disease. (Later dominant inheritance has also been reported; however, it is rather infrequent.) In 1956 Franceschetti regarded the extinguished electroretinogram as a fundamental diagnostic sign at the early stage of the disease.

Incidence: Leber congenital amaurosis (LCA) is a group of diseases, leading to blindness, the incidence of which is 3:100 000 worldwide. (Though it is very rare, 6–20 % of children attending the schools for the blind have LCA.)

Genetic background: heterogeneous. 7 LCA genes have been revealed since 1996 (Marlhens et al. 1997), 5 of which is expressed in photoreceptors, whereas one is expressed mainly in the pigment epithelium (RPE65). Mutations in the known genes are responsible for disease development in 40 % of the affected individuals. (The number of potential disease causing genes in this group is suggested to be around 20.) The variability of clinical appearance in LCA is almost endless. All degrees of impaired visual acuity may occur between 0.1 and complete loss of light sensation. The refractive errors include severe myopia and hypermetropia, and fundoscopic findings vary between normal and severely pigmented retinopathy. Keratoconus and cataract may also develop, and associations with systemic diseases are common.

Diagnosis: The task of an ophthalmologist diagnosing a blind infant is complex. The following considerations may be of help:

- Ophthalmological and systemic diseases masking the primary disease have to be excluded (Koenekoop 2004)
- Traditional (Ganzfeld) ERG examination is needed before the age of 1 year (Foxman et al. 1985). Evaluation of the results of ERG examinations on infants requires cautiousness; the first examination should be performed around the age of 6 months and should be repeated at the age of 1 year (Fulton et al. 1996)

- The mode of inheritance is to be clarified if possible
- Molecular genetic diagnosis is needed (Zernant et al. 2005), which is now readily available, and its result is of help for the GP and ophthalmologist (for definitive diagnosis, prognosis, therapeutic possibilities), the parents and family (carrier state recognition during pregnancy)
- It is important to predict the expectable visual abilities of the child to help planning the future

The Genotype–Phenotype Associations Are the Most Comprehensively Studied in Case of the RPE65 Gene Defect

According to an LCA microarray study published in 2006 by Zernant et al., RPE65 gene mutations (which basically inhibit the vitamin A cycle) are responsible for 2.4% of LCA cases. The retinal pigment epithelium represents the primary location of gene expression (Hamel et al. 1993); however, more recently its expression has been revealed in mammalian cones (Znoiko et al. 2002) as well (but not in rods).

The retinal dystrophy present is of rod–cone-type. The affected infant is usually taken to an ophthalmologist at the age of 3–4 months with the suspicion of blindness. Nystagmus is the characteristic feature, and fundoscopy reveals mild granular appearance of the pigment epithelium and narrow arterioles. The rather poor vision might improve to reach a score of 0.1 at the age of 5 years; however, bull's eye maculopathy gradually develops and the previously detectable cone responses disappear from the retinogram. A slow, progressive deterioration of vision will subsequently occur during the patient's life.

Gene therapy: The RPE65 knockout mouse and the Swedish Briard dog (as a natural 'knockout' model) have proved to be appropriate for phenotype examinations and therapeutic interventions. The news of the successful gene supplementation therapy in Briard dogs spread worldwide (the normal RPE65 gene was transfected into the eye by a virus vector in form of subretinal injection). The treatment resulted in a remarkable improvement in the vision of the treated eyes, and the previously extinguished ERG responses were replaced by an activity corresponding to 16% percent of normal values (Acland et al. 2001). It was reported in an international scientific forum (ARVO 2007) that in February 2007, in Moorfield's Eye Hospital, London, a 17 and a 23-year-old patient with LCA due to RPE65 gene mutation received gene supplement therapy following the above detailed method.

Best Vitelliform Macular Dystrophy

This is a disease with autosomal dominant inheritance, and its familial occurrence has been described by Friedrich Best in 1905. It was Zanen and Rausin, two Belgian ophthalmologists who first used the expression 'vitelliform' (vitellus = egg-yolk) to describe the characteristic appearance on fundoscopy.

Clinical course: the bilateral, sharp-edged alteration that unequivocally resembles an egg-yolk and has a diameter 1–3 times that of the optic disc is usually recognized between the 3rd and 15th year of life (however, it has already been reported in infants with few weeks of age).

Visual acuity of the affected individuals is surprisingly good at that time, often 0.8 or even better. The fundoscopic appearance of the regular yellow macular spot is changing over time (Fig. 36.2); the accumulated substance becomes fragmented and resembles a hypopyon as it sinks towards the bottom of the cystic lesion ('psudohypopyon' stage). Subsequently, the wall of the cyst disrupts (vitelliruptive stage) and a fibrotic scar develops, in some cases with choroidal neo-

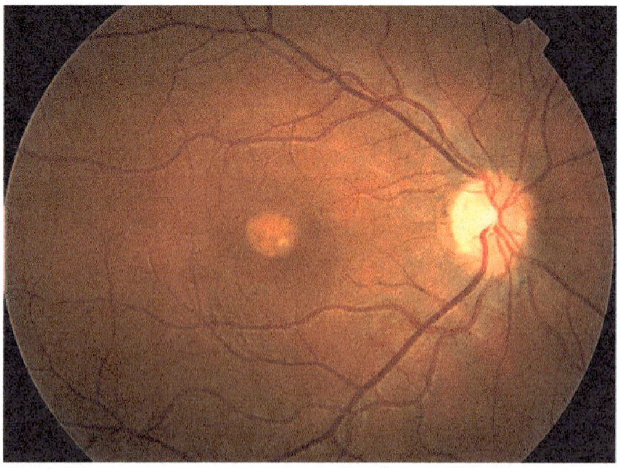

Fig. 36.2 Best vitelliform dystrophy in the right eye: fragmentation is already apparent within the cystic lesion

vascularization and/or subretinal hemorrhage. The patients have no or minimal complaints about their vision until 40–50 years of age (Fishman et al. 1993). Even in more advanced stages, vision is generally not worse than 0.5. (The peripheral edges of the visual field are normal.) The relatively well-preserved visual acuity is explained by the fact that the process primarily affects the pigment epithelium (with intracellular accumulation of lipofuscin-like substance), and the more internal layers of the retina are not affected (Francois et al. 1967).

Electrophysiological examinations: Electrooculography (EOG) is of diagnostic value, which definitely confirms the diffuse damage to the retinal pigment epithelium. The Ganzfeld-ERG shows normal cone and rod functions.

Differential diagnosis: Based on the fundoscopic appearance at the fibrotic stage, the disease needs to be differentiated primarily from Stargard disease and cone dystrophies. Apart from the EOG findings (which are unequivocally pathological in cases with Best disease only) the finding of the 'silent choroid' sign supports the diagnosis of STGD. In cone dystrophies the characteristic features include pathological photopic ERG response, photoaversion and color vision deficiency. At the later stages of chorioretinitis of different origin and of central serous choroidopathy, EOG is the primary differential diagnostic method of choice. Adult-onset foveomacular vitelliform dystrophies also exist, with normal EOG-results in most of the cases. In such cases, optical coherence tomography helps the differential diagnosis.

Genetic aspects: in patients with Best dystrophy mutations have been found in a new retina-specific gene (Lotery et al. 2000). This gene encodes a protein (bestrophin) consisting of 585 amino acids, which is selectively expressed in the retinal pigment epithelium.

Diseases of the Outer Retinal Layer

Retinitis Pigmentosa

The pigmented alteration of the retina observable on fundoscopy was first described by van Trigt in 1853. The name retinitis pigmentosa originates from Donders. The traditional name is still used worldwide due to its simplicity; however, it does not reflect the pathomechanism of the disease. Symptoms are caused by the progressive death of the photoreceptors. The objective assessment of retinal functions is possible by electroretinography, which may prove the degeneration of photoreceptors years before the onset of the first symptoms. (The fact that molecular genetic examinations are becoming more and more routinely available may enable us in the future to register patients based upon their genetic mutation.)

The incidence of retinitis pigmentosa (RP) is suggested to be around 1:4000 worldwide. The inheritance can be autosomal dominant (AD) 20%, autosomal recessive (AR) 20% and X-linked recessive (XR) 10%. The reminder are isolated ('simplex' RP), no known family history. In sporadic or 'simplex' cases the mode of inheritance cannot be established; however, these cases are most probably recessive as well. In general, the AD form is associated with the latest onset of symptoms, and is relatively less progressive. Clinically the most malignant of the disease is the XR form, which presents with early onset of symptoms and rapid progression. According to the data from a number of large rehabilitation centers (Japan, Kuwait, Denmark), RP represents the cause of blindness in 25–29% (Hartong et al. 2006). In most cases, retinitis pigmentosa selectively affects the visual organ; however, in 20–30% of the cases, it associates with the involvement of other organs. (The latter ones have AR inheritance.)

Syndromes Associated with Retinitis Pigmentosa

Usher syndrome: RP+sensoryneural hearing impairment (10–15% of RP patients) is the most frequent among these syndromes, and it represents the most severe condition as it affects the two most important sensory organs. At present 11 Usher gene is known.

Bardet-Biedl syndrome: RP is associated with obesity, mental retardation, polydactylia, hypogonadism and renal failure. From the rest of the infrequent syndromes associated with ritinitis pigmentosa, we discuss three syndromes due to their clinical importance: Bassen-Kornzweig syndrome (abetalipoproteinemia), Refsum syndrome (phytanic acid oxidase deficiency) and the familial isolated vitamin E deficiency (tocopherol transfer protein deficiency). In case, these conditions are recognized at a young age, supplementation of the deficient substances can save the patient from losing the vision.

Symptoms

Rod-Cone Dystrophy

This is the significantly more frequent form. The primary entity is the development of rod dysfunction, which is later accompanied by the dysfunction of cones as well. The onset and progression of symptoms is rather variable. In certain patients develop marked visual loss as early as childhood, whereas others remain more or less asymptomatic until reaching adulthood. (Impaired function of rods may remain unrevealed for a long period of time as lights, e.g. in offices or shopping centers, as well as the intensive street-lighting provide the opportunity for the cones to function even after getting dark). In most patients the appearance of symptoms and signs has a pattern:

- impaired dark adaptation, night blindness in childhood or adolescence,
- concentric visual field constriction (loss of the mid-periphery) in young adulthood,
- loss of the peripheral part of the visual field occurs as well, 'tunnel vision' develops, and subsequently the central part will also be lost at around 60 years of age. Different degrees of pigmentation in the mid-periphery, pale disc, narrow arterioles and relatively well-preserved posterior pole are seen on the fundi (Fig. 36.3).

Cone-Rod Dystrophy

Significantly more infrequently the development of cone dysfunction precedes that of the rods, in such cases impaired central and colour vision, and light sensitivity are the characteristic symptoms (Birch et al. 1999). Decrease of the 180° horizontal visual field to 50° does not interfere with binocular vision and with routine daytime activity. Patients can lose more than 90% of foveal cones without impairment of the visual acuity. Difficulties with reading and daily activity generally appear at a visual acuity of 0.5 (Geller et al. 1993). Fundoscopic findings can change from fine macular pigmentation to a roughly pigmented, and later atrophic form. Lack of the pigmentation and/or pigment deposits can be observed in the periphery. Pale optic disc and narrow blood vessels are also characteristic (Fig. 36.4). In advanced cases, rod function is also impaired that makes the differentiation from the RP difficult. In uncertain cases, disturbance of the central vision, the coarse macular pigmentation, the photoaversion, lack of nyctalopia and the predominance of cone dysfunction on ERG support the diagnosis of cone–rod dystrophy. The majority of the patients – suffering from either

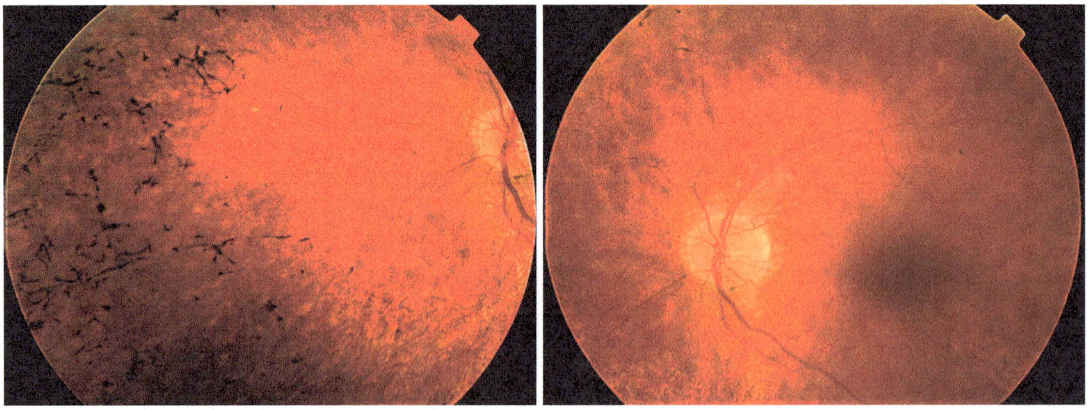

Fig. 36.3 Fundi of retinitis pigmentosa: typical pigmentation in the mid-periphery, the posterior pole is preserved

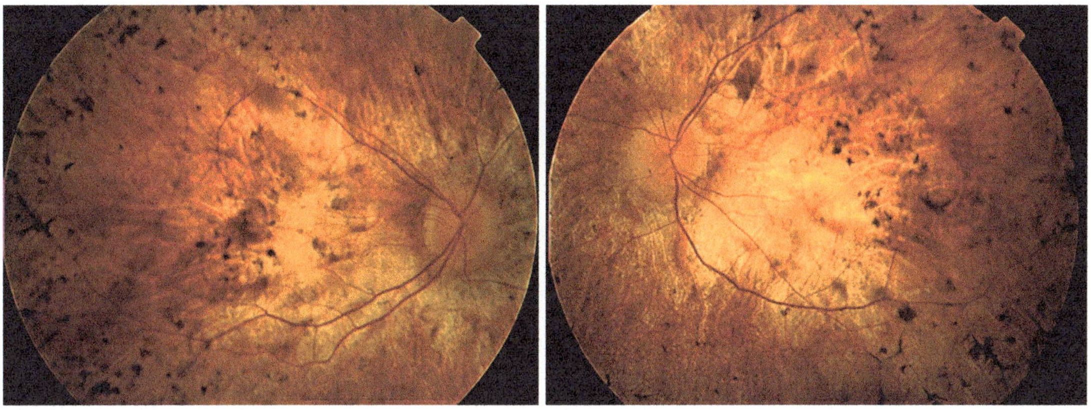

Fig. 36.4 An advanced state of cone–rod dystrophy: coarse pigmentation throughout the fundus, pale discs and scars in the posterior poles

form of the disease – can be regarded as legally blind at the age of 40. Histological examination reveals that the outer nuclear layer – containing the nuclei of cones and rods – is significantly thinner in RP. The internal nuclear layer (with horizontal, amacrine and bipolar cells) and the ganglion cell layer preserve their structure significantly longer, however, these layers will also be impaired in later stages of the disease.

Examination of Visual Functions

Visual acuity: central vision may remain intact even in advanced RP in the small preserved island of the central visual field. Patients with poor vision are grateful for the tiniest improvement that can be achieved by optical correction. Nevertheless, the refractive error often may characterise the mode of inheritance. In X-linked RP, for instance, a myopia of 2.0 D (or higher degree), whereas in dominant forms, hypermetropia is characteristic.

Visual field: the first scotomata typically present in the mid-periphery. In advanced cases, only small islands of visual field remain in the extreme periphery and in the center. Later on these islands disappear as well.

Colour vision: in addition to the Ishihara plates, the use of the Farnsworth D 15 panel is recommended even in the presence of relatively good visual functions. Colour vision in RP is generally preserved, or a decrease can be observed in the function of blue cones (acquired tritanopia). The occurence of X-linked inherited red-green colour blindness is about 5–8 % of males in this group of disease as well; however, it may indicate cone-rod or cone degeneration.

Dark adaptation: it is recommended to measure the rod adaptation threshold (the smallest detectable white light intensity after 30 min spent in the dark). If this intensity is at least hundred times higher than that in healthy population (i.e., the measured threshold value increased at least with 2 log units), a severe rod dysfunction is present, and it is not recommended to drive in dim light, irrespective of the patient's visual acuity and fields. A significant increase of the threshold indicates a decrease in the sensitivity of cones as well.

Contrast sensitivity: decrease in contrast sensitivity frequently occurs in RP, which explains the subjectively experienced poor vision in patients with good visual acuity under strong contrast conditions.

Ophthalmological-Morphological Examinations

Biomicroscopy, fundoscopy: in an approximately 50 % of RP patients, some degree of posterior cortical cataract can be observed. The presence of cellular components and posterior detachment are common phenomena in the vitreous body in this disease. Obligate signs include the narrowed retinal blood vessels and the waxy pallor of the optic disc. In typical cases, diffuse bone spicule-like (or other forms of) intraretinal pigmentation is apparent in the mid- and/or the extreme periphery. The pigment deposits originate from elements of the pigment epithelium migrating to the neuroretina due to the death of photoreceptor cells.

Optical coherence tomography: is a state-of-the-art non-invasive examination method, providing information among *in vivo* conditions about retinal (primarily macular) structure in a resolution comparable to that provided by histological examination. It is especially useful in RP to measure the thickness (and volume) of the macula, to assess the pigment epithelium and photoreceptor layer, as well as to diagnose macular edema. Fundus autofluorescence imaging revealed elevated concentration of lipofuscin in the retinal pigment epithelium in a proportion of RP patients. (The affected areas corresponded with those exhibiting decreased amplitudes on multifocal ERG examination.) (Robson et al. 2006).

Electroretinography (ERG): this is the only method that enables the objective characterization of the functional condition of the external and middle retinal layers. The Ganzfeld method enables to record the summed response of cones and rods as isolated signals (under scotopic or photopic adaptation). In this examination, the amplitude and the 'implicit time' (i.e., peak latency) of the recorded potentials are measured. This method is unequivocally appropriate to diagnose the disease (based on the decreased amplitude and prolonged implicit time) (Berson et al. 1969); however, it does not enable to detect the remaining function in cases with a few number of functioning cells (for instance, electrical response cannot be recorded from an eye with a very small central visual field even with full central acuity). In the past decade, the so called multifocal ERG has become widely applied in the clinical practice. This method is able to examine the function of the central retinal area of 60° diameter presenting the function of the cones as a map. This method enables the objective detection of a small (central) field in advanced retinitis pigmentosa (under photopic conditions).

Time course: The onset of the disease usually cannot be determined exactly. ERG studies suggest that the degeneration of photoreceptors can be detected as early as 6 years of age in patients who are otherwise asymptomatic until adulthood. No individuals with normal ERG findings at year 6 were subsequently diagnosed with typical retinitis pigmentosa in later ages (Berson et al. 1985). Retinitis pigmentosa is a progressive disease; the parameters related to the visual fields and the ERG tests exponentially deteriorate over time (Sahel 2005). The functional loss can be associated with a number of factors (degree of retinal functional loss, environmental and nutritional factors, type of gene defects, etc.). Clinical studies consider the visual field and the ERG tests to be the most appropriate methods for follow-up the disease progression. In contrast, the subjective experience of the patients – regarding visual impairment – is characterized more by the central acuity.

A complaint of a sudden deterioration of vision during the common course of the disease is to be taken seriously – as an association of retinitis pigmentosa with Coats' disease may underlie the abrupt deterioration especially in case of young adults (Figs. 36.5 and 36.6); furthermore, vascular catastrophes may also occur. Early detection and intervention may prevent the patient from a complete loss of visual abilities.

Genetic background: The genetic background of the disease is extremely heterogeneous. The majority of the cases is monogenic. At present 45 genes have been identified in RP, the mutations of which lead to the development of symptoms by interfering with different retinal mechanisms and structures, such as the phototransduction cascade, phagocytosis, vitamin A metabolism and metabolism of the connecting cilia. These genes are responsible for disease development in an approximately 60 % of known cases, the remaining 40 % is due to mutations in currently unknown genes. The majority of RP-related genes are infrequently affected. Exceptions include the rhodopsin gene (RHO), which is affected in 25 % of the dominant forms; the USH2A gene,

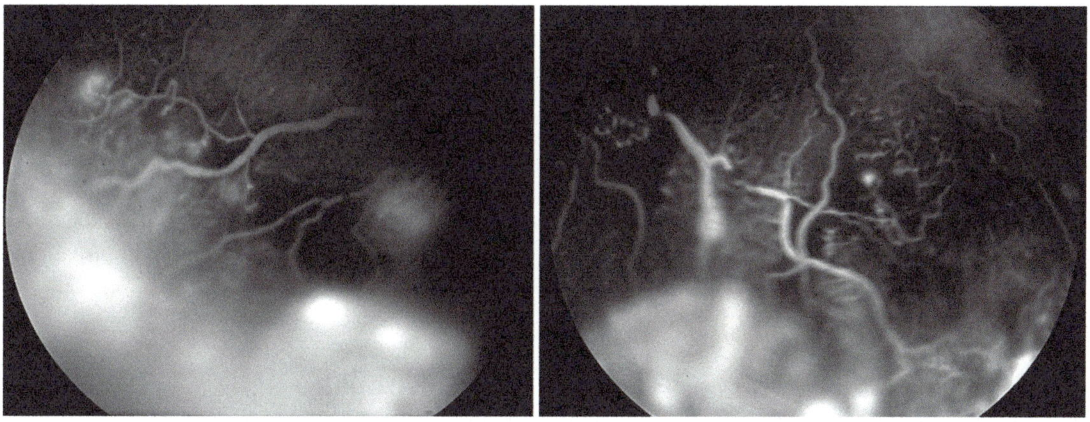

Fig. 36.5 A form of retinitis pigmentosa associated with Coats' disease Colored image: bulk *yellow* exudate in the posterior pole. *Red-free* image: bone spicule-like pigment deposits in the upper half of the retina (right eye)

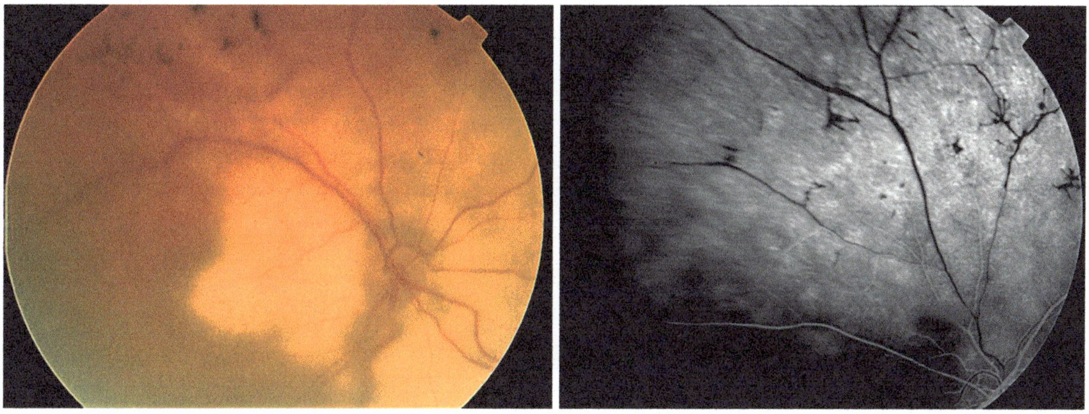

Fig. 36.6 FLAG photographs present serous retinal detachment and pathological neovascularization in the lower halves of the retina in both eyes of the patient presented in Fig. 36.5

which is affected in 20 % of the recessive forms; as well as the RPGR gene, which is affected in the 70 % of X-linked cases. Mutations of these three genes are responsible for a total of 30 % of RP cases (Hartong et al. 2006). How mutations in a gene exclusively expressed in rods can lead to an irreversible loss of function of both types of photoreceptors, is unknown at present. Understanding the interactions between rods and cones and revealing the factors that originate from rods and support the survival of cones may help in the revelation of therapeutic opportunities (Berson et al. 1993).

Infrequent Conditions with Atypical Presentation

RP sine pigmento: a form without pigmentation, which is not equivalent with the poorly pigmented cases occurring at early stages of the typical form.

Sector RP: the atypical fundoscopic alterations and the corresponding loss of function affect only a part of the retina (often the lower half of the retina) in both eyes, symmetrically (the image presented in Fig. 36.7 was taken of the right eye of the patient). *Unilateral RP:* in rather rare cases, the clinical picture can only confirm the involvement of only one of the two eyes (injury, inflammation or other causes can be

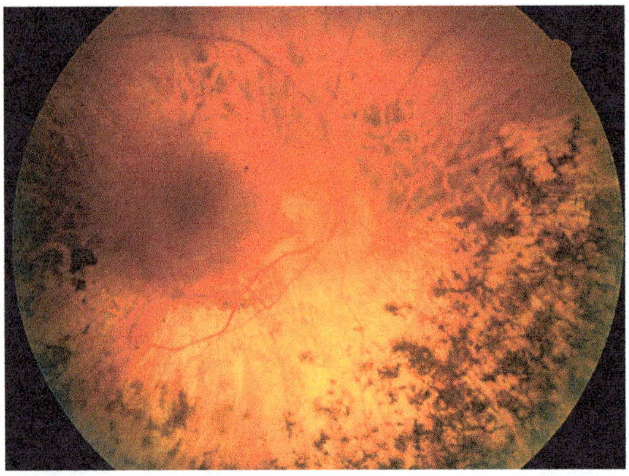

Fig. 36.7 Sector retinitis pigmentosa in the lower half of the retina in the right eye (A similar abnormality can be observed symmetrically in the left eye)

excluded in the eye that appears to be affected). The true existence of this form can only be clarified by genetic studies.

Therapeutic possibilities: According to the findings of large studies on dietary supplements (Berson), regular consumption of vitamin A palmitate (15.000 IU daily) with regular medical follow-up can decrease the progression of the damage to the visual field. (Vitamin A cannot be replaced by beta-carotene.) The same studies did not find any additional beneficial effect of vitamin E if administered in addition to vitamin A (Berson et al. 1993). The regular consumption of docosahexaenoic acid, DHA (omega-3 fatty acid, which can be found in sea fishes such as tuna, mackerel and salmon) has also been found beneficial (Hoffman et al. 2004). This molecule is present in high concentrations in photoreceptors, and is probably necessary for their normal function. In the above mentioned 3 rare syndromes (Bassen–Kornzweig, Refsum's syndromes and familial vitamin E deficiency) the deficient substances need to be supplemented regularly. Data indicate that it is especially important to protect the eyes from light (primarily from UV radiation); however, neither retrospective nor prospective studies on larger cohorts of patients have been conducted to confirm this. It is necessary to perform timely cataract surgery in RP patients as well. Carbonic anhydrase inhibitors can be useful in the treatment of macular edema. Optical tools (manual magnifiers, computer-associated magnifier tools) can help preserving the ability to read and to maintain personal connections even at an advanced stage of the disease. (See Part VI for details.) In the future, application of gene supplementation therapy, transplantation of pigment epithelium, photoreceptor cells and stem cells, as well as the epiretinal/subretinal implantation of electronic devices (chips) based on appropriate indications will hopefully able significantly improve the patients' quality of life.

Cone Dystrophies

A heterogeneous group of diseases, in which several specific gene mutations have been identified. The clinical appearance is variable in terms of the onset of symptoms, the fundoscopic appearance, and even in terms of the findings of electrophysiological examinations with diagnostic value. Typical symptoms and signs: decreased and non-correctable visual acuity, light-sensitivity, various degrees of disturbances in color vision, as well as nystagmus (in cases with early manifestation). These symptoms are usually not spontaneously mentioned by the patients. The predominant finding on ERG is cone dysfunction. *Stationary conditions:*

Congenital achromatopsia (rod-monochromacy) or congenital complete color blindness: a rare disease with autosomal recessive inheritance, characterized by the loss of cone function, with preserved function of the rods. This results in the development of the predominant symptoms, which include decreased visual acuity (generally not better than 0.1), light sensitivity and nystagmus, and the complete lack of color, discrimination.

Fundoscopic appearance is not characteristic, it can be completely intact; however, variable degrees of maculopathy can be observed, especially in older ages (Fig. 36.8). Epidemiological studies estimate the incidence of the disease to be approximately 1:30,000–50,000. In 2005, a study reporting on 9 Hungarian families (12 patients with achromatopsia and 24 asymptomatic relatives) has been published. The patients included 7 children and 5 adults (Varsányi et al. 2005). There is only a rather limited number of studies

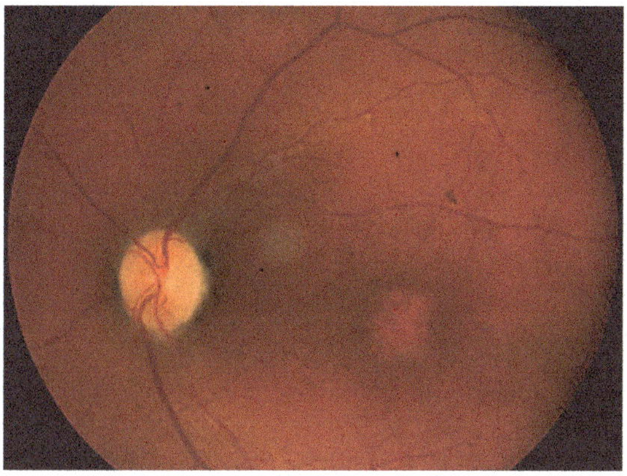

Fig. 36.8 Congenital achromatopsia: maculopathy (hypopigmentation in hyper-pigmented surroundings) in the left eye of a 40-year-old patient (VA ou: 0.1)

about the retinal condition available. The genetic background of congenital complete color blindness is known since the end of the 1990s. Mutations of genes encoding cone-specific proteins that play roles in phototransduction processes, lead to a deficient amount and decreased function of the affected proteins. To date, the role of a cGMP-regulated cation channel present in the cones (the CNGB3 gene encoding one of the subunits of this channel, and the cone-specific GNAT2 gene encoding the transducin protein) has been confirmed in patients with achromatopsia. Mutations of these genes can be detected in 75–80 % of patients with achromatopsia as the etiological factor. Molecular genetic examination confirmed the clinical diagnosis in each of the Hungarian patients: in 6 patients from 4 families the pathogenic mutation was found in the CNGA3 gene, whereas in 6 patients from 5 families the pathogenic mutation was found in the CNGB3 gene (Varsányi et al. 2005).

Blue cone monochromacy: It is a less severe condition compared to achromatopsia, as the blue cones preserve their ability to function. Autosomal dominant (AD), autosomal recessive (AR) and X-linked recessive (XR) forms are known. The age of onset is variable, the symptoms generally appear between the age of 10 year and young adulthood. (Visual acuity of patients with the XR form, generally varies between 0.1 and 0.7).

Fundoscopy: all degrees between minimal macular pigment deposition and atrophic scar may occur, including the 'bull's eye' maculopathy. Phosphorescent sheen has been described in both the XR and AD forms (Mizuo-Nakamura's phenomenon). Temporal optic disc pallor and peripheral pigment deposition are also characteristic. Though the fundoscopic appearance suggests the predominant involvement of the macula, a diffuse degeneration of photoreceptors is present. The decrease in photopic ERG response confirms the dysfunction of the cones, which can be observed even more convincingly by the use of 30 Hz flicker stimulation. ERG response of the rods is normal or slightly subnormal. The function of both types of photoreceptors will further deteriorate (Kellner et al. 1993). In 1983, Gouras et al. described a novel type of cone-dystrophy with nyctalopia and supernormal rod response. The pathogenic mutations have recently been found in the KCNV2 gene (Wu et al. 2006).

Diseases of the Inner Retinal Layers

X-Linked Iuvenile Retinoschisis

X-linked juvenile retinoschisis (XLRS) is one of the most frequent, recessively inherited, progressive ***vitreoretinal dystrophies.*** The disease affects only male children, and is at present non-treatable. The worldwide incidence is suggested to be approximately 1:5000–25,000. The penetrance is 100 % among the affected boys; however, the symptomatic onset, the phenotype and the course are highly variable, which makes the diagnosis rather difficult. At the beginning, the characteristic clinical picture includes the cystous foveal retinoschisis accompanied by different degrees of spoke-wheel pigmentation (Fig. 36.9). The schisis is due to radially oriented microcysts within the inner layers of the retina (nerve fiber and ganglion cell layer). Macular involvement is almost 100 % (with variable onset), and retinoschisis in the lower temporal retinal quadrant leading to peripheral visual field defect can be observed in almost 50 % of the cases, which is progressive in childhood. The non-correctable visual impairment of the little boys is usually detected between 5 and 10 years of age. Their vision progressively dete-

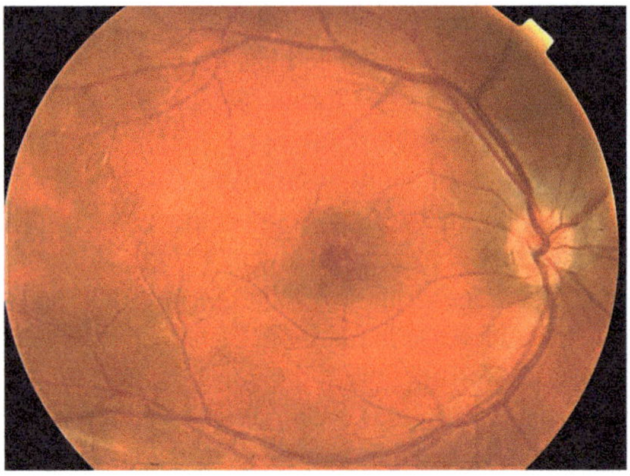

Fig. 36.9 Characteristic picture of moderately pigmented cystic foveal retinoschisis in a spoke-wheel pattern in the right eye of 6-year-old boy

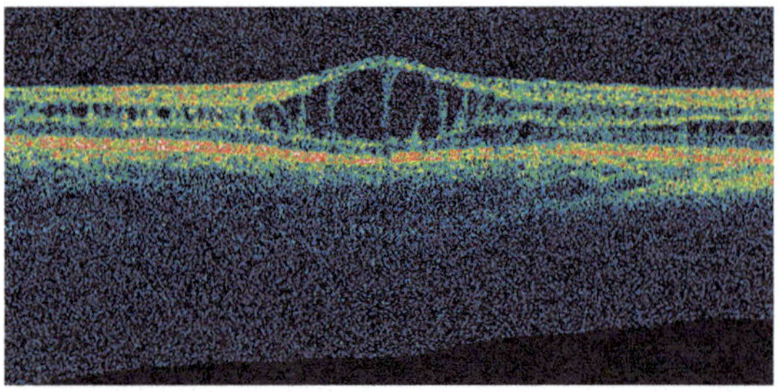

Fig. 36.10 In the macular OCT image of the patient presented in Fig. 36.9, the majority of the cysts are localized between the outer and the inner plexiform layers; however, in the right side of the picture a few cysts are visible in the photoreceptor layer as well

riorates (with variable rate), the central cysts become confluent, the spoke-wheel formation disappears and an atrophic scar develops. Findings of the ERG test are of differential diagnostic value; the *b*-wave evoked by intense light stimulus is significantly subnormal, whereas the *a*-wave amplitude is normal or only slightly reduced (negative-type ERG) (Janáky et al. 1991; Lesch et al. 2006). The multifocal ERG reveals a predominantly central dysfunction with subnormal amplitudes and prolonged implicit times. Most of the heterozygous carrier women are without symptoms and signs (including the retinogram). The pathogenic retina-specific XLRS1 gene encoding the retinoschisis (RS1) protein was identified by Sauer et al. in 1997 (Sauer et al. 1997). The phenotype is caused by the lack of the retinoschisis as well as its pathological intra- or extracellular accumulation. At early stages of XLRS, fundoscopic appearance of the macula is not distinctive. If ERG was not performed, the early diagnosis in most of such children used to be Stargardt's disease. The golden retinal sheen reflex that disappears after vitrectomy (Mizou phenomenon) and is characteristic of Oguchi's disease has also been described in such patients, which is suggested to be due to extracellular accumulation of potassium as a consequence of the defect of Müller cells.

The non-invasive OCT examination brought an important change for both the patients and the ophthalmologists, as it enables the establishment of the correct diagnosis in a matter of minutes, and can be used for the continuous follow-up of the patients. Though an effective treatment is at present unavailable, the exact diagnosis in the affected families is essential for family planning in the future. The spreading of the routine use of OCT turned the attention to this disease again in Hungary as well, and in 2006, a report about a phenotype-genotype study of 27 XLRS patients from 5 independent Hungarian families was published (Lesch et al. 2006). The study – according to recent data from the literature – provided evidence for the appearance of schisis in multiple retinal layers (inner nuclear layer, photoreceptor layer and ganglion cell layer) (Fig. 36.10). Furthermore, it confirmed the need of OCT in every case of visual impairment in childhood with unclarified origin and a probable background of maculopthy. (Reports can be found in the literature about a few female children with a phenotype corresponding to XLRS.)

Congenital Stationary Dark Adaptation Disorders

A very rare group of diseases, which deserves attention because of its leading symptom, the night blindness is suspicious of retinitis pigmentosa at first sight. The correct diagnosis, meaning a relatively benign, stationary condition, is essential for the patient. In the past few years, a number of genes with pathogenic mutations have been identified, which – together with the analyses of visual functions and the electrophysiological examinations – helped the understanding of the underlying pathomechanisms and the classification of related diseases as well.

The most frequent diseases:

- Congenital stationary night blindness
- Fundus albipunctatus
- Oguchi's disease

A common diagnostic feature of these diseases is the negative scotopic ERG response evoked by intense light stimulus (the amplitude of *a*-wave is higher than that of the *b*-wave).

Congenital Stationary Night Blindness (CSNB)

Recessive (Schubert-Bornschein-type) (Schubert et al. 1952), X-linked (XR), autosomal recessive (AR) and dominant (AD). The differential diagnosis is based on subjective and objective tests of rod functions (dark adaptometry and rod responses on ERG). Based on the lack of rod function in the complete form and the decreased but detectable rod function in the incomplete form, the two subtypes appeared to be two different clinical entities. This suggestion was later confirmed by findings of molecular genetic studies. Most of the patients complain about decreased visual acuity, which is between 0.1 and 1.0 in both groups. Disturbance of dark adaptation was mentioned spontaneously only by few patients in both groups.

Clinical symptoms and signs: Fundus picture is basically normal in both groups, different degrees of optic disc pallor may occur. In the complete form, the refractive error can be moderate or severe myopia, whereas rod adaptation is completely absent. In the incomplete form, mild myopia or hypermetropia can occur, the threshold value of dark adaptation is higher compared to that in healthy population.

Electroretinography (ERG): In the complete form, the isolated rod response is extinguished, and the oscillatory potentials are mostly absent, whereas in the incomplete form, the isolated rod response is subnormal, and oscillatory potentials can be detected. The scotopic response using intense light stimulus is negative, with normal *a*-wave and reduced *b*-wave amplitudes, in both groups. This result indicates that the pathological process involves higher order neurons associated with the rods. The use of prolonged light stimuli (with measurement of ON and OFF effects) enables the differentiation between the two forms of the disease. In the complete form, ON responses are definitely pathologi, whereas OFF responses are normal. In the incomplete form, both, the ON and OFF responses are pathological.

Elecotrooculography (EOG): normal in both forms of the disease, which enables the differentiation from progressive diseases.

Molecular genetics:

- The gene (NYX) encoding the protein called nyctalopin responsible for the development of complete CSNB was identified in 2000 (Bech-Hansen et al. 2000; Musarella et al. 1989).
- The gene (CACNA1F) encoding a calcium channel was identified in the background of the incomplete form of CSNB (Bech-Hansen et al. 1998). Dysfunction of this protein results in a decreased flow of calcium into photoreceptors, which pathologically influence the neurotransmitter release.

The dominant form of CSNB is rare, myopia and decreased visual acuity are not characteristic. One type of the dominant forms was named after the first member of a family affected through 11 successive generations (Nougaret).

Fundus Albipunctatus

The AR form of CSNB is a stationary condition. It was distinguished from 'retinitis punctata albescens' (progressive retinal dystrophy) by Lauber in 1910. Typical fundoscopic signs include the numerous, small, round or oval, yellowish–white patches in the pigment epithelium, which become pale over time. Nyctalopia is present from the early childhood. Cone-related functions (visual acuity, color vision, visual field, cone responses on ERG) are normal. Unusually long dark adaptation is needed to obtain the maximum normal scotopic ERG responses and normal EOG light rise.

Molecular background: the mutant gene is RDH5 (11-cis-retinol dehydrogenase gene), the mutation of which leads to a decreased production of 11-cis-retinal in the pigment epithelium, resulting in an inhibition of photoreceptor regeneration after light stimuli (Cideciyan et al. 2000).

Oguchi's Disease

The disease has been described by Oguchi in 1907 as an unusual form of CSNB who observed a prominent grayish-white discoloration of the fundus. In 1913 Mizuo reported the observation that the unusually discoloration of the retina disappears after spending a longer time in the dark (Mizuo phenomenon). Dark adaptation cannot be detected neither by a subjective method (adaptometry) nor by ERG after 30 min, but after 2–3 h spent in the dark.

Molecular background: the genes arrestin and rhodopsin kinase are suggested to be responsible for the disease. Mutations of these genes are supposed to inhibit the phototransduction cascade. The disease is extremely rare and mostly observed among Japanese patients. The underlying mechanism of Mizuo phenomenon has not been clarified yet.

References

Acland GM, et al. Genetherapy restores vision in canine model of childhood blindness. Nat Genet. 2001;28:92–5.

Allikmets R. Further evidence for an association of ABCR alleles with age related macular degeneration. Am J Hum Genet. 2000;67:487–91.

Bech-Hansen NT, et al. Loss-of-function mutation in a calcium-channel alpha-subunit gene in Xp11.3 cause incomplete X-linked congenital stationary night blindness. Nat Genet. 1998;19:264–7.

Bech-Hansen NT, et al. Mutations in NYX, encoding the leucine-rich proteoglycan nyctalopin, cause X-linked complete congenital stationary night blindness. Nat Genet. 2000;26:319–23.

Berson EL. Retinitis pigmentosa. Invest Ophthalmol Vis Sci. 1993;34:1659–76.

Berson EL, et al. Temporal aspects of the electroretinogram. Arch Ophthalmol. 1969;81:207–14.

Berson EL, et al. Natural course of retinitis pigmentosa over a three-years intarval. Am J Ophthalmol. 1985;99:240–51.

Berson EL, et al. Randomized trial of vitamin A and vitamin E supplementation for retinitis pigmentosa. Arch Ophthalmol. 1993;111:761–72.

Birch DG, et al. Yearly rates of rod end cone functional loss in retinitis pigmentosa and cone-rod dystrophy. Ophthalmology. 1999;106:258–68.

Cideciyan AV, et al. Rod and cone visual cycle consequences of a null mutation in the 11-cis-retinol dehydrogenase gene in man. Vis Neurosci. 2000;17:667–78.

Cutler CW. Drei ungewöhnliche Fälle von Retino-Choroideal-Degeneration. Arch Augenheilkd 1895;30:117–122. (Cit. Weleber RG: Gyrate atrophy of the choroid and retina. In: Heckenlively JR, Arden JB, editors. Principles and practice of clinical electrophysiology of vision. 2nd ed. Chapt 60. MIT Press; 2006. p. 705–15.

Eagle Jr RC, et al. Retinal pigment epithelial abnormalities in fundus flavimaculatus: a light and electron microscopic study. Ophthalmology. 1980;87:1189–200.

Fishman GA, et al. Visual acuity loss in patients with Stargardt's macular dystrophy. Ophthalmology. 1987;94:809–14.

Fishman GA, et al. Visual acuity in patients with best vitelliform macular dystrophy. Ophthalmology. 1993;100:1665–70.

Foxman SG, et al. Classification of congenital and early-onset retinitis pigmentosa. Arch Ophthalmol. 1985;18:1502–6.

Franceschetti AJ, et al. Fundus flavimaculatus. Arch D'Ophthal. 1965;25:505–30.

Francois J, et al. Electrooculography in vitelliform degeneration of the macula. Arch Ophthalmol. 1967;77:726–33.

Fulton AB, et al. Vision in Leber congenital amaurosis. Arch Ophthalmol. 1996;114:698–703.

Geller AM, et al. Assessment of foveal cone photoreceptors in Stargardt's macular dystrophy using a small dot detecting task. Vision Res. 1993;33:1509–24.

Hamel CP, et al. Molecular cloning and expression of RPE65, a novel retinal pigment epithelium-specific microsomal protein that is post-transcriptionally regulated in vitro. J Biol Chem. 1993;268:15751–7.

Hartong DT, et al. Retinitis pigmentosa. Lancet. 2006;368:1795–809.

Hoffman DR, et al. Randomized placebo controlled clinical trial of docosahexaenoic acid supplementation for X-linked retinitis pigmentosa. Am J Ophthalmol. 2004;137:704–18.

Janáky M, et al. AzX-hez kötött juvenilis retinoschisis klinikuma és elektrofiziológiai jellegzetességei [The clinical signs and electrophysiological appearance of X-linked juvenile retinoschisis]. Szemeszet. 1991;128:49–52 (In Hungarian).

Kaiser-Kupfer MI, et al. Gyrate atrophy of the choroid and retina: early findings. Ophthalmology. 1985;92:394–401.

Kellner U, et al. Pattern in dysfunction in progressive cone dystrophies: an extended classification. Ger J Ophthalmol. 1993;2:170–7.
Kennaway NG, et al. Gyrate atrophy of the choroid and the retina: characterisation of the mutant ornithine aminotransferase and mechanism of response to vitamin B6. Am J Hum Genet. 1989;44:344–52.
Koenekoop RK. Major review: an overview of recent developments in Leber congenital amaurosis: a model to understand human retinal development. Surv Ophthalmol. 2004;49(4):379–98.
Lachapelle P, et al. The electroretinogram in Stargardt's disease and fundus flavimaculatus. Doc Ophthalmol. 1990;73:395–404.
Lesch B, et al. Az X kromoszómahoz kötötten öröklődő juvenilis retinoschisis korszerű komplex vizsgálata [Advanced complex examination of X-linked juvenile retinoschisis]. Szemészet. 2006;143:165–74. (In Hungarian).
Lotery AJ, et al. Allelic variation in the VMD2 gene in Best disease and age-related macular degeneration. Invest Ophthalmol Vis Sci. 2000;41:1291–6.
Marlhens F, et al. Mutations in RPE65 cause Leber's congenital amaurosis (letter). Nat Genet. 1997;7:139–41.
Mata NL, et al. Delayed dark-adaptation and lipofuscin accumulation in abcr +/– mice: implications for involvement of ABCR in age-related macular degeneration. Invest Ophthalmol Vis Sci. 2001;42:1685–90.
Musarella MA, et al. Assignment of the gene for complete X-linked congenital stationary night blindness (CSNB 1) to Xp 11.3. Genomics. 1989;5:727–37.
Robson AG, et al. Functional characterisation and serial imaging of abnormal fundus autofluorescence in patients with retinitis pigmentosa and normal visual acuity. Br J Ophthalmol. 2006;90:472–9.
Sahel JA. Saving cone cells in hereditary rod disease: a possible role for rod-derived cone viability factor (RdCVF) therapy. Retina. 2005;25:38–9.
Sauer GS, et al. Positional cloning of the gene associated with X-linked juvenile retinoschisis. Nat Genet. 1997;17:164–70.
Schubert G, et al. Beitrag zur Analyse des menschlichen Elektroretinograms. Ophthalmologica. 1952;123:396–412.
Sengers RCA, et al. Gyrate atrophy of the choroid and retina and ornithine-ketoacid aminotransferase deficiency (abstract). Pediatr Res. 1976;10:894.
Simell O, et al. Raised plasma-ornithine and gyrate atrophy of the choroid and retina. Lancet. 1973;1:1031–3.
Stargardt K. Über familäre, progressive Degeneration in der Makulagegend des Auges. Graefes Arch Clin Exp Ophthalmol. 1909;71:534–50.
Takki K. Gyrate atrophy of the choroid and retina associated with hyperornithinaemia. Br J Ophthalmol. 1974;58:3–23.
Varsányi B, et al. Clinical and genetic features of Hungarian achromatopsia patients. Mol Vis. 2005;11:996–1001.
Weleber RG, et al. Clinical trial of vitamin B6 for the gyrate atrophy of the choroid and retina. Ophthalmology. 1981;88:316–24.
Wu H, et al. Mutations in the gene KCNV2 encoding a voltage-gated potassium channel subunit cause "cone dystrophy" with supernormal rod electroretinogram in humans. Am J Hum Genet. 2006;79:574–9.
Zernant J, et al. Genotyping microarray (disease chip) for Leber congenital amaurosis: detection of modifier alleles. Invest Ophthalmol Vis Sci. 2005;46:3052–9.
Znoiko SL, et al. Identification of RPE65 protein in mammalian cone photoreceptors. Invest Ophthalmol Vis Sci. 2002;43:1604–9.

37 The Roles of Electroretinography (ERG) and Visual Evoked Potential (VEP) Examinations in the Diseases of the Retina and/or the Optic Nerve

Márta Janáky

Contents

Both ophthalmologists and neurologist can encounter diseases of the retina and/or the optic pathway which – with or without fundoscopic abnormalities – are associated with visual field deficits, consequent afferent pupillomotor dysfunction as well as nystagmus and double vision suggestive of sensorimotor dysfunction besides the involvement of the sensorium. Electroretinography and visual evoked potential tests are sensitive and objective tools for the examination retinal and optic pathway functions. Two symptomatologies can be distinguished in the diagnostics of diseases affecting the retina and the antechiasmal optic nerve: constrictions affecting the isopters of the field of vision and island-like visual field deficits (scotomata).

M. Janáky, M.D., PhD, habil
Electrophysiological Unit, Department of Ophthalmology, Faculty of Medicine, University of Szeged, Szeged, Hungary
e-mail: janaky@opht.szote.u-szeged.hu

Constrictions Affecting the Isopters of the Field of Vision

Three types are known: concentric constriction of the visual field, vascular-type visual field defect and nerve fiber bundle visual field defect.

The most frequent ophthalmological cause of concentric constriction of the visual field is congenital retinal dystrophy, which is also known as degeneratio pigmentosa retinae (DPR) and more recently, retinitis pigmentosa (RP) (Fishman 1978; Kanski 1984; Bird 1981). This disease is the most frequent cause of night blindness. Impaired vision at dusk with intact visual acuity in daylight represents the early complaint. Later, the progressive constriction of the visual field interferes with daytime orientation. Finally, the central vision becomes impaired as well. In a proportion of patients, impairment of central vision develops as early as childhood. In this case, night blindness is usually not mentioned by the patients, such complaints fade into background. In the presence of typical fundoscopic appearance (pale optic disc, narrow arterioles, bone spicule-like pigment deposits), the diagnosis is clear-cut, and the role of electrophysiological examinations is limited to the assessment of the degree of dysfunction and the stage of disease.

J. Somlai, T. Kovács (eds.), *Neuro-Ophthalmology*, DOI 10.1007/978-3-319-28956-4_37

One of the atypical forms of RP, the sine pigmentosa form, is characterized by the above mentioned complaints of the patient presenting on examination, as well as the fundoscopic findings of pale disc and narrow arterioles without evidence of pigment deposits. Due to the pale optic disc and the lack of retinal pigment deposits in the fundus, intracranial causes are among the differential diagnoses. Notably, however, the ERG response is extinguished in this disease, whereas the VEP findings can be normal or pathological, therefore, the findings of electrophysiological examinations are of differential diagnostic value.

The other atypical form of RP is retinitis punctata albescens, in which point-like white irregular alterations can be observed in the deep layers of the retina. The retina appears to be 'moth-eaten'. Sometimes a few regular bone spicule-like pigment deposits can be observed in the periphery. This disease is also characterized by night blindness, progressive deterioration of vision and constriction of the visual field. The ERG is extinguished, whereas the VEP is either normal or pathological depending on the progression of the disease.

Fundus albipunctatus is the stationary form of this disease. Its appearance on fundoscopy resembles that of retinitis punctata albescens, and the patients experience difficulties in orientation at dusk; however, retinal functions improve or even become normal after spending a few hours in the dark. The ERG is subnormal or negative, but not extinguished.

The congenital form of RP is called Leber's congenital amaurosis. The major clinical sign is progressive deterioration of vision or possibly blindness by 1–2 years of age. The affected infant or little child does not follow the shown objects with the eyes, and searching nystagmus and photophobia are often observable. The fundoscopic appearance is variable: it frequently appears normal in the beginning, and the characteristic pigmentation develops only by 1–2 years of age or even later. The disease is frequently accompanied by mental retardation or a generalized neuromuscular disorder. Distinction of the disease from other neurological diseases or injury due to intrauterine infections (such as toxoplasmosis) may represent a differential diagnostic challenge.

In Leber's congenital amaurosis, the ERG is always extinguished! (Vaizey et al. 1977; Mizuno et al. 1977). Therefore, VEP examination on its own is insufficient when infants or little children present with a suspicion of blindness, and an ERG test is to be done, as it can be of differential diagnostic value.

In unilateral RP, the characteristic symptoms and signs affect only one eye, and the other eye can be completely intact. It is extremely rare. Furthermore, typical symptoms may develop in the other eye months or years later, refuting the early diagnosis. Therefore, a follow-up through years is necessary.

All other diseases associated with concentric constriction of the visual field have to be excluded before the establishment of the exact diagnosis. The ERG is extinguished on one side, whereas it is intact on the other side. The VEP is intact or pathological on the affected side, and it is intact on the other side.

Progressive cone–rod dystrophy represents another condition that also results in a concentric constriction of the visual field. The symptoms and signs appear in young adulthood. The visual acuity decreases, color vision disorder (achromatopsia) and photophobia also occur, and a gradual concentric constriction of the visual field develops. Fundoscopic findings include macular hyperpigmentation, mild arteriolar narrowing, moderate pallor of the optic disc and chorioretinal atrophy, and pigment deposits are frequently observed in the lower half of the retina (pupil dilation!). The disease is characterized by an extinguished or subnormal photopic ERG and a subnormal scotopic ERG.

The distinction of degenerative myopia from degenerative alterations due to a severe myopia is of differential diagnostic significance. Most of the patients suffering from severe myopia (above −10 D) have a certain degree of visual field constriction and some decrease in ERG amplitudes. However, myopia on its own never leads to an extinguished ERG response. In the event of an extinguished ERG, other generalized retinal dystrophies associating with myopia have to be considered.

In inverse retinitis pigmentosa, pigment deposits can only be observed in the macula and in the perimacular areas. Peripheral areas of the retina are intact. There is a central scotoma in the visual field, whereas the peripheral isopters are intact. The ERG is subnormal, sometimes extinguished, and the VEP is pathological. In later stages, rod dystrophy can also develop, therefore, certain authors questioned the existence of this disease as an independent entity, and do not distinguish it from cone-rod dystrophies.

In case of sector RP, the process is localized to one retinal quadrant, often in a symmetrical manner, e.g., affecting the lower nasal or temporal quadrants. The ERG is subnormal.

In pericentral RP, the degeneration is localized to a small retinal area, and the ERG can be intact. In paravenous RP, both the ERG and the field of vision can be intact. Angio-scotoma may be detected due to degenerations developing along the blood vessels. Visual field constrictions in the latter mentioned types are not exclusively associated with the characteristic concentric constriction; their presence in the list merely serves differential diagnostic purposes.

Certain diseases can present with a clinical picture resembling RP, therefore, they have high significance in differential diagnostic point of view. Causes of pseudoretinitis pigmentosa include certain infectious diseases evoking 'salt and pepper' pigmentation in the retina, which can be confused with RP. This entity most frequently develops as a consequence of rubella infection; however, it may occur after any sort of childhood viral infections associating with rashes and high fever. In this case, the ERG and the VEP are both normal, with no functional impairment. Disseminated chorioretinitis is a consequence of (syphilic) infection, and may be accompanied by deafness and dementia. The severe form can be associated with extinguished ERG, but the intact optic functions documented in the history prior to the infection may help the diagnosis. The ERG usually reveals a marked functional difference between the two eyes.

Exudative diseases, such as the Harada's disease may be associated with mental involvement and deafness. Their differentiation from RP is an important and difficult task. The intact or only moderately subnormal ERG together with the other clinical symptoms may help the establishment of the diagnosis. The retinal pigmentation occurring after the absorption of exudation in a form of gestational toxemia associated with retinal exudation can also be classified into this group. Fortunately, this condition does not result in true dysfunction.

Among drugs, phenothiazines can evoke a metabolic dysfunction in melanin-containing retinal pigment epithelial cells, and may induce a degenerative process. Through such mechanisms, thioridazine (Melleril) leads to a diffuse pigmentation disorder, whereas chloroquine (Delagil) evokes a macular lesion (bull's eye retinopathy). The ERG and the VEP may be pathological in proportion to the degree of damage.

Retinal diseases of vascular origin may also represent differential diagnostic challenges. Occlusion of the ophthalmic artery as well as that of the central retinal artery results in a sudden loss of vision. The subsequent generalized retinal atrophy with pigment deposits in the fundus develops later. Occlusion of the ophthalmic artery results in an extinguished ERG, whereas occlusion of the central retinal artery results in a negative ERG. Therefore, if choroidal circulation remains intact (in the case of a central retinal artery occlusion), the layer of cones and rods does not degenerate as indicated by the preservation of the a-wave in ERG. The VEP is extinguished in both cases. In the event of a sudden loss of vision, therefore, the ERG examination may help the differential diagnosis.

The toxic effects exerted on retinal cells by metal foreign bodies (iron, copper and aluminium) that got in the eyes are well known. Observations suggest that the critical period is 3–4 months. If the ERG response does not become extinguished, then it is not expected to be extinguished later either. The toxic effect of a foreign body to the retina is indicated by the appearance of a supernormal a-wave and a subnormal b-wave in ERG, and later the amplitude of the a-wave becomes reduced.

Vascular-Type Visual Field Defects

In the differential diagnosis of vascular-type visual field defects, the significance of electrophysiological methods is not that high as in the prior group of diseases. This sort of deficit in the field of vision generally develops due to impaired blood supply as a consequence of vasculitis or atherosclerosis. However, the condition called AION (Anterior Ischemic Optic Neuropathy), the development of which is based on impaired autoregulation, is not negligible. The incidence of this disease is increasing, and it leads to irreversible deterioration of vision.

The degree of dysfunction is indicated by a moderate prolongation of the VEP latency, as well as a significant decrease in the amplitude. The progression can be followed by PERG examination, which shows the retrograde axonal degeneration.

Nerve Fiber Bundle Visual Field Defects

Injury of the optic nerve due to optic neuritis, impaired blood supply or compression result in the development of nerve fiber bundle visual field defect. Among ophthalmological causes, the most frequent ones include glaucoma, oblique entry of the optic nerve (tilted disc) and optic nerve hypoplasia.

Ganglion cell damage due to glaucoma can early be detected by PERG. For the sake of early diagnosis, more recent electrophysiological methods have been elaborated (glaucoma program based on flicker ERG, multifocal VEP, etc.).

In compressive optic neuropathy, the PERG becomes pathological only after the development of retrograde degeneration. The oblique entry of the optic nerve (tilted disc) may result in a bitemporal loss of visual field. If the visual field defect is only detected in adulthood, the possibility of chiasmal lesion should be considered. Optic nerve hypoplasia itself may result in a bitemporal loss of visual field, which may also indicate a possible central nervous system process in the midline. In this case, central vision can be intact, and the crossing fibers of the optic nerves are not affected. In severe cases, both the crossing and non-crossing fibers are damaged, which is associated with blindness. This can be a part of a complex developmental disorder. It can be associated with septo-optic dysplasia and porencephaly. In such cases, the presence of nystagmus is almost obligatory. The ERG might help the differentiation from blindness of retinal origin. In hypoplasia, the ERG is intact, whereas in Leber's amaurosis (blindness due to retinal degeneration) the ERG is extinguished.

In case of retrobulbar neuritis due to multiple sclerosis, the prolongation of VEP latency is not only pathognomonic but indicates the severity of demyelination as well. In the event of retinal detachment, the reproducibility of a good VEP indicates a good prognosis.

Island-Like Visual Field Deficits

Scotomata

Two types of them are known: central scotoma and centrocecal scotoma.

Central scotoma can develop as a result of diseases of the center of the retina (macula lutea) as well as of the optic pathway. Acquired macular diseases are among the most important diseases of the macula (the fundoscopic appearance is characteristic): central chorioretinitis, senile macular degeneration, cystoid maculopathy, macular hole, myopic maculopathy. The VEP and the PERG indicate the degree of cellular degeneration.

Characteristic manifestations of inherited macular diseases include the Best's vitelliform macular degeneration and the macular and generalized forms of cone degenerations. Apart from these, macular alterations accompanied with systemic diseases are also known.

Though the fundoscopic appearance of Best's vitelliform macular degeneration is characteristic, the function remains intact for long time, and the PERG and VEP findings become pathological only in a later stage by which the degeneration of the cells actually developed. In the early stage, even the central scotoma is absent.

The generalized cone dystrophy can be a stationary or a progressive disease. Rod monochromacy and cone monochromacy are not progressive. Progressive conditions include the cone dystrophy and cone-rod dystrophy. A decreased visual acuity is accompanied with nystagmus, photophobia and color vision disorder. The detection of the central scotoma is difficult because of the presence of nystagmus. Different forms of this condition can be distinguished by electrophysiological examination. The inherited form affecting merely the cones is called Stargardt's macular degeneration, which disease is characterized by childhood onset and progressive deterioration in vision, without nystagmus and photophobia. In case the child can cooperate during the examination, the detection of central scotoma is possible.

Cone degeneration can also develop as a part of systemic diseases or certain neurological disorders. The cherry-red macula (cherry-red spot) syndrome can be caused by sphingolipidoses (Tay–Sachs and Niemann–Pick diseases). The bull's eye macula syndrome can be noticed in ceroid lipofuscinosis (Batten's disease). Considerations regarding the electrophysiology of diseases evoking central scotoma by affecting the optic nerve and optic pathway will be discussed in another chapter.

The most frequent causes of centrocecal scotoma include toxic optic neuropathies, Leber's optic atrophy and optic disc pit. All three diseases are characterized by progressive deterioration in vision. The onset of toxic neuropathy is about 30–40 years of age, whereas Leber's optic atrophy most frequently manifests in 18–30 years of age. All three diseases are characterized by reduced amplitudes of visual evoked potential response. In Leber's disease, the PERG is significantly pathological and hardly detectable (the mitochondrial dysfunction affects the retinal ganglion cells, and an anterograde axonal degeneration develops subsequently).

The Role of Electrophysiology in Diseases That Cause Nystagmus

Nystagmus is a frequent sign of neurological symptoms, but it may occur as a consequence of a congenital eye disease as well. Certain developmental abnormalities associated with nystagmus are apparent and can be immediately diagnosed with ophthalmological examination, whereas in other conditions, the fundoscopic appearance is not characteristic and the electrophysiological examination has a central role in the establishment of the diagnosis (Marek 1971; Good et al. 1989).

Hereby, groups of retinal and/or optic nerve abnormalities will be listed that can partially be diagnosed by ophthalmological examination, and where the ERG and/or VEP examination can be informative for the clinician. In case of congenital opacities of the refractive media of the eye (opacities in the cornea, lens or vitreous body), electrophysiological examination can inform us about the functional state of the optic nerve. These examinations have prognostic significance, as they might represent surgical indication or contraindication (Mashima et al. 1988).

The objective assessment of functions in the event of diseases or developmental abnormalities affecting the optic nerve has therapeutic and sociological importance. For instance, in case of an optic nerve hypoplasia, the papillomacular bundle is mostly intact or only slightly affected, and the fundoscopic appearance is disproportionate to the degree of actual injury to the bundle (Frisen and Holmegard 1978). There can be a difference between the function of the two eyes, which results in amblyopia ex anopsia (deprivation amblyopia). The findings of the electrophysiological examination can provide indication for orthoptic therapy. The objective knowledge of the degree of visual dysfunction in case of optic nerve atrophy or an optic nerve coloboma may be helpful in career choice as well as in shaping the lifestyle.

In macular diseases, the ERG can be intact, whereas the alterations in amplitude and latency in the VEP reflect the degree of dysfunction. In such cases, the practical usefulness of the PERG examination is questionable. The response that is hardly a few μV in extent can become skewed due to the presence of nystagmus, and thus may not be appropriate for evaluation. In the presence of nystagmus, the diagnosis of macular hypoplasia is always difficult and sometimes impossible. The condition can be idiopathic; however, it is always present in albinism and aniridia, further reducing the vision of the eye that is already light sensitive and decreased in value. In case the fundoscopic appearance is not characteristic, the ERG examination has differential diagnostic significance, and the VEP indicates the degree of visual dysfunction.

Leber's congenital amaurosis is the congenital form of RP. The primary pathology is the neurosensory retinal degeneration, which is followed by the degeneration of the pigment epithelium and subsequently the choroid. Blindness develops at birth or soon after. Pendular or searching nystagmus and photophobia are frequent. The condition can be associated with mental retardation and a generalized neuromuscular disease or other neurological disorder. As the fundoscopic appearance is often not characteristic (it can be intact in the beginning, the course pigmentation in the fundus develops by 1–2 years of age), the ERG examination has central role in the differential diagnosis when blindness is suspected in a little child (Vaizey et al. 1977; Mizuno et al. 1977).

Rod monochromacy (the term is confusing) means the extensive (not merely macular) degeneration of cones. The cone degeneration can be progressive or non-progressive. In the non-progressive form, the dysfunction of the cones can be complete or partial. The leading symptoms include nystagmus, photophobia and color vision disorder. In the complete form, macular abnormality is present, whereas in the incomplete form, it is absent. The VEP reflects the degree of visual dysfunction, the scotopic ERG is intact, whereas the photopic one is hardly detectable or extinguished. Electrophysiology has central role in the three forms of congenital stationary night blindness (CSNB) (Miyake et al. 1986; Peachey et al. 1992).

In type I nystagmus, photophobia or decreased visual acuity are absent. The field of vision and the fundus are intact. The validity of complaints related to hemeralopia can be confirmed by a negative ERG. In type II, fundoscopic abnormalities are present. Diseases in this group include Oguchi's disease and fundus albipunctatus. Type III is associated with myopia, nystagmus and non-progressive deterioration of visual acuity. The patients do not complain about night blindness, as their vision is poor even in daylight.

The diseases associated with nystagmus can be differentiated based on the abnormalities observed in the ERG. In case of CSNB-III, the ERG is negative. The alterations found in the VEP reflect the degree of visual dysfunction. A congenital nystagmus can only be regarded as idiopathic if all other causes are excluded.

Electrophysiological methods examining the visual system enter the ophthalmological practice in the present days. Their knowledge and use may protect the patients from several unnecessary examinations, and may be of help for them in the formation of adequate lifestyle by the establishment of exact diagnosis, even in case of an untreatable disease.

References

Bird AC. Retinal receptor dystrophies. Trans Ophthalmol Soc UK. 1981;101:39–47.

Carr RE, Siegel IM. Visual electrodiagnostic testing. A practical guide for the clinician. Baltimore: Williams and Wilkins; 1982. p. 45–101.

Fishman GA. Retinitis pigmentosa gene tic percentages. Arch Ophthalmol. 1978;96:922–6.

Frisen L, Holmegard L. Spectrum of optic nerve hypoplasia. Br J Ophthalmol. 1978;62:7–15.

Good PA, Searle AET, Campbell S, Greys SJ. Value of the ERG in congenital nystagmus. Br J Ophthalmol. 1989;73:512–5.

Kanski JJ. Clinical ophthalmology. London: Butterworths and Co; 1984. p. 13.2–13.17.

Marek P. Adatok a külső szemizmok elektrophysiologiájához. Candidate dissertation; 1971. (In Hungarian).

Mashima Y, Matsuhashi M, Oguchi Y. Simultaneous recording of visual evoked potentials and electroretinograms in patients with unilateral opaque media. Acta Ophthalmol. 1988;66:47–53.

Miyake Y, Yagasaki K, Horiguchi M, Kawase Y, Kanda T. Congenital stationary night blindness with negative electroretinogram. A new classification. Arch Ophthalmol. 1986;104:1013.

Mizuno K, et al. Leber congenital amaurosis. Am J Ophthalmol. 1977;83:32.

Peachey NS, Fishman GA, Kilbride PE, Alexander KR, Kechan KM, Derlacki DJ. Form of congenital stationary night blindness with apparent defect of rod phototransduction. Invest Ophthalmol Vis Sci. 1992;31:237–46.

Vaizey MJ, Sanders MD, Wybar KG, Wilson J. Neurological abnormalities in congenital amaurosis of Leber. Arch Dis Childhood. 1977;152:399–402.

Congenital Diseases of the Optic Nerve

38

Márta Janáky

Contents

Congenital diseases of the visual pathway include developmental abnormalities and hereditary diseases. The recognition of developmental abnormalities, i.e., congenital optic disc anomalies is of great significance. On the one hand, they are not rare; on the other hand, they can cause a differential diagnostic challenge: they can be confused with papilledema, they can cause visual field defects, they can be accompanied by central nervous system malformations, but they can also cause dysfunctions in the retina and macula lutea.

M. Janáky, M.D., PhD, habil
Electrophysiological Unit, Department of Ophthalmology, Faculty of Medicine, University of Szeged, Szeged, Hungary
e-mail: janaky@opht.szote.u-szeged.hu

Developmental Abnormalities

Congenital Optic Disc Pit

A gray, round or oval patch, which is darker than its surrounding, located most frequently in the lower temporal quadrant of optic disc. The disc can be larger compared to the contralateral one. Consequence: serous macular detachment. Differential diagnosis: central serous retinopathy.

Tilted Disc

The condition is characterized by an oblique entry of the optic nerve to the eyeball. The optic disc is oval, its vertical axis is oblique, therefore, the upper nasal part of the disc can be blurred and the lower temporal part is depressed (inferior crescent). Hypopigmentation is frequently observed in the lower nasal quadrant of the retina. Severe myopia and oblique astigmatism are frequently present. Consequence: bitemporal upper quadrantanopia. Differential diagnosis: papilledema, chiasmal compression.

J. Somlai, T. Kovács (eds.), *Neuro-Ophthalmology*, DOI 10.1007/978-3-319-28956-4_38

Optic Nerve Hypoplasia

Optic nerve hypoplasia is not a rare condition. It can affect either one or both eyes, and its severity is variable. The optic disc is surrounded by a small, hypopigmented ring formed by concentric choroidal and pigment epithelial abnormalities (double ring sign). Despite the small diameter of the optic head, the size of the vasculature is normal. The foveal reflex is frequently absent. The condition can also be accompanied by aniridia, and the optic canal can be narrow. The disease can occur as a separate developmental abnormality, but can also be accompanied by other central nervous system alterations as well, such as the absence of septum pellucidum or septo-optic dysplasia, also referred to as de Morsier's syndrome. It can also be accompanied by hydranencephaly, anencephaly. The consequence depends on the severity and the accompanying central nervous system malformations. In certain isolated cases, the visual acuity can be preserved or greatly decreased, depending on whether the central crossing fibers developed in time or not. This determines the extent and type of the visual field defect as well, such as binasal or bitemporal quadrantanopia; however, arcuate or vascular-type scotomas, or rarely central scotoma can occur. The hypoplasia of the fibers of the central visual field is often accompanied by nystagmus. Afferent pupillomotor dysfunction develops as a consequence of an antechiasmal optic fiber lesion. The accompanying neurological abnormalities lead to the development of endocrine syndromes, such as low levels of growth hormone, which can be appropriately treated by substitution therapy. It is more frequent among children of diabetic mothers, and among those who took antiepileptic drugs, quinine or LSD during gestation.

Coloboma of Optic Nerve

It is a result of improper closure of embryonal eye fissure. Large excavation can be observed in the optic disc, mostly in its lower part, and it can be accompanied by choroidal coloboma. This developmental abnormality leads to visual impairment and different forms of visual field defects. Differential diagnosis: it can be confused with glaucomatous excavation based on its fundoscopic appearance.

Morning Glory Syndrome (Dysplastic Coloboma of the Optic Disc)

A rare and generally unilateral condition. The optic disc appears larger, and the vitreous body contains remnants of the hyaloid artery. Blood vessels can be observed radiating in the edge of the optic disc to from a characteristic spoke-wheel pattern. Furthermore, the optic disc is surrounded by a slightly prominent ring developed due to chorioretinal pigment deposits. It is often associated with retinal detachment. This severe developmental abnormality results in a complete blindness in the affected eye.

Megalopapilla

The optic disc is larger than normally (Normal variant).

Myelinated Optic Fibers (Fibrae Medulläres)

During the process of myelination, the nerve fibers become covered by myelin sheath as they develop. The process starts at the lateral geniculate body in the seventh gestational month and stops by reaching the cribriform plate. As a form a developmental anomaly, myelination can propagate to the inside of the eyeball, passing the lamina cribrosa layer of the physiological optic nerve. The process can follow the pattern of the fibers, but it can appear in the periphery of the retina as well, in a form of small white spot. This can result in an enlarged blind spot in the field of vision accompanied by intact visual functions.

Hyaline Deposition (Optic Disc Drusen, Hyaline Bodies)

A congenital abnormality occurring in approximately 1 % of the population. There are abnormal deposits of protein-like material and calcium salts in the front part of the disc. The condition often runs in the family, and the abnormality can be observed in the fundus of both eyes. In children, the alteration is located below the surface of the optic disc, deep in the tissue of the optic head. After 10 years of age, it can be observed more easily (these are deep drusens). Blood vessels exhibit abnormal branching. In the beginning, visual functions are intact, whereas the alterations can cause visual field defects and decreased visual acuity over time. From differential diagnostic point of view, the fact that it can hardly be distinguished from the early fundoscopic appearance of papilledema is of high significance. The presence of spontaneous venous pulsation in 80 % of cases can help in the differential diagnosis, as it is absent in papilledema. The optic disc is generally not hyperemic, the veins are not congested and tortuous. Ocular ultrasound can aid in the diagnosis.

Melanocytoma

A rare and generally unilateral abnormality, usually occupying the lower half of the optic disc. It is considered to be the manifestation of congenital ocular melanosis. Congenital anomalies of the optic nerve can be accompanied by other malformations, such as midfacial malformation and encephalocele, but the most frequent associating conditions are hypertelorism, cleft palate or cleft lip (Fig. 38.1).

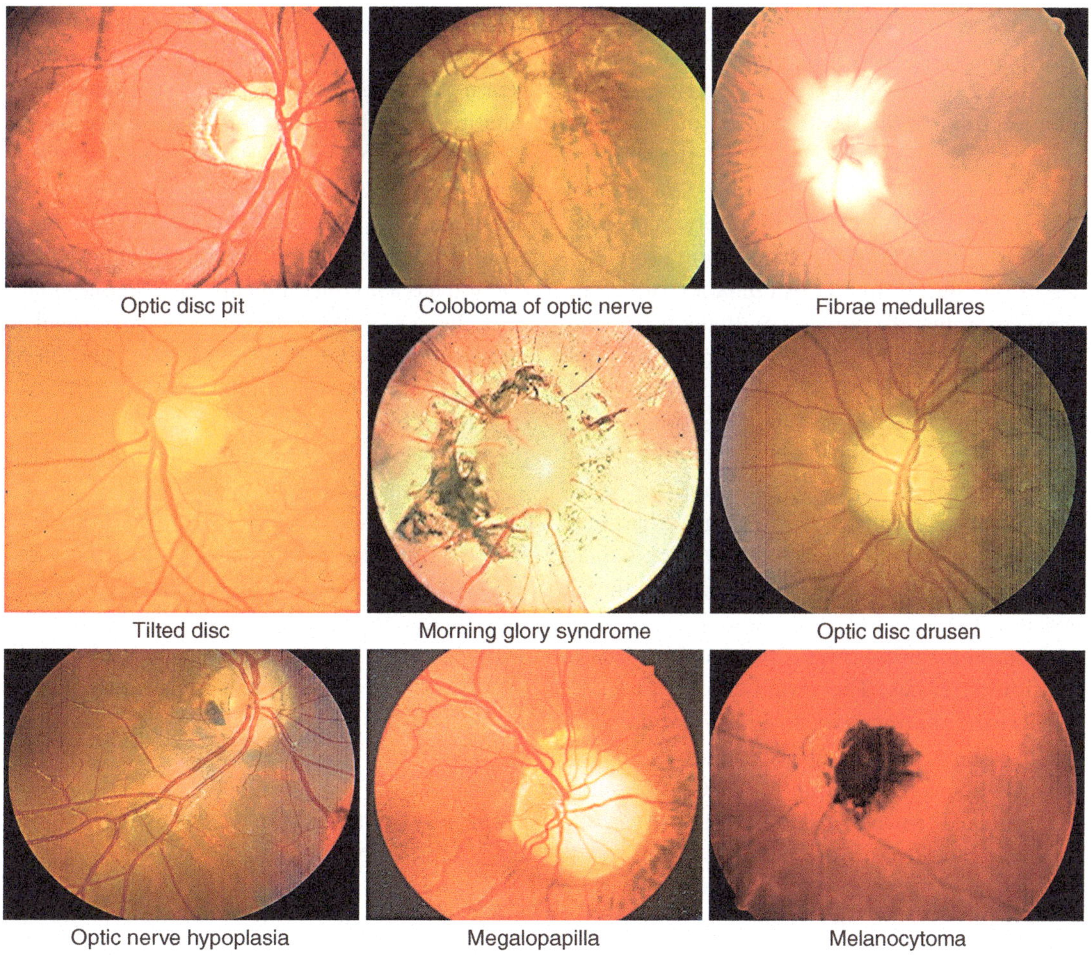

Fig. 38.1 Fundoscopic appearance of optic disc developmental abnormalities

Hereditary Optic Nerve Atrophies

They are rather rare as isolated conditions, and they more frequently occur as a part of heredodegenerative syndromes. Visual dysfunction can be mild or very severe, the first symptoms can appear in early childhood or adulthood. The diseases can be distinguished according to the type of inheritance, and the time of appearance of the syndromes. Additionally, inherited diseases with primarily neurologic or systemic manifestation, such as the multisystem degenerations can include optic atrophy.

Leber's Hereditary Optic Neuropathy (A Hereditary Mutation of Mitochondrial DNA) (LHON)

The first symptoms appear in early adulthood with painless unilateral deterioration of vision, which reaches its maximum severity in 1–2 months time. The development of complete blindness is infrequent. The deterioration of vision in the other eye occurs weeks or months later. The condition can rarely improve. Diagnostic criteria: pseudopapilledema (no leakage of dye during FLAG examination, microangiopathy around the optic disc). In the beginning, it can mimic the appearance of papillitis, and hemorrhage can also be seen temporarily. Subsequently, partial or complete optic nerve atrophy develops. The peripapillary blood vessels can be ensheathed. A characteristic visual field defect is centrocecal scotoma. *Signs and symptoms of Leber's syndrome*: cataract, keratoconus, possibly headache, vertigo and Uhthoff's phenomenon.

Differential diagnosis: optic neuritis due to multiple sclerosis. The visual evoked potential (VEP) examination is of differential diagnostic value, which is practically extinguished. So is pattern electroretinogaphy (PERG), which is extinguished as well. The PERG alteration drew the attention to the primary involvement of retinal ganglion cells, which leads to an optic atrophy via anterograde axonal degeneration.

Juvenile Optic Atrophy (Kjer-Type), Dominant Optic Atrophy (DOA)

In childhood, the deterioration of vision has an insidious onset, and is characterized by a sneaky progression. The decrease in visual acuity is not or merely moderately severe. It manifests in optic neuritis; subsequently, an atrophy affecting primarily the temporal half of the optic disc develops. The retinal arteries and veins are rather tortuous, pigment epithelial destruction and choroidal sclerosis can be observed. Central, paracentral or centrocecal scotomacan be detected by visual field test. Besides the visual disturbances nystagmus can be the first sign in severely affected individuals. The primary pathology is abiotrophy, which results the degeneration of ganglion cells, and subsequently an anterograde axonal degeneration develops.

In 10 % of patients, the condition is accompanied by mental retardation, whereas in 80 %, by neural hearing impairment. The recessively inherited form begins in 3–4 years of age, and is characterized by severe deterioration of visual acuity as well as optic disc pallor, similarly to the dominant form. The form of optic atrophy that is accompanied by central nervous system demyelination has a dominant inheritance. In this condition, the optic disc appears to be subnormal in size, it is pale and grayish in color. The blood vessels are also narrow. In the beginning, the disease resembles optic neuritis, but the atrophy of the optic nerve develops over time despite therapy. The condition associates with limb weakness, ataxia, hemiparesis and dysarthria. The form of optic atrophy that associates with cataract and neurological symptoms has a dominant inheritance. The condition resembles in its symptoms those of the recessively inherited Behr's, Marinesco's, Sjogren's and Friedreich's syndromes.

Behr's Syndrome (Optic Atrophy and Ataxia Syndrome)

The condition has an autosomal recessive inheritance. The infantile form is rare, occasionally a certain extent of progression can be observed; subsequently, the condition becomes stationary. It does not progress after childhood. The optic atrophy results in a decrease in visual acuity, but scotoma and horizontal nystagmus are also characteristic ocular symptoms of the disease. The form manifesting in 6–14 years of age can be associated with diabetes mellitus, but we should not expect the development of retinopathy in this case. The accompanying neurological abnormalities include ataxia, brisk tendon reflexes, positive Babinski sign, impaired coordination and mental impairments. It can also be associated with the weakness of the urinary bladder sphincter muscle. Other symptoms and signs can also be observed, such as progressive spastic paraplegia, dysarthria, club foot and a nodding movement of the head. The optic atrophy associating with acoustic nerve degeneration is recessively inherited and is often associated with a progressive polyneuropathy.

Spastic paraplegia syndrome is a sex-linked recessively inherited disease (ex-linked inheritance), manifesting in spastic paraplegia and optic atrophy. This condition is a neurodegenerative disease in the central nervous system. The 'non-Leber-type' optic atrophy is characterized by early childhood onset. The disease may be associated with mental retardation, increased patellar reflex, dysarthria and tremor. Optic atrophies occurring in **neurodegenerative syndromes** may be associated with Charcot–Ma-rie–Tooth-type hereditary progressive polyneuropathy. The first symptoms appear between 10 and 20 years of age, followed by the development of a characteristic calf atrophy associating with preserved muscles of the thigh, also known as 'stork leg'. Friedreich-ataxia can also be accompanied by optic atrophy as well as with retinitis pigmentosa.

Further Readings

Hamptan Ray F. Ocular syndromes and systemic disease. 3rd edn. Lippincott, Williams and Wilkins, A Wolters Kluver Company; 2002.

Holder GE. Pattern electroretinography (PERG) and an integrated approach to visual pathway diagnosis. Prag Retinal Eye Res. 2001;20:531–61.

Kanski J. Chapter 21. Neuroophtholmology. In: Clinical ophthalmology – a systematic approach. Edinburgh: Butterworth-Heinemann; 2007.

Miyake Y. Electrodiagnosis of retinal diseases. Tokyo: Springer; 2006.

Phacomatoses

39

Judit Somlai

Contents

The term phacomatosis was first used in 1920 by *van der Hoeve* to collectively describe the groups of diseases in which *hamartomata* can be simultaneously noticed in:

- the eye,
- the central nervous system,
- the visceral organs
- and the skin.

J. Somlai, M.D.
Unit of Neuro-Ophthalmology, Department of Neurology & Stroke, Military Hospital, Budapest, Hungary

Neuro-Ophthalmology Section, Hungarian Ophthalmological Association, Budapest, Hungary

Trustee, NOSZA Foundation (for the Prevention and Screening of Ocular Storke), Budapest, Hungary
e-mail: dr@somlaijudit.hu; http://somlaijudit.hu

A hamartoma is a benign, tumor-like bump, which originates from erroneous tissue production (dysgenesis). The incidence of either benign or malignant tumors is higher among patients suffering from phacomatosis. The most relevant phacomatoses for the clinicians:

- Neurofibromatosis (von Recklinghausen's disease)
- Tuberous sclerosis (Bourneville's disease)
- Angiomatosis of the retina and cerebellum (von Hippel–Lindau's disease)
- Encephalotrigeminal angiomatosis (Sturge–Weber–Krabbe syndrome)
- Ataxia teleangiectasia (Louis–Bar syndrome)

Neurofibromatosis: Von Recklinghausen's Disease

The syndrome is an autosomal dominantly inherited disease. The symptoms manifest in forms of dermatological, neurological and ophthalmological diseases. **Dermatological symptoms** can be noticed in 99 % of patients suffering from neurofibromatosis. *Cafe au lait spots* can be observed throughout the body since birth. *Neurofibromata* of variable size, occasionally reaching the size of a nut, can be seen along the peripheral nerves. These can be solitary and plexiform, with fibrotic elements predominating in the histology, also containing parts with Schwann cells. They can cause pain when invading the nerve root. In terms of **neurological symptoms**, *neurofibromata* can

J. Somlai, T. Kovács (eds.), *Neuro-Ophthalmology*, DOI 10.1007/978-3-319-28956-4_39

be observed in part on the peripheral nerves, in part on the spinal roots and on the cranial nerves. The clinical presentation depends on their localization. For instance, a *bilateral acoustic neurinoma* can present with cranial nerve symptoms, a syndrome of increased intracranial pressure, as well as with brainstem symptoms. Among **ophthalmological** symptoms and signs, besides the solitary or plexiform neurofibromatosis of the eyelid (Fig. 39.1), the ***orbital neurofibromatosis*** is of clinical significance. The neurofibroma that stems from Schwann cells can originate from the oculomotor nerve, the abducens nerve or the first branch of the trigeminal nerve. If located in the orbital apex, the neurofibroma leads to the development of ***Terrien's syndrome***, also known as ***superior orbital fissure syndrome***, the most important sign of which is a slowly progressing axial exophthalmos. An additional ophthalmological sign in patients suffering from von Recklinghausen's disease can be the **pulsating exophthalmos**, which is caused by a congenital defect in the orbital wall (mostly in the greater wing of the sphenoid bone). The sign can be provoked by leaning the head forward or by compressing the jugular vein. An additional bone anomaly can be the *bilateral, symmetrically enlarged optic foramen*, which should be considered during the differential diagnosis of optic tumors as well (discussed in more details in Chap. 62. from page 340).

Optic glioma can develop as and independent condition but also as a part of this disease (with an approximate frequency of 15%). This astrocyte-derived tumor appears in childhood, manifesting in an early decrease in visual acuity as well as in exophthalmos. The disease process affects the optic nerve and the optic chiasm. This often bilateral disease results in irregular visual field defects, decreased vision and an asymmetrical enlargement of one or both optic foramina. The findings of asymmetrical enlargement of the optic foramen in case of a glioma and the characteristically symmetrical enlargement in von Recklinghausen's disease are of significance as regards the differential diagnosis. On the other hand, the onset of deterioration of vision precedes the development of exophthalmos in optic glioma, whereas the order is just the opposite in case of optic nerve sheath meningiomas. The characteristic *fusiform enlargement of the optic nerve* apparent in CT or MRI scans of optic gliomas is helpful in the differential diagnosis (discussed in more details in Chap. 62, from page 340) The main principle of the treatment is that the patient has to be regularly followed up after the initial investigation in order to detect the development and consequences of solitary and multiple neurofibromata in time. Pedigree analysis and genetic counseling is recommended because of the dominant inheritance of the disease. In case of an acoustic neurinoma, neurosurgical intervention can be recommended.

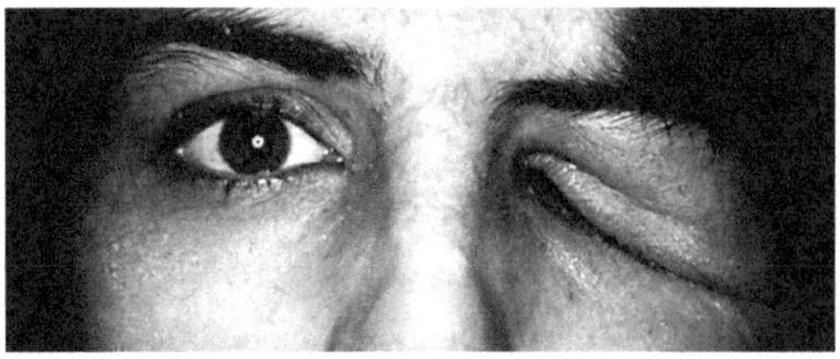

Fig. 39.1 Neurofibroma of the left upper eyelid is one of the ocular symptoms of von Recklinghausen's disease (The picture is courtesy of the Archives of the Department of Ophthalmology and Neuro-ophthalmology of the National Neurosurgical Scientific Institute in Hungary, for which we hereby express my gratitude. Permission granted by Judit Somlai, the editor of Neuro-Ophthalmologia, Literatura Medica Publishing, 1996)

Tuberous Sclerosis (Bourneville's Disease)

The disease was described the nineteenth century by *Bourneville*, following Recklinghausen. The most characteristic symptoms and signs of the disease:

- epilepsy
- facial sebaceous adenoma (Pringle's nevus)
- oligophrenia, dementia

Neurological symptoms and signs related to the central nervous system are caused by dysgenetic tumors in the cerebral cortex, subcortical ganglia as well as in the cerebellum, which begin to proliferate in early childhood. Intracranial calcification becomes apparent after the second–fourth year of life. The most frequent presenting symptom is epilepsy, which begins with infantile spasms, and the disappearing spasms are subsequently replaced by generalized convulsions as the child grows up. Choreiform movements as a rare symptom may appear independently of convulsions. Mental retardation is present in some 60% of patients suffering from tuberous sclerosis. If the dysgenetic tumor is located close to the wall of the ventricular system (subependymal giant cell astrocytoma), it may cause an occlusion of the flow of cerebrospinal fluid, and may lead to mental retardation and chronic papilledema via a permanent increase in intracranial pressure. *Sebaceous adenoma*, a *dermatological sign* of tuberous sclerosis, presents with reddish-brown papular eruptions (angiofobromata) in a butterfly distribution, which are most pronounced in late childhood and in adolescence. Among **ophthalmological symptoms and signs**, the typical ***retinal hamartoma*** can be observed in almost half of the patients suffering from tuberous sclerosis. It is localized within the area of the optic disc or in the peripapillary region, and is characterized by blurred margin, a grayish–yellow color and the shape of a strawberry (Fig. 39.2). The alteration develops in the superficial layers of the optic disc, therefore, it mostly covers the blood vessels going inside it. In contrast, optic disc drusen that presents with a similar fundoscopic appearance is a harmless papillary anomaly, which is caused by hyaline deposits. These deposits are located in the deeper layers of the optic disc, therefore, blood vessels can be observed above them. Therapy of tuberous sclerosis includes antiepileptics in case epilepsy is present. The intracranially located sclerotic nodules are histologically benign, therefore, the small and yet asymptomatic nodules merely require MRI follow-up. To prevent complications, surgical excision of hamartomata that cause an occlusion of the flow of cerebrospinal fluid is recommended.

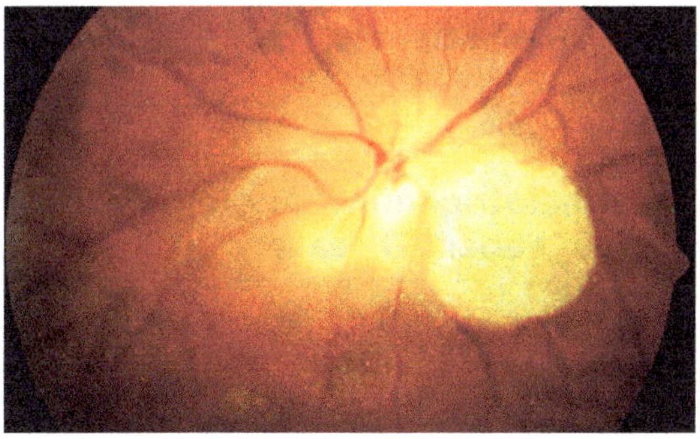

Fig. 39.2 Peripapillary located hamartoma observable on the fundus of a patient suffering from tuberous sclerosis (The picture is courtesy of the Archives of the Department of Ophthalmology and Neuro-ophthalmology of the National Neurosurgical Scientific Institute in Hungary, for which we hereby express my gratitude. Permission granted by Judit Somlai, the editor of Neuro-Ophthalmologia, Literatura Medica Publishing, 1996)

Angiomatosis of the Retina and Cerebellum (Von Hippel–Lindau's Disease)

The association between cerebellar angioma and the retinal tumor previously described by *von Hippel was* recognized by *Lindau* in 1926. This phacomatosis is generally asymptomatic until the end of the second-third decade of life. Its **ophthalmological manifestation** is retinal ***capillary angioma***, which usually appears in late childhood or during adolescence, and is at that time mostly asymptomatic. Welch distinguished different stages in their development, which are not only of diagnostic significance, but have prognostic and therapeutic implications, similarly to that seen in retinopathies.

In *stage 1*, the early stage, merely a tiny reddish-gray angioma or a capillary glomerulus can be observed, with supplying blood vessels of normal size. Fluorescein angiography (FLAG) does not yet reveal defects on the wall of the blood vessels or a subsequent leakage of the dye.

In *stage 2*, blood vessels supplying the capillary angioma become dilated over time, and an arteriovenous shunt develops.

In *stage 3*, the capillary glomerulus becomes more and more circumscribed as it proliferates. As a consequence of pathological flow conditions, the permeability of blood vessel walls increases and a lipid-rich exudate leaks into the surrounding retinal areas. Due to the dysfunction of blood vessel walls, a number of hemorrhagic lesions may also develop (Fig. 39.3). In *stage 4*, the subretinally accumulated lipid exudate may result in retinal detachment during the progression of the process. In this stage, complications leading to severe deterioration of vision may develop. If the growing amount if lipid accumulates in the area of the macula, macular degeneration may develop with irreversible loss of vision. Hemorrhages can penetrate the vitreous body as they advance, which apart from a complete loss of vision may lead to even more severe complications. In *stage 5*, the persistent uveitis, the pharmacologically intractable secondary glaucoma and the complete amaurosis are associated with intractable pain and phthisis bulbi, which will sooner or later necessitate the removal of the eye. As the capillary glomerulus grows, it may bulge into the vitreous body (also known as ***endophytic angioma***) and may become a source of vitreous hemorrhage. In contrast, blood vessel tumors with exophytic proliferation do not protrude, but make the optic disc blurred, and the subretinal fluid may lead to serous retinal detachment (***exophytic capillary angioma***).

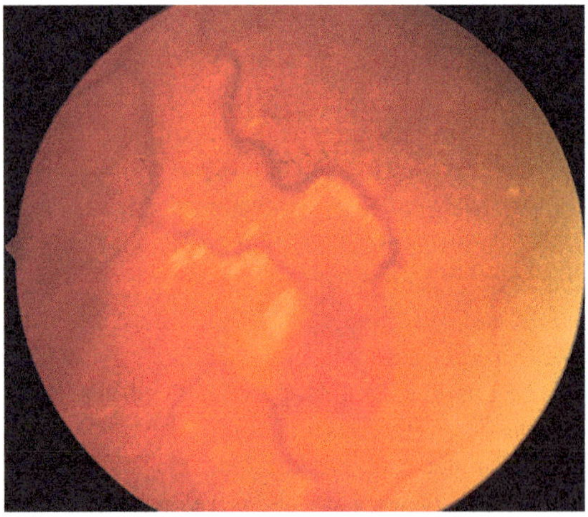

Fig. 39.3 Retinal capillary hemangioma in von Hippel–Lindau's phacomatosis (The picture is courtesy of the Archives of the Department of Ophthalmology and Neuro-ophthalmology of the National Neurosurgical Scientific Institute in Hungary, for which we hereby express my gratitude. Permission granted by Judit Somlai, the editor of Neuro-Ophthalmologia, Literatura Medica Publishing, 1996)

The frequently occurring central nervous system manifestations include the *infratentorial hemangioblastoma*, which can occur mostly in the cerebellum, and less frequently in the brainstem and spinal cord. The cerebellar tumor results in headache, increased intracranial pressure, chronic papilledema as well as cerebellar signs. Syringomyelia and syringobulbia can develop in the spinal cord and brainstem, respectively, either cranially or rostrally to the hemangioblastoma. During the treatment of retinal angiomatosis, the recognition of the disease in a most early stage, the follow-up, and the genetic counseling are essential. Photocoagulation and cryopexy treatments are recommended in the therapy of the retinal processes. The Department of Ophthalmology in the University of Debrecen performs local ruthenium application therapy in the past 20 years. The proper timing of laser photocoagulation therapy is still difficult. Preserving the older approach, a delayed treatment is recommended, waiting with the use of this sort of therapy until the appearance of the first exudate. In the presence of complications, anti-ablation surgery, or if needed, vitrectomy is recommended. Neurosurgical removal of a cerebellar hemangioma is undoubtedly recommended. The therapeutic tool of this century in the treatment of brainstem and spinal cord tumors is the gamma knife (The latter is described in details in Chap. 8 from page 33).

Encephalotrigeminal Angiomatosis-Sturge-Weber's Disease

This disease has three main group of symptoms: *dermatological manifestation*: **vascular naevus** *ophthalmological manifestations*: **glaucoma,choroidal angiomatosis** *neurological manifestations*: **epilepsy and dementia** In the development of the fundamental symptoms, the pathogenetic roles are probably played by congenital anomalies of pial, choroidal and facial (located along the trigeminal nerve) supplying blood vessels in the central nervous system, eye and face, respectively. Dermatological manifestations include the development of vascular naevus or naevus flammeus along one or more branches of the trigeminal nerve. This spreads toward the upper part of the skin of the neck and chest as well (Fig. 39.4). The lesion is observable from birth, and it becomes more and more protruded and dark; however, it does not change in size.

Among *neurological symptoms*, the *pial angioma* has to be highlighted, which is a tortuous conglomerate of dysgenetic blood vessels, and which can also be found inside the brain beneath it, and represents the source of secondary circulatory disorder. This is associated with calcium deposition in the upper part of the cerebral cortex, and the simultaneous calcification of the capillaries is also a part of the process, leading to the

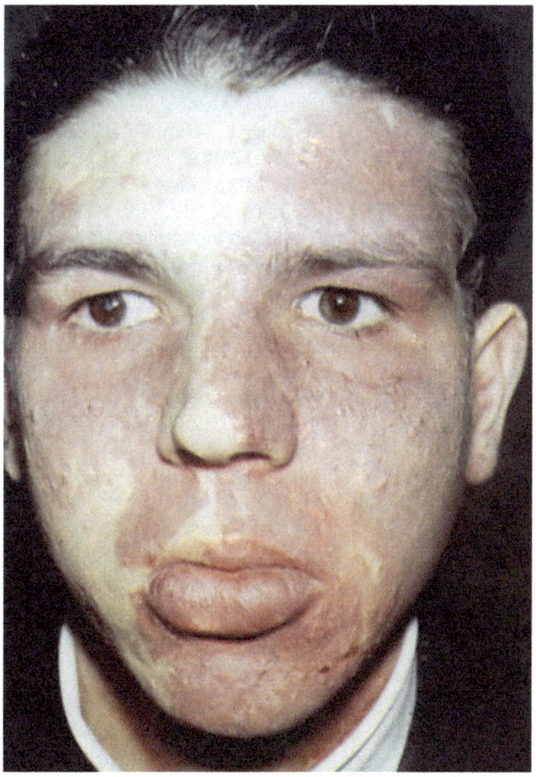

Fig. 39.4 Nevus flammeus seen in the face in Sturge–Weber syndrome (The picture is courtesy of the Archives of the Department of Ophthalmology and Neuro-ophthalmology of the National Neurosurgical Scientific Institute in Hungary, for which we hereby express my gratitude. Permission granted by Judit Somlai, the editor of Neuro-Ophthalmologia, Literatura Medica Publishing, 1996)

development of shadows with the characteristic '*tram track*' appearance on radiological examination. Smaller angiomas commonly cause epilepsy. **Ophthalmological symptoms** can be noticed as early as birth. The characteristic clinical signs of ***congenital glaucoma*** (***buphthalmos***) include the megalocornea, the untreatable increased intraocular pressure, and a consequent lesion to the optic nerve fibers with marked loss of visual function and the corresponding morphological sign, the excavation of the papilla. Choroidal angiomas may occur in 30% of the patients. Fundoscopy reveals an abnormality resembling 'red velvet' (also known as 'tomato–catsup fundus').

In contrast with the capillary angioma of von Hippel-Lindau's disease, the blood vessel tumor in this sort of phacomatosis is composed of *cavernous blood vessel* and it is not located within the retinal layer but in the choroid layer benath is retina. The therapy of *ophthalmological symptoms* of encephalotrigeminal angiomatosis is rather difficult, since the congenital glaucoma is almost intractable by conservative approaches, and the risk of expulsive hemorrhage is high in case of a surgical intervention. Pharmacological and surgical treatments of epilepsy are both possible. Dermatologists do not recommend surgical treatment of skin alterations.

Ataxia Teleangiectasia: Louis-Bar Syndrome

The signs and symptoms of the disease are attributable to congenital, highly severe immune system processes. Leading symptoms include ***cerebellar ataxia***, ***skin*** and ***eye teleangiectasia***, as well as ***eye movement disorders*** and ***recurrent pulmonary infections***.

The development of movements in early childhood begins without any disturbance; however, the gait of the child begins to deteriorate over time due to cerebellar ataxia. Teleangiectasia can develop in the ear, the soft and the hard palate, as well as in the facial skin.

Among ocular symptoms, the teleangiectasia of the conjunctiva does not cause visual impairment but can turn our attention to the disease

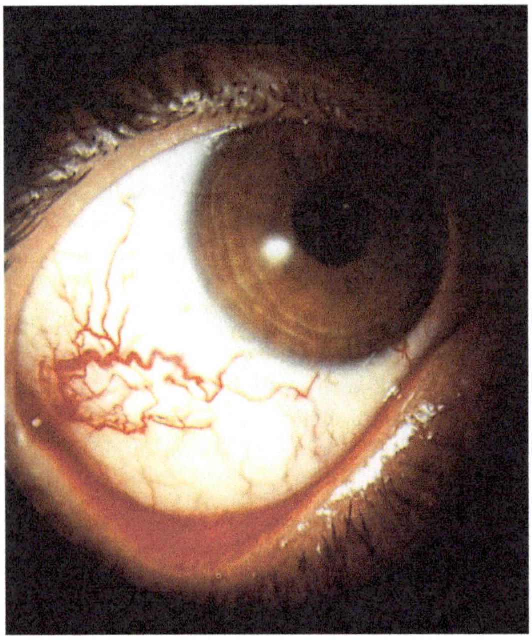

Fig. 39.5 Teleangiectasia of the conjunctiva in Louis–Bar syndrome (The picture is courtesy of the Archives of the Department of Ophthalmology and Neuro-ophthalmology of the National Neurosurgical Scientific Institute in Hungary, for which we hereby express my gratitude. Permission granted by Judit Somlai, the editor of Neuro-Ophthalmologia, Literatura Medica Publishing, 1996)

(Fig. 39.5). An early ocular sign eye movement disorders can be the ***apraxia of smooth pursuit***, thus the patient becomes unable to follow the shown objects with the eyes. A ***complete ophthalmoplegia*** can develop over time. By the child becomes older, the susceptibility to respiratory infections increase, which are hard to treat and the prognosis is poor.

Phacomatoses are infrequent diseases; however, the long-term treatment and a joint caregiving by the affected medical specialties are inevitable because of the severe clinical picture and the often unpreventable complications.

Acknowledgements The pictures are courtesy of the Archives of the Department of Ophthalmology and Neuro-ophthalmology of the National Neurosurgical Scientific Institute in Hungary, for which I hereby express my gratitude (4).

Further Readings

Balázs E, Berta A, Rózsa L, Kolozsvári L, Rigó G. Haemodynamicai változások Hippel angiomatosis ruthenium irradiációja után. Szemészet. 1989;126:79 (In Hungarian).

Berta A, Kolozsvári L, Rigó G, Damjanovich J, Alberth B. Intraocularis tumorok ruthenium irradiációjával szerzett tapasztalataink. Szemészet. 1991;128:16 (In Hungarian).

Gass JDM. Differential diagnosis of Intraocular tumors. St. Louis: CV Mosby; 1974. p. 266.

Hajda M, Korányi K, Remenár L. A jóindulatú orbitadaganatok. Szemeszet. 1988;125:213–7 (In Hungarian).

Halász P. Ataxia-teleangiectasia (Louis–Bar-syndrome). Confin Neurol. 1966;28:50–61.

Kerrison JB. The phacomatoses. In: Miller NR, Newman NJ, editors. Wlash & Hoyt's: clinical neuro- ophthalmology, vol 2. 6th ed. Philadelphia: Lippincott Williams & Wilkins, p. 1821–98.

Michels VV. Investigative studies in von Hippel-Lindau-disease. Neurofibromatosis. 1988;3(1):159–63.

Walsh FB, Hoyt WF. Phacomatosis. In: Clinical neuroophthalmology, vol. 3. 4th ed. Baltimore: Williams & Wilkins; 1985. p. 1747–820.

Welch RB. Von Hippel Lindau disease. Trans Am Ophthalmol Soc. 1970;68:367–424.

Retrobulbar Optic Neuropathy: From the *Neurologist's* Approach

40

Gábor Lovas

Contents

As a practicing clinician, diseases affecting the optic nerve are most frequently seen by manifesting in unilateral blurred vision or loss of vision. Fundoscopy is usually negative (this is the case when 'neither the patient nor the doctor can see anything'). The possible underlying causes can include demyelination, compression, infiltrative process, inflammation, trauma or ischemia. A common feature of all of these conditions is that the optic nerve is injured behind the optic disc: within the intraorbital, the intracanalicular or intracranial space.

G. Lovas, M.D., PhD
Department of Neurology, Délpesti Jahn Ferenc Hospital, Budapest, Hungary
e-mail: lovasgab@hotmail.com

Symptomatology and Clinical Work-Up

The degree of the deterioration of vision is widely variable. From a simple color vision deficit or a monocular visual field defect might be presented in association with a 20/20 (complete) vision, but the disease can manifest in partial or even in complete loss of vision as the other end of the spectrum. The injury to the optic nerve is always associated with an injury to the afferent pupillomotor fibers. Either not or only merely a decreased, short-term myosis can be evoked from the affected side. This results in the characteristic clinical sign of *Marcus-Gunn's* pupillary phenomenon: the direct pupillary response is absent or decreased, whereas the consensual response is intact. If we move the bright light of the pupillary lamp from the unaffected side to the affected side and back (so called, the "*swinging flashlight test*"), the pupil of the affected eye will appear to dilate despite bright light shining to it (this is because the constriction caused by the consensual response vanishes and the direct stimulation of the affected side does not result in remarkable constriction). The decrease or absence of pupillary response is so characteristic

J. Somlai, T. Kovács (eds.), *Neuro-Ophthalmology*, DOI 10.1007/978-3-319-28956-4_40

to demyelination that in case of a well-preserved direct light response one should consider retinal injury (Balcer 2006).

Fundoscopy reveals no abnormality in 65 % of the cases. For alternative fundoscopic appearances see Chap 42 from page 212.

In retrobulbar neuritis, the damaged optic disc gradually degenerates over time. Pallor and atrophy develops (in characteristic temporal localization). Visual field test can reveal special visual field defects monocularly, which are rarely observable in neurological clinical practice: in forms of altitudional, arcuate or centrocecal scotoma (The comprehensive examination of ocular symptoms and the evaluation of clinical signs are discussed in Chap. 42 from page 212). As far as imaging examinations go, optical coherence tomography, orbital MRI and CT scans can assess the structural alterations of the retinal nerve fibers, the optic nerve itself and the bones, respectively.

The sensitivity of the VEP is 70–95 % in retrobulbar neuritis. The prolongation of conduction velocity and the reduction of amplitude (the P100 wave is delayed) are characteristic features. Since the VEP measures the nerve conduction ability, it will reveal any the lesion independently of the etiology (sensitive, but noe specific). Besides multiple sclerosis (MS) the VEP can be positive in other diseases, such as Friedreich's ataxia, vitamin B12 deficiency, neurolues, sarcoidosis, compressive optic neuropathy, vasculitis, etc. as well. However, the positive VEP result can be a sign of spatial dissemination in the McDonald's criteria (McDonald et al. 2001) that helps the establishment of the diagnosis of MS, as its sensitivity is higher than that of the MRI examination in the assessment of optic nerve integrity.

Etiology

Though a number of etiological factors can result in the development of retrobulbar optic neuropathy, the most frequent cause is optic neuritis (retrobulbar neuritis), which frequently appears as the first symptomatic manifestation of multiple sclerosis.

Idiopathic Optic Neuritis (Retrobulbar Neuritis)

A visual impairment with subacute onset (develops within 1–2 days) and inflammatory origin, which is almost exclusively (92 %) associated by retrobulbar pain provoked by eye movements. Characteristic features include a blurred vision in the center of the visual field (*central scotoma*) and decreased color vision (most frequently the sensation of the red light is impaired, in some cases the patient can see only in 'black and white'). The patient can experience increasing vibration or other photopic phenomenon in warm temperature or during physical exercise (app. 30 %). A visual impairment begins to improve in 1 or 2 weeks, but the complete process of recovery can take up to 5–6 months. The prognosis is rather good, with 95 % of the patients having a vision better than 20/40 and 69 % of them having a 20/20 vision after 12 months (see *Optic Neuritis Study Group Studies*). Reminiscent symptoms include mostly mild deficits in association with spatial vision and the sensation of moving objects.

Relationship with Multiple Sclerosis

Acute demyelinating optic neuritis remains a separate disease entity until the presence of inflammatory alterations characteristic of multiple sclerosis (MS) in other regions of the white matter of the central nervous system is confirmed. The relationship with MS is well represented by the fact that in a 60 % of monosymptomatic cases when the first manifest clinical symptom is the deterioration of vision (also known as isolated optic neuritis) the MRI examination reveals inflammatory signs in the white matter.

In such cases, the MRI has predictive value regarding the development of clinically definite MS (CDMS). A negative and a positive MRI result associate with 5–10 % and 65–85 % risk to convert into clinically definite MS within the upcoming 10 years, respectively (Beck et al. 2004a, b). Studies of the *Optic Neuritis Study Group* (The 5-year risk of MS after optic neuritis: experience of the optic neuritis treatment trial 1997) revealed that among untreated patients (the placebo arm of the study) the disease with negative MRI associates with 3 %, whereas in the presence of at least two accompanying lesions with 36 % risk for the development of definite SM within 2 years. This ratio corresponds to that seen in case of patients suffering from a clinically isolated syndrome (CIS) with other clinical manifestation. In case both the MRI and the CSF analysis are negative (there is no intrathecal oligoclonal gammopathy – OGP) the risk of conversion is only 0–4 %, whereas in case of a negative MRI and positive OGP this risk is 27 % (Beck et al. 2003; Arnold 2005; Cole et al. 2000; Cleary et al. 1997).

In 15 % of multiple sclerosis patients optic neuritis is the initial sign in 50 % of patients. The injury to the optic nerve develops during the course of the disease in most cases (The 5-year risk of MS after optic neuritis: experience of the optic neuritis treatment trial 1997; Beck et al. 1993). The optic neuritis can recur. According to data of the optic neuritis study, relapse occurred in a total of 31 % of the cases during the 10-year follow-up. The frequency of recurrence is higher among patients with confirmed diagnosis of multiple sclerosis (48 % vs. 24 %) (Beck et al. 2003).

Thus MRI examination supports the establishment of the diagnosis of MS primarily by the revelation of the accompanying demyelinating lesions (signal-intense lesions in T2 and FLAIR sequences that are larger than 3 mm and are predominantly located scattered in the periventricular white matter). Besides, it has a prognostical significance as well (see above).

During CSF analysis, signs of intrathecal immunoglobulin synthesis as well as CSF oligocloncal gammopathy are looked for (representing an ongoing immune response within the central nervous system). As regards multiple sclerosis, the predictive value of a positive CSF finding can be used in case of a negative MRI or in the presence of white matter foci atypical of MS.

Therapy

In case of an acute demyelinating optic neuritis, short- and long-term therapy can be distinguished. When visual impairment is present, the *administration of highdose parenteral corticosteroid* speeds up the recovery and has a mid-term influence on the course of the disease. The combined, parenterally initiated and orally continued, corticosteroid therapy is also effective (1 g methylprednisolone iv for 3 days followed by 1 mg/kg oral administration for 11 days, which is gradually tapered off in the last 4 days) (Beck et al. 1993), improvement can be expected within days following the initiation of the therapy. The contrast sensitivity and color vision of patients who underwent such therapy is measurably better at 6 months post treatment, compared to untreated patients. In addition to the actual improvement, the results of the study indicate that the therapy delayed the conversion into definite MS by 2 years. However, no benefit, can be observed after 10 years. Given that relapses affecting the optic nerve were more frequent in patients treated with oral steroid, oral administration as well as retrobulbar injection of steroids are not recommended.

Long-term *immunomodulatory therapy* has been documented to decrease progression (Jacobs et al. 2000; McDonald et al. 2001). Double-blind, randomized, multicenter clinical studies indicate the efficacy of early immunomodulatory therapy in delaying the development of definite MS (Balcer 2006). In the everyday practice, however, this knowledge cannot be converted into a therapeutic guideline routinely, as in case of a patient with CIS (*clinically isolated syndrome*, see above) the development of a clinically definite MS cannot be predicted. The appearance of new or enlarging white matter lesions on MRI can help to decide whether or not to establish an immunomodulatory treatment, as missing the opportunity to slow down the conversion into CDMS might have bad impact on long term prognosis, but the initiation of an immunomodulatory therapy in a patient who would not convert into MS anyway is of concern as well.

Differential Diagnostic Considerations

Factors questioning the diagnosis of retrobulbar neuritis (‘*Red Flags*’)

- Age above 50 years
- Bilateral loss of vision
- Lack of pain
- Continuous progression of pain and deterioration of vision for weeks or months
- Further deterioration of vision after 1 week or no improvement of symptoms after 4 weeks,
- Febrile disease, alterations in complete blood count, hemostatic abnormality, dysfunction in other organ systems (suspicion of systemic disease).
- In these cases, an alternative diagnosis can be suggested (Table 40.1) (Balcer 2006).

Posterior Ischemic Optic Neuropathy (PION)

Within the orbit, blood supply of the optic nerve is provided by posterior ciliary arteries through the pial vascular plexus, whereas intracranially the supply is provided by the internal carotid artery, via the superior hypophyseal arteries, the A1 segment of the anterior cerebral artery and the anterior communicating artery. Damage to these blood vessels can develop primarily (vascular risk factors) or secondarily, e.g., via the compressing effect of a space-occupying lesion. The diagnosis of PION is difficult as loss of vision and normal fundoscopy are characteristic similarly to that seen in retrobulbar neuritis. Furthermore, ischemia might be associated with mild pain (whereas on the other side the course of retrobulbar neuritis is painless in 10 % of the cases). Patients with PION are characteristically elderly, have vascular risk factors and the onset of symptoms is acute (and not subacute). The prognosis of PION is significantly worse than that of retrobulbar neuritis (discussed in more details in Chap. 45 from page 226).

Table 40.1 Differential diagnosis of acute demyelinating optic neuritis

Metabolic diseases	Vitamin A-, Bi-, B_{12} deficiencies Methanol intoxication Alcoholic optic neuropathy Heavy metal intoxication
Diseases with autoimmune mechanism	Sjögren’s syndrome SLE Behcet’s disease Sarcoidosis, Antiphospholipid syndrome, Giant cell arteritis, Sarcoidosis, Wegener’s granulomatosis, Inflammatory bowel disease
Infections	
Viral:	HIV, Varicella, EBV, Coxsackie, Adenovirus, CMV, Mumps, Rubeola
Bacterial:	Lyme’s disease Neurolues (neurosyphilis) TBC
Gomba:	Cryptococcus, Aspergillus, Mucormucosis Postinfectious optic neuritis
Genetic diseases	hereditary ataxias and paraplegias Leber’s hereditary optic neuropathy and other mitochondrial diseases Leukodystrophies (primarily X-linked adrenoleukodystrophy) CADASIL
Tumorous diseases	
Primary tumors:	Glioma, Ganglioglioma, Capillary/cavernous hemangioma Melanocytoma
Secondary tumors:	Metastatic carcinoma, lymphoma Leukemia, Nasopharyngeal tumors, paraneoplastic diseases
Multiple sclerosis variants	ADEM, Marburg’s disease CIS (clinically isolated syndrome) Schilder’s disease Neuromyelitis optica (Devic’s syndrome or opticospinal demyelination)

Systemic Diseases

In case fever, rashes, arthralgia, hematological and hemostatic disorders can be observed as well, a comprehensive investigation of systemic diseases is recommended with special focus on autoimmunity and thrombophilia.

Neuromyelitis Optica (NMO) and NMO Spectrum Disease (Discussed in Details in Chap. 41 from Page 207)

NMO can be suggested if brain MRI shows no abnormality or there is a history of a spinal cord lesion with extensive signal abnormality (even years before the onset of optic symptoms and signs). Severe residual symptoms are characteristic of NMO. It most frequently affects both eyes (bilateral optic neuritis). NMO can be suggested also if relapsing optic neuritis can be observed in association with severe residual symptoms. There is no OGP in the CSF; however, NMO antibody (antibody against aquaporine 4, water channel protein) can be detected from the serum in 60–90 % of the cases.

Compressive Retrobulbar Optic Neuropathy

Meningeoma, pituitary tumor and aneurysm are among the most frequent causes of compressive neuropathy. Obscure onset of symptoms is characteristic, and papilledema is frequent. The patients often complain about visual impairment occurring during a certain eye movement or about double vision (discussed in more details in Chap. 47 from page 240).

Infiltrative Lesions

Tumorous and inflammatory (e.g., sarcoidosis) processes can result in a significant thickening of the optic nerve that is detectable with MRI. Though in the beginning a classical clinical appearance of an optic neuritis can be observed, the longitudinal follow-up reveals the correct etiology. The bilateral involvement, the recurrent relapse at the end of steroid therapy, and manifestations of the involvement of other organs are characteristic features.

Trauma

Traumatic optic nerve injury is unequivocally revealed by the history. Besides accidents, traumatic injury of the optic nerve also can occur as an unexpected complication of paranasal sinus surgeries (discussed in more details in Chap. 48 from page 247).

Leber's Hereditary Optic Neuropathy (LHON)

A disease caused by the mutation of the mitochondrial genome, therefore, characterized by familial accumulation (maternal inheritance).

Metabolic Causes

Bilateral loss of vision can be the first sign of methanol intoxication. Besides a precise taking of the medical history, Kussmaul breathing and metabolic acidosis with anion gap can help the recognition of the disease from clinical and laboratory aspects, respectively.

Childhood Cases

Childhood acute optic neuritis is different from the adult form, as it is often bilateral and it is frequently accompanied by papillitis. In general, the course of inflammation is more aggressive, and it is many times associated with residual deficits.

References

Arnold AC. Evolving management of optic neuritis and multiple sclerosis. Am J Ophthalmol. 2005;139:1101–8.

Balcer LJ. Clinical practice. Optic neuritis. N Engl J Med. 2006;354:1273–80.

Beck RW, Cleary PA, Trobe JD, Kaufman DI, Kupersmith MJ, Paty DW, Brown CH. The effect of corticosteroids for acute optic neuritis on the subsequent development of multiple sclerosis. The Optic Neuritis Study Group. N Engl J Med. 1993;329:1764–9.

Beck RW, Trobe JD, Moke PS, Gal RL, Xing D, Bhatti MT, Brodsky MC, Buckley EG, Chrousos GA, Corbett J, Eggenberger E, Goodwin JA, Katz B, Kaufman DI, Keltner JL, Kupersmith MJ, Miller NR, Nazarian S, Orengo-Nania S, Savino PJ, Shults WT, Smith CH, Wall M. High- and low-risk profiles for the development of multiple sclerosis within 10 years after optic neuritis: experience of the optic neuritis treatment trial. Arch Ophthalmol. 2003;121:944–9.

Beck RW, Smith CH, Gal RL, Xing D, Bhatti MT, Brodsky MC, Buckley EG, Chrousos GA, Corbett J, Eggenberger E, Goodwin JA, Katz B, Kaufman DI, Keltner JL, Kupersmith MJ, Miller NR, Moke PS, Nazarian S, Orengo-Nania S, Savino PJ, Shults WT, Trobe JD, Wall M. Neurologic impairment 10 years after optic neuritis. Arch Neurol. 2004a;61:1386–9.

Beck RW, Gal RL, Bhatti MT, Brodsky MC, Buckley EG, Chrousos GA, Corbett J, Eggenberger E, Goodwin JA, Katz B, Kaufman DI, Keltner JL, Kupersmith MJ, Miller NR, Moke PS, Nazarian S, Orengo-Nania S, Savino PJ, Shults WT, Smith CH, Trobe JD, Wall M, Xing D. Visual function more than 10 years after optic neuritis: experience of the optic neuritis treatment trial. Am J Ophthalmol. 2004b;137:77–83.

Cleary PA, Beck RW, Bourque LB, Backlund JC, Miskala PH. Visual symptoms after optic neuritis. Results from the Optic Neuritis Treatment Trial. J Neuroophthalmol. 1997;17:18–23.

Cole SR, Beck RW, Moke PS, Gal RL, Long DT. The National Eye Institute Visual Function Questionnaire: experience of the ONTT. Optic Neuritis Treatment Trial. Invest Ophthalmol Vis Sci. 2000;41:1017–21.

Jacobs LD, Beck RW, Simon JH, Kinkel RP, Brownscheidle CM, Murray TJ, Simonian NA, Slasor PJ, Sandrock AW. Intramuscular interferon beta-1a therapy initiated during a first demyelinating event in multiple sclerosis. CHAMPS Study Group. N Engl J Med. 2000;343:898–904.

McDonald WI, Compston A, Edan G, Goodkin D, Hartung HP, Lublin FD, McFarland HF, Paty DW, Polman CH, Reingold SC, Sandberg-Wollheim M, Sibley W, Thompson A, van den NS, Weinshenker BY, Wolinsky JS. Recommended diagnostic criteria for multiple sclerosis: guidelines from the International Panel on the diagnosis of multiple sclerosis. Ann Neurol. 2001;50:121–7.

The 5-year risk of MS after optic neuritis: experience of the optic neuritis treatment trial. 1997. Neurology. 2001;57:S36–45.

Neuromyelitis Optica (Devic's Disease): A New Concept for an Old Disease

41

Zsolt Illes

Contents

Paradigm Shift and Clinical Phenotypes

Neuromyelitis optica (NMO) is a central nervous system disease, characterized by demyelination, necrosis and inflammation. The disease was described by Eugene Devic and Fernand Gault in the late nineteenth century and was defined as a monophasic fulminant disease caused by inflammation of the spinal cord (myelitis) and the optic nerve (optic neuritis, ON) at the same time. For almost a century, the disease that was later named after Devic was considered as previously defined: an infrequent monophasic form of multiple sclerosis (MS), even though atypical cases including that with relapsing course were reported in the first decades of the twentieth century. It has since then been revealed those the relapsing form is the more frequent one, being responsible for almost 80 % of the cases; however, relapses can characteristically occur within a short period of time, in 'clusters'. Affection of CNS areas beside the optic nerve and spinal cord has been also well established by clinical, pathological and neuroimaging data. In 2004, a specific IgG was isolated from the sera of patients, which was named NMO-IgG. The target of the antibody soon became identified, which proved to be the main water channel of the central nervous system (CNS), the aquaporin-4 (AQP4) molecule. This resulted in a reclassification of NMO as one of the antibody-mediated channelopathies, which fundamentally changed the concept of its therapy as well. Though NMO is an autoimmune inflammatory demyelinating disease of the CNS, its pathogenesis is more reminiscent of myasthenia gravis (MG), the antibody-mediated channelopathy of the neuromuscular junction. NMO is not always associated with the presence of anti-AQP4 antibody, seronegative forms are also known; however, similar to MG, pathogenic role of additional antibodies can be suspected. Indeed, antibodies against myeline oligodendrocyte

Z. Illes, M.D.
Department of Neurology, University of Pécs, Pécs, Hungary
e-mail: zsolt.illes@ouh.regionsyddanmark.dk; zsolt.illes@rsyd.dk;
http://illeszsoit.hu

J. Somlai, T. Kovács (eds.), *Neuro-Ophthalmology*, DOI 10.1007/978-3-319-28956-4_41

glycoprotein (MOG) have been recently detected in the sera of patients with AQP4-seronegative NMO. According to the present international diagnostic classification, both optic neuritis and myelitis are required for the diagnosis of NMO. The diagnosis and therapy is however, complicated by the atypical or abortive forms, which are also referred to as NMO spectrum diseases (NMO-SD). The most important forms among them include the 'spatially limited' forms, in which the two main CNS targets, the optic nerve and the spinal cord are differentially involved: (i) the recurrent isolated optic neuritis (RION) or the bilateral optic neuritis (BON) without myelitis, as well as (ii) the longitudinally extensive transverse myelitis (LETM) with a typical MRI appearance of T2 hyperintense signal with a length ≥3 vertebral segments. The spatially limited spectrum diseases can convert into definite NMO in case the missing symptom appears during a consequent relapse. This, however, can take years or even decades. The clinical complexity and the rapid increase in the knowledge have promoted several recent international guidelines and consensus papers. Considering the problem of NMO-SD, a novel international classification and consensus diagnostic criteria of NMO is also under way.

Epidemiology

The disease is rare in the white Caucasian population, representing 1–2 % of the demyelinating diseases of the CNS. According to a population-based Italian study, MS is about 40-times as frequent. However, it more frequently occurs in other ethnic groups, especially among Asians, where MS is rare. It is more frequent in women: according to a Hungarian database established in Pecs, the female frequency is 5 times higher compared to male, and even higher in AQP4-seropositive NMO. The disease begins approximately a decade later than MS, generally in the late 30s – early 40s; however, forms with childhood or late onset NMO are also known. Relapses are characteristically more severe and less prone to improve than in MS. Disability is predominantly attributed to residual symptoms from relapses and not to secondary progression in contrasting to MS. According to the Hungarian database, NMO patients are in more severe condition within an average duration of 5 years compared to MS. Though the different prevalence in the different ethnic groups emphasizes the role of a genetic background, familial forms are rare, and at present no well-established, confirmed genetic association is known. A mitochondrial genetic background has not been confirmed either.

Pathogenesis

AQP4, the target antigen of the disease, is the main water channel of the CNS. The molecule in expressed in border zones where the parenchyma communicates with fluid (blood or CSF): the subependymal region of the ventricules, the cortex-white matter interface and the perivascular areas. It is predominantly expressed by astrocytes within the central nervous system. Although the AQP4 molecule is expressed in other organs as well (e.g., parietal cells of the stomach, muscle and kidney), damage of those organs has not been established; differential expression of AQP4 isoforms may play a role in this distinct pathology. The antibody-mediated pathogenesis involving anti-AQP4 antibodies has been indicated by a number of clinical and experimental data since 2004. NMO-IgG/anti-AQP4 antibodies can be detected in up to 80 % of patients and differentiate NMO/NMO-SD from other inflammatory demyelinating diseases with high specificity. Serum levels of NMO-IgG/anti-AQP4 and the frequency of IL-6-dependent plasmablasts are increased shortly before and during relapse in some studies. The presence of AQP4-antibodies predicts the disease course in NMO-SD and may be associated with a distinct phenotype. Treatments resulting in B cell depletion are effective in NMO and results in a decreased concentration of AQP4-antibodies. NMO lesions are characterized by deposition of IgG, IgM, complement and loss of astrocytic AQP4 at the sites of AQP4 expression in the CNS. The vanishing of AQP4 molecules is primarily attributable to antibody-mediated complement activation and an increased endocytosis of AQP4 molecules crosslinked by bivalent IgG1 molecules (antigen modulation); however, it is not entirely clear whether the antibodies interfere with water channel functions. Patients with NMO have higher levels of complement products in the blood, and the three complement pathways are functionally abnormal even during remission. AQP4 antibodies mainly belong to the complement-activating IgG1 subclass, and astrocytes transfected by AQP4 are susceptible to cell death by IgG and IgM AQP4-antibodies in the presence of complement. Inhibition of the complement pathway and selective inhibition of anti-AQP4-mediated effector pathways are beneficial in animal models. Passive transfer experiments also provided evidences for the pathogenic role of NMO-IgG by reproducing the neuropathological features of NMO with the appearance of neutrophil and eosinophil granulocytes.

Recently, another antibody against myelin oligodendrocyte glycoprotein (MOG) has been indicated to play a role in the pathogenesis of NMO/NMO-SD. These MOG-antibodies are predominantly of the IgG1 subtype, activate the complement, and are present mostly in AQP4-seronegative patients. A distinct phenotype from AQP4-NMO has been also suggested. Presence of AQP4- and MOG antibodies may also differentially affect the outcome of isolated optic neuritis.

Persistence of AQP4 antibodies for years and even decades without clinical disease has been indicated in a few cases, which may suggest a "second hit" in the evolution of the disease. Indeed, additional immune mechanisms including a T and B cell collaboration may contribute to the generation of pathogenic autoantibodies and also to the evolution of relapses.

Antibody Diagnostics

The detection of anti-AQP4 antibodies is highly specific and can be performed via multiple methods, recently compared by an international collaborative study (results of another study is under way). Indirect immunofluorescence assay (IFA) is the classical method: the serum of the patient is incubated with a rodent brain tissue, and the bound antibody is detected by fluorescein-labeled secondary anti-human IgG. The cell-based assay (CBA) is a more sensitive and appropriate method for quantitative evaluation: mammalian cells are transfected with AQP4 molecules, then the addition of the serum is followed by the use of fluorescein-labeled secondary antibody and detection via flow cytometry (fluorescence-activated cell sorting, FACS) or immunofluorescence. A commercially available cell-based assay applies fixed transfected cell. ELISA seems to be less sensitive than the cell-based assays. Depending on the application of the method, the sensitivity (positivity) is about 60–95 % in NMO, but less in LETM and RION/BON. The specificity is almost 100 %, which means that the antibody is almost exclusively associated with NMO spectrum: it is not or very occasionally present in fulminant, steroid-resistant demyelinating syndromes of the central nervous system. In a prospective study, ON occurring in association with MS was not AQP4-seropositive. The background of seronegativity is not known: the potential role of other antibodies can be suggested. This has been supported by the recent recognition of anti-MOG antibodies in AQP4-seronegative NMO with a distinct phenotype.

Diagnostic Considerations

The diagnosis of the disease is based on the clinical picture, the imaging examinations and the detection of the antibody (Wingerchuk's criteria, table). The sensitivity and specificity of the diagnostic criteria are above 80 %. In typical cases, the definitive diagnosis does not require the presence of the anti-AQP4 antibody: if the patient had episode(s) of both optic neuritis and myelitis during the course of the disease (two mandatory clinical criteria), the myelitis was longitudinally extensive (LETM) on spinal cord MRI, and the cranial MRI is not characteristic of MS or typical of NMO (two radiological criteria), the diagnosis can be established. Diagnostic difficulties generally appear because of the spectrum diseases: in such a case, the AQP4-antibody analysis is necessary and CSF results with pleiocytosis during attack, elevated protein and absence of oligoclonal bands (OCB)/elevated IgG index may be supportive.

Diagnostic Criteria of Neuromyelitis Optica (Wingerchuk's)

Mandatory clinical criteria

- Optic neuritis
- Spinal cord inflammation (myelitis)

Two out of three following (radiological and serological) criteria:

- Cranial MRI: not characteristic of multiple sclerosis
- Spinal cord MRI: T2 hyperintensity corresponding to myelitis extending over 3 vertebral segments
- Serum: anti-AQP4/NMO-IgG positive

1. A relapsing optic neuritis may raise the suspicion of NMO spectrum if the symptoms are severe or do not improve, and the cranial MRI does not indicate a morphology corresponding to multiple sclerosis: i.e., periventricular, infratentorial and corpus callosal lesions. Although OCT indicates a more pronounced axonal destruction in NMO than in MS, its application in clinical routine is not clear.
2. In all cases of bilateral optic neuritis (inflammation of both optic nerves simultaneously) the possibility of NMO spectrum has to be considered.
3. In case of severe myelitis or myelitis presenting with symmetrical lower limb weakness the suspicion of NMO spectrum can be raised. Relapses often begin with thoracic or radicular pain in areas corresponding to the localization of myelitis. Cervical myelitis spreading towards the brainstem may result in respiratory paralysis. Involvement of lower segments and conus has been suggested in NMO with anti-MOG antibodies. Spinal cord MRI predominantly reveals the appearance of a LETM. It is of note, that despite the severe symptoms spinal cord MRI can be negative in early stages, and the appearance of LETM may be accompanied by milder symptoms. Myelitis evolving during multiple sclerosis is generally characterized clinically by asymmetrical symptoms and a frequent predominance of sensory symptoms, MRI lesions localized to the posterior funiculus and extending less than two vertebral segments. LETM can be seen in other diseases as well: if AQP4 antibody is absent, usually another disease is responsible for LETM.
4. In case of an optic neuritis or myelitis associating with known SLE or Sjogren's disease (SLE/Sjogren's myelopathia) an accompanying NMO is highly suspected, therefore, antibody analysis is required.

It is of note that AQP4-seropositivity can be least expected in spectrum diseases. In such cases, the absence of oligoclonal gammopathy supports the diagnosis of NMO spectrum disease as opposed to MS; in 50 % of cases when CSF samples were obtained during a relapse elevated levels of total protein and pleiocytosis occurs, which is not characteristic of MS. Evoked potential examinations do not provide remarkable help in the diagnosis except for a few special cases. For example, VEP can be useful in LETM cases where the complaints of the patients raise the suspicion of prior optic neuritis, but at that time no examinations were performed. Abnormal response in the VEP can confirm the recent optic neuritis. In the Hungarian database, RION/BON cases were never associated with a positive SEP. In contrast, however, an approximately 20 % of LETM cases, the VEP was positive. The cranial MRI is essential primarily in terms of the NMO-SD differential diagnosis. Four types of morphology can be expected: negative (in most of the cases), aspecific T2 hyperintensities (in some 20 % in the Hungarian database), NMO-like (e.g., signal alterations in the hypothalamus and the brainstem; infrequent in the Hungarian database), MS-like (rare, but may occur in long-lasting NMO).

How to Diagnose NMO/NMO-SD in the Clinical Practice (Fig. 41.1)?

- In case the AQP4-antibody analysis gives a negative result (seronegative NMO), it does not have an influence on the therapeutic decision: the initiation of immunosuppressive therapy is mandatory.
- Isolated ON is more likely occur as a manifestation of MS (clinically isolated syndrome,

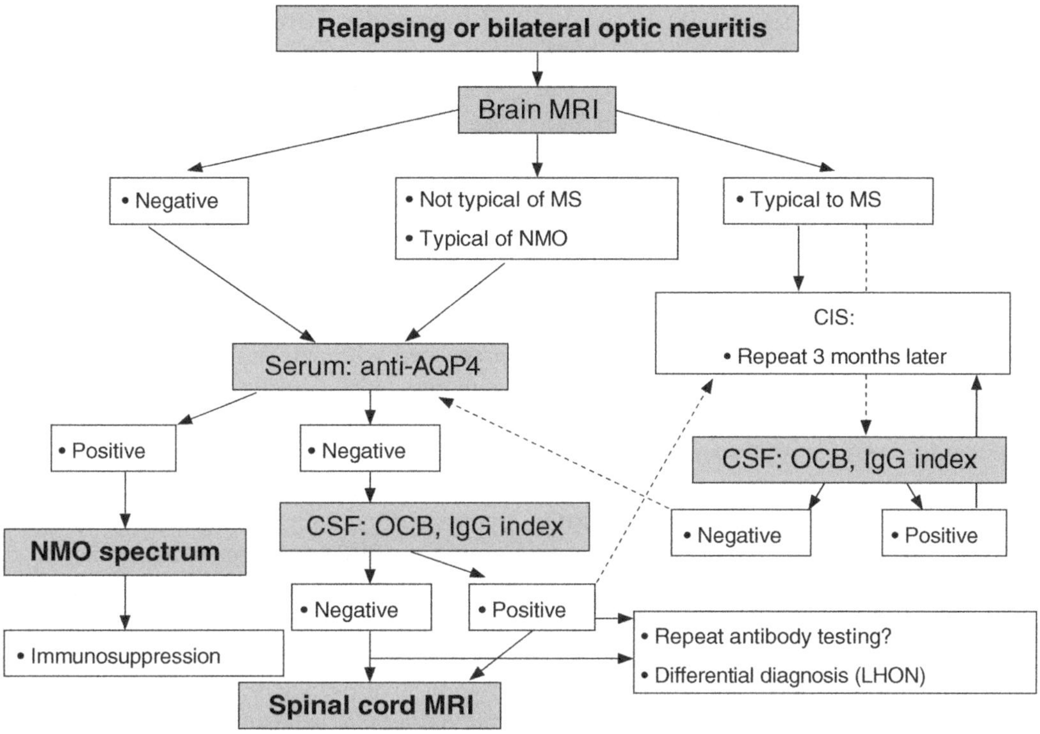

Fig. 41.1 Diagnostic thinking in case of relapsing or bilateral optic neuritis. Brain MRI and anti-AQP4 testing are core diagnostic steps along the clinical, serological and neuroimaging follow-up. (1) Brain MRI examination can reveal typical MS lesions; in this case the subsequent diagnostic steps should be made towards this direction, if anti-AQP4 is negative (clinically isolated syndrome, CIS or definite MS). (2) In case the brain MRI detects no abnormality or the findings are not characteristic of MS or they are characteristic of NMO, AQP4 antibody testing is mandatory. In the event of a positive serum, the disease corresponds to NMO spectrum, and the initiation of immunosuppressive therapy is recommended. (3) If the serum is negative for AQP4-antibodies and brain MRI is not fully informative, examination of the CSF can be helpful: the presence of oligoclonal bands (*OCB*) and elevated IgG index supports the diagnosis of CIS/MS. Repeated testing for anti-AQP4 antibodies, brain and spinal cord MRI is recommended: partial T2 hyperintensity(ies) in the spinal cord may support the diagnosis of CIS/MS. Additional differential diagnosis (e.g., LHON, sarcoidosis, etc.) should be also considered

CIS) or idiopathic ON, therefore, the antibody analysis is not necessary except severe ON. Brain MRI may support CIS.

- In case of a bilateral ON (BON; bilateral optic neuritis evolving at the same time), AQP4-antibody analysis is mandatory, and it is recommended in RION (relapsing optic neuritis).
- If AQP4 antibody cannot be detected in RION/BON, cranial MRI and CSF examination are recommended; the latter should be performed during a relapse if possible. A negative or aspecific MRI, the lack of OCB, elevated protein or the presence of pleiocytosis in the CSF are suggestive of NMO spectrum, and the initiation of immunosuppressive therapy in the patient should be considered, depending on the clinical picture. Spinal cord MRI may help differential diagnosis, especially if cranial MRI is negative, but OCB is present in the CSF: a partial T2 hyperintense lesion supports the diagnosis of MS.
- In case of a LETM, antibody analysis is mandatory.
- If antibody cannot be detected in LETM, cranial MRI and CSF examination are recommended, and extensive differential diagnostic steps are usually required.

In case of NMO/NMO-SD, systemic or other organ-specific autoimmune diseases may be considered, especially if relapses occur in association with fever, the patient is anemic, leukopenic or thrombocytopenic (e.g., TSH, ANA, anti-dsDNA, ENA, anticardiolipin and antiphospholipid antibodies). Antinuclear antibodies have been reported in 44 % of patients with NMO and LETM. Cases with clinical and radiological characteristics of NMO during the course of SLE have been reported, sometimes with alarmingly high number of myelitis and optic neuritis. Besides, a number of organ-specific and non-organ-specific antibodies and autoimmune diseases have been described to be associated with NMO, including neural autoantibodies. Since AQP4-antibodies were exclusively detected in patients with rheumatologic diseases only in the presence of NMO-associated syndromes, a co-existing condition in patients with susceptibility to multiple autoimmunity was suggested. In Hungary, about one third of NMO/NMO-SD are accompanied by other antibody-mediated disease, especially in female patients.

Analysis of the CSF for anti-AQP4 antibodies is not routinely recommended, the titer is several hundred times lower. In our database, the elevation of intrathecal antibody levels was a consequence of a decreased integrity of the blood-CSF barrier. The association of the antibody titer with treatment effect and activity of the disease is not clear in individual patients. The elevation of antibody levels is supposed to begin weeks before the relapse. Treatment with steroid, azathioprine, plasma exchange and rituximab (anti-CD20) decreases the antibody levels. It is reasonable to take the serum sample during a relapse and before the initiation of immune therapy (high-dose steroid, plasma exchange) for AQP4-antibody analysis. Data indicate that the presence of AQP4 antibody is associated with an increased frequency of relapses and cranial MRI alterations, a larger extension of myelitis and more severe residual symptoms. Although AQP4-seronegative NMO also responds to plasms exchange, seropositivity of patients was associated with a significantly higher need for plasma exchange, and an increased occurrence of a relapse number above 3 in the Hungarian database.

Therapeutic Considerations

Similarly to other autoimmune diseases, the therapy of NMO is based on three pillars: acute treatment of relapses, chronic immunosuppression to prevent relapses and symptomatic therapy. No prospective controlled trials have been done, but two consensus papers (2012, 2013) and an EFNS guideline (2010) have been published. In seronegative NMO, treatment is the same as NMO associated with anti-AQP4 antibodies. In NMO with anti-MOG (myelin oligodendrocyte glycoprotein) antibodies, treatment consideration is the same as in AQP4-NMO, but it may change in the future. The aim of treatment is to achieve remission first with pulse steroid and/or plasma exchange (PLEX), and maintain remission first with chronic steroid; then steroid is gradually removed and replaced by long-term immunosuppression. Immunomodulation, which is generally used in multiple sclerosis (MS) worsens NMO: interferon-beta, natalizumab and fingolimod are contraindicated in NMO/NMO-SD. Chronic immunosuppressive treatment of NMO and NMO-SD is mandatory: inadequately treated or untreated patients have poor prognosis. Given the increased relapse rate following delivery, rapid introduction of prophylactic therapy could be warranted; however, the benefits of these therapies should be balanced against the benefits of breastfeeding. To data there is no evidence that the maternal anti-AQP4 attack human fetal CNS. Pediatric NMO should be treated the same way as in adults.

First-line therapy for acute treatment is high-dose intravenous methylprednisolone (IVMP): 1 g MP daily for 5 days. Combination with PLEX may be more efficacious than IVMP monotherapy. IVMP should be followed by oral prednisone (or methlyprednisolone) 1 mg per kg body weight for 1 month. Then oral steroid should be gradually tapered off over 6–12 months. Plasma exchange (PE, 1–1.5 plasma volume every second day up to 7 times) is recommended in case of severe relapse, deterioration despite the MP treatment, or if previous relapses responded well to PLEX. Significant improvement is expected in 44–75 % of cases. Plasma exchange is also effective in AQP4-seronegative patients. Experience with intravenous immunoglobulin (IVIG) in relapse is limited, therefore IVMP or PLEX is preferred. No improvement was found in steroid-resistant cases with IVIG: in those cases PLEX is recommended. Cyclophosphamide is suggested as a 2nd line relapse treatment if steroid and PLEX is not efficacious.

Chronic immunosuppression is mandatory in all AQP4-seropositive NMO and NMO-SD. Immunosuppression should be build up during the tapering off of steroid treatment after relapse. Immunosuppression has to be effective by the time the oral steroid dose is low: this may take 3–6 months depending on treatment: e.g., azathioprine longer, mycophenolate and methotrexate shorter. Azathioprine can be a convenient first choice: recent larger retrospective case series have been published. In case of relapse, possible escalation can be oral mycophenolate mofetil or methotrexate if azathioprine is not tolerated; as next step in escalation, iv. rituximab, or iv. cyclophosphamide pulse can be applied. Other options, e.g., cyclospirine, tacrolimus, and PLEX at regular intervals can be also considered. Clinical trials interfering with complement and IL-6 pathways are running, potential options in the future are already established anti-B cell therapies (e.g., ocrelizumab, ofatumumab) and hematopoietic stem cell transplantation. A number of data suggest efficacy of antigen-specific experimental treatments. Combination therapy has not been yet established, except steroid combined with azathioprine, mycophenolate mofetil, methotrexate or cyclosporine; and regular PLEX with immunosuppression. If the patient develops a relapse during chronic immunosuppression, transient high-dose oral steroid is recommended after the acute administration of high-dose IVMP because relapses often occur in clusters. Afterwards, escalation can be considered, but if treatment without immediate effect is introduced, it should be combined with oral steroid until it is surely effective (e.g., azathioprine, mycophenolate mofetil).

The gradual dose escalation of azathioprine should be paralleled with high-dose MP therapy, as its effect is late, being effective after 6–12 months. This practically means that high-dose intravenous MP treatment of a relapse should be followed by oral administration of 1 mg/kg body weight oral MP (or prednisone) every day and subsequently every second day. Sustaining this high-dose oral steroid therapy for at least 4–6 weeks we initiate the escalation of azathioprine therapy: by increasing the dose with 25–50 mg every week with weekly follow-up of complete blood count and liver function. Steroid can cause leukocytosis, whereas azathioprine can cause leukopenia. The dose of azathioprine needs to be escalated to a maximum daily dose of 2.5–3 × 1 mg/kg body weight (this corresponds to a daily dose of 200 mg azathioprine in case of 70–80 kg body weight). The slow tapering of steroid therapy should be started after 4–6 weeks, with a maximum decrease of 4 mg every 2 weeks; however, this period should be prolonged in case of lower doses. After 8–12 months, the patient is left on full-dose azathioprine monotherapy. Ten percentages of the population lacks thiopurine methyltransferase (TPMT): either test patients for deficiency or start with low dose.

Chronic steroid therapy requires potassium supplementation, and, especially in postmenopausal female patients, calcium and vitamin D supplementation, ulcer prevention (proton pump inhibition), and a low sodium, high protein diet. Regular laboratory follow-up (blood sugar, ions, blood count, liver function) is recommended. Azathioprine is a safe and comfortable immunosuppressant: it can be administered also during pregnancy if necessary, severe side-effects (severe infection, tumor) are extremely rare. Annual oncological screening is recommended.

In case of mycophenolate mofetil the dosis should be at least 2 × 1000 mg/day and should be given orally. Gastrointestinal side effects may occur. Methotrexate should be given at least in a dosis of 17.5 mg (up to 25 mg) once a week orally. Folic acid 1 mg should be given daily except methotrexate-day. Rituximab is an option in refractory NMO. A convenient administration is 1 g intravenously twice, 14 days apart. It should be repeated every 6–12 months, or based on monthly monitoring of CD19 B cells (redosing above 2 %); another frequently used strategy is beginning with 4 weekly doses of 375 mg/m^2 followed by 2 biweekly doses of 1 g. Two small clinical trials showed different results with cyclophosphamide. It can be used as an induction treatment with monthly intravenous pulse for 6 months, repeated if necessary, and change to oral immunosuppression thereafter. Although two small case report series with mitoxantrone indicated benefits, it should be avoided due to high risk of leukemia.

Whom to Treat with Chronic Immunosuppression?

- Every case of definite NMO should be treated, regardless if the patient is AQP4-seropositive or seronegative. The risk of a relapse is 50–60 % in the first year, and 90 % in the first 3 years following the diagnosis.
- Chronic immunosuppression is also recommended in AQP4-serpositive RION/BON and LETM. The risk for NMO spectrum to convert into definite NMO within 3–7 years is 50–100 %; therefore, there is a high chance for a severe relapse. In case of LETM, this occurs within the first year, a relapse will occur in almost two third of patients. Half of seropositive RION cases convert within 5 years.
- Treatment issues are more complex in AQP4-seronegative RION/BON and LETM. Commercial anti-MOG antibody testing is not available for AQP4-seronegative patients. These cases, especially LETM require extensive differential diagnosis. Based on recent case series, the ultimate diagnosis is not NMO-SD in the majority of AQP4-seronegative LETM cases. Therefore, these cases require individual assessments.

Further Readings

Axtell RC, Raman C, Steinman L. Type I interferons: beneficial in Th1 and detrimental in Th17 autoimmunity. Clin Rev Allergy Immunol. 2012;44:114–20.

Bakker J, Metz L. Devic's neuromyelitis optica treated with intravenous gamma globulin (IVIG). Can J Neurol Sci. 2004;31:265–7.

Barnett M, Prineas J, Buckland M, Parratt J, Pollard J. Massive astrocyte destruction in neuromyelitis optica despite natalizumab therapy. Mult Scler. 2012;18:108–12.

Bedi GS, et al. Impact of rituximab on relapse rate and disability in neuromyelitis optica. Mult Scler. 2011;17:1225–30.

Bichuetti DB, Lobato de Oliveira EM, Oliveira DM, Amorin de Souza N, Gabbai AA. Neuromyelitis optica treatment: analysis of 36 patients. Arch Neurol. 2010;67:1131–6.

Bichuetti DB, Oliveira EM, de Boulos FC, Gabbai AA. Lack of response to pulse cyclophosphamide in neuromyelitis optica: evaluation of 7 patients. Arch Neurol. 2012;69:938–9.

Bonnan M, Cabre P. Plasma exchange in severe attacks of neuromyelitis optica. Mult Scler Int. 2012;2012:787630.

Bonnan M, et al. Plasma exchange in severe spinal attacks associated with neuromyelitis optica spectrum disorder. Mult Scler. 2009;15:487–92.

Collongues N, Marignier R, Zéphir H, Papeix C, Blanc F, Ritleng C, Tchikviladzé M, Outteryck O, Vukusic S, Fleury M, Fontaine B, Brassat D, Clanet M, Milh M, Pelletier J, Audoin B, Ruet A, Lebrun-Frenay C, Thouvenot E, Camu W, Debouverie M, Créange A, Moreau T, Labauge P, Castelnovo G, Edan G, Le Page E, Defer G, Barroso B, Heinzlef O, Gout O, Rodriguez D, Wiertlewski S, Laplaud D, Borgel F, Tourniaire P, Grimaud J, Brochet B, Vermersch P, Confavreux C, de Seze J. Neuromyelitis optica in France: a multicenter study of 125 patients. Neurology. 2010;74:736–42.

Costanzi C, et al. Azathioprine: tolerability, efficacy, and predictors of benefit in neuromyelitis optica. Neurology. 2011;77:659–66.

Cree BA, et al. An open label study of the effects of rituximab in neuromyelitis optica. Neurology. 2005;64:1270–2.

Elsone L, et al. Role of intravenous immunoglobulin in the treatment of acute relapses of neuromyelitis optica: experience in 10 patients. Mult Scler. 2014;20:501–4.

Greenberg BM, et al. Idiopathic transverse myelitis: corticosteroids, plasma exchange, or cyclophosphamide. Neurology. 2007;68:1614–7.

Greenberg BM, et al. Rituximab dosing and monitoring strategies in neuromyelitis optica patients: creating strategies for therapeutic success. Mult Scler. 2012;18:1022–6.

Höftberger R, Sepulveda M, Armangue T, Blanco Y, Rostásy K, Cobo Calvo A, Olascoaga J, Ramió-Torrentà L, Reindl M, Benito-León J, Casanova B, Arrambide G, Sabater L, Graus F, Dalmau J, Saiz A. Antibodies to MOG and AQP4 in adults with neuromyelitis optica and suspected limited forms of the disease. Mult Scler. 2014. pii: 1352458514555785. [Epub ahead of print].

Illes Z. Pathogenesis, diagnosis and treatment of neuromyelitis optica: changing concept of an old disease. Clin Exp Neuroimmunol. 2010;1:103–23.

Izaki S, et al. A case of neuromyelitis optica spectrum disorder developing a fulminant course with multiple white-matter lesions following fingolimod treatment [Japanese]. Rinsho Shinkeigaku. 2013;53:513–7.

Jacob A, et al. Treatment of neuromyelitis optica with rituximab: retrospective analysis of 25 patients. Arch Neurol. 2008;65:1443–8.

Jacob A, et al. Treatment of neuromyelitis optica with mycophenolate mofetil: retrospective analysis of 24 patients. Arch Neurol. 2009;66:1128–33.

Jacob A, McKeon A, Nakashima I, Sato DK, Elsone L, Fujihara K, de Seze J. Current concept of neuromyelitis optica (NMO) and NMO spectrum disorders. J Neurol Neurosurg Psychiatry. 2013;84:922–30.

Jarius S, Wildemann B. AQP4 antibodies in neuromyelitis optica: diagnostic and pathogenetic relevance. Nat Rev Neurol. 2010;6:383–92.

Jarius S, Wildemann B, Paul F. Neuromyelitis optica: clinical features, immunopathogenesis and treatment. Clin Exp Immunol. 2014;176:149–64.

Kalluri SR, Illes Z, Srivastava R, Cree B, Menge T, Bennett JL, Berthele A, Hemmer B. Quantification and functional characterization of antibodies to native aquaporin 4 in neuromyelitis optica. Arch Neurol. 2010;67:1201–8.

Kim SH, et al. Repeated treatment with rituximab based on the assessment of peripheral circulating memory B cells in patients with relapsing neuromyelitis optica over 2 years. Arch Neurol. 2011;68:1412–20.

Kim SH, et al. Does interferon beta treatment exacerbate neuromyelitis optica spectrum disorder? Mult Scler. 2012;18:1480–3. PubMed: 22354738.

Kim SH, et al. A 5-year follow-up of rituximab treatment in patients with neuromyelitis optica spectrum disorder. JAMA Neurol. 2013;70:1110–7.

Kimbrough DJ, et al. Treatment of neuromyelitis optica: review and recommendations. Mult Scler Relat Disord. 2012;1:180–7.

Kitley J, et al. Methotrexate is an alternative to azathioprine in neuromyelitis optica spectrum disorders with aquaporin-4 antibodies. J Neurol Neurosurg Psychiatry. 2013;84:918–21.

Kitley J, et al. Catastrophic brain relapse in seronegative NMO after a single dose of natalizumab. J Neurol Sci. 2014;339:223–5.

Kleiter I, et al. Failure of natalizumab to prevent relapses in neuromyelitis optica. Arch Neurol. 2012;69:239–45.

Magraner MJ, Coret F, Casanova B. The effect of intravenous immunoglobulin on neuromyelitis optica. Neurologia. 2013;28:65–72.

McKeon A, Fryer JP, Apiwattanakul M, Lennon VA, Hinson SR, Kryzer TJ, Lucchinetti CF, Weinshenker BG, Wingerchuk DM, Shuster EA, Pittock SJ. Diagnosis of neuromyelitis spectrum disorders: comparative sensitivities and specificities of immunohistochemical and immunoprecipitation assays. Arch Neurol. 2009;66:1134–8.

Merle H, et al. Treatment of optic neuritis by plasma exchange (add-on) in neuromyelitis optica. Arch Ophthalmol. 2012;130:858–62.

Min JH, Kim BJ, Lee KH. Development of extensive brain lesions following fingolimod (FTY720) treatment in a patient with neuromyelitis optica spectrum disorder. Mult Scler. 2012;18:113–5.

Miyamoto K, Kusunoki S. Intermittent plasmapheresis prevents recurrence in neuromyelitis optica. Ther Apher Dial. 2009;13:505–8.

Okada K, Tsuji S, Tanaka K. Intermittent intravenous immunoglobulin successfully prevents relapses of neuromyelitis optica. Intern Med. 2007;46:1671–2.

Palace J, Leite MI, Nairne A, Vincent A. Interferon beta treatment in neuromyelitis optica: increase in relapses and aquaporin 4 antibody titers. Arch Neurol. 2010;67:1016–7.

Papadopoulos CM, Bennett LJ, Verkman SA. Treatment of neuromyelitis optica: state-of-the-art and emerging therapies. Nat Rev Neurol. 2014;10:493–506.

Papeix C, Vidal JS, de Seze J, Pierrot-Deseilligny C, Tourbah A, Stankoff B, Lebrun C, Moreau T, Vermersch P, Fontaine B, Lyon-Caen O, Gout O. Immunosuppressive therapy is more effective than interferon in neuromyelitis optica. Mult Scler. 2007;13:256–9.

Paul F, Jarius S, Aktas O, Bluthner M, Bauer O, Appelhans H, Franciotta D, Bergamaschi R, Littleton E, Palace J, Seelig HP, Hohlfeld R, Vincent A, Zipp F. Antibody to aquaporin 4 in the diagnosis of neuromyelitis optica. PLoS Med. 2007;4:e133.

Petzold A, Pittock S, Lennon V, Maggiore C, Weinshenker BG, Plant GT. Neuromyelitis optica-IgG (aquaporin-4) autoantibodies in immune mediated optic neuritis. J Neurol Neurosurg Psychiatry. 2010;81:109–11.

Pittock SJ, et al. Eculizumab in AQP4-IgG-positive relapsing neuromyelitis optica spectrum disorders: an open-label pilot study. Lancet Neurol. 2013;12:554–62.

Saadoun S, Waters P, Bell BA, Vincent A, Verkman AS, Papadopoulos MC. Intra-cerebral injection of neuromyelitis optica immunoglobulin G and human complement produces neuromyelitis optica lesions in mice. Brain. 2010;133:349–61.

Sellner J, Boggild M, Clanet M, Hintzen RQ, Illes Z, Montalban X, Du Pasquier RA, Polman CH, Sorensen PS, Hemmer B. EFNS guidelines on diagnosis and management of neuromyelitis optica. Eur J Neurol. 2010;17:1019–32.

Shimizu J, et al. IFNß-1b may severely exacerbate Japanese optic-spinal MS in neuromyelitis optica spectrum. Neurology. 2010;75:1423–7.

Trebst C, et al. Update on the diagnosis and treatment of neuromyelitis optica: recommendations of the Neuromyelitis Optica Study Group (NEMOS). J Neurol. 2014;261:1–16.

Warabi Y, Matsumoto Y, Hayashi H. Interferon beta-1b exacerbates multiple sclerosis with severe optic nerve and spinal cord demyelination. J Neurol Sci. 2007;252:57–61.

Watanabe S, et al. Low-dose corticosteroids reduce relapses in neuromyelitis optica: a retrospective analysis. Mult Scler. 2007;13:968–74.

Wingerchuk DM, Lennon VA, Lucchinetti CF, Pittock SJ, Weinshenker BG. The spectrum of neuromyelitis optica. Lancet Neurol. 2007a;6:805–15.

Wingerchuk DM, et al. A secondary progressive clinical course is uncommon in neuromyelitis optica. Neurology. 2007b;68:603–5.

Yaguchi H, et al. Efficacy of intravenous cyclophosphamide therapy for neuromyelitis optica spectrum disorder. Intern Med. 2013;52:969–72. PubMed: 23648715.

Acquired Inflammatory Diseases of the Optic Nerve: From the Neuro-Ophthalmologist's Approach

42

Judit Somlai

Contents

Multiple sclerosis is the most frequent inflammatory disease of the central nervous system, frequent initial symptoms of which develop due to the involvement of the visual system. Neuropathological and neurological characteristics of inflammatory diseases of the central nervous system and up-to-date information about Devic's disease are discussed in Chap. 1.1.2 as well as in Chaps. 40 and 41, respectively. Subacute unilateral deterioration of vision in young adulthood is most frequently caused by retrobulbar neuritis developing in the antechiasmal segment of the optic nerve. According to an English study, the visual pathway lesion is the first sign of multiple sclerosis in 50–98 % of the cases. The other ocular symptom of MS that starts with loss of visual acuity and double vision together with other neurological signs indicating the functional impairment of the eye movement system is less frequently noticed in the clinical practice.

J. Somlai, M.D.
Unit of Neuro-Ophthalmology, Department of Neurology and Stroke, Military Hospital, Budapest, Hungary

Neuro-Ophthalmology Section, Hungarian Ophthalmological Association, Budapest, Hungary

Trustee, NOSZA Foundation (for the Prevention and Screening of Ocular Storke), Budapest, Hungary
e-mail: dr@somlaijudit.hu; http://somlaijudit.hu

Clinical Features of Optic Neuritis

The first symptoms that make the patient seek the ophthalmologist or neurologist include the unilateral central *blurred vision* or central 'blinding white light' and subsequently a *central defect in the visual field*, which predominantly results in a deterioration of near vision, and a disturbance of the recognition of letter. In contrast with the subjective complaints due to circulatory disorders, the symptoms are not transient but gradually increase and can lead even to complete amaurosis in the absence of therapy. The degree of visual loss ranges from blurry central vision to the most severe deterioration of visual acuity, the *slight light perception in the periphery*. The ability to perceive some light generally remains, which has a differential diagnostic significance since in case of traumatic optic lesions and the embolization of central retinal artery the remaining light perception can also vanish. At the early stage of this inflammatory disease, as a consequence of the deterioration of colour perception, the patients perceive their environment as grayish and dim,

J. Somlai, T. Kovács (eds.), *Neuro-Ophthalmology*, DOI 10.1007/978-3-319-28956-4_42

and the contours of the objects become blurred in the pathological side. The impairment of binocular vision leads to a disturbance in depth perception. The patients often complain of a change in the intensity of light in the affected side, for instance they feel as if the lighting of the room were dim in the affected side.

The deterioration of vision is accompanied in 90 % of the cases by acute pain increasing due to eye movement and radiating to the rim of the orbit. In such a case, the exclusion of local causes (e.g., iridocyclitis) or periorbital paranasal sinusitis is essential. The appearance of symptoms due to conduction disturbance or conduction block provoked by sun bathing, fever or physical exercise is a common sign in demyelinating diseases, which may also be associated with impaired vision (*Uhthoff's sign*, cannot be regarded as a relapse). It is generally accepted that symptomatic therapy is sufficient in such cases because of the different pathomechanism.

Clinical Signs and Their Appropriate Tests

The ocular complaints of the patient can be confirmed or excluded by instrumental examinations. The decrease in ***visual acuity for distant*** can be examined even bedside by asking the patient to read our fingers from a few meters distance, whereas ***near vision*** can be examined by making the patient read a newspaper. The ophthalmological examination starts with the assessment of visual acuity for distant by the use of a vision chart viewed from five meters. The near vision can be examined by the most widely used traditional Csapody chart, making the patient read its lines written with a gradually decreasing font size. (Csapody XIII-VI). A quantitative decrease in visual acuity can be the first sign of the disease, whereas an increase can be the first sign of symptomatic relief. However, impaired conduction of the visual pathway as well as an improvement in the disease can be tested by a more sensitive and rather precise method, the measurement of the ***critical fusion frequency*** (***CFF***) value. A value below 20–25 Hz (the normal value is 40 Hz) is sure sign of dysfunction due to inflammatory symptoms. Whereas the increase of Hz value during treatment is a clear sign of improvement. The ***Visual Evoked Potential*** (***VEP***) ***test*** is the most sensitive method to assess the conduction disturbance of the optic nerve. The records can be used to adequately document the changes in both the latency and amplitude values of the waves during the clinical events. The clinical significance and the methodological basis of VEP examination is discussed in details in Chaps. 16 and 37).

Acquired disorders of ***colour vision*** can vary from a decreased tone to complete color blindness. Its widely available screening tools are the color vision charts (e.g., Ishihara chart). The examination of ***pupillomotor function*** requires minimal instrumental background. Lesions of any origin affecting the fibers of the antechiasmal segment of the optic nerve cause the dysfunction of the afferent pupillomotor pathway passes next to the optic nerve up until the chiasm. Therefore, a conduction disturbance in the afferent pupillomotor fibers can predict the progressive antechiasmal optic nerve disease. The slightest degree of papillary dysfunction can be detected by the ***swinging flashlight test***. The two eyes are flashed in an alternating manner and the initial pupillary constriction is followed by a re-dilation in the affected side still shone into by direct light. (The dysfunction results in an inability to keep the pupil constricted in the absence of incoming stimulus.) The occurrence of the phenomenon not only due to swinging flashlights but even due to an alternating covering of the eyes may indicate a marked optic injury (Fig. 42.1).

This is called ***Marcus-Gunn's phenomenon***, and its degree can be scored from the slightest +1 to a more severe +3 value. The most severe injury, the complete amaurosis, is indicated by the ***amaurotic fixed pupil***, associating with absent direct and intact indirect pupillary responses. The diagnostic inventory of pupillomotor dysfunctions and diseases of the pathway system are discussed in details in Chaps. 23 and 52. In optic neuropathies due to inflammatory processes, **visual field defects** are typically found within 30°, and are also known as ***central*** (***or centrocoecal***) ***scotomata*** of the visual field. The clinical signs are

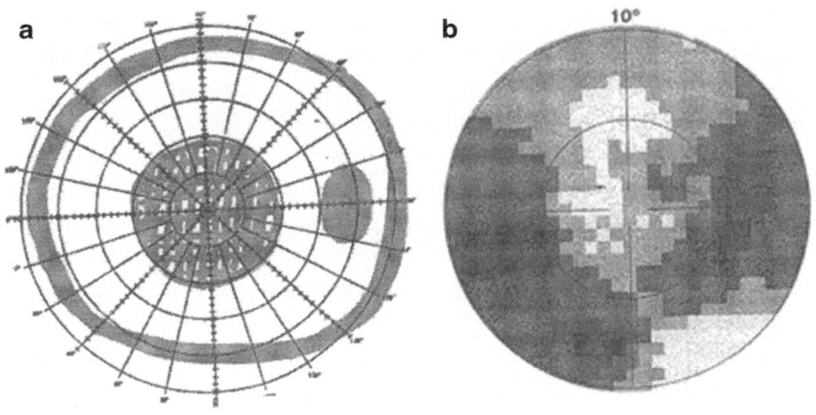

Fig. 42.1 Characteristic perimetry result of optic neuritis: central and subsequently centrocoecal scotoma as a consequence of a dysfunction in macular and subsequently papillomacular nerve fibers. (**a**) Central scotoma on Bjerrum's screen. (**b**) Central scotoma precisely detected by computer perimetry

caused by the rapidly developing dysfunction of macular and papillomacular nerve fibers as a consequence of the underlying disease.

Regression of the central scotoma is a measure of adequate therapy. If no change occurs, examinations should be extended to look for compressive or circulatory etiologies. The distinction of optic neuritis from prechiasmal optic or chiasmal lesions by ophthalmological methods is essential in differential diagnostic point of view. The latter can develop due to the compressive effect a slowly enlarging frontobasal meningioma or a tuberculum sellae meningioma. While optic neuritis mostly leads to a relative and later absolute central scotoma, prechiasmal/chiasmal lesions are characterized by a unilateral central scotoma accompanied by a simultaneously appearing visual field defect in the upper temporal quadrant of the contralateral eye (also known as junction scotoma) in the beginning of the chiasmal lesion. Therefore, examinations of the central and peripheral fields of vision should always be performed in both eyes! The precise diagnostics of visual field defects are discussed in details in the chapter reviewing compressive optic neuropathies, found in Chap. 47. Clinical signs leading to bilateral central blindness are characterized by symmetrical bilaterally present centrocecal absolute scotomata, which is mostly a consequence of toxic amblyopia. This is discussed in details in Chap. 49. If inflammation of the papilla starts in the area of the optic disc, the blurred disc is associated with blind spot enlargement and rapid loss of vision. In case these symptoms are bilaterally present with preserved visual functions and an almost equal bilateral blind spot enlargement, the possibility of papilledema due to intracranial hypertension should be considered. Optic neuritis can temporarily present with a similar visual field defect as seen in an optic lesion of vascular origin, i.e., a unilateral defect of the lower nasal quadrant. However, the central field of vision is mostly preserved in case of a circulatory disturbance, whereas in case of an inflammation, the central loss of vision is present and progresses from the onset in combination with an absolute central scotoma. The possibilities of the differentiation of central es peripheral alterations by perimetry examinations are discussed in details in Chap. 17.

On fundoscopic examination, according to the classical definition, 'neither the patient nor the examining doctor can see anything', which means that in the acute phase, the optic disc has sharp margins, it still appears to be hyperaemic and does not protrude. Therefore, the patients' complaints can only be confirmed or excluded by the above mentioned functional examinations. During the subsequent chronic and recurrent processes of the disease, a temporal pallor or after several acute exacerbations the ***pallor papilla*** of the complete surface of the optic disc can be noticed. In such cases, signs of significant nerve fiber destruction can be observed, manifesting in both visual dysfunction and in the records of the electrophysiological test (VEP; prolonged latency, reduced amplitude).

However, care should be taken during the assessment of fundoscopic findings. Fundoscopic appearance of a physiologically paler myopic optic disc or childhood discs misdiagnosed as 'atrophy' or 'pallor of MS origin' in the absence of comprehensive examinations cause a life-long and erasable stigmatisation for our patients. Therefore, the application of sound and most objective examination methods of the most up-to-date functions are essential before establishing any diagnosis.

If the pathomechanism involves the intraocular segment of the optic nerve in the clinical entity called ***inflammation of the optic nerve head*** ('papillitis nervi optici'), the dysfunction reminiscent of that above is accompanied by a slightly prominent disc, and funduscopy can also reveal neuroretinitis as a consequence of the process spreading in the peripapillar area. Perimetry result of 'enlarged blind spot' visual field defect with or without central scotoma indicates an inflammatory process ongoing within the optic disc. Such a clinical course can be seen bilaterally in childhood, most probably due to a more pronounced susceptibility to develop edema. Papillitis can be accompanied, though infrequently, by an inflammation ongoing also in the peripheral part of the retina, which is characterized by sheathing of the peripheral segments of retinal venules, and the presence of peripheral inflammatory foci (lesions resembling snowballs and snowbanks, etc.), collectively termed pars planitis. It is mostly seen as an ocular symptom in autoimmune diseases of the young. The precise diagnosis and the most up-to-date and still unique local therapy of this disease were first introduced in Europe by the late Janos Gal MD, head of department. (OSZI issue 1984). In addition to the functional measurements of fundoscopic alterations, the novel ophthalmological examinations (e.g., FLAG, ICG, OCT, HRT, etc.) and the evolution of electrophysiological methods represent an enormous help in the differential diagnosis for the clinicians. Among neuroradiological procedures, the novel methods of cranial MRI can help the clinicians in the confirmation or exclusion of demyelinating processes with monosymptomatic onset (See in Chap. 31).

Differential Diagnosis of Antechiasmal Optic Pathway Diseases

The differential diagnosis includes optic pathway diseases in the background of which systemic diseases can often be revealed. The main groups of antechiasmal optic diseases:

1. Hereditary optic atrophies (Table 42.1)
2. Heredodegenerative syndromes (Fig. 42.2)
3. Acquired antechiasmal optic lesions (Table 42.2)

The most frequent causes of retrobulbar neuritis and the most frequent diseases leading to consequent optic atrophy -differential diagnosis:

- Demyelinating diseases (MS, NMO)
- Complication of autoimmune diseases (SLE, antiphospholipid syndrome)
- Complications of childhood viral infections (chicken pox, rubella, mumps)
- Postinfectious neuritis (herpes zoster, infectious mononucleosis)
- Meningitis, orbital inflammation and paranasal sinusitis
- Complication of granulomatous inflammations (TBC, sarcoidosis, HIV infection)
- Consequence of intraocular inflammation
- Unknown origin

Diseases with similar clinical symptomatic onset leading to optic atrophy:

- Leber's hereditary optic atrophy (LHON) and relevant heredodegenerative optic atrophies
- Anterior ischemic optic neuropathy (AION)
- Optic lesions of nutritional and toxic origin

Exploration of pathological processes leading to antechiasmal optic fiber lesions is frequently rather difficult, requires the cooperation of several specialties and is, therefore, a rather time-consuming task. This may result in a delay in the initiation of adequate therapy, which may lead to an irreversible deterioration of vision. Therefore, the significance of differential diagnostic

Table 42.1 The most important hereditary optic atrophies

Etiology	Dominant	Recessive		Cytoplasm disease
Type	Juvenile	Behr's type	Diabetes mellitus	Leber's type (LHON)
Age (years)	4–8	1–9	6–14	18–30
Visual acuity	0.1–0.5	0.1	HMV – 0.05	HMV – 0.1
Nystagmus	None	present (50 %)	None	None
Optic disc pallor	Temporal	Temporal	Complete	Complete
Colour vision disturbance	+/–	+/–	+++	Centrális++
Progression	Mild	None	Significant	Stationary/progression

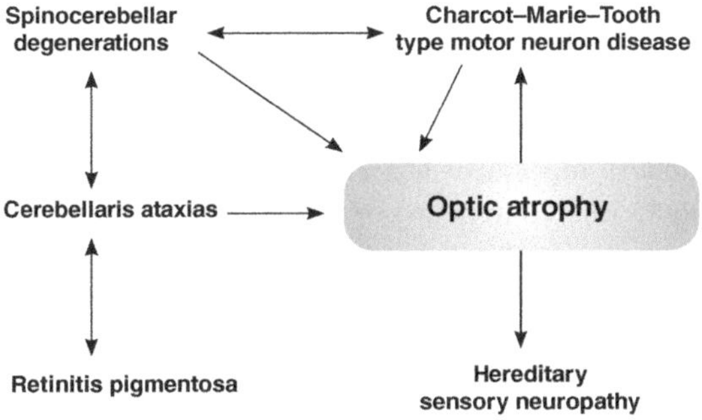

Fig. 42.2 The connection between heredodegenerative syndromes and optic atrophies

approaches is high in this group of diseases, even though the ocular symptoms are similar or almost equivalent. Retrobulbar neuritis is a manifestation of ***multiple sclerosis*** in the vast majority of patients younger than 40 years, which may as well be the first symptom.

In the group of ***autoimmune diseases***, the involvement of the optic nerve can be noticed in the primary and secondary forms of systemic lupus erythematosus (SLE) and antiphospholipid syndrome, and in many cases the ocular symptom was the first warning sign of the beginning of a systemic disease. In addition to these, uni- or bilateral involvement of the optic nerve has been described and we have also noticed in our own patients in association with Sjogren's syndrome, Hashimoto's thyreoiditis and ulcerative colitis (inflammatory bowel diseases).

Among ***infectious diseases***, retrobulbar neuritis can develop as a consequence of chicken pox, mumps, herpes zoster and infectious momonucleosis. The deterioration of vision appears approximately 10–14 days following the onset of skin symptoms. Papillitis is frequently present in the second stage of Lyme borreliosis in association with chorioretinitis (also known as posterior uveitis). Serological positivity, however, does not per se represent a diagnosis. Papillitis of the optic nerve can also develop due to Toxoplasma or Toxocara infection in association with extensive chorioretinitis.

Optic neuritis developing as a consequence of inflammations infiltrating the orbit can also evolve as a complication of untreated, late-recognized ***severe purulent inflammation of the orbital cavity, the paranasal sinuses and/or the meninges***. It is highly important from differential diagnostic point of view and cannot be overemphasized that symptoms of chronic inflammations can mask the underlying slowly enlarging compressive processes, which may continuously enlarge for decades. We should think of such underlying diseases in case of every obscure therapy-resistant processes, e.g., paraclinoid aneurysm, tuberculum sellae meningioma and parasellar pituitary tumor. The compressive optic processes are discussed in details in Chap. 47.

Leber's hereditary optic neuropathy (***LHON***) is a maternally inherited disease, which (predominantly) affects male patients, and is characterized by optic atrophy evoked by mitochondrial dysfunction. The atrophy is not accompanied by other neurological signs or symptoms and is almost exclusively bilateral. It irreversibly and severely deteriorates the central vision and is not influenced by steroid therapy. In the early stage, fundoscopic findings include peripapillary telangiectasias as well as an enlargement of optic the nerve fibers; however, papilledema cannot be observed (pseudoedema), which can be confirmed by angiography, as there is no leakage of dye from the blood vessel walls. Subsequently, the pallor of the optic disc extends to its whole surface due to the excessive degeneration of nerve fibers. This is by then accompanied by centrocecal scotoma in the field of vision as a progression of central scotoma, which causes an irreversible deterioration of central vision in both eyes. Being a genetic disease, neurogenetic examination has differential diagnostic value. Characteristics of the most important hereditary optic atrophies that are essential in differential diagnostic point of view and their interconnections are presented in Figs. 42.2 and are discussed in Chap. 6.

The differentiation of an antechiasmal optic nerve abnormality due to ***anterior ischemic optic neuropathy*** (*AION*) from that due to an inflammatory process can be based on clinical signs, e.g., the multiple occurrence of amaurosis fugax – transient losses of vision – as opposed to a progressive loss of central vision. Contrasting with the central scotoma due to inflammatory processes, the circulatory disorder of the retina and optic nerve head, following an initial central loss of vision, leads to a lower nasal quadrant anopsy that is essential for reading; therefore, it results in difficulties in recognition, reading and near manipulations. This group of disease is discussed in details in Chap. 45. Similarly to the papillitis of the optic nerve, intracranial hypertension begins with the development of papilledema. The ocular symptoms are discussed in details in Chap. 50 (Table 42.2).

Optic lesions of nutritional and toxic origin may mostly be caused by nicotine and/or alcohol, and frequently by illicit drug abuse. The patient's general history, the characteristic visual field defect (bilateral centrocecal scotoma), and the intractable deterioration of central vision together with the ineffectiveness of steroid therapy support the toxic origin. This group of diseases is discussed in details in Chap. 4.2.5 from page 254.

The differential diagnosis of ocular symptoms indicating an inflammatory process of the antechiasmal optic nerve and the identification of the underlying cause are among the most difficult tasks related to neuro-ophthalmological diseases. Symptomatology of inflammatory optic disc diseases and disorders with similar appearance are presented in (Table 42.2) and are discussed extensively the next chapter about diseases of the antechiasmal optic nerve.

In the past decades, therapeutic principles of retrobulbar neuritis due to multiple sclerosis were equivalent with the therapeutic protocol of neurological diseases due to systemic demyelination. This is true for high-dose steroid therapy as well as the combined, yearly updated and more and more modern immunosuppressive therapies that were established to decrease the frequency of acute exacerbations and to maintain remission. These therapies are discussed in details in the

Table 42.2 Differential diagnosis: optic neuritis, papilledema and anterior ischemic optic neuropathy

	Optic neuritis	Papilledema	Anterior ischemic optic neuropathy (AION)
Loss of vision	Central	None	Progressive
Other symptoms and signs	Pain on eye movement	Headache, vomiting, obscuration	Headache, pain in the eye
Laterality	Unilateral	Bilateral	Uni- then bilateral (pseudo-Foster–Kennedy syndrome)
Pupillary signs	+/– Marcus-Gunn	Normal responses	+/– Marcus-Gunn
Visual acuity	Significantly decreased	Intact for a long time	Significantly decreased
Fundoscopic appearance	*Neuritis*: normal *papillitis*: edematous	Progressive prominent papilla	Acute: mild papilledema chronic: optic disc pallor
Field of vision	*Neuritis*: central scotoma *papillitis*: enlarged blind spot	Significant blind spot enlargement	Quadrantanopia +/– centrocecal scotoma
Prognosis	Vision returns	Intact visual functions	Irreversible loss of vision

review prepared by heads of neuroimmunological centers (See in Chaps. 40 and 41).

Similarly to optic diseases of vascular, compressive or traumatic origin, the diagnosis, the therapy and the often lifelong caregiving of the patient can only be realized by a *team* of specialists, such as neurologist, ophthalmologist, electrophysiologist, neuroradiologist and internal medicine specialist-immunologist.

Further Readings

Beck RW, et al. The effect of corticosteroids of acute optic neuritis on the subsequent development of multiplex sclerosis. N Engl J Med. 1993;329:1764–9.

Clanet RQ, Hintzen Z, Illes X, Montalban RA, Du Pasquier CH, Polman PS, Sorensen B. Hemmer: EFNS guidelines on diagnosis and management of neuromyelitis optica, EFNS guidelines/CME article Journal compilation 2010 EFNS (1019).

Fazekas F, Komoly S, et al. Intravenous immunoglobulin in relapsing-remitting multiple sclerosis: a dose-finding trial. Neurology. 2008;71(4):265–71.

Gal RL, Vedula SS, Beck R. Corticosteroids for treating optic neuritis. Cochrane Database Syst Rev. 2012;(4):CD001430.

Glaser JS. Neuritis retrobulbaris. In: Neuroophthalmology. Philadelphia: JB Lippincott Comp; 1990. p. 69–110.

Goodin DS, Frohman EM, Garmany Jr GP, et al. Disease modifying therapies in multiple sclerosis: report of the Therapeutics and Technology Assessment Subcommittee of the American Academy of Neurology and the MS Council for Clinical Practice Guidelines. Neurology. 2002;58:169–78.

IFNB Multiplex Sclerosis Study Group: interferon beta 1b is effective in relapsing-remitting multiplex sclerosis. Clinical results of a multicenter, randomized, doubled-blind, placebo-controlled trial. Neurology. 1993;43: 655–61.

Lublin FD, Reingold SC. Defining the clinical course of multiple sclerosis: results of an international survey. National Multiple Sclerosis Society (USA) Advisory Committee on clinical trials of new agents in multiple sclerosis. Neurology. 1996;46:907–11.

McDonald WI, Compston A, Edan G, et al. Recommended diagnostic criteria for multiple sclerosis: guidelines from the International Panel on the Diagnosis of Multiple Sclerosis. Ann Neurol. 2001;50:121–7.

Rieckmann P, Toyka KV, Bassetti C, et al. Escalating immunotherapy of multiple sclerosis – new aspects and practical application. J Neurol. 2004;251: 1329–39.

Sellebjerg F, Barnes D, Filippini G, et al. EFNS guideline on treatment of multiple sclerosis relapses: report of an EFNS task force on treatment of multiple sclerosis relapses. Eur J Neurol. 2005;12:939–46.

Vascular Diseases of the Optic Nerve: Internal Medicine Aspects

43

György Pfliegler

Contents

Blood vessels supplying ocular structures originate from the internal carotid artery, so the blood supply of the eyes and the brain are closely connected. The various branches of the ophthalmic artery (central retinal artery, short and long posterior ciliary arteries, lacrimal artery, anterior ciliary artery) originating from the internal carotid artery and the corresponding veins are responsible for supplying the region indicated by their name. In rare cases, when the ophthalmic artery is absent, the medial meningeal artery performs the same task. The uvea is supplied by the ciliary artery, and the retina gets its blood supply from the branches of the central retinal artery. The posterior ciliary arteries (that supply the optic disc) and the central retinal artery (that supplies the medial two-thirds of the retina) are the first arteries to branch off the ophthalmic artery that enters through the optic foramen. The central retinal artery divides into superior temporal, inferior temporal and nasal branches. The next vessels to branch off are the long posterior ciliary arteries that supply the peripheral parts of the choroidea, the ciliary body and the iris. The last branch is that of the anterior ciliary arteries. Venous drainage from the retina is carried out by the central retinal vein and its smaller branches that have the same name and course as the corresponding arteries. The vorticose veins drain the choroidea towards the inferior and superior ophthalmic vein and the cavernous sinus. The capillary network between the retinal arteries and veins serves to ensure overly efficient oxygen and nutrient exchange. It is only the macula lutea (responsible for acute vision) and the fovea centralis that have no capillaries. Another special feature of these vessels is that retinal blood vessels have the same structure as cervical ones, and it is also true for uveal and extracranial vessels. These veins and arteries are located very close to each other, sometimes in the same adventitia sheath.

Syndromes developing as a result of circulatory disorders of the eyes (***ocular ischemic syndromes***) are rather difficult to review, especially for those not specialized in ophthalmology. Therefore, first we should interpret the terminology used in scientific literature (Table 43.1). However, in order to set up the differential diagnosis, we have to emphasize that the symptoms do not only mean loss of vision due to circulatory disorders of hematological or hemostaseological

---

G. Pfliegler, M.D., med. habil.
Department of Rare Diseases, 2nd Department of Internal Medicine, Institute for Internal Medicine, Medical and Health Center, University of Debrecen, Debrecen, Hungary
e-mail: g.pfliegler@gmail.com

J. Somlai, T. Kovács (eds.), *Neuro-Ophthalmology*, DOI 10.1007/978-3-319-28956-4_43

Table 43.1 Ophthalmological diseases of vascular origin

Severity and duration of the symptoms	(a) Transient blurred vision (b) Amaurosis fugax (c) Permanent loss of vision (infarction of the optic nerve)
Consequences	(a) Anterior ischemic optic neuropathy (AION) Arteritic (AAION) Non-Arteritic (NAION) (b) Posterior ischemic optic neuropathy (PION)
Etiology (cause of occlusion)	(a) Thrombosis/embolism (b) Damage to vessel wall (vasculitis: autoimmune, infection, arteriosclerosis, diabetes, etc.)
Affected vessel	(a) Retinal artery Central retinal artery occlusion (CRAO) Occlusion of arterial branch (CRABO: temporal or nasal branch) (b) Short posterior ciliary artery AAION, NAION (c) Long posterior ciliary artery PION (d) Retinal artery Central retinal vein occlusion (CRVO) Occlusion of venous branch (CRVBO: temporal or nasal branch)

origin. Sudden loss of vision can develop, for example, as a result of cholesterol crystals (Hollenhorst's plaque) getting stuck at arterial bifurcations. Emboli of septic or tumorous origin may also obstruct vessels, and there are also local causes, e.g., glaucoma. Rarely, loss of vision can also be caused by the orbital compartment syndrome (long-lasting spinal anesthesia, surgeries performed in the Trendelenburg's position), which leads to the development of tamponade due to increased orbital pressure. Circulatory disorders (e.g., the occlusion of fundal veins) can develop in hematological diseases associated with paraproteinemia (multiple myeloma, Waldenstrom's macroglobulinemia, hyperlipidemia, multiple sclerosis, cryoglobulinemia). We have to consider blindness caused by a blunt blow to the eyeball (e.g., ball) and pseudoblindness in psychiatric diseases.

Ocular ischemic syndrome (OIS) is a collective term for ocular signs and symptoms that usually develop as a result of chronic circulatory disorders. *As a general rule, we can say* that damage to the anterior segment is associated with cataract, inflammation and neovascularization of the iris, while damage to the posterior segment is accompanied by narrow retinal arteries, dilated but not spiral fundal veins, hemorrhages, cotton wool spots and neovascularization of the optic nerve. Symptoms are usually painless.

Sudden Loss of Vision

A frequent descriptive term (group of symptoms) that does not refer to the cause. There are various degrees of severity based on the symptoms: *transient blurred vision* (*transient visual obscuration*; *TVO*) that lasts for a few seconds, papilledema usually the result of increased intracranial pressure. *Amaurosis fugax* means an episode of partial or complete *blindness* that is usually unilateral and lasts for seconds or minutes. In case of *transient visual loss* (TVL), the episode is more severe; the developing blindness is complete, and it lasts for some minutes or longer. TVL can affect only one (monocular) or both eyes (binocular). The most severe, irreversible loss of vision is caused by *infarction of the optic nerve*.

From an *etiological* point of view, similarly to other organs, circulatory disorders of the fundus can be classified according to the type of the blood vessel that has been affected by the occlusion/circulatory disorder (arterial: anterior or posterior ciliary arteries, central retinal artery or one of its branches; venous: central retinal vein or one of its branches).

Anterior ischemic optic neuropathy (*AION*): two forms are known. *Non-arteritic optic neuropathy* (*NAION*) more commonly affects older patients of European origin, while giant cell *arteritic* (*temporal artery*) *optic neuropathy* (*AAION*) tends to develop in younger patients. If we consider case numbers, the incidence of NAION is higher than that of AAION. The female:male ratio is only slightly higher in NAION, but it is 2:1 in AAION. NAION usually manifests as a sudden, painless loss of vision in the early morning hours. Its annual incidence over 50 is 1/10,000. AAION; however, is of inflammatory origin, thus the affected blood vessel (temporal artery) is painful to touch and the patient also experiences difficulty chewing and fever. According to observations, in prolonged cases of AION several blood vessels can be affected and the aneurysm of the abdominal aorta is more common. The condition is caused by *occlusion of the posterior ciliary arteries* and it is characterized by pale papilledema, hemorrhages and cotton wool exudates. The loss of vision develops suddenly and improvement cannot be expected in the first weeks or months. Regardless of the trigger factor, the blood supply of the posterior ciliary arteries that supply the optic nerve decreases, which will eventually lead to the atrophy of the nerve. As here, at the exit, the nerve is surrounded by glia only, its volume can increase (edema) and this phenomenon can be noted on ophthalmoscopy. The background of NAION contains both hereditary (certain HLA constellations, Scandinavian origin, thrombophilia, glucose-6-phosphate dehydrogenase deficiency, sickle cell anemia, etc.) and acquired (vasculitis; autoimmune diseases including the rare Susac's syndrome; systemic diseases, such as diabetes mellitus, hypertension, arteriosclerosis, polycythaemia vera, shock; medications like phosphodiesterase-5 inhibitors, such as sildenafil; cryoglobulinaemia, paraproteinaemia, etc.) factors. In a young female patient of ours we detected NAION associated with chronic hepatitis C. The most likely factor is the combined effect of coagulation, inflammation, atherosclerosis and sometimes infections. The contribution of these components varies from patient to patient just like the actual *trigger factors*. In spite of this, a significant number of cases is still termed 'idiopathic' even today.

In ***posterior ischemic optic neuropathy*** (***PION***) the lesion affects the deeper ciliary arteries; therefore, papilledema usually remains hidden for ophthalmoscopy. However, regardless of whether the edema is inside or outside the bony foramen, it will still hinder blood flow thereby causing a vicious circle.

Occlusion of the central retinal artery (**OCRA**) can be caused by embolism, thrombosis or endothelial inflammation. It is characterized by pain on the affected side and *sudden loss of vision*, which is often preceded by attacks of transient blindness (*amaurosis fugax*). The resulting loss of vision covers almost the complete field of vision; sometimes there are some remaining peripheral or paracentral islands of vision and patients can also perceive light and hand movements. The ophthalmoscopic view features narrow arteries, thick sludge, cherry-colored macula and the retina is initially normal-appearing, then becomes pale, greyish-white and swollen. If there is a cilioretinal artery, the area supplied by it (papillomacular region) is spared. The embolus can originate from the carotid artery, aortic arch or chambers of the heart but the occlusion may also be caused by tumor cells. Thrombosis can develop locally, and it is not uncommon to find congenital and/or acquired thrombophilia in the background. Vasculitis can also be the cause of the occlusion, regardless of its etiology (e.g., giant cell, autoimmune, infectious, etc.). Unfortunately – just like in venous thromboembolism – iatrogenic cases are becoming more frequent (e.g., carotid angiography, angioplasty, chiropractic adjustment, retrobulbar injection, irradiation, etc.). The symptoms of ***arterial branch occlusion*** (***RABO***) depend on which branch has become occluded. Afferent pupillary defect is typical. The ophthalmoscopic view is similar to that in OCRA but the extent is smaller. The most likely trigger factor is embolism.

Occlusion of the central retinal vein (***CRVO***) mostly develops at the level of or behind the lamina crimrosa, as here the vein runs together with the central retinal artery in the same, narrow adventitia sheath, thus its damage (e.g., high blood pressure, rigidity due to arteriosclerosis, thickening of the wall) hinders normal blood flow. Apart from that, thrombi or emboli can cause occlusion as well. The clinical picture is characterized by painless loss of vision, diffuse fundal hemorrhages, dilated, tortuous veins, soft cotton wool exudates and papilledema. The hemorrhage affects the macula as well. Later typical neovascularization will develop in the optic disc, retina or iris. Late complications can be secondary glaucoma, vitreous body bleeding or even retinal detachment. We can distinguish between severe (multiple soft foci, extensive hemorrhages, areas with no circulation) and mild, non-ischemic forms, which are also called impending occlusion, partial or venous stasis retinopathy in scientific literature. ***Occlusion of venous branches*** (***OVB***) has a less severe course. Venous occlusions are similar to diabetic retinopathies; sometimes there are overlaps as well. For the differential diagnosis we have to remember that venous occlusion is bilateral and associated with dot- or pool-like hemorrhages. Lesions caused by hypertension also tend to be bilateral and characterized by markedly narrow arterioles and hemorrhages that do not respect areas supplied by certain vessels and spread horizontally. According to Hayreh's survey, the most common systemic diseases in occlusion of the central or hemicentral retinal vein are hypertension, diabetes mellitus and ischemic heart diseases. If only one of the branches is obstructed the order of trigger factors is the following: arterial hypertension, cerebrovascular diseases, chronic obstructive pulmonary diseases, peptic ulcer, juvenile diabetes and thyroid disorders.

Diagnostic Tasks

Diseases affecting ocular blood vessels — even if they are prominent – always have to be treated as *symptoms*, and a thorough internal medicine and neurological examination has to be performed besides the detailed ophthalmological one (intraocular pressure, ophthalmoscopy with dilated pupils, fluorescein angiography, electroretinogram, etc., — for detailed description see other chapters). For an easier overview of the recommended algorithm see Table 43.2. Naturally, not every patient needs all examinations. The assessment always has to be tailored to the individual patient and situation. So, for example in a young, otherwise healthy patient with a positive family history and/or contraceptive use thrombophilia has to be in the focus, older, female patients with migraine should be assessed for giant cell arteri-

Table 43.2 Additional investigations to be performed in case of an ophthalmic vascular event

Investigations to be performed in every patient	
History taking	Hereditary diseases/tendency, previous incidents/diseases, medications, etc.
Physical examination	Obesity, circulatory disorder, aneurysm, blood pressure (bilateral!), arrhythmia, cardiac murmur, carotid bruit, etc
Routine laboratory tests liver- and kidney function tests, glucose (diabetes)	Blood count (leukemia, anemia), ESR, CRP (inflammation)
Instrumental investigations	Blood pressure measurement (both arms), EKG, echocardiography (transthoracic) and carotid Doppler (source of embolism), chest X-ray, cervical and abdominal ultrasound (cancer screening)
Targeted investigations:	
Special laboratory investigations (if a certain syndrome is suspected)	Tumor markers, hormone levels (thyroid disorders, immunoglobulins, electrophoresis, antibodies, infections (e.g., toxoplasmosis, viruses), etc.
Screening for thrombophilia (in predisposed patients: young age, family history, use of contraceptives)	*Congenital thrombophilia*
	Prothrombotic factors: FII polymorphism, FV Leiden, FVIIIC, Lp(a), homocysteine (MTHFR), 'sticky platelet syndrome'
Endogenous anticoagulants	AT, PC, PS deficiency, *Acquired thrombophilia*
	Lupus anticoagulant, anticardiolipin antibodies, etc
Instrumental investigations, imaging scans (in case of suspicion)	Blood pressure monitoring (ABPM; non-fixed hypertension),
	Holter monitoring (paroxysmal arrhythmia), CT, MRI (cerebral accidents, tumor, developmental abnormalities), CTA (carotid stenosis, plaque), echocardiography (transesophageal if malformations or thrombus in the auricle is suspected), temporal artery biopsy (if giant cell arteritis is suspected)

tis, while atrial fibrillation *mainly* warrants a cardiological and endocrinological evaluation. However, we must never forget that a detected cause or disease does not provide protection against other causes, and the combination of congenital and acquired factors is not uncommon. Similarly to most diseases, vascular disorders of the eyes are ***multicausal***. No matter what modern technologies are available, a careful and thorough ***history*** is still the most important element of the diagnosis. It has to cover family history (thrombosis, diabetes, hypertension, hereditary diseases), environmental factors (visit in tropical countries, hygiene, occupation, pets) lifestyle (diet including nutritional supplements, vitamins, trace elements, potency pills (!), previous or current concomitant diseases, surgeries, infections, sport/injuries, accidents, etc.) ***Physical examination*** will give us information about blood pressure, arrhythmia, heart murmur or some typical anatomical changes, etc.

Treatment, Prevention

Unfortunately, there is no single way of management that would certainly be successful. However, just like in all other diseases, it is important to treat all recognized underlying diseases and reduce risk factors. Ophthamological management procedures (eye massage, paracentesis of the anterior chamber, local thrombolysis, intravenous acetazolamide, carbogen therapy, hyperbaric oxygen therapy, osmotic diuretics, beta blockers, sympathomimetic drugs, steroids, decompression and other surgical interventions, etc.) are not going to be described in this chapter, partly because they are applied in the first session of ophthalmological care, and partly because they are beyond the author's competence. The continuous care of the patient needs the close cooperation of the internist, family physician, cardiologist (or other specialists) and ophthalmologist in order to monitor and control blood pressure, glucose and lipid levels, diet and lifestyle, and to perform plasmapheresis if necessary. As regards anticoagulant and antiplatelet therapy and secondary prevention, based on previous cooperation with ophthalmologists and favorable experience, we think that if ischemic/thrombotic origin is obvious, prophylactic, low molecular weight heparin and antiplatelet therapy (e.g.,. 100 mg aspirin or 75 mg clopidogrel) is justified as initial therapy. Later, if severe thrombophilia is confirmed (e.g., FV Leiden homozygous mutation, AT, PC or PS deficiency) or if there are other thrombotic events in the history and there are no contraindications, oral anticoagulant can be given as a form of secondary prevention, but in case of vitamin K-antagonists (VKA) INR has to be checked regularly. As for the new oral, targeted anticoagulants (NOAC, IIa-, or Xa-inhibitors) no systemic data are yet available but is seems plausible that they can be used as well. In case of mild thrombophilia or arterial circulatory disorder, the above mentioned antiplatelet prophylaxis may be continued. However, we always have to aim for individual therapy, as guidelines are optly called GUIDElines — you have to know them, they give you some guidance but it is always the responsibility of the attending physician(s) what they describe to a given patient and for how long time.

Fundal Hemorrhages

Surgical interventions performed during anticoagulant therapy

If the INR is under 2.0, oral anticoagulant treatment with VKA need not be switched to LMWH or UFH prophylaxis ("bridging") in case of *smaller ophthalmological operations* (blepharoplasty, interventions performed on the conjunctiva or cornea) and phacoemulsification performed with the help of eye-drop anesthesia via a small incision on the cornea. The same is true for NOACs.

In case of more major ophthalmological operations, anticoagulation can be temporarily stopped or if anticoagulant therapy cannot be interrupted, e.g. in patients with mechanical heart valves it has to be switched to LMWH in order to decrease the risk of intraocular or hard-to-stop bleeding. Such operations include: intrabulbar surgeries (artificial lens implantation), if the incision is carried out on vascularized tissue, or if normal intraocular pressure cannot be maintained during surgery (corneal transplant, glaucoma, retinal detachment, vitrectomy), major blepharo- or facioplasty, removal of large tumors, dacryocystorrhinostomiy, evisceration, enucleation, exenteration.

Aspects to be considered on switching:

- *Antiplatelet drugs* have to be stopped 7 days before the surgery. If justified, the original therapy can be resumed the day after the surgery
- *Patients on oral anticoagulants*
  1. *in low thrombotic risk patients* (no stroke or transitoric ischemic attack in history, following deep vein thrombosis or pulmonary embolism with more than 12 months, bileaflet/bicuspid/aortic valve with no other risk factors) smaller ophthalmological operations may be performed on prophylactic dose of LMWH* or on VKA* (INR:<2), or no bridging at all, as in most cases in patients with NOAC*.
  2. in high thrombotic risk patients (any mitral mechanical valve, earlier type aortic mechanical valve, stroke or transitoric ischaemic attack <3 months, venous thromboembolism <3 months, atrial fibrillation patients with high risk score) oral, VKA-anticoagulants have to be stopped at least 4 days prior to surgery and substituted by therapeutic and – on the day of the surgery prophylactic – doses of LMWH. If the INR is under 2.0, the surgical intervention has no severe risks. One day after the surgery, LMWH has to be supplemented with oral anticoagulants until the desired level of INR is reached (in view of the underlying disease). In cases of patients with NOAC shorter period of stop and bridging with heparin is necessary due to the shorter half-life of these drugs.

  If even the transient interruption of anticoagulant therapy seems hazardous from an internal medicine (i.e. original anticoagulant indication) point of view, anticoagulation has to be continued.

Alternative options of anesthesia and surgery in patients on anticoagulants:

If local anesthesia is used (retro- or parabulbar injection), shorter needles and a single shot seems safer than a conventional needle. Eye-drop anesthesia has proved even safer.

The preferred method of cataract surgery is phacoemulsification performed with the help of eye-drop anesthesia via a small incision on the cornea.

Further Readings

Atkins EJ, Bruce BB, Newman NJ, Biousse V. Treatment of nonarteritic anterior ischemic optic neuropathy. Surv Ophthalmol. 2010;55:47–63.

Balogh Z, Berta A, Pfliegler G, Nagy V. Bilateral central retinal vein occlusion caused by malignant hypertension in a young patient. Clin Experiment Hypert. 2011;33:53–5. IF: 1.147.

Brown G. Retinal artery occlusive disease. In: Guyer DR, editor. Retina-vitreous-macula, vol 1. WB Saunders; 1999, p. 271–85.

Fodor M, Facskó A, Berényi E, Sziklai I, Berta A, Pfliegler G. Transient visual loss triggered by scuba diving in a patient with petrous epidermoid and combined thrombotic risk factors. Pathophysiol Haemost Thromb. 2007;36:311–4.

Fodor M, Nagy V, Berta A, Tornai I, Pfliegler G. Hepatitis C virus presumably associated bilateral consecutive anterior ischaemic optic neuropathy. Eur J Ophthalmol. 2008;18:313–5.

Fraunfelder FW, Pomeranz HD, Egan RA. Nonarteritic anterior ischemic optic neuropathy and sildenafil. Arch Ophthalmol. 2006;124:733–4.

Hayreh SS. Non-arteritic ischaemic optic neuropathy and thrombophilia. Graefes Arch Clin Exp Ophthalmol. 2009;247:577–81.

Hayreh SS. The role of aspirin in non-arteritic anterior ischaemic optic neuropathy. Neuro Ophthalmol. 2010;34:1–5.

Hayreh SS, Zimmerman B, McCarthy MJ, Podhajsky P. Systemic diseases associated with various types of retinal vein occlusion. Am J Ophthalmol. 2001;131:61–77.

Kasza M, Berta A, Pfliegler G, Nagy V. Az Eales-betegség klinikai tünetei, differenciáldiagnosztikai problémái, kezelése. [Clinical symptoms, differential diagnosis and treatment of Eales disease]. Szemészet [Ophthalmologica Hungarica]. 2007;144:92–4.

Kesler A, Irge D, Rogowski O, Bornstein N, Berliner S, Shapira I, Shani ST, BenAssayag E. High-sensitivity C-reactive protein measurements in patients with non-arteritic ischaemic optic neuropathy: a clue to the presence of a microinflammatory response. Acta Opthalmol. 2009;87:216–21.

Mike A, Gaál V, Németh A, Kövér F, Komoly S, Illés Z. Susac-szindróma: egy ritka autoimmun kórkép neurologiai, pszichiátriai, szemészeti, fül-orr-gégészeti és neuroradiológiai vonatkozásai. [Susac syndrome: neurological, psychiatric, ophthalmological, oto-rhino-laryngological and neuroradiological aspects of a rare autoimmune disorder]. Orv Hetil [Hungarian Medical Journal]. 2007;148:897–905.

Nagy V, Facskó A, Takács L, Balázs E, Berta A, Balogh I, Édes I, Czuriga I, Pfliegler G. Activated protein C resistance in anterior ischemic optic neuropathy. Acta Ophthalmol Scand. 2004;82:140–3.

Nagy V, Steiber Z, Takács L, Vereb G, Berta A, Bereczky Z, Pfliegler G. Thrombophilic screening for nonarteriitic anterior ischemic optic neuropathy. Graefes Arch Clin Exp Ophthalmol. 2006;244:3–8 (Epub 2005 Apr 15).

Nagy V, Balogh ZS, Kasza M, Ujhelyi B, Csutak A, Reznek I, Damjanovich J, Berta A, Pfliegler G. Cardiovascular and thrombophilic risk factors in retinal vein occlusion. Exp Clin Cardiol. 2014;20:238–44.

Pfliegler G, editor. A thromboemboliák kockázatának csökkentése és kezelése [Reducing the risk of thromboembolism and its treatment] Professional guidelines of the Ministry of Health. Orv Hetil [Hungarian Medical Journal]. 2009;52:331–2403.

The Cardiovascular Background of 'Intracerebral Small Vessel Disease'

44

Éva Nieszner

Content

Abbreviations

ABPM	Ambulatory blood pressure monitoring
ACE	Angiotensin-converting enzyme
AgII	Angiotensin II
CADS	Carotid artery duplex scanning
CCA	Common carotid artery
CRP	C-reactive protein
CTA	Computed tomography angiography
DSA	Direct angiography
ECA	External carotid artery
ECHO	Echocardiography
EKG	Electrocardiogram
FLAG	Fluorescein angiography
ICA	Internal carotid artery
ICAM	Intravascular cell adhesion molecule
IL-6	Interleukin-6
LDL	Low density lipoprotein
MA	Microalbuminuria
MRI	Magnetic resonance imaging
NO	Nitrogen monoxide
PAI-1	Plasminogen activator inhibitor-1
PTA	Percutaneous transluminal angioplasty
PTCA	Percutaneous transluminal coronary angioplasty
TNF-α	*Tumor necrosis factor*-α
US	Ultrasound
VCAM	Vascular cell adhesion molecule
x-ray	x-ray

É. Nieszner, M.D., PhD
Internist, Cardiologist, Diabetology Specialist, Angiology Specialist, Military Hospital, Budapest, Hungary
e-mail: nieszner.eva@gmail.com

Intracerebral vascular pathologies of cardiovascular origin cover all *structural and functional* disorders that develop as a result of *morphological or functional changes* in the heart and in the vessels located between the heart and the affected vascular segment.

The most important task of consultants is to give their opinion concerning the *dynamism of the cardiovascular condition and the expected progression*, together with the therapeutic recommendation after reviewing their subspecialty in a thorough and accurate way and *recording the data found* on the examination of the physical status. The neuro-ophthalmological assessment will reveal the intracerebral cause of visual loss and its topographic-anatomical location, thereby clarifying the nature of the lesion (arterial/capillary occlusion or venous circulatory disorder). Occlusion of medium-sized cerebral arteries may be caused by an embolus that becomes dislodged from a thrombus situating in the dilated chambers of the heart, calcified valvular deposits originating from an inflammation or a septic conglomerate of

J. Somlai, T. Kovács (eds.), *Neuro-Ophthalmology*, DOI 10.1007/978-3-319-28956-4_44

acute endocarditis. Atrial fibrillation or other high-frequency arrhythmias play a significant role in the development of cerebral embolism, as thrombus of various size existing in the leftheart chambers can become dislodged and reach cerebral end arteries this way. The causal role and significance of these emboli can be evaluated based on the general symptoms of neurological, neuro-ophthalmological and concomitant *cardiological diseases*, historical data, and findings of instrumental investigations *(EKG, ECHO, Holter, angio/ventriculography, x-ray, CTA, MRI)*.

Carotid artery duplex scanning (CADS), which is part of screening protocols today, meant a great step forward in the detection of *vascular embolism sources* as it could be used in the non-invasive diagnosis of *vulnerable atherosclerotic plaques* in the aortic arch and in the extracranial parts of the carotid arteries (CCA, ICA, ECA) (Fig. 44.1). As regards cerebral embolism, in contrast with stable plaques, cholesterol-rich, soft, fragile plaques can be a source of microembolism and may even predispose patients to thrombosis. For hemodynamic reasons, the anterior and medial cerebral arteries are the most commonly affected medium cerebral arteries that become obstructed by emboli (60 %).

The evaluation of cerebral and ocular microcirculation needs a much more precise and detailed differential diagnosis, as apart from microemboli (calcium particles, fibrin, cholesterol crystals, fibrin filaments) originating from the above mentioned morphological changes, *functional changes, stimulus-generated reactions, and inflammatory conditions of the vascular system can result -in vascular obstruction, spasm, infiltration, perivascular edema, rheological or fluid dynamic changes*, which can *lead to definite changes* in the metabolism of the retina, even if only temporarily. The morphological basis of this phenomenon is partly determined by the *reactivity of arterioles and capillaries*, but the *terminal branch feature of the retinal blood supply* (ciliary arteries and central retinal artery originating from the ophthalmic artery, first branch of ICA) also contributes to it.

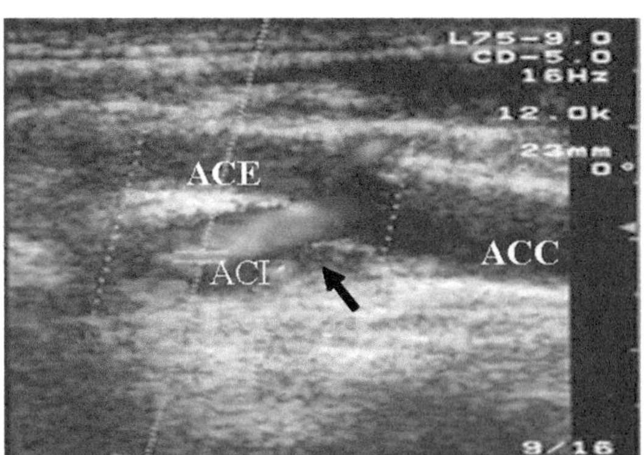

Fig. 44.1 A plaque of soft morphology leading to stenosis in the proximal part of the internal carotid artery (ICA)

The *endothelium*, a separate organ system in our body, weighs 1.5 kg and plays a role in vascular *fluid dynamics*. It has both *mechanical and neuroendocrine* functions (Fig. 44.2). The vascular system has a modulated response to the disorder of other organs, e.g., vasoconstriction protects peripheral organs in hypertension, hyperkinesis ensures surplus oxygen in anemia, vasodilation, impaired expansion and increased fragility develop in metabolic disorders (e.g., hyperlipidemia, diabetes mellitus), and polycythemia is characterized by slow flow parameters and increased viscosity. Its system-like organization is proved by the fact that the change of microcirculatory reactivity can be followed clinically according to the organs with the help of US, laser-Doppler, MA, and FLAG. However, the correlation of the various organic manifestations is not fully clarified. Cerebral microcirculation has a special characteristic feature, namely the *increased tendency to stasis* in the hypoxic areas beyond the ischemic stroke, which means that the survival of retinal cells is rather limited.

Our vascular system has a magnificent design, as it can serve two functions at the same time: it can both maintain flow ("*conduit*") and decrease it ("*cushing*") in order to protect certain organs. The powerful, *pulsatile flow* of the blood coming from the heart will slow down in the *major blood vessels* and smaller arterioles, and in the periphery, at the level of the capillaries the flow is almost steady-state. Owing to the *conduit function*, the mean arterial pressure decreases by <1 mmHg only between the ascending aorta and the peripheral arteries (e.g., radial artery).

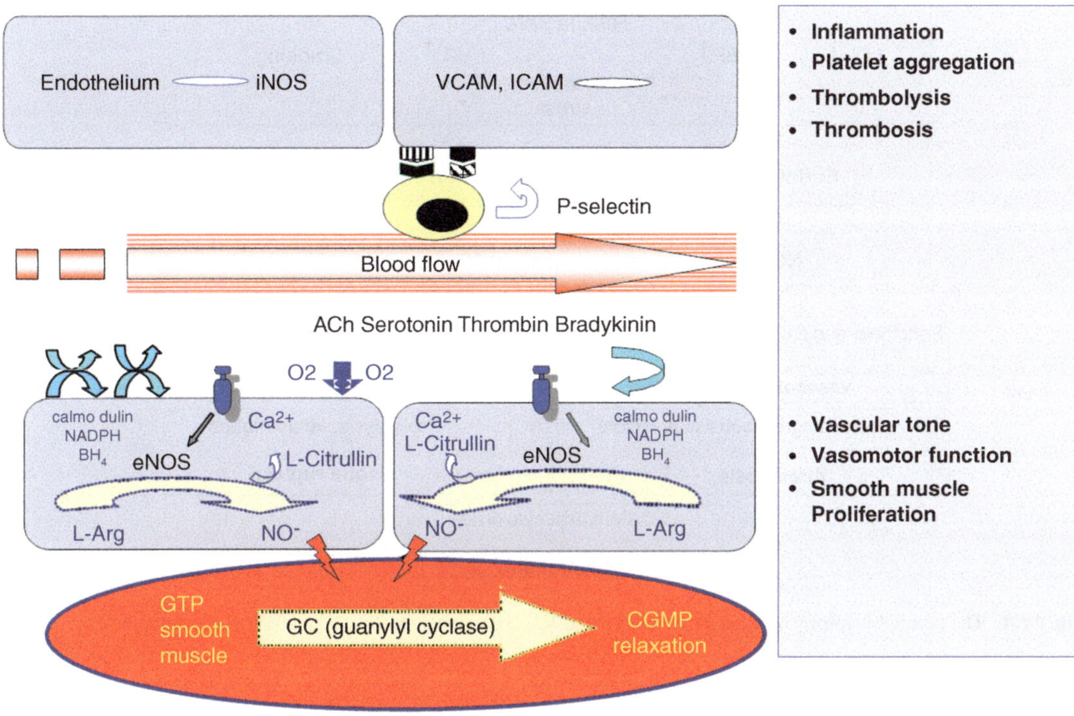

Fig. 44.2 The physiological role of the endothelium

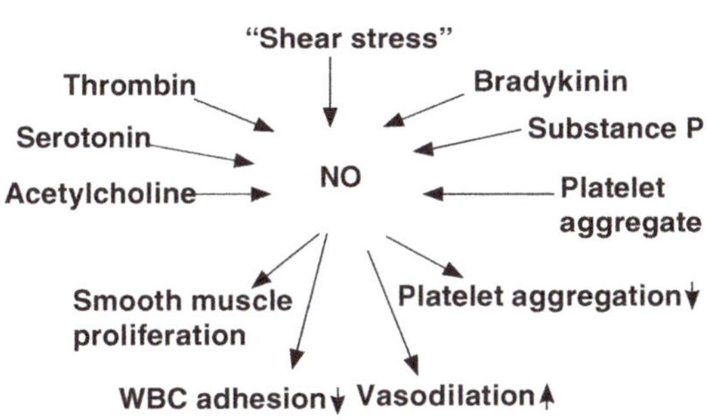

Fig. 44.3 The role of nitrogen monoxide (*NO*) in the local regulation of circulation

Pulsation in the major arteries uses <10% of energy, while *flow at the level of arterioles and capillaries is continuous* due to the viscosity of blood and vessel walls. Circulation is primarily regulated by NO (nitrogen monoxide), which is produced in the endothelium (Fig. 44.3). Pathological endothelial function leads to accelerated atherosclerosis, which will result in damage -of major vessels and microcirculation aswel (Fig. 44.4).

While the vasoconstriction of arterioles provides the capillary system with a certain degree of protection in other organs, the low resistance of cerebral arterioles will mean a passive flow, that is, a potent pulsatile effect will be present in the underlying microcirculation during systole and diastole. The degeneration of the elastic lamellae in major blood vessels over time leads to an increase in the elastic modulus, thus, the aorta will become less flexible, and its stiffness value will increase. This way the average intravascular pressure may increase four-fold even in unchanged flow conditions, which will increase both the *pulsatile (circumferential stress and longitudinal shear force) and shear stress effect* in the vessels.

As a result, increased pulsatile stress damages cerebral endothelial and smooth muscle cells, which may lead to vasodilation, stasis, microaneurysm, rupture of small vessels, lipohyalinosis and fibrinoid necrosis. This microcirculatory damage can explain the rapid loss of function and the development of definite lesions in tissues with high oxygen demand, such as the retina. As

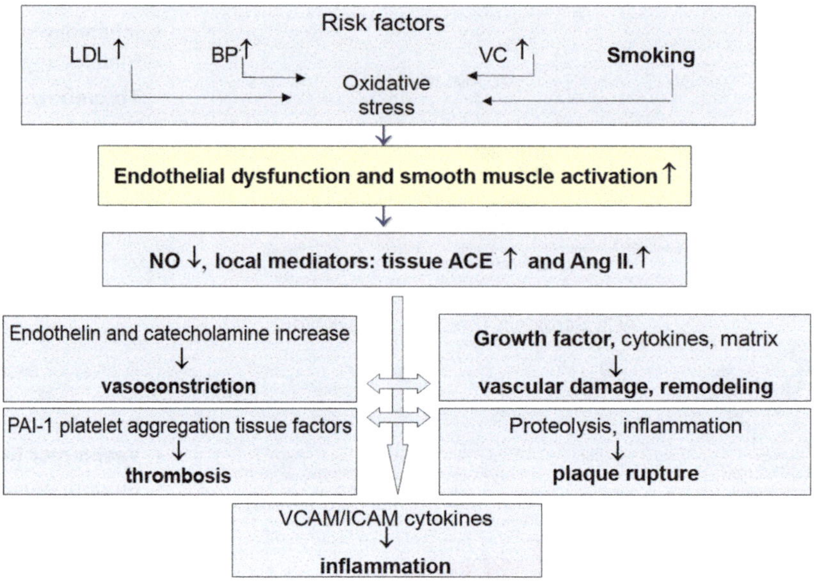

Fig. 44.4 The pathophysiology of atherosclerosis (Dzau VJ, Hypertension, 2001; 37:1047–1052. -alapjan)

Table 44.1 Pathophysiological changes in diabetic blood vessels

Aorta:	Rigidity
Flexible arteries:	Rigidity
Resistance vessels:	Decreased endothelin-dependent vasodilation
Arterioles:	Hyalinosis
	Loss of autoregulation
	Decreased endothelin-dependent vasodilation
Capillaries:	Hyperemia at rest decreased peak flow
	Pressure dysregulation increased
	Permeability
Venous system:	Increased tone and vasoconstrictor
	Response decreased compliance

Table 44.2 Characteristic features of endothelial dysfunction in diabetes mellitus

Decreased endothelial nitric oxide synthase (eNOS) activity
Decreased endothelial reactivity to NO
Increased adhesion molecule expression (ICAM-1, VCAM-1)
Increased thrombocyte and monocyte adhesion
Increased procoagulant activity
Decreased fibrinolytic activity
Impaired plasmin degradation
Decreased prostacyclin release
Increased endothelin-1 synthesis, expression

the flexibility of small vessels plays a key role in the protection of underlying circulatory units, patients suffering from metabolic disorders (diabetes mellitus, hypercholesterolemia, thyroid disorders, etc.) have to be considered as high risk groups. Increased fragility of smalls vessels and damage to the vulnerable microcirculation, which are attributed to metabolic stress (Table 44.1) and the effect of free radicals lead to progressive visual impairment (Table 44.2).

Evidence supports that in diabetes mellitus, a 1 % improvement in metabolic state can result in a 37 % improvement in microcirculation (UKPDS retinopathies).

Therefore, if a patient presents with the symptoms of amaurosis fugax, cardiologists – together with physicians representing other specialties – have to assess the complete circulatory system, evaluate the actual condition of blood vessels and the heart, perform instrumental investigations (ECHO, CADS, ABPM, Holter, stress test, telemetry), *detect and treat embolus sources and conditions that predispose patients to embolism/thrombosis – hyperkinesis, hypertension, arrhythmias – as well as evaluate and normalize metabolic conditions* (endocrinological causes, lipid and carbohydrate metabolism). As a sudden visual disorder raises the suspicion of both an intracerebral arterial accident and the increased tendency to venous thrombus formation, we have to assess coagulatory functions (hematological diseases, essential or secondary thrombocytosis, antiphospholipid syndrome) and exclude inflammatory and autoimmune syndromes. In several cases, microembolism occurs as a complication of significant volume loss, anemia, surgery, invasive diagnostic or therapeutic interventions (coronary angiography, PTCA, DSA, PTA), and it is detected with some delay.

As the time factor is of considerable importance in the regression of neuro-ophthalmological symptoms, rapid initiation of the therapy is a must.

Immediate and double anticoagulant therapy has to be started: an acute ocular stroke and loss of vision may necessitate the administration of transient anticoagulants besides *aggressive and multi-target antiplatelet agents*. Unfortunately no official guidelines have been published for the use of the former agents. Although the administration of *double platelet aggregation inhibitors* is already accepted in angiology, cardiology and in major ischemic neurological diseases, their daily use in small intracerebral vessels is still an issue of professional debate. It can be a sound argument for *double platelet aggregation inhibitors* that sudden visual impairment or ocular stroke often develops in patients who take anticoagulants or aspirin as secondary prevention for some prior cardiovascular event or arrhythmia or who receive antiplatelet therapy as primary prevention for their underlying disease. The regression of the visual disorder can be promoted by antiplatelet therapy combined with *plenty of fluids* (*to avoid hypovolemia*!), *normalization of blood pressure and the metabolic status* (*normal levels of glucose, uric acid, cholesterol, triglycerides, LDL*) and treatment of arrhythmias.

This group of patients needs a comprehensive neuro-ophthalmological, cardiological, angiological, ophthalmological, immunological and internal medicine treatment. Their vision can be improved or at least the progress of the condition can be halted with the help of multidisciplinary follow-up, and they also need regular meetings and a close bond with their attending physician.

Further Readings

A guideline from the American Heart Association/American Stroke Association Stroke Council, Clinical Cardiology Council, Cardiovascular Radiology and Intervention Council, and the Atherosclerotic Peripheral Vascular Disease and Quality of Care Outcomes in Research Interdisciplinary Working Group. Circulation. 2007;115:e478–534.

Choudhri TF, Hoh BL, Zerwes HG, Prestigiacomo CJ, Kim SC, et al. Reduced microvascular thrombosis and improved outcome in acute murine: stroke by inhibiting GP IIb/IIIa receptor-mediated platelet aggregation. J Clin Invest. 1998;102:1301–10.

Developed with the special contribution of the European Heart Rhythm Association. Eur Heart J. 2010. doi:10.1093/eurheartj/ehq278.

ESC guidelines for the diagnosis and treatment of acute and chronic heart failure.

Esper RJ, Nordaby RA, Vilarino JO, Paragano A, Cacharr6n JL, Machadp RA. Endothelial dysfunction: a comprehensive appraisal. Cardiovasc Diabetol. 2006;5:4, 1–18.

Guidelines for the early management of adults with ischemic stroke.

Guidelines for the management of atrial fibrillation. The Task Force for the Management of Atrial Fibrillation of the European Society of Cardiology (ESC).

Morillas P, Pallarés V, Llisterri JL, Sanchis C, Sánchez T, et al. Prevalence of atrial fibrillation and use of antithrombotics in hypertensive patients aged ≥65 years. The FAPRES Trial. Rev Esp Cardiol. 2010;63(8):943–50.

Nicolucci A, De Berardis G, Tognoni G. AHA/ADA vs ESC/EASD recommendations on aspirin as primary prevention strategy in people with diabetes: how the same data generate divergent conclusions. Eur Heart J. 2007;28:1925–7.

O'Rourke M, Safar ME. Relationship between aortic stiffening and microvascular disease in brain and kidney: cause and logic of therapy. Hypertension. 2005;46:200–4.

The Task Force for the Diagnosis and Treatment of Acute and Chronic Heart Failure 2008 of the European Society of Cardiology. Developed in collaboration with the Heart Failure Association of the ESC (HFA) and endorsed by the European Society of Intensive Care Medicine (ESICM). Eur Heart J. 2008.

Watson K. Managing cardiometabolic risk: an evolving approach to patient care. Crit Pathw Cardiol. 2007;6:5–14.

Vascular Diseases of the Optic Nerve: The Neuro-Ophthalmologist's Approach

45

Judit Somlai

Contents

J. Somlai, M.D.
Unit of Neuro-Ophthalmology, Department of Neurology & Stroke, Military Hospital, Budapest, Hungary

Neuro-Ophthalmology Section, Hungarian Ophthalmological Association, Budapest, Hungary

Trustee, NOSZA Foundation (for the Prevention and Screening of Ocular Storke), Budapest, Hungary
e-mail: dr@somlaijudit.hu; http://somlaijudit.hu

Ocular stroke, i.e., the thromboembolism of the visual system is a syndrome which causes a mostly irreversible, painless, unilateral, complete loss of vision that develops over the course of a few minutes or hours and which, over time, will affect the other eye as well. The condition primarily affects the function of the central field of vision, thereby rendering reading and working impossible. Among the most common causes of blindness, circulatory disorders of the eyes are only preceded by senile glaucoma and macular degeneration. As an ocular stroke can be the precursor or part of a systemic cardio- and/or cerebrovascular disorder, an etiology-specific treatment can not only prevent loss of vision in the other eye but it can also prevent the development or progression of systemic thromboembolism and cerebrovascular circulatory disorders (stroke).

The significance of anatomical and physiological connections in the vascular diseases of our visual system:

- in the visual system (and in the central nervous system as well) *the retina has the highest*

J. Somlai, T. Kovács (eds.), *Neuro-Ophthalmology*, DOI 10.1007/978-3-319-28956-4_45

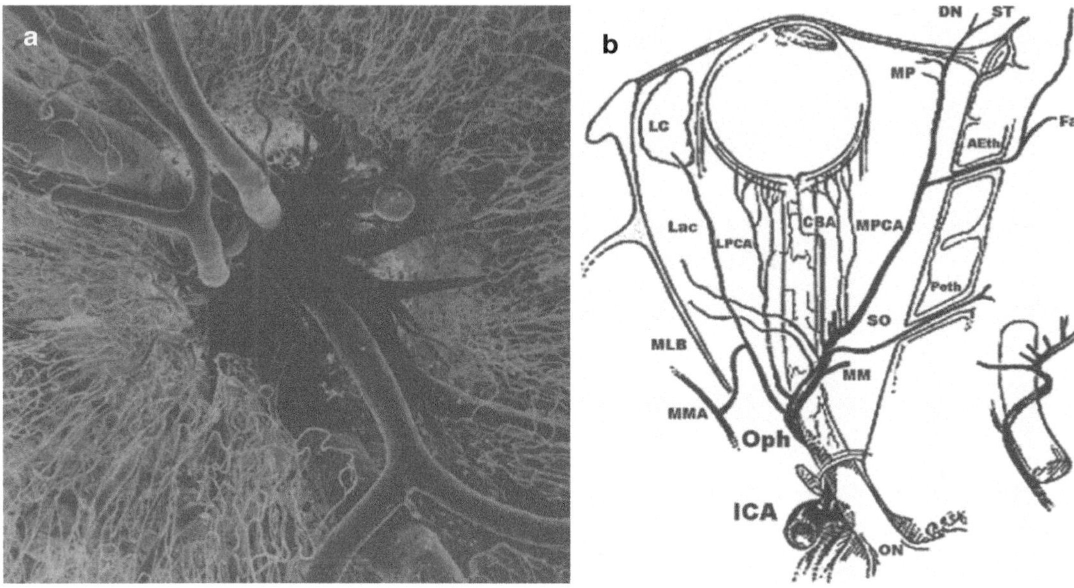

Fig. 45.1 (**From**: **Dr. H.A. Quigley**). (**a**) Electron microscope image of the retinal vascular system: it has the highest perfusion due to its rich vascular network; (**b**) Illustration of optic disc blood supply, the ophthalmic artery branching off the internal carotid artery (Miller and Newman (2005). Published by Lippincott Williams & Wilkins)

perfusion, therefore, it can be a sensitive indicator of cerebral circulatory disorders (Fig. 45.1a);

- arteries supplying the retina and the optic disc are *end-arteries*, so physiological shunt mechanisms cannot be utilized when these small vessels are occlusion;
- the ophthalmic artery that supplies the optic disc, first branches off the internal carotid artery (ICA), so both microemboli from the heart and eroded plaques from the ICA can serve as embolus sources in the circulatory disorders of the visual system (Fig. 45.1b) (Holló 1966; Kupersmith et al. 1994; Hungarian Society of Thrombosis and Haemostasis Thromboembóliák megelözèse is kezelèse 1998).

Ocular Symptoms: Ocular Stroke

As you can see in the table, amaurosis fugax was not only the early symptom but also the most common clinical sign of a circulatory disorder of the optic nerve among our patients. Apart from that, we noted the symptoms of circulatory disorders of the prae- and retrochiasmal optic nerve among our 'ocular stroke' patients (Fig.45.2).

The Definition of Amaurosis Fugax (AF, Transient Monocular Blindness/TMB/) and so Called 'Ocular Stroke'

Amaurosis fugax – also abbreviated as TMB (transient monocular blindness) based on its English term – refers to a transient circulatory disorder in the visual system because of the following features:

- it lasts for a few seconds or max. half an hour;
- it mostly affects one eye, sometimes both;
- patients report being disturbed by strange light spots on the periphery of visual field, jagged or zigzag line of light, blurred vision or some 'foggy vision' or curtain coming down in from of one eye;
- if the central field of vision is affected as well, patients usually consult an ophthalmologist, even though the specialist examination

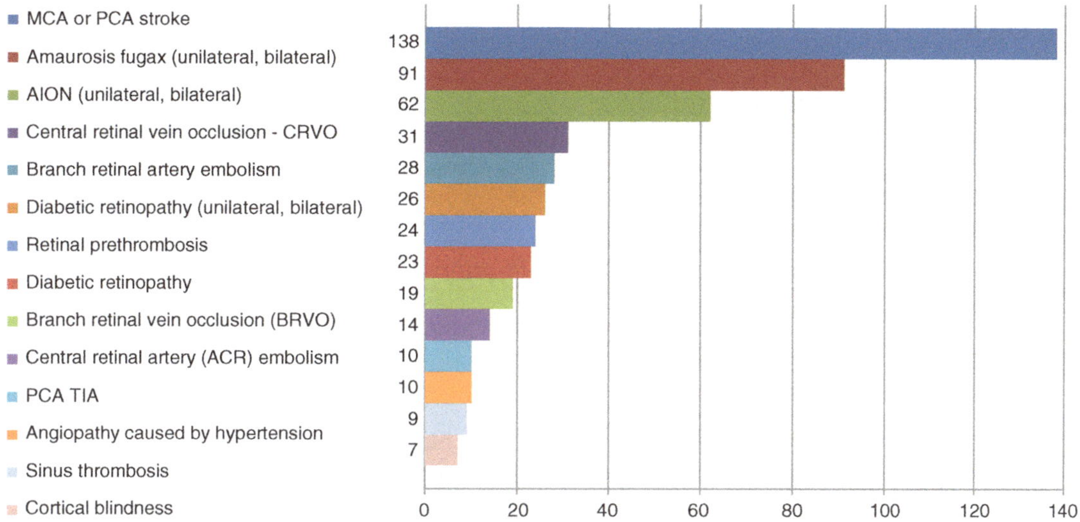

Fig. 45.2 Distribution of ocular symptoms in 514 patients suffering from ocular stroke

- will usually find no abnormalities as the phenomenon lasts only for a few minutes;
- sometimes it can be perceived in front of both eyes; on direct questioning they will mention the homonymous parts of the visual field, but in this case it is considered less disturbing as the central field of vision is spared;
- if this transient visual disorders occur again more and more frequently, it suggest progression of the circulatory disorder: this warning has to be taken it seriously;
- regarding its etiopathomechanism, only the theory of multiple microembolism and vasospasm has been proved;
- it is the task of the ophthalmologist to differ flashlight vision that caused by vitreoretinal changes from an ocular stroke syndrome

As an ocular stroke can be the initial symptom or part of a systemic cardio- and/or cerebrovascular disorder, the eye symptoms can indicate or precursor an imminent cerebrovascular process which is mostly due to some vascular or intravascular disorder causing cardiovascular microembolism. The microvascular circulatory disorder (in international terminology a.k.a. 'lacunar infartcs disease' or Small vessels occlusive disease') caused by some circulatory abnormality in the end arteries of the central nervous system shows an analogy with circulatory disorders in the end arteries of the visual system, as arteries supplying the visual pathways and the retina are part of the same vascular system (Fig. 45.3).

The Arterial Circulatory Disorders of the Visual Pathway System

The etiopathomechanism of central nervous system multiple microembolism shows an analogy with thromboembolism in the visual pathway system. Partial or complete occlusion of blood vessels supplying the visual system can be caused by either atherothrombotic processes in the ICA or fibrin thromboembolism originating from the heart.

Embolism in the trunk or branches vessels of the central retinal artery (ACR) leads to rapid loss of central vision accompanied by extensive visual field defects. Ocular symptoms are usually due to the occlusion of the trunk artery or end arteries of the retina. The ophthalmoscopic image is not informative enough if we consider the rapid and practically irreversible loss of vision. The actual detection of a

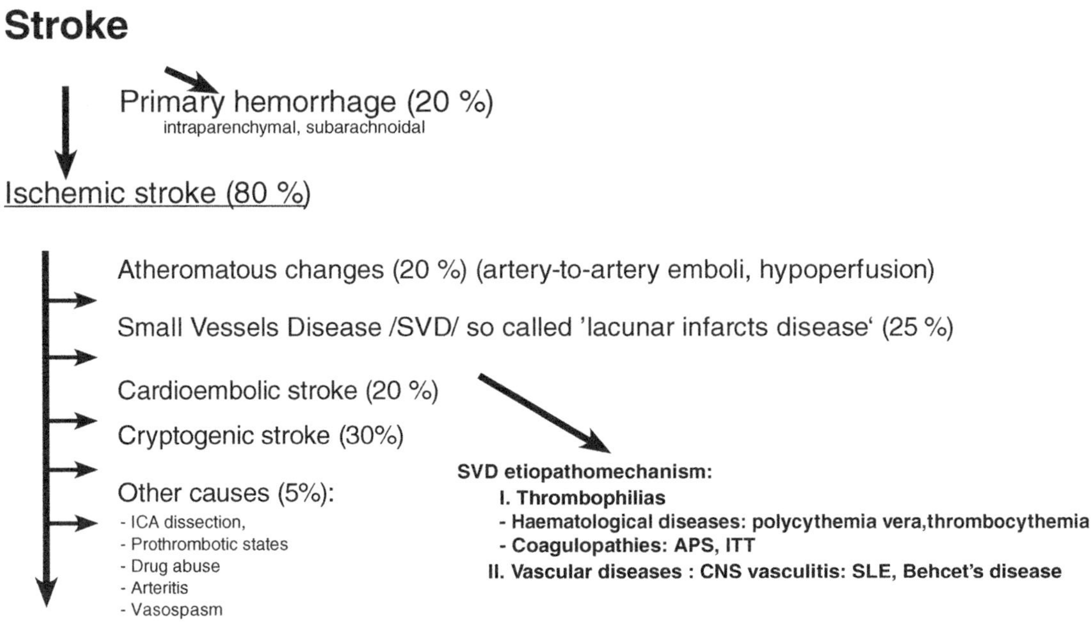

Fig. 45.3 Etiological-didactic classification of strokes (*redrawn*) (Miller and Newman (2005). Published by Lippincott Williams & Wilkins, vol 2, p. 1971, Fig. 40.1)

cholesterol or fibrin particle in the retinal artery is rare. Short-lasting retinal edema is followed by the pale, non-excavated apperance of the papilla, which is indicative of loss of function. Among our patients, 42 cases (7.7 %) were caused by retinal microembolism, which probably had a cardiogenic origin or was due to eroded plaque migration.

Figure 45.4 shows one of our young patients (32 years), who had an incomplete ACR – retinal trunk embolism. In the initial phase of the dominant hemisphere stroke, right-sided hemiplegia was accompanied with almost complete motor aphasia. A severe vascular disorder affecting the internal carotid artery resulted in stenosis and multiple microembo-lism leading to the almost complete occlusion of the central retinal artery. The remaining central and paracentral vision of some degrees was provided via the residual circulation of an cilioretinal segment coming from the direction of the choroid. Prior to the development of the neurological symptoms and the severe stroke, the young patient regularly experienced transient loss of vision on the left eye.

Anterior Ischemic Optic Neuropathy (AION) The embolism of end-arteries of retina, papilla antechiasmal optic nerve, leads to incomplete amaurosis by rapid loss of central vision. Multiple embolisms occurring in the lateral end branch of the posterior ciliary artery, i.e., the artery that supplies the optic disc is most likely to play a central role in the development of the condition (Fig. 45.5a–c, d-1, d-2).

The blood supply of the optic disc is provided by the circle of Haller Zinn, which is formed by the end branches of the short ciliary arteries as well as choriocapillary and pial branches. Disorders of blood supply to the optic disc can be divided into two groups, based on the location of the lesion in the above mentioned system.

RETINAL blood supply to the innermost layers (i.e., closest to the vitreous humor) is provided by the main branch of the ophthalmic artery, the central retinal artery (CRA). Its occlusion leads to a complete loss of vision, which is called retinal trunk embolism (*see:red narrows*). The outer layers of the retina (photoreceptor and pigmented epithelium layers) are supplied by the choriocapillary network via diffusion (*see:blue narrows*). The perimacular and submacular parts of the retina get their blood

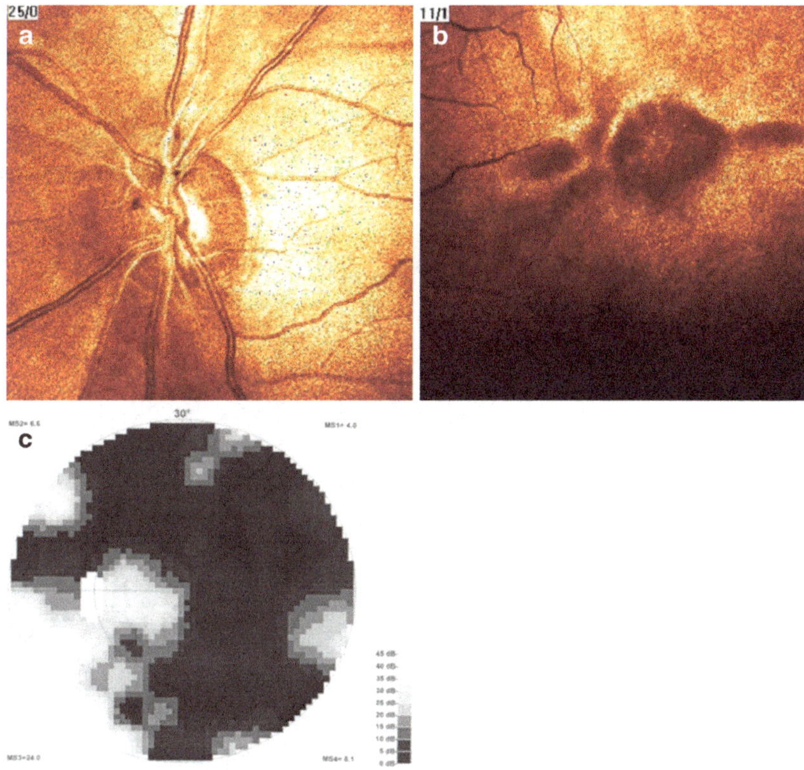

Fig. 45.4 Trunk occlusion in the main branch of the central retinal artery (left) with consequent maculopathy and severe loss of visual field leading to incomplete amaurosis Primary disease: status p. stroke of MCA l.s. (Occlusion of ICA and MCA l.s). (**a**) Image of the optic disc: Surrounded chronic edema of peripapillary region. (**b**) Perimacular region: Pigment migration due to organised edema. (**c**) Octopus (D1) perimetry: residual visual field in papillomacular region by the salvaging effect of cilioretinal arteria from choroidea

supply from the **short branches posterior ciliary artery**. Multiple microembolism in these areas leads to blood supply deficit in the perimacular region of the retina, thereby causing rapid loss of function in the center of vision (Fig. 45.5a–c)

The blood supply of the OPTIC DISC is provided by the Circle of Zinn-Haller, which is formed by the end branches of the short ciliary arteries as well as choriocapillary and pial branches. Disorders of blood supply to the optic disc can be divided into two groups, based on the location of the lesion in the above mentioned system (Fig. 45.5d).

Blood supply to the **INTRAORBITAL section** of the optic nerve is partly provided by the ***radial arteries of the pial arterial system***, while the posterior third gets its blood supply from the ***ophthalmic artery***. Occlusion of the latter artery results in **posterior ischemic optic neuropathy** (**PION**).

Clinical signs of anterior ischemic optic processes (**AION**): Branch or trunk embolism in the end arteries that supply the antechiasmal optic pathway and the retina leads to incomplete amaurosis via the loss of central vision.

It can develop in both eyes with a time shift of some months or even years. When the condition affects the fellow eye, fundoscopy of the previously affected eye reveals a well-circumscribed, pale optic disc (decoloratio papillae (*lat*)), while the fellow eye features a slightly prominent, edematous optic disc with ill-defined – blurred margins. In this stage the function of the fellow eye deteriorates rapidly. The fundus image shows a clear resemblance to the ocular symptoms of Foster–Kennedy syndrome, which is a well-known neurological condition associated with increased intracranial pressure. However, contrary to the space-occupying intracranial process, bilateral AION is accompanied by rapid and progressive loss of vision in the fellow eye. Due to

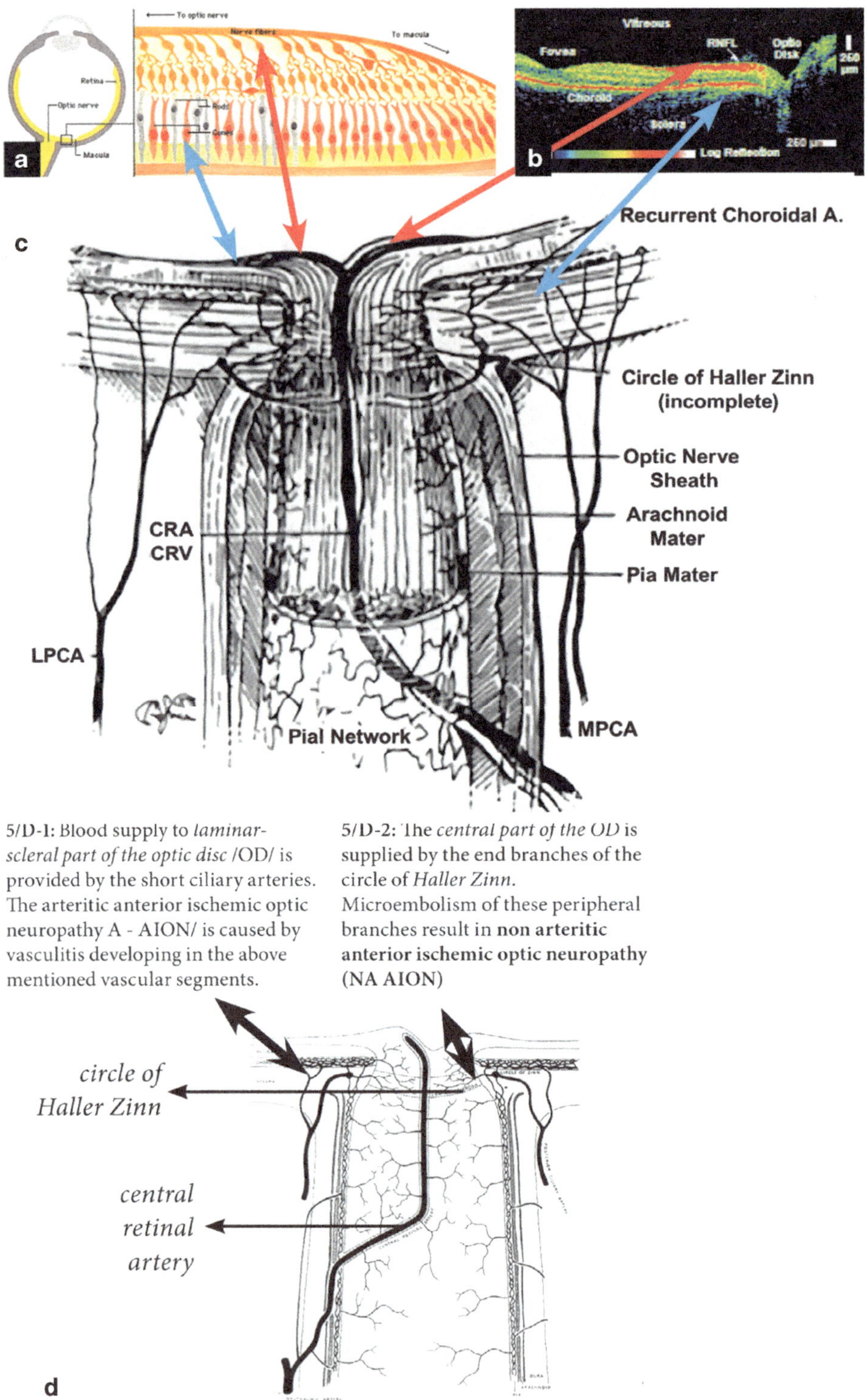

Fig. 45.5 (From Kupersmith (1993)). Retinal blood supply with arterial circulate system of papilla demonstrate the peri-papillare, macular regions of retina by a schematic drawing and OCT photo. (**a**) Schematic drawing of retinal layers. (**b**) OCT photo of retinal layers. (**c**) Schematic drawing of the retina and the optic disc. *CRA* Central Retinal Artery, *CRV* Central Retinal Vein, *LPCA* Lateral Posterior Ciliary arteries, *MPCA* Medial Posterior Ciliary arteries (Miller and Newman (2005). Published by Lippincott Williams & Wilkins, vol 1. p. 31, Fig. 1.30) (**d**-**1**, -**2**) Blood supply of the optic disc (Miller and Newman (2005). Published by Lippincott Williams & Wilkins, vol 2. p. 1908, Fig. 39.12)

the similarity of the ophthalmoscopic view, the latter syndrome was aptly named ***pseudoFoster-Kennedy syndrome***

Regarding its etiopathomechanism and clinical course, AION can be divided into two big groups: A partial phenomenon of vasculitis, **arteritic AION (A-AION)** (arteritic anterior ischemic optic neuropathy) may be the ocular symptom of a systemic autoimmune process. Systemic necrotizing vasculitis in the central nervous system usually affects medium and big arteries, thus end arteries are rarely affected. As a result, it is not accidental that short ciliary arteries are affected only in a very small proportion (~5%) of giant cell arteritis (GCA) cases. The disease usually develops around the age of 50 and the fellow eye soon becomes affected. Warning symptoms are headache, polymyalgia rheumatica, i.e., intense pain in the jaw while chewing and strong pain in the temporal region. In addition, patients may also report the swelling of the temporal artery during the headache. Characteristic laboratory findings and altered immune parameters may also be of assistance. Ocular symptoms are rapid and significant loss of vision (first in one eye only, but later in the other one as well) that primarily affects the central field of vision. As a result, patients cannot read or focus on near objects and they frequently suffer from headaches. As a result of multiple infarcts affecting the optic disc, fundoscopy will reveal an edematous, ill-defined optic disc and the retina will also manifest signs of ischemia, namely cotton wool exudates and intraretinal bleeding. In untreated cases the optic disc will become well circumscribed and pale, at the level of the retina. In later stages the optic disc will become pale papilla as a result of the severe loss of fibers, and severe, irreversible, almost complete blindness will develop.

Differential diagnosis is assisted by a histological sample taken from the temporal region to confirm vasculitis in the temporal artery (Fig. 45.6).

Angiography of the fundus*, i.e., *fluorescein angiography: In cases of arteritic AION, the bigger arteries of the retina are already filled with the dye, while the optic disc and the *peripapillary region fill more slowly from the direction of the choriocapillaries*. Differentiation can be assisted by the fact that in non- arteritic AION cases, the *dye comingfrom the direction of the peripapillary choroidea will appear simultaneously with the filling of the retina*. (For differential diagnosis assisted with angiography see Chap.19).

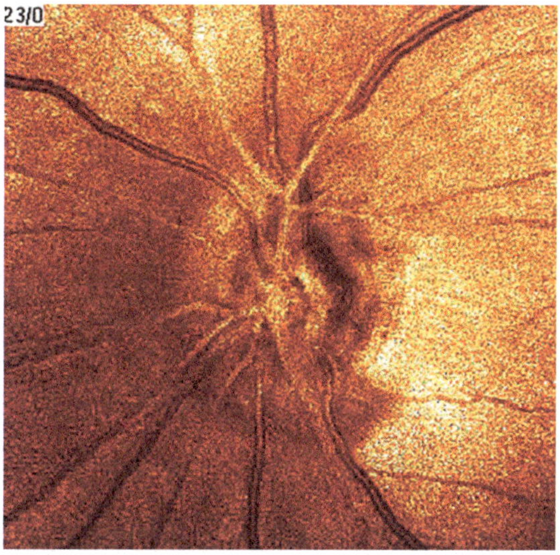

Fig. 45.6 Ophthalmoscopic view of unilateral arteritic AION of a patient suffering from SLE. Flat, pale optic disc with narrow arteries, bordered with peripapillary edema

Non-arteritic anterior ischemic optic neuropathy/NA-AION/: in the vast majority of cases it causes bilateral circulatory disorder of the optic disc over time, just like its arteritic form. The underlying diseases are usually untreated hypertension, diabetes mellitus and most frequently atherosclerosis. Besides the most common, multiple risk factors our patients also had congenital thrombophilia, sickle-cell anemia, polycythemia vera and other diseases.

The initial symptoms were painless loss of central or near central vision (sometimes associated with occipital headache) in the morning with no other neurological symptoms. Besides the significant deterioration of antechiasmal optic nerve functions (both near and distant vision, critical fusion frequency) the acute phase is also characterized by ill-defined papilledema that shows prominence of +1, +2 diopters. Over time, the optic disc will lose this prominence and it will

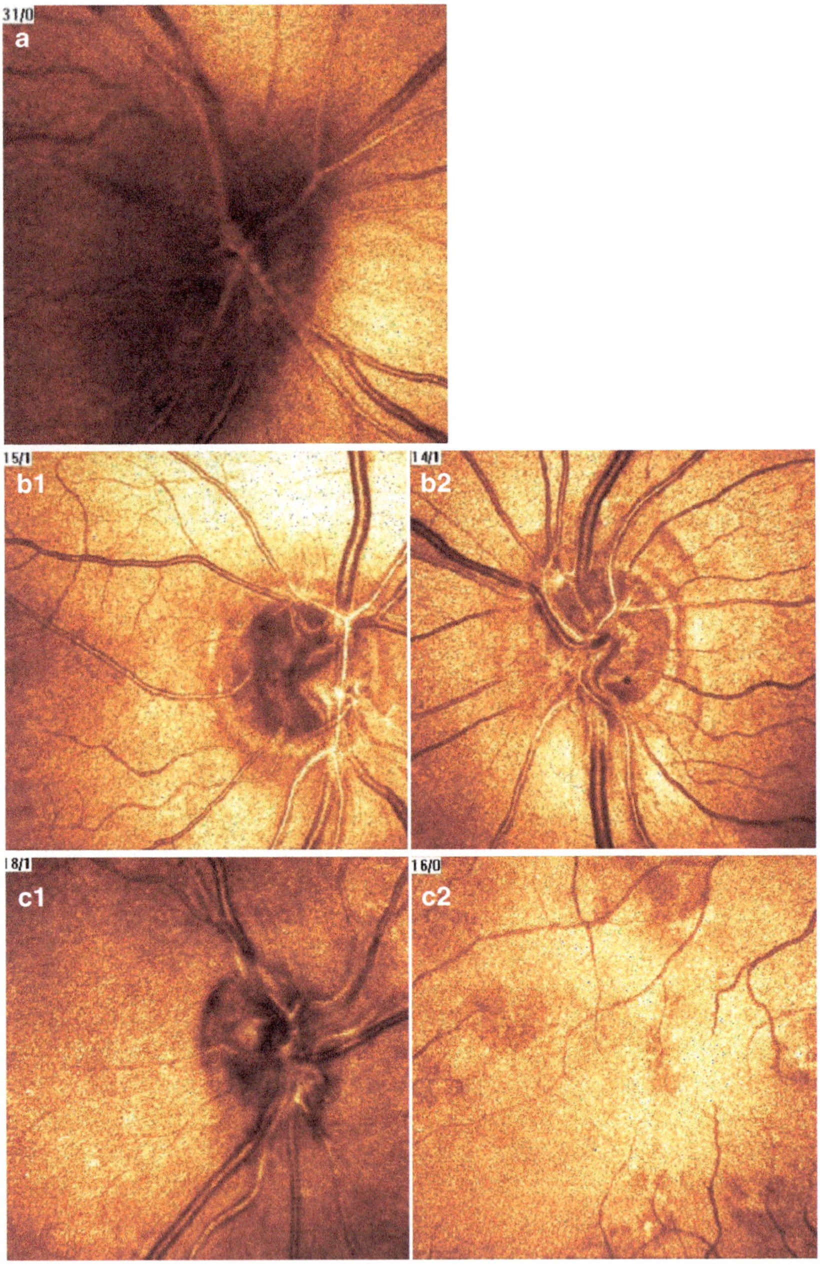

Fig. 45.7 Ophthalmoscopic view of non-arteritic AION: (**a**) early signs of AION: moderate papilledema, mild prominence; (**b**1,**b**2) Bilateral, non-simultaneous chronic AION the optic disc is surrounded by organized edema (**c**1,**c**2) Papillary image of chronic NA-AION (right side) perimacular image: organized edema at the end of the perimacular branches with pigment leak (background disease: antiphospholipid syndrome – APS)

appear pale but not porcelain-white and non-excavated. This latter feature can be explained by the difference in etiopathomechanism. In untreated patients or when the condition is detected late, the circulatory disorder of the perimacular small vessels is visible in the form of organized edema and pigment leak (Fig. 45.7).

The circulatory disorder of the fundus is well demonstrated by the ***defects of the visual field***. At first, the blind spot seems bigger due to papilledema as a *big blind spot sign*. The persistence of the circulatory disorder leads to the spread of the process in the direction of the papillomacular bundle and the macular region, which causes *centrocecal scotoma* associated with an increasing loss of the central field of vision. In the chronic phase of the condition, the ineffective treatment leads to significant

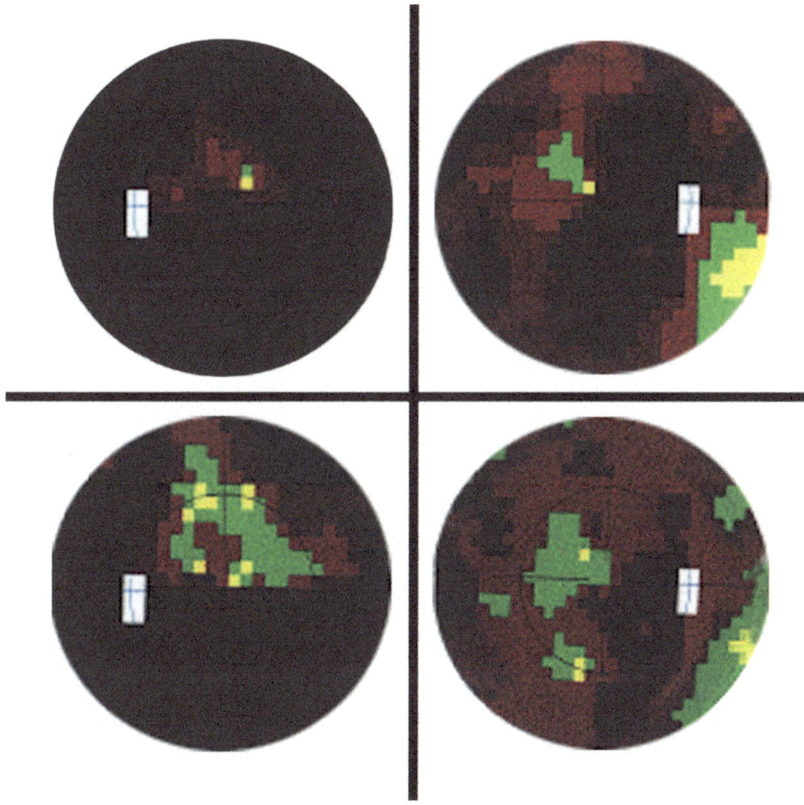

Fig. 45.8 The visual field defect of a patient with bilateral nonarteritic AION, pseudoFoster–Kennedy syndrome in chronic phase, with a severe central visual field defects, namely: bilateral central and centrocecal scotomas. (*The defects of he visual field in this case: before therapy-top images and after treatment–bottom images*)

and irreversible damage to the long temporal fibers accompanied by nasal – inferior quadrantopia. This latter phenomenon will persist as a residual symptom. The patient will be unable to read and recognize faces. Figure 45.8 shows a bilateral process that can no longer be improved with late treatment: perimetry test detected bilateral, *severe loss of central visual field* (more severe on the left side of the visual field defects).

When *fundus fluorescein angiography* (*FLAG*) is performed, in AION of non-vascular origin the dye coming from the direction of the peripapillary choroidea will appear simultaneously with the filling of the retina. For more details see Chap.18.

In most cases of AION, when the ocular symptoms develop, *at the same time* there are already several small infarcts in the central nervous system, which can confirm the possible same etiopathomechanism of multiple microvessel circulatory disorder. ('Lacunar infarcts disease' or 'Small Vessels occlusive Syndrome'/SVD/)

Ocular symptoms of strokes and TIA affecting the retrochiasmal visual system: Abnormal function of the optic radiation (in areas supplied by the MCA and PCA) caused by stroke was found in 138 (27 %) of our patients.

Circulatory disorder of the retrochiasmal optic tract developing as part of a cerebrovascular event (stroke) causes bilateral transient or permanent loss of vision, and it can be characterized by *incomplete or complete homonymous hemianopia*. The most common clinical sign of vertebrobasilar circulatory disorder (VBI-TIA) is vertigo, balance problems as well as *short, bilateral, frequently blurred vision*and/or transient diplopia. Patients are often frightened by the visual disorder that affects both eyes simultaneously and lasts for a few seconds; later the visual field defect may becomes permanent. Progressing disorder of consciousness and disorientation are common initial symptoms of circulatory disor-

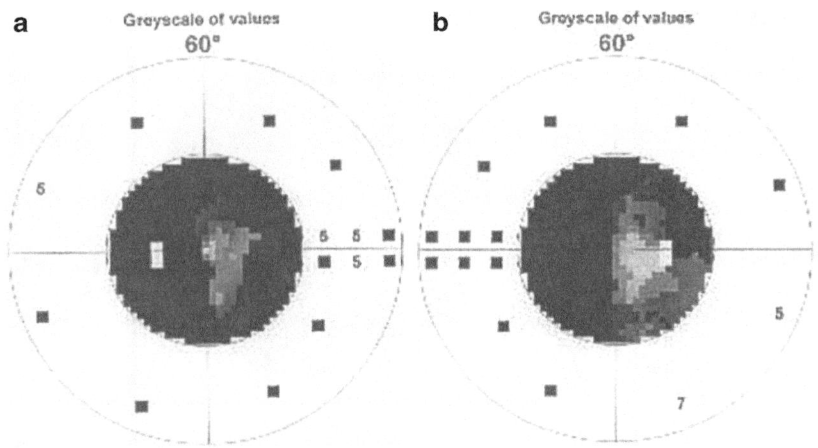

Fig. 45.9 Left homonymous hemianopia due to occlusion of the right posterior cerebral artery

ders in the vertebrobasilar artery. If it affects the area supplied by one of the branches of the posterior cerebri artery, the result will be homonymous hemianopsia, which is illustrated by Fig. 45.9.

Venous Circulatory Disorders of the Visual System

Prethrombosis of Retinal Veins ('Enlarged Blind Spot Syndrome')

According to our observations, *prethrombosis of retinal veins (enlarged blind spot syndrome)* – is the first sign of venous blood supply disorder in the retina and the part of the optic disc. In later stages or untreated cases, more severe venous disorders are manifest itself as a branch or trunk thrombosis. The incidence or retinal prethrombosis was 4.6 % (24 cases) among our patients. Its initial symptoms are unilater headache, higher blood pressure and amaurosis fugax that can repeat more and more frequently. The ophthalmoscopic view shows incipient papilledema with small peripapillary hemorrhages, without bigger perivenous hemorrhages at this time period.

Branch or Trunk Thrombosis of Retinal Veins

Branch or trunk thrombosis of retinal veins indicate of the further worsening of the venous disorders of the papilla.

Ophthalmoscopic view shows a more and more hyperemic and prominent papilla/measurement of papilla prominentia by ophthalmoscopy/, with tortuos veins, perivenous, small intraretinal hemorrhages. It is an important element of differential diagnosis that in contrast with the swelling of the optic discs caused by the higher intracranial pressure. In cases of retinal thrombosis is characterized by perivenous hemorrhages that reach the periphery, and antechiasmal visual functions deteriorate rapidly. The deterioration of visual functions is not so rapid (hours, days) as in the case of embolism of the retinal arteries. In later stages the inability to read that can causes the central vision loss and it is probably the consequence of circulation disorders of macular area.

The lack of preventive laser therapy can results in the most severe ophthalmological complication. Namely they are: either simultaneous neovascularization of the retina, iridocorneal angle and iris. The latter can lead to almost uncontrollable secondary glaucoma and bleeding in the vitreous body (see below) (Figs. 45.10 and 45.11). In acute phase of retinal thrombosis only, we tried to prevent these untreatable complications by the systemic anticoagulant and adjuvant therapies.

Ocular Symptoms of Intracerebral Sinus Thrombosis

The first predictor sign of the increased intracranial pressure (HIP) the bilateral papilledema, with normal optic functions for a long time (except of a visual filed defect by bigger blind spot). The intracerebral venous thrombosis may begin the same ocular sign, namely by uni- or bilateral papilledema with different etiopathomechanism. Early ocular signs can draw our attention to the intracerebral venous circulatory disorders. The tardive recognize of these disorders (venous stasis or thrombosis in the transverse or sigmoid sinuses, as well carotid-cavernous fistulas, etc.) can lead to the most serious cerebrovascular events. (For more details on modern diagnostics and treatment see Chaps.9 and 48).

Stroke Epidemiology: International and Hungarian Data

According to Hungarian statistical data, stroke is the third most common cause of mortality following tumorous and cardiovascular diseases (American Heart Association (AHA) 1996). According to WHO data, 700,000 cases of stroke

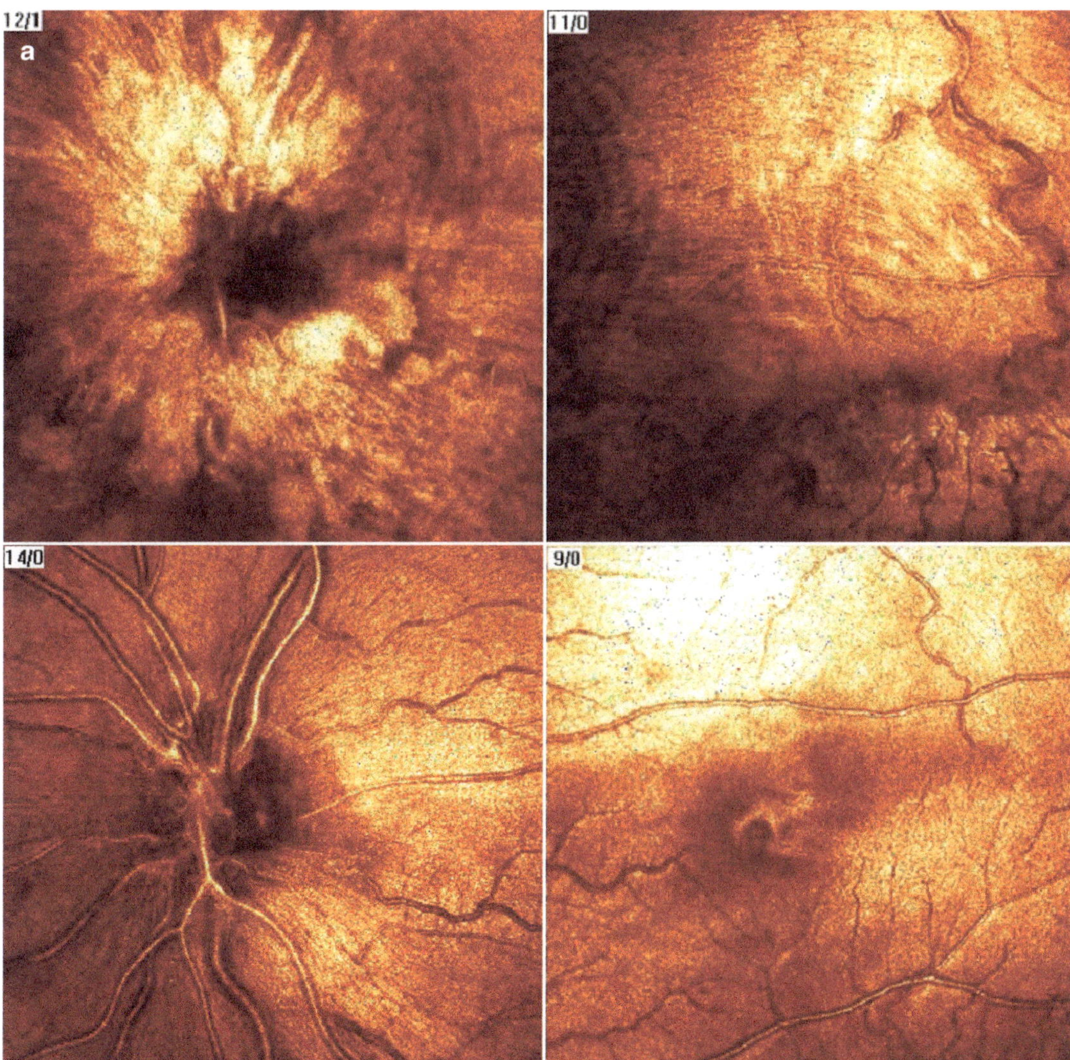

Fig. 45.10 (**a**) *Top photos*: left retinal trunk thrombosis with consecutive –peripillar and perimacular retinal edema and haemorrhages *bottom photos*: papilla and perimaculararea after systemic treatment. (**b**) Visual filed defects views before and after systemic therapy by comuter perimetry (G2)

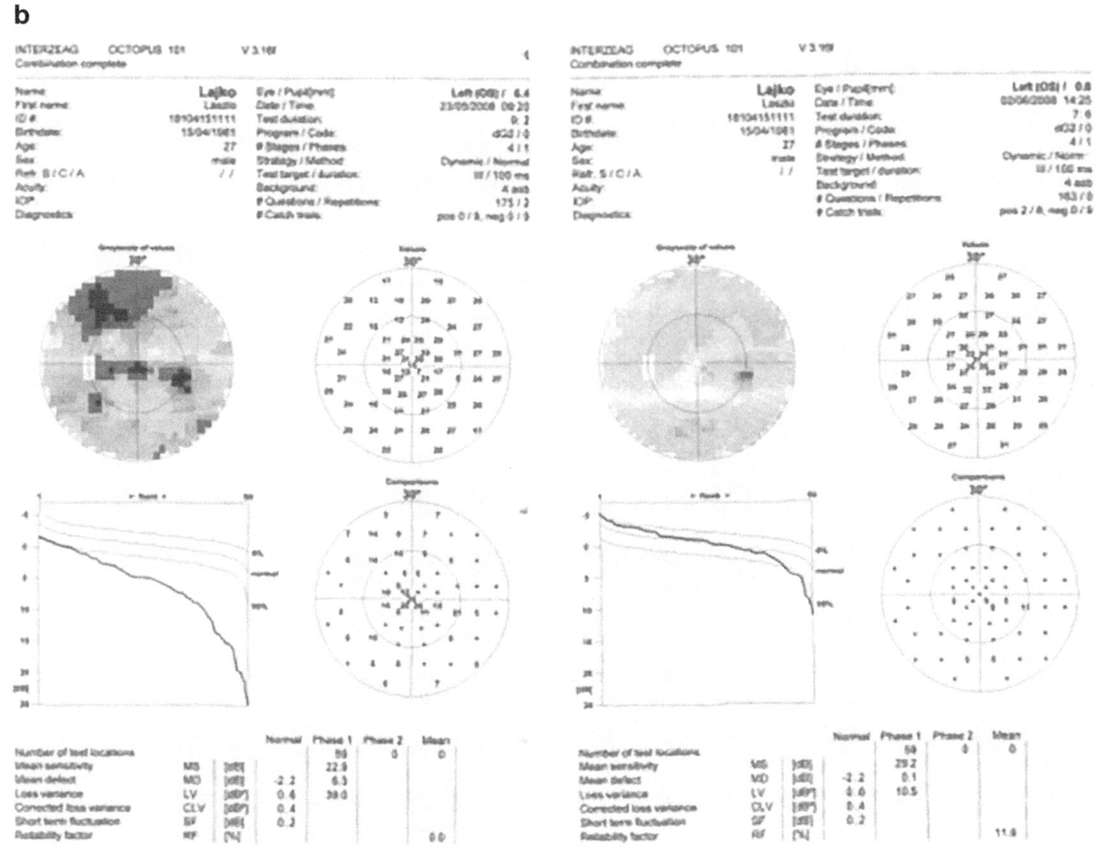

Fig. 45.10 (continued)

are registered in the USA every year, which means an incidence of 25/10,000 people (about 300 million being the total population of the USA). Stroke is endemic as it causes the mortality of almost 5 million people every year, and with the continuous increase in life expectancy this number may double by 2020.

The number of cerebrovascular diseases is 40–60,000 in Hungary. It means the morbidity rate of 40/10,000; however, according to recent surveys it is closer to 60/10,000 (the total population of Hungary is approximately 10 million). Thus, the morbidity rate in Hungary is about two-three times as high as that in the USA (as per 10,000 inhabitants).

According to Hungarian mortality data, out of the annual 40 cases of stroke, 18 end in death, which means that the mortality rate is nearly 50 %. Eighty percent of stroke cases in Hungary is caused by some ischemic change, half or even two-thirds of which are the result of microembolism due to atherosclerosis.

The Epidemiology of Ocular Strokes: National and International Data

The incidence of anterior ischemic optic neuropathy (AION) is about 6000/year in the USA (Objectives of the Hungarian Public Health Program & Stroke 2001). Extrapolated calculations based on this figure give us an annual case number of 250–300 in Hungary. In our patient group, out of 514 ocular strokes 62 were caused by either unilateral or bilateral AION, which accounts for 12.5 % of all cases.

The *fellow eye* often becomes affected; the rate of unilateral and bilateral cases was 26.3 %

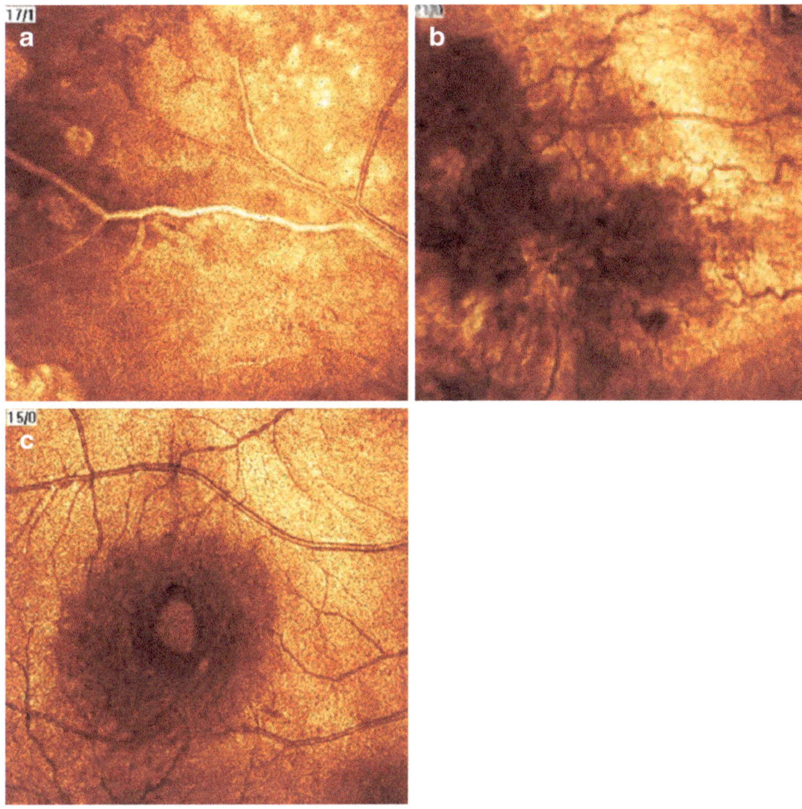

Fig. 45.11 The most frequent complications of thrombosis of retinal vessels in untreated cases. (**a**) Image of complete branch vein occlusion (untreated case): 'empty vein': there is no circulation in the venous branch following complete occlusion by thrombus). (**b**) Retinal neovascularization that affected a major part of the posterior perimacular pole, with hemorrhages, signs of serious ischemic degeneration. (**c**) Characteristic maculopathy as a frequent complication of retinal trunk thrombosis with serious central vision loss

and 73.7 in our care, while the rate of males and females was about the same. The mean age of patients was *57.7 years*, which indicates a *shift towards younger ages. MRI* examinations detected a high rate of intracranial parenchyma lesions already at the development of ocular symptoms (*54.6 %*). As for the etiology, we noted the combined and simultaneous occurrence of common and rare causes as well as risk factors. Undetected or *untreated hypertension* (Primary and secondary prevention of cerebrovascular diseases 2001) is one of the most important underlying diseases among patients suffering from ocular stroke. The most common trigger factors seem to be vascular diseases, *atheromatosis* and arterial microembolism, all of which are caused by disorders of carbohydrate (DM) and fat metabolism (*hypercholesterinaemia, mixed hyperlipidemia*). Congenital coagulopathies were rare, while the combination of fat metabolism disorder and lesions that can result in cardiac embolism was common (Bousser 2001).

Predisposing Factors

According to the databases of the Hungarian Stroke Centers, Stroke departments the rates of risk factors and background diseases of the stroke disease are very similar to the those of microembolism sources of our ocular stroke patients.

When comparing the data on the source of microembolism in stroke and ocular stroke, we found very similar rates of f.e. ubtreaated hypertension and ICA stenosis, while the rate of fat metabolism disorder was much higher at the onset of ocular stroke.

We tried to focus on the screening of the cardiological disorders as a microembolism'sources, especially atrial fibrillation and cardiac rhythm problem as a serious and frequent origin of the fibrin microembolism. The efficient screening program of our lipid clinic is supported by the high proportion of ICA atheromatosis (57.1 %) in initial phase of hyperlipidaemia. Compared to the risk factors' data of stroke patients, we found a

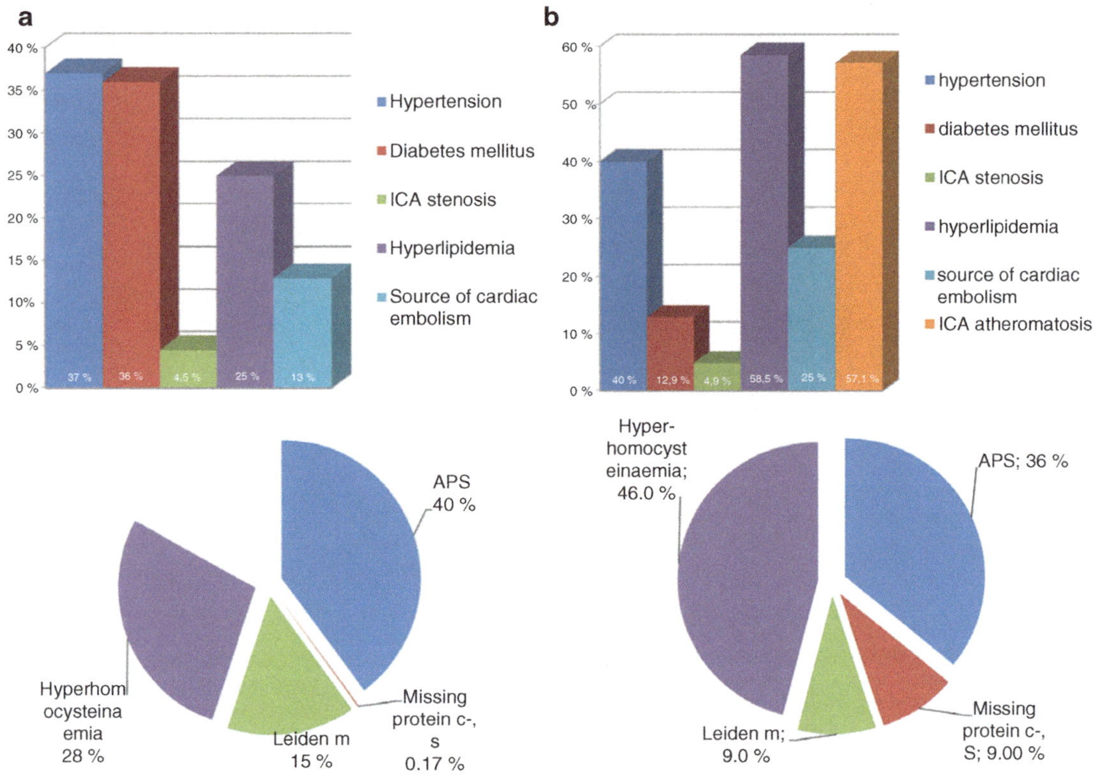

Fig. 45.12 Rates of predisposing factors and background diseases in cerebrovascular disorders. (**a**) Databaseof the Stroke Centers at the former Hungarian Psychiatric and Neurological Institution (OPNI)) and (**b**) from our ocular stroke patients' database

similar rate of antiphospholipid syndrome (APS) but a higher rate of thrombophylia and hematological disorders (Leiden mutation, protein C and S deficiency, hyperhomocysteinemia) as the possible source of microembolism (Fig. 45.12).

Basic Principles of Treatment

– **recommendations for a consensus *on comprehensive, local and systemic treatment***

Local therapeutic procedures:

The laser and vitreoretinal surgical interventions :prevent the development of severe complications (e.g., secondary glaucoma, neovascularisation). Laser treatment and vitreous body surgical interventions are mostly performed in the advanced and complicated stage of the vascular optic disease: This period means that optic fibers have already significant lesion. In consequence the results of the improvement of visual acuity are really poorly.

The aim of the systemic-, etiology-specific therapy is causal treatment, namely :

- ocular symptoms draw the attention to the potential of multiple embolism;
- ocular symptoms can help to decide what kind of systemic treatment is necessary;
- patients with acute ocular symptoms have to be treated in an appropriate healthcare center as soon as possible in order that the process can be reversed (Bohdanecka et al. 1999).

We would also like to emphasize the protection of the fellow eye, so very important the prevention of the ocular stroke on the fellow eye. In our APC stroke (541) patients had a unilateral ocular stroke 26.3 %, while 73.7 of them had bilateral ocular thromboembolism. This high proportion might be attributable to the high rate of numerous patients, who suffered from retrochiasmal vascular lesions in cases of APCstroke.

However, in 30 % of our ocular stroke cases were strated by NA-AION (62 patients), and 30 % of these patients had bilateral NA-AION, namely thay had so called pseudo-Foster Kennedy syndrome.

Among our patients, the cranial MR detected ischemic disorders particularly lacunar infarcts, as a vascular encephalopathy of our cases about 54.6 %, it was observable near at the same time as the initial signs of ocular stroke.

Prevention of Systemic Microembolism

The risk factors and background diseases do not caused ocular stroke by an isolated factor. In the clinical practice the ocular vascular diorders are caused by multifactorial effects, mostly cardiovascular and metabolic effects as an overlapping way, to promote loss of vision.

Multifactorial pathomechanism is seems probably, because of the in the time period of recognition of the ocular signs other organs (kidney, cardiocasular system, etc.) has been affected by background disease.

Systemic therapy may not be carried out without consulting the relevant specialists and considering the methodological regulations of fellow specialties. Etiology-specific therapy is efficient only if it fits the indications and dosing criteria, and if its long-term application can be effective and void of side effects. The treatment has to be performed according to the uniform therapeutic principles stipulated by the methodological newsletter of the Hungarian Society of Thrombosis and Hemostasis (Bohdanecka et al. 1999). Similarly to the treatment of cerebro- and cardiovascular diseases, these conditions need the cooperation of a professional TEAM to diagnose the disease and to carry out lifelong therapy and care.

Treatment Options

Antiplatelet Therapy

- aim of therapy: to prevent increase of aggregation of platelet and development of microthrombus, prevention of the development of soft-vulnerable plaque and intima lesions of vessels;
- it is widely accepted in the primary and secondary prevention of cerebro- and cardiovascular diseases;
- aggregometry: measures the increase in platelet aggregation ability, while stress tests evaluate the efficiency of appropriate medical therapy (Costa et al. 2003).

Anticoagulant Treatment

- isolated
- can be followed by antiplatelet therapy
- etiological causes: atherothrombosis, venous occlusion:
  - to prevent the enlargement of the thrombus;
  - to prevent further spread of embolism from the source;
  - to prevent the development of fibrin thrombus (European Stroke Initiative (EUSI) 2000; Flammer et al. 2001).

The patient whose case is illustrated by Fig. 45.13 underwent the first neuro-ophthalmological assessment when the right eye was already amaurotic. The evaluation of the left eye – previously with good visual function – was initiated because of the massive hemianopia involving the center, visual impairment and other neurological symptoms. Underlying disease: secondary antiphospho-lipid syndrome: severe autoimmune disease with central nervous system manifestations. Adequate

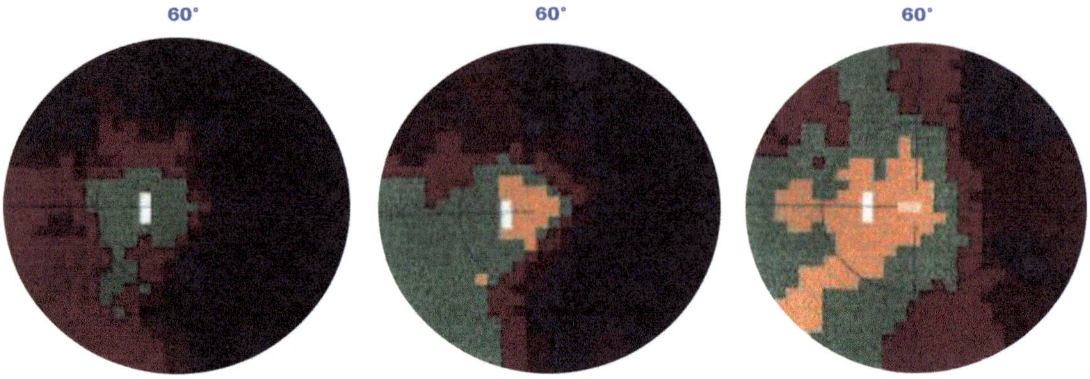

Fig. 45.13 Visual field defects series made by computer perimetry: improvement of the left visual field defect of a monocular patient by anticoagulant therapy. Background disease: antiphospholipid syndrome (APS)

anticoagulant therapy resulted in the improvement of the visual field (middle and right image) and other visual functions.

Thrombolysis

Only a very low number of cases have been reported in ophthalmology, but the significant loss of vision caused by arterial occlusion – practically complete amaurosis with some light perception – will sooner or later neccessitate the development of a consensus with the relevant specialties (rapid improvement is evident in the field ofthrombolysis) (Heinze 2000).

Supplementary Treatment

- hemodilution: improvement of microcirculation, isovolemic hemodilution;
- neuroprotetive treatment: corticosteroids, reduction of celebral edema, diuretics (Mannitol, etc.), reduction of edema in the macula. EUSI: it has no effect on stroke outcome, there are no guidelines whether it is recommended following an ischemic stroke or not;
- vasodilators: vasospasm, microcirculation +/– improvement of metabolic processes appropriate therapy of disorders of carbohydrate and fat metabolism (Hacke et al. 2000; Haefliger et al. 1999).

Recommendations for the Systemic Therapy of Ocular Stroke

(based on the recommendations of EUSI–, AHA and the Hungarian Stroke Society)

<u>**Anticoagulant treatment**</u>

Non arteritic anterior ischemic opticopathy (NA–AION)
- monocular NA- AION in acute phase:
- NA AION in pts history with known etiology
- pseudoFoster–Kennedy syndrome: bilateral NA AION with time lag

Retinal thrombosis
- acute unilateral thromboembolism +/– known etiology
- acute unilateral thrombosis + previous ocular stroke of the fellow eye
- in the background : untreated hypertension or coagulopathies (younger age)

Cardiological source of embolism + OCULAR symptoms
- ocular stroke and its source was 25 % of our cases

ICA–, vertebral artery dissection + OCULAR symptoms

in cases of dissection of large vessels absolutely

Thrombophilia + OCULAR symptoms

Leiden–mutation (1.4 %), protein C and S deficiency (1.4 %)

enzyme defect leading to a disorder in homocysteine synthesis.

APS+OCULAR symptom+

it affects many organ systems (CNS, lungs, heart, kidneys, venous thrombosis in the lower limbs)

our patients showed a 5.5 % increase in APA titer when the ocular symptoms presented

autoimmune disease, the majority of patients need anticoagulant therapy

Contraindications of anticoagulant treatment

Uncooperative patient
Malignant–, uncontrolled hypertension
Dementia
Skull trauma, risk of falling
Local–ophthalmological causes:

- vitreous body bleeding
- Diabetic retinopathy +/– neovascularization

Indications of platelet aggregation therapy in ocular stroke:

- **Embolism of the central retinal artery**
  - + atherosclerosis (our own patients: 51.7 %)
  - + diabetes mellitus (our own patients: 12.9 %)
  - + fat metabolism disorder (our own patients: 58.5 %)
    - Previous bilateral AION – pale optic disc/pseudo–Foster–Kennedy syndrome
    - AION + severe ICA atheromatosis
    - complicated cases of retinal thromboembolism (pale optic disc, macular degeneration)
  - *despite the lack of systemic indication*
- Antiplatelet therapy is indicated instead of anticoagulation:
  - intracranial "small vessel disease" +/– ocular symptoms
  - cardiac syndrome X with a low risk of stroke +/– ocular changes
  - severe ICA stenosis +/– ocular symptoms

Dilemmas and Questions

The etiopathomechanism of the clinical signs and symptoms of ocular stroke is still unclear. The complications of severe, untreated hypertension and vascular encephalopathy frequently manifest in the form of venous circulatory disorders of the retina, while the atherosclerosis of cervical blood vessels more commonly leads to the embolism of the retinal arteries. The separation and interpretation of venous and arterial thromboembolism is a task for the future.

Time factor: in the vast majority of cases, ocular strokes result in an irreversible decrease in visual acuity in a matter of hours or even minutes. Hemorrheologic and neuroradiological investigations are time-consuming. If the leading and only symptom affects the eye, is it advisable to start systemic (e.g., anticoagulant) therapy following blood count and some acute neuroradiological investigations? The decision needs tailored consideration! (cryptogenic stroke – 40 %)

Thrombolysis? Acute care is efficient if it is performed within 3 h in a well-equipped cerebrovascular healthcare center that works in a synchronized way, following methodological regulations rigorously.

TEAM: This activity has to be performed within a network that applies uniform diagnostics, therapeutic and nursing principles. According to the data of the stroke centers, there are 32 stroke centers in Hungary (since 1991). Based on the relevant system of conditions (Doppler, CT, etc.) their activity covers the whole population. The consultant team participating in the care of ocular stroke patients would like to assist the work of these centers.

References

American Heart Association (AHA). Guidelines for thrombolytic therapy for acute stroke. A supplement to the guidelines for the management of patients with acute ischemic stroke. Circulation. 1996;94:1167–74.

Biousse V. Chapter 40. Cerebrovascular disease. In: Miller NR, Newman NJ, editors. Walsh & Hoyt: clinical neuro-ophthalmology. Lippincott Williams & Wilkins; 2005. p. 1967–2168.

Bohdanecka Z et al. Influence acquisition parameters on haemodynamic measurements with the Heidelberg

retina flowmeter at the optic disc. J Glaucoma. 1998;7:151–7.
Bohdanecka Z et al. Relationship between blood flow velocities in retrobulbar vessels and Laser Doppler Flowmetry at the optic disc in glaucoma patients. Ophthalmologica. 1999;213:145–9.
Bousser MG. Antithrombotic strategy in stroke. Int Soc Thrombosis & Haemostasis (IHTS), XVIIIth Word Congr, Paris; 2001.
Costa VP et al. The effects of antiglaucoma and systemic medications on ocular blood flow. Progr Retin Eye Res. 2003;22:769–805 (international study).
Erb C, et al. Confocal scanning laser Doppler flowmetry of the optic nerve in smokers. Neuroophthalmology. 1999;21.
European Stroke Initiative (EUSI). Recommendations for stroke management. Cerebrovascul Dis. 2000; 10(Suppl 3).
Flammer J et al. Susac syndrome: a vasospastic disorders? Eur J Ophthalmol. 2001;11(2):175–9.
Hacke W et al. Acute treatment of ischemic stroke. Cerebrovascul Dis. 2000;10:22–33.
Haefliger IO, et al. Modulation of Heidelberg retina flowmeter parameter flow at the papilla of healthy subjects: effect of carbogen, oxygen, high intraocular pressure and B-blockers. Surv Ophthalmol. 1999;43(Suppl 1).
Heinze KG. Molecular risk factor for thrombosis & risk factors in venous thrombotic diseases. Clin Lab. 2000;46:191.
Holló G. A szem vèrkeringèse glaukomdban.[Ocular circulation in glaucoma] Klinikai vizsgálati lehetösègek, eredmènyek ès azok gyakorlati èrtelmezèse.[Clinical investigation options, results and their practical interpretation]. Szemèszet [Ophthalmologia Hungarica]. 1966;133.
Hungarian Arteriosclerosis Society Összefoglalás: a hyperlipoproteinaemiák kezelèsi irányelvei [Summary: management guidelines of hyperlipoproteinemias]. Agyèrbetegsègek [Cerebrovascular Diseases]. 2002;3.
Hungarian Society of Thrombosis and Haemostasis Thromboembóliák megelözèse is kezelèse. [Prevention and management of thromboembolism]. Magyar Konszenzus Nyilatkozat. [Consensus statement]. 1998, 2001.
Killer HE. Bilateral non-arteritic anterior ischemic optic neuropathy in a patient with autoimmune thrombocytopenia. Eur J Ophthalmol. 2000;10(2):180–2.
Kupersmith MJ. Neurovascular – neuro-ophthalmology. New York: Springer; 1993.
Kupersmith Y, et al. Cerebrovascular neuroophthalmology. New York; 1994.
Levin LA. Update on anterior ischemic optic neuropathy. 4th annual ocular drug symposium; 2002.
Miller NR, Newman NJ, editors. Walsh & Hoyt's clinical neuro-ophthalmology. 6th ed. Philadelphia: Lippincott Williams & Wilkins; 2005.
Objectives of the Hungarian Public Health Program, Stroke (2001–2010) [Cerebrovascular diseases]. 2001;1.
Óváry CS. Epidemiológiai vizsgálatok [Epidemiological studies] OPNI Agyèrbetegsègek Országos Központja, Adatbank, [Database of the Center for Cerebrovascular Diseases at the former Hungarian Psychiatric and Neurological Institution (OPNI)]. 2001.
Primary and secondary prevention of cerebrovascular diseases. Recommendations for the management of acute ischemic stroke. Cerebrovascular Diseases. 2001;1.
Schmidt D et al. Stage dependent efficacy of intraarterial fibrinolysis in CRAO. Neuroophthalmology. 1998;20:125–41.
Wong KS et al. Risk factors for early death in acute ischemic stroke and intracerebral hemorrhage. A prospective hospital-based study in Asia. Stroke. 1999;30:2326.

Diseases Causing Compression of the Optic Nerve: The Neurosurgeon's Perspective

46

János Vajda

Contents

Diseases causing compression of the optic nerve encompass pressure-related diseases of the oral (cisternal) part of the optic nerve-chiasm-tract. These entities include trauma-related, oncological, and vascular diseases, but traumatology is discussed in a separate section of this book. Compression of the optic nerve may have several different causes of similar pathomechanism. In most regions of the body, compression emerges when a process exerts pressure on normal organs. The characteristics of the visual pathway's regional anatomy create special conditions. A lesion growing in the proximity of the optic nerve may cause symptoms of compression even in a way that the direct damage to the nerve is induced and maintained by surrounding normal structures: bony and dural elements. This is important from the aspect of surgical strategy. The upper side of the aperture of the optic canal is sharp-edged, while its lower wall forms an arc in the direction of the sella, thus a process dislocating the optic nerves in a downward direction pushes the nerve against the smooth surface of the sellar dura (similar to the general mechanisms of compression), in contrast to a mass lifting the nerve upwards, because in this case the optic nerve is damaged by the sharp rim of the canal, which blocks the small vessels of the nerve. Thus it can be understood, why the visual functions of patients with frontobasal meningioma have improved dramatically more after surgery, compared to optic lesions caused by suprasellar space occupying masses. The physical size of the compression is not proportional to the resulting deterioration of function. The correspondence is better, if we also consider the temporal dynamics of the process as velocity. Segments of the optic nerve are capable to retain their function while being considerably tapered to a surprising extent, enduring the slow deformation. At the same time, due to certain chronic changes, in contrast to fast deterioration, slowly developing clinical presentation may have smaller chance for improvement after decompression. Malignancies or lesions causing sudden, gradual compression (saccadic dilation of aneurysms) result in more severe disturbance.

J. Vajda, M.D., PhD
National Institute of Neurology, Budapest, Hungary
e-mail: janosvajda@gmail.com; http://www.oiti.hu

J. Somlai, T. Kovács (eds.), *Neuro-Ophthalmology*, DOI 10.1007/978-3-319-28956-4_46

However, rapidly developing compression, and short but significant ischemia most often cause permanent damage, since the structures of the visual pathway are extremely sensitive, the chance of functional restitution is minimal. Adaptation to the compression of benign, slow processes may also easily become perturbed, when the tension exceeds a certain limit, followed by a disturbance in the circulation of the neural elements.

Neurosurgical Diseases Causing Compression of the Optic Nerve

Pathologies affecting the visual pathway and requiring surgery are practically classified according to their etiology.

Tumors (The Most Frequent Cause)

The most important extraparenchymal tumors are meningiomas, pituitary adenomas, craniopharyngiomas, and teratomas. Tumors involving the oral segment pertain to processes around the sella, and result in a diversity of defects in visual acuity and/or visual field, depending on the origin and direction of expansion. All these can be reversible even in case of severe functional disturbance: it is the surgery of tumors that may be the most spectacularly successful. To restore the function of the optic fibers, certain rules of manipulation should be followed:

- If dislocation or later consequent compression can be predicted in advance in the proximity of the optic canal, the first phase of the surgery should be decompression at the level of the optic canal. Thus mobilization due to the removal of the tumor preserves the nerve trapped into the canal. It is recommended to identify and open the optic canal as a first step, unless the nerve is lifted by a cyst, the puncture of which results in an immediate, spectacular decompression.
- The greatly stretched segments of the optic nerve gradually loose their color and shape, becoming similar to the tissue maintaining the compression, moreover, they may become involved in the capsule of the tumor. The direction and extent of the optic nerve deviation have to be considered based on the findings of the CT, MRI and angiography. It is practical to first find structures that serve as reference to their identification: anterior clinoid process, internal carotid artery and the edge of the tentorium, or at best all these structures together.

The individual tumor types possess few neuro-ophthalmological characteristics, there are fewer differences between a meningioma and a pituitary adenoma of the same location and size, etc. than between tumors of different location and size, but of the same histological type.

However, it has to be noted that:

Nowadays, thanks to endocrinology, the majority of pituitary **adenomas are recognized before the development of severe damage to the visual pathway**. Their suprasellar growth endangers the chiasm and the optic nerves, but bigger tumors are also generally eligible for transnasal removal, as the sellar cavity filled by the tumor is easily accessible from the nasal cavity, and removing the abnormal tissue gradually opens space within the tumor for aspiration of its expansive parts, or their traction into the sellar cavity (Fig. 46.1).

Due to the restricted visibility, radicality affecting the suprasellar parts, thus complete decompression of the optic nerve may be occasionally questionable. Of techniques recommended for achieving the most favorable radicality, the use of endoscopy and several management strategies have to be mentioned. As the injury of the perichiasmatic arachnoid mater with consequent leakage of the cerebrospinal fluid is the most frequent surgical complication of adenomas causing suprasellar compression, it is practical to approach the oral parts at the end of the procedure. During the reduction of the posterior part of the intrasellar tumor, the dorsum sellae comes into view, and the posterior lobe of the pituitary gland may also be occasionally preserved. The transnasal approach is also successful in case of parasellar tumor growth, in which case blind recognition of the location of the gently pulsating intracavernous carotid artery may provide guidance. The transnasal approach puts a significantly lower load on the patient,

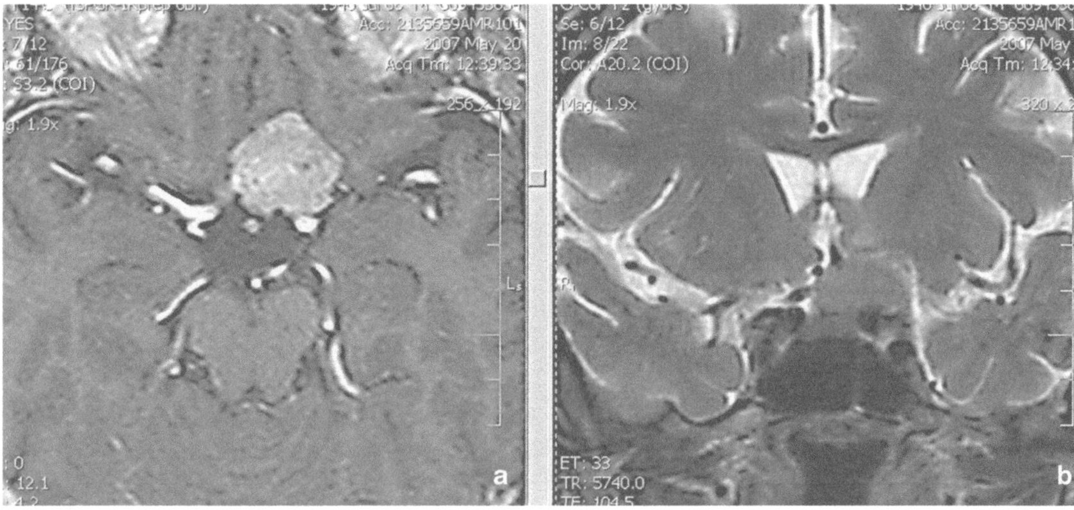

Fig. 46.1 (**a**) On the left side, an axial, contrast-enhanced, T1-weighted MR scan of an optic foramen–tuberculum sellae meningioma. (**b**) T2-weighted coronal MR image, showing the clinoid segment of the carotid artery within the tumor, suggesting significant dislocation of the optic nerve

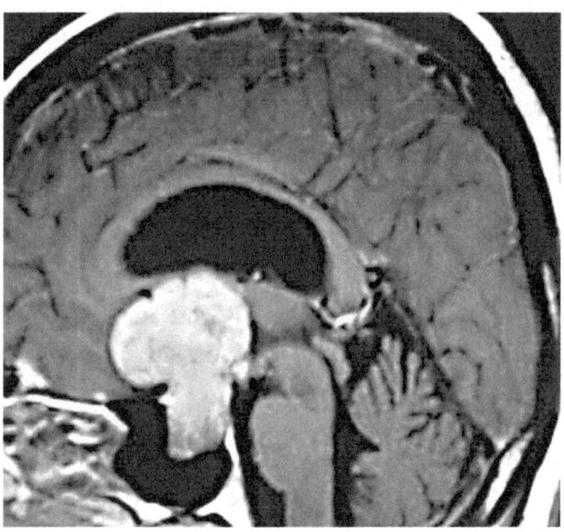

Fig. 46.2 This image depicts a pituitary adenoma causing compression of both optic nerves and the chiasm with its suprasellar growth. The sagittal T1-weighted, contrast-enhanced scan shows the sphenoid sinus with the intruding tumor, the location of which helps in transnasal approach to resect the part of the tumor that is located in the 3rd ventricle and maintained the occlusive hydrocephalus, by penetrating the tumor itself

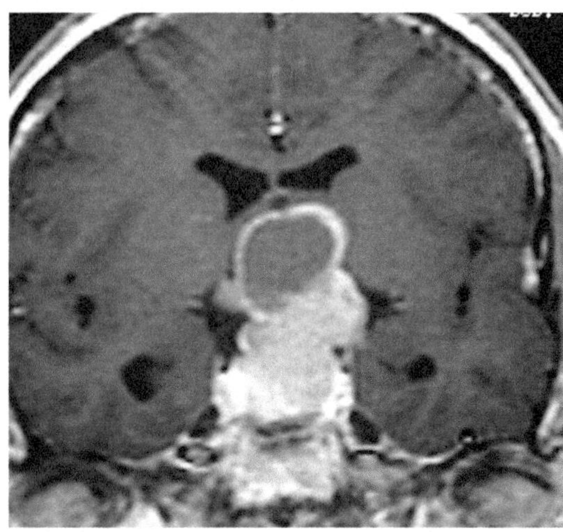

Fig. 46.3 The MR image shows the cystic and solid parts of a craniopharyngioma. The coronal MR image of a tumor compressing the visual pathway shows the obliteration of the 3rd ventricle (preoperative image)

therefore, it is also recommended in case of severe deterioration of visual functions. If the expected improvement is not achieved after transnasal surgery, reoperation from frontotemporal approach is recommended. In rare cases, due to smaller or greater intratumoral hemorrhages, pituitary adenomas may result in acute functional impairment of the optic pathway associated with amaurosis developing in a few days or hours. In our opinion, acute decompressive surgery should be performed from frontotemporal approach. Although it depends on the fundoscopic appearance and the visual functions, considerable improvement can be achieved in all such acute cases (Figs. 46.2 and 46.3).

Meningiomas

Since meningiomas may be broadly attached to the dura forming the most variable shapes, the optic nerves and their vessels may be deformed and take the most unpredictable positions. Tumor removal is speeded up and facilitated by terminating the tumor's blood supply. At the same time, during the coagulation of the basal dura, the optic nerves may be overheated, and increased attention should be paid to the ophthalmic artery. Optic canal meningiomas take a special place in this group, as they may significantly damage the blood supply of the optic nerve even before surgery, to which the effect of the surgical intervention should also be added. This explains why results are frequently less favorable. Sphenoid plane meningiomas often expand towards the dura of the optic canal (predominantly ventrally). These small tumor fractions are covered by the optic nerve, and are often left behind during surgery, because they remain unrecognized, and result in early recurrence and deterioration in vision. Optic foramen meningioma should be suspected if there is a significant difference between the two eyes in the extent of the deterioration in vision, and in the length of the medical history. Opening the optic canal also has the advantage of making these parts of the tumor visible. In those cases, when a tumor mass relatively big compared to the size of the optic canal had protruded into the canal, and it has already resulted in amaurosis, no relevant improvement has been achieved in visual functions.

Craniopharyngiomas

According to our experience, surgery of craniopharyngiomas is the most dangerous regarding pre- and postoperative visual functions. This group involves the highest number of unsuccessful cases and postoperative deterioration of the condition worldwide. This can be explained with the simultaneous effect of several factors, like frequently occurring prefixed chiasm, close contact of the protruding surface of the tumor and the chiasm, and identical course of the normal optochiasmatic vessels and the vessels of the tumor.

As a proof of these factors, it can be mentioned that resection from the direction of the corpus callosum and the 3rd ventricle by approaching the superior–posterior surface of the tumor is accompanied by fewer complications affecting the visual pathway. The poorer results are explained by the frequently questionable radicality and the threatening recurrence even after complete resection of the adamantinomatous type, but maybe above all, the damaging effect of the sharp-pointed, calcified tumor mass. This is even spontaneously a far coarser morphological trauma compared to other tumors, but almost cuts the fibers stretched on the crystals during mobilization.

The recidiva may occur in the disease process of all **extraparenchymal tumors**, and its surgical cause is not always detectable. Regarding the outcome of the visual pathway, recurrence is an absolutely negative factor, because of the multiple adhesions, circulatory disturbances, and surgical decompression postponed to later stages.

Intraparenchymal tumors are optic and chiasmatic gliomas pertaining to the absolutely benign spongioblastoma (pilocytic astrocytoma) group and representing no differential diagnostic problem nowadays in the era of the CT and MRI. Recently research is going into the identification of visual pathway segments, where the tumor leaves the axis of the neural elements and gains a pseudo-extraparenchymal character, that is, its location can be exactly determined: thus which part of the tumor can be surgically removed without any risk. Even nowadays, in case of a purely axial, diffuse, infiltrating type, there is no other option left, only bony, dural decompression, and in case of the chiasm, the incision of the tense capsule. In special cases, when the unilateral amaurosis is permanent due to the lateralized progression, to save the remaining vision, transsection of the nerve is recommended in a segment determined by functional rules (Figs. 46.4 and 46.5).

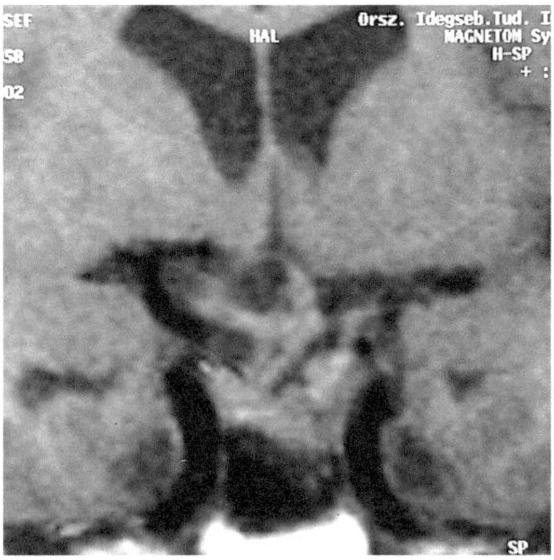

Fig. 46.4 Control MR image of the tumor removed from a transcallosal approach (postoperative scan)

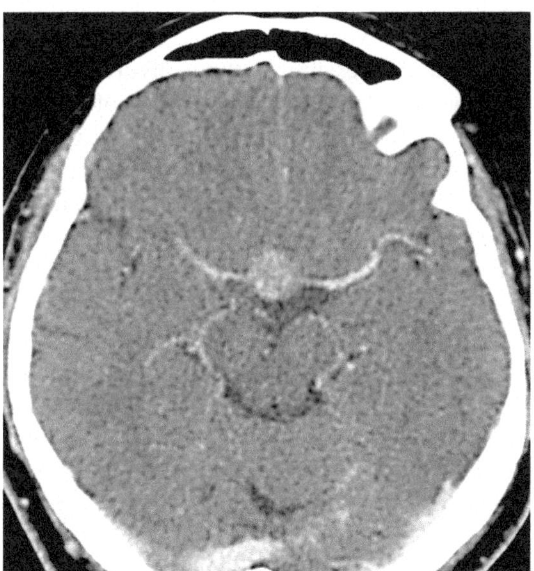

Fig. 46.5 The contrast-enhanced axial CT scan reveals that an anterior communicating artery aneurysm stands in the background of the compression of the chiasm

Vascular Compression-Related Diseases of the Optic Nerve

Vascular compression-related diseases of the visual pathway are dominated by giant aneurysms of the anterior part of the Willis circle. Sellar location is a separate clinical entity due to its characteristic symptoms. Abnormalities of the optic nerve (can be bilateral, even if to a different degree) and the chiasm may be caused by giant sacs originating from the distal cavernous and the entire supraclinoid segments of the internal carotid artery on both sides, or the horizontal segment of the anterior cerebral artery, or the anterior communicating artery. Lateralized opto-chiasmatic lesions are of the highest incidence and are caused by aneurysm of the ipsilateral ophthalmic artery-carotid artery junction, and the symptoms of a chiasmatic lesion due to the downward protruding sac from the anterior communicating artery. The clinical problem starts with differential diagnostics, as today the first line diagnostic tool is the CT: but it cannot decisively differentiate between extracerebral suprasellar tumors and aneurysms. As the latter ones are much less frequent than the previous ones, angiography is not suggested in all cases, thus the presence of an aneurysm has to be proposed consciously, and MR followed by MR angiography should be recommended. In those rare cases, when the giant aneurysm originates from the contralateral carotid artery and angiography gives false negative results even under compression of the contralateral common carotid artery, attention should be called to the necessity of bilateral carotid artery angiography.

Angiography provides help choose the method with which the aneurysm can be obliterated the easiest way. Now there is a wide range of endovascular solutions providing possibility for intervention without opening the skull.

Giant aneurysms of the internal carotid artery and the ophthalmic artery are in very close contact with the bony and dural components of the skull base, frequently these components may considerably cover the origin of the sac, thus transcranial surgery begins with extradural removal of the anterior clinoid process, the roof of the optic canal, already during the preparation of the surgical trajectory. The dural sheath of the carotid artery is incised as well. The relatively big distance of the aneurysm neck from the stretched nerve facilitates the treatment of the aneurysm, but the wall thickness of the neck may occasionally render their clipping similarly difficult as that of other giant sacs. In several cases, the surgeon is forced to create a real neck with the clips used to obliterate the aneurysm, parallel with the supplying vessel.

Some aneurysms of the ophthalmic artery stemming quite close and medial to the origin of the ophthalmic artery, have the interesting strategic characteristic that they lift the nerve and push it rather in a lateral direction, resulting in an easier and safer possibility to approach them from the contralateral side. In most cases the direction of the dislocation of the optic nerve cannot be detected before surgery, thus it may also occur, that the operation has to be continued from a contralateral approach. Theoretically, the obliteration of the neck is not sufficient for the desired therapeutic effect in case of compression of the visual pathway, the sac expanding the nerve has to be evacuated, but the good functional outcome of endovascular aneurysm obliterations suggests that the cessation of the blood flow pulsation already leads to improvement. The bony-dural decompression of the optic nerve is naturally enhanced by the space gain, related to the evacuation of the blood content of the sac. For the absence of the desired improvement or the deterioration, impairment of the flow in the ophthalmic artery (the giant sac may easily push the metal clip closing the neck against the origin of the thin vessel), the forced interruption of the close contact between the mobilized wall of the sac and the nervous components, or the too long compression, and the irreversible consequences of the microcirculatory disturbance can be blamed.

Generalized Hypertension

Symptoms of the visual pathway associated with generalized intracranial hypertension develop as a result of the pressure exerted by the tense 3rd ventricle on the chiasm, and the damaging effect of the consequent fundus congestion on the circulation of the visual pathway. This is generally known by ophthalmologists and neurologists. It has to be kept in mind that on the one hand, certain types of increased intracranial pressure may theoretically require different neurosurgical interventions, thus they have to be discussed according to these groups, and on the other hand that the timing of the intervention and the evaluation of emergency predominantly depend on the ophthalmological condition, thus it is also a field where the cooperation of the ophthalmologist and the neurosurgeon is indispensable.

Generalized intracranial hypertension affecting the visual pathway may be caused by accumulation of cerebrospinal fluid or relative increase in the cerebral blood volume. Solving the chronic hydrocephalus by a ventriculoatrial or a peritoneal shunt renders reversible the deterioration of visual acuity recognized in time. Naturally, the triggering factor is decisive in the treatment method of hydrocephalus: the goal is to treat the obliterating tumor, cyst or membrane, etc. as the first step in the treatment of occlusive ventricular dilations. Increased intracranial pressure without hydrocephalus may be maintained by a disorder of permanently decreased absorption of cerebrospinal fluid or consequent disturbance in the circulation of cerebrospinal fluid, when drainage of the spinal cerebrospinal fluid via a lumboperitoneal shunt results in improvement of the visual function. The permanent relative increase of the cerebral blood volume is mainly caused by high venous pressure maintained by the large draining veins, such as the basal sinuses and in particular arteriovenous fistulas in the confluence of the sinuses, thus the main point of the treatment in cases revealed by angiography and MRI is the closure of the fistula, necessitated not only by the ophthalmological status, but also the prevention of hemorrhage from the fistula.

The empty sella symptom complex is a local form of increased pressure affecting the visual pathway, in which case the dilated 3rd ventricle protrudes into the sellar cavity and causes deformation of the chiasm and presumably circulatory disorder. In certain severe cases, shape reconstruction of the sellar cerebrospinal fluid space is necessary with the use of muscle tissue from a transsphenoidal approach.

Neuro-Ophthalmological Aspects of Tumors Causing Compression of the Visual Pathway System

47

Bernadett Salomváry

Contents

Tumors may cause injury to the visual pathway at any point between the retina and the visual cortex. The generally gradual and progressive loss of vision is the leading symptom in compression-related diseases of the different segments. The location can be deduced by the evaluation of the loss of visual field and the accompanying neurological symptoms.

B. Salomváry, M.D.
Head of Department, Head Physician Ophthalmologist, Neuro-ophthalmologist, Orbital Surgeon, National Institute of Neurology, Budapest, Hungary

Neuro-Ophthalmology Section, Hungarian Ophthalmological Association, Budapest, Hungary
e-mail: salom.betty@gmail.com

Intraocular Tumors

Seventy-five percent of intraocular tumors pertain to the group of uveal melanomas, 20 % are retinoblastomas and 5 % metastases. In Hungary, 80 out of 10 million inhabitants get these diseases per year. The location, size and type of the tumor determine which part of the eye is damaged. The nearer the tumor is to the macula, the earlier it causes disturbance of the central vision. Ophthalmological ultrasound, FLAG, ICG, CT and MR of the orbit are the diagnostic options. Two-thirds of intraocular tumors can be treated with radiotherapy, and the enucleation of the eye can be avoided.

Intraorbital Tumors

Tumors of the optic nerve, that is optic gliomas and optic nerve sheath meningeomas cause optic lesion early in the course of the disease (Fig. 47.1a, b). Tumors growing in the proximity of the optic nerve, mainly those spreading into the orbital apex cause compression of the optic nerve. Hemangiomas, neurinomas, neurofibromas, lymphomas, and malignant tumors as melanomas, hemangiopericytomas and metastatic tumors belong to this group. Damage to the optic nerve is partially due to ischemia, and partially to impairment of the axonal transport.

Other diseases causing compression of the optic nerve:

J. Somlai, T. Kovács (eds.), *Neuro-Ophthalmology*, DOI 10.1007/978-3-319-28956-4_47

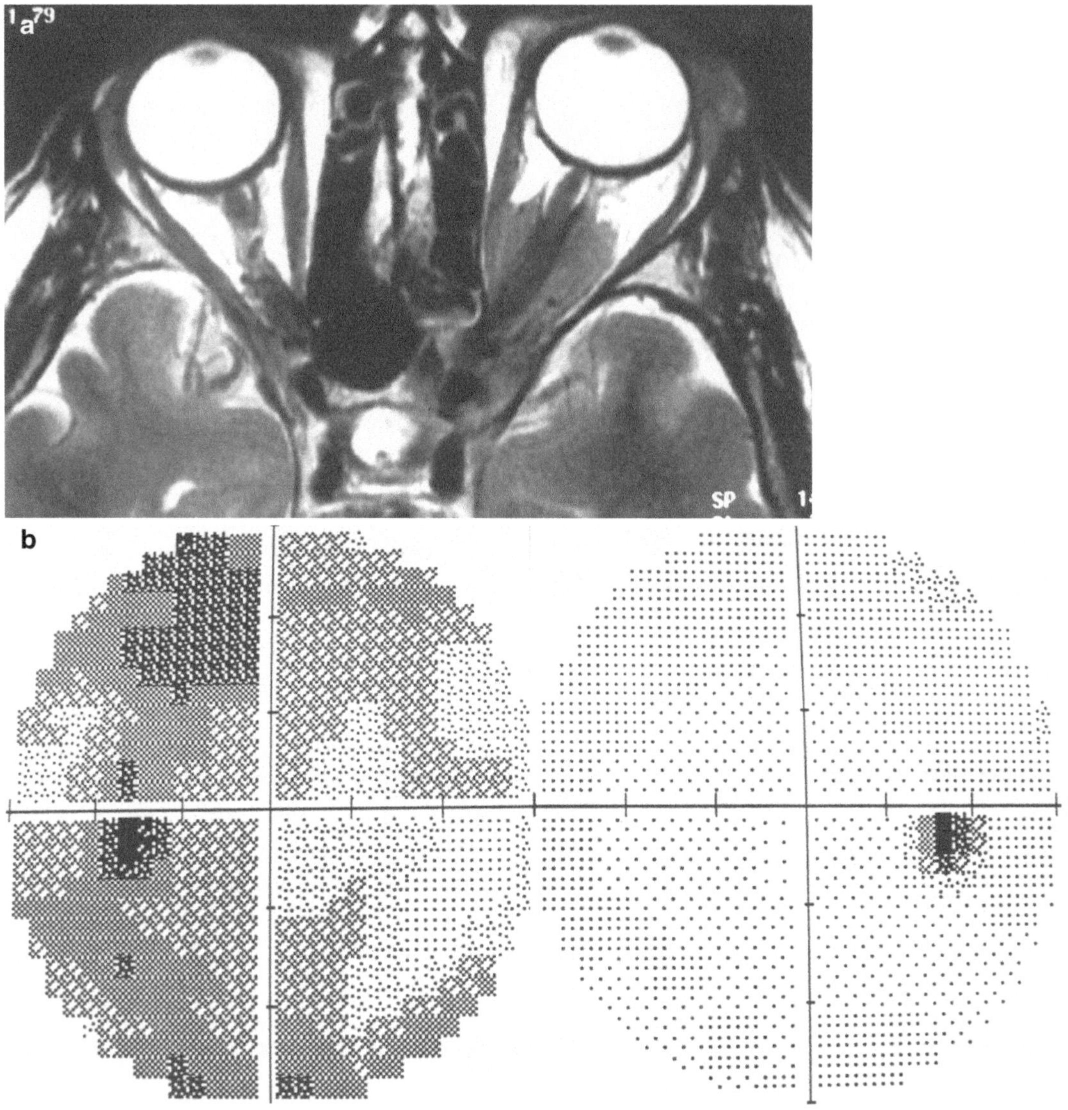

Fig. 47.1 (**a**) T2-weighted axial MR image of a meningeoma of the left optic nerve sheath. (**b**) Diffuse decrease in the threshold sensitivity on the left side of the field, mainly in the temporal segment

- inflammatory or infiltrative diseases: Crowded apex syndrome, granuloma, sarcoidosis,
- primary bone diseases: craniofacial fibrous dysplasia, Paget's disease,
- spontaneous or traumatic hematoma of the orbit.

Primary symptoms of the diseases of the orbit are those developing as a consequence of the mass effect in the orbit, exophthalmus, dislocation of the bulb, eye movement disturbances and resistance to retropulsion of the globe. Congestion or decoloration of the papilla, opticociliary shunt veins in case of meningeoma (Fig. 47.2), and folding of the retina in case of tumors in contact with the eye-ball, may occur.

Tumors of the orbit are discussed in more details in the chapter on 'Diseases of the orbit'.

Chiasmal and Parasellar Tumors

Even nowadays, when modern diagnostic procedures are available, ophthalmologists still play a

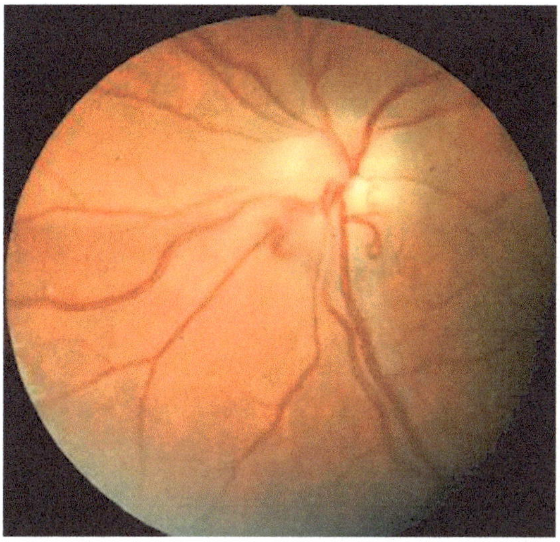

Fig. 47.2 Fundoscopic appearance of optociliary shunt veins in optic nerve sheath meningeoma

significant role in the diagnostics of diseases affecting the chiasmal region. According to statistical data, almost every fourth brain tumor is located in the sellar region, and the initial and frequently single symptom of more than half of these tumors is visual disorder. Thus patients first visit an ophthalmologist with their complaints. Early diagnosis is of decisive importance regarding the further prognosis of the patients, particularly in the aspect of visual functions. This is also important because the majority of tumors located in the sellar region are benign, and patients are curable if surgery is performed in time. The subjective complaints of the patients are quite variable. They report decrease in visual acuity in one or both eyes. Loss of visual field is rarely mentioned. In most cases, they suppose that they need new glasses. Frequently it is an incidental recognition that their vision is poorer in one eye. The loss of vision is generally progressive, but slight temporary improvement may occur.

Important factors influencing the chiasm lesion:

- the direction of tumor growth,
- anatomical factors, the position of the chiasm relative to the sellar diaphragm –it is located above the pituitary gland in 80 % of cases, found above the tuberculum sellae, that is prefixed in 9 %, and located above the dorsum sellae, that is postfixed in 11 % of the cases.
- the size of the tumor, and the extent of mechanical compression,
- blood supply of the chiasm and circulatory disturbance caused by the tumor.

Perimetry is of decisive importance in the diagnostics of perisellar pathologies. Symmetric, classical bitemporal hemianopia is a typical symptom at the beginning and during the progression of the disease, and it is a consequence of the injury of the nasal fibers crossing in the midline in the chiasm. It is also called heteronymous hemianopia, in contrast to the homonymous loss of visual field, characteristic to the injury of the retrochiasmal segment.

Classification of the loss of visual field depending on the damaged segment

1. *prechiasmal optic lesion*: presellar tumors: most frequent in case of olfactory meningeomas, tuberculum sellae meningeomas, and aneurysms (aneurysms of the anterior cerebral artery, anterior communicating artery). The earliest sign is a central or centrocecal scotoma in the visual field as a consequence of damage of the central fibers of the optic nerve (Fig. 47.3a, b).
2. *prechiasmalchiasm lesion*: most frequently it is caused by tuberculum sellae meningeoma. It is characterized by ipsilateral optic lesion with central scotoma (junctional scotoma), accompanied by contralateral superior temporal quadrantanopia. It is caused by the injury of the lower nasal fibers (Willebrand's knee) crossing first in the chiasm and forming a loop in the contralateral optic nerve. The superior temporal quadrantanopia in the contralateral eye frequently remains unrecognized, therefore, the possibility of chiasm lesion is not considered (Fig. 47.4a, b).
3. *Medial chiasm lesion*: it is mainly caused by pituitary adenomas with suprasellar spread. In a typical case symmetric bitemporal hemianopia can be detected, in addition to the initially intact visual acuity (Fig. 47.5). In case of pathological processes compressing the chiasm on its lower surface, fibers originating from the nasal lower quadrant and crossing at the bottom of the chiasm are damaged

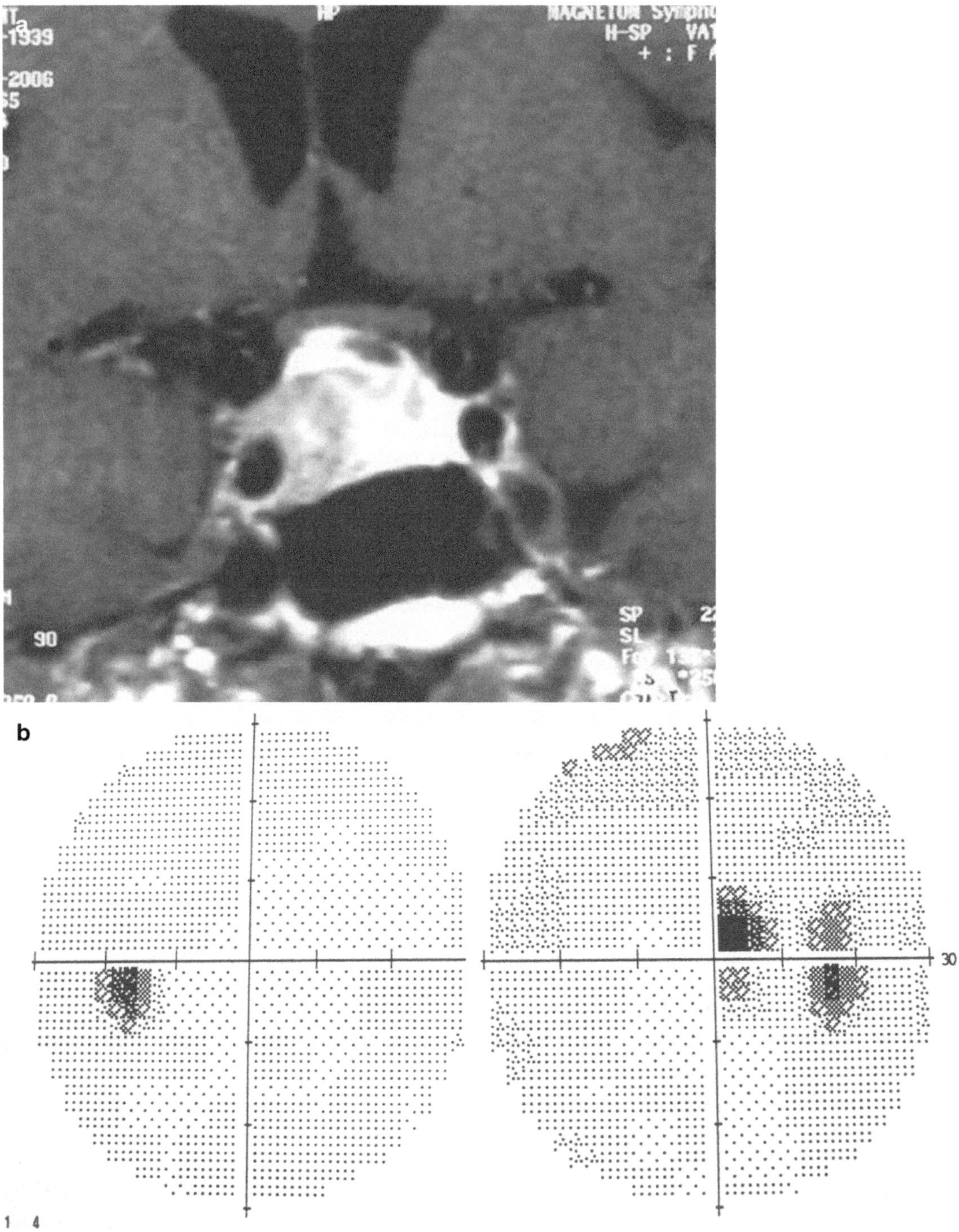

Fig. 47.3 (**a**) Coronal MR image of a pituitary adenoma. (**b**) Initial prechiasmal optic lesion: with central superior temporal quadrant scotoma on the right side

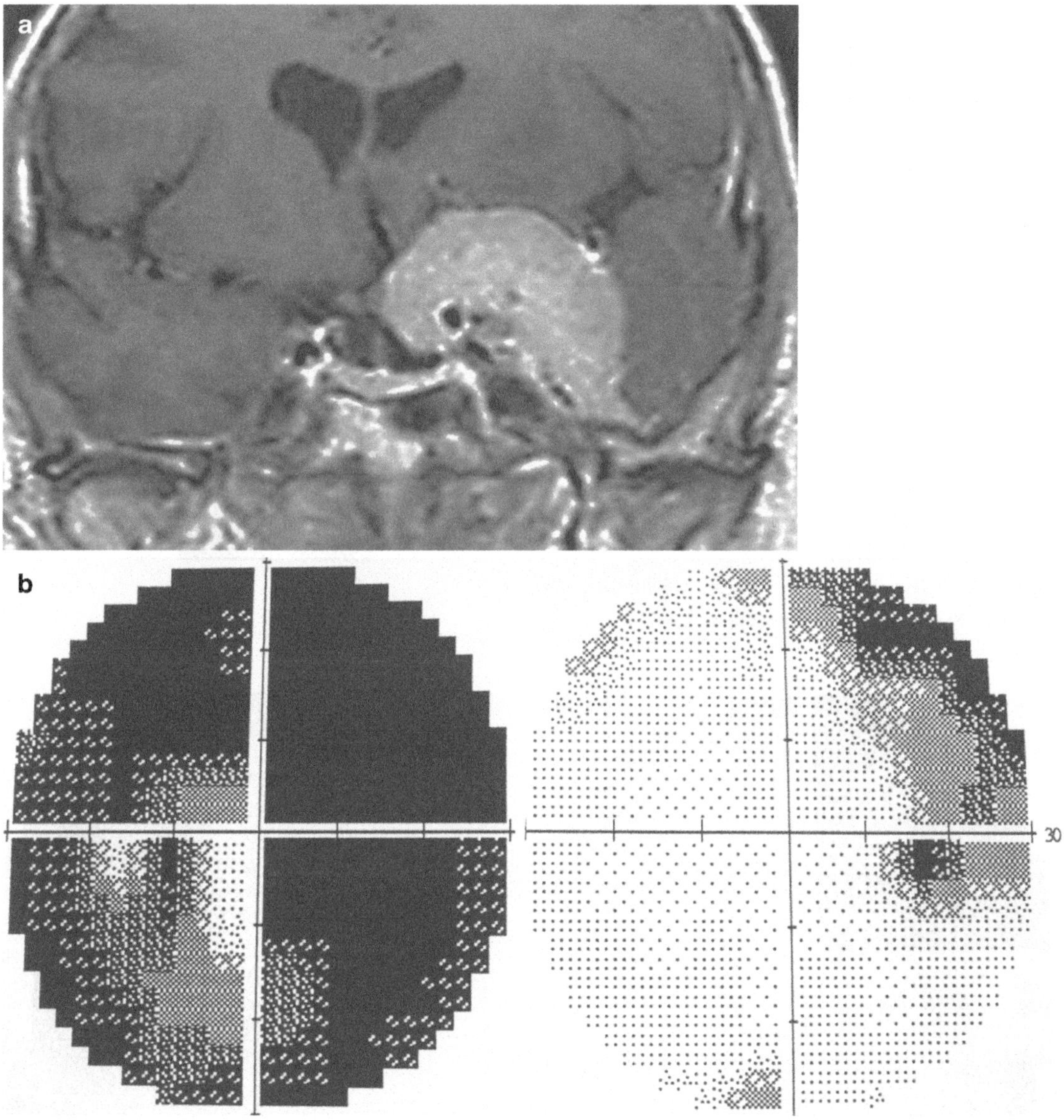

Fig. 47.4 (**a**) Coronal MR image of a left sided parasellar meningeoma. (**b**) Visual field defect caused by a prechiasmal chiasm lesion (junctional scotoma): left sided optic lesion + contralateral superior temporal quadrantanopia

first, therefore, the loss of visual field starts in the superior temporal quadrant, and the progression proceeds clockwise in the right eye, while in the opposite direction in the left eye (Fig. 47.6). In case of pathological processes compressing the chiasm on its upper surface, upper-nasal fibers are injured first, leading to bitemporal inferior quadrantanopia (Fig. 47.7). This is most frequent with gliomas and germinomas.

4. Posterior chiasm lesion may be caused by craniopharyngiomas, chordomas, tumors of the 3rd ventricle and hydrocephalus, but it may also develop in case of prefixed chiasm in pituitary tumors. Macular fibers crossing posterio-superiorly in the chiasm are injured first, causing central scotoma with bitemporal hemianopia.
5. Lateral chiasm lesion: it has low incidence, and may be caused by a heavily calcified and dilated carotid aneurysm in the cavernous

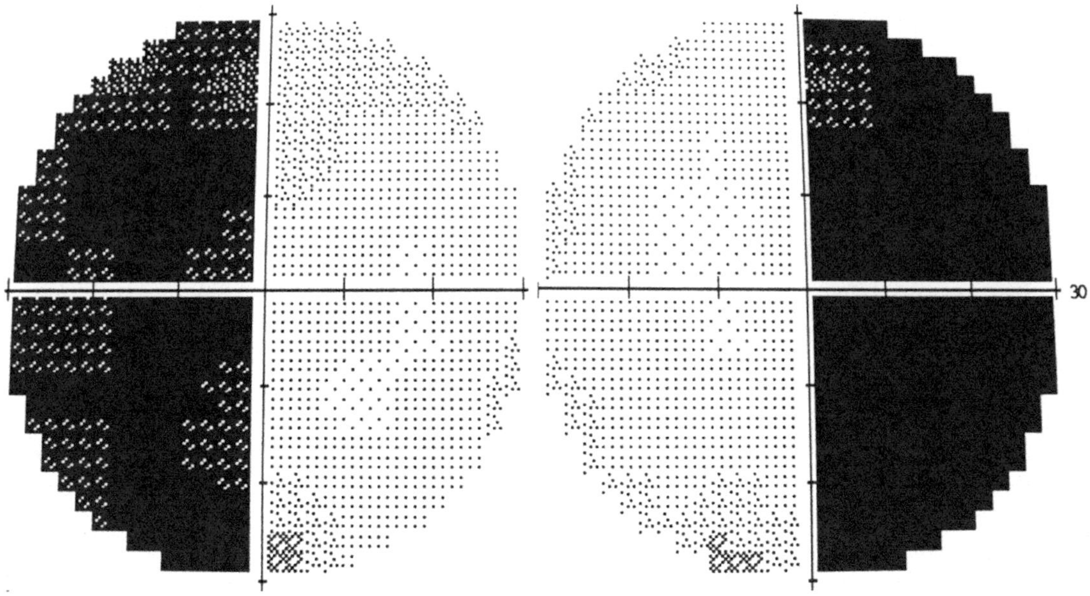

Fig. 47.5 Symmetrical bitemporal hemianopia

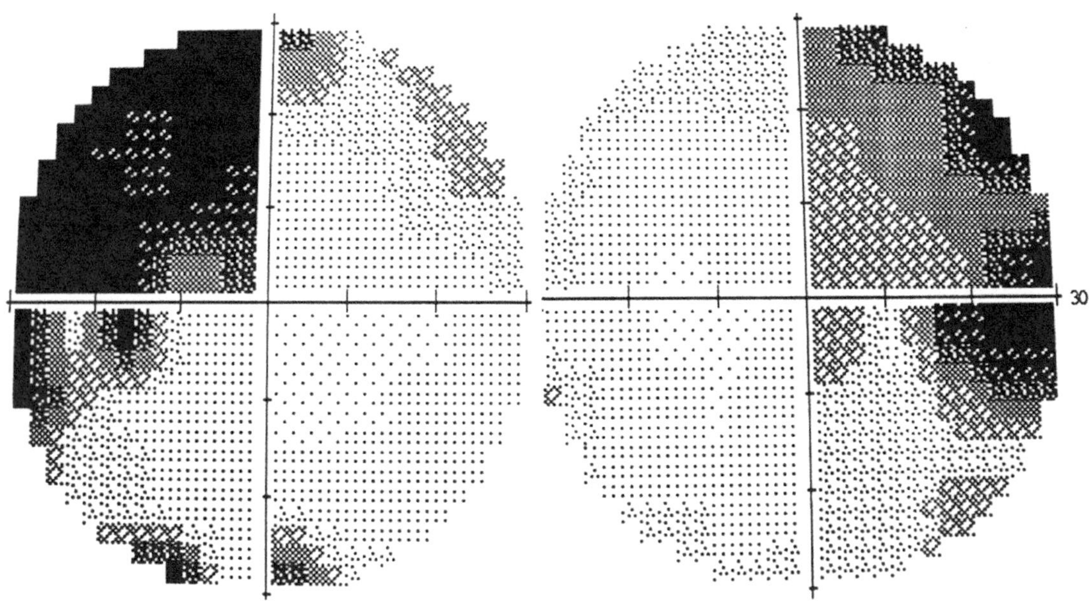

Fig. 47.6 Bitemporal superior quadrantanopia

sinus. However, the ipsilateral nasal visual field defects due to the injury of the uncrossed temporal fibers are rarely seen, regarding the nearness of the contralateral crossing nasal fibers, generally it is associated with temporal defects in the other eye. Sometimes bilateral carotid aneurysms cause binasal visual field loss. Lateral chiasm syndrome is mainly characteristic to parasellar meningeomas, but it can also be detected in case of laterally expanding pituitary tumors. It is characterized by an ipsilateral optic lesion, associated with contralateral homonymous hemianopia, the ipsilateral uncrossed temporal fibers and the

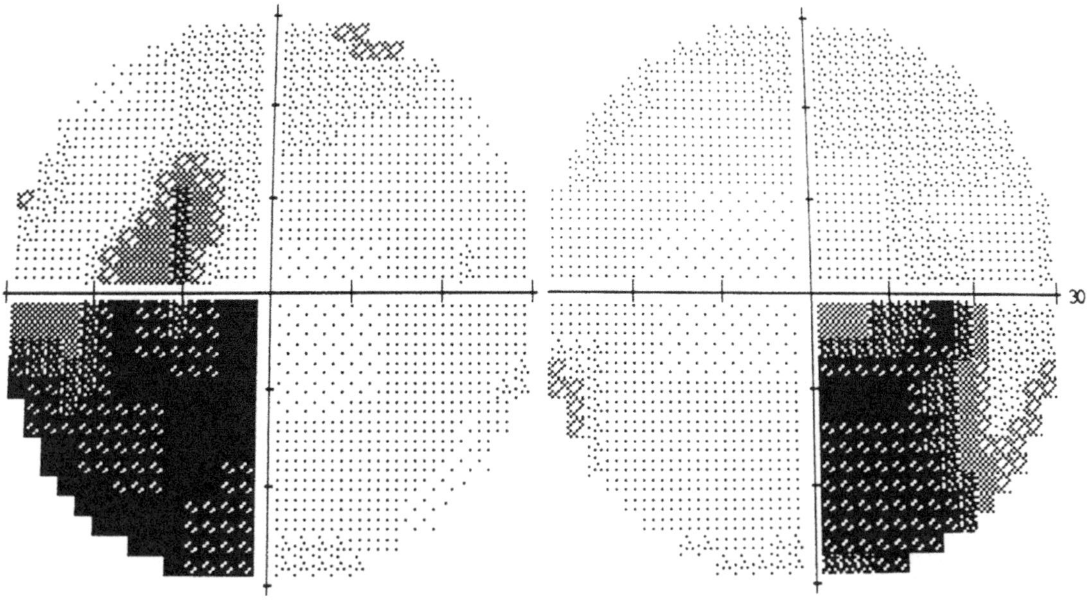

Fig. 47.7 Bitemporal inferior quadrantanopia

contralateral crossed nasal fibers (optic tract lesion) are also injured (Fig. 47.8a, b).

Visual field defect in the form of a *scotoma can be considered as an early sign of chias compression*. It occurs in association with tumors of relatively rapid growth. Patients recognize central and paracentral scotomas earlier, it disturbs them more, thus they visit an ophthalmologist earlier, which means a better prognosis.

The optic disc on the fundus is initially normal, later the different extent of optic disc decoloration indicates the damage of the optic nerve. However, the visual acuity impairment is not always proportional to the appearance of the optic disc seen on the fundus. The loss of vision and the loss of visual field occur earlier, compared to the decoloration of the optic disc which is delayed. The development of the descending atrophy takes more time.

The preoperative state of the optic disc is of prognostic value. Even in case of poor vision and severe loss of visual field an intact or slightly decolorated optic disc suggests a recent damage, thus improvement of the visual acuity can be expected after surgery. If severe decoloration of the optic disc is detected, the damage to the optic nerve and the vision loss is frequently already irreversible. In certain cases, however, vision may show improvement even in spite of the decoloration of the optic disc. Decoloration of the optic disc is not a contraindication of surgery.

Papilledema is not characteristic to intra-suprasellar tumors, as these tumors are extradural and the sellar diaphragm is intact. However, retrochiasmal suprasellar tumors and tumors of the 3rd ventricle may cause papilledema at an early stage, because of the consequent occlusive hydrocephalus. Foster–Kennedy syndrome may develop in subfrontal meningeomas, consisting of optic atrophy in the ipsilateral eye and papilledema in the contralateral eye. Diplopia may be caused by tumors of the chiasmal region spreading laterally into the cavernous sinus, oculomotor palsy occurs most frequently. Headache is a common symptom, it generally affects the forehead and it is caused by the strain of the sellar diaphragm. Hormone producing pituitary adenomas may result in symptoms of endocrine dysfunction.

I would like to highlight, that neuro-ophthalmological examination is primarily expected to yield diagnosis regarding the location, but it rarely provides qualitative diagnosis.

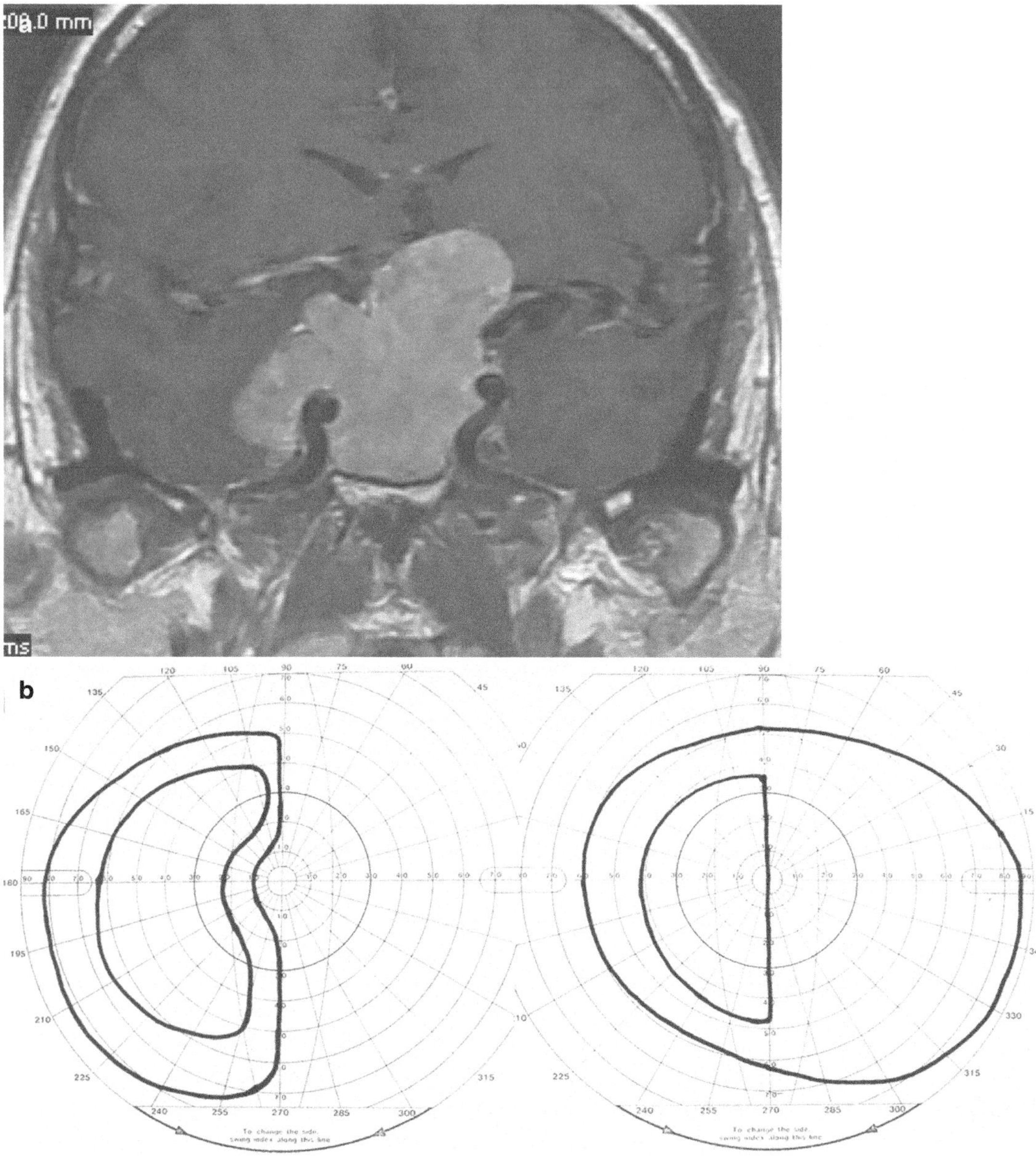

Fig. 47.8 (**a**) Coronal MR image of a giant pituitary adenoma. (**b**) Visual field defect corresponding to left sided lateral chiasm lesion

The most frequent tumors causing compression of the chiasm:

Pituitary adenoma (50–55 % of the cases)

Characteristics:

- hemianopia on chart reading, intact visual acuity at the beginning,
- symmetrical bitemporal hemianopia, beginning in the superior quadrant,
- endocrine symptoms.

Pituitary apoplexy is an acute clinical syndrome, which involves:

- sudden headache,
- rapidly worsening visual acuity impairment,
- nausea, vomiting, signs of meningeal irritation,
- ophthalmoplegia.

In the background of the symptoms may stand hemorrhage or hemorrhagic necrosis of the pituitary adenoma, leading to compression of the parasellar structures as a result of the acut expansion of a pituitary adenoma. General and neurological symptoms often predominate, masking the severe ophthalmological abnormalities. Therefore, prompt establishment of the diagnosis is not always easy. Apoplexy develops generally in pituitary tumors with a longer history, but it may be the first presenting sign of the pituitary adenoma. In case of early diagnosis, it may be successfully cured by transsphenoidal surgery.

Skull base meningeomas (10 % of the Cases)

Asymmetry is typical, thus loss of vision of one eye precedes the development of chiasmatic or contralateral optic lesion by years. Unilateral optic lesion with central scotoma is a characteristic early symptom. The typical appearance develops much later: unilateral amaurosis with optic atrophy, contralateral temporal visual field loss (prechiasmal chiasm lesion). Visual acuity impairment is often the only symptom. The establishment of the correct diagnosis is postponed by the lack of focal neurological and endocrine symptoms. Patients are often treated for several years with the diagnoses of retrobulbar neuritis, vascular optic lesion, glaucoma, macular degeneration or central retinitis.

Symptoms of *tuberculum sellae meningeomas*:

- initially unilateral decrease in visual acuity with central or paracentral scotoma in the visual field, or temporal defect (ipsilateral nasal fibers are damaged)
- later asymmetrical chiasm lesion, frequently amaurosis in one eye and temporal defect of the visual field on the other.

Symptoms of *olfactory meningeoma*:

Initial symptoms like ansomia, increased intracranial pressure and psychoorganic syndrome frequently precede ophthalmological symptoms. The tumor may reach a considerable size before compression of the optic nerve or the chiasm develops.

- initially papilledema (bilateral or unilateral, Foster–Kennedy syndrome may occur)
- central or paracentral scotoma,
- atypical, asymmetrical, incomplete bitemporal hemianopia

Symptoms of *meningeomas of the lesser sphenoid wing*:

- unilateral optic lesion with central scotoma,
- unilateral nasal defect,
- lateral chiasm syndrome,
- extraocular muscle palsies, diplopia,
- unilateral exophthalmus

Slowly developing, unilateral, mild exophthalmus, eye movement disorder, and diplopia are predominantly characteristic to parasellar meningeoma, may be followed by the development of a gradually progressing unilateral optic or chiasm lesion only after several years.

Craniopharyngioma (20–25 % of the cases)

Symptoms in childhood:

- choked disk (the chronic type is frequent),
- visual impairment (rapid progression),
- endocrine symptoms,
- symptoms of hypothalamus lesion,
- suprasellar calcification in 90 % of the patients.

Symptoms of increased intracranial pressure dominate the picture.

Symptoms in adulthood:

- loss of vision, initially often unilateral,
- asymmetrical bitemporal hemianopia,
- posterior or lateral chiasm lesion,
- rarely paresis of the 3rd cranial nerve,
- suprasellar calcification in 40 % of the patients.

In adulthood the loss of vision, the asymmetrical bitemporal hemianopia starting in the inferior quadrant are the most frequent initial ophthalmological symptoms.

Optic glioma (7 % of the cases)

It occurs in childhood, and is frequently associated to Recklinghausen neurofibromatosis.

- uni- or bilateral loss of vision,
- irregular bitemporal hemianopia,
- alternating nystagmus,
- endocrine symptoms,
- symptoms of hypothalamus lesion

Other tumors causing chiasm lesion:

- chordoma
- cholesteatoma
- dermoid tumor
- tumor of the 3rd ventricle
- lymphoma, plasmocytoma
- arachnoid cyst
- metastasis

Chiasm lesions of non-neoplastic origin:

- inflammatory process, e.g., posterior ethmoid or sphenoid mucocele, pituitary abscess,
- hydrocephalus,
- trauma,
- empty sella,
- aneurysm, carotid sclerosis

Supratentorial Space Occupying Processes- Retrochiasmal Optic Lesion

In contrast to the heteronymous hemianopia caused by the chiasm lesion, lesions of the retrochiasmal segment of the visual pathway are typically associated with homonymous hemianopia, that is, the same side of the visual field is lost in both eyes, contralateral to the lesion. The loss of visual field always preserves the vertical midline. Complete, congruent, homonymous hemianopia, with macular splitting may occur in lesions of any segment of the retrochiasmal pathway, it has no importance regarding the establishment of the location. However, incongruency is typical to lesions of the anterior parts of the pathway (optic tract, lateral geniculate body, initial segment of the optic radiation).

Vision is usually intact, except for the case when the compression causes chiasm and optic lesion in addition to the lesion of the optic tract, or in case when the compression is bilateral, for example in bilateral occipital lesions. The loss of visual field generally splits the macula. The center may be intact in case of injuries of the occipital pole. Pupil reactions are intact, except for the segment distal to the lateral geniculate body (optic tract), where pupillomotor fibers run together with the fibers of the visual pathway. Accompanying neurological symptoms are mainly present in case of temporal and parietal lesions. Optic atrophy may develop in 3–6 months in case of optic tract lesion.

Optic Tract Lesion

Incongruous, incomplete homonymous hemianopia is typical in this case. Hemianopia is complete in total lesions of the optic tract. Isolated optic tract lesion is a rare finding. Because of the proximity of the structures, tumorous space occupying processes usually result in injury of the chiasm and the optic nerve parallel with the lesion of the optic tract, therefore, it is more appropriate to speak of an *optic tract syndrome*, than an optic tract lesion which can be characterized by ipsilateral reduced central visual acuity and contralateral incongruous homonymous hemianopia.

The most frequent pathologic entities leading to this syndrome are : craniopharyngiomas, pituitary tumors, supraclinoid carotid aneurysms, gliomas and demyelinating diseases.

Pupillary signs characteristic to the lesion of the optic tract:

- RAPD ipsilateral to the lesion.
- Wernicke's homonymous hemianopic pupil reaction: pupil reactions are absent when light is directed to the blind half of the retina, but when light is directed to the intact half of the retina, the pupil constricts.
- Behr's sign: anisocoria with the larger pupil on the side of the hemianopia.

Characteristically asymmetrical descending optic atrophy may develop. It is more pronounced ipsilateral to the hemianopia (contralateral to the lesion), since the proportion of crossing fibers in the chiasm is higher, than the uncrossing ones, the ratio is 3:1. Accompanying symptoms: endocrine disorder is possible due to damage of the neighboring hypothalamus.

Lesion of the Lateral Geniculate Body

The isolated lesion of the CGL has a very low prevalence. The lesion of this nucleus produces moderately to completely congruent homonymous hemianopia. No pupillary signs develop, regarding that pupillomotor fibers leave the optic tract before the lateral geniculate body. Optic atrophy is possible, similarly to optic tract lesions. It is usually of vascular origin, evoked by occlusion of the anterior and lateral choroid arteries. Tumor, arteriovenous malformations, trauma and demyelination may be further causative factors. Accompanying neurological symptoms: lesion of the neighboring thalamus may cause hemihypesthesia, injury to the pyramid pathway may result in contralateral hemiplegia.

Lesion of the Optic Radiation

Fibers leaving the lateral geniculate body run partially through the temporal and partially through the parietal lobes towards the occipital lobe. Fibers from the upper half of the retina run through the parietal lobe to the upper part of the occipital lobe, while fibers from the lower retinal half course through the temporal lobe (Meyer's loop) to the lower part of the occipital lobe. Macular fibers are located in the part of the visual cortex near to the occipital pole.

Lesion of the Temporal Optic Radiation

The nasal lower fibers of the contralateral eye and the fibers of the temporal lower quadrant of the ipsilateral eye are damaged, therefore, in temporal lesion a characteristic loss of visual field develops, contralateral superior quadrant homonymous hemianopia. The defect is mostly incongruent; the nasal defect is more severe than the temporal. The vertical boundary always follows the midline, the horizontal boundary is parallel to the midline or bending upward (Fig. 47.9a, b). It is generally accompanied by severe neurological symptoms, hemiplegia, hemihypesthesia, aphasia, alexia, agraphia, and epilepsy may occur. It is most frequently caused by tumors. The ratio of neoplasms and ischemia is 9:1.

Lesion of the Parietal Optic Radiation

Fibers from the upper retina are injured, therefore, contralateral inferior quadrant homonymous hemianopia is typical, but the complete homonymous hemianopia with macular splitting is even more frequent, as these processes are generally extensive. Damage to the anterior radiation leads to incongruent defect, while lesions of the posterior segment cause congruent defect. Among its causes the ratio of vascular and neoplastic (meningeomas, gliomas, metastases) processes is nearly similar. The accompanying neurological symptoms are predominant:

Non-dominant (right) hemispheric lesions result in hemihypesthesia, apraxia, neglect of the left visual field and the left half of the body. In case of visual neglect, by simultaneous examination of the visual fields of the left and right eyes (examination of extinction) the patient does not perceive stimuli of one side, while on isolated examination of one or the other eye, no hemianopia can be detected.

In the presence of a lesion in the dominant hemisphere, aphasia, finger agnosia, left–right confusion, acalculia and agraphia may occur.

Occipital Lesion

The main symptoms are visual loss and visual field defect. It is characterized by monosymptomatic homonymous hemianopia in a patient without neurological symptoms. Fibers of the visual pathway show a completely symmetrical spatial arrangement on reaching the occipital cortex, therefore, the hemianopia is exquisitely congruous in all cases.

It may be:

- complete homonymous hemianopia with macular splitting (Fig. 47.10a, b), or with intact center,
- quadrantanopia,
- congruent scotoma.

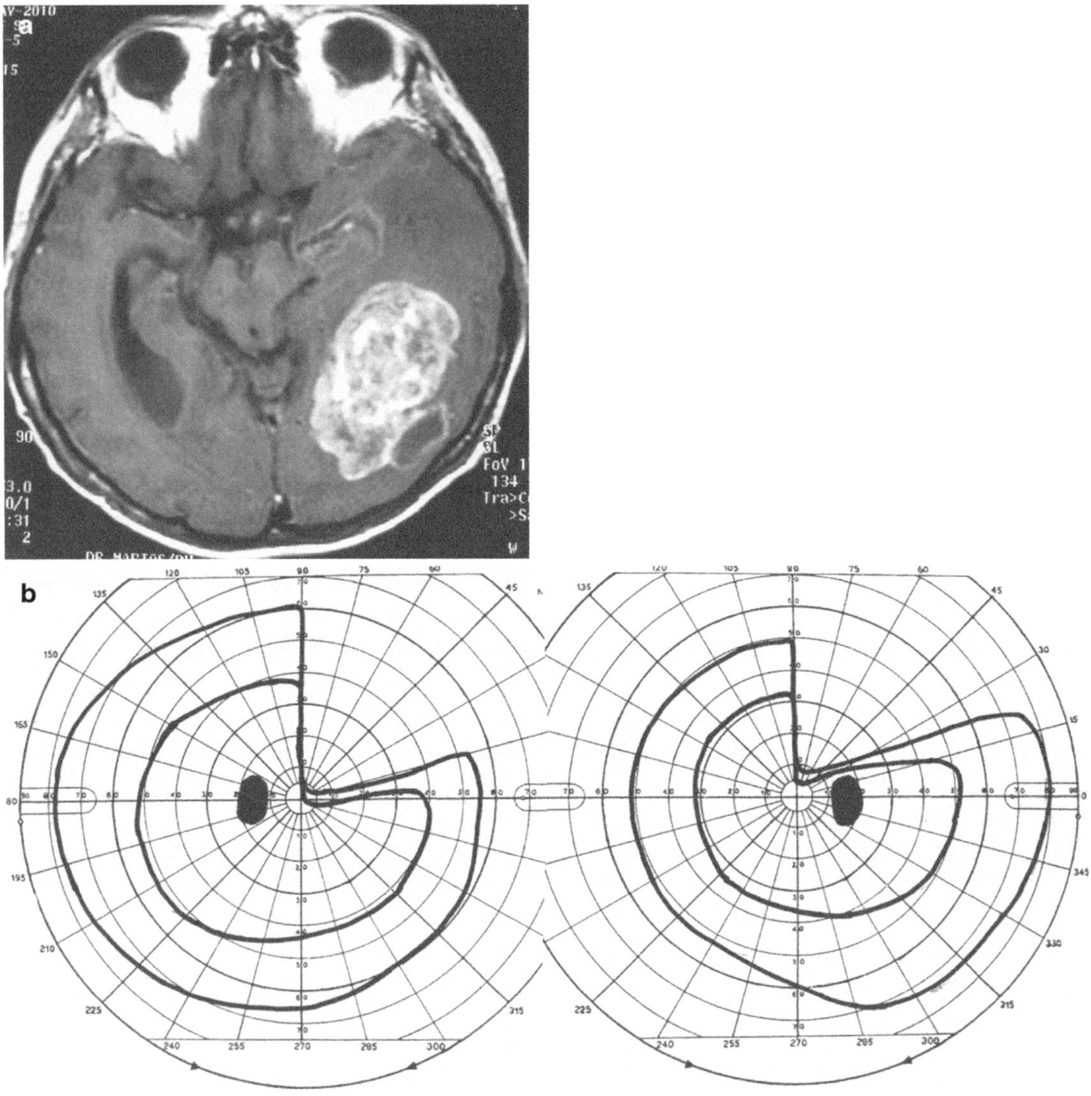

Fig. 47.9 (**a**) MR image of left temporal glioblastoma. (**b**) Right sided superior quadrant homonymous hemianopia

One explanation for the macular sparing is that the occipital pole has dual arterial blood supply, from posterior and middle cerebral arteries or bilateral retinal ganglion cell projection to the macular region. In case of superior quadrant homonymous hemianopia, the lower lip of the calcarine fissure is damaged, while in inferior quadrant homonymous hemianopia the upper lip of the calcarine fissure is affected. An island of vision between 60° and 90° in the most nasal retinal area within the temporal defect in the contralateral visual field may be characteristic to lesions of the occipital lobe. The anterior part of the calcarine fissure representing the nasal retina of the contralateral eye may remain intact after an infarction affecting the occipital lobe. Destruction of both occipital lobes may result in cortical blindness. Vision is lost with intact fundoscopic appearance and normal pupillary reflexes. It is caused by simultaneous circulatory disturbance of the posterior cerebral arteries on both sides, possibly being a result of the basilar artery occlusion (basilar apex syndrome). It may be caused by trauma, CO toxic-

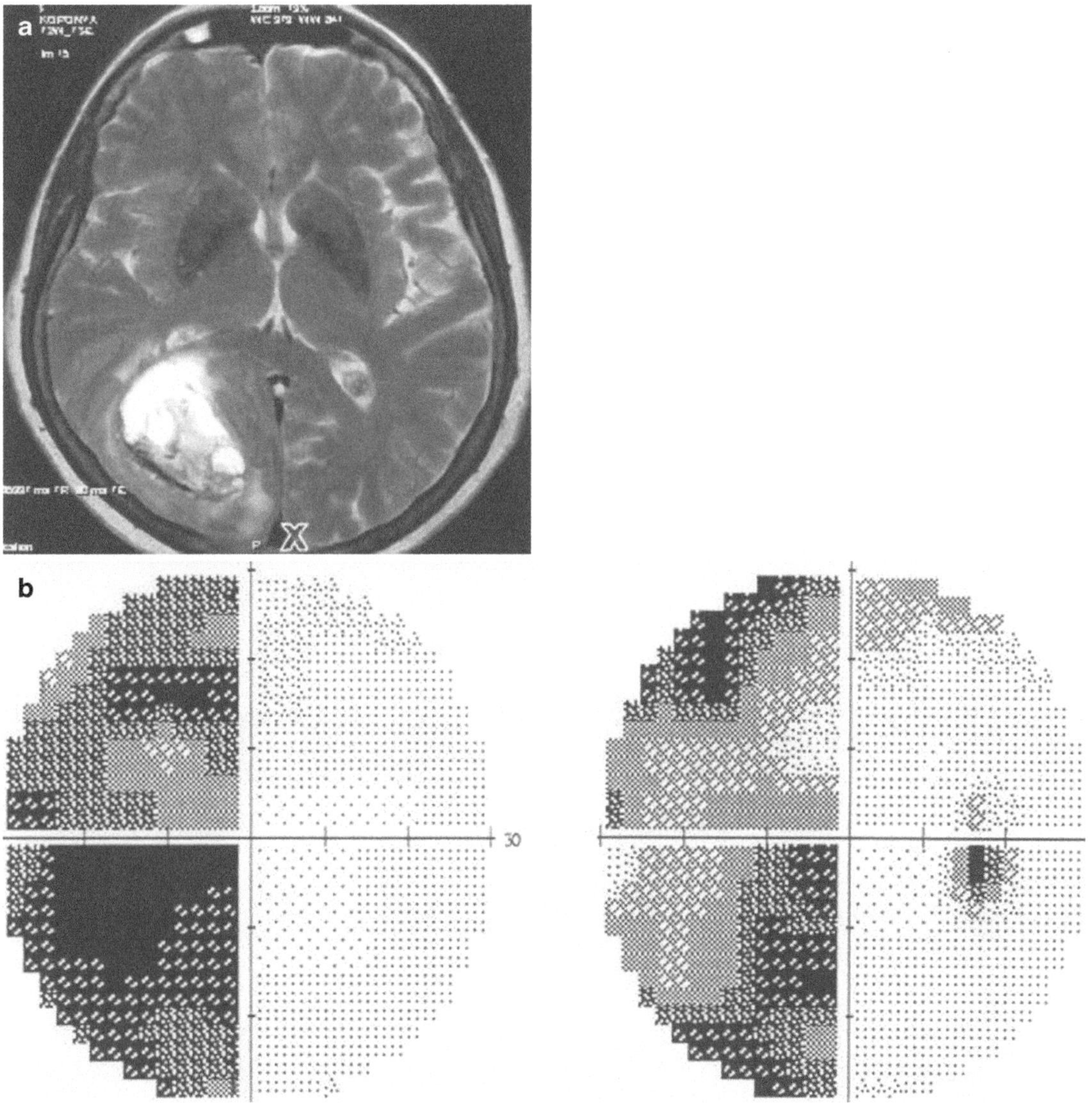

Fig. 47.10 (**a**) MR image of a right sided occipital tumor. (**b**) Left sided central homonymous hemianopia

ity, severe hemorrhage, and toxemia of pregnancy. In Anton syndrome, patients with cerebral blindness (bilateral occipital lesions) are not aware of their visual loss and insist that they can see, neglets the blindness, employs confabulations and reports visual experience. cy. Bilateral occipital lesion may also result in bilateral homonymous hemianopia with sparing of the macula, causing tunnel vision. Macular lesion in the visual cortex may develop in case of injury to the pole of the visual cortex. It is characterized by contralateral hemianopic central scotoma with disturbance in reading and recognition of faces. The Riddoch sign means that the patient recognizes only the moving object in the blind field, where static stimuli remain unrecognized (statokinetic dissociation). The phenomenon is a favorable prognostic sign, forecasting the regression of hemianopia. It can be examined the simplest way by Goldmann perimetry, the patient does not perceive the static sign, only if it begins to move. Palinopsia is the continuation of visual sensations after the stimulus has been removed or intermittent reappearance of images. The images are brief and incorporated into the actually seen optical environment. It usually appears in the region of the homonymous hemianopic defect. The more common lesions of the occipital lobe are vascular from either intraparenchymal hemorrhage or ischemic infarction. Only 20 % of the cases are of neoplastic origin (meningeoma, metastasis).

Further Readings

Burde RM, Savino PJ, Trobe JD. Clinical decision in neuro-ophthalmology. 2nd ed. St. Luis: Mosby-Year Book; 1992.

Duke-Elder S. System of ophthalmology, vol. XII. London: Henry Kimptom; 1971.

Gaini SM, Tomei G, Arienta C, Zavanone M, Giovanelly M. Optic nerve and chiasm gliomas in children. J Neurosurg Sci. 1982;26:33–9.

Hajda M, Pásztor E. A szemfenéki kép prognosztikai jelentösége a látásfunkciók javulásában hypophysis adenomák mütétje után [Prognostic importance of fundoscopic appearance in the improvement of visual functions following surgery of pituitary adenomas.]. Szemészet [Ophthalmology]. 1981;118:209–17.

Huber A. Eye symptoms in brain tumors. Saint Luis: Mosby; 1971.

Pásztor E. Operálhato idegbetegségek [Operable diseases of the nervous system]. Budapest: Medicina; 1985.

Somlai J. Neuroophthalmologia [Neuro-ophthalmology]. Literatura Medica Publishing; 1996.

Somlai J. Neuroophthalmologia [Neuro-ophthalmology]. PressCon Publishing; 2007.

Townssend JC, Selvin GJ, Griffen JR. Visual fields. Clinical case presentations. 1st ed. Boston: Butterworth-Heinemann; 1991.

Walsh TJ. Neuroophthalmology: clinical signs and symptoms. 3rd ed. Philadelphia: Lea and Febiger; 1992.

Walsh FB, Hoyt WF. Clinical neuroophthalmology, vol. 3. 4th ed. Baltimore: Williams and Wilkins; 1985.

48 The Significance of Neuro-ophthalmology in the Diagnosis and Therapy of Cranial Trauma

György T. Szeifert and Judit Somlai

Contents

G.T. Szeifert, M.D., med. habil. (✉)
Unit for Neurosurgical Injuries, Péterfy Accident Center, Semmelweis University, Budapest, Hungary
e-mail: gszeifert@yahoo.co.uk

J. Somlai, M.D.
Unit of Neuro-Ophthalmology, Department of Neurology and Stroke, Military Hospital, Budapest, Hungary

Neuro-Ophthalmology Section, Hungarian Ophthalmological Association, Budapest, Hungary

Trustee, NOSZA Foundation (for the Prevention and Screening of Ocular Storke), Budapest, Hungary
e-mail: dr@somlaijudit.hu; http://somlaijudit.hu

> The eternal dilemma concerning which is harder: to imagine a world one has never seen or to lose a world that has once been familiar with and to accept that it will never return? We must never decide, just let empathy guide us.

Neurosurgical and neurological diseases can be accompanied, especially at young ages, by severe and irreversible loss of vision. An intracranial hemorrhage developed either as a consequence of a cranial trauma (e.g., due to a traffic accident or a sport injury) or a ruptured aneurysm can lead to the loss of consciousness in seconds. On returning from a shorter or longer period of unconscious state, the patient can experience a loss

J. Somlai, T. Kovács (eds.), *Neuro-Ophthalmology*, DOI 10.1007/978-3-319-28956-4_48

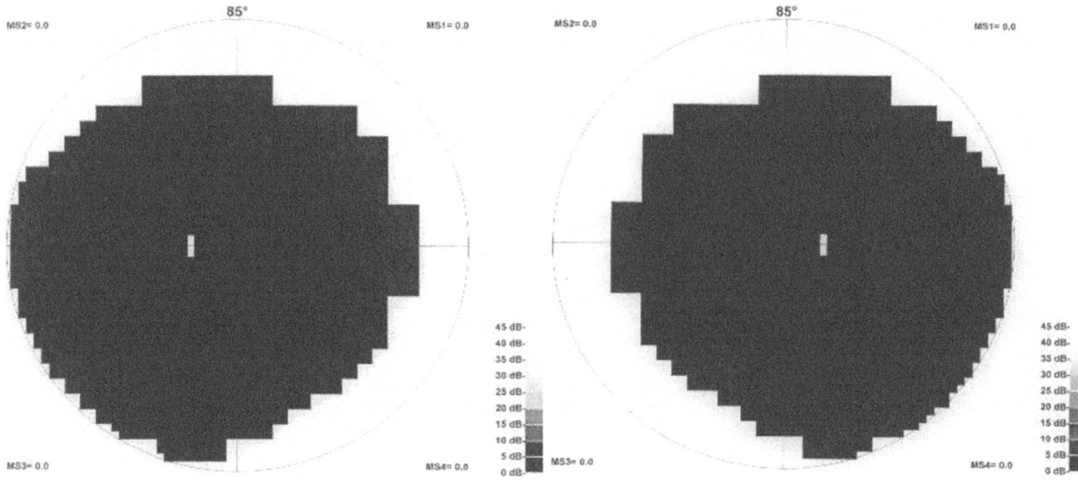

Fig. 48.1 *Computer perimetry (CP) examination: (LVC–LVP programs within 85°)* Bilateral complete amaurosis on both eye, caused by traumatic antechiasmal optic lesion, it was tested by CP with low vision central and low vision peripheral programs

ofvision, even in form ofa complete blindness in both eyes. This is when the handling of the true tragedy indeed begins for both the patient and the family, as in most cases of optic nerve injuries only a small residual island of vision remains, or even less (Fig. 48.1). The ophthalmologist has to do everything in order to prevent such a severe final state; however, in case of the development of such a severe condition, we should be an aid for the patient in the complex rehabilitation.

The Most Frequent Causes of Traumatic Optic Nerve Lesions – Direct or Indirect Injuries

Traumatic injury is the leading cause of death at young ages and in childhood in our own patient population as well. In addition to (car, motorcycle, bicycle, sport, etc.) accidents, this can develop as a consequence of a generalized epileptic seizure as well. A significant proportion of accidents associated with loss of consciousness is due to polytrauma. This may be accompanied by surgical shock due to thoracic or abdominal hemorrhages in association with a rapid hypotension, tachycardia with frequent and hardly palpable pulse and elevating respiratory rate. In case of a cranial trauma occurring in association with polytrauma or separately, brain edema and intracranial hypertension (HIP) can develop, which may result in a life-threatening condition. It is associated with the distinctive triad of increased blood pressure, slow-periodic breathing and decreasing pulse rate.

Clinical Forms of Traumatic Optic Neuropathies

Direct Optic Nerve Injuries and Blunt Orbital Trauma

- injuries associated with basal skull fracture
- orbital fractures and its tissue dislocation (***'blow-out' fracture,*** orbital and periorbital injuries)

The most threatening conditions include *avulsion of the distal part of the optic nerve,* suddenly developed bleeding within the optic nerve sheath, fracture of the optic canal, as well as *intracanalicular bleeding* and *edema.*

These require immediate decompression of the optic nerve because an irreversible optic nerve lesion can develop. Swelling of the eyelids and *periorbital hematoma* represent typical signs of base of the basal skull and orbital injuries. These may be accompanied by *nasal liquorrhea* and *otorrhea.* Injury to the skull base should always be considered in case these signs occur, and the

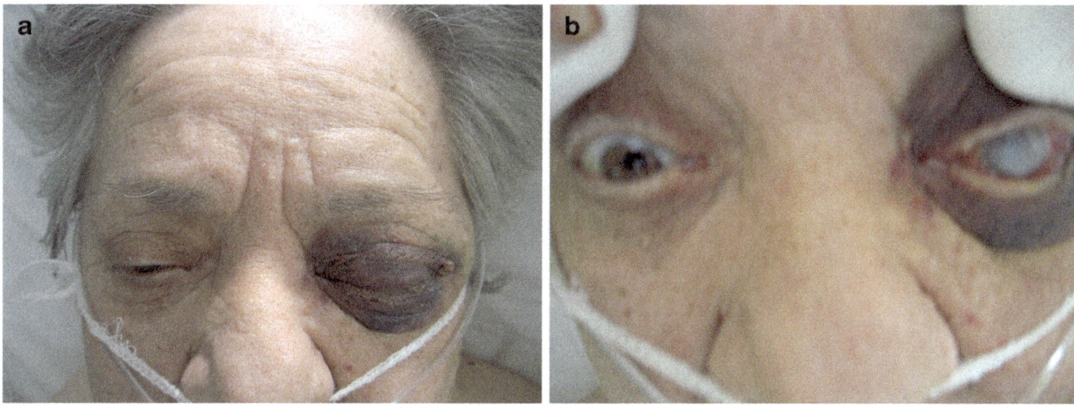

Fig. 48.2 (**a**) Left periorbital haematoma caused by periorbital injury (**b**) After the careful opening of the eyelids: corneal leukoma developed due to an old injury, which makes it impossible to assess the pupillomotor functions from the left side

source of liquorrhea, i.e., the site of injury of dura mater injury has to be identified. At the bedside, after the careful opening of the eyelids of periorbital hematomas, we look for some chance of the perforating ocular lesion. Following of injuries to the anterior and posterior segments of the eye should be looked for by slit lamp if possible. At the same time, pupillomotor responses are to be examined, which is not an easy task in certain forms of local ocular injuries (Fig. 48.2).

Indirect Optic Nerve Injuries

The consequencies of cranial trauma can result in an acute space-occupying process caused by epidural or subdural hematomas, and they indicate the largest threats of an increasing intracranial space occupying process with midline dislocation and higher and higher intracranial pressure.

Anisocoria is the first alarming ocular sign of transtentorial herniation in cases of cranial trauma, too. The trauma of the superficial pupillomotoric fiber lesion of the nervus oculomotorius can results in the effect of higher intracranial pressure. The consequence of this process is a functional lesion of the efferent pupillomotoric pathway and an indirect reaction of the pupillomotoric pathway can be extinguished, as well on the affected side the pupil becomes more and more dilated (the indirect response is absent on flashing into the contralateral side). (Discussed in more details in Chap. 50.)

In these cases, an **urgent neurosurgical intervention** is required, namely evacuation of epi- or subdural hematomas, at the same time the decompression of the brainstem is promoted by an excision of the uncus and parahippocampal gyrus. In case the patient's level of consciousness declines to a GCS below 8, the insertion of a ventricular drain is recommended, and permanent monitoring of intracranial pressure is needed. In case intracranial hypertension cannot be influenced by conservative therapy (ICP>20 mmHg), a CSF drainage needs to be established by means of a ventricular puncture, which simultaneously enables a permanent decrease of intracranial pressure.

In addition to performing fundoscopy and establishing the diagnosis ofa papilledema, precise continuous monitoring ofpupillomotor functions is essential in such patients, and it should be documented in an hourly basis if necessary. Therefore, pupil-dilating drops are contraindicated not only before neurosurgical interventions but also during the postoperative monitoring of the patient. Chronic subdural hematoma primarily affects the elderly, commonly alcoholic, prostrate people. Predisposing factors include associated brain atrophy and the stretched tiny veins, the tears of which can be evoked by frequent falls or minor hits on the head and result in the development of long asymptomatic chronic subdural hematoma with acute hemorrhage (Figs. 48.3c and 48.4). As revealed by fundoscopy, the condition leads to chronic papilledema, optic nerve

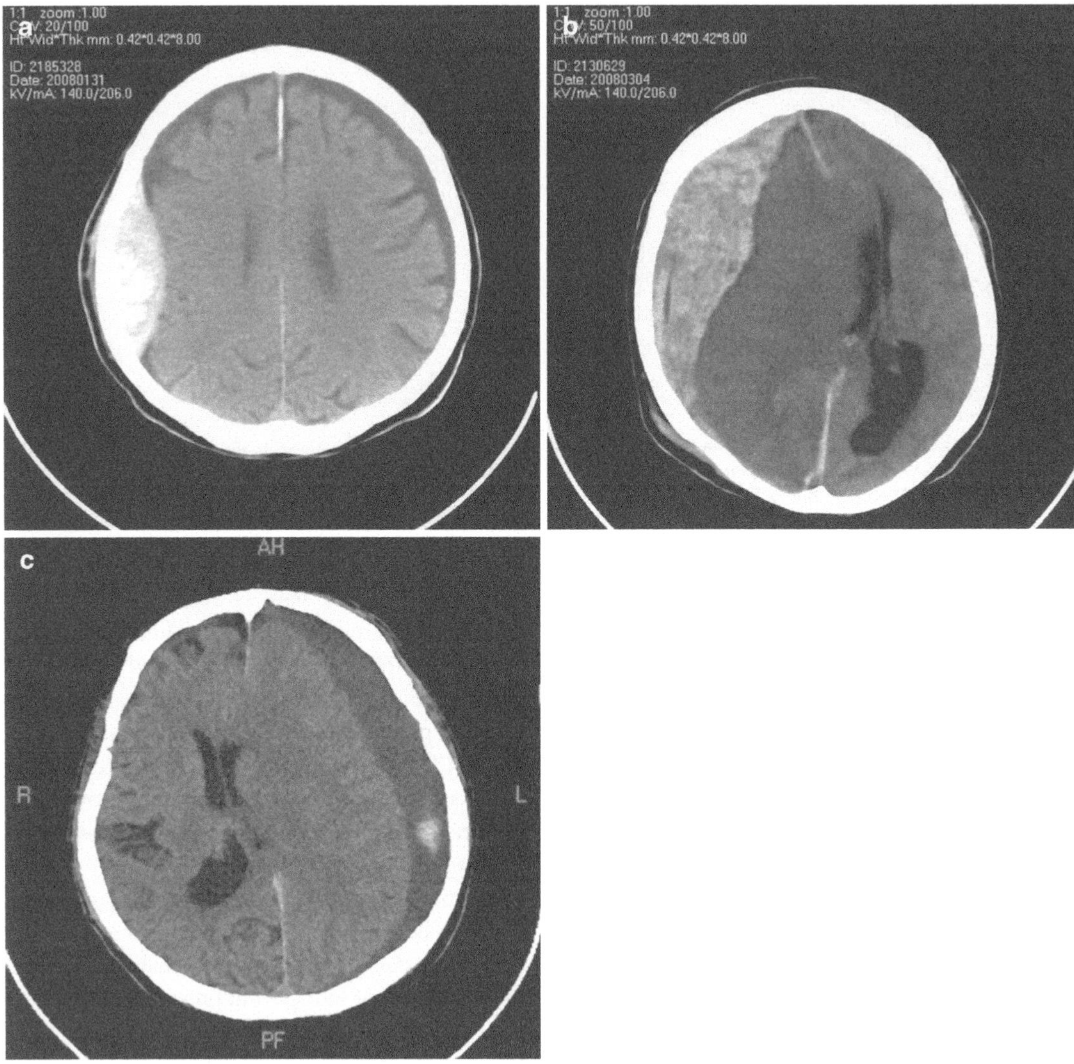

Fig. 48.3 (**a**) Epidural hematoma (**b**) acute subdural hematoma (**c**) chronic subdural hematoma with acute bleeding

fiber atrophy in late-diagnosed cases and an irreversible loss of vision. (Chronic papilledema is discussed in more details in Chap. 50.).

The conservative management of indirect optic nerve injuries is the same as the systemic treatment of cerebral edema; however, patients often do not receive the adequate therapy in time. Visual functions may improve with high-dose corticosteroid therapy; however, according to our own experience and the consensus of the scientific literature, conservative therapy does not provide much hope if administered late. In case of an acute subdural hematoma accompanied by diffuse malignant cerebral edema, decompressive craniectomy should be performed, when the evacuation ofthe hematoma and the conservative intensive treatment are not sufficiently effective, and the intracranial pressure cannot be managed.

Neuro-ophthalmological Complications of Basal Skull Fracturas

Traumatic Injuries of the Chiasm and the Parasellar Regions

The optic nerve can be.irreversibly damaged within 24 h. In case of blunt cranial injuries, damage can occur to the antechiasmal optic

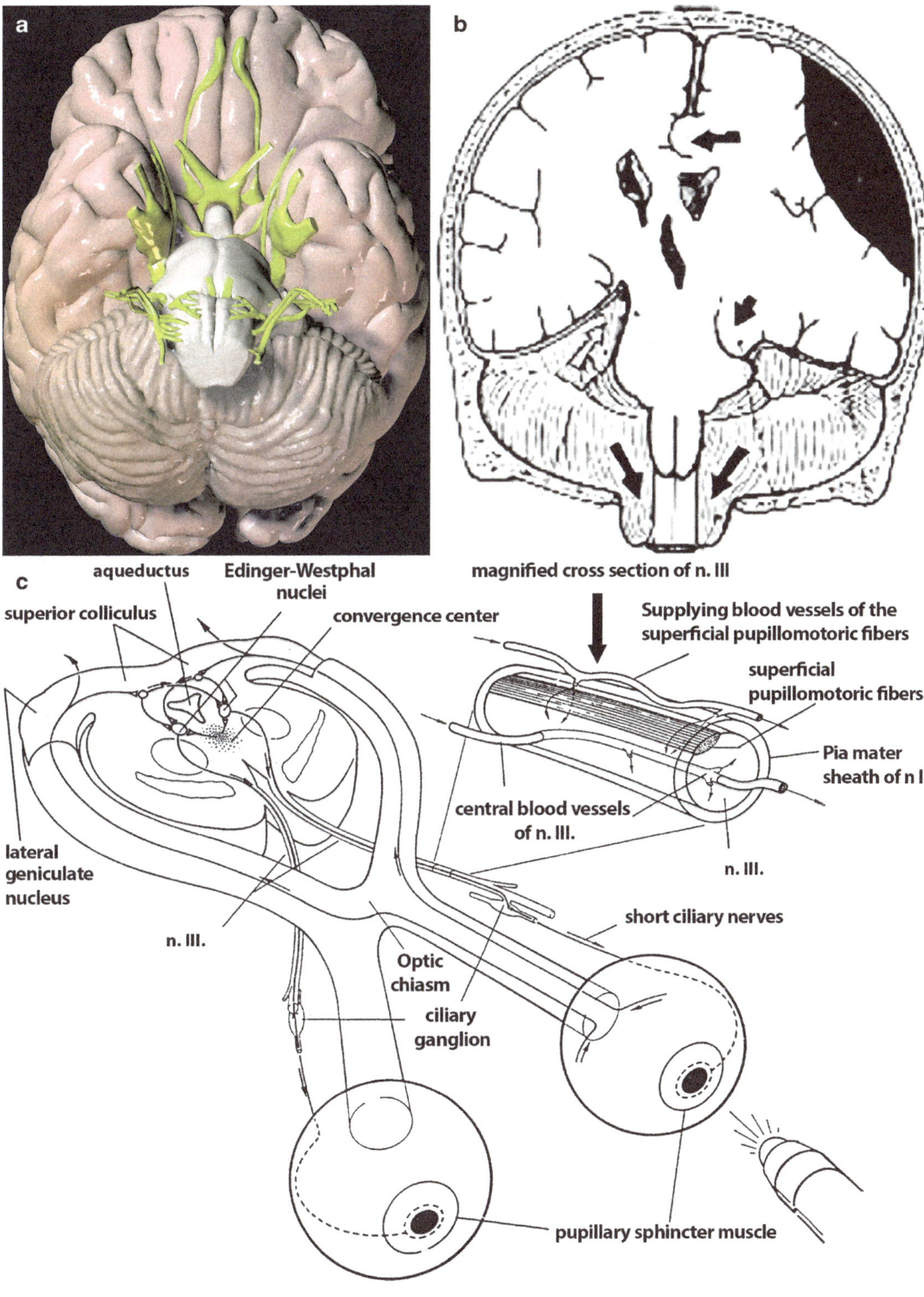

Fig. 48.4 (**a**) Basis of the brain with the cranial nerves. (**b**) Transtentorial herniation of the uncus of hippocampal gyrus (schematic figure). (**c**) Anisocoria the pupillomotor efferent nerve fibers are superficially located within the oculomotor nerve, and are therefore, most sensitive to compression. Therefore, anisocoria, the unilateral dilation of the pupil caused by pupillomotor dysfunction, i.e., compression, represents an early sign of rapidly increasing intracranial pressure

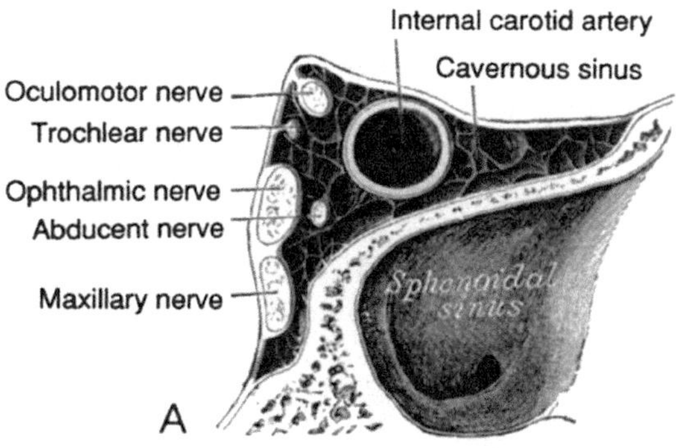

Fig. 48.5 The wall of the internal carotid artery can rupture within the cavernous sinus as a consequence of trauma. Cross section of the three cranial nerves that control eye movements and also travel within the cavernous sinus can be observed as well, the dysfunctions of which lead to an eye movement disorders

nerve fibers, to the cranial nerves involved in eye movements running aside the lateral part of the chiasm as well as to the lower brainstem cranial nerves. Basal skull fractures can lead to an injury to the chiasmal region of the optic nerve, uncontrolled forms of which can result in *an irreversible damage to the optic nerve within 24 h.* In addition to the optic pathway, all three nerves (namely the oculomotor nerve, the trochlear nerve and the abducens nerve) which control eye movements and travel along the skull base, can be injured, which may lead to characteristic eye movement disorders. Characteristic neurological symptoms can be noticed in trigeminal, facial and vestibulocochlear nerve injuries occurring as a result of skull base injuries. In consequence of dural injury can develop the *leakage of liquor.*

Traumatic carotid-cavernous fistula (tFCC) syndrome can develop upon acute blood vessel injury in those elderly patients whoseinternal carotid artery is already significantly damaged by atherosclerosis. As a consequence of the accident, the arterial blood of theinternal carotid artery enters directly the cavernous sinus. The mixing of arterial blood with venous blood leads to a disturbance invenous drainage, and it results in the development of the characteristic characteristic ocular signs of FCC (See Fig. 48.5). Due to the severe general condition of the patient, the tFCC is generally not recognized immediately following the injury, and theprogression of the condition is frequently marked by the ocular symptoms.

Characteristic ocular signs and symptoms:

1. unilateral edema of the lower and upper eyelids without any skin hyperemia
2. *conjunctival chemosis* caused by marked edema and their developing in the palpebral fissure as well – (Fig. 48.6b.)
3. *progressive protrusion* of the eyeball (the difference in Hertel value between the two eyes can be even 6–8 mm)
4. fundus examination reveals *papilledema,* peripapillary and *perivenous hemorrhages* due to congestion, stasis of venous blood in the ophthalmic vein (Fig. 48.7).
5. *double vision* due to eye movement disorder, even total ophthalmoplegia can develop (Fig. 48.8).
6. *pulse-synchronous lokomotive bruits* can be heard above the orbit on auscultation.

A neurosurgical investigation is necessary (CT-AG, DSA), which can be followed by the occlusion of the fistula by means of endovascular approaches. Symptoms and signs developing in the ocular muscles evoked by the carotid–cavernous fistula are discussed in details in Chap. 60 in subchap. 1.2.3.

Algorythm of the Neuro-Opthalmological Examination in Cases of Traumatic Ocular and Optic Nerve Injures

Is There a Local – Ocular Sign of Trauma?

The most characteristic traumatic signs are periorbital hematoma, skin wound, or a local injury. The assessment of the visual acuity, pupillary reflex responses and injuries to the orbit is difficult as the patient is unable to open the eye because of the extensive periorbital hematomas in the skin and the conjunctiva. These examinations should, however, be performed as soon as possible by cautious exploration of the affected area.

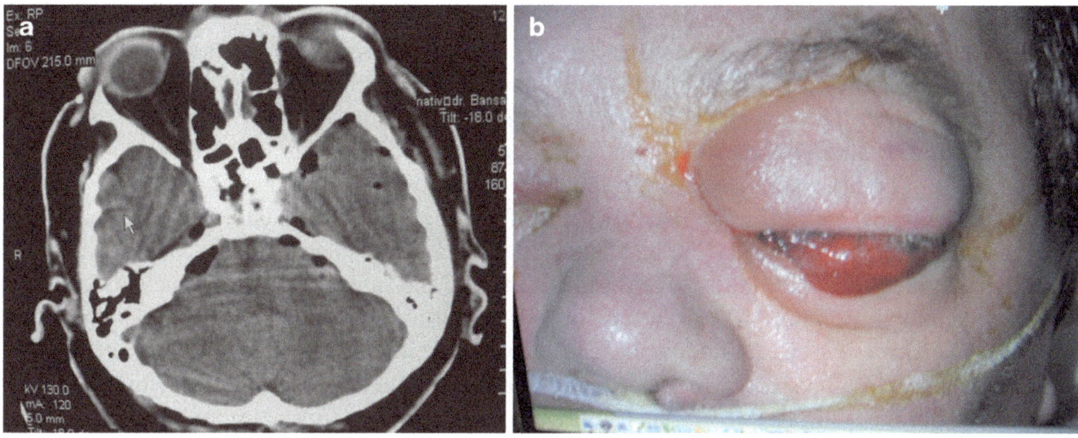

Fig. 48.6 (**a**) CT image: A traumatic carotid–cavernous fistula developed in consequence of a basal skull fracture. (**b**) Characteristic swelling eyelid edema caused by the fistula, in serious phase of FCC the eyelids can barely be opened, and the highly edematous chemotic conjunctival parts bulge into the palpebral fissure due to the extensive protrusion of the eyeball

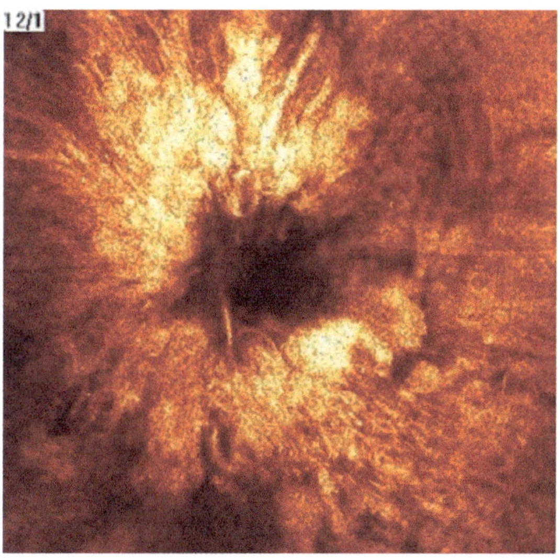

Fig. 48.7 Fundoscopic appearance due to impaired flow in the ophthalmic vein caused by mixing of arterial and venous blood: prominent, edematous optic disc several peripapillary, perivenously hemorrhage (per diapedesim)

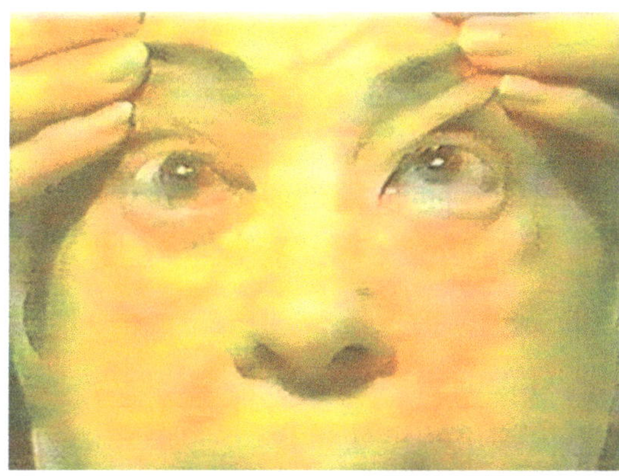

Fig. 48.8 Right paralysis of the right eye upon upward gaze: simultaneous paresis of the three cranial eye movement nerves in the cavernous sinus caused by a traumatic carotid-cavernoid fistula

Is the Patient Able to Open the eye?

If the patient can open the eye to command, we have to assess if the degree of eye opening and closing is equal or not. Furthermore, it is essential to check if the patient has difficulty closing the eye as a consequence of facial palsy, as in such a case a risk for ***keratoconjunctivitis e lagophthalmo*** is imminent, and pharmacological prevention as well as physical prevention (a glass that seals and protects the eye) have to be arranged for to prevent anterior segment of the eye from getting dry as keratoconjuncitis. If an injury to lower brainstem cranial nerves might have occurred, we should consider the injury to the first branch (V/1) of the trigeminal nerve as well. It is of importance because *corneal* *hypesthesia due to trophic disturbances* can be a source of severe and intractable ***corneal ulceration,*** and in most severe cases it may lead to ***corneal perforation.*** The disease is known as ***neuroparalytic keratoconjunctivitis.*** The underlying causes can be neurosurgical interventions and space-occupying processes localized in the skull base. In addition to locally applied eyedrops therapy, the only solution to prevent serious complications is intermittent partial or complete *blepharorrhaphy.* Difficulty in eye opening is measured on a scale, which needs to be regularly checked during the patient follow up: E4: spontaneous, E3: to command, E2: to pain E1: no eye opening.

Does the Patient Have Ptosis?

Ptosis can be uni- or bilateral. Unilateral ptosis can appear as part of oculomotor nerve palsy. If ***unilateral ptosis*** is not accompanied by eye movement disorder but ipsilateral myosis, i.e., a constricted pupil, the disorder may be caused by central or peripheral ***Horner's syndrome.*** These clinical syndromes are discussed in details in Chap. 52.

Examinations of the Pupil Reflexes

On first inspection, it should be precisely described whether the ***pupils are equal and round.*** The first examination should always include the examination of ***direct and indirect pupillary responses,*** and if the patient is conscious, bilateral miosis should be examined by forced convergence and by evoking the ***consensual pupillary responses.***

Anisocoria the size of the pupils is different. Unilateral mydriasis can develop as a consequence of a local trauma. In such case, other signs of an injury to the eyeball are present. Anisocoria with unilaterally dilated but not fixed pupil accompanied by decreased indirect pupillary response is mostly the first sign of an oculomotor lesion, and it can be the consequence of increased intracranial pressure. An indirect pupillomotor lesion on one or both sides is one of the most important alarming signs of direct and indirect cranial injuries, as it can indicate intraparenchymal hemorrhage of sudden onset or a hemorrhage expanding to the intraventricular space, as well as cerebral edema and subsequent midline dislocation. These are discussed in details in Chap. 52. A fixed and dilated pupil is suggestive of tentorial or axial cerebral herniation, which requires immediate neurosurgical intervention. The difference in pupillary size should be recorded in mm in each examination.

Marcus Gunn pupil **and/or** *relative afferent pupillary defect* (*RAPD*) **sign** Decreased direct pupillomotor response indicates an injury to the afferent pupillomotor pathway, which is measured on a 1+ −4+ scale and is called Marcus Gunn sign. Marked injury of the uni- or bilateral afferent pupillomotor pathway refers to complete or incomplete amaurosis, therefore to marked antechiasmal optic nerve injury and consequent loss of visual functions, and it is called the ***amaurotic pupil.*** No anisocoria is present in such injuries as the indirect pupillary response is intact. The precise assessment of it has a practical significance mainly in unconscious, polytraumatized patients. Characteristic symptoms of injuries to the pupillomotor pathway are discussed in details in Chap. 52.

Is There or not any eye Movement Disorder? What are eye Movements Like?

Are there any spontaneous eye movements? In ***primary position,*** absence of optokinetic reflex: these may develop as a consequence of brainstem injury in the pons-midbrain region.

What can be observed in primary position? Are the eyes aligned parallel? Is there any horizontal and/or vertical pathological misalignment or ***conjugate deviation*** due to paralytic strabismus? It is extremely important to observe and record these signs in unconscious patients, and continuous follow-up is recommended. If necessary, the ***oculocephalic reflex*** can also be examined, and an otoneurological examination can also be considered. It is discussed in details in Chap. 56.

It is recommended to examine, observe and precisely describe whether the eyes movements are conjugated or dysconjugated the consequence of neurogen strabism. Subsequently, depending on the general condition of the patient, an ***analysis of double vision*** and the initiation of possible treatment options are necessary. They are discussed in details in Chap. 24.

Why is the Injury of the Optic Nerve Rarely Recognized in the Acute Phase of the Traumatic Optic Nerve Injury?

1. Unconscious state (even permanently) can results in remain hidden the other neurological symptoms
2. Severe respiratory and circulatory disorders
3. Immediate neurosurgical intervention is needed

Diagnostic Possibilities

Local Examinations at the Bedside - in Case of the Unconsciousness Patients

Fundoscopy examination mostly insufficient because the findings on fundoscopy view are not informative by itself, apart from the case of papilledema. In acute phase of traumatic optic neuropathy not indicated by ophthalmoscopy. In this phase papilla view is normal, but the local functional test of the optic nerve can reveal in initial phase of the optic nerve lesions. Therefore, the following basic examinations are recommended to be performed and documented in acute phase of polytraumatic patients:

Examinations of the Functions of the Pupillomotor Pathway

Evoking the direct, i.e., afferent pupillary response by shining a light into the eyes one after the other, or in the absence of a light source by covering them: the first sign of a lesion in the afferent pupillomotor pathway is when the pupil first constricts as a response to direct light or covering; however, it subsequently redilates ('as if it could not maintain the constricted state of the pupil'): it is recorded on the scale as MG1 +4+. In the most severe cases, the pupil does not even constrict on the affected side (+4 MG sign). Since the pupillomotor pathway runs together with the antechiasmal fibers of the optic nerve, they can be both damaged during an antechiasmal injury. It is the most sensitive diagnostic sign in traumatic optic nerve injury.

Examination of the indirect pupillomotor response pupillary constriction is absent on the affected side when shining a light into the contralateral eye. If the eyes of the patient are shone in an alternating manner, the affected side remains more dilated, it is also known as anisocoria. Its size in millimeters (PD diameter) is recommended to be documented in the patient chart. The most severe form of it is dilated and fixed pupil, which is a definite sign of increased intracranial pressure.

We should NEVER administer a eye-drop to dilate the pupil of a patient presenting with cranial injury, however,examination of the pupillomotor response is essential.

Tests of the eye Movements

In case of an unconscious patients, abnormalities in the eyelid, e.g., ptosis, lagophthalmus, and the observation eyes alignment in primary position is recommended. Spontaneous eye movements need to be observed as they have differential diagnostic value. (The are discussed in more details in Chap. 24.).

Test by Ophthalmoscopy

Papilledema can be the first sign of increased intracranial pressure. The absence of papilledema does not (!) exclude the possibility of intracranial hypertension! Retinal and peripapillary bleedings and sometimes hemorrhages expanding towards the vitreous body are not exclusively caused by increased intracranial pressure, but they can also occur as a consequence of intraventricular bleeding as a part of intracranial subarachnoid bleeding. This is also referred to as ***Terson's syndrome*** in the neuro-ophthalmological scientific literature. ***Papillary decoloration*** can caused by marked loss of optic fibers in the late phase of chronic higher intracranial pressure.

Local Examinations at the Bedside - in Case of Intact Consciousness Patients

- *visual acuity* : what distance can the patients count our fingers from? (fc)
- *confrontation visual field examination:* it can be used for the detection of severe hemianopia, the same can be used in non-cooperative patients and in young children.
- bedside examination of *pupillary responses* and *eye movements.*
- thorough *examination of the fundus*

The first examination should be performed precisely in ambulatory screening, and the the collected data need to be documentated and the patient be informed in case of a life-long care as well.

The Importance of the Topography in the Differential Diagnosis of Traumatic Optic Neuropathy

Neuro-radiological examination and diagnosis of antechiasmal optic nerve diseases are often difficult. This is due to the limited possibility to examine the orbital fat and the intracanalicular segment of the optic nerve even by the most modern MRI methods. On the other hand, severe cranial injuries result in so extensive morphological and functional alterations that injuries to the optic nerve may remain undetected or late-detected. Therefore, the most precise and objective assessment of the visual functions is of high significance.

The significance of visual field tests in cooperative patients after regaining their consciousness:

- it refers to the location of the lesion (ante-, retrochiasmal lesion, cortical blindness, etc.),
- it shows the degree of damage (initial state, assessment of change),
- the type of the disease determines the long-term prognosis at the same time,
- it represents a crucial decisive point regarding the nature of therapy and rehabilitation.

Antechiasmal optic nerve lesion it is very difficult to diagnose as such lesions are detected very late. This is well presented by the case of a young man who had a basal skull fracture and a subsequent bilateral antechiasmal optic nerve lesion as a result of polytrauma due to a car accident. Visual acuity and VEP examinations both revealed only a small peripheral island of visual field, finger count of 1 m on the left side and other pupillomotor signs (See perimetry images of Fig. 48.9).

Traumatic injuries of the *chiasm and the parasellar region* are less frequent, whereas compressive injuries due to tumors are more common. Visual field defect accompanying uni- or bilateral loss of vision, as well as diplopia and eye movement disorder in association with unilateral loss of vision, can frequently be detected.

Traumatic injury to *the optic tract and optic radiation* is less common in the young; therefore, visual field defects developing due to such lesions

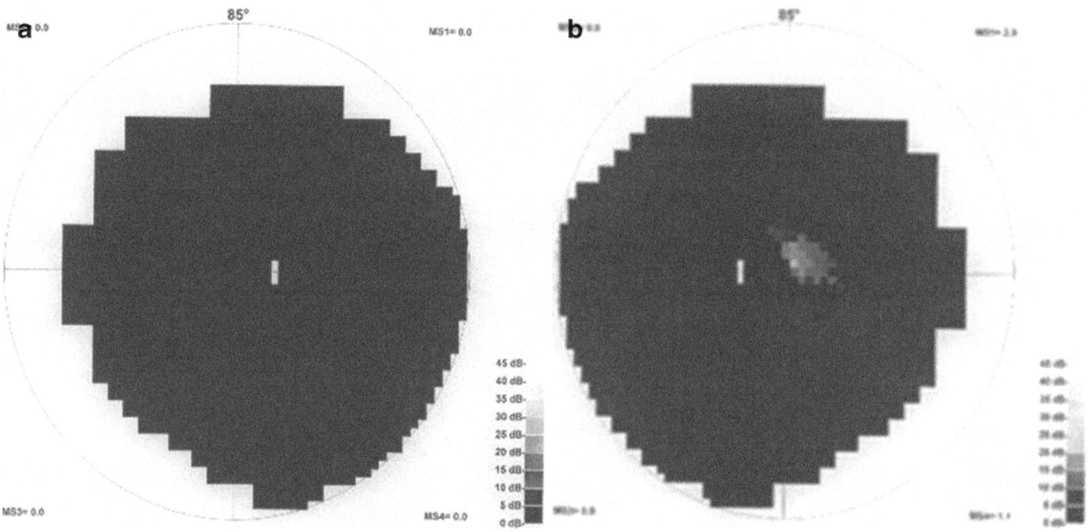

Fig. 48.9 (**a**) In addition to a complete amaurosis on the right side (absence of light vision). (**b**) A small remaining peripheral island of vision can be seen in the perimetry chart of the left eye, which results in a small peripheral vision remaining instead of complete blindness

are predominantly attributable to a compressive process or stroke. The presence of hemianopia, a defect halving the center or some defect present also in the intact halves of the visual field are all rather embarrassing during reading and street traffic, especially, if the defect manifests in the form of an absolute scotoma.

Testablishment of the diagnosis of incomplete and complete *cortical blindness,* as well as the care-giving and rehabilitation of such patients are among the most difficult tasks of the ophthalmologist. In addition to the preserved fundus and intact pupillomotor functions, the history of the patient can be helpful. Cortical blindness is frequently seen after resuscitation, and as a neurological complication of cardiac microembolisation (e.g., after cardioversion in a patient with cardiac shock due to marked arrhythmias).

However, incomplete or complete cortical blindness can frequently be observed as a complication after long-term coma, intraparenchymal hemorrhages, or cerebral edema. Cranial MRI does not always reveal any morphological abnormality in these patients. Neuropsychological support, primary rehabilitation and the empathic help of the ophthalmologist plays an important role in the care of these patients.

Optic agnosias develop as a consequence of damage to cortical areas that are responsible for the acquisition and processing of visual experience, and which provide the coupling of seen and memorized signs as well as the harmonization of other sensory and cognitive functions. (Such as visual neglect syndrome.) The are discussed in details in Chap. 67. from page 394. Neuropsychologists have been providing valuable help in the complex rehabilitation of patients with their essential cooperative work for decades.

In an event of an injury affecting either segment of the visual pathway system, the visual field test provides the most valuable information in cases of cranial traumas as well. The most severe defects are detected in this group of patients. Figure 48.10 guides us in the topographic localization of the defect based on the different types of visual field defects.

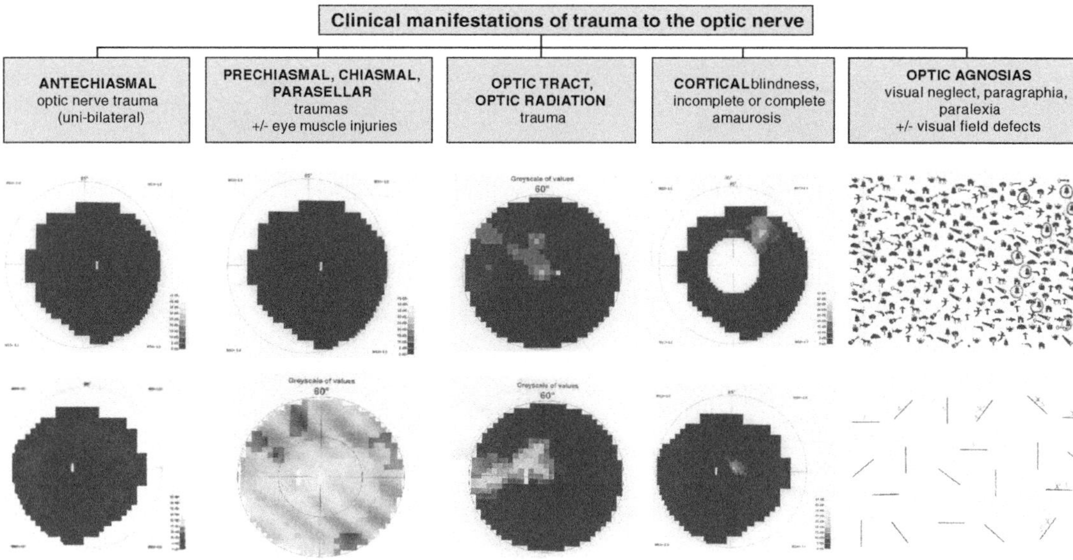

Fig. 48.10 Characteristic visual field defects due to traumatic injuries developed in different sites of the optic pathway system. It mostly provides useful information in terms of localizing the diasese

Further Readings

Hamill MB. Ophthalmologic injuries in the head injured patients. In: Narayan RK, Wilberger Jr JE, Povlishock JT, editors. Neurotrauma. New York: McGraw-Hill; 1996. p. 239–53.

Keidel M, et al. *Head trauma. Intensive care in neurology*. In: Brandt T et al., editors. Neurological disorders. Course and treatment. San Diego: Academic Press; 1996. p. 531–45.

Kenneth D, et al. Traumatic optic neuropathy. In: Walsh and Hoyt's: clinical neuro-ophthalmology. Lippincott: Williams & Wilkins; 2005. p. 431–47.

Pásztor Emil – Vajda János: Idegsébeszet. Medicina, Budapest; 1995. (In Hungarian)

Wang S. Clinical treatment of traumatic brain injury complicated by cranial nerve injury. Injury. 2010;41: 997–1002.

Toxic and Deficiency Optic Neuropathy

49

Vera Klein

Contents

These diseases primarily affect the optic segment of the visual pathway. The damage of optic nerve develops owing to the neurotoxic effect of exogenous substances and/or due to nutritional factors. In etiological point of view, the much more common group of optic nerve diseases originating from dietary insufficiencies and nicotine-alcohol abuse should be distinguished from direct opticopathies caused by medications/chemicals.

Nutritional Optico Neuropathies

(frequent synonyms: toxic opticopathy, toxic amlyopia, deficiency amblyopia, alcohol–tobacco amblyopia) The clinical picture is characteristic, the establishment of the diagnosis is easy in most of the cases.

V. Klein, M.D.
Ophthalmologist, Neuro-ophthalmologist,
Budapest District 13, Health Care Nonprofit Ltd,
Budapest, Hungary
e-mail: Fiume@cheiio.hu

Characteristics

- exclusively bilateral, though it generally presents with unequal degree of gradually progressing painless deterioration of vision in the two eyes, which can decrease below one tenth, down to finger count vision;
- acquired-type of color vision disturbance, decreased critical fusion frequency value (CFF) and pathological visual evoked potential record (VEP) are always present;
- centrocecal scotoma develops in the field of vision corresponding to the damage of the papillomacular bundle (this can be well detected by kinetic perimetry) with intact peripheral vision;
- the optic disc is initially intact, subsequently a temporal pallor appears, rarely hemorrhage may appear radiating from the sharp optic disc margins;
- it does not lead to complete blindness even in untreated cases.

Etiology

- the most frequent etiology is the combination of tobacco and alcohol abuse, but it occurs also in isolated tobacco or alcohol abuses as well;

J. Somlai, T. Kovács (eds.), *Neuro-Ophthalmology*, DOI 10.1007/978-3-319-28956-4_49

- exclusively nutritional causes, such as complex dietary deficiency, low levels of vitamin B-1 or B-12, absorption disorders, folate deficiency;
- any combination of the above.

Any of the listed etiologies result in a clinically identical entity. The cause of hypovitaminosis in alcohol-induced ambylopia is dual. On the one hand, alcoholic individuals a priori consume less amount of food, because a part of their energy demand is covered by alcohol; on the other hand, malabsorption in the gastrointestinal tract develops in advanced stages. We learned from experience that the disease becomes manifest only in a small proportion of exposed individuals, and that toxic neuropathy can also occur as one of the symptoms of chronic alcoholism as well as the solitary sign of alcohol disease. It is hard to explain why the disease manifests in a well-nourished otherwise healthy excessive drinker, and why the visual functions are almost completely intact in a chronic alcoholic patient with several episodes of delirium in the past medical history. The need for a genetic predisposition for the development of the disease in addition to the above described multifactorial etiology is probable.

Pathology

According to Winken, a symmetrical bilateral demyelination can be observed in the central fibers of the optic nerve, which correspond to the axially located papillomacular bundle, and it can be followed as an arrow-like abnormality from the retrobulbar part of the optic nerve through the optic chiasm and the optic tract until the lateral geniculate body. The site of the primary damage is proposed to be in the retrobulbar segment of the optic nerve. Winken considers the degeneration of the macular ganglion cells as secondary.

Therapy and Prognosis

The key point of the therapy is the adherence to abstinence, the vitamin and protein abundant diet. Kanski (2007) recommends the administration of 1000 mcg inj. Hydroxocobalamine once a week for 10 weeks in addition to these. In case of a cooperative and abstinent patient, the prognosis is generally good, the visual acuity can improve from the level of a finger count vision to 1.0. The centrocecal scotoma in the field of vision gradually decreases, divides into two parts, subsequently the central defect disappears and the blind spot becomes normal in size. The regression is rather slow; therefore, the patients need to be encouraged not to lose their patience.

The complete recurrence of vision generally requires months or even a year. The acquired dyschromatopsia is definitive. Without treatment, the severe deterioration of vision becomes permanent; however, it never leads to complete blindness as the peripheral vision is preserved. In milder degrees of toxic amblyopia, spontaneous regression can also occur, which may be explained by an improvement of living conditions. Notably, the characteristically beer-consuming countries have rather low frequencies of toxic optic neuropathy.

We are aware that alcoholism is an epidemic, and it is rather difficult to asses the frequency of toxic amblyopia among alcoholic patients. According to our own experience, the imminent loss of vision forces a remarkable proportion of patients to cooperate, and therefore, in a paradox manner, helps the patients getting out from the vicious circle of alcoholism.

Drug-Induced Optic Neuropathy

Several medical drugs/chemicals can cause toxic optic nerve lesion. The following substances are mentioned, without being exhaustive: ethambutol, chloramphenicol, streptomycin, isoniazid, amiodarone, vigabatrin, as well as, lead, antimony, arsenic and mercury among the heavy metals. In extreme rare cases of acute alcohol toxicity, the direct opticotoxic effect of ethyl alcohol results in a severe, acute-onset deterioration of vision lasting for a couple of days. (Duke Elder). Optic nerve damage due to methyl alcohol intoxication is definitive. Hereby, we discuss in more details the adverse effects related to optic nerve functions of drugs used in the everyday practice.

Ethambutol

An anti-TB drug used in combination.

It can cause a dose- and time-dependent toxic optic neuropathy. The incidence of optic neuropathy is 6 % with doses higher than 25 mg/kg body weight per day, and it generally manifests in the 3rd–6th month of the treatment. The disease is extremely rare if the drug is used in doses less than 15 mg/kg body weight per day. The disease can be screened by regular preventive ophthalmological examination: an early decrease in CFF value can be an introductory sign turning our attention to an imminent deterioration of optic nerve functions. A typical centrocecal scotoma or constriction of the visual field, together with a severe deterioration of vision and an acquired color vision disturbance are characteristic. The prognosis is generally good after the cessation of administration; however, the complete recovery may take up to 12 months. Definitive deterioration of vision in association with optic atrophy remains only in a small propoportion of patients. The recommended frequency of screening: once in every 4 weeks if the dose is higher than 15 mg/kg/day, and once in every 3–6 months if the dose is lower. Administration of the drug should be ceased as soon as the first signs appear.

Amiodaron

A known and practically harmless side effect of this frequently indicated antiarrhythmic drug is 'vortex keratopathy'.

Less widely recognized is the fact that optic lesion occurs in 1–2 % of the patients, the signs and symptoms of which include bilateral mild papilledema, deterioration of vision and variable visual field defects. From differential diagnostic point of view, it has to be distinguished from the bilateral, non-arteritic anterior ischemic optic neuropathy (NAION), which is reminiscent of amiodarone-induced optic nerve lesion. It is not dose-dependent. Screening is not obligatory, as the group of patients that are at risk cannot be predicted in any way. The prognosis is questionable, the cessation of drug administration does not result in an improvement of vision in all cases.

Vigabatrin

A frequently used antiepileptic drug in complex partial epilepsy in adults and in childhood epilepsy (West's syndrome). A gradually developing bilateral concentric constriction of the visual field may develop as a drug adverse effect, with intact visual acuity. The patient is asymptomatic due to the slow progression and the intact visual acuity. Fundoscopy reveals no abnormality, possibly mild atrophy can be noticed. The color vision is preserved, the CFF value is normal. The constriction of the visual field will remain unchanged after the cessation of drug administration. Due to the absence of symptoms, the regular ophthalmological check-up is extremely important, including the kinetic perimetry, performed once in every half year in the first year, then once a year, following the internationally accepted recommendation.

Reference

Kanski Jack J. Clinical ophthalmology. Oxford: Butterworth Heinemann; 2007. p. 845–6.

Ocular Symptoms and Signs of Intracranial Hypertension

50

Judit Somlai

Contents

J. Somlai, M.D.
Unit of Neuro-Ophthalmology, Department of Neurology and Stroke, Military Hospital, Budapest, Hungary

Neuro-Ophthalmology Section, Hungarian Ophthalmological Association, Budapest, Hungary

Trustee, NOSZA Foundation (for the Prevention and Screening of Ocular Storke) Budapest, Hungary
e-mail: dr@somlaijudit.hu; http://somlaijudit.hu

In the clinical practice, increased intracranial pressure can drive the patient towards a severe and life-threatening condition. According to a number of clinical observations, the three leading clinical symptoms *(headache, vomiting, papilledema)* are NOT early symptoms of emergency, since according to the observations, these symptoms can only be detected in 50% of patients with a cerebral tumor that needs to be operated on. The ophthalmologists are mostly asked to examine the fundus; however, alarming pupillary signs and eye movement disorders can indicate or even precede an increase in intracranial pressure that could evoke the development of a papilledema. Ocular symptoms leading to

J. Somlai, T. Kovács (eds.), *Neuro-Ophthalmology*, DOI 10.1007/978-3-319-28956-4_50

papilledema are rather poor, as there are no alarming symptoms apart from obscuration (transient darkening of the sight in both eyes for short periods of time). Edema of the optic nerve head developed due to different etiologies show the same clinical signs both in intracranial hypertension and in other systemic diseases (such as inflammation, circulatory disorder). Therefore, in such cases, the significance of differential diagnosis is especially high.

The Pathomechanism and Most Frequent Causes of Intracranial Hypertension

Papilledema mostly develops as a consequence of increased intracranial pressure. Causes of intracranial hypertension are different; however, their pathomechanism can be interrelated, such as:

- intracranial mass
- disturbances in CSF production, circulation and/or absorption
- cerebral edema (of metabolic, traumatic, inflammatory as well as circulatory disorder-related origin)
- spatial disproportion between the skull volume and intracranial content (developmental abnormality)
- intracranial circulatory disturbance (disturbed cerebral venous flow: e.g., sinus thrombosis)

Overcome by the space-occupying process, the brain can only be dislocated within the bony skull in directions that are allowed by:

- the falx,
- the tentorium,
- and the skull open from below (foramen magnum).

Acute Neurological Consequences of Increased Intracranial Pressure (Intracranial Hypertension, IH)

The slowly enlarging space occupation is initially not accompanied by an increased pressure, due to the effect of compensatory processes. Thus the occupation of space happens at the expense of cerebral and cerebrospinal fluid (CSF) volume. However, reaching the limits of compensatory processes, the intracranial pressure begins to increase rapidly. The relationship between the expansion of the space-occupying process and intracranial pressure is non-linear, and in the end even a small amount of tissue enlargement will result in a rapid and high degree of increase in intracranial pressure. (This is supported by the fact that the drainage of even a small amount of CSF is sufficient to restore the pressure.) Brainstem dysfunction evoked by processes associated with rapidly increasing intracranial pressure, inintracranial hypertension (IH) lead to respiratory disorder, which triggers a further increase in pressure as a vicious circle. This is due to the phenomenon that respiratory disturbance is accompanied by an increased CO2 concentration in the blood, leading to subsequent vasodilation and hyperemia, which result in an increase in cerebral, i.e., total volume inside the enclosed intracranial space. Increased intracranial pressure leads to a progressive deterioration of circulation owing to an immediate decrease in arterial perfusion pressure. This is due the fact that cerebral autoregulation does not work below 50 mmHg (also known as critical cerebral perfusion pressure) and therefore, the cerebral circulation passively follows the cerebral pressure, which leads to a subsequent deterioration of perfusion. If intracranial pressure reaches the mean arterial pressure, the perfusion will be zero, i.e., the cerebral circulation stops. Increased intracranial pressure leads to an increased venous pressure and an increased venous resistance. This plays an important role in the development of cerebral edema.

Suddenly Developing Increased Intracranial Pressure due to Local Circulatory Disturbance

Pathological processes leading to double vision and/or the development of a papilledema are not exclusively caused by space occupation but can

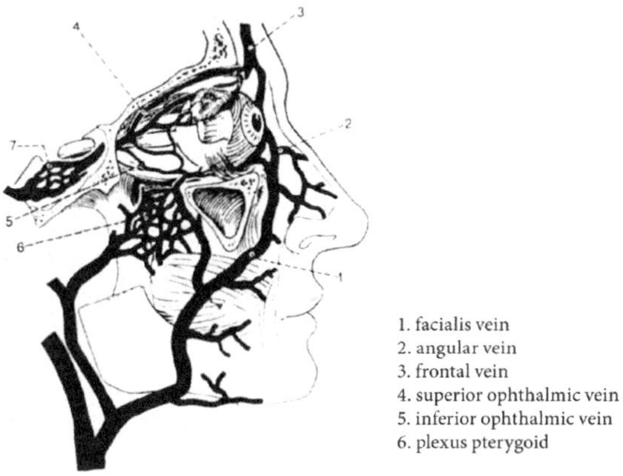

Fig. 50.1 Venous drainage of the optic nerve is in a rather close functional interconnection with the venous sinuses of the skull base that play the most important role in the venous drainage of the brain. Kayenbuhl et al. (1968)

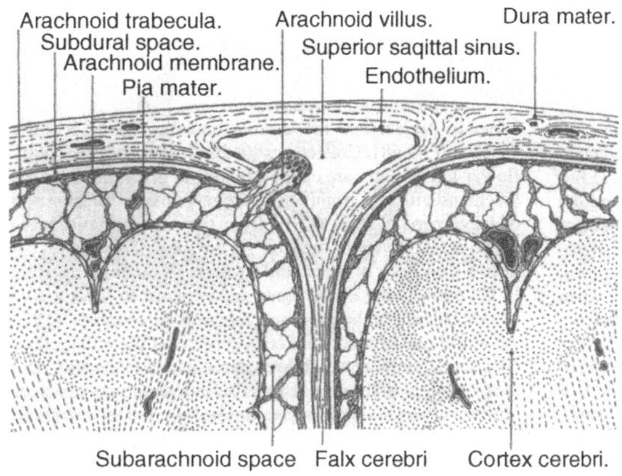

Fig. 50.2 Due to the close physiological and therefore, pathophysiological relationship between venous sinuses and the circulation of CSF, disturbances either in the circulation of CSF or in the venous drainage can lead to ocular symptoms. Weed (1923)

also be induced by intracranial circulatory disturbance. For instance, the arteriolization of venous blood (carotid-cavernous fistula, CCF) or a progressive venous congestion (e.g., cerebral sinus thrombosis), which lead to local volume translocation and thus to a subsequent alteration in one of the three components that determine the intracranial pressure. Venous drainage of the optic nerve is in a rather close functional interconnection with venous sinuses of the skull base that play the most important role in the venous drainage of the brain (Fig. 50.1). Therefore, a circulatory disturbance, stasis or thrombosis of these venous sinuses leads to a disturbed venous drainage of the eye in a retrograde manner. Such conditions include the pre-thrombosis of the optic disc accompanied by papilledema and/or eye movement disorder. Figure 50.2 presents the close physiological and therefore, pathophysiological relationship between venous sinuses and the circulation of CSF. Due to this close interconnection, disturbances in the circulation of CSF and in the venous drainage within the central nervous system (CNS) can lead to ocular symptoms. The peculiar blood supply of the brainstem as well as the special cerebral venous network play essential roles in the development of eye movement disorders caused by brainstem dysfunctions due to increased intracranial pressure. (Circulatory disorders of the retina and the visual pathway are discussed in more detailsin Chap. 43.).

Types of Herniation as a Consequence of Intracranial Hypertension

Central (Axial) Herniation

This is most frequently caused by a space-occupying process located in the medial fossa or close to the midline, associated with increased production of edema or a general cerebral edema. Together with a direct downward displacement of the brainstem, increased supratentorial pressure shifts to the posterior fossa and the cerebellar tonsils can be pushed into the foramen magnum. The major causes include non-communicating hydrocephalus, meningitis, diffuse cerebral edema and midline tumors (predominantly that are located in the region of the diencephalon) (Fig. 50.3).

Lateral (Hemispheric) Herniations

Hemispheric i.e., lateral space-occupying processes dislocate the brain medially. In the beginning, the pressure affects merely the diencephalon, similarly to that seen in axial herniation. Further displacements can result in two different forms of herniation:

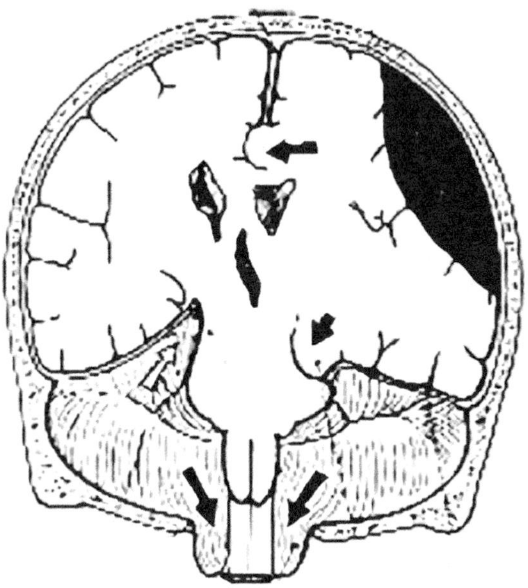

Fig. 50.3 Depiction of the different types of cerebral herniations. Pasztor (1983)

- *uncal herniation* (Fig. 50.3) The further increase in intracranial pressure results in the herniation of the medial part of one of the temporal lobes (uncus and hippocampal gyrus) in the tentorial incisura. This may lead to the development of one of the characteristic ocular symptoms due to the compression of the oculomotor nerve running there. Anisocoria and ophthalmoparesis due to eye movement disorder.
- *cingular herniation:* (Fig. 50.3) In case of a lateral increase in intracranial pressure, the paramedian structures can herniate beneath the falx (subfalcine herniation).

The most frequent causes of lateral herniation include intracranial, e.g., subdural and epidural hemorrhages, tumors and sudden intratumoral bleedings.

Infratentorial Space-Occupying Lesion

In case of an infratentorial herniation, the space-occupying process within the posterior fossa leads to a impaction of the anterior-superior part of the cerebellum in the tentorial incisura from below (where the tentorium merges with the falx – straight sinus), whereas in case of a foraminal herination, the process in the posterior fossa herniates into the foramen magnum as a consequence of mass effect.

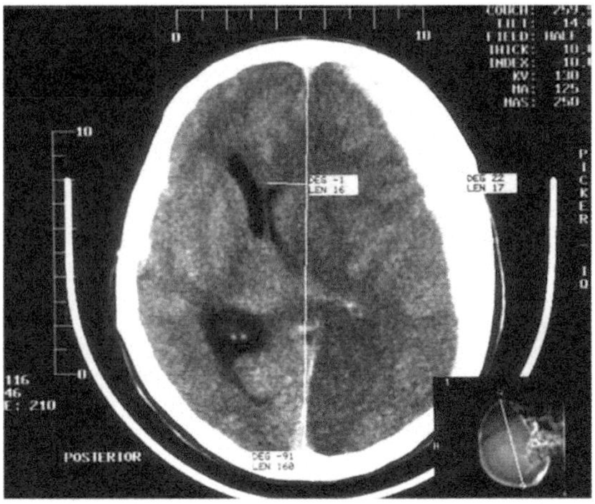

Fig. 50.4 CT image of a lateral herniation caused by subdural hemorrhage

Foraminal Herniation (Herniation into the Foramen Magnum)

Cerebellar tonsils reach the plane of the foramen magnum in most of healthy individuals. Space-occupying processes growing in the posterior fossa result in the displacement of the tonsils into the foramen magnum, which leads to the compression of the lower brainstem region (Fig. 50.3). The major causes include processes in the posterior fossa such as tumors, hemorrhages, space-occupying lesions of the cerebellar lobes and that expanding towards the central structure, as well as status epilepticus – progressive cerebral edema. Ocular symptoms are not that much informative due to the rapid deterioration of autonomic functions. Only the presence or absence of oculocephalic reflex checked during the careful examination of neck stiffness can provide some additional information (Fig. 50.4).

Symptoms and Signs of Intracranial Hypertension – Papilledema (Synonyms: Swollen Disc or Chocked Disc)

Though the mechanism of the development of papilledema is not known, we may come closer to understanding intracranial hypertension if we make an attempt to think about the factors determining intraocular pressure as an analogy. Intraocular pressure is determined by the relationship of the actual characteristics of the aqueous humor in terms of quantity, production, drainage and absorption; furthermore, the stability or imbalance in the physiological equilibrium developed between the intraocular space-occupying lesion and the arterial–venous circulation of the eye plays a role as well. Within the completely closed intracranial space, an increase in pressure can develop in different pace, of different origin and with different etiopathomechanism.

Table 50.1 The most frequent causes of papilledema

Space-occupying processes
Intracranial tumor, pseudotumor cerebri, disorders in CSF dynamics
Congenital optic disc anomaly
Hyaline bodies – optic disc drusen
Uveitis, hypotension, occlusions of retinal veins
Inflammatory diseases of the optic nerve
Papillitis of the optic nerve
Papillophelebitis, neuroretinitis
Tumors of the optic nerve
Hemangioma, glioma, metastasis
Vascular optic nerve lesions
Anterior ischemic optic neuropathy (AION), pre-thrombosis or branch or trunk occlusion of retinal blood vessels, diabetic retinopathy or hypertensive retinopathy
Infiltrative diseases
Lymphoma, reticuloendotheliosis
Systemic diseases
Anemia, hypoxia, hypertension, uremia
Orbital tumors
Optic sheath meningioma, optic glioma, metastases
Endocrine orbitopathy
Vascular encephalopathy
Hypertonia, lipid and carbohydrate metabolic disorders

The Most Frequent Causes of Papilledema

The most frequent causes of papilledema (synonyms include swollen disc or papilledema) are summarized in the table below. Edema of the optic nerve head most frequently develops as a result of intracranial or intraorbital spaceoccupying processes, local vascular processes, and, rarely, inflammatory processes (Table 50.1).

The Clinical Features of Papilledema

Visual Acuity (Vision) and a Decrease in Critical Fusion Frequency (CFF) Value

At the initial, acute stage, increased pressure expanding towards the subarachnoid space does not result in a loss of visual functions, as the numerous small arteries supplying the optic nerve head (e.g., pial end arteries, terminal branches of short ciliary arteries) provide compensatory blood supply despite the increasing pressure and consequent disturbance in venous drainage. With time, however, the permanent increase results in a situation analogous to a pre-thrombotic retinal circulatory condition due to the disturbance of venous drainage, naturally with different etiologies. When a secondary blood supply disorder is permanently present, the decrease in CFF in both eyes will develop as first sign, and the transient episodes of blurred vision subsequently lead to a permanent decrease in visual acuity (Fig. 50.5).

Visual Field Defects: 'Blind Spot Enlargement syndrome'

The evaluation of fundoscopic appearance is rather difficult in case of an early papilledema. In case the cooperation of the patient enables, the detection of abnormal size of the blind spot via visual field examination provide the most objective measure of early edema of the optic disc as

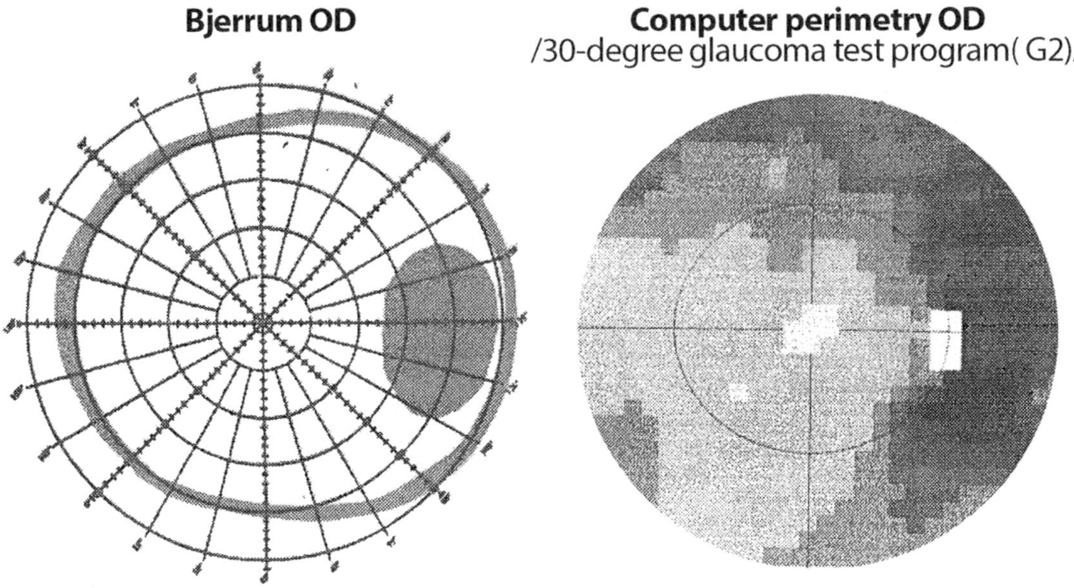

Fig. 50.5 Blind spot enlargement due to papilledema on Bjerrum's screen and computer perimetry

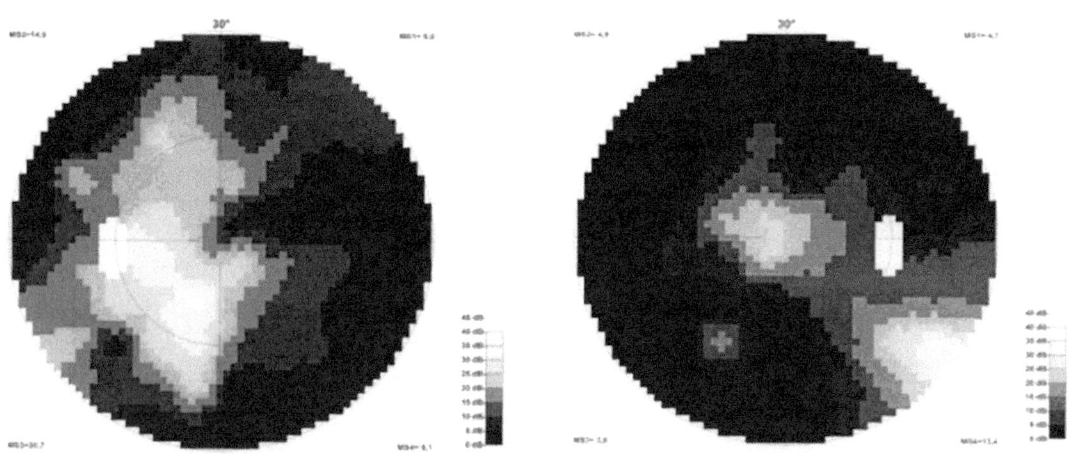

Fig. 50.6 Visual field defect developed as a consequence of persistent papilledema presents in a right-dominant bilateral concentric constriction of the field of vision, computer perimetry, program G2

well as the consequent functional impairment. The enlargement of the diameter of the optic nerve head is caused by the hyperemia of the optic disc, and the subsequent edema developed due to a circulatory disturbance. Due to the subsequent circulatory consequences (obliterated vascular funnel, and later the protrusion of the optic disc also known as prominent optic disc, and finally the presence of peripapillary abnormalities) the diameter of the optic disc and correspondingly that of the blind spot become enlarged. Enlargement of the blind spot can be well tested in a plane surface, i.e., via the examination of the central part of the field of vision by the use of a Bjerrum's screen and/or computer perimetry (Fig. 50.6).

The deterioration of the visual field defect is a sensitive marker of untreated or late-diagnosed cases. Permanent intracranial hypertension results in an irreversible loss of nerve fibers manifesting in form of a temporal and subsequently concentric constriction of the visual field. Finally even a 'tunnel vision' can develop accompanied by optic disc pallor.

Characteristic Fundoscopic – Ophthalmoscopic Appearance (Frisén's Scale)

The enlargement of the diameter of the optic disc is caused by the edema of the optic nerve head, which is indicated, in addition to the subjective assessment, by the enlargement of the blind spot as measured by visual field test. Hyperemia of the optic disc is an early sign indicating capillary dilation and a disturbance in circulation. Progressive edema due to a disturbance in venous drainage pushes the papillary nerve fibers apart, which in the beginning gives the optic disc a 'fibrous' appearance, and subsequently elevating above the level of the lamina cribrosa the optic disc becomes 'filled'. Due to the increasing edema, the optic disc progressively protrudes into the vitreous body. The prominence can be assessed by the use of an ophthalmoscope via the measurement of the difference between the diopter value the peripapillary (base) and highest intrapapillary blood vessel (peak) – a difference of 1 mm corresponds to a prominence of three diopters (Fig. 50.7).

Signs of venous circulatory disorder will appear as a consequence of rapidly increasing intracranial pressure due to shifting of increased intracranial pressure to the subarachnoid space surrounding the intraorbital segment of the optic nerve. This results in a subsequent deceleration of the reflux of venous blood from the retina, leading to a stasis in intraocular retinal veins.

This can be observed through the tortuosity of veins surrounding the choked disc, which subsequently become accompanied by signs of perivenous hemorrhages and metabolic disturbance. Disturbance of venous drainage can be so severe as the process deteriorates that the margins of the optic disc can be covered by the bleeds leaking from the damaged veins.

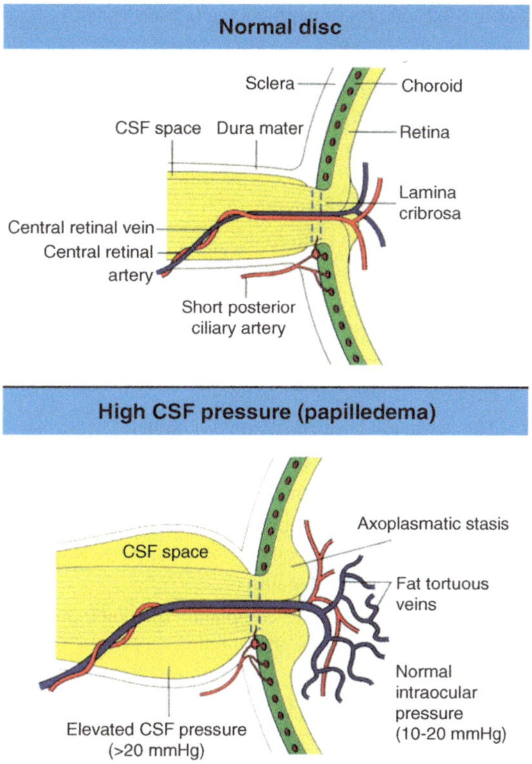

Fig. 50.7 Normal state of subarachnoid space surrounding the intraorbital segment of the optic nerve, and tissue abnormalities caused by increased intracranial pressure, which secondarily lead to disturbed cerebral venous drainage (redrawn). Rosen et al. (1998)

In the event of a central retinal vein (trunk) thrombosis, hemorrhages expand towards the peripheral segments of the venous branch as well, which is an essential sign from differential diagnostic point of view. As a consequence of long-lasting untreated intracranial hypertension, exudates and soft degenerative foci appear on fundoscopy, which are already associated with nerve fiber damage. On fundoscopy, the disturbance in retinal blood supply is indicated by the presence of perimacular folds (also known as 'Spritz figur' in the German terminology). In chronic papilledema, the margins of the optic nerve head become almost sharp, surrounded by organized edema.

At the same time, the optic disc becomes pale, i.e., porcelain-white, and the visual functions

Table 50.2 Stages of papilledema (Frisén's scale)

St. 0.: normal optic disc	
The nasal margin of the optic disc is blurred (occasionally the superior and inferior margins are as well)	Infrequently, a segment of a blood vessel is obscured (mainly in the upper pole)
The peripapillary radial nerve fiber layer arrangement is preserved	
St. 0.: minimal papilledema	
The nasal margin is blurred	Concentric or radial chorioretinal folds
No prominence can be observed yet	The temporal optic disc margin is intact
The perpapillary radial nerve fiber layer regionally shows grayish opacity	Early signs of peripapillary halo temporally (blurred small grayish splits)
St. II.: mild papilledema	
Concentrically blurred margins	The nasal margin is elevated
The peripapillary halo becomes complete	
St. III: modern papilledema	
Concentric obscuration of optic disc margins	Concentric elevation of the optic disc margins
The diameter of the optic nerve head is increased	A proportion of blood vessels radiating from the optic nerve head becomes obscured
St. IV.: marked papilledema	
The optic disc becomes completely filled and prominent, the prominence can be measured in diopters	Concentric obscuration of the optic disc margins
Blood vessels radiating from the optic nerve head becomes totally obscured	The peripapillary halo becomes irregular with finger-like
	Extensions
St. V.: severe papilledema	
Dome-shaped protrusion of the optic nerve head	The peripalliary halo becomes narrow and evenly demarcated
A segment of blood vessel becomes blurred or totally obscured	The complete obliteration of the optic nerve head
Supplementary fundoscopic signs:	Hyperemia
Tortuosity of the veins	Hemorrhages
Exudates	Cotton wool spots
Optic disc pallor	

Redrawn after Frisén (1982)

severely deteriorate, which is followed by a concentric constriction of the field of vision (Table 50.2).

Stages of Papilledema (Frisén's Scale)

In the next two figures, fundoscopic images of early papilledema highly characteristic of Frisén stage one can be seen with blurred nasal optic disc margin and intact temporal optic disc margin (Fig. 50.8).

Whereas in the fundoscopic image highly characteristic of Frisén stage three, the concentrically blurred and elevated (prominent) optic disc is accompanied by obscured blood vessels coursing in and out of the optic disc, and the peripapillary halo becomes irregular with finger-like extensions (Fig. 50.9).

Differential Diagnosis of Papilledema

In the early and acute phase of papilledema developed as a consequence of intracranial hypertension, the visual functions remain intact for a long period. However, antechiasmal optic neuropathies caused by circulatory

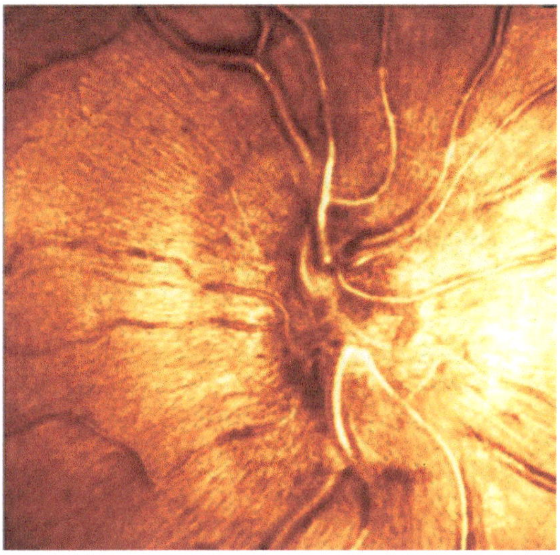

Fig. 50.8 Frisen stage two papilledema. Concentric blurred margins and the diameter of the optic nerve head is increased

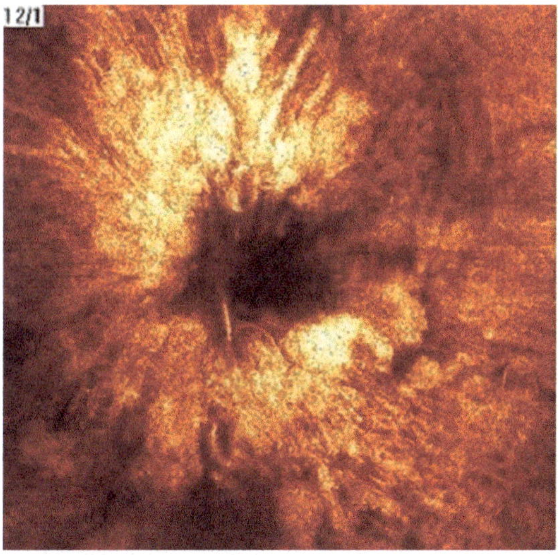

Fig. 50.9 Frisén stage three papilledema. Concentric obscuration of a proportion of blood vessels radiating from the optic nerve head and of all borders of the optic disc can be observed, the margins of the optic disc become concentrically elevated, the diameter of the optic nerve head is increased

disorder such as anterior ischemic optic neuropathy (AION) as well retinal trunk thromboses do not only present with a similar initial fundoscopic appearance but also with a remarkable deterioration of vision at the onset. (This is discussed in more details in Chap. 43.).

In inflammatory processes (such as multiple sclerosis) – except for papillitis – the deterioration of visual functions is not accompanied by any sort of fundoscopic abnormality. In addition to a comprehensive ophthalmological and neurological medical history, the sound and long-term examination documentation represents a true support for the examiner.

Among diseases resulting in intracranial hypertension, *benign intracranial hypertension (BIH)* also known as *pseudotumor cerebri* has a special position. Its diagnostic criteria include narrow cerebral ventricles in the absence of intracranial spaceoccupying lesion on CT or MRI scan, in addition to a bilateral papilledema and the general symptoms and signs of increased intracranial pressure (abducens palsy, headache) (Table 50.3).

Besides, the CSF pressure is mostly increased. Cerebral venous circulatory disorders (sinus thrombosis or stasis) as well as primary and secondary pathologies of CSF dynamics comprise the main syndromes in this group.

Symptoms and Signs of Intracranial Hypertension – eye Movement Disorders

The aligned gaze of eyes looking straight ahead can be assessed in the outpatient clinic as well as in unconscious patients (this is called primary position) The precise documentation of pupil size, their difference in size as well as the pupillary responses are, however, essential during the bedside examination of an inpatient. This is because an initial anisocoria or the clinical signs of a unior bilateral afferent or efferent pupillomotor pathway lesion can be the most important warning signs of initial or even progressive cases of intracranial hypertension associated with different degrees of impaired consciousness. Eye movement disorders and/or pupillary symptoms and signs may have an alarming role especially if they precede the

Table 50.3 Differential diagnosis of systemic and local diseases causing papilledema

	Papilledema	Optic neuritis	Anterior ischemic optic lesion (aion)	Retinal vein thrombosis
Visual symptoms and signs	Acute phase: Intact visual functions, obscuration	Rapid central loss of vision	Episodes of amaurosis fugax progressive acute deterorioration of vision and visual field	'Descending curtain' (AF)
	Chronic phase progressive deterioration of vision	Periorbital and ocular pain provoked by eye movement	Ischemic pain in the eyeball	Slower but progressive deterioration of vision. unilateral deterioration of spatial vision
Distant and near visual acuity	Acute phase: intact	Deterioration of vision, distant < near	Deterioration of both distant and near vision	Acute phase: unilateral deterioration of spatial vision
	Chronic phase decreased visual aculty	Color vision disorder		Chronic phase central deterioration of vision (secondary maculopathy)
Visual field defects				Branch thrombosis: quadrantanopia
	Blind spot enlargement syndrome	Central absolute scotoma	Unilateral lower nasal quadrantanopta	Central (trunk) thrombosis: blind spot enlargement syndrome
Uni-or bilateral ophthalmo-logical abnormality	Bilateral	Bilateral in adulthood, bilateral but infrequent in childhood	Unilateral'pseudo-Foster-Kennedy syndrome (AION on the contralateral eyes as well)	Unilateral, the involvement of the contralateral eye is frequent (in case of an untreated underlying disease)
Neuro-logical and other symptoms and signs	Eye movement disorder, headache, nausea, focal neurological signs	Headache, periorbital pain radiating from the eyeball, sensory distrurbance	Generally NAD, occasionally signs of vascular encephalopathy	Vascular encephalopathy (untreated hypertension ICA atherosclerosis, cardiac mkrembolization
Pupillary Symptoms and signs	Intact pupillomotor responses or anisocoria (IH)	Afferent pupillomotor lesion: Marcus Gunn sign +1<+2<+3	Afferent pupillomotor lesion: Marcus Gunn sign +1<+2<+3	Afferent pupillomotor lesion: Marcus Gunn sign +1<+2<+3
Fundoscopic appearance	Progressive (+5 – 6D) papilledema, peripapillary hemorrhages, exudates	Neuritis: intact fundus papillitis: papilledema	Moderate papilledema: scattered hemorrhages, optic disc pallor	Marked papilledema, striate hemorrhages, exuadate, maculopathy

development of a papilledema. Therefore, in the everyday clinical practice the examination of the eye movement system is a task for the ophthalmologist, in addition to fundoscopy. Signs of eye movement system dysfunctions are classified hereby based on the typical associating type of herniation, which may be of help in the localization diagnosis. The particular types of eye movement disorders are discussed in details in Chaps. 54 and 55, respectively.

Central–axial herniation is most frequently caused by a space-occupying process located in the medial fossa or close to the midline associated with increased production of edema or a general cerebral edema. This is associated with a direct downward displacement of the brainstem.

Major causes:

- non-communicating hydrocephalus
- meningitis
- diffuse general edema
- midline tumors (especially in the region of the diencephalon)

Symptoms and Signs

The efferent parasympathetic (pretectal region of the mesencephalon) fibers and the trineuronal sympathetic pathways can damage separately or jointly (sympathetic–central fibers originating from the diencephalon descend through the midbrain, the pons and the dorsolateral part of the medulla towards the lateral funiculus of the cervical spinal cord, where they synapse; the preganglionic nerve fiber originating from here and traveling along the superior thoracic motor nerve root synapses in the superior cervical ganglion, from where the fibers run with the carotid plexus and eventually reach the pupillary sphincter muscle located in the iris in the eyeball.

Eye Movement Disorders Caused by Central Herniation

In central herniation, the brainstem suffers direct or indirect compression, and, therefore, brainstem dysfunctions predominate. Diencephalic syndrome

- Pupils (sympathetic effect): constricted, responsive
- In case of a diencephalic compression, a moderate response to light and slightly constricted pupils can be seen. The pathological background is in part the absence of pupil-dilating effect of sympathetic fibers, with intact a pupil-constricting parasympathetic functions
- Increased oculocephalic reflex: the doll's eye phenomenon: the head is tilted backward and to the side. If the brainstem is intact, the eyeballs move towards the contralateral direction, whereas if the brainstem is damaged, the eyeballs move towards the direction of the tilting, passively following its direction
- Eye movement disorder: upward gaze palsy – downward gaze of the eyes
- Injury to nuclei controlling vertical eye movements and their internuclear fibers: functional interconnections between the diencephalon and midbrain are also affected. Bell's phenomenon: on forced closing of the eyelids, the bulbs roll upward and to the lateral side corresponding to a normal innervation
- Injury to the upward gaze center: Bell's sign is intact or is absent only in cases when the afferent fibers or the nucleus itself or its surrounding is damaged

Midbrain Damage

Pupillary symptoms and signs:

- midbrain tectum: bilaterally dilated, unresponsive pupils with hippus
- lesions of upper brainstem tectal and midbrain nuclei and fibers (with predominant involvement of parasympathetic fibers but affecting the sympathetic fibers as well) lead to the development of fixed, dilated, unresponsive pupils
- in case of an isolated compressive injury to the midbrain, pupils remain midsize, but are unresponsive on both sides, which is probably due to the damage of both sympathetic and parasympathetic fibers
- cranial nerve (uncal herniation): unilaterally dilated, unresponsive
- oculocephalic reflex: decreased

Signs of Medullary – Pontine Lesions

- pupill: pinpoint
- in case of a pontine compressive lesion, pinpoint – myotic – pupils develop because the parasympathetic pathway already exited from the brainstem and only the sympathetic fibers travel

along this region, which due to the extended injury of the sympathetic fibers results in the predominance of the parasympathetic effect.

Injury to the Lower Pons-Medulla Oblongata

- coma, irregular respiration, and severe autonomic symptoms and signs are accompanied by:
- eye movement disorder – the characteristic 'ocular bobbing': a rapid downward movement of the eye followed by a return to the midline
- oculocephalic reflex: lost
- pupillary sign: unilateral central Horner's syndrome, i.e., unilaterally constricted pinpoint pupil can be observed in case of a lateral pontomedullary brainstem compression (as well as in case of a cardiovascular origin as a part of Wallenberg's syndrome)

Different Forms of eye Movement Disorders due to Lateral Hemispheric–Uncal Herniation

They are mostly observed in association with hemispheric space-occupying processes.

Most frequent causes

- intracranial hemorrhage
- subdural, epidural hemorrhage
- tumor, intratumoral hemorrhage

Ocular symptoms:

- Oculomotor palsy: The oculomotor nerve exiting from the brainstem gets under compression due to the mass effect of the herniating brain part. Lateral herniation is most frequently associated with oculomotor nerve compression, by means of the herniation of the uncus of the hippocampal gyrus beneath the edge of the tentorium. This is the characteristic uncal – downward transtentorial herniation. Its signs include miosis, which is followed by a slightly responsive pupil, and in the end of the process, a pupil unresponsive to contralateral lighting, this is anisocoria. Pupillomotor fibers traveling superficially within the cranial nerve are highly exposed to suffer injury due to compression; therefore, the first sign of a direct impact on the oculomotor nerve is the decrease in pupillary response (Fig. 50.10 – depiction).
- abducens nerve palsy: long-lasting intracranial hypertension can cause uni- or bilateral compression of the abducens nerve – the etiopathomechanism is not entirely clear, but they most frequently occur in slowly enlarging skull base tumors
- nystagmus and cerebellar symptoms and signs can be observed as a consequence of brachium pontis compression

Initial neurological symptoms: nausea, headache, vomiting, and then apathy. Subsequently, long tract symptoms, pyramidal signs and paresis occur. The later signs include decerebrate (extensor) posturing and cerebellar fits due to brainstem herniation (these are already signs of central herniation).

Foraminal Herniation (Herniation into the Foramen Magnum)

Cerebellar tonsils reach the plane of the foramen magnum in most of the healthy individuals. Space-occupying processes growing in the posterior fossa result in the displacement of the tonsils into the foramen magnum, which leads to the compression of the lower brainstem region.

Major causes:

- tumors, hemorrhages located in the posterior fossa
- space-occupying lesions of the cerebellar lobes and that expanding towards the central structure
- status epilepticus – progressive cerebral edema.

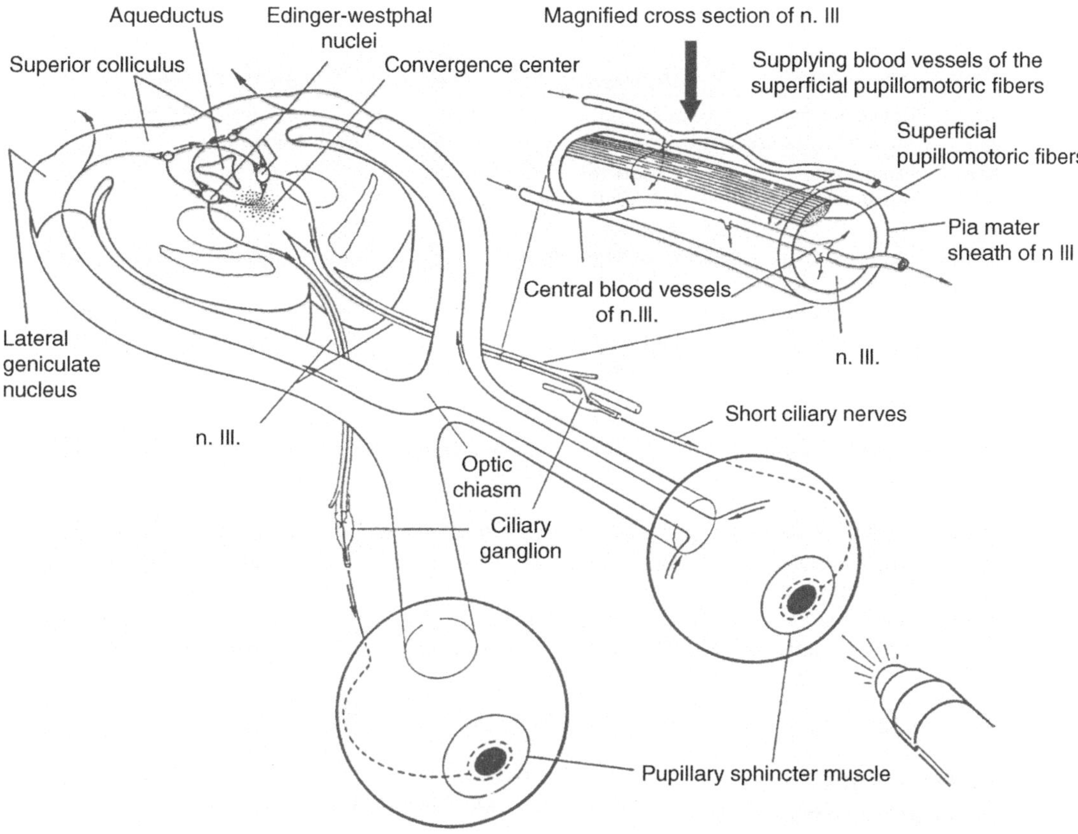

Fig. 50.10 The afferent and efferent routes of the parasympathetic pupillomotor pathway. In the upper-right quadrant of the Figure: magnification of a section the oculomotor nerve emphasizing the external therefore, more vulnerable pupillomotor fibers (Redrawn after Peter 1989)

Ocular symptoms are not that much informative due to the rapid deterioration of autonomic functions. Only the presence or absence of oculocephalic reflex checked during the careful examination of neck stiffness can provide some additional information.

As a continuation of supratentorial herniation, the tonsils of the cerebellum herniate into the foramen magnum. The upper part of the brainstem suffers damage, and subsequently, the compression of the medulla oblongata leads to the following signs: the irregular respiration becomes shallow, the pulse is irregular and filiform. The infratentorial process can evoke sudden respiratory paralysis. In the beginning, the consciousness is preserved. However, later, the diffuse occipital headache may be accompanied by neck stiffness and an abnormal posture of the head.

General Therapeutic Guidelines in Intracranial Hypertension

The potential therapeutic tools include the monitoring of intracranial pressure (it has prognostic significance), ventilation, oxygen supplementation, decreasing hypercapnia, the application of osmotics, diuretic treatments, the use of hyperosmotic Mannitol solution.(it increases the osmolality of the blood while decreasing the edema and the viscosity of the blood), the administration of corticosteroids (they decrease vasogenic edema and the production of CSF), neurosurgical interventions, decompression surgeries, the application of ventricular or lumbar drain). The most frequent causes of intracranial hypertension and their therapeutic options are summarized in Table 50.4.

Table 50.4 The most frequent causes of intracranial hypertension and their therapeutic options

Etiology	Excess tissue	Hydrocephalus	Arterial/venous congestion	Specific therapy
Trauma, severe head injury	Hematoma (epi-, subdural, intracerebral)		Arterial, in the early phase	Neurosurgical (midline dislocation)
Intracerebral hematoma	Parenchymal hematoma	Obstructive, intraventricular neoplasm, communicating neoplasm	Secondary elevation of blood pressure	Neurosurgical
Tumor	Space-occupying tumor	Obstructive, intraventricular neoplasm, communicating neoplasm		Neurosurgical, ventricular drain
Venous thrombosis	Secondary diffuse edema		Secondary hemorrhage, therapeutic complication	Anticoagulation, ventricular drain
Subarachnoid hemorrhage	Intraventricular, intraparnechymal hemorrhage	Late, obstructive	Secondary hemorrhage	Vasospasm, antihypertensive therapy, ventricular drain
Intracranial infection	Abscess, empyema, parasitic cyst	Obstructive, malabsorption	Septic venous thrombosis	Casual therapy, ventricular drain

The Most Frequent Causes of Intracranial Hypertension and Their Therapeutic Options

Edema of the optic nerve head and pupillomotor signs can indicate (or even predict) the early intracranial hypertension, i.e., they may have an alarming role. Timely examinations and the differential diagnostic approaches do not only lead us to adequate medical therapy and a neurosurgical intervention if necessary, but may also prevent the development of potentially life-threatening conditions. Furthermore, we can save our patients from the development of an irreversible loss of vision or bilateral blindness caused by a late diagnosis.

References

Frisén L. Swelling of the optic nerve head: a staging scheme. J Neurol Neurosurg Psychiatry. 1982;45: 13–8.

Kayenbuhl H, Yasargil M. Cerebral angiography Ed. 2. 1968. In: Miller N, Neman N, editors. Walsh & Hoyt's: clinical neuro-ophthalmology, 1956. 2005.

Pasztor E. Operalhato idegsebeszeti betegsegek. 60. Medicina; 1983.

Peter D. Topical diagnosis in neurology. Thieme; 1989.

Rosen ES, et al. Neuroophthalmology. London: Mosby Ltd; 1998.

Weed LH. The absorption of cerebrospinal fluid into the venous system. Am J Anat. 1923; 31: 191–221. Miller N, Neman N. Walsh & Hoyt's: clinical neuro-ophthalmology, 1950. 2005.

Further Readings

Albright A, et al. Occult hydrocephalus in children with cerebral palsy. Neurosurgery. 2005;56(1):93–7.

Brandt T. Vertigo: its multisensory syndromes. London: Springer; 1991. p. 233–77.

Brandt T, et al. Neurological disorders (course and treatment). San Diego: Acad Press; 1996. p. 571–2.

Crassare I, et al. Cerebral venous thrombosis. J Neuroophthalmol. 2004;24(2):156–63.

EwerbackH.Gyermekkorielkülönítődiagnosztika[Pediatric differential diagnostics]. Budapest: Medicina; 1989. p. 181–4 (In Hungarian).

Glaser JS. Neuroophthalmology. Philadelphia: Lippincott; 1990. p. 115–23.

Korányi K. A pangásos papilla jellemzői és differenciáldiagnosztikája [Characteristics and differential diagnoses in congested papilla]. In: Somlai J, editor.

Neuroophthalmologia. Budapest: Literatura Medica; 1996. p. 129–34 (In Hungarian).

Maródi L, et al. Gyermekgyógyászat [Pediatrics]. Budapest: Medicina; 1998. p. 666–9 (In Hungarian).

Miller N, Neman N. Walsh & Hoyt's: clinical neuro-ophthalmology. 1950. p. 2005.

Miller NR, Newman NJ. Papillaoedema. In: Walsh & Hoyts clinical neuro-ophthalmology. VIth ed. Philadelphia: Lippincott; 2005. p. 237–92.

Minns RA, et al. Cerebrospinal fluid pressure in pyogenic meningitis. Arch Dis Child. 1989;64:814–20.

Pásztor E. Operálható idegsebészeti betegségek [Operable neurosurgical diseases], 60. Medicina; 1985 (In Hungarian).

Rabinstein AA. Treatment cerebral edema. Neurology. 2006;12(2):59–73.

Somlai J, Kollár Gy, Szeifert Gy. Gyermekkori papillaoedema differenciál diagnosztikája [Differential diagnostics in pediatric papilloedema]. Gyermekorvos Továbbképző Szemle. 2006; IV (In Hungarian).

Somlai J et al. A koponyaűri nyomásfokozódás figyelmeztető tünetei: jellegzetes szemmozgászavarok és pupillomotoros funkciózavarok [Warning signs in increasing intracranial pressure: characteristic disorders of eye movements and pupillomotor dysfunctions]. Balatonaliga: Magyar Szemorvos Társaság; 2003 (In Hungarian).

Big Blind Spot Syndrome (Papillophlebitis)

51

Gyula Gács and Ildikó Szilvássy

Contents

The presence of papilledema without a decrease in vision is always an alarming sign, especially if bilateral (Table 51.1). A unilaterally papilledema may also be secondary to an early yet asymmetrical intracranial hypertension. However, unilateral papilledema can also occur without intracranial hypertension accompanied by an enlarged bind spot as the only functional abnormality.

This Chapter aims to draw attention to the latter syndrome and to its differential diagnostic significance

G. Gács, M.D., PhD
Budapest City Council Péterfy Sándor Street Hospital and Outpatient Department, Budapest, Hungary
e-mail: gacs.gyula@peterfykh.hu

I. Szilvássy (✉)
Districts 2 and 14 Outpatient Department, Budapest, Hungary
e-mail: gacs.gyula@peterfykh.hu

Case Report

A 33-year-old female patient presented with a history of two episodes of treated bilateral iridocyclitis in the past. Three weeks before admission, uncertain complaints about a spot in the visual field appeared. On examination, vision was 1.0 OU, the visual field was complete OD with objects I/4 and I/2, a 20° blind spot was detectable with I/2, no scotoma was indicated. The visual field was complete OS with object I/4 and I/2, the size of the blind spot was normal, no scotoma was indicated. CFF: 42 Hz OU. Fundoscopy revealed a hyperemic swollen optic disc OD with blurred margins, congested veins and striate peripapillary hemorrhages of different size (Fig. 51.1a). No abnormality was detected on neurological, internal medicine and laboratory examinations. The papilledema OD gradually decreased on parabulbar steroid therapy, completely disappearing after 2 months (Fig. 51.1b). Pathological alteration

Table 51.1 Visuscsökkenés nélküli papilladuzzanatok

I. Bilateral
Papilledema due to intracranial hypertension
II. Unilateral
1. Early yet asymmetrical papilledema due to intracranial hypertension
2. Unilateral papilledema without intracranial hypertension, with the only functional impairment being the enlarged blind spot

J. Somlai, T. Kovács (eds.), *Neuro-Ophthalmology*, DOI 10.1007/978-3-319-28956-4_51

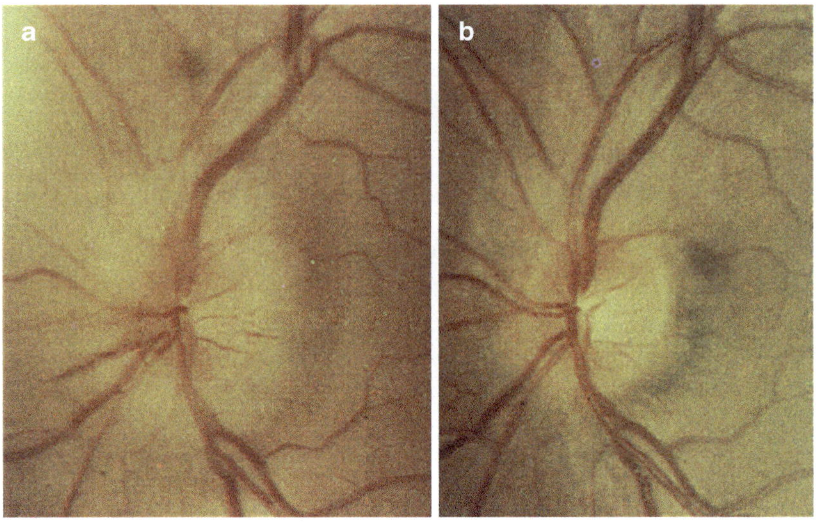

Fig. 51.1 Fundoscopic image of the right eye of a 33-year-old female patient. (**a**) On admission, the optic disc had blurred margins and a hyperemic and edematous appearance, together with congested veins and a few peripapillary striate hemorrhages. (**b**) Two month later, following local steroid therapy, the optic disc on the right side was flat, it showed sharp margins and normal color, the hemorrhages were reabsorbed and the venous congestion ceased

could not be detected by fundoscopy OS either in the first or subsequent examinations. Since then, until the publication of the current edition, seven additional patients with similar presentation and disease course have been examined and treated by our group. The most important data of the 8 cases are summarized in Table 51.2. The above data well demonstrate the characteristics of 'blind spot enlargement syndrome'.

Discussion

The disease was first drawn attention to by Lyle and Wybar in 1961 (LyleTk 1961) in relation to 7 cases. Since then different authors have called this condition various terms: retinal vasculitis (LyleTk 1961), papillophlebitis (Lonn and Hoyt 1966; Ellenberger and Messner 1978) benign retinal vasculitis (Hart et al. 1971), 'optic disc vasculitis' (Hayreh 1972) big blind spot syndrome (Miller 1977).

The currently widely applied term (Acute Idiopathic Blind Spot Enlargement Syndrome, AIBSE) is based on the most appropriate early nomenclature used by Miller (1977). The fundoscopic appearance of blind spot enlargement syndrome undoubtedly suggests a venous circulatory disorder, which is most probably caused by an underlying autoimmune mechanism.

The presence of autoimmune diseases in the past medical history of some of our patients is of note (i.e., recurrent bilateral iridocyclitis, thrombocytopenia recovering with steroid therapy, hay fever). It should be pointed out, however, that a similar syndrome can occur, though rather infrequently, in association with a well-defined underlying disease. Such conditions include papilledema without decreased vision in juvenile diabetes, but unilateral papilledema without a deterioration of vision has also been described in severe iron deficiency anemia as well as in anemia perniciosa. These conditions are more probably due to a local vascular abnormality than to a direct inflammation.

Since the first edition of this book section, our group identified among similar cases two patients that presented with an upper quadrant defect involving the blind spot in addition to its enlargement. These two patients underwent complete recovery as well, and their visual field defect disappeared without any residual optic disc pallor (Rózsa et al. (In press) (Table 51.3).

The latter cases raise the question whether the blind spot enlargement syndrome represents the mildest manifestation of venous circulatory disorders of the retina, which would be followed in the order of severity by the 'blind spot enlargement syndrome' associated with visual field defect, the partial central retinal vein occlusion, and finally

Table 51.2 The most important characteristics of our patients

Age, Gend	Vision	CFF	Field of	Subjective complaints	Fundoscopy	Status		Laboratory abnormalities	Past medical history	Disease course
	on the affected side					Neurol.	Internal			
33, F	1.0	42Hz	Normal, 20° blind spot OD	Spot in the visual field OD	Typical papilledema OD (Fig. 51.1a) intact OS	NAD	NAD	–	Recurrent iridocyclitis OU	Local steroid Complete recovery ofter 2 months (Fig. 51.1b)
21, F	1.0	45Hz	Normal, 20° blind spot OD	Blurred vision OD	Papilledema OD Intact OS	NAD	NAD	–	NAD	Local steroid Complete recovery ofter 2 months
18, F	1.0	42Hz	Normal, 20° blind spot OS	Headache, spot in the visual field OS	Intact OD, papilledema OS (Fig. 51.2a, b)	NAD	NAD	-	Thrombocytopenia recovered with steroid therapy 10 years ago	Spontaneous recovery within 3 months (Fig. 51.2c)
47, M	1.0	42Hz	Normal, 20° blind spot OD	Spot in the visual field OD	Papilledema OD (Fig. 51.3a), l.s. intact	NAD	NAD	Immunoelectrophoresis Elevated IgA, IgM	Hay fever, mild hypertonia	Local steroid Complete recovery ofter 2 months (Fig. 51.3b)
42, F	1.0	38Hz	Normal, 10–20° blind spot OD	A few-day history of spot in the visual field OD	Papilledema OD (Fig. 51.4a), intact OS	NAD	NAD	–	NAD	Systemic and local steroid Recovery after 6 weeks (Fig. 51.4b)
46, M	1.0	42Hz	upper quadrant defect involving the blind spot OD (Fig. 51.5a–b)	Spot in the visual field OD	Papilledema OD (Fig. 51.6a), intact OS	NAD	NAD	Mild hypertension	Neg.	Spontaneous recovery within 6 months (Figs. 51.5c, 51.6b)
23, M	1.0	40Hz	Normal, enlarged blind spot OD	Spot in the visual field OD	Papilledema OD, intact OS	NAD	NAD	NAD	NAD	Local steroid Recoverey after 7 weeks
36, M	1.0	42Hz	upper quadrant defect involving the blind spot OD	Spot in the visual field OD	Papilledema OD, intact OS	NAD	NAD	NAD	NAD	Oral steroid Recovery after 6 months

CFF critical fusion frequency, *F* female, *M* male, *OD* in the right eye, *OS* in the left eye, *OU* in both eyes, *NAD* no abnormality detected

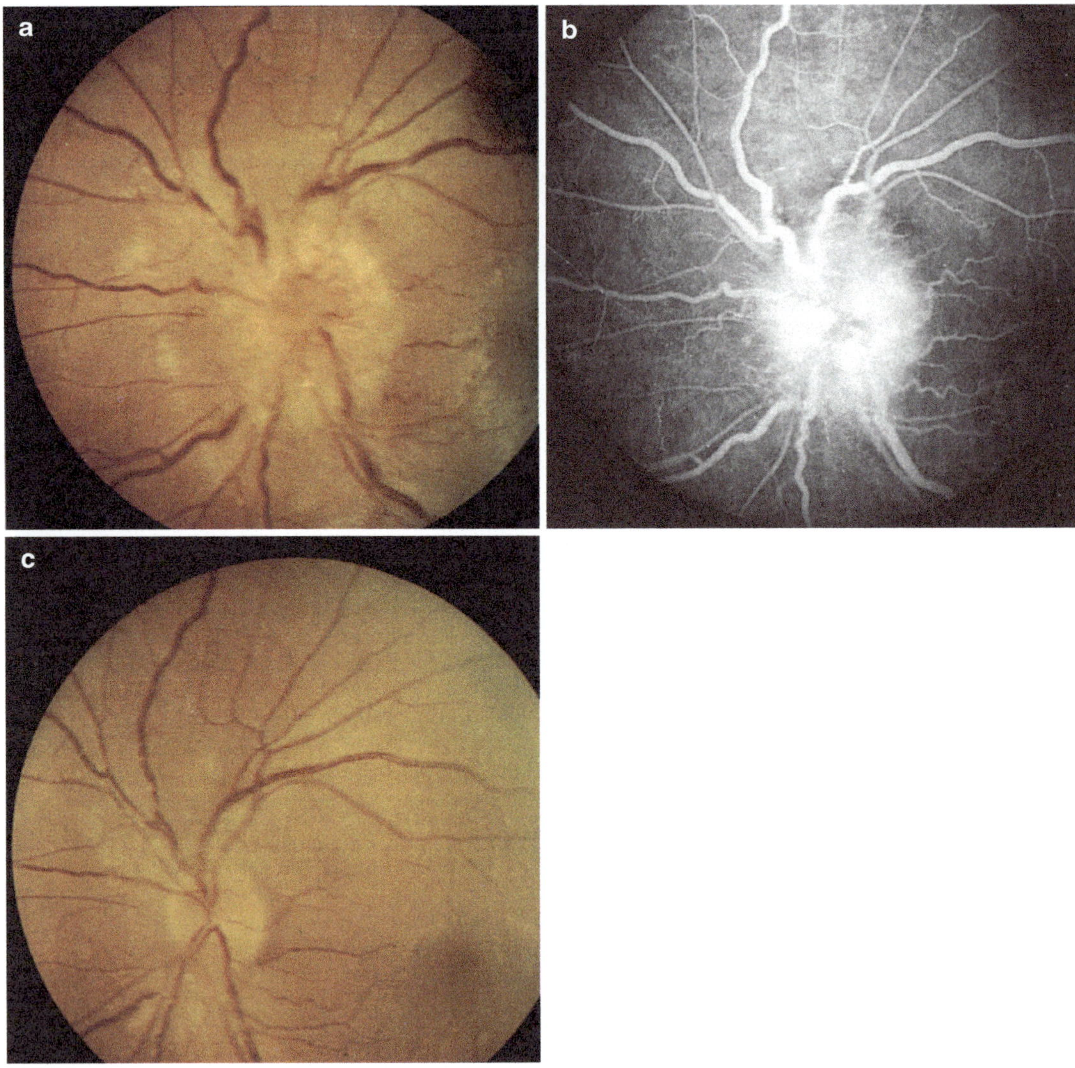

Fig. 51.2 18-year-old female patient. (**a**) On admission, typical papilledema could be observed OS with congested tortuous veins and several dilated peripapillary capillaries and a scattered appearence of peripapillary intraretinal hemorrhages. (**b**) Fluorescein angiogram OS. Papilledema is characterised by hyperfluorescence, peripapillary leakage of the dye and dilated veins. (**c**) The left-sided optic disc 2 months later. The swelling of the disc and the pathological congestion of the veins spontaneously disappeared and the hemorrhages got spontaneously absorbed

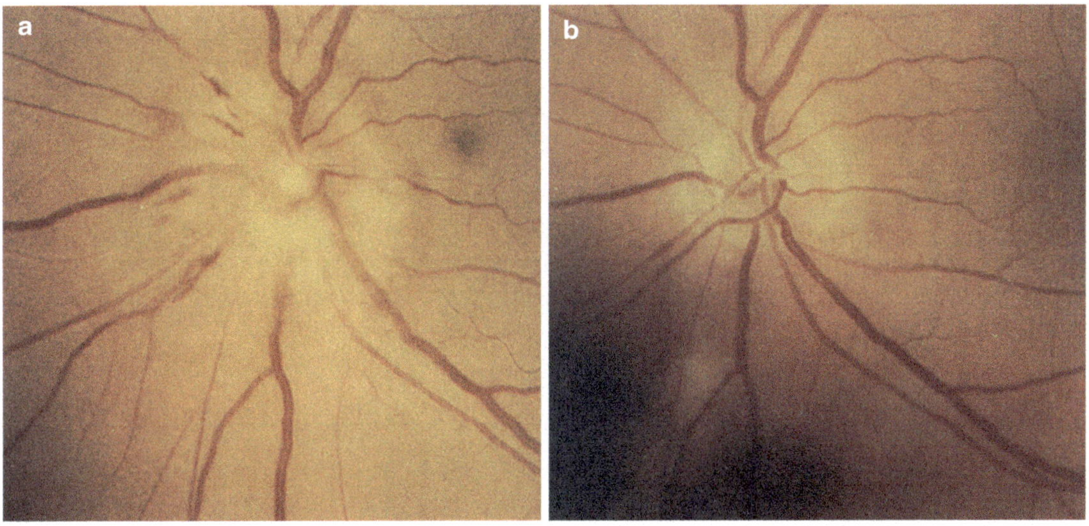

Fig. 51.3 47-year-old male patient. (**a**) The optic disc has blurred margins OD, it is significantly edematous and prominent, the blood vessels are embedded in the edema, and a number of striate hemorrhages can be noticed. (**b**) Complete recovery of the optic head after 6 weeks following steroid therapy

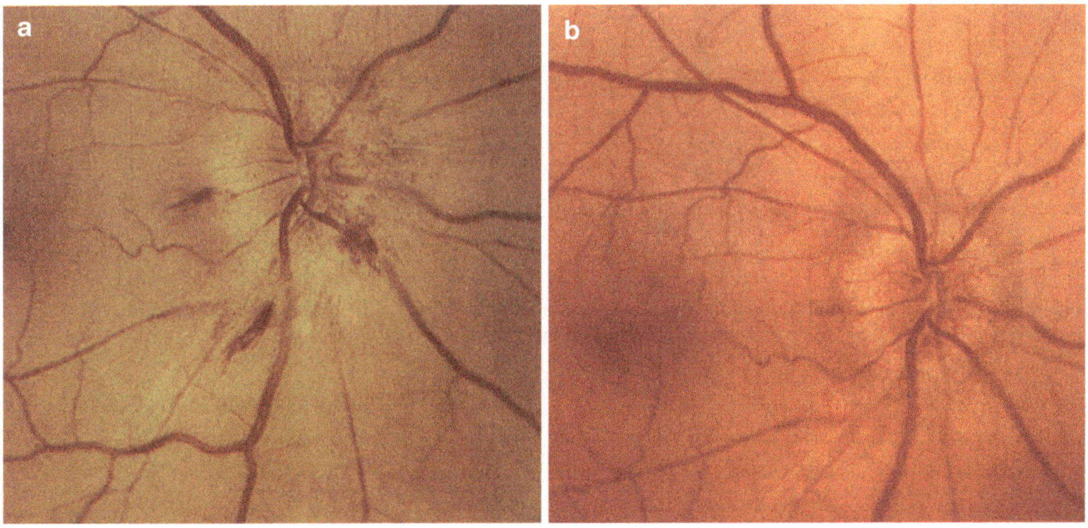

Fig. 51.4 42-year-old female patient. (**a**) Papilledema OD with several peripapillary hemorrhages and pronounced swelling (**b**) After 4 weeks on local steroid therapy, the swelling of the optic head OD dramatically decreased, the hemorrhages are reabsorbed, hyperemia is present due to the still dilated capillaries

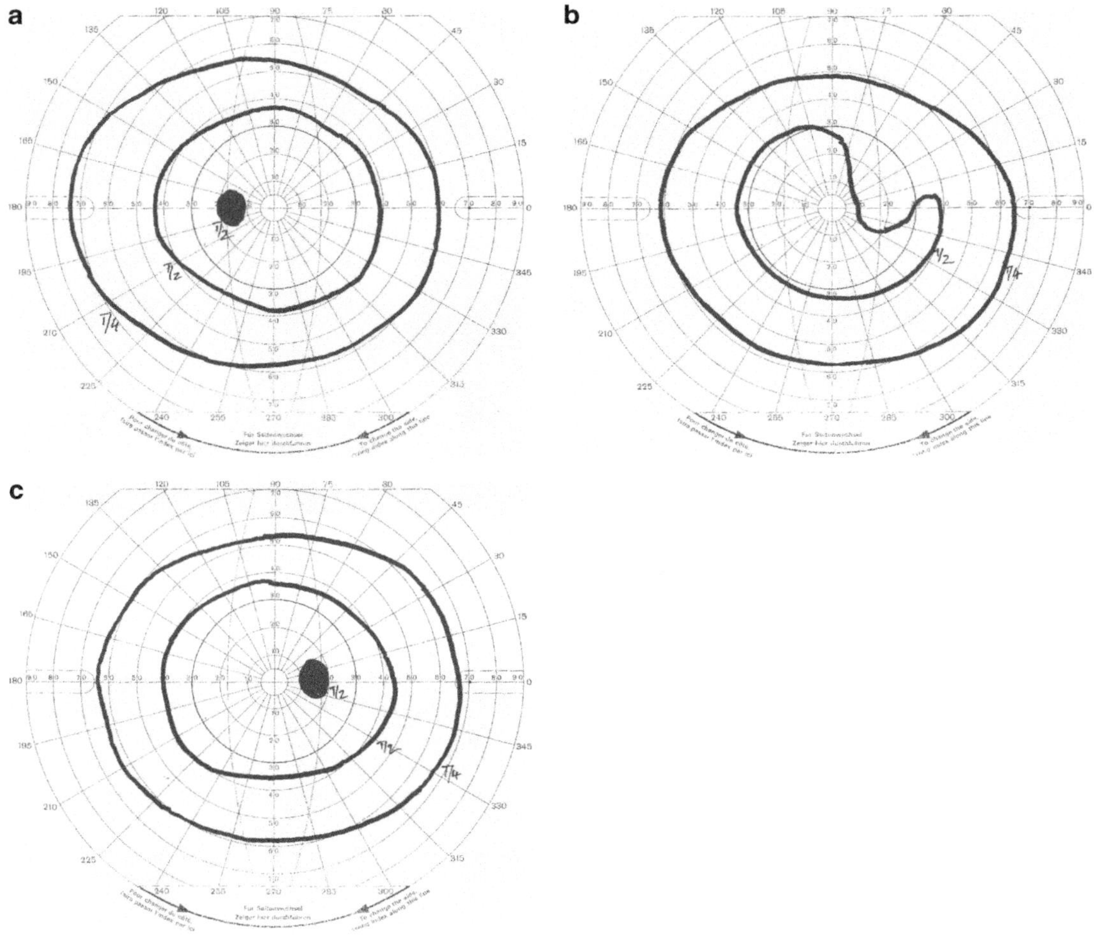

Fig. 51.5 (**a**) 46-year-old male patient, complete visual field OS (**b**) enlarged blind spot associated with an upper quadrant defect OD. (**c**) The visual field is complete after 6 months in OD as well

the complete central retinal vein occlusion accompanied by a severe deterioration of vision. The identification of further transient cases might help clarifying this issue. The question whether bilateral blind spot enlargement syndrome exists is currently impossible to answer; however, its possibility cannot be excluded. Considering the case with bilateral 'papillophlebitis' in a patient suffering from severe coagulopathies described by Savir et al. (1977) as such a condition is at least questionable. Nevertheless, it is highly likely that a proportion of idiopathic benign intracranial hypertension syndromes are in fact manifestations of bilateral blind spot enlargement syndrome. This may be an explanation for the existence of patients with pseudotumor cerebri (benign intracranial hypertension) who have no complaints indicative of intracranial hypertension and the CSF pressure is not significantly elevated either. If this conclusion could be objectively confirmed in some way, we could distinguish between three forms of papilledema associated with intact visual acuity:

1. Papilledema due to intracranial space-occupying processes
2. Papilledema due to other causes of intracranial hypertension (sinus thrombosis, vitamin A overdose, lead intoxication, etc.).
3. Optic disc abnormality presenting with all features of papilledema (fundoscopic appearance, enlarged blind spot, intact vision, normal CFF and FLAG findings) in the absence of intracranial hypertension (blind spot enlargement syndrome)

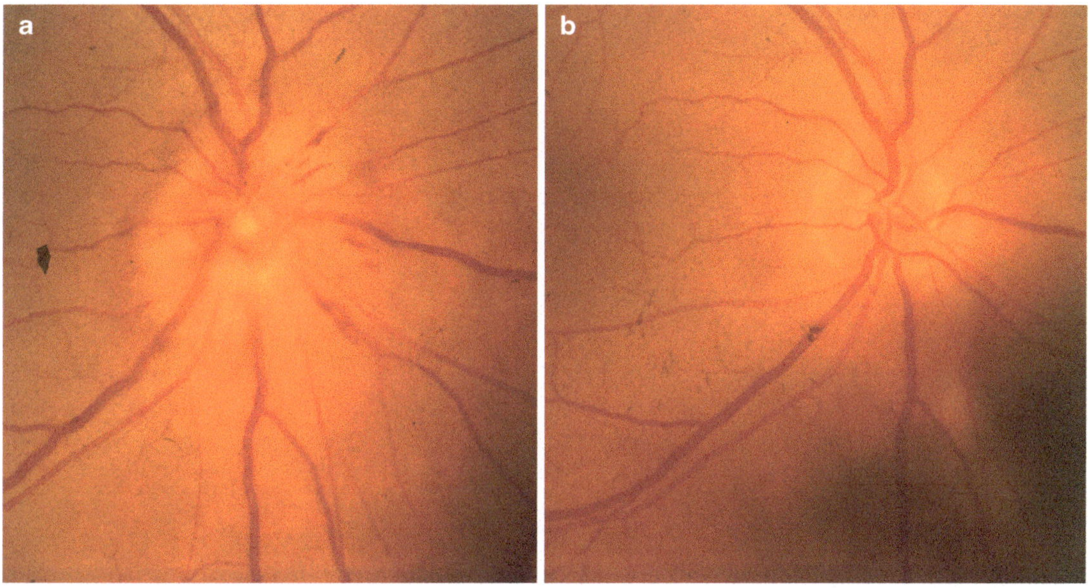

Fig. 51.6 (**a**) 46-year-old male patient. One diopter of papilledema, peripapillary striate hemorrhages. Mild venous congestion. (**b**) Flat optic disc with sharp margins, normal color and normal venous congestion

Table 51.3 Characteristics of blind spot enlargement syndrome

Mostly young adults, more frequently female individuals are affected
Unilateral papilledema with pronounced venous congestion and the peripapillary appearance of striate (flame-shaped) hemorrhages of different size
Good optic nerve functions except for the enlarged blind spot
No abnormality detected on neurological and internal medicine examinations
Benign course: spontaneous recovery in a few months, probably accelerated by steroid therapy, with no residual pallor
Certain cases can be accompanied by a visual field defect larger than the blind spot that is also associated with complete recovery

Summary

Though the etiology of blind spot enlargement syndrome is not yet clarified (also referred to as acute idiopathic blind spot enlargement syndrome, AIBSE), we should consider the possibility of this disease in the event of a unilateral (or possibly bilateral) papilledema not associated with a deterioration of vision in otherwise healthy young adults, in case other causes can be excluded.

References

Ellenberger C, Messner KH. Papillophlebitis: benign retinopathy resembling papillaedema or papillitis. Ann Neurol. 1978;3:438–40.

Hart CD, Sanders MD, Miller SIH. Benign retinal vasculitis. Br J Ophthalmol. 1971;55:721–33.

Hayreh SS. Optic disc vasculitis. Br J Ophthalmol. 1972;56:652–70.

Lonn LI, Hoyt WT. Papillophlebitis. A cause of protracted yet benign optic disc edema. Eye Ear Nose Throat Mon. 1966;45:62–8.

LyleTk WK. Retinal vasculitis. Br J Ophthalmol. 1961;45:778–88.

Miller NR. The big blind spot syndrome: unilateral optic disc edema without visual loss or increased intracranial pressure. In: Smith IL, editor. Neuro ophthalmology update. New York: Masson; 1977. p. 163–9.

Rózsa A, Kovács K, Boór K, Vagyóczky Á, Szilvássy I, Gács Gy. Nagy vakfolt szindróma szokatlan látótérkieséssel. [Blind spot enlargement syndrome with unusual visual field defect] Ideggy Szemle. In press. (In Hungarian)

Savir H, Wender T, Creter D, DjaldettiM SR. Bilateral retinal vasculitis associated with clotting disorder. Am J Ophthalmol. 1977;84:542–7.

Part V

Neuro-Ophthalmologic Aspects of the Ocular Motor System

The Most Important Disorders of the Pupillomotor Pathway in the Clinical Practice

52

Judit Somlai

Contents

Diagnostic Opportunities of the Neurological Examination

The proper evaluation of the functions of the pupillomotor pathway, like that of the external components of the oculomotor system, is an instrumental part of the examination of the cranial nerves. Either with a direct ophthalmoscope or the strong and focused beam of an indirect ophthalmoscope or even with a simple pocket pupil lamp, the physician can test the pupil reflexes. It is recommended that the tests be performed in a dimly lit or dark examination room. Regarding the most important tests the reader is referred to Chap. 23.

In the clinical practice the following parameters and findings should be evaluated and registered in the management of both inpatients and the out-patients:

- Registration of the difference between the palpebral fissures, the description of the real and virtual ptosis.
- Evaluation and recording of the direct and indirect pupil reactions
- Test of convergence and accommodation upon provocation. Estimation of pupillomotor functions upon fixation on close objects
- In order to increase visual acuity, the synkinesis of three components (convergence, accommodation and pupil constriction) should be observed. The afore-mentioned accommodation triad is examined by asking the patient to focus on the near point, while the physician observes the process of convergence, the consensual constriction of the pupils and estimates the visual acuity.
- The additional eye-drop tests for localization purposes are described on pages …

J. Somlai, M.D.
Unit of Neuro-Ophthalmology, Department of Neurology & Stroke, Military Hospital, Budapest, Hungary

Neuro-Ophthalmology Section, Hungarian Ophthalmological Association, Budapest, Hungary

Trustee, NOSZA Foundation (for the Prevention and Screening of Ocular Storke), Budapest, Hungary
e-mail: dr@somlaijudit.hu; http://somlaijudit.hu

J. Somlai, T. Kovács (eds.), *Neuro-Ophthalmology*, DOI 10.1007/978-3-319-28956-4_52

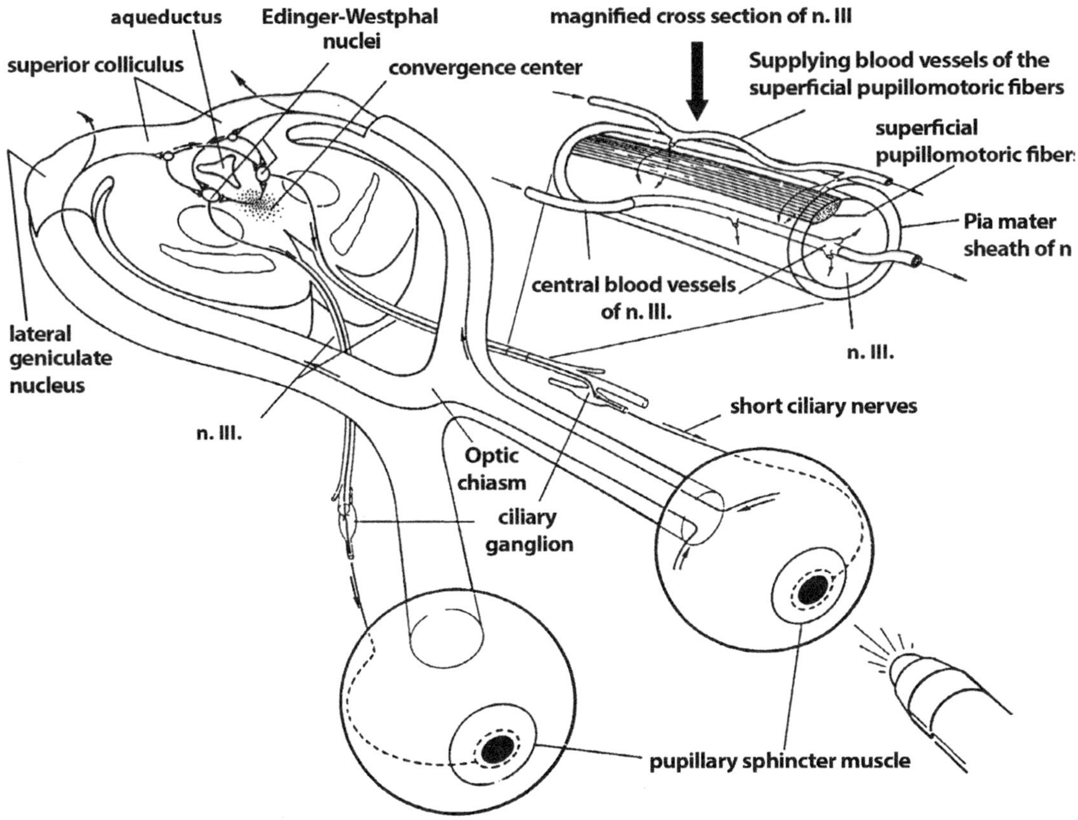

Fig. 52.1 The afferent and efferent routes of the parasympathetic pupillomotor pathway. In the upper-right quadrant of the Figure: magnification of a section the oculomotor nerve emphasizing the external therefore, more vulnerable pupillomotor fibers. *(Redrawn after Peter Duus: Topical Diagnosis in Neurology, Thieme 1989, Springer 1999.)*

Disorders of the Parasympathetic Pupillomotor Pathway

Group of Symptoms

- Anisocoria
- The characteristics of the amaurotic pupil
- The Marcus-Gunn, or "swinging flash-light" pupillary sign.
- The "light-near dissociation" sign.
- The Argyll-Robertson syndrome
- The differential diagnostic significance of the unilaterally fixed and dilated pupil.
- The Adie's tonic pupil

Anisocoria

In neurological disorders, the examination of the pupillomotor pathway is most frequently requested upon the observation of an abrupt onset of **anisocoria**. It means unilateral wider pupil, which does not respond to light. It is worth checking previous photos, certain asymmetries of the face and the eyes themselves to exclude inborn conditions. The local strictly ophthalmological causes have to be excluded (Fig. 52.1).

Features Upon straight gaze the pupil is wider of at least 2–3 mm on the affected side, its direct and indirect reaction are protracted, but the responses of extraocular optic muscles innervated by the oculomotor nerve are completely spared and retained. The absolute pupillary sign is the most severe form of the above symptom: neither the direct nor the indirect pupillary response can be evoked. See for details the chapter on *"The syndrome of unilateral fixed and dilated pupil"*.

Diagnosis Undiluted Pilocarpin test, Cocaine test, Paredrin eye-drop test, Epinephrine test. For more details the reader is referred to Chap. 23. A pathologically wider pupil, usually sign of the paresis of oculomotor nerve with retained optic nerve functions. A pathologically narrower pupil generally refers to the decreased activity of the dilator muscle innervated by the sympathetic pathway system and usually represents a component of the *Horner's syndrome* accompanied by slight ptosis.

The Characteristics of the Amaurotic Pupil

The **amaurotic pupil** represents the clinical pupillary symptoms of amaurosis, that is means no light perception on affected side, caused by complete lesion of antechiasmal optic nerve. Simultaneously happens the afferent pupillomotoric nerve complete lesion

Features The blind eye does not show direct pupil reactions since the affected pupillomotor fibers do not transmit stimuli. In the clinical practice the trauma of the skull base leads to such destruction of antechiasmal optic nerve fibers with the afferent pupillomotor pathway.

- Indirect response cannot be detected on the intact side since the amaurotic side does not convey information, which would evoke the contralateral reaction.
- Obviously the spared eye shows direct response and the affected eye indirect response since the intact afferent pupillomotor fibers evokes the indirect reaction.
- Anisocoria does not develop on the affected side since the indirect reaction keeps the affected pupil in contraction Severe lesion of the afferent pupillomotor pathway can develop due to the trauma of the optic nerve or the embolism of the main supplying arteries of the retina and the optic disc. Although it is painless, it usually goes with complete blindness.

The Marcus-Gunn or Relative Afferent Pupillary Defect (RAPD) Sign

The Marcus–Gunn (MG) or relatív afferent pupillary defect (RAPD) sign as "swinging flash-light" pupillary sign is one of the most important harbinger of the injury of the afferent pupillomotor pathway. In practice it serves as a semi-quantitative tool to assess the impairment of the conduction of the antechiasmal optic nerve of the visual pathway mainly at the bedside in the case of disorders of consciousness.

Features Upon examination of ***the Marcus-Gunn sign or RAPD sign***, the physician alternately covers the eyes observing the physiological pupil response.

Rapid alternations lead to a pathological re-dilation in the affected eye. Since, due to impaired innervation, the pupil cannot be kept completely constricted. The stages from the mildest to the most severe are: from 1+ to 4+. In stage 4+ the pupil cannot be constricted at all, it represents the complete loss of the direct pupil response, which is consistent with the amaurotic pupil. This is the most characteristic pathological response caused by the lesion of the afferent pupillomotor pathway. The swinging flash-light pupillary sign virtually represents the same examination but the test relies on the alternated illumination of the eyes.

Diagnosis Evoking of the direct and indirect pupil reactions with pupil lamp. For more details the reader is referred to Chap. 23. Since the afferent pupillomotor pathway runs together with the antechiasmal visual pathway, they often show simultaneous impairment in the most different pathological conditions of the optic nerve. Therefore, the dysfunction of the pupillomotor system represents as a very sensitive predictor of any diseases of the antechiasmal optic nerve.

The Tectal or "Light-Near Dissociation" Pupillary Sign

In the case of the "**light-near dissociation**" pupillary sign, the pupil reactions to light differ upon fixation on distant objects or evoking convergence. This pupillary sign is most frequently the consequence of the impairment of those upper brainstem regions, which control both the pupillomotor functions and the eye movements.

Characteristics The direct and indirect pupil reactions are considerably limited or cannot be triggered, while upon convergence the pupil constrict so the consensual pupil reaction remains intact. The visual functions are usually preserved. The most important cause of the disease is decompensated diabetes mellitus (tabes diabetica). The most important differential diagnostic question in this case whether this pupillary sign is isolated or accompanied by other eye movement disorders. If this sign is combined with eye movement disorders, the syndrome is referred to "rostral mesencephalon syndrome" as it is elicited by a dysfunction of the mesencephalon and the neighbouring neural structures. In the background, usually pinealoma or a tumour of the third ventricle can be found in the clinical practice. Upon progression of midline tumors, the severe general condition of the patient is accompanied by wide and fixed pupils. The tectal pupils are also characterized by vertical gaze weakness, then upward gaze palsy, retraction of the eyelids *(Collier-sign)*, nystagmus retractorius, and rarely upon upward gaze tonic or clonic convergence. It is the most frequent brainstem eye movement disorder, which can be accompanied by the skew deviation, which ocular movement disorder causes vertical and asymmetrical shift of the image seen by the patient. For more details the reader is referred to Chap. 3.2.5.

Argyll-Robertson-Pupillary Sign

The **Argyll-Robertson pupillary sign** is characterized by fairly intact visual acuity and small, irregularly dilating pupils on one or both sides.

Characteristics The direct and indirect pupil reactions are lost. The pupil dilates with difficulty even upon administering eye-drops. However, upon convergence, a proper reaction can be seen like in the case of the tectal pupillary sign. Once it was seen most frequently as the consequence of neurosyphilis. The lesion is presumably located around the cerebral aqueduct (Sylvii) and ruins the afferent pathways of the Edinger-Westphal nucleus, while the nucleus itself and the efferent pathways remain intact. Atypical the Argyll- Robertson pupillary sign can develop due diabetes mellitus, alcoholism, multiple sclerosis, tumors of the mesencephalon and encephalitides. ***PseudoArgyll-Robertson pupillary sign*** is related to the abnormal regeneration process of the oculomotor nerve (n III.). On the affected side the pupil does not show direct reaction but constricts upon convergence.

The Unilateral Fixed – Dilated Pupil (Ophthalmoplegia Interna: "Hutchinson's Pupillary Sign")

The **unilateral fixed dilated pupil** or **anisocoria** is the most important alarming neuro-ophthalmologic sign, which can be caused by:

- increased intracranial pressure (uncus herniation)
- aneurysm (abrupt dilation or rupture which may lead to the compression of the oculomotorius nerve).
- due to the pathological regeneration of the oculomotor nerve
- Adie's tonic pupil reaction

It is characterized by *the loss of both the direct and indirect pupil reactions on the affected side.* It is very important to consider the anatomical characteristics of the oculomotor nerve, that is the pupillomotor fibers run superficially in the nerve, therefore, any sort of compression always impairs first the pupillomotor functions, and only later and more pronounced lesions can results in the dysfunction of the extraocular muscles. That is why in the clinical practice, the observation of oculomotor palsy without pupillary sign is regarded as a far less ominous sign as the anisocoria. For more details the reader is referred to Chap. 54).

Differential diagnosis 2 % Pilocarpin eye-drop test. For more details the reader is referred to Chap. 23.

The Unilateral Fixed – Dilated Pupil Sign Can Occur in the Following Syndromes

- Midriatic ***eye-drop*** or the injuries of the central parasympathetic pathway.
- Hutchinson's pupil is characteristically a unilateral, dilated and fixed pupil which is usually the consequence of tentorial herniation due subdural hematoma. The supratentorial space occupying process leads to the herniation of the uncus of the hippocampal gyrus and the direct compression of the oculomotor nerve. However, the paresis of the internal oculomotor nerve is only the initial symptom of the "***clivus edge***

syndrome". When complete plegia develops, it is usually accompanied by cardio-respiratory depression, pyramidal signs and disorder of consciousness. Then it harbingers the end-stage of the increased intracranial pressure elicited condition. Tumors of the temporal lobe cause unilateral, dilated pupil not only due to the increased intracranial pressure but also the direct pressure exerted on the nerve itself.

- One of the symptoms of the ***pathological regeneration of the oculomotor nerve*** is the unilaterally fixed and dilated pupil. In adults it is usually caused by the aneurysm of the internal carotid artery or the posterior communicating artery or slowly progressing meningeoma. Besides the pupillary sign, further symptoms and signs of the pathological regeneration process of the oculomotor nerve: the *pseudoGraefe's sign;* upon downward gaze the patient produces Graefe's sign. The symptom is related to the pathological re-innervation process when the regenerating oculomotor fibers predominantly and mistakenly targeted the levator palpebrae superioris muscle instead of the pupillary sphincter muscle. Upon vertical gaze, the *dyskinesis* develops due to the fact that the pathologically innervated levator muscle is activated together with those muscles, such as the medial rectus, which normally carry out the adduction, therefore, the palpebral fissure will be wider. The pathological retraction of the eyelids and, at the same time, the pathological adduction of the eyeballs also result from the defective reinnervation. Upon upward gaze, due to the pathological regeneration the medial, the inferior and the superior rectus muscles are activated simultaneously. Therefore, besides upward gaze, the retraction toward the retro-orbital space will develop (nystagmus retractorius)

Adie's Tonic Pupil

Adie's tonic pupil is characterized by unilateral and fixed pupil, which is most frequently observed in female patients of 20–30 years. Presumably it is related to the disorder of the ciliary ganglion due to inflammatory or traumatic reasons, although neither theory is confirmed.

Features Both the direct and indirect pupil reactions are slow and tonic, or even they cannot be evoked at all. Upon seeing the close point (e.g., the tip of a pen), the patient's pupil slightly constricts, then upon fixing the far point the pupil again shows the slow and tonic redilation. Repeating the same examination, under the magnification of a slit-lamp, the irregular fine movements of the edges of the pupils can be seen.

Diagnosis Diluted pilocarpine test. Positivity reflects hypersensitivity to cholinergic agents, as *ten times diluted, 0.1 %, Pilocarpin* does not elicit reaction in physiological circumstances, while the Adie's pupil usually constricts. It has differential diagnostic value: if undiluted 1 % pilocarpine also evokes constriction the condition refers to the paresis of the oculomotor nerve.

According to our clinical observations, administration of ten times diluted, 0.1 % Humacarpin to the affected eye, 2–3 times daily for months will result in a sort of pharmaceutical training. Consequently either the anomaly completely disappears or the accommodation problem, which interfered with both near and far vision, considerably decreases. Obviously, this goes specifically for Adie's pupillomotor disease, but often such treatment proved effective in residual pupil anomalies due to the injuries of the oculomotor nerve related to polytraumas.

Disorders of the Sympathetic Pathway

When the pupillomotor fibers of the sympathetic pathway get injured at any level of the system, Horner's syndrome develops, which is characterized by *three symptoms, therefore, it is Horner's triad.* The subdivision of the sympathetic pathway system into three neuronal sections is essential due to localization purposes.

The most important function of these sympathetic fibers and the consequences of their injuries. Innervation of *several ocular muscles*: **Horner's syndrome**

- The *superior tarsal muscle,* which elevates the upper eyelid.
  Its dysfunction leads to moderate **ptosis**.

- The *orbitalis muscle of Müller.* It maintains the proper orbital tone of the eyeball.
  Its dysfunction leads to depression of the eyeball, i.e., **enophthalmos**.
- The *dilator muscle of the pupil,* which dilates the pupil.
  Its injuries lead to very narrow pupil, i.e., **myosis**

Since these fibers also provide *vasomotor functions* constricting the blood vessels of the **conjunctiva, hyperemia** develops on the affected side in the case of their dysfunction.

Their injuries also impair the *sudomotor functions* leading to **ipsilateral anhidrosis** in the affected side.

A draft of the parasympathetic and the "three-neuron" sympathetic innervation of the internal ocular muscles (this figure can be found in the chapter of the diagnostics of the pupils (Chap. 23).

The 1st neuron. The first part of the central or preganglionar section

The central neuron starts from the posterior-lateral region of the hypothalamus and projects through the reticular formation downward to the C8-Th2 segments of the spinal cord. Then it synapses in the *ciliospinal or Budge's centre.*

The 2nd neuron. The second part of the central or preganglionar section.

It represents the pathway between the *ciliospinal center and the paravertebral superior cervical ganglion.* The fibers of the ciliospinal center reside in the lateral horn of the gray matter, leave the spinal cord through the anterior fascicle, go upwards via the rami communicates in the sympathetic chain and connect to the neurons of the superior cervical ganglion. Here the sympathetic chain gets to close proximity of the pleura of the apex of the lungs, and the fibers also circumvent the subclavian artery.

The 3rd neuron. The peripheral or postganglionar section.

This section establishes connection between *the superior cervical ganglion and the intraorbital ciliary ganglion.* The fibers leaving the superior cervical ganglion follow the internal carotid artery and enter again the skull. In this second intracranial section, they get to the orbit through the cavernous sinus. In the orbital cavity, the fibers form the sympathetic root of the ciliary ganglion. Here these peripheral sympathetic fibers do not make further synapses but directly project to the eyeball.

Diagnostics (for more details the reader is referred to Chap. 23) Eye drop test with 4 % cocaine

- 0.1 %, i.e., diluted epinephrine test.
- 0.1 % i.e., diluted hydroxyamphetamine (Paredrin) test

The Most Frequent Causes of Horner's Syndrome (Fig. 52.1)

1. *Injuries of the 1st section of the sympathetic pathway*
   - Extended cerebral infarction of a given hemisphere.
   - The symptoms of brainstem cerebrovascular disorders, multiple sclerosis, encephalitis, Wallenberg's syndrome, pontine tumors and hemorrhages are the followings: Ipsilateral Horner's sign and contralateral hypalgesia and caloric hypesthesia.
   - Cervical spinal cord processes, such as syringomyelia, hematomyelia, multiple sclerosis, tumors (ependymoma, glioma)
   - They feature the following symptoms and signs: Horner's syndrome on both sides and loss of reflexes and analgesia of both upper extremities.
2. *Injuries of the 2nd section of the sympathetic pathway are usually caused by:*
   - Lesions of the Th1 segment due to injuries of the proximal part of the cervical ribs, aneurysm of the subclavian artery or the internal carotid artery or the compression exerted by mediastinal lymphatic nodes or tumors.
   - Pancoast's syndrome related to the cancer of the apex of the lung. Beside the pupillary sign blood and lymphatic fluid circulatory problems will develop in the arm, which is later accompanied by paralysis of the brachial plexus.
   - The lesions of the sympathetic chain results usually from the tumors of the thyroid

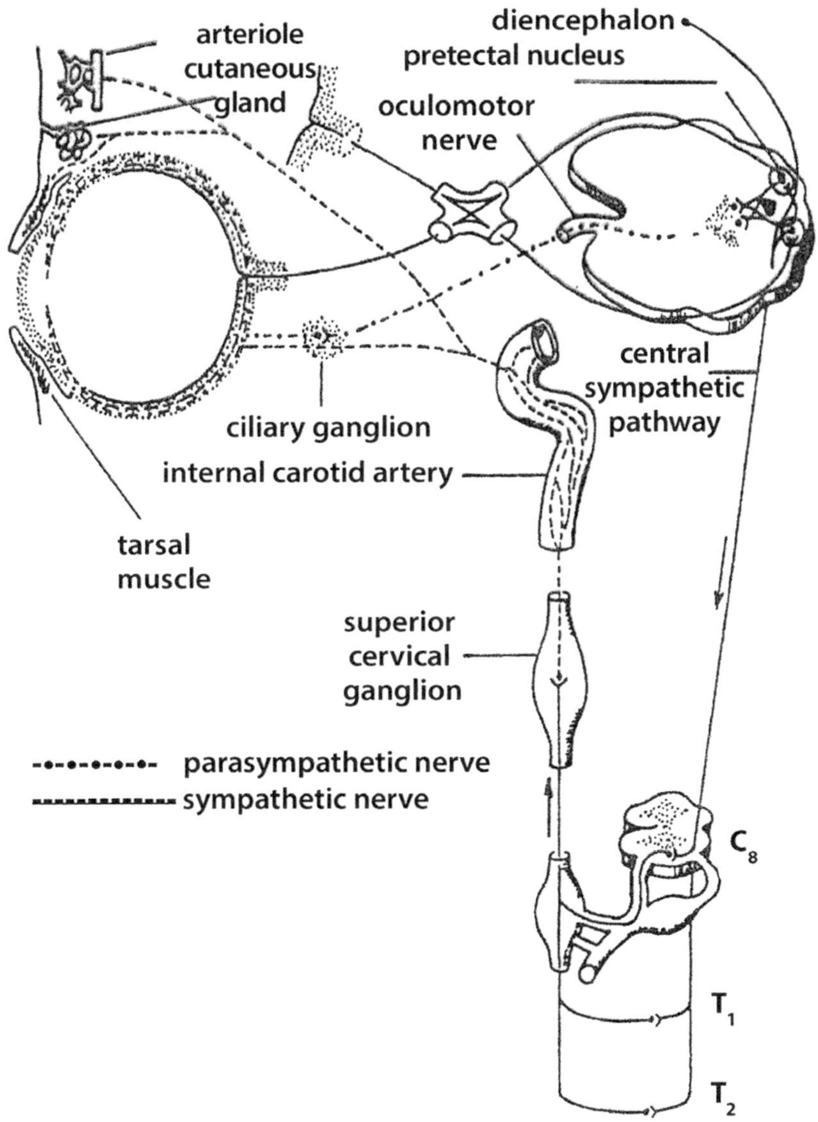

Fig. 52.2 A draft of the parasympathetic and the "three-neuron" sympathetic innervation of the internal ocular muscles (this figure can be found in the chapter of the diagnostics of the pupils *(Redrawn after Peter Duus: Topical Diagnosis in Neurology, Thieme 1989, Springer 1999.)*

gland, complications of the surgical interventions performed on the thyroid gland, cervical sympathectomy, puncture of the jugular vein or the carotid artery.

3. *Injuries of the 3rd section of the sympathetic pathway are usually caused by:*

In the extracranial, cervical region if the past history does not reveal earlier traumas or surgical interventions, the most frequent reason of the Horner's syndrome is usually a malignant process. Namely, compression exerted by cervical lymphatic nodes, nasopharyngeal carcinomas, esophageal tumors, goiter, paranasal-sphenoidal sinusitis, herpes zoster of the trigeminal nerve, purulent otitis media.

In the intracranial-intracavernous region the diseases of the cavernous sinus, namely, the superior orbital fissure syndrome, when the both the sympathetic and the parasympathetic fibers are afflicted, therefore, the size of the pupil is normal. Besides, it can be the complication of basilar skull fractures, parasellar processes propagating into the orbit, neurosurgical interventions on the Gasser's ganglion or Raeder's paratrigeminal syndrome mostly due to migraine or stroke (see Chap. 65 from page 374).

The Most Important Pupillary Signs in Coma

Regarding the eye movement disorders of the comatose patient the reader is referred to page 304 in Chapter, which deals with the disturbances of eye movement disorders of brainstem origin.

References

Arruga J, et al. Chronic isolated trochlear nerve palsy produced by intracavernous internal carotid artery aneurysm. J Clin Neuroophthalmol. 1991;11(2):104–8.

Baker RS, et al. Vertical ocular motility disturbance in pseudotumor cerebri. J Clin Neuroophthalmol. 1985;5:41–4.

Borchert MS. Priciples and techniques of the examination of ocular motility and alignment. In: Miller NR, Newman NJ, editors. Walsh & Hoyt's: clinical neuro-ophthalmology. Philadelphia: Lippincott Williams 2005. p. 887–906.

Brandt TH, et al. Different types of skew deviation. J Neurol Psychiatry. 1991;54:549–50.

Brandt T, et al. Skew deviation with ocular torsion: a vestibular brainstem sign of topographic diagnostic value. Ann Neurol. 1993;33:528–34.

Burde RM, et al. Clinical decisions in neuro-ophthalmology. St Louis: Mosby; 1985.

Calvert PS. Disorders of neuromuscular transmission. In: Miller NR, Newman NJ, editors. Walsh & Hoyt's: clinical neuro-ophthalmology. Philadelphia: Lippincott Williams 2005. p. 1041–84.

Cogan D. Neurology of the ocular muscles. Springfield: Ch Thomas; 1956.

Davis SL. Modeling Uhthoff 's phenomenon in MS patients with internuclear ophthalmoparesis. Neurology. 2008;70(13 Part 2):1098–106.

Dietrich M, et al. Wallenberg syndrome: lateropulsion, cyclorotation and subjective visual vertical in thirty-six patients. Ann Neurol. 1992;31:399–408.

Dietrich M, et al. Ocular torsion and tilt of subjective visual vertical use sensitive brainstem signs. Ann Neurol. 1993;33:292–9.

Dieterich M, Brandt TH. Vestibular syndromes and vertigo. In: Bogousslasky J, Caplan L, editors. Stroke syndromes. Cambridge/New York: Cambridge University Press; 2001. p. 129–43.

Frohman EM, et al. The utility of MRI in suspected MS. Report of the Therapeutics and Technology Assessment Subcommittee of the American Academy of Neurology. Neurology. 2003;61:602–11.

Guy JR, et al. Paraneoplastic downbeating nystagmus (a sign of occult malignancy). J Clin Neuroophthalmol. 1988;8(4):269–72.

Halmágyi GM. GM aid coll tonic contraversive ocular tilt reaction due to unilateral meso-diencephalic lesion. Neurology. 1990;40:1503–9.

Herzau V. Myasthenia gravis. Supplementum of course of strabismus and neuro-ophthalmology on IXth congress of the European Society of Ophthalmology. Brussels; 1992.

Jay WM, et al. Pseudo-internuclear ophthalmoplegia with downshoot in MG gravis. J Clin Neuroophthalmol. 1987;7(2):74–6.

Kawasaki A. Disorders of pupillary function, accommodation, lacrimation. In: Miller NR, Newman NJ, editors. Walsh & Hoyt's: clinical neuro-ophthalmology. Philadelphia: Lippincott Williams 2005. p. 739–805.

Keane JR. Internuclear ophthalmoplegia: unusual causes in 114 of 410 patients. Arch Neurol. 2005;62(5):714–7.

Kennard C. The supranuclear control of eye movements. Supplement of IXth EUPO Course. 1992.

Korányi K és mtsa. Az ophthalmoneurológiai diagnosztika és a szemészeti terápia MG és endocrin ophthalmopathia együttes előfordulásakor [Diagnostics in ophthalmology and ophthalmological therapy in concomitant MG and endocrine ophthalmopathy]. Szemészet. 1986;123:132–8.

Pierrot- Deseilligny CH. Eye movement abnormalities. In: Bogousslasky J, Caplan L, editors. Stroke syndromes. Cambridge/New York: Cambridge University Press; 2001. p. 76–86.

Sargent JC. Nuclear and infranuclear ocular motility disorders. In: Miller NR, Newman NJ, editors. Walsh & Hoyt's: clinical neuro-ophthalmology. Philadelphia: Lippincott Williams 2005. p. 907–68.

Judit S. Az agytörzsi eredetű szemmozgászavarok vizsgálatának új irányzatai. Ideggyógy Szeml. 1999;52:5–6.

Szobor A. Myasthenia gravis. Budapest: Akadémia Kiadó; 1990.

Szobor A, et al. Myasthenia gravis: Plasmapheresis kezelés hatása [Myesthenia gravis: the effect of plasmapheresis]. Ideggyógy Szeml. 1983;36:385–90.

Szobor A, et al. Myasthenia gravis: thymectomia eredménye 550 betegen [Myasthenia gravis: the effect of thymectomy in 550 patients]. Orv Hetil. 1990;131(46):2519–24.

Zee DS, Newman-Toker DE. Supranuclear and internuclear ocular motility disorders. In: Miller NR, Newman NJ, editors. Walsh & Hoyt's: clinical neuro-ophthalmology. Philadelphia: Lippincott Williams & Wilkins; 2005. p. 907–68.

Congenital Eye Movement Disorders

53

Andrea Deák

Contents

Congenital Eye Movement Disorders

- Congenital esotropia
- Congenital paralysis of the oculomotor nerve
- Double elevator palsy
- Double depressor palsy
- Isolated palsy of the inferior oblique muscle
- Brown's syndrome
- Congenital retraction syndrome (Stilling-Turk-Duane)
- Trochlear nerve palsy
- Plagiocephaly
- Congenital oculofacial paresis (Mobius's syndrome)
- Fibrosis syndromes
- Generalized fibrosis syndrome
- Congenital fibrosis of the inferior rectus muscle
- The quantitative diagnosis of strabismus

The importance of ophthalmological examinations in childhood in the recognition of congenital eye movement disorders cannot be overestimated. Their differential diagnosis and the initiation of the appropriate therapy without delay is a huge responsibility. After the overview of the most important diseases, the chapter covers the diagnostic options.

Congenital Esotropia

The syndrome is also known as infantile esotropia. In 50–70 % of the cases, it is apparent at birth but in 30–50 % it becomes obvious only after some months after delivery. Characteristically the angle of convergence is wide and does not change over time. High proportion of newborn patients with brain injury has congenital esotropia, but in these cases, the angle of strabismus changes with age and can even progress to exotropia. Congenital esotropia should be differentiated

A. Deák, M.D.
Orthoptic Unit, Department of Ophthalmology, Albert Szent-Györgyi Clinical Center, University of Szeged, Szeged, Hungary
e-mail: antalpetermiklos@gmail.com

J. Somlai, T. Kovács (eds.), *Neuro-Ophthalmology*, DOI 10.1007/978-3-319-28956-4_53

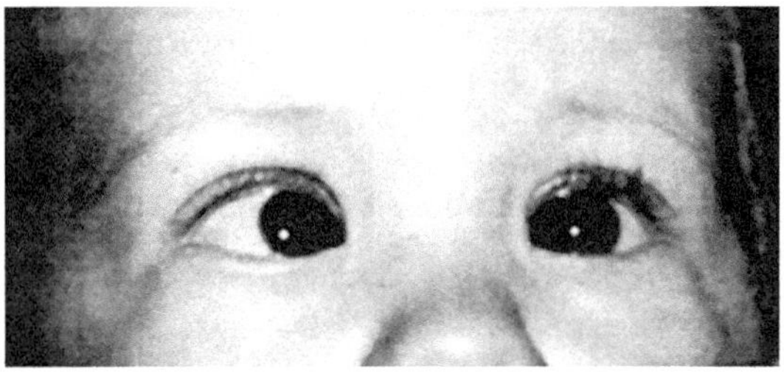

Fig. 53.1

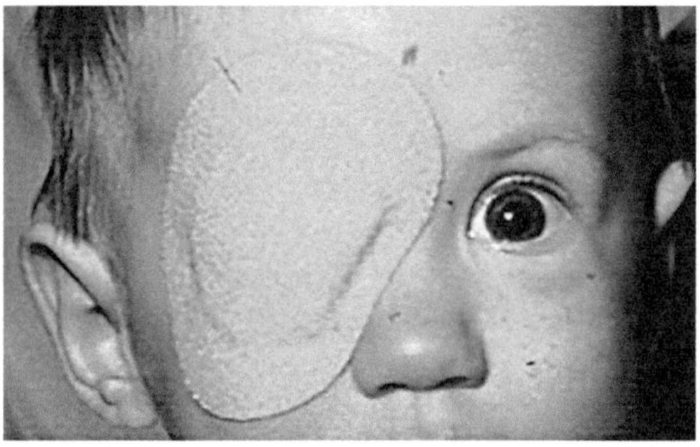

Fig. 53.2

from the early onset accommodatinge esotropia, which consists of wide angle esotropia, changing level of deviation and hypermetropia of +3.75 to 7.5 D.

Diagnosis The majority of the infants suffering from congenital esotropia alternately cross fixate (Fig. 53.1). A smaller proportion of them eventually develop amblyopia with overt eccentric fixation. The examiner should pay attention to this and the lack of abduction as well. The disease should be clearly differentiated from the bilateral abducens palsy, Duane's syndrome and Mobius's syndrome. The congenital esotropia is accompanied by dissociated vertical deviation (DVD) in 62–72 % of the cases, which latter condition manifests itself usually between 2 and 3 years. Early surgical intervention of the congenital esotropia does not decrease the incidence of this cycloverti-cal disorder. DVD becomes apparent upon the elevation and extorsion of the fixed eye. Its extent is difficult to estimate before surgical correction of the horizontal disorder. The change in the angle of strabismus on up- and downward gaze (A and V pattern incomitance) can also be observed usually around the age of 3 years. Both eyes have the same refraction values, which can encompass a rather wide range. Hypermetropia does not show progression over time. Astigmatism is a common feature, the axis of which is asymmetrically oblique. Over time the asymmetry decreases, and the axes take on TABO values of 45° and 135°, respectively. Latent nystagmus characterizes 55–90 % of the cases. In adduction the nystagmus is minimal. Covering either eye or abduction triggers it. Sometimes torticollis can be noticed, when the patient tilts his head toward the side of the leading eye while the other eye is in adduction. The differential diagnosis relies on two tests:

1. The child sits on the lap of the assistant, who holds the patient's head and turns it to the right, and then to the left. The examiner sits in front of them looking for a short movement of abduction on the opposite side of the direction of the turn.
2. Applying an eye occluder on either eye, and after some days on the opposite one, abduction can be observed. The traction test is negative. In deep anesthesia, the patient's eyes diverge from each other.

Treatment is surgical. But the prevention of amblyopia is essential even before the operative intervention. Since the foveal fixation begins around the 3rd month and becomes permanently stabilized around the 5th month, the facial occlusion has to be started in this period (Fig. 53.2) Its extent and length should be determined according to the past history, the patient's physical status and the parents' reliability. In the English literature, more and more frequently reports can be read about the successful surgical treatment performed between the 6th and 18th months.

The actual surgical intervention is bilateral recession of the medial rectus depending on the angle of strabismus determined by the Krimsky's test. However, it appears that bilateral global laminotomy, performed on both medial rectus muscles, gives better results. This procedure was introduced in Hungary in 1986 and retains intact the innervation circle. However, only one intervention rarely provides optimal solution for congenital esotropia. If necessary, a second operation should be performed between the ages of 3 and 4 years. The horizontal deviation should not be corrected completely. In the clinical practice a 5–7°

under compensation proved to be sufficient. This approach significantly decreases the probability of the development of secondary exotropia 10–30 years later. The A and V syndromes can be solved with the vertical transposition of the horizontal rectus muscles together with the surgical treatment of the horizontal deviation. In the case of sursoadductorius strabismus and DVD, the over activity of the inferior oblique muscles can be corrected also together with the treatment of horizontal deviation performing the uni-or bilateral myotomy, myectomy or recession of the muscles. The later operation performed between the ages of 3 and 4 years will rely on the traditional approach. The exact values of the close and distant angle of strabismus will determine the extent of resection on the lateral rectus muscle and recession on the medial rectus muscle. After both interventions the patients' attention should be called for the following therapeutic consequences.

1. Certainly a second surgical intervention should be necessary.
2. The therapy of amblyopia has not been finished yet

Sensorium Unfortunately in this condition, complete correction of binocular vision cannot be achieved even with earliest and most determined therapy. The alternating occlusion treatment is essential in the prevention of amblyopia, but it cannot stop the development of suppression and the anomalous retinal correspondence (ARC). The peripheral fusion should satisfy us since it usually keeps the eyes in parallel direction.

Congenital Paralysis of the Oculomotor Nerve

The paralyses of the 3rd cranial nerve manifest themselves in variable clinical conditions. The intraocular muscles are rarely affected in the case of congenital paralysis, although sometimes pathological regeneration can lead to pupil constriction upon adduction maneuvers. The congenital paralysis is of unknown etiology, perhaps it represents a developmental disorder. In this case, the disorder impairs those motor centers of the nuclear complex oculomotor nerve, which innervates the four extraocular and the levator muscles. It represents a rather common eye movement disorder, and most often it appears unilaterally. The nuclear complex innervates the ipsilateral muscles apart from the superior rectus muscle, which receives bilateral innervation. Since those fibers, which supply the superior rectus muscle already cross in the nuclear complex a unilateral central paralysis will also result in the paresis of the contralateral superior rectus muscle. Since the nuclei are very close to each other, but the nerves run fairly separately from each other, central lesions represent themselves as bilateral disorder while the peripheral ones go with unilateral symptoms. The possibility of oculomotor palsy should always be considered in the case of ptosis if either eye is exotropic and hypotropic. The lack of adduction makes it difficult to assess the function of the ipsilateral trochlear nerve. Observation of the crypts of iris, while the affected eye is in abduction, can help the diagnosis. The patient is instructed to look upwards and downwards. If the trochlear nerve is intact, the crypts of iris reflect in torsion upon infraduction and extorsion upon supraduction. The traction test is unexceptionally negative in the case of oculomotor palsy, which excludes any form of adhesion (Fig. 53.3).

Treatment Basically it depends on the severity of the paresis. Mild cases do not need surgical intervention. In contrast, complete congenital oculomotor palsy necessitates surgery to correct the exotropia, hypotropia and ptosis. To correct hypotropia, the tendon of the superior oblique muscle is detached from the eyeball since it is tight and contracted. The maximum recession of the external rectus muscle and the resection of the internal rectus muscle usually provide satisfactory primary alignment for the eye. Obviously adduction cannot

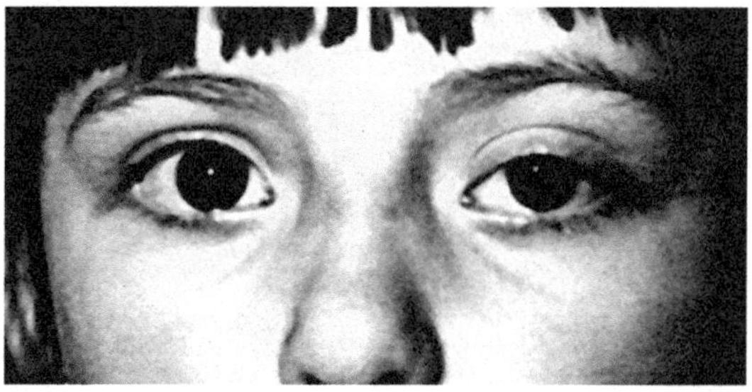

Fig. 53.3

be expected in this case. Elston recommended maximum recession of the lateral rectus muscle and resection of the internal rectus muscle together with the simultaneous transposition of the insertion to the superior rectus muscle. This procedure is considered to provide the best cosmetic results. The resection of the superior oblique muscle either with or without trochleotemy should be avoided according to Sanders and Rogers. In the first case, hyperdeviation and paradoxical eye movements while in the latter one adherence syndrome was observed. The traditional surgical solution of the ptosis is not recommended, either. An alternative option is bringing upward the ptotic eyelid frontally with 4-0 Supramid suture. Therefore, the potential corneal disorders, which may develop due to the lack of the Bell phenomenon, can be cured by the removal of the sutures. The pathologic regeneration of the oculomotor nerve can be established with more certainty from the positions of the upper eyelid in different gaze positions. Since the levator muscle of the upper eyelid is essentially innervated by the neurons which supply the medial rectus muscle and the inferior rectus muscle, upon downward gaze, the levator does not relax and the palpebral fissure remains wider than that of a healthy eye. Closing the eyes, sulcus becomes apparent on the upper eyelid of the affected side owing to the retraction of the bulb elicited by the pathological regeneration and the lack of the Bell phenomenon (Fig. 53.4).

Double Elevator Palsy

A mild form of the congenital oculomotor palsy. It affects only the elevator muscles. Characteristically it features ptosis and pseudoptosis as the position of the upper eyelid follows the orientation of the eyeball. Upon fixation with the hypotropic eye, pseudoptosis completely disappears. The traction test is negative.

Treatment is surgical. Knapp's method is recommended in the case of negative forced duction (traction) test and is based upon the transposition of the insertions of the external and internal rectus muscles to that of the superior rectus muscle. This procedure usually results in 19° correction in primary alignment and allows 25° movement into the direction normally controlled by the paretic muscle. In the case of positive traction test, Scott and Jackson recommends the recession of the inferior rectus muscle as initial intervention. In some patients binocularity is preserved due to torticollis. Without such compensation, however, amblyopia can develop on either eye (Figs. 53.5 and 53.6)

Double Depressor Palsy

Very rare disorder. Depression is hindered due to the mild paresis of the inferior rectus and the superior oblique muscles. The traction test is negative (Figs. 53.7 and 53.8).

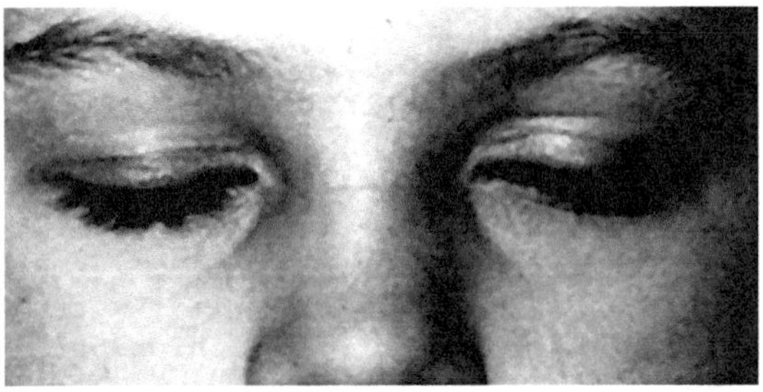

Fig. 53.4

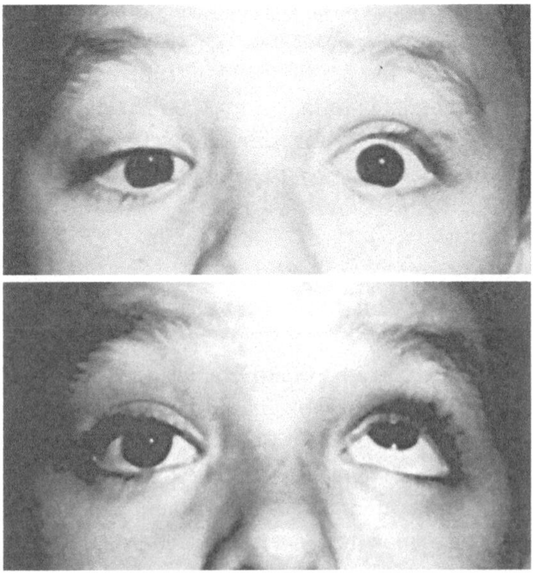

Figs. 53.5 and 53.6

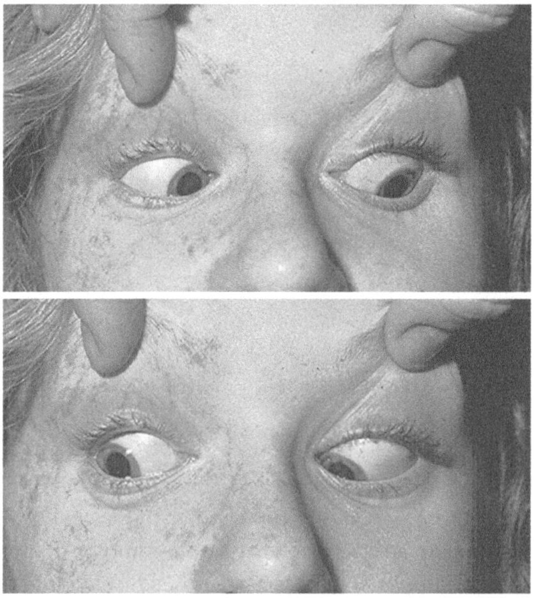

Figs. 53.7 and 53.8

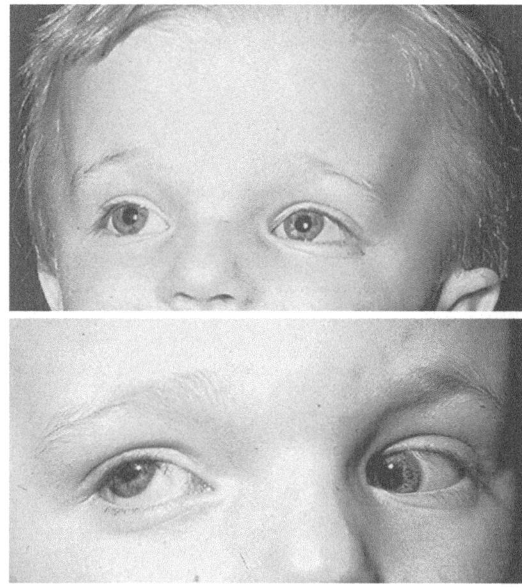

Figs. 53.9 and 53.10

Isolated Palsy of the Inferior Oblique Muscle

Much more frequent abnormality than it is generally assumed. It can be diagnosed as an unexpected finding even in the case of perfect binocular vision. However, it can be accompanied by horizontal deviation and severe amblyopia, as well. Rarely does it cause torticollis. According to our observations the hypofunction of the inferior oblique muscle frequently goes together with an abnormal whorl between scalp and the forehead. This suggests that the two abnormalities are rooted in a common developmental disorder. Only should the accompanying horizontal deviation, anisometropia or amblyopia be treated (Figs. 53.9 and 53.10).

Brown's Syndrome

In the congenital form, a pathological connection is formed between the trochlea and the tendon of the superior oblique muscle. It has to be differentiated from the hypofunction of the inferior oblique muscle by forced duction test, which is positive in Brown's syndrome. In adduction both the elevation and the depression are limited. Brown first suspected the paresis of the inferior oblique muscle, but later he proved by electromyography that the muscle is completely healthy. Most of the patients have parallel alignment in primary alignment. Despite the mild restriction of the eye movements, perfect fusion can be noticed upon downward gaze. Therefore, the patient raises his chin (Figs. 53.11 and 53.12). Therapy: Surgical intervention is rarely advisable. Helveston reserves it for such cases, when the upward tilt causes cosmetic problems or the hypotropia of the affected side is extreme.

Secondary Brown's syndromes due to injuries or surgical interventions call for individual therapies. The true congenital abducens palsy is very rare. It can be easily mistaken for congenital esotropia, Duane's syndrome or Mobius's syndrome. It is still debated whether obstetrical traumas are the most important reasons for the disorder. Reisner et al. have documented 35 cases of transient abducens palsy among 6360 newborns. The abnormality

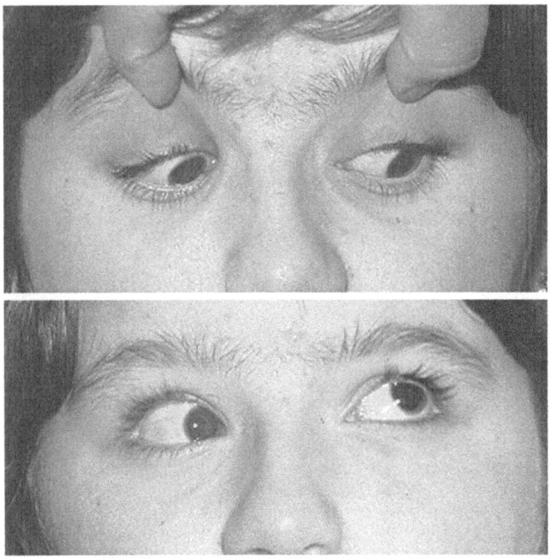

Figs. 53.11 and 53.12

spontaneously healed in 97% of the cases in 6 weeks. True abducens paresis is usually results from the hypoplasia of the abducens nucleus, the anomaly of the abducens nerve and the hypoplasia or lack of the abducens muscle itself.

Treatment Non-invasive: correction of hypermetropia; in the case of binocular vision and torticollis: prism eyeglasses; amblyopia: occlusion.

- Surgically: weakening of the medial rectus muscle according to the methods of Hummelsheim or Jensen

Congenital Retraction Syndrome (Stilling-Türk-Duane)

Due to the inborn defect of the abducens nerve, the hypofunction of the abducens neurons is partially compensated by the oculomotor nerve Figs. 53.11 and 53.12.

Electromyography provided evidence of it. The pathologic innervation of the lateral rectus muscle explains the following symptoms.

1. The abduction and/or the adduction are restricted.
2. In adduction the bulb retracts and secondary blepharospam develops.
3. Binocular vision can be achieved by slightly turning the head.

The actual clinical picture of the eye movements depends on the versatile pathological innervation possibilities.

- The innervation potential of the abducens itself.
- The extent of the innervation provided by the oculomotor nerve.
- The volume of the denervated, fibrotic musculature.

The individual cases will show different clinical picture depending on whether the lateral rectus muscle is innervated by the oculomotor fibers, which supply the medial rectus muscle or the ones which are responsible for the vertical eye movements. These differences lead to the A and V symptoms, which are classified according to Huber in the following way:

Type I.	Abduction	Considerably limited
	Adduction	Mildly limited
Type II.	Abduction	Considerably limited
	Adduction	Considerably limited
Type III.	Abduction	Considerably limited
	Adduction	Limited

The most frequent is the Type I (Figs. 53.13 and 53.14) with severely limited abduction and mildly impaired adduction. Then the fibers supplying the medial rectus muscle also innervate the lateral rectus muscle. Therefore, upon adduction, both the medial rectus muscle and the lateral rectus muscle contract, therefore, the bulb retracts and the palpebral fissure narrows.

Treatment Correction of the refractive error, in the case of severely abnormal head posture, surgical intervention might be necessary. It means simultaneously performed recession of the medial and lateral rectus muscle, which alleviates the retraction of the eyeball. Sometimes loosening of the contralateral medial rectus muscle can be considered. The resection of the pathologically innervated lateral rectus muscle and transposition surgeries should be avoided.

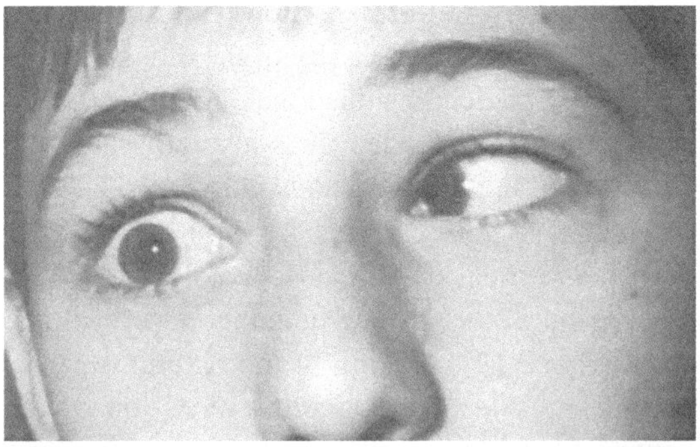

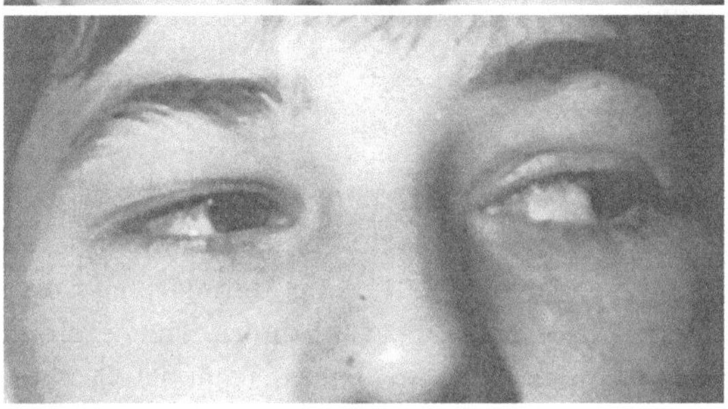

Figs. 53.13 and 53.14

Trochlear Nerve Palsy

It is the most frequent cyclovertical paralysis. In both congenital trochlear paresis and in the one which develops in early childhood, the vertical deviation is approximately the same upon elevation and depression. It is in sharp contrast with the findings that the difference is bigger in adduction than is abduction. Therefore, the infantile form of the trochlear paresis resembles the non-paralytic strabismus sursoadductorius. However, they can be separated with the help of the Bielschowsky's head tilt test. It is positive only in trochlear palsy. Tilting the head towards the affected side results in the elevation and intorsion of the ipsilateral eye. In normal circumstances, due to activity of the vestibular system, tilting the head leads to counter rotation of the eyes. This counter rotation mainly relies on the activity of the oblique ocular muscles. Therefore, paralysis of the superior oblique muscle results in loss of intorsion and depression leading to excyclotorsion. It is compensated by turning the head into the opposite direction and tucking the chin in (Figs. 53.15 and 53.16). This way the

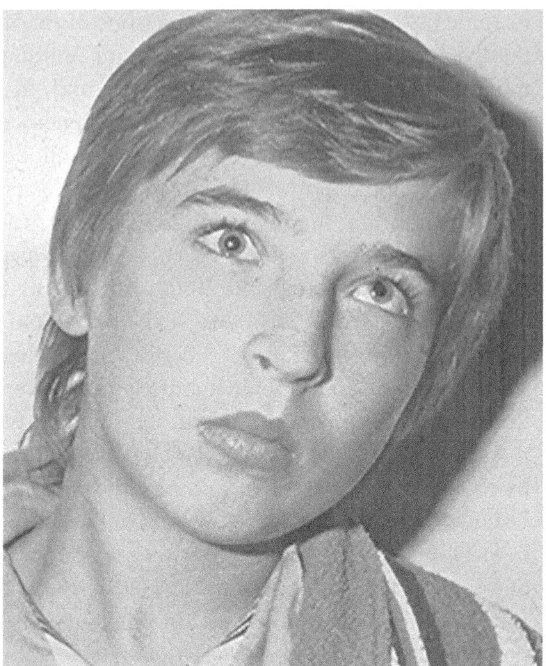

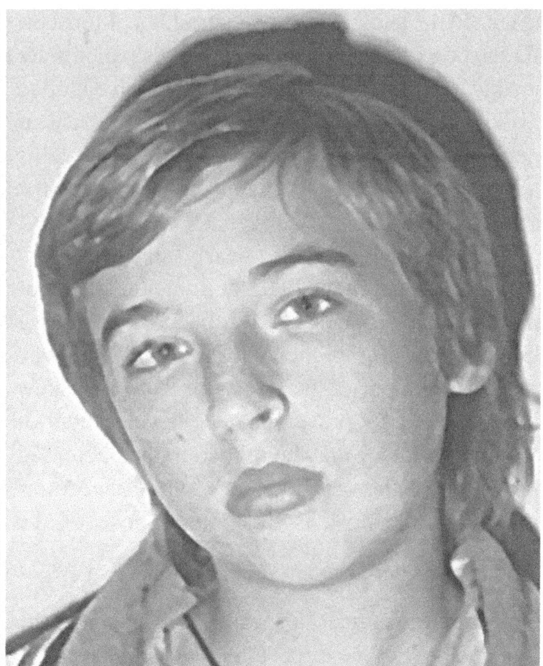

Figs. 53.15 and 53.16

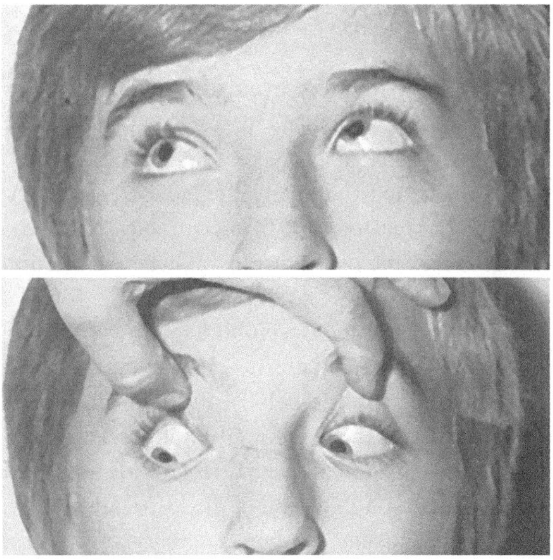

Figs. 53.17 and 53.18

patient can achieve binocular vision. The above abnormality can be missing or sometimes paradoxical posture of the head can be observed. Frequent finding is the hyperactivity of the ipsilateral antagonist, the inferior oblique muscle, which can be attributed to increased innervation (Figs. 53.17 and 53.18). The paradoxical torticollis can be explained by the fact that the patients are unable to maintain the fusion and they give it up to avoid double vision. The congenital trochlear nerve palsy in some of the cases causes torticollis and apparent vertical strabismus as early as by the 6th month.

With certain diagnosis, early surgical intervention is recommended to facilitate the development of fusion to increase the chance of achieving binocular vision without torticollis. This way the development of facial asymmetry and skew distortion can be prevented. The development of facial asymmetry may be related to the decreased perfusion of the carotid artery, while the deformation of the nose is the consequence of the gravity.

Treatment Surgical according to Knapp. If the hyperactivity of the direct antagonist can be established then the first option is the weakening of the inferior oblique muscle. This can be accomplished by recession or, based upon our experience, by the myotomy of the inferior oblique muscle according to McNeer-Scott-Jampolsky as modified by Dunlap. As the hyperactivity subsides, the torticollis disappears and the Bielschowsky test becomes negative. When hyperactivity of the direct antagonist cannot be demonstrated tucking of the paretic muscle is recommended. It is also advisable the recession of the inferior rectus muscle.

If the vertical deviation does not exceed 12°, weakening of the ipsilateral antagonist develops, while above 12°, tucking of the paretic superior oblique muscle and/or gradual recession of the contralateral synergistic muscle occurs.

Plagiocephaly

The syndrome which can mimic trochlear nerve palsy is brought about by the untimely and unilateral fusion of the coronal suture. The outcome is flattening of the ipsilateral frontal bone and the protrusion of the contralateral one (Figs. 53.19, 53.20, and 53.21). In plagiocephaly the affected orbital plate of the frontal bone becomes shorter, and due to the retroposition of the trochlea, the section of the superior oblique muscle spanning between its origin and the trochlea also shortens. Therefore, it can generate less force than the contralateral superior oblique muscle, but the function of the ipsilateral inferior oblique muscle remains intact. The clinical picture mimics the paresis of the superior oblique muscle on the affected side. Both torticollis and Bielschowsky test positivity can be found. Obviously the activity of superior the rectus muscle remains intact since it directly radiates to the sclera. In primary alignment, the segment of the superior oblique muscle, which connects the trochlea and the sclera forms, like the inferior oblique muscle 51° with the optical angle of the eye. Obviously, a change to either angle will definitely tip the balance of muscles according to the principle of sagittalisation. In plagiocephaly the segment of the superior oblique muscle after the trochlea form an angle with the optical axis of the eye, which exceeds 51°. This condition is

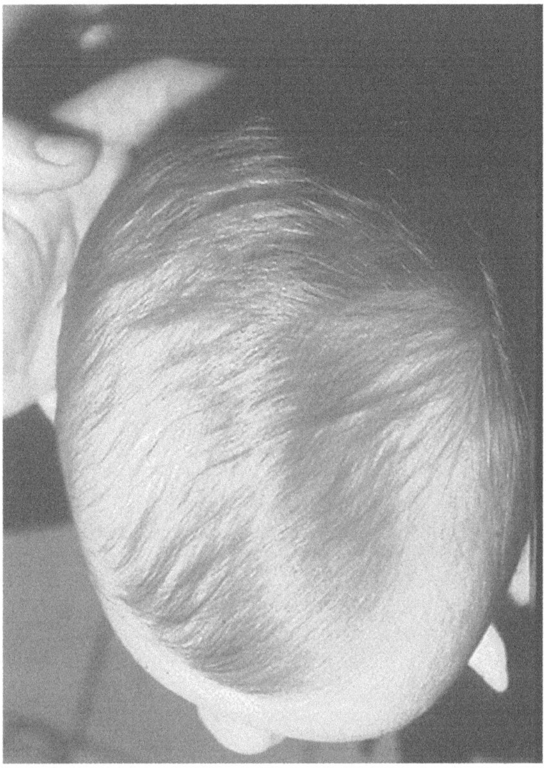

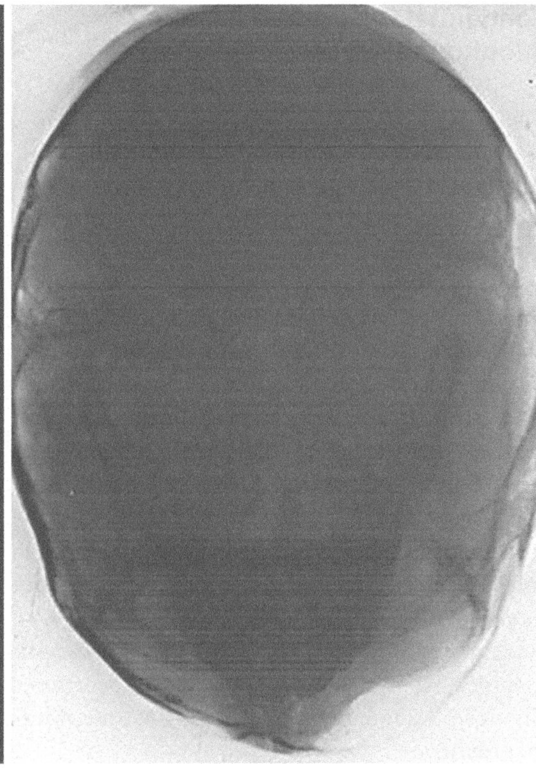

Figs. 53.19 and 20

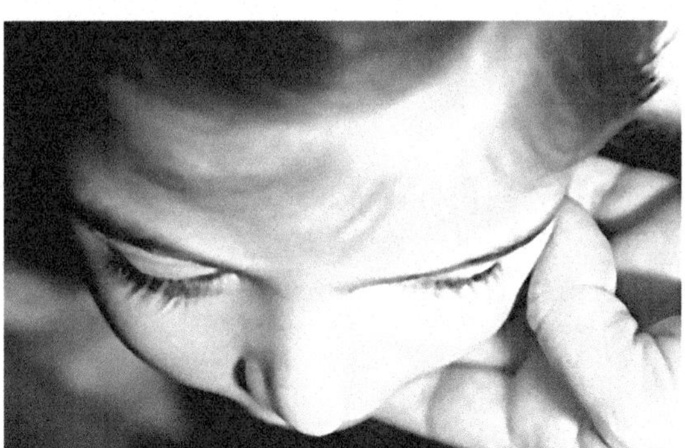

Fig. 53.21

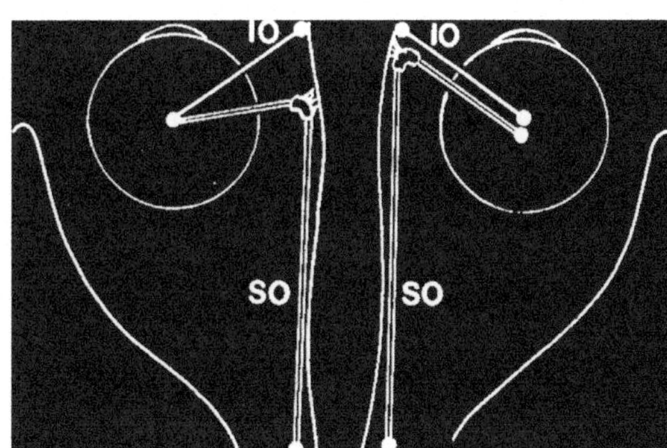

Fig. 53.22

called "desagittalisation" (Fig. 53.22). This way the vertical pull of the muscle decreases while the torsion increases. Due to the decreased depression, it results in the relative over activity of the antagonistic inferior oblique muscle; therefore, the condition does not represent true paralysis. To achieve binocular vision, the patient frequently compensates with torticollis similarly to true trochlear nerve palsy. The treatment is surgical. The procedures are identical with those applied in trochlear nerve palsy. Surgery eliminates the over activity of the affected inferior oblique muscle, the positive Bielschowsky test and the torticollis.

Congenital Oculofacial Paresis (Mobius's Syndrome)

The most important ophthalmological symptoms are esotropia and inability of abduction. Bilateral facial nerve paralysis is reflected most conspicuously by the dysfunction of the orbicularis oculi muscles. The lower eyelid relaxes and the tear accumulates. The face is smooth, expressionless, the mouth is round, and smiling is difficult. An accompanying defect is the paralysis of the tongue, which leads to difficulties in swallowing and disorders of speech development. Mental retardation of some extent and skeletal abnormalities can also be apparent. The disorders of the eye, face and tongue and their movements are related to the aplasia or hypoplasia of the nuclei of the abducens, facial and glossopharyngeal nerve. The severity of the innervation disorder shows a wide clinical spectrum. Figures 53.23, 53.24, and 53.25 illustrate mild disorders.

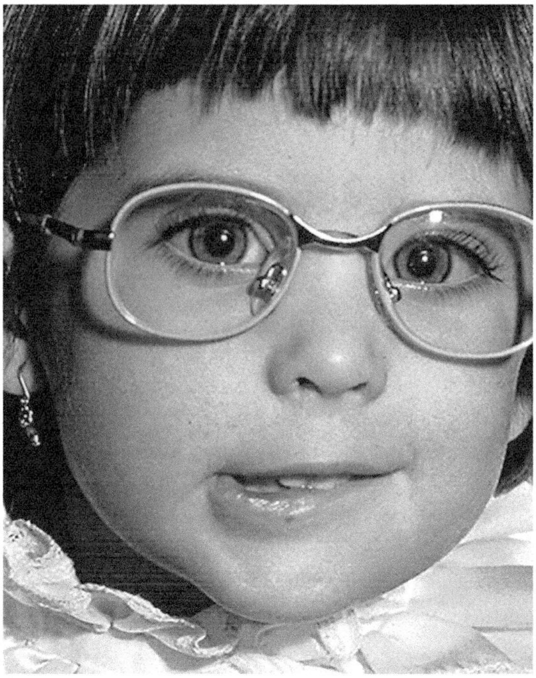

Fig. 53.24

Fibrosis Syndromes

Due to fibrosis of the extraocular musculature, the normal eye movements are severely restricted. It is partly due to the rigidity of the fibrotic mass, partly due to lack of tension provided by the affected muscle and the abnormal constriction of the antagonist.

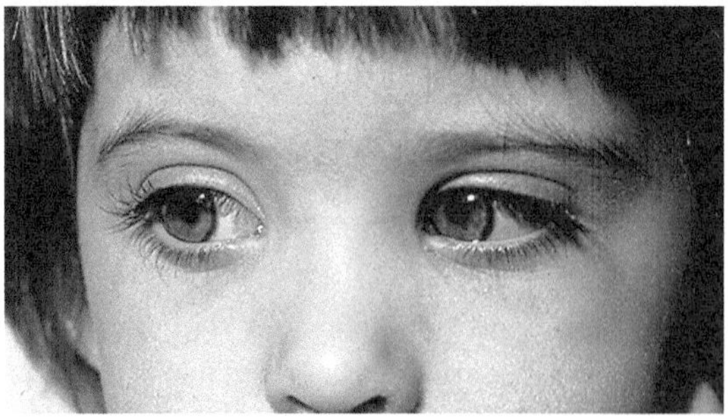

Fig. 53.23

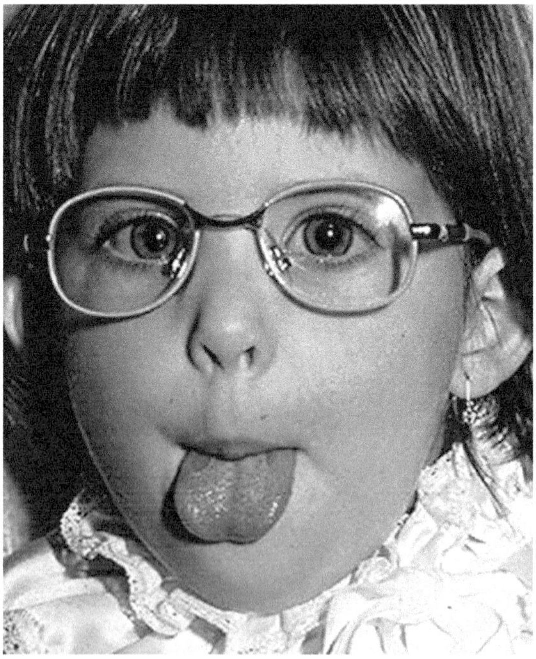

Fig. 53.25

Generalized Fibrosis Syndrome

Every external ocular muscle is afflicted, even the levator muscle. Although the disorder is bilateral slight differences can be noticed between the two sides. The muscles usually show fibrosis of various extent. The inferior rectus muscles are affected. The eyes look downward and ptosis can be seen!

Congenital Fibrosis of the Inferior Rectus Muscle

It is a variant of generalized fibrosis syndrome, which impairs only the inferior rectus muscle. It can be either uni- or bilateral, usually it is asymmetric. It causes vertical strabismus. Binocular vision can be achieved only by lifting the chin. It must be separated from the double elevator palsy. In fibrosis the eyes cannot be elevated.

Treatment is surgical. The maximum recession of the inferior rectus muscle(s).

Further Readings

Bagolini B, et al. Plagiocephaly causing superior oblique deficiency and ocular torticollis. Arch Ophthalmol. 1982;100:1093.

Baker JD, Parks MM. Early-onset accommodative esotropia. Am J Ophthalmol. 1980;90:11.

Balkan R, Hoyt CS. Associated neurologic abnormalities in congenital third nerve palsies. Am J Ophthalmol. 1984;97:315.

Burian HM, et al. Absence of spontaneous head tilt in superior oblique musde palsy. Am J Ophthalmol. 1975;79:972.

Chink NB, et al. Iris cysts and miotis. Arch Ophthalmol. 1964;71:611.

Deák A, et al. Mit Plagiocephalie vergeseUschaftete Hypofunkti on des Musculus obliquus superior. Augenklinik der Albert Szent- G y ö r g y i Medicinischen Universitat, Szeged.

DelMonte MA, et al. Denervation and extirpation of the inferior oblique. Ophthalmology. 1983;90:1178.

Ernest JT, Costenbader FD. Lateral rectus muscle palsy. Am J Ophthalmol. 1968;65:721.

Fells P. Management of paralytic strabismus. Br J Ophthalmol. 1974;58:255.

Gradenigo G. A special syndrome of endocranial otitic complications (paralysis of the motor oculi externus of otitic organ). Am Otol. 1904;13:637.

Harada M, et al. Surgical correction of cyclotropia. Jpn J Ophthalmol. 1964;8:88.

Hoyt WF, Nachtigaller H. Anomalies of ocular motor nerves. Am J Ophthalmol. 1965;60:443.

Hummelsheim E. Weitere Erfhrungen mit partie Uer Schnenuber pflanzung an den augenmuskeln. Arch Augenheilkd. 1909;62:71.

Jensen CDF. Rectus muscle union: a new operation for paralysis of the rectus muscle. Trans Pac Coast Otoophthalmol Soc Annu Meet. 1964;45:359.

Knapp P. The surgical treatment of double elevator paralysis. Trans Am Ophthalmol Soc. 1969;67:304.

Meloff KL, et al. Conversion 6th nerve palsy in a child. J Psychosomat. 1980;21:769.

Miller NR. Solitary oculomotor nerve palsy in childhood. Am J Ophthalmol. 1977;83:106.

Miller MT, et al. Superior oblique palsy presenting in late childhood. Am J Ophthalmol. 1970;70:212.

Mitchell PR, et al. Surgery for bilateral superior oblique palsy. Ophthalmology. 1982;89:484.

Molnár K. Másodlagos kontaktúrák kísérő kancsalságban és egy szelektív kontraktúra oldó műtét: Laminotomia globalis [Secondary contracturesin accompanying squinting and a selective surgical intervention to treat contracture. Global laminotomy]. Doktori disszertáció; 1993.

Molnár K. Újítások és állásfoglalások az orthoptikában [Advances and opinion in orthoptics] (kandidátusi értekezés). Budapest; 1977, p. 57.

Molnár K, et al. Szemészet. 1970;3:198.

Parks MM. Isolated cydovertical musde palsy. Arch Ophtalmol. 1958;60:1027.

Parks MM. A study of the weakening surgical procedures for eliminating overaction of the inferior obliques. Trans Am Ophthalmol Soc. 1971;69:163.

Parks MM. The weakening surgical procedures for eliminating overaction of the inferior oblique muscle. Am J Ophthalmol. 1972;73:107.

Parks MM. The overacting inferior oblique muscle: the XXXVI de Schweinitz Lecture. Am J Ophthalmol. 1974;77:787.

Rucker CW. The causes of paralysis of the third, fourth and sixth cranial nerves. Am J Ophthalmol. 1966;61:1293.

Rush JA, et al. Paralysis of cranial nerves m, IV and VI, cause and prognosis in 1000 cases. Arch Ophthalmol. 1981;99:76.

Saunders RA, et al. Superior oblique transposition for third nerve palsy. Ophthalmology. 1982;89:310.

Seat WE, et al. Double elevator palsy: the significance of inferior rectus restriction. Am Orthopt J. 1977;27:5.

Shrader EC, et al. Neuroophthalmologic evaluation of abducens nerve paralysis. Arch Ophthalmol. 1960;63:84.

Victor DI. The diagnosis of congenital unilateral third nerve palsy. Brain. 1976;99:711.

54 The Most Important Clinical Syndromes of Acquired Nuclear and Infranuclear Eye Movement Disorders, and Their Diagnostic and Therapeutic Options

Judit Somlai

Contents

In the central nervous system, the coordination of the eyes is provided by *the ocular motor system, which consists of three units* and connect the cortical centers with the muscles of the eyes. The cooperation between the ocular **motor** and the **visual** pathway systems results in the proper cortical processing of the two separate images of the eyes.

J. Somlai, M.D.
Unit of Neuro-Ophthalmology, Department of Neurology & Stroke, Military Hospital, Budapest, Hungary

Neuro-Ophthalmology Section, Hungarian Ophthalmological Association, Budapest, Hungary

Trustee, NOSZA Foundation (for the Prevention and Screening of Ocular Storke), Budapest, Hungary
e-mail: dr@somlaijudit.hu; http://somlaijudit.hu

The Ocular Motor System

I. **The peripheral ocular motor system:** *ocular muscles – brainstem.*
   (oculomotor nerves: n. III., n. IV., n. VI.)
II. **The ocular motor system of the brainstem:** *periphery – eyeball – eye movement centers of the brainstem.*
   (nuclei of the cranial nerves, eye movement gaze centers and internuclear pathways)
III. **Supranuclear ocular motor systems:** *brainstem centers – cortical eye movement centers* fast eye movements (FEM), slow eye movements (SEM)

The peripheral eye movement controlling neural pathways establishes connection between the intraorbital eye muscles and the nuclei of the ocular motor nerves.

The following cranial nerves control the eye movements:

- **oculomotor nerve (n.III.) –** *(nervus oculomotorius/Latin/)*
- **trochlear nerve (n. IV.)** – *(nervus nerus trochlearis/Latin/)*
- **abducens nerve (n. VI.).** – *(nervus abducens/ Latin/)*

Eye-related symptoms of peripheral ocular muscle palsies can be observed in the case of the isolated lesion of the oculomotor cranial nerves. The clinical picture depends on whether the func-

J. Somlai, T. Kovács (eds.), *Neuro-Ophthalmology*, DOI 10.1007/978-3-319-28956-4_54

tional impairment is localized in the *intraorbital* or the *intracranial segment.* Peripheral pareses can be of either **neurogenic** or **myogenic origin.** Obviously neurogenic paresis is related to injuries of the nerve, while the myogenic form is due to the disease of the muscle itself, and the function of the nerve remains intact. The oculomotor nerves can suffer isolated injuries on their peripheral part before reaching the brainstem, which is responsible for conjugated eye movements. This dysconjugate gaze disorder is unilateral and afflicts only a given phase of the eye movements. **Peripheral neurogenic paresis** presents with the dysfunction of the ipsilaterally innervated ocular muscle(s) and the overactivity of the contralateral synergistic muscles leading to severe disparity of the retinal images, narrowing of the visual field also due to the eye movement disorder. The shift of the borders of the visual field makes the fusion impossible. Diplopia is so frustrating that the patient immediately closes his either eye. The disorders of the central regulation of the ocular movements lead to the impairment of the complex conjugated motor mechanisms. This results in almost symmetrical displacement of the perceived images causing mild diplopia or the impairment of stereopsis (Table 54.1 and Fig. 54.1).

Case History – In the Case of Abrupt Onset of Double Vision

- Eye symptoms – *double vision: How is better your vision: monocular or binocular?*

Table 54.1

Peripheral paresis	Central (brainstem) paresis
Marked double vision – either eye: exclusion	Mild diplopia
Heterotropia – monocular strabismus isolated ophthalmologic symptom	Heterophoria – only the fusion is affected accompanying neurological symptoms
Ophthalmologist	Neurologist or if necessary oto-neurologist

- Onset – *when: some days, hours or months?*
- The characteristics of image displacement.
  - *permanent or transient?*
  - *has it intensified over time, increasing of the degree of the double vision?*
- In which plane can be the shift of the images observed?
  - *vertically*
  - *horizontally*
  - *skew deviation?*
- Can *tilt* of the pictures be noticed?
- Daily *fluctuation?*
- +/– *ptosis,* closed eyes, spastic closure of the eyelids?
- *Strabismus* – infantile, amblyopia, hidden?

Additional Symptoms Suggesting Systemic Disorder

- headache, confusion, vertigo?
- difficulties of swallowing and breathing? (alarm signs of myasthenia gravis)
- disturbances of stereopsis, walking stairs?
- further neurological symptoms?
- Have the neurological symptoms intensified (headache, onset of disorder of consciousness)?

Oculomotor Nerve (n. III.) Palsy

The oculomotor nerve innervates the majority of the ***extraocular eye muscles*** (which attach to the external layer of the bulbs) and the levator palpebrae superioris muscle. The dysfunction of the latter and those which elevate the gaze, ***elevator*** (e.g., the **superior rectus muscle** and **levator palpebrae superioris muscle** lead to ptosis). The ***depressor*** of the gaze is achieved through the action of the **inferior rectus muscle,** whereas the adduction through the action of the **internal rectus muscle,** adductor. The ***upward gaze in adduction*** is carried out by the **inferior oblique muscle.** Partial or complete palsy of them leads to the unilateral paresis of the upward and downward gaze in adduction (Fig. 54.4).

The oculomotor nerve together with the trochlear nerve performs the adduction and abduction,

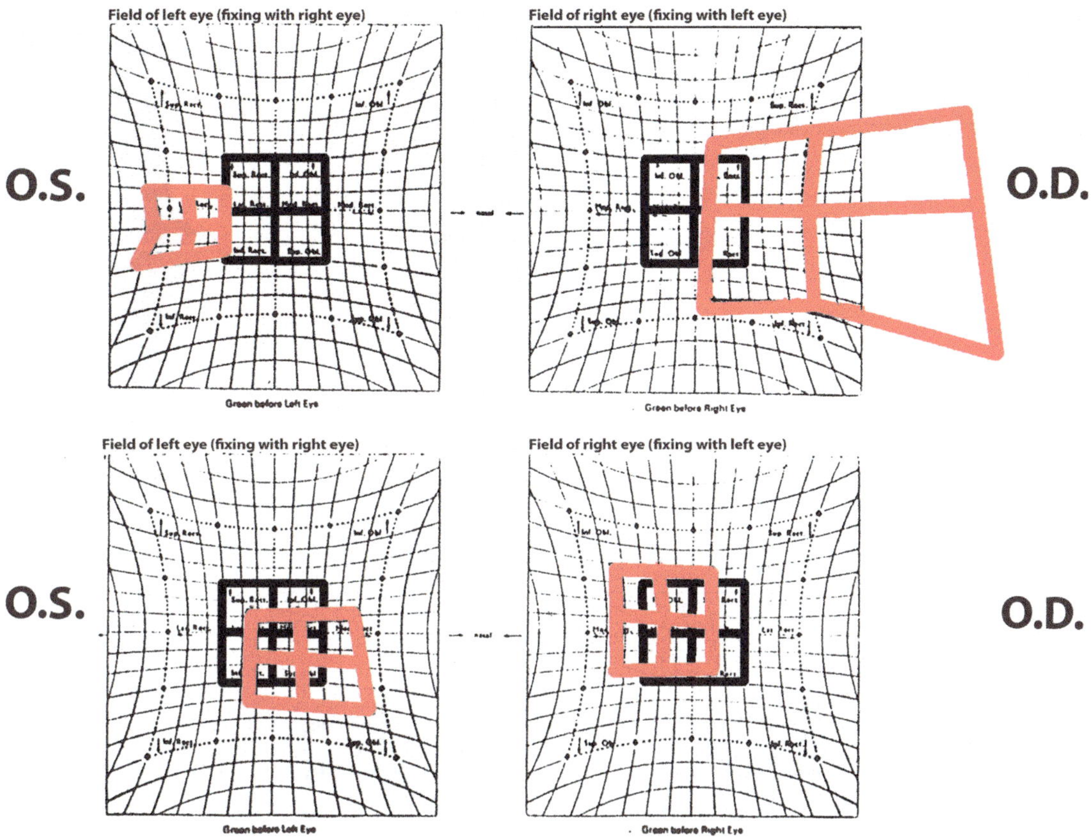

Fig. 54.1 Illustration by Hess-chart of the image displacements in peripheral and central ocular muscle palsies

which are accompanied by the simultaneous torsional movement of the eyes. The dysfunction of rotation can be usually noticed as torsional nystagmus using ***Frenzel goggles*** or ***during fundoscopy.*** During fundoscopy, it is reflected by the pathological rotation of the virtual axis of the papillomacular bundle. Serial fundoscopic images will reflect the pathological change in the angle of the rotational movement, (Figs. 54.2, 54.3, and 54.4).

The nerve also innervates the pupillary sphincter muscle from the intraocular muscles, (**muscle sphincter pupillae**) which constricts the pupil. It plays a role both in adaptation and accommodation (the accommodation triad consist of accommodation itself, convergence and miosis). The *complete paralysis of the third cranial nerve (n. III.)* – due to the unbalanced activity of the muscles innervated by the n.IV. and n.VI. cranial nerves- leads to downward gaze of the affected eye, complete ptosis and wide fixed pupils. The actual clinical picture varies according to the presence of pupillomotor symptoms and the number and extent of the affected muscles innervated by the dysfunctioning oculomotor nerve (Fig. 54.3).

Clinical manifestations Internal oculomotor nerve palsy: anisocoria and sluggish indirect pupil reactions on the affected side.

The most superficial fibers of the oculomotor nerve are the pupillomotor ones; therefore, the dysfunction of them and that of the pupils is the most sensitive predictor of the injury of the nerve, related to uncus herniation and increased intracranial pressure (for more details the reader is referred to Chap. 24).

External oculomotor nerve palsy: the eye movements are limited upon upward, downward gaze and and/or adduction (i.e., looking toward the nose) due to the innervation disorder of the extraocular muscles. That is, apart from

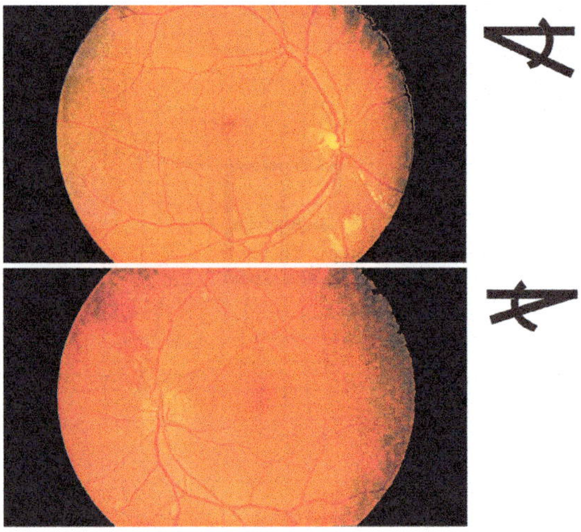

Fig. 54.2 The observation of the pathological cyclorotation on the fundus: the change in the acute angle formed by the horizontal line running through the macula and the line running through the optic disc; the options of measurement and detection of changes

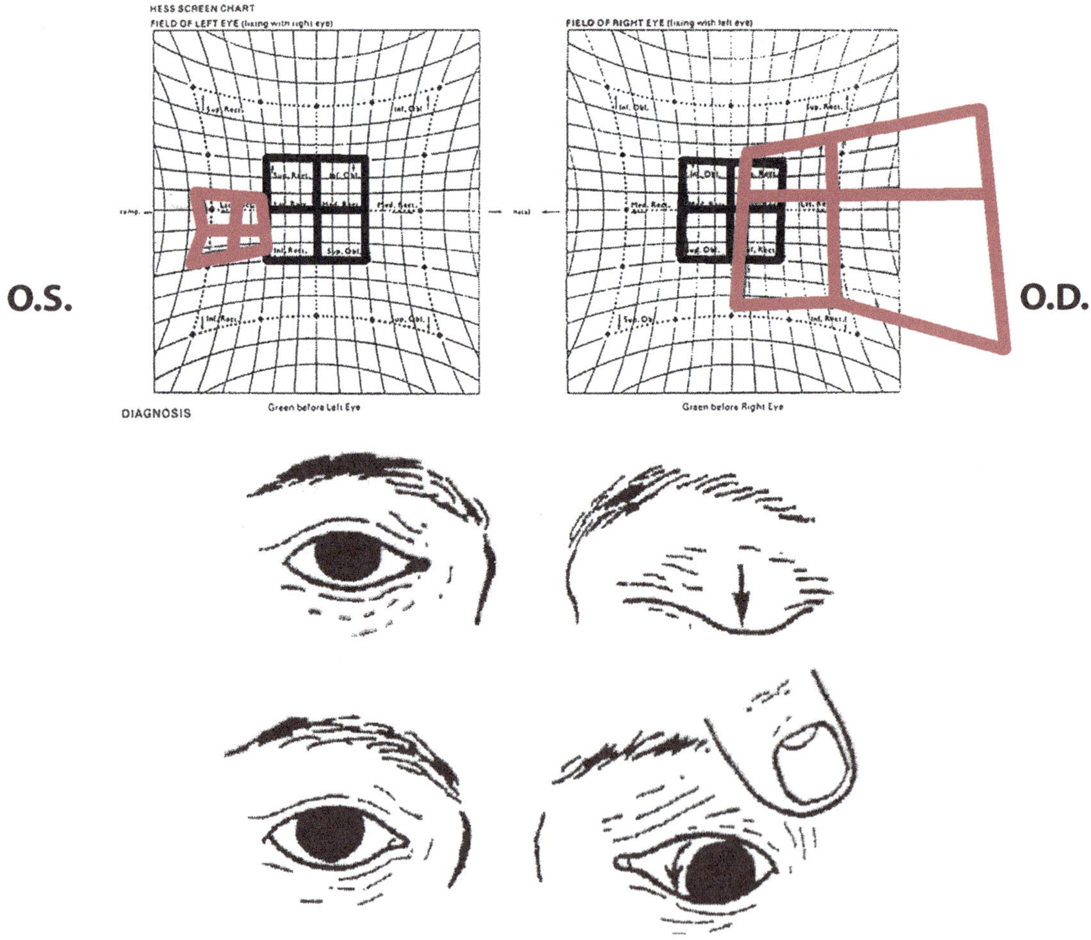

Fig. 54.3 *Up*: The pathological alignment due to eye movement disorder evoked by oculomotor nerve palsy is illustrated in a Hess chart *Down*: Graphical representation: the pathological alignment due to left-sided oculomotor nerve complete palsy

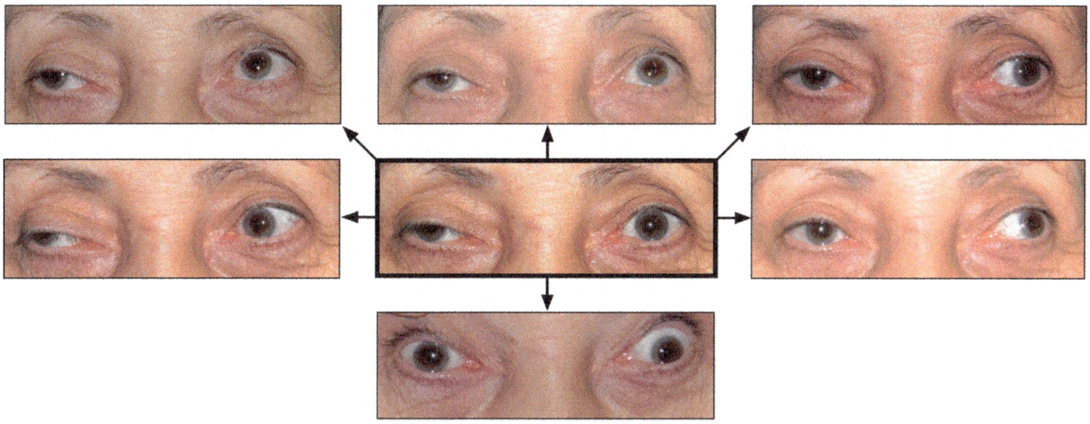

Fig. 54.4 Near complete oculomotor nerve (n. III.) plegia owing to the trauma of the skull **In primary position** (*in the middle*): divergent alignment of the right eye (due to uncompensated activity of the abducens nerve) and incomplete ptosis **Upon right and right-upward gaze** elevation plegia (due to the paresis of the elevator muscles innervated by the affected oculomotor nerve) **Upon left and left-upward gaze**: Adduction paresis accompanies the elevation plegia (the paresis leads to the dysfunction of the right medial rectus muscle) Incomplete paresis **upon downward** gaze due to the dysfunction of the inferior rectus muscle

abduction, gaze disorder develops into every direction on the affected side.

External-internal oculomotor nerve palsy: anisocoria and gaze disorder into every aforementioned direction.

Complete plegia of the oculomotor nerve: fixed, dilated pupils and the eyeball is dislocated and locked in downward and abducted position.

The most frequent causes of the oculomotor nerve palsy:

1. **Reasons of the *isolated* oculomotor nerve (n. III.) paresis:**
   - *aneurysm:* dilated pupil – the progressing anisocoria is the first and also alarming symptom The most frequent locations of the eye muscles paresis eliciting aneurysm are the internal carotid artery and the posterior communicating artery.
   - *increased intracranial pressure:* lateral herniation – tentorial compression -, the pupil dilates first on one side then on both sides
   - *laterally progressing pituitary tumor* – the anisocoria is an early symptom
   - *Skull injury* (in 23 %)
   - *Circulatory disorders of the brainstem:* as part of cerebrovascular incidents, characteristically the pupillary functions are spared, while the extraocular muscles are affected
   - *Disorders of the cavernous sinus* (aneurysm, fistula, carcinoma, meningeoma, intracavernous thrombosis)
   - *Pathological regeneration* – usually due to space occupying processes
   - *Intracranial inflammations:* herpes infection, Hodgkin's disease, extended sinusitis
   - *Congenital oculomotor nerve palsy*

Patients present with spared pupillary responses in 80 %. The most important systemic reasons of such disorder are diabetes, uncontrolled hypertension, hypertensive encephalopathy and generalized atherosclerosis.

Alternated Neurological Syndromes with Oculomotor Paresis (Paresis n.III.)

- *Benedikt's syndrome*: hemitremor + **oculomotor paresis (paresis n.III.)**

- $$\left.\begin{array}{r}\text{Weber's syndrome: contralateral hemiplegia}\\ \text{central paresis of the hypoglossal}\end{array}\right\} + \text{oculomotor paresis (paresis n.III.)} +/- \text{facial nerve}$$

- *Tumors of the skull base:* chordoma, metastatic carcinoma + **oculomotor paresis (paresis n.III.)**
- *Skull base fracture* + **oculomotor paresis (paresis n.III.)**
- *Tolosa-Huntsyndrome* + **oculomotor paresis (paresis n.III.)**
- *Diseases of the cavernous sinus* + **oculomotor paresis (paresis n.III.)**
- *Supraclinoid aneurysm of the ICA, tuberculum sellae meningeoma* + **oculomotor paresis (paresis n.III.)**
- *Syndrome of the superior orbital fissure* + **oculomotor paresis (paresis n.III.)**
- *Syndrome of the orbital apex* + **oculomotor paresis (paresis n.III.)**

Trochlear Nerve (n. IV.) Palsy

The most important clinical aspect of the anatomy of the trochlear nerve is that it is the only oculomotor nerve, which leaves the brainstem dorsally then circumvents the cerebral aqueduct, crosses the contralateral trochlear nerve and penetrating the dura mater enters the cavernous sinus. Therefore, any trauma of the vertex leads to the injury of this specifically vulnerable portion of the nerve leading to trochlear nerve paresis. The trochlear nerve innervates only one eye muscle, the superior oblique muscle. The function of this muscle is to pull the eye, in adducted position, downward (i.e., in opposite direction of the trochlea). Therefore, the activity of the right trochlear nerve turns the eyes to the left and in that adducted position, it depresses the gaze. Therefore, one can expect maximum image displacement due to the neurogenic paresis in the most remote point of the extent of the eye movement normally evoked by the muscle. Therefore, right-sided trochlear nerve palsy leads to skew deviatio (horizontal-vertical image displacement) in the left, infero-temporal visual field. During incyclotorsion torsional nystagmus can also be noticed upon smooth pursuit eye movements. The patient try to decrease or eliminate his-her double vision by the compensatory head tilting: slightly backwards and into the opposite direction of lesion. On the paretic side due to the vertical disorder of the bulb assumes higher position, which leads to hyperphoria in primary position.

The most important ocular symptoms of the unilateral trochlear nerve palsy:

- the patient tilts his head into the opposite direction of the lesion. In primary position the bulb is elevated on the affected side (hyperphoria)
- the punctum maximum of the image displacement can be observed infero-temporally, in the opposite direction of the lesion.
- the image displacement is skew deviation (horizontal-vertical) accompanied by torsional nystagmus.
- *(The typical eye positions are illustrated by photos in* Chap. 53 in Figs. 18 and 19. *Further information and photos is available for the reader on the subject in* Chap. 21.)

The typical diagnostic results obtained by Hess screen in Fig. 54.5.

Clinical manifestations

- unilateral trochlear nerve palsy
- unilateral trochlear nerve palsy with further neurological symptoms.
- bilateral trochlear nerve (n. IV.) palsy

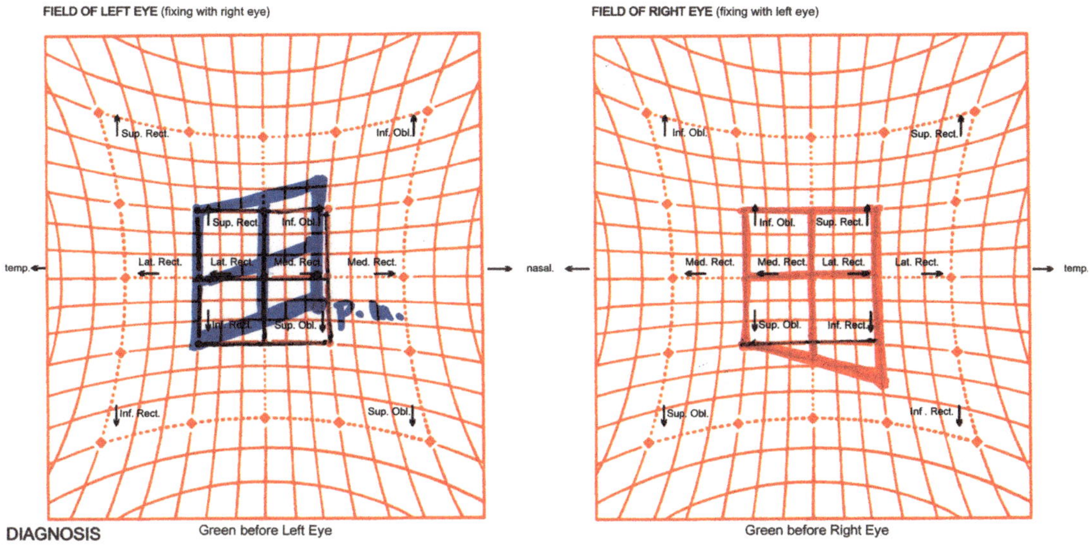

Fig. 54.5 Trochlear nerve (n. IV.) palsy. The image displacement caused by a left trochlear nerve palsy registered on a Hess chart. *Blue lines* indicate the eye movement disorder elicited by the disease of the left superior oblique muscle. Therefore, the patient is unable to adduct (i.e., turn it toward the nose) his left eye and enable to look downwards in adduction plane. The patient realizes double image with punctum maximum contralaterally temporally and inferiorly

The most frequent causes of the trochlear nerve palsy:

- Trauma of the tip of the calvaria: the fibers which leave the brainstem dorsally and circumvent advancing forwardly are rather vulnerable.
- Processes located around the tectum can exert compression.
- Cerebrovascular disorders.
- Aneurysm of the basilar artery.
- The congenital form can be assessed by childhood photos. If the vertical strabismus is not so obvious, the compensatory torticollis is usually apparent.
- herpes zoster ophthalmicus: 2–4 weeks after the appearance of rashes.

In the differential diagnosis the case history, the abrupt onset of vertical diplopia, the Camsilon test, cranial CT, cranial MR and detailed neurological examination proved to be the most helpful.

Diagnostic opportunities: Parks-Bielschowsky test, examination by a Hess screen (more details in Chap. 21 and in Chap. 53.)

Abducens Nerve (n. IV.) Palsy

The abducens nerve innervates the **lateral rectus muscle,** which abducts the eyeballs, that is, evokes temporal eye movement in the horizontal plane. It also takes part in the elevation as a depressor together with the vertical ocular muscles. The fibers leaving the nucleus of the nerve form important anatomical and functional connections with the pontine gaze center (pontine paramedian reticular formation, PPFR; for more details the reader is referred to Chap. 55). Leave the brainstem, the two abducens nerves run parallel on both sides of the clivus upward and then penetrate the dura mater, below the processus clinoideus. This long extracranial section is rather vulnerable and frequently can injure consequence of the traumatic basilar skull fractures-, the growth and penetration of tumors- and higher intracranial pressure. The most characteristic ocular symptom of the abducens paresis is double vision because of movement of the eyeball is restricted in the abduction during the lateral gaze in the horizontal plane. In the case of complete plegia, the affected eye shows convergent strabismus and will not move the eyeball outward at all.

The characteristic eye-related symptom

- on the affected side esotropia
- on the affected side to the lateral gaze, the abduction movement is restricted
- the patient reports the largest image displacement upon looking to the direction of abduction palsy.

Clinical manifestations

- Unilateral isolated abducens nerve palsy
- Unilateral paresis with horizontal-vertical eye movement dysfunction.
- Bilateral isolated abducens palsy with horizontal-vertical eye movement dysfunction (Fig. 54.6).

The most frequent causes of the abducens nerve palsy:

- Early alarming symptom of higher intracranial pressure (HIP), caudes by
  - axial herniation
  - due to trauma
  - subdural hematoma
  - sinus thrombosis
- Tumorous processes of the skull base or the sphenoid bone
- Basilar skull fracture
- It represents a component of the conjugated horizontal paresis
- Multiple sclerosis (under 40 years)
- Circulatory disorders of the brainstem – part of the VBI
- Brainstem tumors, mainly due to gliomas together with pyramidal and cerebellar symptoms (Fig. 54.7).

Abducens Nerve Palsy: Non – Isolated Forms

- *Millard-Gubler syndrome:* abducens and facial nerve paresis together with contralateral hemiplegia.
- *Foville's syndrome:* abducens and facial nerve paresis together with ipsilateral conjugated gaze paresis.
- *Gradenigo's syndrome:* combination of abducens and trigeminal nerve lesions (due to meningeoma of the apex of the pyramid of the temporal bone)

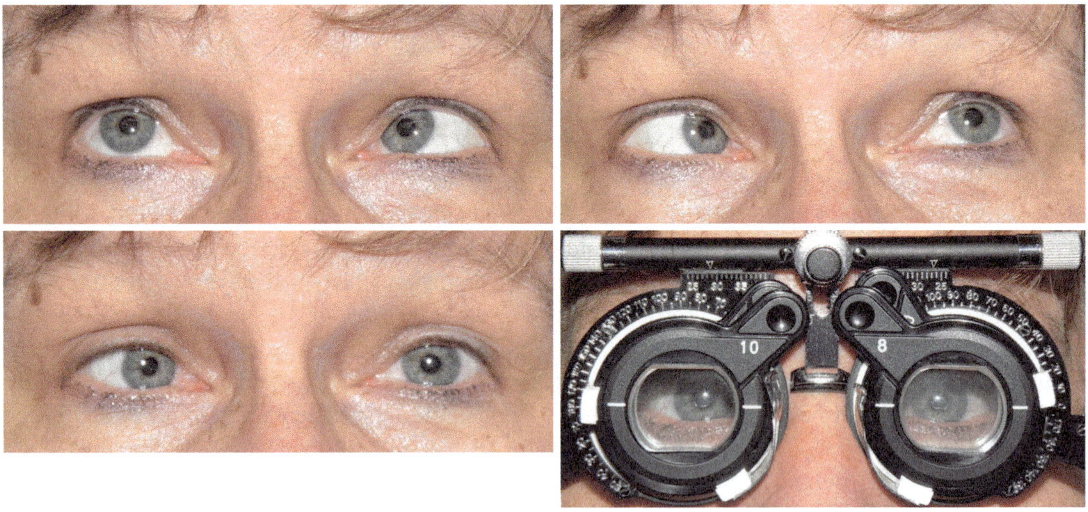

Fig. 54.6 Bilateral abducens nerve (right>>left) palsy. Upon straight gaze (in primary position): Convergent strabismus of the right eye: owing to the abduction plegia of the right nervus VI. The consequence of its is the right eye incapable of turning to temporal direction). Upon right upward gaze: The elevation of the right eye in abduction lags behind the parallel movement of the left eye. Upon left upward gaze. The movement of the left eye lags behind the concomitant movements of the right eye. Although the first therapeutic option is surgical in such a severe strabismus, with prism correction the vision problems of the bilateral, but dominantly right abduction weakness. Vertical misalignment cannot be observed in either direction

- *acoustic neurinoma:* concomitant paresis of the abducens, the trigeminal, the facial and the vestibulocochlear nerves.
- *disorders of the cavernous sinus* (aneurysm, fistula, carcinoma, meningeoma, intracavernous thrombosis).
- *intracranial sinus thrombosis*
- *syndrome of the superior orbital fissure.*
- *syndrome of the orbital apex*

Differential diagnosis

Duane's syndrome (or Duane's retraction syndrome)

(the most of them frequent congenital eye movement disorders, that can mimic bilateral abducens palsy in childhood)

- it is diagnosed in childhood and it does not cause diplopia
- on the affected eye, the abduction manoeuvre can not be to execute
- Upon abduction the bulb retracts and the palpebral fissure narrows.
- Upon adduction the palpebral fissure widens.
- Etiopathomechanism: due to inborn paradoxical innervation, even the external rectus

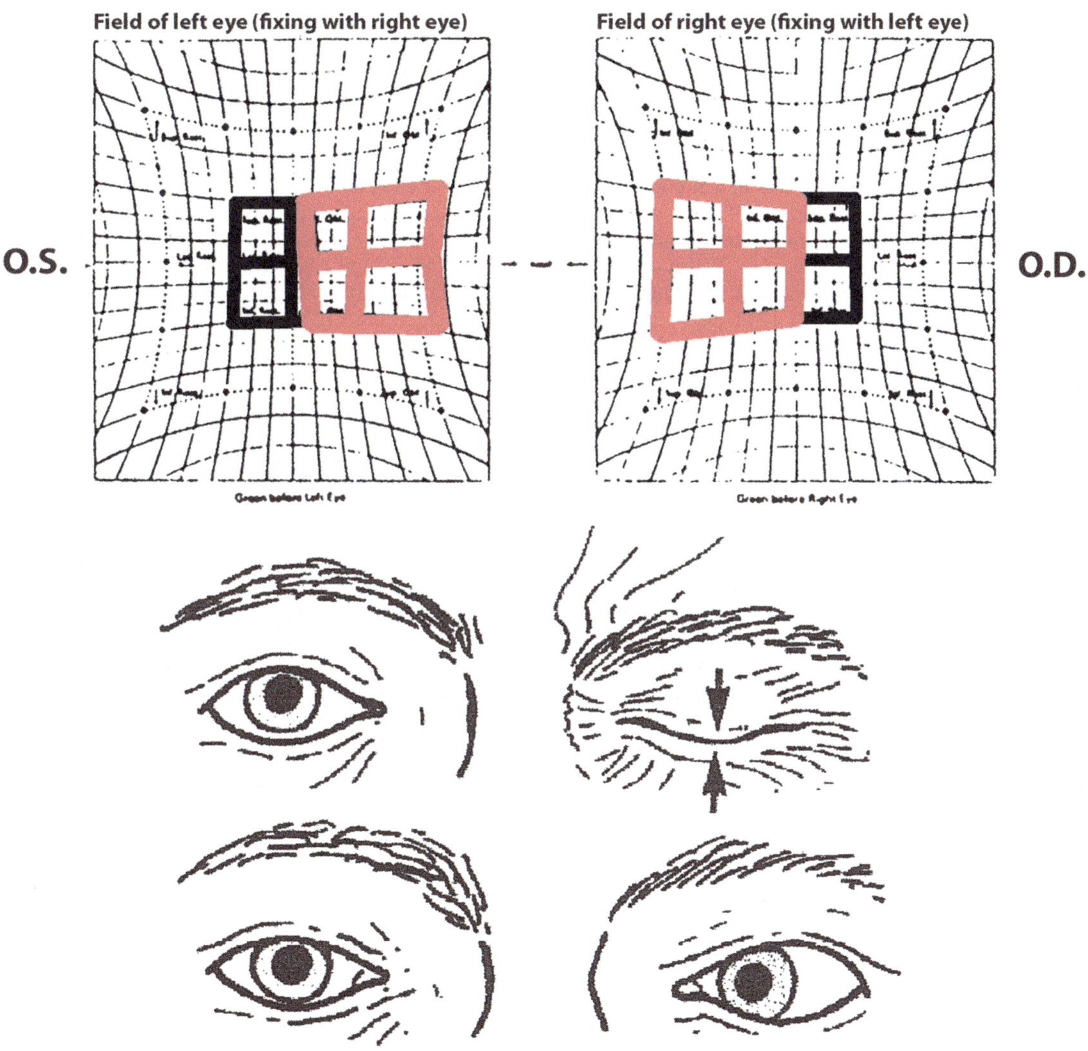

Fig. 54.7 *Up*: Hess screen chart: the figure represents the image displacement reported by the patient in the case of bilateral abducens nerve palsy with left over right side *Down*: Graphical illustration of the ocular signs of the bilateral abducens nerve palsy with left side dominance

muscle is pathological innervated by the oculomotor nerve. *(for more details the reader is referred to* Chap. 23.)

Further Readings

Arruga J, et al. Chronic isolated trochlear nerve palsy produced by intracavernous internal carotid artery aneurysm. J Clin Neuroophthalmol. 1991;11(2):104–8.

Baker RS, et al. Vertical ocular motility disturbance in pseudotumor cerebri. J Clin Neuroophthalmol. 1985;5:41–4.

Borchert MS. Principles and techniques of the examination of ocular motility and alignment. In: Miller NR, Newman NJ, editors. Walsh & Hoyt's: clinical neuro-ophthalmology. Philadelphia: Lippincott Williams 2005. p. 887–906.

Brandt T, et al. Different types of skew deviation. J Neurol Psychiatry. 1991;54:549–50.

Brandt T, et al. Skew deviation with ocular torsion: a vestibular brainstem sign of topographic diagnostic value. Ann Neurol. 1993;33:528–34.

Burde RM, et al. Clinical decisions in neuroophthalmology. St Louis: Mosby; 1985.

Calvert PS. Disorders of neuromuscular transmission. In: Miller NR, Newman NJ, editors. Walsh & Hoyt's: clinical neuro-ophthalmology. Philadelphia: Lippincott Williams 2005. p. 1041–84.

Cogan D. Neurology of the ocular muscles. Springfield: CH Thomas; 1956.

Davis SL. Modeling Uhthoff's phenomenon in MS patients with internuclear ophthalmoparesis. Neurology. 2008; 70(13 Part 2):1098–106.

Dietrich M, et al. Wallenberg's syndrome: lateropulsion, cyclorotation and subjective visual vertical in thirty-six patients. Ann Neurol. 1992;31:399–408.

Dietrich M, et al. Ocular torsion and tilt of subjective visual vertical use sensitive brainstem signs. Ann Neurol. 1993;33:292–9.

Dieterich M, Brandt TH. Vestibular syndromes and vertigo. In: Bogousslasky J, Caplan L, editors. Stroke syndromes. Cambridge/New York: Cambridge University Press; 2001. p. 129–43.

Frohman EM, et al. The utility of MRI in suspected MS. Report of the therapeutics and technology assessment subcommittee of the American Academy of Neurology. Neurology. 2003;61:602–11.

Guy JR, et al. Paraneoplastic downbeating nystagmus (a sign of occult malignancy). J Clin Neuroophthalmol. 1988;8(4):269–72.

Halmágyi GM. GM aid coll tonic contraversive ocular tilt reaction due to unilateral meso-diencephalic lesion. Neurology. 1990;40:1503–9.

Herzau V. Myasthenia gravis. Supplementum of course of strabismus and neuroophthalmology on IXth congress of the European Society of Ophthalmology. Brussels; 1992.

Jay WM, et al. Pseudo-internuclear ophthalmoplegia with downshoot in MG gravis. J Clin Neuroophthalmol. 1987;7(2):74–6.

Kawasaki A. Disorders of pupillary function, accommodation, lacrimation. In: Miller NR, Newman NJ, editors. Walsh & Hoyt's: clinical neuro-ophthalmology. Philadelphia: Lippincott Williams 2005. p. 739–805.

Keane JR. Internuclear ophthalmoplegia: unusual causes in 114 of 410 patients. Arch Neurol. 2005;62(5): 714–7.

Kennard C. The supranuclear control of eye movements. Supplement of IXth EUPO Course. 1992.

Korányi K, et al. Az ophthalmoneurológiai diagnosztika és a szemészeti terápia MG és endocrin ophthalmopathia együttes előfordulásakor [Diagnostics in ophthalmoneurology and ophthalmological therapy in concomitant MG and endocrine ophthalmopathy]. Szemeszet. 1986;123:132–8.

Pierrot- Deseilligny CH. Eye movement abnormalities. In: Bogousslasky J, Caplan L, editors. Stroke syndromes. Cambridge/New York: Cambridge University Press; 2001. p. 76–86.

Sargent JC. Nuclear and infranuclear ocular motility disorders. In: Miller NR, Newman NJ, editors. Walsh & Hoyt's: clinical neuro-ophthalmology. Philadelphia: Lippincott Williams 2005. p. 907–68.

Somlai J. Az agytörzsi eredetű szemmozgászavarok vizsgálatának új irányzatai [New ways in examining eye movement disorders of brain stem origin]. Ideggyógy Szeml. 1999;52:5–6.

Zee DS, Newman-Toker DE. Supranuclear and internuclear ocular motility disorders. In: Miller NR, Newman NJ, editors. Walsh & Hoyt's: clinical neuro-ophthalmology. Philadelphia: Lippincott Williams & Wilkins; 2005. p. 907–68.

Eye Movement Disorders Related to Brainstem Dysfunctions -Types, Clinical Significance of Vertical Localization, Modern Therapeutic Principles

55

Judit Somlai

Contents

The **brainstem** as a *"sending-receiving relay station* " connects the periphery (the oculomotor cranial nerves and their nuclei of the brainstem to the highest cortical supranuclear systems. It is here that conjugated eye movements are first coordinated. The most important anatomical and physiological aspects of the brainstem and supranuclear control of the eye movements are available in details in Chapter 5.4. In the case of injuries to the oculomotor systems of the brainstem the eye movements become disconjugated in the vertical and/or horizontal planes. At the same time, torsional movements can also be affected. Beside its several physiological functions of vital importance, the brainstem plays a role in the coordination of balance and movements. This process is based upon the activity of the oculovestibular pathway system. This system consists of a vestibular part which controls the body position and its activity is coordinated with that of the regulatory neurons, which regulate the postural skeletal muscles and the eye movements. Therefore, eye movement disorders of brainstem origin are frequently associated with vertigo, imbalance, unsteady gait and walk and diplopia upon changing head and body posture.

J. Somlai, M.D.
Unit of Neuro-Ophthalmology, Department of Neurology & Stroke, Military Hospital, Budapest, Hungary

Neuro-Ophthalmology Section, Hungarian Ophthalmological Association, Budapest, Hungary

Trustee, NOSZA Foundation (for the Prevention and Screening of Ocular Storke), Budapest, Hungary
e-mail: dr@somlaijudit.hu; http://somlaijudit.hu

J. Somlai, T. Kovács (eds.), *Neuro-Ophthalmology*, DOI 10.1007/978-3-319-28956-4_55

Options in the Differentiation of Peripheral and Central Eye Movement Disorders

Peripheral neurogenic ocular muscle palsies present with so disturbing diplopia that usually the patient immediately turns to a physician. In contrast, the central disconjugated eye movement disorders lead to a much milder image displacement; it is also accompanied by other neurological symptoms, and therefore they are generally first recognized by the neurologist. Even the proper description of the symptoms related to the perception of outlines and depth and the visual signs brought about by changing head and body posture appear to be difficult for the patients, mainly due the frustrating but very elusive characteristics of the symptoms. The most typical complaints reflect disturbance of stereopsy, vertigo upon gaze changes, transient blurred vision and frequent disability to walk stairs. These symptoms are related to the physiological activity of the brainstem, which serves as a subcortical "preprocessing" center of the conjugated eye movements. Therefore, its functional impairment severely impairs the basics of the whole organization process leading to disconjugated eye movements. In the majority of the cases, several eye muscles are afflicted simultaneously. Therefore, the syndromes usually present with symmetrical image displacement in both the horizontal and/or vertical plane. Disorders of fixation due to dysfunction of torsion are not rare findings either.

Narrowing of the visual field is illustrated by a pair of Hess charts (Fig. 55.1). In peripheral neurogenic paresis while narrowing of the field of vision is accompanied by borderline shift brought about by the overcompensated activity of the contralateral synergistic muscles. The displaced images cannot be fused and the disturbing diplopia is eliminated by the central nervous system. Central eye movement disorder leads to an almost symmetrical and much less frustrating image disparity. This milder diplopia does not lead to visual impairment or only causes a moderate one which patients have difficulty describing.

The clinical characteristics observed in eye movement disorders are summarized in the following Table.

Differential diagnosis	
Peripheral paresis	Central eye muscle paresis
Large image disparity the patient immediately turns to ophthalmologist It cannot be corrected even by the largest prism dioptry (PD) Causal treatment – surgical intervention on the eye muscles Then the residual deviation should be corrected by PD	Symmetrical image displacement better tolerated double vision Then the patient turns to neurologist It may be corrected by PD (below 10 PD) By prism can be corrected in the horizontal and/or the vertical plane but the torsion problem cannot be corrected

**PD* prism dioptry eye glass-correction

Central eye movement dysfunctions caused by brainstem disorders are usually in the background of the following diseases:

- cerebrovascular,
- traumatic and
- demyelinization processes.

In the clinical practice, a small lacunar infarction or plaque (which remains invisible even by MR) can result in brainstem dysfunction impairing in some phases of the multistep mechanism of the eye movements (e.g., uni- or bilateral paresis of adduction and abduction). However, more extended brainstem lesions will lead to uni- or bilateral complete gaze palsy.

The Most Frequent Clinical Syndromes of the Eye Movement Disorders Caused by Brainstem Diseases

For didactic purposes, these eye movement disorders of the brainstem will be classified by a topographic localization: We tried to classify the level

Fig. 55.1 Graphical representations of the Hess screen. Comparative illustration of the typical image displacements between peripheral and central ocular muscle palsies result in double vision. The *black lines* depict the normal alignment, and the *red lines* reflect the image displacement reported by the patient

IMAGE DISPLACEMENTS AND DIPLOPIAS IN PERIPHERAL AND CENTRAL EYE MUSCLE PALSIES RECORDED BY A HESS SCREEN

IN PERIPHERAL AND CENTRAL EYE MUSCLE PARESIS

Dg.: OCULOMOTOR NERVE PALSY
on the leftSaccular aneurysm rupture
and subarachnoid hemorrhage
of the internal carotid artery on the left

Left Eye

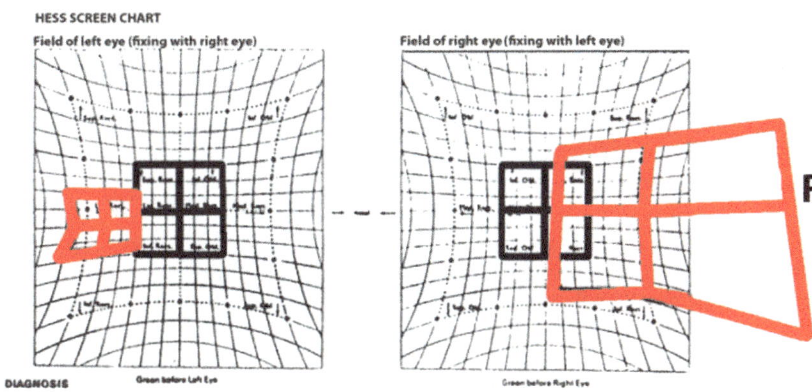

Right Eye

CENTRAL EYE MUSCLE PARESIS

Dg.: ABDUCENS NERVE PALSY on both sides
and SKEW DEVIATION
Superior, homonymous central quadrantanopia on the right.
Ischemic lesion in the territory of the left occipital lobe

Left Eye

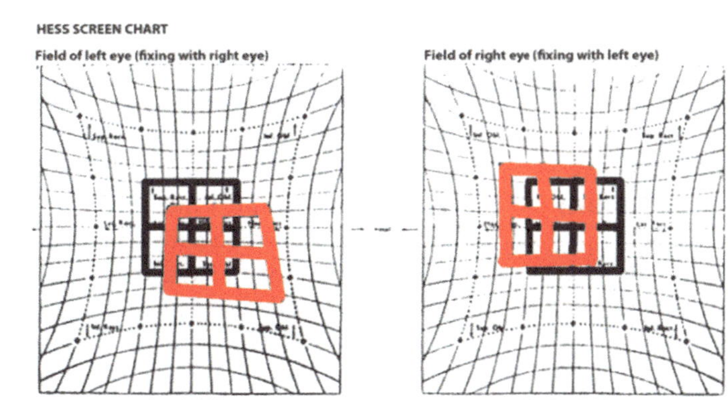

Right Eye

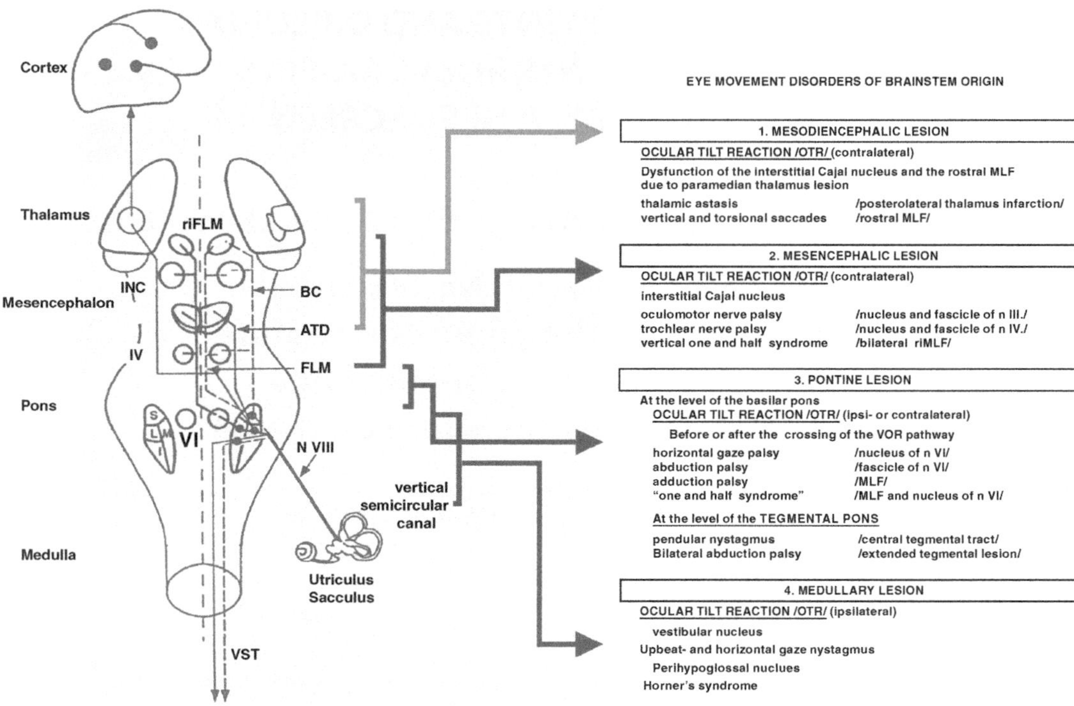

Fig. 55.2 Classification in Table and graphical illustration of the topographic localization of eye movement disorders of brainstem (Redrawn after Brandt et al. (1993))

of the brainstem injury leading to the typical functional disorders of the eye movements. For example horizontal eye movement disorders are related to the injuries of the pontine regions, which coordinate the horizontal and conjugated horizontal-vertical eye movements. However, it is the oculovestibular system which begins in the pontomedullary region and crosses the complete brainstem vertically that coordinates the vertical eye movement. Therefore, vertical eye movement disorders are the consequence of injuries in the oculovestibular system and can be classified into a completely different group (see Fig. 55.2).

Horizontal Eye Movement Disorders of the Brainstem

- conjugated gaze palsy
- classical internuclear ophthalmoparesis (INO)
- WEBINO syndrome
- the so-termed "one and a half" syndrome
- conjugated gaze palsy

Horizontal Eye Movement Disorders of the Brainstem

In ***conjugated gaze palsies (conjugate deviation)*** the patient cannot look into the direction of the lesion, *"looks away from the side of the lesion"* – a sign of more extended brainstem injuries. The most frequent causes are the thrombosis of the basilar artery, multiple sclerosis, pontine gliomas or Wernicke's encephalopathy.

In everyday clinical practice, internuclear ophthalmoplegia (INO) develops in the population of under 40 mainly due to demyelinization processes, while in the elder generations due to cerebrovas-cular disorders.

Etiopathomechanisms should focus on the fact that the syndrome indicates the uni- or bilateral dysfunction of one of the most primordial pathway systems, the *medial longitudinal fasciculus (MLF)* of the brainstem. This pathway system is one of the most important coordinators of the horizontal conjugated eye movements. When looking in a lateral direction, impulses will run

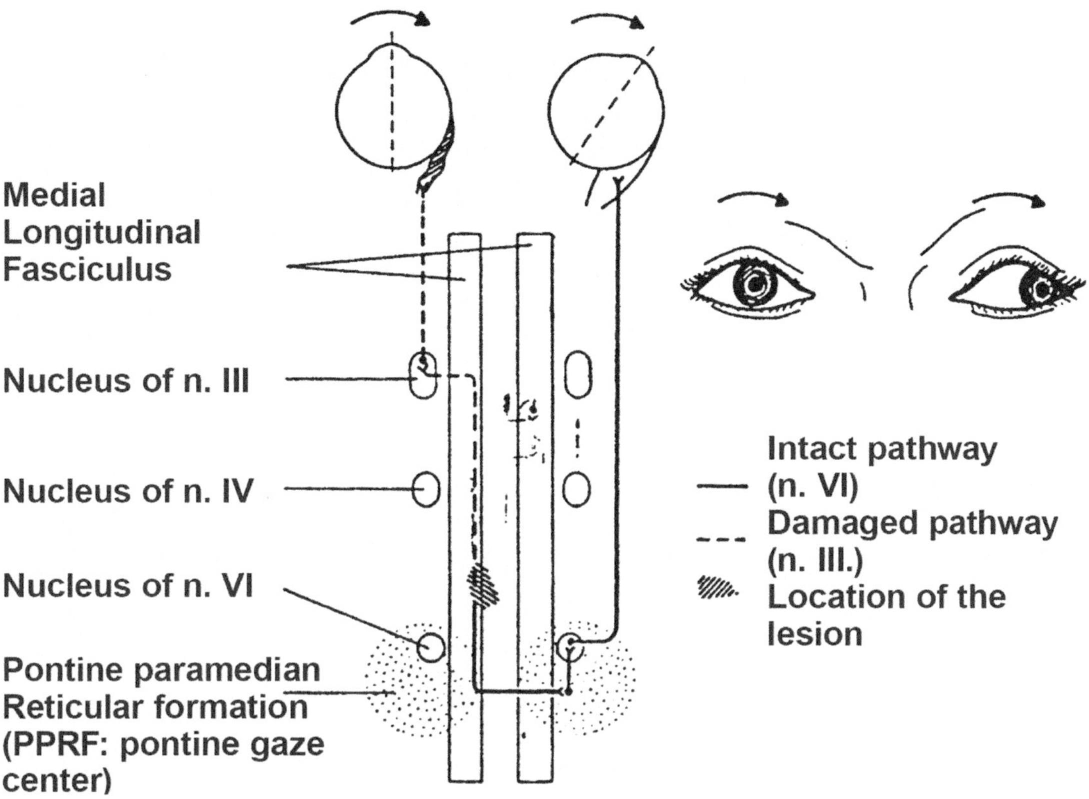

Fig. 55.3 The graphical representation of the presumed pathomechanism of the internuclear ophthalmoplegia (INO) and the disorder of eye alignment upon conjugated leftward gaze

from the *pontine gaze center (Pontine Paramedian Reticular Formation, PPRF)* to the ipsilateral *abducens nucleus,* evoking ipsilateral abduction and, at the same time, the pontine medial longitudinal fasciculus activates the contralateral *oculomotor nucleus* leading to the adduction of the opposite eye (see the graphical illustration of Fig. 55.3).

Clinical Manifestations of INO

1. Unilateral internuclear ophthalmoplegia (INO): Due to the *unilateral lesion of the MLF*. Unilateral weakness of adduction and preserved capabilities of abduction and convergence. It develops mainly due to cerebrovascular disorders, as the blood supply of the brainstem is symmetrically unilateral and end-arterial till the territory of the paramedian system. In contrast, asymmetrical forms often develop multiple sclerosis (see Fig. 55.4).
2. Bilateral INO: Making the patient look into both directions in the horizontal plane, the adduction movements are paretic, while the abduction is spared. However, when the convergence also becomes affected; even upon straight gaze a *"divergent misalignment"* can be noticed. This is the "Wall-Eyed Bilateral Internuclear Ophthalmoplegias" (WEBINO) syndrome, when upon straight gaze both eyes are in "divergent misalignment".
3. The "one and a half" syndrome: The name derives from the fact that beside intact vertical eye movements, the patient's eye on the *affected side cannot move into either horizontal direction*. Furthermore, the *contralateral eye only can abduct in the horizontal plane*. According to the proposed pathomechanism, bilateral MLF lesion

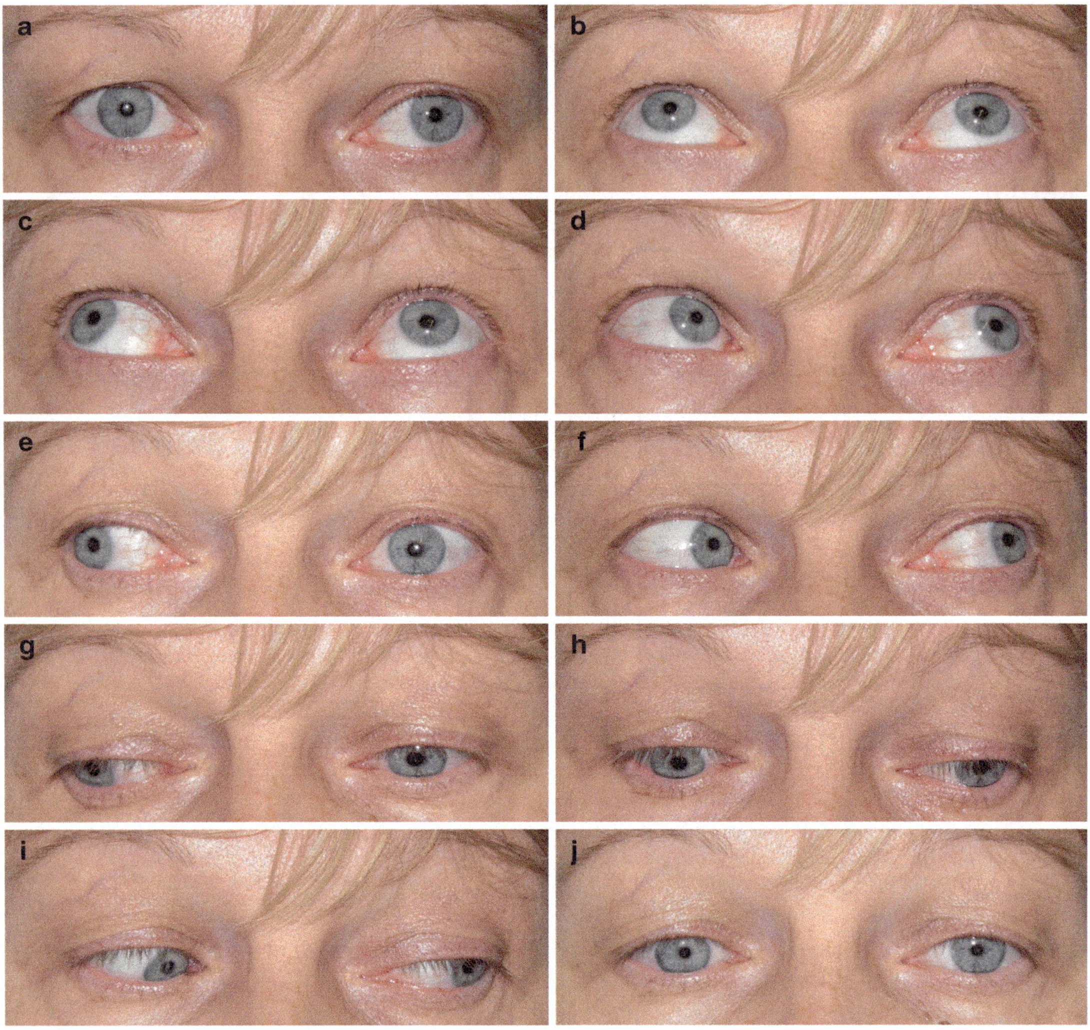

Fig. 55.4 Left-sided internuclear ophthalmoplegia. (**a**) in primary position: divergent strabismus of the left eye (adduction paresis) (**b**) in the direction of upward gaze: divergent strabismus of the left eye (adduction paresis) (**c**) right upward gaze: left eye adduction paresis of the left eye (**d**) left upward gaze: conjugated alignment (**e**) leftward gaze: horizontal gaze adduction paresis of the left eye (**f**) rightward gaze: horizontal gaze conjugated alignment (**g**) right downward gaze: adduction paresis of the left eye (**h**) vertical downward gaze: divergent strabismus of the left eye (adduction paresis) (**i**) left downward gaze: conjugated alignment (**j**) convergence paresis of the left eye

leads to *bilateral adduction paresis*, accompanied by the *dysfunction of the pontine gaze center (PPRF)* (see Figs. 55.5 and 55.6).

1. **Anterior internuclear ophthalmoplegia (ant-INO).**

   It is characterized by bilateral adduction weakness, convergence paresis or complete plegia, which is often accompanied by vertical eye movement disorder. The latter is also asymmetrical, with one eye moving upwards while the other one downwards. In the most critical cases a "see–saw nystagmus" can be observed, which reflects the alternated, opposite, vertical jerks of the eyes. The most frequent reasons are brainstem hemorrhage due to a hypertensive crisis or multiple sclerosis.
2. **Posterior internuclear ophthalmoplegia (post – INO):**

   The pathological process as classical INO can develop between the pontine nucleus of the nerve abducens and the nucleus n. III. in

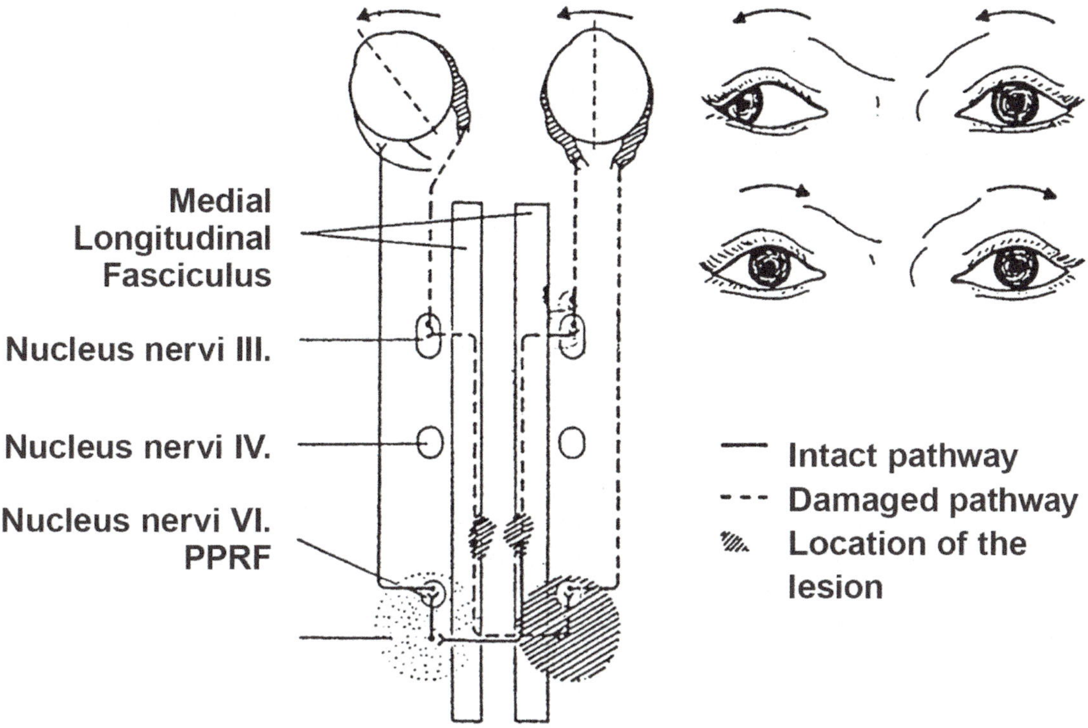

Fig. 55.5 The graphical representation of the pathomechanism of the "one and a half" syndrome, and the depiction figure: pathological eye alignments in horizontal eye movements

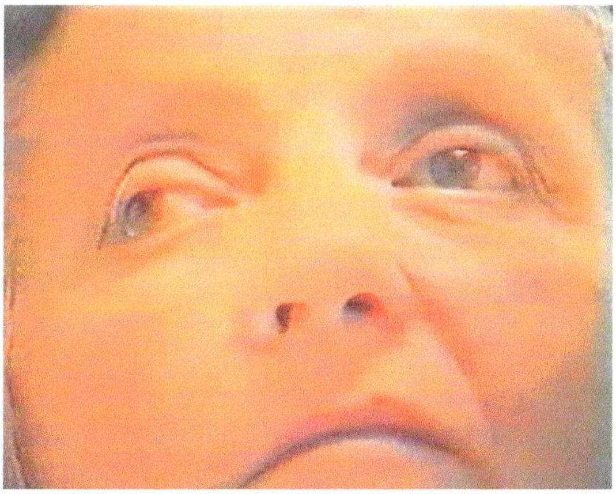

Fig. 55.6 "One and a half" syndrome: In primary position the right eye is fixated in abduction, as it cannot adduct. Therefore, it looks into nasal direction upon horizontal leftward gaze. The left eye remains in mid-alignment upon horizontal gaze in both directions. It caused by bilateral internuclear ophthalmoplegia (INO) and left conjugated gaze paresis: right INO (1/2) + left complete horizontal gaze paresis (Arruga et al. 1991)

the mesencephalon. It is characterized as an "ataxic nystagmus with INO". During horizontal smooth pursuit eye movements in the extreme abduction, we can observe a violent abductive nystagmus and a mild adductive nystagmus; a so-termed end point nystagmus, which may be bilateral and caused by multiple sclerosis and pontine glioma (Recklinghausen neurofibromatosis in childhood).

In neurological clinical practice "transient bilateral INO with end point nystagmus of the abduction eye position" was described as a side effect of some antiepileptic medicines.

3. Inverz INO: During conjugated horizontal movement we can observe abduction paresis with intact adduction. The etiopathomechanism is unknown.
4. **Bilateral abduction paresis:**
   A syndrome supposedly similar to inverse INO, bilateral abduction paresis is characterized by *bilateral abduction weakness* in the

horizontal eye movement. Frequent reasons of this syndrome are as follows:

- Higher intracranial pressure with different origins (earlier onset than papilledema)
- Brainstem glioma in childhood with facial paresis and abducens paresis
- tumors in the posterior cranial fossa
- tumors of the posterior cranial fossa
  - in childhood: rapidly progressing cerebellar tumors
  - in adults: primarily ependymomas
  - slowly progressing posterior fossa tumors(chordomas, cholesteatomas and meningeomas)
  - metastatic processes
- Brainstem cerebrovascular events often result in brainstem abduction paresis. Most frequently it is caused by pontine paramedian infarction, which later may also be accompanied by conjugated gaze palsy.
- Transient brainstem symptoms and signs can be elicited by the atherosclerotic ectasia and aneurysm of the basilar artery which can lead to a compression of the anterior surface of the brainstem. (*neurocompression of the brainstem*)

Vertical Eye Movement Disorders of the Brainstem

Vertical gaze palsy develops due to the dysfunction of the upper brainstem regions (i.e., the rostral portion of the medial longitudinal fasciculus (MLF) and the region of the interstitial nucleus of Cajal) and the pathways which connect them. The studies of great clinical and practical significance by professor Th. Brandt and professor M. Dieterich (Brandt et al. 1991, 1993; Dietrich et al. 1992, 1993; Dieterich & Brandt 2001) revealed that the lesion of the mesodiencephalic and paramedian thalamus regions results in the disorder of the integration of the cyclo-vertical conjugated eye movements. The etiopathomechanism of the vertical eye movement disorders of brainstem origin may reveal such conditions as the diseases of the extrapyramidal motoric system, cerebrovascular disorders and less frequently midline space-occupied processes.

Clinical Manifestations and the Most Frequent Syndromes

1. **Parinaud's syndrome (DMB): Upward and/or downward gaze paresis**

Parinaud's syndrome ***(Dorsal MidBrain syndrome, DMB)*** is an eye movement disorder which most frequently develops due to the dysfunction of the pontomesencephalic region and associates with the direct compression elicited by midline tumors (pinealoma, periaqueductal astrocytoma, etc.) or the indirect effect exerted by occlusive hydrocephalus. Clinical symptoms:

- *Upward gaze palsy*, *"upbeat nystagmus"*: At the beginning, as the introductory sign of the *upward gaze palsy*, *"upbeat nystagmus"* develops when the elevation is possible but, at the upper limit of the movement, a nystagmus with upward quick phase reflects the beginning of the upward gaze paresis.
- *Upward gaze weakness*: Upon smooth pursuit eye movements symmetrical or asymmetrical *upward gaze weakness* of one or both eyes.
- *Convergence weakness*: It can also be noticed and upon provocation convergence spasm develops.
- Ophthalmoplegia interna: Also early symptoms of the syndrome are the *paresis* and finally *the plegia of the pupil indirect reactions*
- *Anisocoria, "light-near dissociation"*: usually reflects a rather advanced stage of the disorder, however upon the examination of convergence the pupils still constrict; that is the *"light-near dissociation"* (see Chap. 52.)
- *Eye-ball – bulbs retraction:* There is a pathological simultaneous contraction is reflected by the *retraction of the bulbs* upon triggering convergence.
- *Retraction of the eyelids*: The *upward gaze palsy* is frequently accompanied by the *pathological retraction of the eyelids.*

Differential diagnostics of upward gaze palsy:

- P*seudoparesis of the upward gaze* can develop due to isolated myositis or endocrine myopathy

(autoimmune thyroiditis) of inferior rectus muscle and medial rectus muscle
- Consequence of the neurogen pareses (most frequently due to lesion of the oculomotor nerve), regeneration often takes place in muscles other than the ones causing the paresis, often leading to *pathological reinnervation.*

2. **"Symmetrical vertical image displacement" or "skew deviation"**

Vertical eye movement disorders (mainly the internuclear ophthalmoplegias) are frequently accompanied by this eye movement disorder, which leads to ***image displacement in the vertical and oblique planes namely "skew deviation"***.

The symptoms may disturb the daily activity of the patient while driving or walking stairs, and they can impede line shifting during reading. In neurological clinical practice, it is the most frequent consequence of cerebrovascular disorders. Its etiopathomechanism is detailed in connection with the ocular tilt.

3. **"Ocular tilt" syndrome**

The **vestibulo-ocular reflex (VOR) mechanism** establishes an essential function of the brainstem.

The physiology of the VOR:

It represents a synchronizing process, during which changing the position of the head and body posture can be completed by a compensatory eye movement. The functional principle of the pathway, that tilting the head leads to the activation of the receptors in the inner ear by the otholiths. Then the neural pathways will switch in the vestibular nuclei and establish connection with the nuclei and pathways of the oculomotor nerves through the activity of the aforementioned MLF pathway system. This way upon tilting the head the eyes produce ***a conjugated, compensatory eye movement that is in the opposite direction of the head movement and which consists of horizontal, vertical and torsional components.***

The lesion of the vestibulo-ocular reflex (VOR) (see Fig. 55.7) leads to the dysregulation of these complex processes and results in a characteristic triad of symptoms. The symptoms of **pathological head tilt** and the simultaneous eye movement disorder are referred in the literature as "**ocular tilt reactions" (OTR)**.

Characteristics of the Ocular Tilt Reaction (OTR) (Lesion of the Vestibulo-Ocular Reflex (VOR))

I. **Pathological head tilt**, which is of different etiopathomechanism than the compensatory posture of the head related to trochlear nerve palsy.
II. "**Skew deviation"** (i.e., **symmetrical vertical image displacement** due to the dysfunction of the horizontal–vertical eye movements) and/or internuclear ophthalmoplegia (see Fig. 55.8)
III. Upon lateral gaze, a **horizontal–torsional nystagmus**, which reveals the dysfunction of the physiological, rotator eye movements.

Prof. M. Dieterich and ***Prof. Th. Brandt*** (Brandt et al. 1991, 1993) have publicated the most significant volume of publications related to the etiopathomechanism and differential diagnostics of the symptoms of the Ocular Tilt Reaction (OTR) (lesion of the vestibulo-ocular reflex (VOR) diseases. The three forms of symmetrical, oblique image displacement or skew deviation can be elicited by various lesions affecting different levels of the brainstem. (Classification according to Th. Brandt, Fig. 55.9.)

The clinical appearance form of Skew Deviation (SD):

1st FORM OF SD:

In the first form, due to the *disease of the semicircular canals (Tullio phenomenon),* both eyes marked as hyperphoria with higher vertical position by different degrees.

2nd form of SD:

In the second type, usually only either eye is of higher position (hyperphoria) in primary position, usually due to the lesions of the *nuclei and pathways of the vestibular system or the medulla oblongata.*

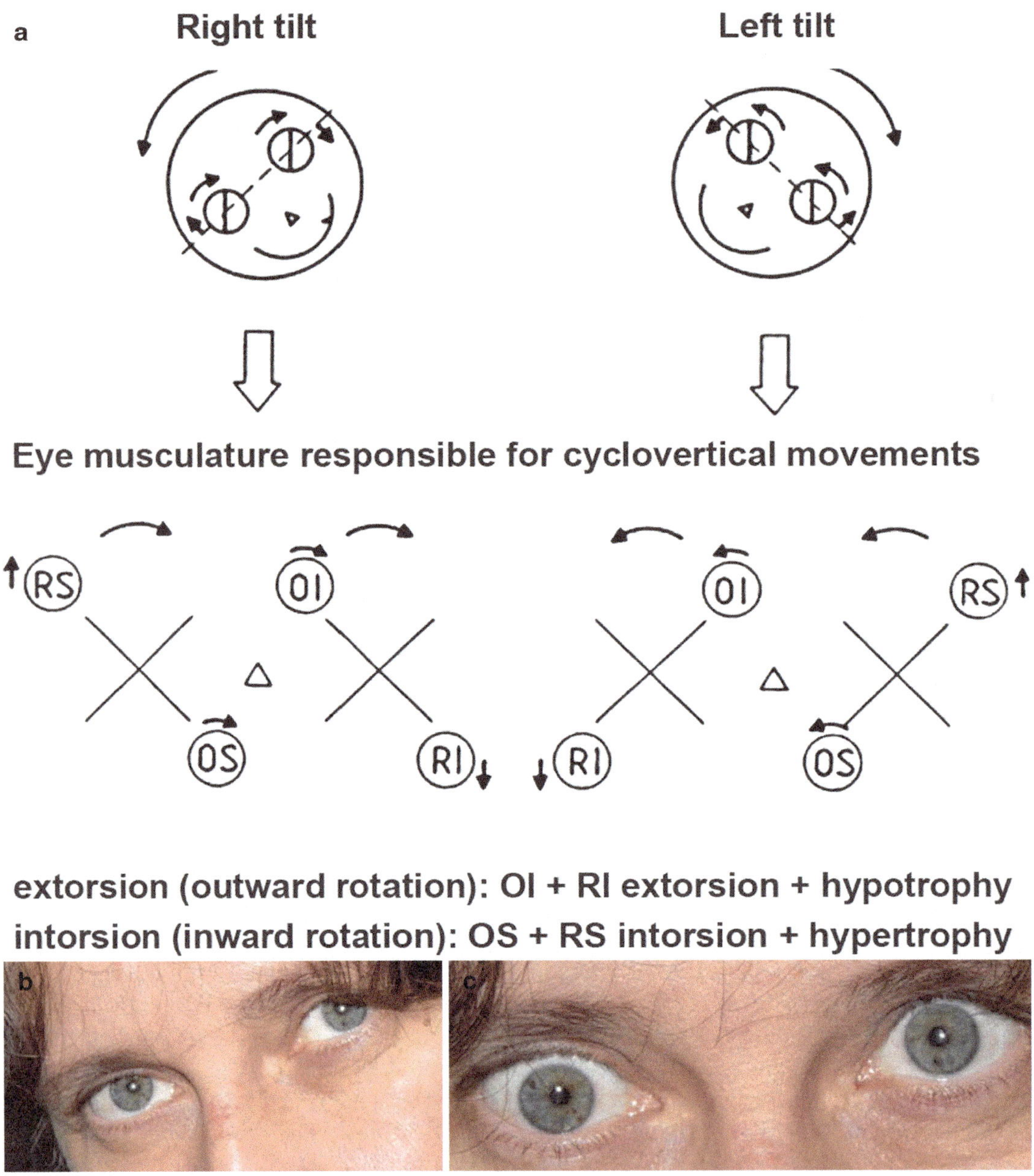

Fig. 55.7 (**a**) The physiological vestibulo-ocular reflex (VOR) is a conjugated, compensatory eye movement that is in the opposite direction of the head movement mechanism upon the head tilt. (**b**) The clinical consequence of the pathological VOR process: pathological head tilt caused by OTR. (**c**) The same patient' eyes position in primary position without pathological head tilt: typical skew deviation of eyes (right hypophoria, left hyperphoria)

3rd form of SD:

In the most frequent third form, one eye is of higher (hyperphoria) and the other is of lower position (hypophoria) due to lesion dysfunction of the *mesodiencephalic regions of brainstem.*

The clinical important of the establishment of OTR in topographic localization of brainstem disorders were concluded by *Th. Brand and M. Dieterich.* They are based upon data compiled from numerous cases of brainstem stroke and provide indispensable help in localisation diagnostics.

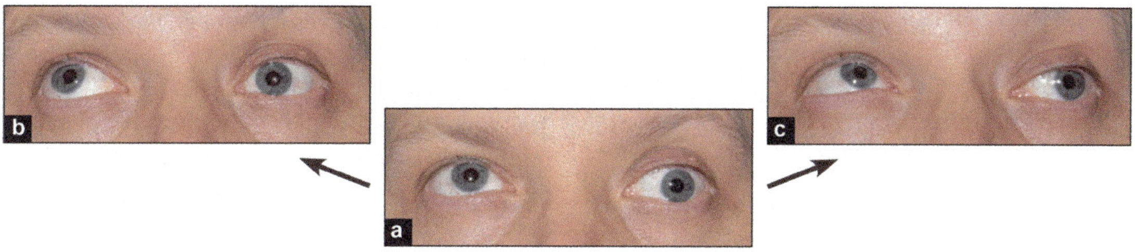

Fig. 55.8 Ocular tilt reaction: skew deviation and bilateral internuclear ophthalmoplegia (INO). (**a**) In primary position: symmetrical skew image displacement, skew deviation with right hyperphoria and left hypophoria (**b**) right upward gaze: weakness of adduction due to bilateral internuclear ophthalmoplegia (INO) with skew deviation (**c**) left upward gaze: weakness of adduction due to bilateral internuclear ophthalmoplegia (INO) with skew deviation

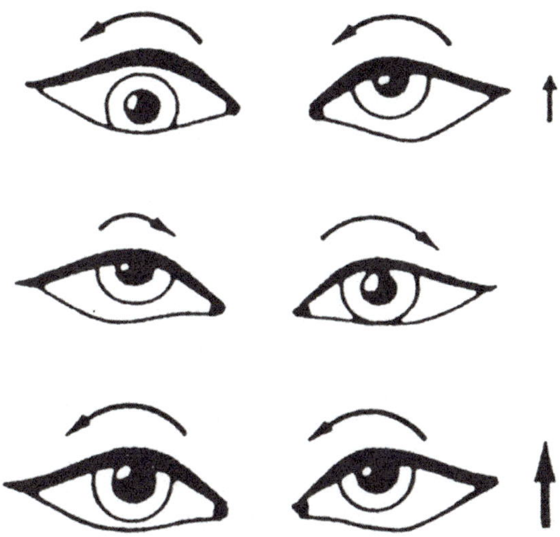

Fig. 55.9 Th. Brandt (Brandt et al. 1991): the different types of skew deviation (Redrawn after Th. Brandt et al. (1991))

1. *Unilateral dysfunction of the VOR marks:* **pontomedullary injury to the VOR pathway.**
2. *Contralateral symptomatic triad of VOR dysfunction maks:* **pontomesencephalic section of the VOR pathway is injured**.

Differential Diagnostics of Eye Movement Disorders of Brainstem Origin

The following syndromes may present with eye movement disorders, which manifest themselves similarly to those of brainstem origin, but are of different etiopathomechanism.

1. The non-isolated forms of ocular muscle palsies can develop due to *intraaxial alternating syndromes* or *extraaxial brainstem lesions* (see details in Chap. 60).
2. In *endocrine myopathy* – myositis: inflammation, scarring and contracture of any ocular muscle leads to secondary dysfunction wich may imitate the clinical symptoms and signs of neurogenic pareses (see Chap. 60.)
3. *Ocular myasthenia gravis* represents the dysfunction of each eye muscles due to the disorder of the neuromuscular junction, which leads to both isolated and conjugated motoric malfunctions. This can be verified with certainty utilizing ocular EMG, diplopia tests and Camsilon test (see Chap. 60.)

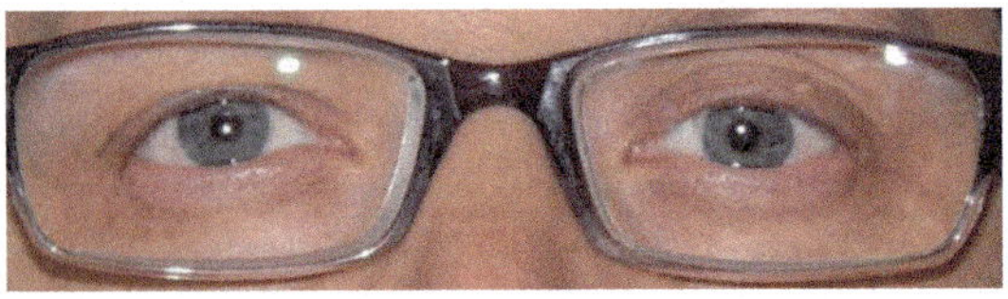

Fig. 55.10 Prism eyeglass correction

Therapeutic Approaches to Eye Movement Disorders of Brainstem Origin

Beside the treatment of the underlying condition, it is strongly recommended to use the prism correction validated in pediatric ophthalmology (see Fig. 55.10). For more details regarding the necessary equipment and the exact determination of the desired correction required for the prescription, the reader is referred to Chapter 22. (Polatest and/or series of prism lenses). This way the necessary prism corrections, which correct the image displacement can be determined in vertical, horizontal and oblique planes. The latter is recommended if the diplopia, due to the eye movement disorder, cannot be cured by pharmaceutical and/or surgical therapy, or the residual image displacement is still not tolerable for the patient and interferes with his/her daily activities. In the case of serious peripheral ocular muscle palsies, which cannot be corrected by prism dioptres, the correctional surgical intervention is the most viable opportunity in the clinical practice. If the patient still complains about diplopia (but it is less than 10 PD), the residual image displacement can be cured by prism correction.

The correction significantly reduces or completely eliminates the considerable skew deviation and alleviates the bilateral adduction weakness. With correction the patient's double vision disappeared for both near and distant and the patient is able to read again even to drive

By the classification of the eye movement disorders caused by brainstem disease is important in our clinical practice, before of **different type of the eye movement syndromes symptomatic constellations refer to specific topographic localization of brainstem, which are characteristic in the determined neurological syndromes.**

For instance, the internuclear ophthalmoplegia, which appears under 40 typically relates to multiple sclerosis, while Parinaud' syndrome is the consequence of midline space occupying processes, which compress the brainstem reflecting their etiology specificity. In addition to by the exact measurement of the degree of the eye movement disorder, the efficiency of the treatment can be better estimated.

References

Arruga J, et al. Chronic isolated trochlear nerve palsy produced by intracavernous internal carotid artery aneurysm. J Clin Neuroophthalmol. 1991;11(2):104–8.

Brandt T, et al. Different types of skew deviation. J Neurol Psychiatry. 1991;54:549–50.

Brandt TH, et al. Skew deviation with ocular torsion: a vestibular brainstem sign of topographic diagnostic value. Ann Neurol. 1993;33:528–34.

Dietrich M, et al. Wallenberg syndrome: lateropulsion, cyclorotation and subjective visual vertical in thirty-six patients. Ann Neurol. 1992;31:399–408.

Dietrich M, et al. Ocular torsion and tilt of subjective visual vertical use sensitive brainstem signs. Ann Neurol. 1993;33:292–9.

Dieterich M, Brandt TH. Vestibular syndromes and vertigo. In: Bogousslasky J, Caplan L, editors. Stroke syndromes. Cambridge/New York: Cambridge University Press; 2001. p. 129–43.

Judit S. Az agytörzsi eredetű szemmozgászavarok vizsgálatának új irányzatai. Ideggyógy Szeml. 1999;52:5–6.

Further Readings

Baker RS, et al. Vertical ocular motility disturbance in pseudotumor cerebri. J Clin Neuroophthalmol. 1985;5:41–4.

Borchert MS. Principles and techniques of the examination of ocular motility and alignment. In: Miller NR, Newman NJ, editors. Walsh & Hoyt's: clinical neuro-ophthalmology. Philadelphia: Lippincott Williams 2005. p. 887–906.

Burde RM, et al. Clinical decisions in neuro-ophthalmology. St. Louis: Mosby; 1985.

Calvert PS. Disorders of neuromuscular transmission. In: Miller NR, Newman NJ, editors. Walsh & Hoyt's: clinical neuro-ophthalmology. Philadelphia: Lippincott Williams 2005. p. 1041–84.

Cogan D. Neurology of the ocular muscles. Springfield: CH Thomas; 1956.

Davis SL. Modeling Uhthoff 's phenomenon in MS patients with internuclear ophthalmoparesis. Neurology. 2008; 70(13 Part 2):1098–106.

Frohman EM, et al. The utility of MRI in suspected MS. Report of the therapeutics and technology assessment subcommittee of the American Academy of Neurology. Neurology. 2003;61:602–11.

Guy JR, et al. Paraneoplastic downbeating nystagmus (a sign of occult malignancy). J Clin Neuroophthalmol. 1988;8(4):269–72.

Halmágyi GM. GM aid coll tonic contraversive ocular tilt reaction due to unilateral meso-diencephalic lesion. Neurology. 1990;40:1503–9.

Herzau V. Myasthenia gravis. Supplementum of course of strabismus and neuro-ophthalmology on IXth congress of the European Society of Ophthalmology. Brussels; 1992.

Jay WM, et al. Pseudo-internuclear ophthalmoplegia with downshoot in MG gravis. J Clin Neuroophthalmol. 1987;7(2):74–6.

Kawasaki A. Disorders of pupillary function, accommodation, lacrimation. In: Miller NR, Newman NJ, editors. Walsh & Hoyt's: clinical neuro-ophthalmology. Philadelphia: Lippincott Williams 2005. p. 739–805.

Keane JR. Internuclear ophthalmoplegia: unusual causes in 114 of 410 patients. Arch Neurol. 2005;62(5): 714–7.

Kennard C. The supranuclear control of eye movements. Supplement of IXth EUPO course. 1992.

Korányi K és mtsa. Az ophthalmoneurológiai diagnosztika és a szemészeti terápia MG és endocrin ophthalmopathia együttes előfordulásakor [Diagnostics in ophthalmology and ophthalmological therapy in concomitant MG and endocrine ophthalmopathy]. Szemészet. 1986;123:132–8.

Pierrot- Deseilligny CH. Eye movement abnormalities. In: Bogousslasky J, Caplan L, editors. Stroke syndromes. Cambridge/New York: Cambridge University Press; 2001. p. 76–86.

Sargent JC. Nuclear and infranuclear ocular motility disorders. In: Miller NR, Newman NJ, editors. Walsh & Hoyt's: clinical neuro-ophthalmology. Philadelphia: Lippincott Williams 2005. p. 907–68.

Szobor A. Myasthenia gravis. Budapest: Akadémia Kiadó; 1990.

Szobor A, et al. Myasthenia gravis: Plasmapheresis kezelés hatása [Myesthenia gravis: the effect of plasmapheresis]. Ideggyógy Szeml. 1983;36:385–90.

Szobor A, et al. Myasthenia gravis: thymectomia eredménye 550 betegen [Myasthenia gravis: the effect of thymectomy in 550 patients]. Orv Hetil. 1990;131(46):2519–24.

Zee DS, Newman-Toker DE. Supranuclear and internuclear ocular motility disorders. In: Miller NR, Newman NJ, editors. Walsh & Hoyt's: clinical neuro-ophthalmology. Philadelphia: Lippincott Williams & Wilkins; 2005. p. 907–68.

The Clinical Significance of Otoneurology in the Diagnosis of Brainstem Disorders

56

Ágnes Szirmai

Contents

Anatomical and Physiological Foundation

The regulatory disorders of balance, gait and posture typically arise as interdisciplinary differential diagnostic problems in the everyday clinical practice. Therefore, as usual, different specialists have their own ways in their clinical approach to the patient. To achieve the optimal therapeutic result, it is essential that they should communicate with each other to share their views in a common language. According to Brandt's concept the vertigo is a multisensory sensorimotor syndrome, with perceptional, autonomic, postural and oculomotor manifestations. While discussing the syndrome, the otoneurologist emphasizes the latter, oculomotor manifestations. Otoneurology, as interdisciplinary subject of otology and neurology deals with vertigo and nystagmus of vestibular origin. The vestibular system is a complex sensory organ. Its receptors are located in the inner ear beside the auditory system and its center is located in the brainstem in the transitional area between the pons and medulla. The 8th cranial nerve consists of two completely separate components (the vestibular and the cochlear nerves). Their common part contains the section between the exit from the brainstem and the internal auditory meatus. The fibers innervating the semicircular canals and the otolith apparatus run to the ganglion Scarpae as vestibular nerve. They reach the lateral recess of the 4th cerebral ventricle then end up in the medial (Schwalbe), lateral (Deiters), superior (Bechterew), and descending spinal (Roller) vestibular nucleus. From these centers important neural pathways arise

- the vestibulospinal and vestibulocervical pathways;
- the vestibulocerebellar pathway;
- the vestibuloocular pathway;
- the vestibuloreticular pathway;
- the vestibulocortical pathway which projects into the temporal cortex.

Á. Szirmai, M.D., PhD
Department of Otorhinolaryngology, Head and Neck Surgery, Faculty of Medicine, Semmelweis University, Budapest, Hungary
e-mail: szirmai.agnes@med.semmelweis-univ.hu; http://drszirmaiagnes.hazipatika.net

J. Somlai, T. Kovács (eds.), *Neuro-Ophthalmology*, DOI 10.1007/978-3-319-28956-4_56

Differential Diagnostics of the Peripheral Vestibular Disorders

The disorders verified by the otoneurological examination as peripheral vestibular lesions belong to the territory of ENT. In the majority of peripheral injuries the nystagmus present as the part of the harmonic vestibular syndrome Caloric stimulation unveils paresis of the semicircular canal, therefore, one ear responds less to both warm and cold stimuli. Except Benign Paroxysmal Positioning Vertigo (BPPV), which typically presents with positional nystagmus. The differential diagnosis is based upon the extent of the vertiginous attack and the accompanying symptoms and signs (Fig. 56.1).

In peripheral injuries, the findings elicited by caloric stimulation show protean clinical picture, which ranges from the complete loss of function to the mild dysfunction. In the acute phase, the caloric reaction can be difficult to assess due to presence of spontaneous nystagmus. As the acute phase subsides, the semicircular paresis becomes readily apparent. Upon warm stimulus on the affected side the spontaneous nystagmus still persists, while on the intact side, it becomes more obvious due to the retained sensitivity. Cold stimulus will stop or even reverse the direction of the spontaneous nystagmus. On the intact side, the caloric reaction can be difficult to assess due to presence of the spontaneous nystagmus (Fig. 56.2). Among peripheral disorders, special attention should be paid from neuro-ophthalmological point of view to BPPV brought about by the canalolithiasis and cupulolithiasis of the semicircular organs. The localization of the disease determines the clinical presentation of the nystagmus. Obviously, the exact analysis raises tremendous

Disease	Length of vertiginous attacks	Head position changes alter the character	Ear discharge	Hearing impairment
Meniére 's disease	hours	no	no	variable
Neuronitis vestibularis	days	no	no	no
Labyrinthitis	minute	no	yes	worsens
Vestibular Schwannoma	weeks	no	no	worsens
Labirynthine infarction	days/no	no	no	sudden
BPPV	seconds	yes	no	no

Fig. 56.1 Differential diagnosis of vertigos of peripheral origin

	Intact vestibular system	*Acute peripheral lesion*	*Compensated peripheral lesion*	*Acute central lesion*	*Chronic central lesion*
Spontaneous nystagmus	*0*	→	*0*	←↔	↔
Vestibulospinal tests	*0*	←	*0*	←	↔
Right warm	←	→	*0*	←←	←
Left warm	→	→	→	→	→
Right cold	→	→→	*0*	→	→
Left cold	←	←,*0*	←	←←	←

Fig. 56.2 The evaluation of vestibular lesions according to the findings of caloric nystagmus test (right sided lesion). *The direction of arrows reflect when the examiner and the physician assume face to face positions*

difficulties to the naked eye, therefore, for differential diagnostic purposes videonystagmography should be recommended. In the everyday practice the varied clinical presentation of the nystagmus represents considerable differential diagnostic problems.

The most frequent form is BPPV of the posterior semicircular canal (over 90% prevalence) the representation of the other ones remain much below 10% each. The canalithiasis of the posterior semicircular canal leads to accumulation of otoconia in the lowest portion of the posterior canal. Dix-Hallpike manoeuvre will elicit ampullofugal flow, which is slightly modified by the gravity. This results in upbeating and counterclockwise torsional nystagmus of the ipsilateral eye and upbeating clockwise torsional nystagmus of the contralateral eye. This represents the most frequent form of BPPV. The disease of the other semicircular canals may result in different nystagmus types which represent considerable diagnostic difficulties.

Diagnostics of Central Vestibular Disorders

From neuro-ophthalmological point of view, the central vestibular disorders are of much higher significance than the peripheral ones. The central vestibular pathways begin in the vestibular nuclei of the brainstem, they form the ipsi- and contralateral medial longitudinal fasciculus and project to the brachium conjunctivum, the system of the oculomotor muscles, the supranuclear integrating centers of the rostral midbrain and the nuclei of the thalamus. Another ascending pathway connects the vestibular nuclei with the cortex through the cerebellum and the fastigial nucleus. Central vestibular symptoms are grouped according to the direction of the vestibulo-ocular reflexes in the 3 dimensional space. The syndromes consist of the vestibulo-ocular symptoms, that is, the eye movement disorders and different forms of nystagmus and the postural symptoms, that is, disorders of gait and body posture. Some diseases such as the demyelinization disorders feature a certain combination of the syndromes.

Central Vestibular Lesion in the Frontal Plane

The balance disorder in the frontal plane may either reflect ipsilateral pontomedullary lesion or contralateral injury at pontomesencephalic level. The medial longitudinal fasciculus is usually affected. The most typical clinical presentation consists of ocular tilt, the asymmetrical position of the bulbs (one looks upward and the other downward) and torsional spontaneous nystagmus.

Central Vestibular Lesion in the Horizontal Plane

Horizontal plane vestibular lesion is a much rarer finding elicited by the damage to fewer brainstem loci. However, this syndrome is yet more frequent in the otoneurologists' practice as it is accompanied by rather few other neurological symptoms. The diagnosis of this syndrome raises the most difficulties for the neurologist, therefore, it represents the most frequent subject of consultations between the neurologist and the otoneurologist. The syndrome is usually caused by the injury of the upper and medial vestibular nuclei, the entry of the eighth cranial nerve or the pontine paramedian reticular formation (PPRF, the integration center of the horizontal eye movements). The most characteristic symptoms are horizontal nystagmus, the lateral-posterior tilt, which is sometimes intensive enough to make the patient fall. The clinical presentation resembles that of vestibular neuronitis. When the entry region of the 8th vestibular cranial nerve is damaged (e.g., by a plaque of multiple sclerosis) even the decreased response to caloric vestibular stimulation can be noticed. The differential diagnosis may take advantage of the observation of the contralateral nystagmus in the direction of the gaze and the incomplete nature of the paresis (upon caloric stimulation) of the semicircular canals. Mainly it is caused by the damage of the medial, less frequently of the lateral vestibular nuclei. Since during the examination of the spontaneous symptoms, signs suggesting harmonic vestibular syndrome can be frequently seen, therefore, in this group of diseases, the detailed investigation by vestibular provocation tests is indispensable.

Central vestibular lesion in the sagittal plane

The balance disorder in the sagittal plane suggests bilateral paramedian functional impairment or flocculus lesion. It is a frequent finding in balance disorders of metabolic or toxic origin.

Main clinical symptoms:

- upbeat or downbeat nystagmus
- head tilt into anterior or posterior direction and concomitant fall

Downbeat Nystagmus

Downbeat nystagmus is a more frequent and permanent phenomenon. Usually it signifies bilateral pontomedullary or flocculus lesions, but it may occur in different pathological conditions of the paramedian craniocervical junction. Generally it renders the gait severely unstable. It is a frequent finding in Arnold–Chiari malformation.

Upbeat Nystagmus

A much rarer and transient finding, which is usually due to pontomesencephalic lesions and is accompanied by severe instability of the gait and oscillopsia The causes involve brainstem tumor, brainstem infarction, brainstem hemorrhage, multiple sclerosis, abscess, Wernicke's encephalopathy and intoxications (this can be still reversible). The pharmacological treatment relies on the administration of dimenhydrinate, scopolamine and baclofen.

Central Vestibular Lesions of Neuro-Ophthalmological Importance Leading to Eye-Related Symptoms in Several Planes

A variety of nystagmus forms can be found in demyelinization or cerebrovascular disorders. At least in 5% of the patients suffering from multiple sclerosis, the first symptom is vertigo. The symptoms may imitate those of vestibular neuronitis and may appear in the form of vertical upbeat or downbeat nystagmus. Sometimes it can be accompanied by eye movement disorders of non-vestibular origin. Torsional spontaneous nystagmus is more frequent than the horizontal one. Gaze induced nystagmus, internuclear ophthalmoplegia may be present. Most often, upon caloric stimulation, vigorous liberated reaction, with strong directional preponderance, can be observed. Upon the observation of certain otoneurologic symptoms; during the examination, the ophthalmologist should consider seriously the possibility of multiple sclerosis. These symptoms are the following ones:

- Vertical, horizontal or pendular nystagmus. One of them is of high frequency or amplitude despite that the case history did not reveal vertiginous attack, which would refer to peripheral disorder.
- Central positional nystagmus, without the presence of spontaneous nystagmus. Upon examining positional nystagmus it may occur only on either eye. To unveil this important symptom, the patient should always be examined by Frenzel"s goggles also then can the electronystagmography be performed.
- Positional nystagmus often resembles that of the typical BPPV, but this cannot be extinguished, that is, when repeating the provocation, its intensity does not decrease. Epley's manoeuvre does not improve it.
- Gaze induced nystagmus into every direction.
- Pathological results upon the examination of smooth pursuit and saccades.
- Internuclear ophthalmoplegia
- Pathological caloric reaction, such as inverted nystagmus, hyperreactivity, directional preponderance.

Visual Impairment and Vertigo

What does the otoneurologist expect form the ophthalmological examination?

In some ophthalmological diseases, vertigo arises due to the lack of visual afferentation.

Patients frequently complain about dizziness in ophthalmological disorders, which (ocular muscle palsies, traumas of the orbit, myopathies, inflammatory diseases) lead to diplopia and neurological disorders, the presentation of which (internuclear ophthalmoplegia, vertical gaze palsy) implies eye-related symptoms. Sometimes improper eyeglasses, when the difference in vision is bigger than 4 diopters, can cause significant vertigo.

Intact vision provides indispensable information to differentiate whether the patient or the environment is moving. The visually impaired learn to compensate very effectively the lack of visual afferentation, but the balance coordination of these patients is much more vulnerable even if they do not complain about dizziness. It is clearly reflected by the movements of the blind person on vehicles. The unpredictable shaking of the vehicle completely interferes with the proprioceptive efforts to determine posture. Therefore, blind patients are restricted to rely on the activity of their vestibular system. However, even its function can be impaired by the movements of the vehicle, which can elicit flow of the endolymph. According to clinical observations blind patients afflicted by vestibular disorders heal with more difficulty and at a much slower rate than similar patients with intact vision.

In the case of some nystagmus forms, it is the ophthalmologist that sends the patient to otoneurological examination, but the opposite is more frequent as the examination schedule of the dizzy patient always involves the ophthalmological examination. The otoneurologist expects answers for the following questions:

- Does the patient have a specific underlying ophthalmological disorder (decreased visual acuity, loss of visual field), which could explain the vertigo and unsteadiness?
- Does the patient have a hidden disorder, which can trigger or alter the nystagmus?
- Presence of choked disk? Choked disk with appropriate clinical symptoms may refer to the tumor of the cerebellopontine angle or intracranial space occupying processes! In the case of intracranial space occupying processes vestibular provocation tests are contraindicated!
- The condition of the blood vessels of the fundus (fundoscopy may reveal untreated hypertension or diabetes)
- The condition of the blood vessels of the fundus directly reflects the condition of cerebrovascular system.
- How can the eye movement disorder be characterized exactly according to neuro-ophthalmological aspects, in the case of central vestibular disorders?

Further Readings

Brandt T. Vertigo (Its multisensory Syndromes). London: Springer; 2000.

Szirmai Á, et al. Tapasztalataink az ICS Chartr ENG computeres electronystagmograph használatával [Results in using ICS Charter ENG computer electronystagmograph]. Fül-orr-gégegyógy. 1998;44:49–55.

Szirmai Á. Szédülés [Vertigo] (Háziorvoslás aktuális kérdési sorozat). Budapest: Therapia Kiadó; 2002.

Szirmai Á. Az egyensúlyzavarok differenciáldiagnosztikája és terápiája [Differential diagnosis and therapy in balance diseases]. Budapest: Semmelweis Kiadó; 2006.

Examination of the Eye Movements of the Patient in Coma

57

György Geréby

Contents

In the diagnostics of the disorders of consciousness (somnolence, sopor, coma) the examination of pupil reactions and the symptoms of the extraocular muscles provide considerable help in localisation. Further, changes in their character, over time, can predict the progress, stagnation or improvement of the condition. This provides indispensable help in those situations, when modern imaging techniques are not readily available or when they are incapable of providing the necessary morphological information in a given clinical condition. The observation and proper evaluation of the symptoms of the comatose patient helps the physician to establish which examination devices should be used and in which order according to professional and/or economical reasons. Despite the patient does not cooperate, the neglectful practice of dismissing the examination of eye movements is unacceptable. Such remarks as "eye movements cannot be examined" are too frequent in medical reports. In such cases, instead of the voluntary – guided and commanded – eye movements, the reflex ones should be checked.

The central neural pathways, which control the innervation the external ocular muscles and the pupil, project from the cortex to the pons spanning several levels of the central nervous system running in close proximity to those centers, which are responsible for maintaining consciousness. Further, even some peripheral components of these pathways still run intracranially. This anatomical distribution explains that symptoms of the external and internal oculomotor systems are of localization value in comatose patients at least to determine the level of damage.

This short chapter will only describe and interpret the symptoms of conditions of clinical relevance omitting the anatomical and pathophysiological intricacies, which otherwise are still not fully clarified. (Further information is available in the recommended and referred literature.) In contrast with the high specificity of the symptoms in localization, they can boast of much less etiological value, therefore, the most frequent causative disorders are given in brackets in the order of incidence.

G. Geréby, M.D.
Department of Neurology and Stroke Center, Budapest City Council Saint John Hospital and United Hospitals of North Buda, Budapest, Hungary
e-mail: idgereby@gmail.com

J. Somlai, T. Kovács (eds.), *Neuro-Ophthalmology*, DOI 10.1007/978-3-319-28956-4_57

Table 57.1 The pupillary signs and the vestibulo-ocular reflexes in hypo- or areactive conditions

Level of lesion or functional impairment	Pupil (reaction to light)	Vestibulo-ocular reflex (caloric test)
Hemispheres	2–3 mm reactive	Tonic, conjugate deviation
Diencephalon	1.5–2 mm reactive	Tonic, conjugate deviation
Uncus herniation	Anisocoria, dilated on the affected side	Symptoms of oculomotor nerve palsy
Mesencephalon	Of moderate patency, irregular, fixed	Difficult to stimulate or internuclear ophthalmoplegia
Pons	Extremely narrow ("pinpoint"), temporarily fixed	Cannot be triggered
Medulla (intact consciousness)	Narrow (circa 2 mm), reactive	It can be triggered to a complete extent
Psychogenic areactive condition	2–3 mm reactive	Nystagmus

Pupillary Symptoms in Coma

Since a separate chapter deals with the function of the pupillomotor pathway, here you can read only about the relevant aspects of the comatose patient's examination discussed in detail with special emphasis on the comprehensive evaluation of the pupillomotor and external oculomotor symptoms and their relationship (Table 57.1).

The diameter of the pupil is determined by the actual balance or imbalance of the sympathetic (dilating) and parasympathetic (constricting) activities. The anatomical or pharmaceutical blockade of one of them leads to uncompensated activity of the other one resulting in severe mydriasis or myosis. In coma beside the native pupil size and shape, the reaction to light and the ciliospinal reflexes can be examined. To observe the frequently hypoactive reactions, the application of a suitably strong light source and magnifying glass are recommended. Such equipment is indispensable in the examination of the extremely myotic pupil, which develops due to sympathetic lesions or metabolic (pharmaceutical) agents. Negligent examination may lead to the diagnosis of fixed pupils, which eventually leads to wrong localization diagnosis. In contrast with conscious patients, the *ciliospinal reflex* of sleeping or comatose subjects is much more conspicuous. In this condition, the transient dilation of the pupil evoked by the nociceptive stimulation of the face or the upper portion of the torso is much more visible. Its presence reflects that the sympathetic pathways of the mildly comatose patient are still intact. Since the connection between the afferent nociceptive pathway and the pupil dilatory efferent sympathetic pathway is probably established at spinal level, the reflex is not a reliable tool in the examination of brainstem functions.

The Evaluation of Pupillary Signs for Localization Purposes

Hypothalamus lesions (ischemia, hemorrhage, tumor) mainly located in the posterior or the ventrolateral regions lead to *ipsilateral myosis*. It is generally accompanied by ipsilateral ptosis and hemianhydrosis, which involves the whole side of the body. (Differential diagnosis: in cervical sympathetic lesions the anhydrosis affects only the face, the neck and the upper extremity) If the above hypothalamus lesion, which elicits central *Horner's syndrome*, is completed with contralateral hemiplegia in more extended damages, the syndrome may be regarded diencephalic syndrome (the descending sympathetic pathway does not cross). Since Horner's syndrome rarely accompanies the occlusion of the internal carotid artery, some assume that it is brought about by a peripheral ischemic insult to the perivascular sheat of the vessel. However, considering that in asymptomatic carotid occlusion Horner's syndrome cannot be observed either, but it is fairly frequent in hypothalamus lesion of different origin, the direct damage of the hypothalamus is more probable.

Detection of unilateral Horner's syndrome (or just narrower pupil) is of vital importance in deepening disorder of consciousness, since it can be the first harbinger of the transtentorial herniation. In the case of diencephalic dysfunctions elicited by *supratentorial space occupying processes*, *myosis is usually bilateral*, but the reaction to light is intact.

In some (dorsal pretectal, tectal) *mesencephalic lesions* (due to transtentorial herniation, hemorrhage, emollition, tumor) the pathway of the pupillary light reflex will be disrupted, but that of the accommodation reflex may remain intact. *The moderately (or a bit more) dilated pupil(s)* show regular contour, they are fixed, but may slightly change in size, they may show hippus, and the ciliospinal reflex is intact. Minute tectal lesions can damage the reticular formation of the periaqueductal region eliciting coma. Therefore, the aforementioned symptoms are of importance in the localization of the lesion, which is responsible for the coma.

The *mesencephalic lesions* (transtentorial herniation, tumor, hemorrhage, ischemia) usually elicit simultaneous sympathetic and parasympathetic damage. This time the *pupils are of moderate diameter*, they are unequal, slightly irregular and fixed. The disorders, damaging the *3rd intracranial nerves* around their nuclei and their exit from the brainstem, manifest themselves by *markedly dilated pupils* and the *paralysis of the external ocular muscles*. In contrast, with the peripheral processes of different etiology, they are usually bilateral. In *pontine damages* (hemorrhage, emollition) both descending sympathetic pathways are affected, therefore, *both pupils are narrow*. Some assume that it is further aggravated by simultaneous parasympathetic excitation (irritation due to the pontine bleeding). This time the pupillary responses are very difficult to examine or they can be virtually missing due to the maximum constriction ("pinpoint pupil"). *Lateral medullary or ventrolateral spinal injuries to the cervical segment* (ischemic vascular lesions, e.g., Wallenberg's syndrome) result in ipsilateral Horner's syndrome with intact pupillary response to light (these lesions, however, usually do not cause disorder of consciousness). *Peripheral damages* can affect both the sympathetic and the parasympathetic systems. In uncus herniation (lateral and temporal space occupying processes) the oculomotor nerve is pressed against the edge of the tentorium or the posterior cerebral artery. Presumably due to their superficial localization, the parasympathetic pupillomotor fibers are more sensitive to compression, therefore, *the pupillary dilation (mydriasis)* frequently precedes the paralysis of the external ocular muscles. *Metabolic disorders*: the action of pharmacons and other exogenous toxic substances being involved, are responsible for the majority of the disorders of consciousness observed in the clinical practice, and they also influence the condition of the pupils. But the pupillary signs of the metabolic encephalopathies are different from those elicited by structural lesions. Since the pupillomotor pathways are relatively insensitive to metabolic effects, *the reaction to light may remain intact*. Even if it is sluggish, it can usually be triggered by the preterminal stage, whereas in the destructive processes the reflex completely disappears. Therefore, the presence or the lack of the pupillary response to light is the most important diagnostic tool to differentiate between comas related to metabolic disorders and structural lesions *Therefore, the patient who shows symptoms of severe mesencephalic lesion (deep coma, corresponding motoric symptoms and breathing pattern), but his/her pupillary reactions are intact must be in metabolic coma.*

However, some differential diagnostic difficulties and exceptions cannot elude our attention.

The anticholinergic agents, mainly larger dose of *atropine* and *scopolamine* may result in disorder of consciousness (delirium or stupor), dilation of the pupils and decrease or lack of the pupillary reactions to light. The dilated pupil of parasympathetic denervation can be constricted by *pilocarpine*, but in atropine intoxication the pupil does not react to pilocarpine. If coma is the consequence of of glutethimid intoxication, the pupils are moderately or slightly more dilated, mild anisocoria can be present, but not even fixed pupils represent necessarily poor prognosis.

Opiates (morphine, heroine) result in "pinpoint" pupils, which strongly resembles the finding of pontine hemorrhages. In such cases, the intact reaction to light is very difficult to demonstrate (strong light and magnifier are needed!).

Hypothermia may also result in fixed pupils. In barbiturate intoxication, when the pupils are already fixed, the patient usually suffers from severe hypotension and does not have spontaneous respiration either.

In anoxia and ischemia (suffocation, asystole) the pupils are dilated and fixed. If the condition persists for longer than some minutes, it usually leads to irreversible brain damage. However, those reanimation attempts, during which the pupillary reactions soon return, are usually successful.

Mydriatics may conceal the pupillary signs and the alterations of them, therefore, the application of mydriatics is not recommended during the examination of patients suffering from the disorders of consciousness. If it is still inevitable, it should be performed with short acting agents.

The pupillary signs are summarized in Table 57.1 and Fig. 57.1

Alterations of the Peripheral Oculomotor System in Coma

The examination of the external oculomotor system starts with the observation of the *position of the eyelids and the globes at rest*, which is followed by the examination of *reflexes of the eyelids and the eye movements*. In the majority of coma cases, the eyelids are closed (they could behave differently in chronic comatose or coma-like conditions: apallic syndrome, and the "locked-in syndrome"). *Upon passive opening of the palpebral fissure* the examiner can feel the

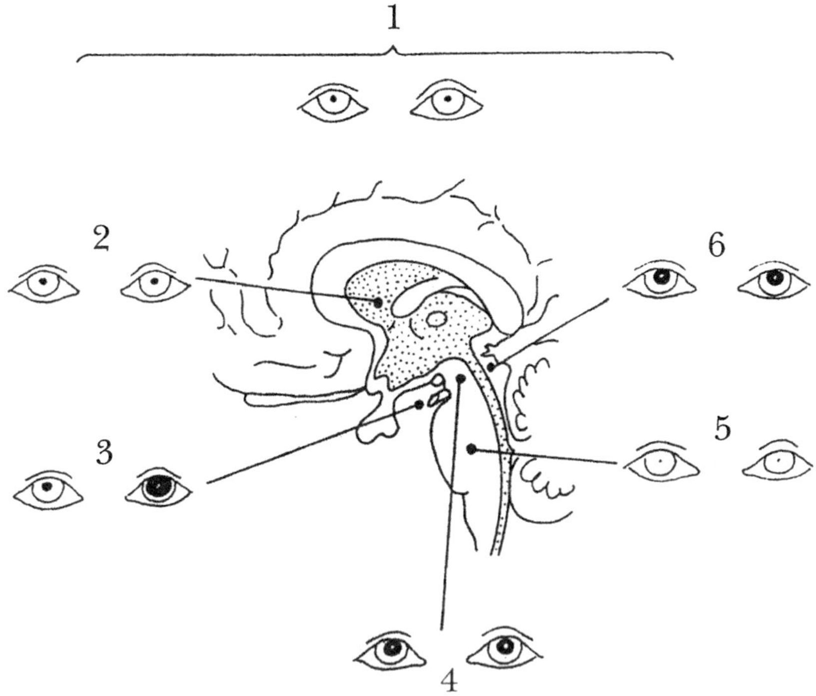

Fig. 57.1 *1*. In metabolic encephalopathies the pupils are usually narrower than average and react to light (variants of, and alterations to the above condition are discussed in the text in detail). *2*. Diencephalic lesion or functional impairment (narrower pupils, they react to light). *3*. Lesion of the oculomotor nerve (frequently unilateral, uncus herniation): dilated fixed pupil. *4*. Mesencephalic lesions: fixed pupils of moderate diameter. *5*. Pontine damage: very narrow ("pinpoint") pupils which seemingly do not react to light. *6*. Mesencephalon tectum lesion: wider, fixed pupils, sometimes hippus

actual tone. When the patient exerts considerable resistance upon and opening attempt and closes the eyelids immediately (except for the reflex blepharospasm), it reflects the psychogenic origin of the areactive condition. In true disorders of consciousness after passive opening, the eyelids close gradually, which practically cannot be imitated. Lack of tone and gradual closure refer to facial paralysis. Uni- or bilateral *ptosis* may be the consequence of hemispheric lesions, as well. Then the ptosis is more pronounced on the side of the hemiparesis. In brainstem lesions, the ptosis presents as the component of the Horner's syndrome. The literature reported cases in which the palpebral fissure remained permanently open due to tonic retraction of the upper eyelid. When either spontaneously or upon visual stimulation (strong light, movement to the eye) the patient *blinks*, this reflects the functionality of the pontine reticular formation and in the case of visual stimulation that of the sensory afferent pathway, as well. Lack of the blink reflex suggests the paresis of the facial nerve, while bilateral deficit argues for bilateral structural lesion of the brainstem or metabolic depression. In unconscious patients, the corneal reflex needs stronger stimuli to be triggered. Upon symmetrical closure of the eyelids, the upward turn of the bulbs (*Bell's phenomenon*) reflects that the pathways connecting the oculomotor and facial nuclei are intact. When the lesions are localized above the mid-pons the Bell phenomenon cannot be elicited. This time upon corneal stimulation the mandible may move to the opposite direction according to the *corneopterygoid reflex*. When the Bell phenomenon is intact but the blink-reflex is missing, the facial nucleus or nerve is injuredt.

Eye Positions at Rest and the Spontaneous Eye Movements

In comas when the external oculomotor system is not affected, the patient's eyes look ahead and they are conjugated or slightly divergent probably due to the simultaneous and equal relaxation of every eye muscle. Divergence of greater than 15° may be the consequence of already existing divergent strabismus or lesion of the oculomotor nerve. The differential diagnosis is based upon the eye movement reflexes (see later).

Even with intact innervation of the external eye musculature, *roving eye movements* are frequent findings. They are slow, random, predominantly horizontal, conjugate or dysconjugate eye movements of changing direction. (roving eye movements are also important is the diagnosis of psychogenic areactive conditions as they cannot be imitated).

Roving eye movements are usually accompanied by vigorous *cephalo-ocular reflexes*. As the coma deepens, the roving eye movements disappear. The periodically alternating, *ping–pong gaze* develops in the horizontal plane. It is a conjugate eyemovement, which alternates between the two end-points every few seconds. It was described in bilateral hemispheric infarction, cerebellar (vermis) hemorrhage, and it seems that it is not related to brainstem lesions, therefore, some consider it the variant of roving eye movements. *Nystagmus* – in strict sense – is an extreme rarity in coma, since the fast compensatory component would require intact vestibuloocular-cortical interactions, but obviously the cortical influences are missing. However, some nystagmuslike spontaneous eye movement can be present, which have diagnostic relevance.

Retraction nystagmus means the eyeballs' non-rhythmic jerk backward to the orbit. It usually accompanies mesencephalic tegmental lesions. It is generally assumed that the liberation from the inhibitory corticomesencephalic impulses results in the simultaneous contraction of the six external ocular muscles. Stimulating any nuclei of the ocular muscles will lead to their simultaneous contraction as it was verified by electromyographic experiments.

In *convergent nystagmus*, the slow divergence of the eyes is followed by fast convergence. According to observations, it can alternate with retraction nystagmus reflecting mesencephalic lesion. *Ocular bobbing* represents a recurring series of usually conjugate eye movements, which last for 5–30 s and consist of two components: a rapid downward beat and a slow return to the primary position. The movement cannot be influenced by caloric stimulation. Usually it develops due to lower pontine lesions (hemorrhages due to hypertension, aneurysm, brain infarction, sometimes encephalitis), but it can be the consequence of transtentorial herniation due to distant processes, brainstem compression owing to cerebellar hemorrhage, anoxia (because of asystole) or sometimes due to severe metabolic encephalopathy. It must be distinguished from ocular myoclonus, the downbeat nystagmus, the downward conjugate deviation or the potential voluntary vertical movements of the "locked in syndrome" (ventral pons lesion).

Sometimes *nystagmoid jerks* of horizontal, vertical or torsional character can be observed on either eye. They are usually irregular (arrhythmic) and refer to pontine lesions. The irregular, rotatory and vertical slow movements alternate on the opposite eyes: the upward moving bulb rotates inward, while the downward moving one outward. The phenomenon in appearance may imitate "see–saw" nystagmus, but they represent different entities; otherwise the latter is a rare finding is coma.

The *disturbances of conjugate gaze* are almost always the consequences of structural lesions. The most frequent form of them is *lateral gaze palsy*, which is related to destructive lesions. Since metabolic disorder and compressions (supratentorial displacements) usually cause bilateral impairment in the supranuclear section of the control mechanism of the conjugate gaze. The sudden abruption of the latter (hemispheric hemorrhage, emollition) due to the uncompensated activity of the contralateral innervation, provided that the brainstem oculomotor systems are intact, leads to *conjugate deviation*. Due to the crossing of the descending supranuclear pathway, the deviation is oriented to the side of the injury (the patient looks toward the side of the lesion). This sort of conjugate deviation goes with contralateral gaze palsy. Conjugate deviation directed away from the focus can, however, develop in epileptic seizures involving the frontal cortical gaze areas. However, the deviation of the bulbs is not tonic but nystagmus-like or consists of clonic jerks. From the acute lesions, the most important reasons are hemorrhages, and they last only for at most 1–2 h, the progresses into conjugate deviation toward the lesion. In chronic epileptic patients, obviously it persists only during the attack, and then, similarly to the postictal pareses, it may progress into transient, ipsiversive conjugate deviation.

When the lesion is located *below the crossing of the supranuclear fibers*, at the level of the abducens nucleus, it also causes conjugate gaze paresis. However, in contrast with the hemispheric processes, it is directed away from the lesion. (in the case of concomitant hemiparesis, "the patient looks at the paretic side"). The deviation, nevertheless, is smaller, and the eyes will not cross the midline to the side of the lesion, even upon turning the head or using caloric vestibular stimulation (this is the most important difference compared to conjugate deviation elicited by hemispheric insults, see later).

From the *vertical gaze palsies*, the most frequent one is *upward gaze paresis* due to destruction or compression of the pretectal region and the posterior commissure. The damage of the medial longitudinal fasciculus together with the surrounding reticular matter may also lead to the weakness or paresis of the upward gaze.

The upward gaze can be examined by mechanical *cornea stimulation* after opening the palpebral fissure. This, provided, the reflex pathway is intact, evokes closure of the eyelids and upward turn of the bulbs (*Bell phenomenon*). In *deeper coma*, vestibular stimulation by *turning the head or caloric stimuli* may be needed.

When the eyes positioned below the horizontal plane, it always signifies a brainstem injury. Most often it refers to the compression of the tegmentum of the mesencephalon, but similar eye position results from extended brainstem destructions. Sometimes it was observed in severe metabolic encephalopathies, primarily in hepatic coma. Conjugate or dysconjugate, tonic, downward deviation, as an atypical reaction to unilateral, cold, caloric stimulus, was observed in patients intoxicated by sedative drugs.

In the *skew-deviation* one eye deviates from the conjugated horizontal position upwards while the other one downwards. In patients, who are able to cooperate to some extent, slight vertical or *see–saw nystagmus* may also be observed. The *skew-deviation* reflects brainstem lesion. According to the neuropathological investigation of the cases, the lesion can be found either in the dorsal portion of the medulla or the brachium pontis, on the side of the eye of lower position, or in the medial longitudinal fasciculus on the side of the eye assuming higher position (for more details regarding the pathomechanism the reader is referred to Chap. 55 on page 292). Skew-deviation should be differentiated from vertical strabismus, and pathological eye positions related orbital processes (e.g., blowout fracture).

Reflex Eye Movements

Conjugate binocular fixation is always maintained, due to the continuous afferentation from the vestibular system and the cervical proprioceptive units, and their connection to the oculomotor systems despite the constantly changing spatial position of the head and the body. The oculomotor systems span from the caudal portion of the pons (vestibular nuclei) to the mesencephalic nuclei of the oculomotor nerve, in close proximity to or partly overlapping with the neighbouring neuronal networks of arousal and consciousness.

The proper analysis of the *eye movements triggered by vestibular stimulation* frequently makes possible the differentiation between the comas due to metabolic reasons and structural damages, and also helps to subdivide the latter group into conditions of hemispheric or brainstem origin.

In physiological circumstances – when the patient is awake – hemispheric influences inhibit the vestibular reflexes. However, when the *hemispheres are damaged* or functionally impaired, obviously the *vestibulo-ocular reflexes becomes pathologically vigorous* and can easily triggered till the brainstem remains intact. These tests do not require special equipment, and the results obtained by a skilled physician are very reliable.

Although in the literature various nomenclatures are used to classify the vestibular eye reflexes, but according to the conventional terminology, only should *"vestibuloocular"* and *"cephaloocular"* be regarded as proper names (in the literature one can find the following, mainly, synonyms: oculovestibular reflex, oculocephalic reflex, doll's eye reflex, proprioceptive head-turn eye reflex). To elicit *flow of the endolymph* in the semicircular organs and trigger the *vestibulo-ocular reflexes* in the comatose, that is, a lying patient, the physician *turns the patient's head from one side to the other*, performs flexion and extension of the neck or relies on *caloric stimulation*. In the first case, the inertia, whereas in the latter one, the temperature difference will result in inhomogeneity in density and turbulent flow of the endolymph. Presumably to the postural head reflex also contributes the proprioceptive afferentation of the cervical anatomical units.

The Examination of the Vestibulo-Ocular Reflexes

The Cephaloocular Reflex

The physician raises the upper eyelids while holding the head of the recumbent patient. Then the head is turned from one side to the other. After each turn at the lateral positions, the physician waits for 1–2 s. When the eye movement systems of the brainstem and the vestibular apparatus are intact upon turning the head, conjugate deviation can be seen into the opposite direction. i.e., upon rightward turn left, upon leftward turn right deviation. The vertical movements can be checked by flexion and extension of the neck. Conjugate upward gaze upon flexion and conjugate downward gaze upon extension correspond to positive response. Upon leaning the neck the eyelids may open temporarily and this reflex may help evaluate the function of the levator muscle, as well. After a complete turn, even if the head remains in the end-position of the manoeuvre, the eyes return to their original position. When neck injury is suspected, the head cannot be turned!

The Examination of the Vestibulo-Ocular Reflexes by Caloric Stimulation

At the beginning of the examination, the patient's head should be raised by 30°, so that the lateral semicircular canal should get into horizontal position. Depending on the intensity of the response (and the depth of the coma), maximum 150 mL of ice-cold water is injected into the external meatus through a thin catheter. The conscious or arousable patient can be tested by 30° water or 1 mL of ice-cold water. When the brainstem is intact and the patient is awaken, the *cold stimulus* elicits rhythmic, horizontal nystagmus of small amplitude, which lasts for about 2–3 min, and the slow component of which is directed to the trigger, while the fast component is directed away from it. In metabolic encephalopathies or hemispheric lesions, the fast component completely disappears and tonic conjugate deviation will develop to the side of the trigger, which can last for 1–3 min. In stupor or superficial coma stages, the tonic ipsiversive deviation can be disrupted by an opposite jerk, which takes the bulbs back to the midline. After the stimulation of one side, a 5 min interval is needed before the stimulation of the other side. The evaluation of the vertical eye movements requires the *simultaneous stimulation of both sides*. Bilateral cold stimulation leads to upward vertical movement, whereas bilateral warm one results in downward vertical gaze. In those disorders of consciousness, where the lesion disrupts the pathway of the vestibulo-ocular reflex, *these eye movements may become dysconjugated or cannot be triggered at all* (see details later), while in metabolic encephalopathies only can it be found in extremely deep comas. Patients who persist in coma (post-traumatic, post-anoxic conditions) or suffer from certain metabolic disorders can react with atypical or paradoxical responses to caloric stimuli (these findings represent exceptions and well exceed the scope of the chapter).

Disorders of the Vestibulo-Ocular Reflexes

The responses evoked by passive turning of the head and by caloric stimulation are quite similar. Apart from some exceptions, only does the caloric stimulus appear stronger than the postural one. This hypothesis is confirmed by the finding that in metabolic coma the postural reflex disappears sooner than the caloric one. By caloric stimuli reflexes can still be triggered when by turning of the head responses cannot be evoked.

In physiologic circumstances, in alert patient and areactive conditions of psychogenic origin, the postural responses are inconsistent and caloric stimuli evokes nystagmus.

In bifrontal or diffuse bilateral hemispheric processes and in diencephalic lesions, even if the patient is alert, by turning the head vigorous reflex responses can be elicited and by caloric stimulation tonic deviation not nystagmus can be evoked.

In superficial coma stages, if supratentorial process is the underlying disorder, the doll's head phenomenon can be triggered and for caloric stimuli the response is usually tonic conjugate deviation not nystagmus. Especially when roving eye movements are present only can strong turning of the head trigger the conjugate deviation.

As the disorder of consciousness gets deeper – if the oculomotor systems of the brainstem remains intact – the activity of the vestibulo-ocular reflexes increases, they can even be triggered by one turn. *The tonic deviation* (toward the lesion) can be overcome in supranuclear (hemispheric) injuries if the stimulus is strong enough, and the bulbs can be moved to the opposite direction. *However in massive, hemispheric lesions, in the beginning*, sometimes combined stimulation may be necessary, that is caloric and postural stimuli should be exerted simultaneously to elicit the desired response.

In metabolic comas the reflex eye movements can be evoked even when the symptoms of the severe depression other brainstem functions, such as decerebrate rigidity and neurogenic hyperventilation became apparent. When the functional impairment progresses, the reflex eye movements become hypoactive, and then disappear: first the doll's head later the caloric response disappears. Those processes, which directly, or indirectly through displacement compress the brainstem (and the oculomotor structures) impair the reflex eye movement. Usually in these instances, the responses become dysconjugate or cannot be evoked at all, depending on the location of the lesion.

The pretectal and mesencephalic tectal lesions cause the paralysis of the upward gaze. Due to the compression or destruction of the oculomotor nucleus or the nerve itself, every ipsilateral eye movement disappears except for the activity of the external rectus muscle, which is innervated by the abducens nerve. Those injuries of the pons and the mesencephalon, which also affect the medial longitudinal fasciculus cause *internuclear ophthalmoplegia*. Then upon postural or caloric stimulation, the reflex horizontal eye movements show characteristic features: the *eye on the affected side will not adduct* together with the abduction of the contralateral eye. Naturally, to set up the correct diagnosis of internuclear ophthalmoplegia, the detection of normal convergence would also be necessary in order to exclude the peripheral plegia of the internal rectus muscle. However, this function cannot be evaluated in coma, but the isolated paralysis of the internal rectus muscles is so rare that in coma, the lack of the adduction of both eyes almost certainly indicates uni- or bilateral internuclear ophthalmoplegia (for more details see internuclear ophthalmoplegia on page 241). The recognition of the internuclear ophthalmoplegia is of vital importance since this symptom usually reflects structural brainstem lesion. In metabolic encephalopathies and narcoses, internuclear ophthalmoplegia is rare. It can be present transiently in barbiturate intoxication or in some other comas of metabolic origin (e.g., hepatic encephalopathy) if the applied stimulus is not strong enough.

The acute or subacute *injuries to the lateral pons*, which involve the abducens nucleus, *lead to conjugate gaze palsy*. Then the spontaneous position of the bulbs points away from the lesion, in contrast with higher (hemispheric) damages, when the conjugate deviation is directed toward the lesion. Further, in the conjugate deviation evoked by damages to the lateral pons, in contrast with the hemispheric damages, neither turning of the head nor caloric stimulation can make the eyes cross the midline to the side of the injury. *Those lateral pons lesions, which affect the vestibular nuclei on both sides*, will extinguish the responses to caloric stimulation, however, the postural responses can be spared as the cervical proprioceptive afferentation may remain intact.

During the evaluation of the vestibulo-ocular reflexes, attention should be paid to the fact that *the normal reflex does confirm that the oculomotor system of the brainstem is intact, but the lack of the reflex does not necessarily imply that the areflexia is evoked by the same condition as the disorder of consciousness. Since, the loss of the vestibulo-ocular reflexes can be be related to previous vestibular disorders, administration of ototoxic drugs (certain antibiotics), neuromuscular blockade (succinylcholine), or due to intoxication by drugs (barbiturates, diphenylhydantoin, tricyclic antidepressants), which specifically impair the vestibular functions.*

The Summary of the External Eye Movement Symptoms in Disorders of Consciousness

The arousable patient's vestibulo-ocular reflexes cannot be triggered in their whole extent; caloric stimuli evoke nystagmus not tonic conjugate deviation.

In those unconscious conditions which were elicited by diffuse or bilateral hemispheric injuries, the eyes look forward, they are in the midline or slightly divergent, sometimes roving eye movements can be observed. *The vestibulo-ocular reflexes are vigorous, and by caloric stimulation tonic conjugate deviation can be triggered.*

In the acute damages to the frontal gaze center the eyes look into the direction of the lesion. The vestibulo-ocular reflexes can be triggered, however with some difficulty in the immediate few hours after the injury.

In metabolic encephalopathies, the vestibulo-ocular reflexes can be easily elicited both by turning the head and by caloric stimulation, and decrease or disappear only in deep coma (substances, barbiturates, hydantoin, which disproportionately depress the vestibular functions, this develops earlier).

Forward aligned gaze does not represent any localization diagnostic values. Conjugate deviation in the horizontal plane may reflect ipsilateral hemispheric injuries or contralateral damage to the lateral pontine areas. When the *conjugate deviation* reaches the extreme of the range, but by turning the head or by caloric stimulation *the eyes can be moved over the midline*, this usually represents *hemispheric* lesion.

When the deviation is partial, but the eyes will *not* cross the midline this suggests *pontine* lesion. *In comas of mesencephalic origin* the eyes assume forward looking gaze and the reflex movements are missing (*complete lack of the vestibulo-ocular reflexes*). In the case of small lesion, which disrupts the medial longitudinal fasciculus, the eyes look forward, but upon vestibular stimulation on *the eye of the affected side, they do not adduct* (uni- or bilateral internuclear ophthalmoplegia).

Lateral pons lesions will elicit *contralateral conjugate deviations* of smaller extent than the hemispheric ones (see above.) Downward conjugate deviation refers to decreased mesencephalic activity due to either metabolic reasons or secondary compressions (direct destructions are rare culprits in this case). When the eyes with reflex manoeuvres can be raised above the horizontal plane, this usually reflects metabolic reasons, whereas in compression cases they will not raise above the horizontal line. Apart from the fairly frequent and mild (maximum 15°) divergence, *the dysconjugate gaze suggestsstructural brainstem lesion* (chronic strabismus, which is independent from the coma, should be excluded!).

When *triggering the reflex eye movements, the lack of the adduction* of one or both eyes reveals the lesion of the medial longitudinal fasciculus, provided, the lack of the pupillary sign does not suggest peripheral oculomotor palsy.

Unilateral *weakness or lack of the abduction* means the peripheral injury to the abducens nerve. In reflex eye movements, dysconjugate vertical gaze is a very rare finding. If it is present, it is the consequence of of brainstem injury.

Further Readings

Brandt T. Coma und Augenbewegungen. In: Brandt T, BücheleW,JungR,editors.Augenbewegungsstörungen. Leipzig: VEB Georg Thieme; 1983. p. 109–16.

Buettner UW, Zee DS. Vestibular testing in comatose patients. Arch Neurol. 1989;46:561–3.

Fischer CM. Neurological examination of the comatose patient. Acta Neurol Scand. 1969;45 Suppl 36:1–56.

Plum F. Organic disturbances of consciousness. In: Critchley M, O'Leary J, Jennet B, editors. Scientific fundations of neurology. London: William Heinemann; 1973. p. 193–201.

Plum F, Posner J. The pathologic physiology of signs and symptoms of coma; pupils, ocular movements. In: Plum F, Posner J, editors. The diagnosis of stupor and coma. 3rd ed. (Contemporary neurology series, Vol 19). Philadelphia: FA Davis; 1980. p. 41–64.

Schiffter R, Pohl P. Zum Verlauf der absteigenden zentralen Sympathicusbahn. Arch Psychiat Nervenkr. 1972;216:379–84.

Schiffter R, Schliack H. Über ein charakteristisches neurologisches Syndrom bei Ischämien der Arteria carotis interna -cerebri media – Strohmbahn. Fortschr Neurol Psychiat. 1974;42:555–62.

Supranuclear Regulation of the Eye Movements and the Significance of Their Disturbances

58

Szilvia Gulyás

Contents

This chapter first discusses the classification of the eye movements, and then reviews the central regulation of the different types till the level of the rostral brainstem structures. To facilitate understanding and due to limitation of space, the descriptions of the individual regulatory pathway systems are simplified, which is followed by the discussion of the eye movement disorders of everyday clinical significance.

S. Gulyás, M.D., PhD
Electrophysiology Unit, Department of Neurology, Faculty of Medicine, Semmelweis University, Budapest, Hungary
e-mail: gulyszi@yahoo.co.uk

Types of the Eye Movements

Eye movements can be categorized into two main groups. One of them is important to shift our gaze from one object to a new one, which raised our attention, whereas the other type ensures to fix the actually interesting object. The first group consists of fast eye movements, saccades while the second group comprises fixation and pursuit. Pursuit can be roughly subdivided into further categories: foveal slow tracking (smooth pursuit eye movement (SPEM)), and the other type involving the whole visual field: the slow phase of optokinetic nystagmus (OKN), the vestibulo-ocular reflex (VOR), and the oculocephalic reflex.

Saccades make it possible for us to change the image, the target of our interest, seen on the fovea responsible for sharp vision. The maximum velocity of the saccades can reach even 700°/s, and even their average speed is about 300–360°/s. Their latency, direction and amplitude but not their speed is under voluntary control. The latter can be modified temporarily by the impact of medicines, addictive substrates (e.g., alcohol) and psychoactive drugs and fatigue. Permanent changes are attributed to the dysfunction of the nervous system. In the young, the latency of the saccades, which is summarized by the duration of retinal image processing, and the information processing of the cortex, superior colliculus, and the cerebellum is about 200 ± 50 ms, and with advancing age, it becomes progressively longer. According to the various

J. Somlai, T. Kovács (eds.), *Neuro-Ophthalmology*, DOI 10.1007/978-3-319-28956-4_58

regulatory mechanisms, different saccade types are known as presented in *s*. The reflexive saccades are triggered by external stimuli (e.g., sudden acoustic, tactile stimuli). The voluntary saccades are elicited by internal motives (e.g., having a look at the source of a sound has been heard for a longer period of time, searching for an object in the ambient space). The voluntary saccades, besides motivation and memory, are under the influence of cognitive processes. The spontaneous saccades are meaningless fast eye movements, which take place in darkness or during speech. The fast component of the nystagmus, which returns the bulbs to their primary position, is also a saccade.

Smooth pursuit fixates the image of object of interest on the fovea and begins 80–120 ms after the image shifted on the retina. Its velocity is usually 15–30°/s, but it can reach 100°/s. The foveal type (i.e., smooth pursuit eye movement (SPEM)) appears when a small object moves slowly, like a prey moves far from the predator. When the predator gets closer to the prey, the other types, the OKN and the VOR are needed to stabilize the image of the prey. The slow phase of OKN develops in stable head position following the movement of the environment, whereas the slow phase of VOR develops when the head or the body is moving. In natural circumstances the two systems complement each other in stabilizing the image.

Vergence represents convergent–divergent eye movements, which are needed to adjust the depth of field. Vergence is a component of the accommodation triad. Without vergence diplopia would develop upon fixation to close objects.

The Supranuclear Areas of Eye Movement Regulation

These areas consist of structures which are located rostrally from the oculomotor nuclei (nucl. III, IV, and VI). According to the classical concept, the cortical gaze center can be found in Brodmann area 8, which regulates both the horizontal and vertical eye movements. From the subcortical areas, paramedian pontine reticular formation (PPRF) is responsible for the horizontal conjugate gaze, while the rostral interstitial nucleus of the medial longitudinal fasciculus (riMLF) controls vertical conjugate gaze. However, according to recent knowledge, regulation is a more complex process. At both cortical and subcortical levels, the regulatory system is significantly more extensive.

The anterior cortical coordinating regions involve the frontal eye field (FEF), the supplementary eye field (SEF), the dorsolateral prefrontal cortex (DLPFC), and the posterior ones consisting of the parietal eye field (PEF), as well as the temporal eye fields (located in the middle temporal gyrus (MT)) and the medial superior temporal area (MST) (Fig. 58.1). In the subcortical regions some nuclei of the thalamus (internal medullary lamina, dorsomedial nucleus, pulvinar), the basal ganglia, practically the whole brainstem (saccade generator cells, the riMLF in the midbrain, the posterior commissure, the superior colliculus, the interstitial nucleus of Cajal, the nucleus of Darkschewitsch, the pontine reticular formation, the vestibular and oculomotor nuclei) and the cerebellum (especially the flocculonodular region and the vermis) play an important role in the regulation of the eye movements.

FEF (Br 8) can be found in the premotor cortex, SEF (Br 6aβ) is located in the superior frontal gyrus, in the anterior portion of the supplementary motor cortex, while the DLPFC covers Brodmann area 46 (Fig. 58.1). FEF represents the primary gaze center, which, beside the horizontal eye movements, regulates the vertical ones presumably as well. SEF plays an important role in the learning of movements through storing motor program, while the DLPFC takes part in the spatial memory and cognitive processes. These cortical areas are interconnected by reciprocal pathways, and all of them project to the superior colliculus. The PEF consists of the Br 39 and Br 40 (Fig. 58.1) and has an impact on the saccades through the coordination of visual attention processes. The temporal gaze centers (MT=V5 and MST=V5A visual areas) are located in the temporal– parietal–occipital junction (Fig. 58.1) in the borderland of Br 19, 37 and 39. The latter regions are responsible for the motion perception, therefore, they primarily take part in the regulation smooth pursuit.

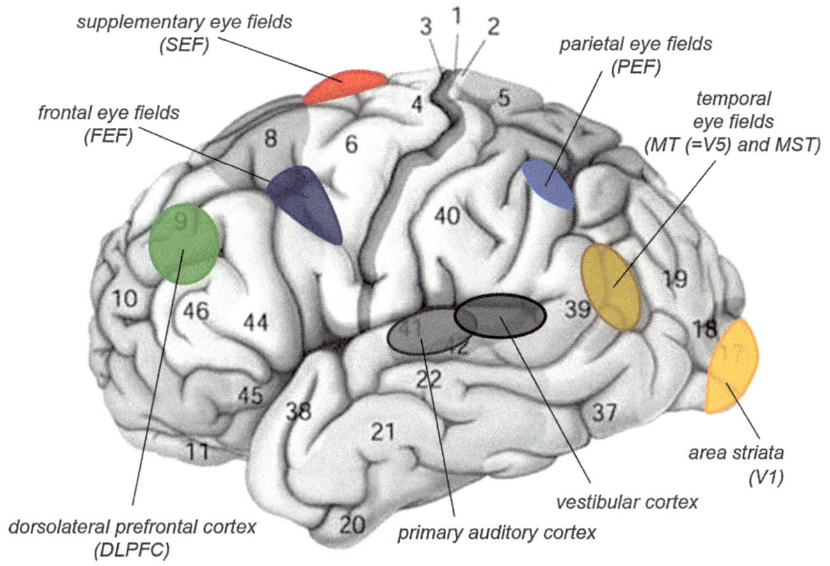

Fig. 58.1 The location of cortical gaze centers

The basal ganglia and thalamus are the essential components of the descending pathways of saccade regulation. The vestibulocerebellum contributes to the adaptation mechanisms and plays a role in the learning of motor programs as well. The brainstem saccade generator cells are located in pontomedullary and mesencephalic reticular formation, and their task is the generation of the ocular premotor command. The riMLF nucleus, in contrast with earlier knowledge, plays a role not only in the vertical but also in the horizontal eye movements. Then the actual oculomotor impulse is transmitted to the extraocular muscles by the n. III, IV and VI. The interconnection between their nuclei is established by the medial longitudinal fasciculus (MLF), the intact function of which is essential to generate conjugate eye movements.

Regulation of the Eye Movements

Regulation of the Saccades

The generation of the saccades is under the control of descending pathways, which originate in the anterior and posterior cortical areas, then either directly or indirectly, synapsing in the thalamus or the basal ganglia reach the superior colliculus and afterwards project to the pontine and mesencephalic saccade generator cells, and finally, end up in the oculomotor nuclei. However, the system is also influenced by the information from the cerebellum and the vestibular nuclei.

The regulatory process is carried out by the contralateral cortical areas (FEF, PEF, SEF and DLPFC). The FEF controls especially the voluntary saccades, while the reflexive ones are under the primary influence of the PEF, which is also in reciprocal interconnection with the FEF. The DLPFC is connected to both the SEF and PEF areas, and due to cognitive and memory processes, it inhibits the reflexive saccades to wrong direction (typically in voluntary antisaccades – see Table 58.1) and controls the saccades which require spatial memory (see predictive saccades, Fig. 58.2). The memory guided processes go together with hippocampal activation. The vestibular information arrives from the vestibular cortex to the FEF regulating the vestibular type of the memory guided saccades, whereas the connections with the auditory cortex are responsible for the control of the reflexive, acoustically guided saccades (Fig. 58.2).

The cortical information reaches the superior colliculus and the lower structures through several parallel pathways. **The direct pathway** (*pedunculopontine*) connects the PEF and the

Table 58.1 Types of the saccades

Main types	Subtypes	Features
1. Reflexive	1. **Visually guided (prosaccade)** 2. **Acoustically guided** 3. Sensorially guided	Fast eye movement triggered by exogenous stimuli **Toward the object which suddenly appeared on the periphery of the retina** **Toward a sudden acoustic stimulus (the examiner snaps his fingers)** Toward a sudden sensory stimulus
2. Voluntary (intentional)	1. Scanning 2. Voluntary, visually guided 3. Voluntary, acoustically guided 4. Predictive 5. Memory guided 6. **To command** 7. Antisaccade	Endogenously triggered, object oriented fast eye movement Exploration of the environment Toward objects which have occupied the periphery of the visual field for a longer time Toward source of sounds which can have been heard for a longer time. Toward a suddenly disappearing object. Visual type: toward the place of a previously seen object which was recalled from the memory. Vestibular type: toward a position which preceded the movement and was recalled from the memory. **Saccades performed on the cue of the examiner ("look to the right")** In the opposite direction of an object which suddenly turned up (look into the opposite direction of the object which comes into sight)
3. Spontaneous		Endogenously triggered but meaningless, scanning eye movement. (e.g., during movements, speaking, at rest, in darkness)
4. The fast phase of the nystagmus		

The saccades most frequently examined in the neurological and ophthalmological practice are italicized (Based on Leigh and Zee (2006))

FEF to the superior colliculi (Fig. 58.3) descending in the posterior limb of the internal capsule, then in the middle the cerebral peduncle and synapses the pontine paramedian reticular formation, and then projects to the abducens nucleus. **The indirect route** is the transthalamic pathway involving the thalamus and the basal ganglia descending to the brainstem structures (Fig. 58.3). The *transthalamic pathway* ends up in the superior colliculus and the periaqueductal gray matter through the internal medullary lamina (IML) and the dorsomedial nucleus of the thalamus (DM). Its projections run to the nucleus of n. III, the ipsilateral riMLF and interstitial nucleus of Cajal. The parallel descending pathway synapses in the basal ganglia. The FEF activates the neurons in the middle of the caudate nucleus, which subsequently exerts phasic inhibition on the pars reticulata of the substantia nigra. This leads to the liberation of the burst neurons of the superior colliculus from tonic inhibition (Fig. 58.3), which is required to generate the appropriate saccade. The electric stimulation of the IML of the thalamus leads to contralateral saccades. The pulvinar, which is connected to the posterior parietal cortex, beside the superior colliculus, also takes part in the regulatory mechanisms, mainly in the control of

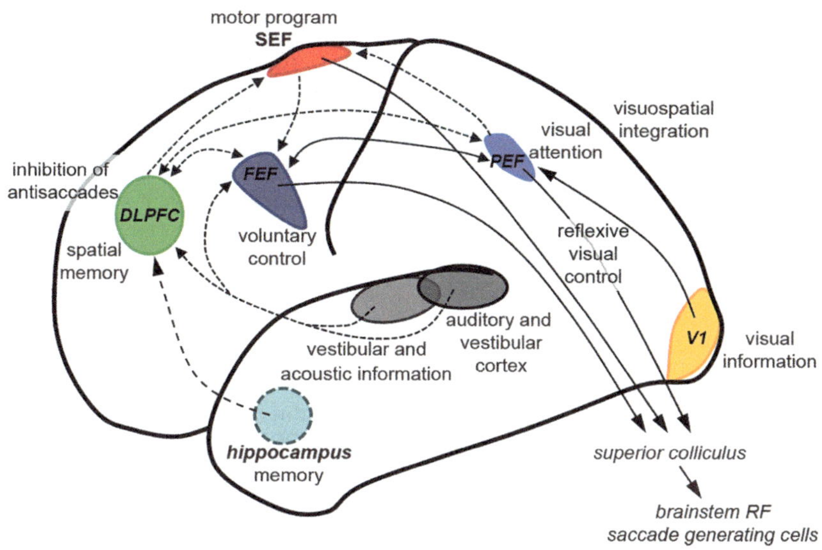

Fig. 58.2 Schematic representation of the saccade regulating centers and their functions and connections

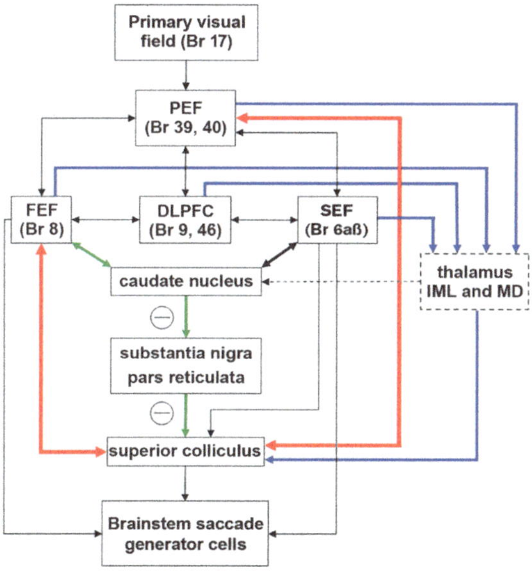

Fig. 58.3 The organizing chart of the regulation of the saccades. *Red line* represents the direct descending pedunculopontine pathway. The indirect pathways reach the superior colliculus through the thalamus (the transthalamic pathway depicted in *blue*) and the basal ganglia (this parallel pathway in *green*). (*IML* internal medullary lamina, *DM* medial dorsal nucleus) (According to Gulyás et al. (2006))

attention and in the generation of the visually guided reflexive saccades. One portion of it guides shifting of visual attention, while the other one is responsible for motion perception.

Through its rostral connections, the superior colliculus is responsible for the selection of the target which the saccade is developed to, the generation of the saccades and the adjustment of their direction and amplitudes. Its main projection lands on the saccade generator cells of the brainstem, which ultimately begin the saccade. The superior colliculus also gives feedback to the saccade regulatory system, as its fibers run back to the thalamus and the FEF.

The saccade generator cells of the brainstem are under the control of the cortical areas, and they generate the premotor impulses for the nuclei of n. III, IV and VI. It is important to emphasize that in contrast with the voluntary, reflexive and spontaneous saccades, the fast phase of the nystagmuses (such as those of the VOR and the OKN) are generated by the saccade generator cells of the brainstem without the control of the cortical gaze centers, relying only on the proprioceptive impulses evoked by the raised tension of the elastic and collagenous components of the orbit, when the bulb reaches the end position. While the horizontal saccade generator cells are located in the caudal portion of the pons (in the PPRF and the medullary RF), and the vertical and torsion saccades can be found in the rostral section of the mesencephalon (in the riMLF and the interstitial nucleus of Cajal). The saccade generator cells can be divided into two general groups: the burst neurons and the omnipause neurons. Their cooperation yields the premotor saccade command, which is transmitted to the oculomotor nuclei. There are several subtypes of the burst neurons; the excitatory and long lead burst neurons generate, maintain and stop the saccades with adequate direction and amplitude. The inhibitory burst neurons inhibit the contralateral abducens nucleus during the ipsilateral saccades, therefore suppress the contralateral eye movement. The premotor regulators of the vertical and torsion saccades can be found in the riMLF. This nucleus also receives inputs from the semicircular canals, therefore, it also plays a role in the regulation of the ocular tilt reaction. Since the regulation of the vertical saccades is bilateral, unilateral damage of the riMLF rarely causes dysfunctions. The vertical inhibitory burst neurons are located in the interstitial nucleus of Cajal. The omnipause cells are discharging continuously, only do they interrupt directly before and during the saccades, and during blinking. The omnipause neurons inhibit the firing of the burst neurons, therefore, they prevent the generation of unwanted saccades (e.g., during fixation). The motor command of the saccade generator cells is transmitted to the nuclei of the oculomotor, trochlear and abducens nerves, which innervate the extraocular muscles.

The Regulation of Smooth Pursuit Movements (SPEM)

During SPEM, the ipsilateral cortical areas control the eye movements. Their inciting stimulus is the shift of the image of a moving object on the fovea. The image of a moving object is projected to the primary visual cortex (Br 17, V1), then the striatal neurons project either directly to the temporal–parietal– occipital junction or through the parastriate cortex (Br 18) (Fig. 58.4). The temporal gaze centers (MT and MST) sense the motion, that is determine the speed and direction of the movement of the visual stimulus in three dimensions, and harmonize the smooth pursuit with the

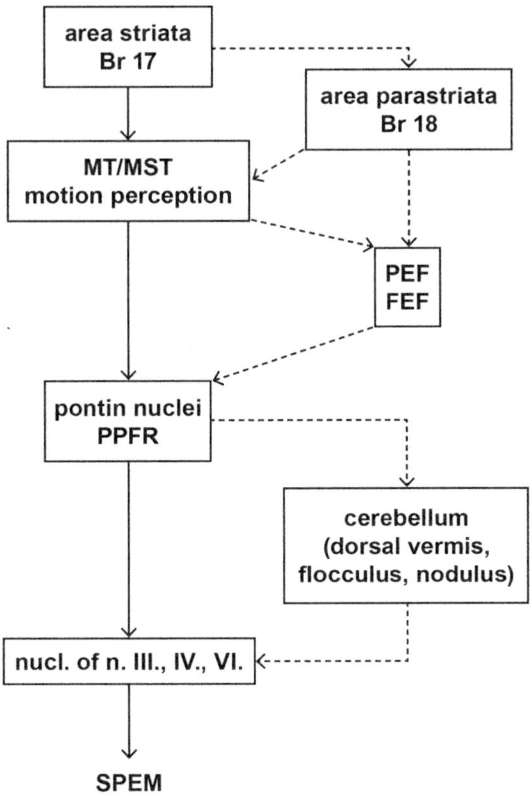

Fig. 58.4 The schematic summary of the the regulatory system of the SPEM

movement of the object relative to the position of the head and the body. The temporal gaze centers project to the posterior parietal cortex (PEF), which are much more important in the maintenance of visual attention (e.g., focus on a small target) than in the actual regulation of motor processes. The FEF also takes part in smooth pursuit (Fig. 58.4). Electric stimulation of FEF elicits slow contralateral deviation of the bulb. Nevertheless, the corresponding area is located slightly posteriorly than in case of stimulation of saccades. For the development of SPEM, the information is transmitted from the cortical areas to brainstem structures via descending pathways. The pathway circumvents the lateral cerebral ventricles in the posterior limb of the internal capsule, then runs through the cerebral peduncle and reaches the dorsolateral and lateral nuclei in the pons.

The contralateral spino- and vestibulocerebellar regions, such as the uvula, vermis, flocculus, nodule and dorsal vermis (Fig. 58.4) play a role not only in the regulation of SPEM but also the slow phase of VOR and OKN. The flocculus sends information through connection with the inferior cerebellar peduncle to the ipsilateral medial vestibular nucleus of Schwalbe. The nucleus of Schwalbe together with the nucleus prepositus hypoglossi, i.e., the neural integrator, summarized the speed and position related inputs and transmits the output to the oculomotor nuclei. The vermis transmits information to the inferior vestibular nucleus of Roller, the lateral vestibular nucleus of Deiters, the lateral nucleus of the dorsomedial pontine nucleus and PPRF surrounding the abducens nucleus. The neurons of the vermis encode and harmonize the movement velocity of the eye with that of the retinal image and the head. Finally, according to the integrated supranuclear information, the nuclei of oculomotor nerves (n. III, IV and VI) carry out the actual SPEM with adequate velocity, direction and amplitude.

The Regulation of VOR and OKN

To stabilize the image of an object, about 70 ms after the oscillopsia elicited by the movement of the head or the object itself, a stabilizing compensatory eye movement will start in the form of SPEM or OKN. Image processing requires the above 70 ms. The vestibulo-ocular is a phylogenetically ancient system, which can be found in some lower species. It generates eye movements at a latency of about 15 ms preventing oscillopsia caused by visual processing. This system connects the semicircular canals via their brainstem centers to the nuclei of the oculomotor nerves. It generates compensatory eye movements to the opposite direction of head turning, which help the fixation of a shifting image on the fovea. For instance upon turning the head to the right, a horizontal slow eye movement to the left can be observed, which is followed by fast repositioning movement (saccade) to the other direction; this is the **vestibulo-ocular reflex** (VOR). In case of its absence, oscillopsia develops when turning the head. The vestibular and oculomotor systems are connected by the vestibular nuclei through the MLF. The MLF makes the relation between not only the nucleus of the n. VI and the contralateral n. III, but it also mediates information toward the pontine reticular formation from the vestibular nuclei and the segments of cervical musculature of the spinal cord. The latter connections are responsible for the oculocephalic reflexes. During head movements of larger extent, VOR can develop several times. When the head moves for a short time, such as rotation of the body, rhythmic, nystagmus like eye movements will develop, and the fast phase is generated by the brainstem saccade generator cells. VOR can be maintained for approximately 40–45 s, then its function is taken over by the OKN in the fixation of the image on the fovea. During permanent rotation, the VOR, which is initially of high gain, over time habituates, and it becomes gradually slower, its frequency gets lower, ultimately extinguishes, and OKN of opposite direction will begin. OKN in physiological circumstances can be triggered not only by vestibular information but also the fast movement of an object in front of the stable head. Physiologically the VOR and the OKN cooperates in the integration of head and eye movements to ensure visual acuity. VOR habituates not only due to permanent challenges but also with practice. This adaptation mechanism can be observed in Sufi whirling dervishes for instance, but it is the mechanism, that is responsible for the gradual decline and disappearance of seasickness. The fixation of one point in the visual field also decreases VOR, vertigo and the accompanying vegetative symptoms, such as the nausea. However, the background of these vestibulo-ocular adaptation processes is not sufficiently clarified yet. Early adaptation relies on visual support (i.e., fixation). The cerebellum recalibrates the vestibular system during adaptation and requires visual reference input for that purpose. However, cognitive control also contributes to these processes. Even the imagination of spinning may evoke the compensatory slow eye movements (slow phase of VOR). Motivation, visual attention and orientation are also crucial in the adaptation. The direction of visual attention to one point of the visual field may reduce the vestibulo-ocular response and vertigo.

OKN or ***railway nystagmus*** is evoked by the movement of the whole visual field or one component (e.g., an object) of it, and due to this compensation, the image gets stabilized on the retina. Its latency is about 80–100 ms, which corresponds to that of the smooth pursuit. Intact retina and visual pathway are needed to elicit this response. The moving image evokes a slow tracking movement, which is directed toward the motion of the object with approximately the same velocity of that of the object in healthy, and can reach maximum about 100°/s. Then the eyes return to their primary position with a fast saccade, which form the second phase of OKN, and then the eyes will look for a new target and follow it again. OKN is classified according to the direction of slow phase, similarly to the smooth pursuit (SPEM). Its characteristic feature is the gain or tracking ratio, which represents ratio of eye tracking velocity to target velocity. In healthy subjects it is about "1". During OKN, the retinal image processing is permanent, therefore, the image is continuously sharp, the movement seems slower, whereas without OKN oscillopsia develops and the movement appears faster. The slow phase of OKN is generated by the SPEM pathway, but the ipsilateral inferior oliva also contributes to it. The fast, saccade phase is induced by the increasing tension of the elastic and collagen components of the orbit, and it is regulated by the brainstem saccade generator cells. In both VOR and OKN, a velocity-storage mechanism maintains the nystagmus even some seconds after the trigger disappears. It develops due to the fact that the neurons of the vestibular nuclei in the brainstem do not cease discharging immediately after the head or the environment stopped moving.

The Regulation of Vergence Eye Movements

The convergent–divergent eye movements together with changing the sphericity of the lens and the diameter of the pupil contribute to maintain sharp vision during accommodation. Similarly to saccade generation, the premotor neurons of vergence eye movements are also located in the reticular formation of the mesencephalon and the pons. Their regulation, however, is not completely clarified yet in details. According to the most popular concept, the Perlia nucleus, which can be found next to the nuclei of the n. III, is the ocular convergence center. Via the corticobulbar fibers, the frontal eye field reaches the Perlia nucleus, which innervates the medial rectus muscle on both sides and generates the convergent eye movement. These can be fast (together with a saccade) or slow (with SPEM) convergent eye movements. The saccade, SPEM and vergence regulatory systems overlap at several levels. The FEF, SEF, the temporal gaze centers, the posterior parietal cortex (including the parietal eye field), the flocculonodular lobe and the vermis of the cerebellum all contribute to the supranuclear regulation of vergence, and the three systems are also interconnected at the levels of the superior colliculi and the mesencephalic and pontine RF neurons such as the saccade generator cells. Although the exact regulatory mechanism is still unknown, it is supposed that motor command of the fast convergent eye movements is generated simultaneously in the frontal eye field (FEF), then via parallel pathways, it reaches the Perlia nucleus and the pontine omnipause cells (i.e., a group of the saccade generator cells), which ultimately harmonize the fast and convergent eye movements. The system of the smooth pursuit eye movements is connected to vergence regulation presumably through the tegmental pontine reticular nucleus. Further components of the system play a role in the fine-tuning of the motor command of FEF, in order to adjust the extent and speed of the vergence to the simultaneous saccade or SPEM.

The Examination of Eye Movements at Bedside

During the examination, the **spontaneous scanning eye movements**, then the **primary position** of the bulbs are observed looking for nystagmus and pathological eye positions. Then in fixed position of the head, we ask the patient to look at our finger or the tip of our pen. In pathological conditions, pathological eye movements can still be noticed even **during fixation** (opsoclonus, ocular flutter). To check **smooth pursuit and the guided eye movements**, the patient is instructed to follow the examiner's finger, which is moved in approximately 50 cm distance horizontally and vertically and stopped briefly at the extreme of movements. We observe whether fast saccadic movements or nystagmus are present, and the range of the movements is complete and conjugated, and also ask the patient about diplopia. To evaluate **the commanded eye movements** (voluntary saccades), we instruct the patient "to look to the right, to the left, up and down". In healthy subjects, conjugated movements of full range can be seen, and no nystagmus can be noticed. In the routine practice, reflexive saccades usually cannot be checked. However, they can be observed, for instance, when the nurse suddenly enters the surgery. When **convergence** is being checked, we advance our finger from about 60 cm towards the nose of the patient and ask him to "look at the tip of the finger". The **vestibulo-ocular reflex** (VOR) can be evoked by the slow turn of the patient's head to one side. With healthy system, the bulbs will deviate conjugately to the opposite direction of the turn, which is followed by fast conjugate movement towards the turn. This reflex can also be tested in non-cooperating, unconscious patients. The vestibulo-ocular system can also be examined by caloric stimulation of the semicircular canals. In healthy subjects, upon cold stimulus (air or water), the eyes show slow conjugated deviation to the side of the stimulation, while upon warm stimulus, they move to the opposite direction. For the investigation of the **optokinetic nystagmus (OKN)**, the striped rotating drum is the most suitable, but a paper with alternating pattern may also make do. OKN is elicited by the movement of an alternating pattern (like the black and white stripes). We can check the patient, while the drum is being turned into the four main directions.

The Most Significant Gaze Disoders in the Neurological Practice

When the lesion is located rostrally from the brainstem, the eye movements remain conjugated, nystagmus does not develop. The regulation of the saccades is contralateral, therefore, unilateral acute frontal lobe (involving the FEF) lesions (such as the occlusion of the middle cerebral artery) lead to overactivity of the intact side, and the patient looks at the focus ("toward the lesion"). In contrast, the excitement of the frontal eye field (such as in an epileptic seizure) results in conjugate deviation to the opposite side (away from of the focus). The dysfunction of the frontal and parietal eye fields (due to vascular or degenerative disease) may augment the latency and modify the accuracy of the contralateral saccades, and it may lend saccadic characteristics to the ipsilateral smooth pursuit movements as well. Dysmetria of saccades means that the amplitude of the saccades is not appropriate, the eyes target behind (hypermetric) or ahead (hypometric) the object. However, these dysfunctions are difficult to percept during bedside examination, their objective analysis can be performed by specific equipment, the electrooculography (EOG). Unilateral parietal damage can lead to contralateral ocular apraxia, e.g., in corticobasal degeneration. In this case, the patient cannot perform the contralateral commanded saccades, but during the examination of the guided eye movements (SPEM), the patient can follow the physician's finger if they are being moved with increasing amplitude.

The lesion of the basal ganglia leads to hypometric saccades and saccadic SPEM similar to the frontal and parietal dysfunctions, for instance in Parkinson's disease, but these alterations are rather difficult to assess upon routine examination. The lesion of the thalamus may result in both horizontal and vertical gaze disorder. In medial thalamic bleedings, the eyes are in conjugate deviation towards the intact side. According to the literature, the hemorrhage irritates the surrounding structures, therefore, despite the fact that the pathway is still before crossing, the eyes look at the healthy side. When the thalamic bleeding compresses the midbrain and the riMLF nucleus inside it, the patient looks downward, the eyes converge, and they are miotic ("the patient looks at his nose"). Similar constellation can be seen in the case of damages to the diencephalic–mesencephalic transition (e.g., pineal tumors, thalamic hemorrhages, midbrain infarction), but they may also lead to convergence spasm. It was also described in disorders affecting the cerebellum and the lower brainstem and even in Wernicke–Korsakoff syndrome. The lesion of the caudal thalamus leads to the palsy of downward gaze, due to the damage of adjacent riMLF and its input. The dysfunction of the middle portion of the thalamus results in saccadic dysmetria, which, however, can be noticed only with difficulty at the bedside. The lesion of mesencephalic riMLF may lead to pseudoabducens palsy, which represents supranuclear abduction weakness. It is a rare condition, but the patient complains about diplopia in certain situations, the cause of which cannot be unveiled by routine neurological tests, only EOG can make the diagnosis possible. Pseudoabducens palsy means that during the horizontal saccades, the abducting eye completely turns to temporal direction, but compared to the adducting one, it moves more and more slowly. Therefore, the eyes gradually diverge, and the patients complain about that during reading they have difficulties in shifting lines. Bilateral pseudoabducens palsy was observed in bilateral paramedial thalamic infarction, which spared the midbrain. The convergence–retraction nystagmus also represents a supranuclear weakness of abduction and convergence. During upward saccades, beside the vertical movement, a fast asynchronic convergent one also appears, which is accompanied by the rhythmic retraction of the bulbs as well. Bilateral riMLF leads to complete vertical and torsion gaze palsy. Beside riMLF, the Cajal nucleus is responsible for the vertical gaze. Its lesion, therefore, decreases the speed and amplitude of the vertical eye movements. When the MLF gets impaired beside the nucleus of Cajal, the vertical "one-and-a-half" syndrome develops. The syndrome essentially represents bilateral downward gaze palsy, which is accompanied by upward gaze palsy on the side of the lesion, but the opposite constellation may also occur.

The lesion of the paramedial pontine RF (PPRF) makes it impossible to generate ipsilateral saccades. Milder dysfunction leads to the decrease of the speed of the ipsilateral saccades such as at the early stage of neurodegenerative progressive supranuclear palsy (PSP). When PSP progresses, besides the Parkinsonian symptoms, vertical and later even horizontal gaze palsy may develop. The lesion of MLF results in internuclear ophthalmoplegia (INO) if it is accompanied by the lesion of the abducens nucleus "one-and-a-half" syndrome ensues (for more details the reader is referred to Chap. 55 on page 292). The impairment of the omnipause subtype of the saccade: generator cells in the PPRF cause disturbance in the harmonization of the function of saccade generator cells. Therefore, they cannot inhibit the involuntary saccades, and slow horizontal and vertical saccades also develop. The first condition is characterized by pathologic oscillations during fixation proven by EOG, which depending on their amplitude and direction can lead to square-wave jerks (amplitude of 1–5°), macro-square-wave jerks (amplitude between 5 and 15°), ocular flutter and in severe cases opsoclonus (oscillation with horizontal, vertical and torsional components). The macro-square-wave jerks and the opsoclonus can be noticed even with the naked eye. These phenomena can also be found in neurodegenerative disorders such as PSP, multiple system atrophy (MSA), and cerebrovascular lesions affecting the PPRF. In brainstem lesions, the ipsilateral OKN is also pathological, the eyes cannot follow the moving stripes adequately, in severe cases OKN cannot be evoked at all. When the vestibulo-ocular connections in the brainstem are disrupted on both sides, doll's head phenomenon develops. Then upon horizontal movements of the head, the eyes remain in their primary position like the painted eyes of a doll. This can be noticed, for instance, in basilar artery occlusions. In the unilateral lesions of the paramedial pontine RF, eye movements induced by vestibular inputs cannot be elicited toward the side of the lesion.

Cerebellar lesions can impair both the SPEM and the saccades and can induce nystagmus. The bulbs may show 10–30° conjugate deviation toward the intact side, and when the patient fixates an object in the midline, the eyes slowly float to this position, then quickly jumps back to the fixated object. In the unilateral lesion of the flocculonodular area, the eye always falls behind the moving object, the smooth pursuit becomes saccadic, while after cerebellectomy smooth pursuit completely disappears. In vermis damages cause principally saccadic dysmetria. The lesions of the inferior cerebellar peduncle and/or the vestibulocerebellum impair the contralateral OKN.

References

Gulyás S, Nagy F, Szirmai I. Összetett szemmozgászavar thalamus ès mesencephalon infarktusban, esetismertetès [Complex eye movement disorder in thalamic and mesencephalic infarctions, a case report]. Clin Neurosci/Ideggy Szle. 2006;59(5–6):193–200.

Leigh RJ, Zee DS. The neurology of eye movements, fourth. New York: Oxford University Press; 2006.

Further Readings

Bucher SF, Dieterich M, Seelos KC, Brandt T. Sensorimotor cerebral activation during optokinetic nystagmus. A functional MRI study. Neurology. 1997;49:1370–7.

Büttner U, Brandt T. The ocular motor disorders of the brainstem. London: Bailliere Tindall; 1992. p. 263–73.

Gaymard B, Pierrot-Deseilligny C. Neurology of saccades and smooth pursuit. Curr Opin Neurol. 1999;12:13–9.

Ilg UJ. Slow eye movements. Prog Neurobiol. 1997;53:293–329.

Ilniczky S, Kamondi A, Vdrallyay G, Gaal B, Palásti A, Gulyás S, Szirmai I. One-and-a-half syndrome – two cases. Clin Neurosci/Ideggy Szle. 2007;60:489–93.

Leigh RJ, Daroff RB, Troost BT. Supranuclear disorders of eye movement. In: Glaser JS, editor. Neuro-ophthalmology. Philadelphia: Lippincott Williams & Wilkins; 1999.

Pierrot-Deseilligny C, Gaymard B, Müri R, Rivaud S. Cerebral ocular motor signs. J Neurol. 1997;244:65–70.

Pierrot-Deseilligny C, Milea D, Müri RM. Eye movement control by the cerebral cortex. Curr Opin Neurol. 2004;17:17–25.

Pierrot-Deseilligny C, Rivaud S, Gaymard B, Müri RM, Vermersch AI. Cortical control of saccades. Ann Neurol. 1995;37:557–67.

Pierrot-Deseilligny C, Rivaud S, Gaymard B, Agid Y. Cortical control of reflexive visually guided saccades. Brain. 1991;114:1473–85.

Scudder CA, Kaneko CRS, Fuchs AF. The brainstem burst generator for saccadic eye movements. A modern synthesis. Exp Brain Res. 2002;142:439–62.

Sparks DL. The brainstem control of saccadic eye movements. Nat Rev Neurosci. 2002;3:952–64.

Szirmai I. Neurológia [Neurology], 2. kiadás. Budapest: Medicina; 2005.

Tusa RJ. Cortical control of eye movements. In: Kennard C, Rose F, editors. Physiological aspects of clinical neuro-ophthalmology. London: Chapman and Hall; 1988. p. 249–64.

Vastagh I, Folyovich A, Arányi Z, Bodrogi L, Tárczy M. Bal oldali thalamuslágyulás ès komplex tekintèsi zavar [Thalamomalacia on the left side and complex gaze disorder]. Clin Neurosci/Ideggy Szle. 1996;49:391–6.

Disorders of the Neuromuscular Junction and Their Diagnostics

59

László Sándor Fornádi

Contents

Introduction

The neuromuscular junction (NMJ) is an especially frequent target of the autoimmune diseases. First, here the blood–brain barrier is open; second, the NMJ is rich in ion channels, which represent considerable extracellular space via which the autoantibodies easily reach the antigens. The following basic processes take place in NMJ (based on John Newsom-Davis's research): The propagating action potential of the nerve is generated by the gradually opening sodium channels. The inactivation of the sodium channels and opening of the voltage-gated calcium channels lead to the repolarization of the membrane. When the action potential reaches the endplate, it opens the P/Q type voltage-gated calcium channels and elicits the local influx of calcium ions. This triggers the exocytosis of the acetylcholine containing synaptic vesicles. Afterwards, the acetylcholine molecules diffuse through the synaptic cleft and bind to the free site of the α2 subdomain of the acetylcholine receptor, which opens the central pore of the ligand-gated channel and leads to the inward current of small ions (mainly sodium). This leads to the generation of the endplate potential, which then triggers the action potential of the muscle. And this ultimately activates the contraction (Newsom-Davis et al. 1986). The blockade of the neuromuscular junction, besides the dysfunction of the skeletal muscles, involves the weakness, fatigue or paresis of the ocular musculature as well, which necessitates the detailed discussion of the topic in a neuro-ophthalmological textbook, most importantly because of the great differential diagnostic importance of the disorder. Numerous, although individually not too frequent, but severe, even life-threatening diseases can mimic the condition and mislead the clinician. Exo- and endogenous intoxications, autoimmune and paraneoplastic disorders may all elicit the pathological or

L.S. Fornádi, M.D.
Department of Neurology, Jahn Ferenc South Pest Hospital, Budapest, Hungary
e-mail: fornadi@t-online.hu

J. Somlai, T. Kovács (eds.), *Neuro-Ophthalmology*, DOI 10.1007/978-3-319-28956-4_59

decreased activity of the *neuromuscular junction*. Further, ophthalmopareses can be also elicited by genetic disorders, several of which (like the mitochondrial diseases) are accompanied by other severe complications, which are often hardly compatible with life. Congenital myasthenias can also go together with eye-related symptoms (ptosis, diplopia). Several *congenital myasthenias* are known, and different genetical defects are responsible for each entity, but the basic problem (insufficient or pathological activity of the neuromuscular junction) and the symptoms are generally the same. *Oculopharyngeal myopathies* are also the consequences of genetical defects, but in these cases, besides the eye-related symptoms, typical nasal dysphonia and dysphagia can also be found.

Myasthenia Gravis, Myasthenia Syndrome, Congenital Myasthenia

Myasthenia gravis (MG) represents the most exactly verified autoimmune disorder. The target organ, the antigen and the autoantibody are all identified. Main characteristics: Treatable, but without therapy, it can be a lethal condition. Before the introduction of the immune-modulating treatments, approximately 1/3 of the cases proved to be fatal. Further, it can mimic other, unfortunately incurable disorders (motoneuron disorders, such as amyotrophic lateral sclerosis, bulbar palsy), therefore, their early differentiation is of vital importance. To diagnose the disorder takes 5–6 years on average. Often three to four physicians meet the patient till the diagnosis is established.

Types of Myasthenia

1. *Autoimmune myasthenia gravis*, which can start spontaneously, may be neonatal (maternal antibodies cross the placental barrier eliciting transient myasthenia) and penicillamine induced.
2. *Hereditary* (*congenital*) *myasthenia*
3. *Lambert–Eaton paraneoplastic myasthenic syndrome* (LEMS)

The Characteristics of Autoimmune Myasthenia Gravis

(a) Increasing weakness and fatigue of the typical target sites (ocular, facial, masticatory, bulbar and other skeletal muscles). The pattern of attacks changes in localization and time, and sometimes it affects only individual muscles (e.g., generalized vs. ocular and bulbar myasthenia). The purely ocular forms make up 20 % of myasthenia cases, and less than 15 % of the latter group becomes generalized during the first 2 years of the course. The primary or secondary generalized forms account for 80 % of the cases. From them 67 % present with ptosis or ophthalmoparesis, 80 % complain about difficulties in chewing and swallowing, 70 % experience weakness of the neck, the trunk and the extremities and in 5 % the respiratory muscles are affected.
(b) Progressive weakening and fatigue of the skeletal muscles develop during the day with normal physical expenditure.
(c) Rest leads to temporary restitution
(d) The course of the disease is periodic and characterized by remissions and relapses.
(e) Upon the administration of cholinesterase inhibitors, immediate and remarkable symptomatic improvement can be noticed in the majority of the cases (edrophonium chloride = *Tensilon test*).
(f) With electromyography, the myasthenic response can be demonstrated: repetitive nerve stimulation of 3 Hz frequency will elicit the typical (more than 10 %) reduction of the compound muscle action potential (CMAP) amplitude (decremental response).
(g) The underlying myasthenic disorder represents a neuromuscular blockade, which develops due to the decrease in the number of acetylcholine receptors. The destruction of the postsynaptic membrane is caused by the autoantibodies targeted against acetylcholine receptors. The antibodies are predominantly of IgG type, and their production begins early intrathymically against the myoid cells. These antibodies in 85–90 % of the myasthenic cases are targeted against the

acetylcholine receptors (AChR) of the neuromuscular junction. Forty percent of the remaining (10–15 %) cases feature antibodies against the muscle specific tyrosine kinase (MuSK). Recent anti-MuSK cases have shown a more malignant course of their myasthenic disease, whereas they are more therapy resistant. Striational antibodies, which react with epitopes on the muscle proteins titin, ryanodine receptor (RyR), and Kv1.4, are frequently found in MG patients with late-onset and thymoma. In purely ocular myasthenia, anti-AChR antibodies can be found in 50 % of the cases.

(h) Spontaneous remission can only be expected in 10 % of the cases. Without medical treatment, 1/3 of the patients will ultimately die, while remission can be achieved in 95 % of the cases with adequate immune-modulating treatment (Rózsa et al. 2006).

Other Disorders Accompanied by MG (Szobor 1985)

MG most frequently goes together with disorders of the thyroid gland (Szobor and Környei 1966a; Csenkèr et al. 1977; Bohaty and Balázs 1984) (hyper- and hypothyroidism) and rheumatoid arthritis, but several cases were reported in association with poly-, dermatomyositis, systemic lupus erythematosus, progressive systemic sclerosis, Sjogren's syndrome, psoriasis, non-Hodgkin-lymphoma and pernicious anemia. The bewildering combination of the symptoms makes the diagnosis a formidable challenge, further, the accompanying disorders will influence the progress of the disease and the therapeutic responses, too. Moreover, a rather frequent finding is the resistance or intolerance to acetlycholinesterase inhibitor therapy (such as Mestinon), but *the immune-modulating therapies* are almost effective in every association of disorders. Sometimes they give satisfactory therapeutic result even alone, but they are certainly effective in combination (e.g., azathioprine and methylprednisolone). Obviously the outlined therapy can be amended according to the requirements of the treatment of the accompanying autoimmune diseases. Thymectomy can also improve the symptoms of the accompanying disorder (e.g., psoriasis) (Szobor and Molnár 1985). *Thymectomy* appears to be effective in young (below 45 years) patients, who are positive for antibodies against the acetylcholine receptor and suffer from generalized myasthenia. In those patients, thymectomy may yield significant improvement, and in 20 % of the cases, complete remission (recommendation level B) is achieved. The chance of complete remission is higher in the case of young female patients, when the surgical intervention is performed at the beginning of the course of the disease. In cases which are negative for antibodies against the acetylcholine receptor, contradictory evidence is available regarding the indication of thymectomy. The published data do not make possible to outline an unequivocal guideline in these cases, while in anti-MUSK positive cases thymectomy is positively contraindicated due to its ineffectiveness (recommendation level C). However in myasthenia cases associated with thymoma, the resection of the tumor must be performed as soon as possible, irrespectively of the type of the myasthenia, since in these cases the goal of the intervention is the removal of the tumor itself (Szakmai Kollègium 2007).

Drug Elicited Myasthenia

Several drugs are infamous for their neuromuscular transmission impairing side effect, which may cause myasthenic symptoms or activate latent myasthenia. Obviously these drugs are strictly contraindicated in myasthenia (Szakmai Kollègium 2007).

Absolutely contraindicated ones are muscle relaxants, the sedato-hypnotic drugs with muscle relaxant side effect (primarily meprobamat and benzodiazepin derivatives), depolarizing antibiotics (tetracyclins, streptomycin, kanamycin, neomycin, bacitracin, colistin, telitromycin etc.), and fluorochinolone derivatives (ciprofloxacin, ofloxacin, norfloxacin etc.). Some drugs represent relative contraindication, therefore, beta-blockers, calcium channel blockers can be used only with care. These drugs *do not cause true myasthenia*, only do they activate the latent form or aggravate the persisting condition. Prolonged dose-dependent myasthenic reaction can develop due to the treatment with D-penicillamine, which is frequently used in rheumatoid arthritis (Szobor et al. 1979). These D-penicillamine treated rheumatoid arthritis cases, which show characteristic antibody production, typical electrophysiological symptoms and HLA-susceptibility background, should also represent latent MG cases. They are activated by the provoking impact of D-penicillamine treatment and similar to those ones, which develop immediately after thymoma surgery or other surgical interventions when attempting to disconnect the patient from the respirator.

Differential Diagnosis of Myasthenia Gravis

MG may produce extremely protean, frequently unilateral, fluctuating ocular (and of other preferred muscular sites, obviously) symptoms, and may even go to remission for years, therefore, it should be clearly separated from other disorders of eye-related symptoms.

1. **Neuromuscular blockade due to toxins**
   From the diseases caused by numerous plant and animal poisons and bacterial toxin, *curare intoxication*, *botulism* and *diphtheria* bear clinical relevance in practice. The antidote of *curare intoxication*, physostigmine, due to the efforts of a young English physician, Mary Walker (1934) became the most important symptomatic treatment of *myasthenia gravis*, a disorder, which until then had been incurable and had frequently proved to be fatal (Walker 1938). Later research proved that in both cases the blockade of the neuromuscular junction is responsible for the symptoms. In botulism, the *toxin deriving from contaminated food or from wounds infected by the anaerobic Clostridium botulinum*, directly inhibits the release of acetylcholine from the neuromuscular junction. Moreover, the toxin impairs the functions of the central nervous system and the peripheral nerves, as well. The clinical picture of botulism (Cherington 1974) is characterized by ocular muscle palsies (e.g., severe bilateral ptosis; so typical of myasthenia, too), impairment of cholinergic innervation (decreased lacrimation, salivation, accomodation paralysis, dilated fixed pupils), bulbar symptoms (dysphagia and dysarthria) and sensory disturbances. The paralysis of the skeletal muscles will affect first the muscles of the head and the neck. This feature clearly distinguishes it from the similarly acute but ascending, Landry-type, polyradiculoneuritic paralysis or Guillain–Barre syndrome. Botulism, finally, may lead to diaphragm and respiratory paralysis. The fatal outcome can only be prevented by early and intensive therapeutic intervention (like the critical cases of Guillain–Barre syndrome and myasthenia gravis). From the rapidly progressing myasthenia, which quickly involves the oculobulbar motor system, the early paralysis of the pupillomotor fibers, and the characteristic bilateral, fixed pupils differentiate it. The thorough and meticulous examination of the patient is rewarded by the differentiation between myasthenia and Guillain-Barre syndrome. Otherwise, the similarities of the conditions such as the early development of nasal dysphonia, dysphagia, respiratory insufficiency and the diffuse skeletal muscle weakness may mislead the physician. Obviously the three syndromes can be easily separated by electromyography and electroneurography. With intensive care, and assisted ventilation, the majority of botulism cases heal with axonal resprouting. The efficacy of polyvalent antiserum treatment is heavily debated by the experts. The toxin of *Corynebacterium diphteriae* causes similar symptoms. The eye movement disorder usually affects the area innervated by the oculomotor nerve, which is accompanied by accommodation palsy, paralysis of the soft palate and sensorimotor neuropathy. Snake, scorpion and spider venom can also cause neuromuscular transmission

disorder. The Hungarian literature published the first and fatal case of the wasp bite associated dermatomyositis and myasthenic neuromuscular transmission disorder in 1979 (Szobor et al. 1985). In our large collection of Hungarian cases, several wasp and tick bite associated myasthenia cases of verified autoimmune origin can be found. Although the exact relationship has not been clarified yet, presumably the toxin initiated immune response goes awry due to antigenic mimicry (i.e., the similarity of surface antigens) and cross-reaction leads autoimmune response.

2. One of the most frequent form of the **paraneoplastic syndromes**, the small-cell lung carcinoma associated *myasthenic syndrome* (*Lambert–Eaton–Rooke*), appears in an obscure form, but even in this case, the cranial motor units (and the eye muscles) are not affected only the pelvic muscles and the proximål muscles of the lower limb. In Lambert–Eaton paraneoplastic myasthenia syndrome (LEMS), anticholinesterase therapy is ineffective. Small cell lung carcinoma (SCLC) associated Lambert–Eaton syndrome is typically of immune origin. The circulating antibodies attack the presynaptic voltage-gated calcium channels (VGCC). Immune modulating therapy, plasmapheresis and guanidine-hydrochloride therapy can be recommended.
3. **Acquired neuromyotonia** (*Isaac's syndrome*, **ANMT**)

   The most important symptoms consist of twitching (myokymia), cramps, sometimes weakness and hypohydrosis. Sometimes paresthesias and symptoms of the central nervous system (disturbance of sleep, mood disorders, hallucinations) can develop. ANMT can be associated with thymoma (in 15 % of the cases), myasthenia gravis and SCLC. Further, like myasthenia gravis, it can be provoked by penicillamine. EMG reveals double, triple or even multiple, repetitive firing activity of the motor units, which also feature high (40–300 Hz) intraburst frequency. The pathological process is associated with the axon terminals of the motoneurons. The activity persists even during sleep and general anesthesia, which clearly differentiates it from the discharges of the Stiff-person syndrome. In several patients the underlying disorder is caused by the attack of autoantibodies against the voltage-gated potassium channels (VGKC).
4. **Disorders of the thyroid gland (hyper- and hypothyroidism) can be accompanied by** both **myopathy and myasthenia**. The clinical evaluation of *endocrine ophthalmopathies* can be rather difficult, since it needs the exact differentiation of the movement limitation due to mechanical constraints of the edematous bulb from true ophthalmoplegia, which most frequently affects the superior rectus muscle.
5. The differentiation between **ocular myopathies** (Bastiansen et al. 1974; Iannaccone et al. 1974; Olson et al. 1972) and myasthenia is of vital importance. The familial, isolated ocular muscle dystrophy progresses extremely slowly and leads to eye-movement limitations and ptosis. About 1/3 of those ptosis cases can be attributed to this genetic disorder. The form which is accompanied by dysphagia and dysarthria and can also appear in myasthenic families is called oculopharyngeal dystrophy (Bastiansen et al. 1974; Iannaccone et al. 1974; Olson et al. 1972). Previously the slowly progressing ocular muscle dystrophies which do not involve the internal eye muscles were classified as Graefe's progressive external ophthalmoplegias, and they were attributed to neurogenic disorder. However, based upon the evaluation of large collection of biopsy specimens, it became apparent, that the majority of the cases are of myogenic origin, with the histological picture of irregular "ragged" red fibers.

Among the *mitochondrial disorders*, some of the clinical syndromes go with ophthalmoplegia and the aforementioned histological alterations. *Mitochondrial disorders are multisystemic diseases due to the defect of the mitochondrial DNA*. Chronic progressive external ophthalmoplegia (CPEO) belongs to the mitochondrial disorders. Their characteristics are weakness of the girdles, retinitis pigmentosa, conduction abnormalities in the heart and the histological picture of "ragged red fibers". Molecular biological investigations revealed the deletions of the mitochondrial DNA in the background as in the case of the closely related but more severe syndrome variant, Kearns-Sayre mitochondrial encephalomyopathy (Berenberg et al. 1977).

Kearns-Sayre characteristics:

- *onset around 15–20 years of age*
- *mainly sporadic occurence*
- *progressive external ophthalmoplegia*
- *retinitis pigmentosa,*
- *weakness of the muscles of the nape and shoulder*
- *dysfunction of the blood-brain barrier*
- *dementia*
- *cerebellar ataxia*
- *hardness of hearing*
- *conduction abnormalities in the heart, which, without implantation of a pacemaker may lead to life-threatening complications.*

6. The second most frequent **hereditary muscle dystrophy**, *myotonic dystrophy (DM)* (Bethlem 1977; Jerusalem 1979), *originally described by Steinert and Curschmann*, manifests itself around 20 years of age. Genetic studies separated two types of it. In type I DM (which represents a tri-nucleotide repeat disorder), besides the typical myotonic reaction, bilateral ptosis, myopathic facies, muscle atrophy of distal onset and weakness, the accompanying symptoms may include cataract, balding, hypothyroidism, hypogonadism and hardness of hearing. The cardiac conduction abnormalities may result in sudden death and even respiratory failure can be an early symptom. Infrequent blinking, convergence spasms and pseudo-Graefe's sign may complement the eye-related symptoms. Genetic analysis is available in Hungary, which is based upon the determination of the extent of CTG-repeats in DMPK (DM protein kinase) gene. The inheritance is autosomal dominant. Type II DM represents a tetra-nucleotide repeat disorder, in which eye-related symptoms are missing, the atrophy is less pronounced, but myalgia and muscle cramps dominate the clinical picture.
7. **Polymyositis**, **dermatomyositis** can itself be responsible for MG-like symptoms and signs, and they can also accompany MG. Especially, the cases with severe dysphagia represent differential diagnostic difficulties, however, EMG–ENG and histological studies make the diagnosis unambiguous. Fortunately in both types of conditions the same range of immuno-therapies is recommended (steroid, azathioprine, plasmapheresis) with similar efficacy in the individual conditions and in their combination, too. A rare condition is idiopathic giant cell polymyositis, which is accompanied by thymoma, myocarditis and sometimes MG-like symptoms and the disorder of the thyroid gland.
8. **Congenital ptoses** can usually be attributed to uni- or bilateral hypoplasia of the nuclei of cranial nerve, and show strong familial aggregation. *Moebius's syndrome* is a congenital hypo- or aplasia of the VI and VII cranial nerves (rarely V and VIII) Beside lateral eye movement inability, difficulty in speaking, swallowing and breathing are the additional symptoms.
9. **Motoneuron disorders** can also be accompanied by MG-like weakness, and even in the Hungarian practice the association of amyotrophic lateralsclerosis (ALS) and MG (Szobor and Samu 1984) has already been described. However, it must be emphasized that the ocular motor system is never affected in ALS! This represents an important differential diagnostic criterion. Interestingly, the cholinergic edrophonium-chloride and other cholinergic drugs used in the treatment of myasthenia can provoke the fasciculations so characteristic of ALS, unveiling the hidden condition. This can also help in differential diagnosis. Cholinergic overdose will lead to

characteristic "twitching" of the eyelids. From the peripheral motoneuron disorders both the Kugelberg–Welander-type pseudomyopathic juvenile spinal muscle atrophy (Kugelberg and Welander 1956) and the Fazio–Londe-type juvenile spinal muscle atrophy (Mátyus et al. 1982), can also be accompanied by ophthalmoplegia. In the latter, the bilateral ptosis and the myopathic facies bewilderingly resembles MG. In this form, besides the motoric cranial nerves, the phrenic nerve is also affected, the life of the child can be prolonged only with respirator. Tensilon test, EMG or muscle biopsy is the suitable tool of separating this neurogenic lesion from MG.

10. **Nuclear, internuclear and supranuclear ophthalmoplegias**. The diverse eye-related symptoms of MG can imitate almost every manifestation of neurogenic ophthalmoplegias. Duane's retraction syndrome develops due to supranuclear innervation disorder and leads to paralysis of the external rectus muscle, which is accompanied by the retraction of the bulb and blepharospasm upon the adduction of the affected eye. EMG reveals the simultaneous activation of the external and internal rectus muscles. In myasthenia a similar retraction syndrome was described by Szobor (1990b). Myasthenia may also be mimicked by Horner's syndrome, the most frequent central reason of which is Wallenberg' syndrome, which usually develops in retro-olivary emollitions due to circulatory disorders of the posterior inferior cerebellar artery (PICA). In Horner's syndrome, besides ptosis and enophtalmos, miosis can also be noticed. It is the pharmacological testing (Paredrin's test) of the latter that could help differentiate whether a preganglionic (central) or postganglionic sympathetic lesion is responsible for the symptoms. In one unilateral form of the congenital ptoses, opening of the mouth and the slight movement of the mandible to lateral direction leads to widening of the affected palpebral fissure, which reflects pathological innervation. This is the Marcus–Gunn phenomenon (or jaw-winking reflex), which is related to the congenital maldevelopment of the internuclear cranial motoric connections.

    Internuclear ophthalmoplegia (Szobor 1990b), which most frequently develops due to unilateral lesions (multiple sclerosis, brainstem vascular disorders, Wernicke's encephalopathy or hemorrhagic superior polioencephalitis) is characterized by adduction palsy of the affected eye upon lateral gaze. While the opposite eye turns properly, the affected one remains in the midline. The abducted eye shows monocular nystagmus. The underlying disorder is the lesion of the medial longitudinal fasciculus (MLF). The "one and a half" ophthalmoplegia develops in the simultaneous damage of the pontine gaze center and the MLF (mostly in multiple sclerosis). Horizontal gaze palsy is accompanied by internuclear ophthalmoplegia. This can also imitate myasthenic oculomotor disorder.

11. **Demyelinisation diseases**. The most frequent and known demyelinization disorder is multiple sclerosis (MS), the eye-related symptoms of which are attributed to the demyelinization of those neural pathways, which connect the oculomotor nuclei with each other and the gaze centers. The diverse symptoms of supra and internuclear opthalmoplegias may also resemble the ocular manifestasions of myasthenias. For instance, obscure, transient diplopias of long case history, years later can prove to be caused by MG or MS with equal feasibility. Nonetheless, the association of these two disorders is rare. However, in that case even without typical case history data and clinical symptoms, the separation is feasible in out-patients by the analysis of visually evoked potentials (VEP) and by cranial MR. (Landry)–Guillain–Barrè–(Strohl) syndrome (Guillan et al. 1916; Haymaker and Kernohan 1949) (poly-ganglio-radiculo-neuritis) resembles the MG not only in several characteristic symptoms, but also in therapeutic considerations. Its sudden onset (frequently associated with viral

infections), the rapidly progressive ascending peripheral paralysis, which often skips the diaphragm supplying C4 segment then involves the cranial nerves causing bilateral ptosis, dysphagia, dysarthria, facial paralysis strongly resembles phenomenologically the foudroyant bulbar form of MG. When diaphragm paralysis also develops, the differential diagnosis relies on Tensilon test and EMG–ENG. Fortunately, in both cases, plasmapheresis represents the life-saving therapy, which causes rapid symptomatic remission. Sometimes retrospective analyses of the case history and the information obtained with palliative treatment help together set up the correct etiologic diagnosis, when the patient arrives to the hospital with the symptoms of respiratory failure without data collected by taking collateral history. One form of the demyelinization polyneuropathies, Miller–Fisher syndrome (Blau et al. 1980; Fisher 1956; Meienberg and Ryffel 1983) afflicts usually the young. The ophthalmoplegia–ataxia–areflexia triad is accompanied by pupillary signs, facial paralysis and the protein content of the cerebrospinal fluid is high. Bell's phenomenon is intact, despite the paralysis of the voluntary upward gaze. This phenomenon and the presence of the Adie's pupil support the impairment of the brainstem. The prognosis is generally good, but in some cases respiratory failure may develop.

Summary

The differentiation of those neurological syndromes, which are accompanied by ocular muscle palsies and other eye-related symptoms represent an especially important chapter of neuro-ophthalmology since their proper diagnosis is often difficult in emergency situations, without sufficient case history data. Frequently they also represent life-threatening conditions, such as curare intoxication, botulism or the critical cases of myasthenia gravis (MG) and Guillain–Barrè syndrome (GBS). In such cases, beside the EMG–ENG some specific diagnostic clues can help (like the fixed pupils of botulism). They are of vital importance to initiate the adequate life-saving therapy (e.g., plasmapheresis in the case of MG or GBS). In some other instances the ophthalmologist's "watchful eye" and the ENT specialist's "flair" provide the necessary additional data to recognize and treat the given neurological condition in time, since the sufferers of myasthenia gravis or multiple sclerosis frequently attend their office first.

References

Bastiansen LAK, et al. Ocular myopathy. A case history with electron microscopy, biochemistry, and review of literature. Ophtalmologica (Basel). 1974;168:325–47.

Berenberg RA, et al. Lumping or splitting? "Ophthalmoplegia-plus" or Kearns-Sayre syndrome? Ann Neurol. 1977;1:37–54.

Bethlem J. Myopathies. Amsterdam: North-Holland Publishing Co.; 1977.

Blau I, Casson I, Liebermann A, Weiss E. The not-so-benign Miller Fisher syndrome – a variant of the Guillain-Barrè syndrome. Arch Neurol (Chic). 1980;37:384–5.

Bohaty I, Balázs C. Az ocularis myasthenia ès Hashimoto thyreoiditis társulása [Association of ocular myasthenia and Hashimoto thyroiditis]. Orv Hetil. 1984;125:2077–80.

Cherington M. Botulism: 10–year experience. Arch Neurol (Chic). 1974;30:432–7.

Csenkèr E, Diószeghy P, Prèkopa A, Mechler F. Hyperthyreosis ès myasthenia társulása [Association of hyperthyreoidism and myasthenia]. Ideggyógy Szle. 1977;30:377–83.

Fisher CM. An unusual variant of acute idiopathic polyneuritis (syndrome of ophthalmoplegia, ataxia and areflexia). N Engl J Med. 1956;255:57–65.

Guillan G, et al. Sur un syndrome de radiculo-nèvrite avec hyperalbuminose du liquide cèphalo-rachidien sans rèaction cellulaire. Bull Soc Med Hop Paris. 1916;40:1462–70.

Haymaker W, Kernohan JW. The Landry-Guillain-Barrè syndrome. Medicine (Baltimore). 1949;28:59–141.

Iannaccone ST, et al. Familial progressive external ophthalmoplegia and ragged-red fibers. Neurology (Minneap). 1974;24:1033–8.

Jerusalem F. Muskelerkrankungen. Stuttgart: Thieme; 1979.

Klinikai irányelvek a myasthenia gravis ès a neuromuscularis transzmisszió zavarával járó egyèb autoimmun betegsègek kezelèsère (Neurológiai Szakmai Kollègium, 2007) dr Csilla Rózsa PhD head physician of the department, Prof. dr. Sámuel Komoly, DSc of the Hungarian Academy of Sciences, chairman of the Hungarian Neurological Society, dr. habil. Pèter Diószeghy PhD head physician of the department.

Kugelberg E, Welander L. Heredofamilial juvenile muscular atrophy simulating muscular dystrophy. Arch Neurol Psychiatr (Chic). 1956;75:500–9.

Mátyus A, Paraicz E, Szènásy J. Csecsemö- ès gyermekneurológia [Pediatric neurology]: Fazio-Londe typusú spinalis izomatrophia. Budapest: Medicina könyvkiadó; 1982.

Meienberg O, Ryffel E. Supranuclear eye movement disorders in Fisher's syndrome of ophthalmoplegia, ataxia, areflexia. Arch Neurol (Chic). 1983;40:402–5.

Newsom-Davis J, Mossman S, Vincent A, Burges J, Wray D. Autoantibodies to non-Acetil-koline Receptor (ACHR) end-plate determinant in anti-ACHR negative myasthenia gravis (MG). Muscle Nerve. 1986;9:Suppl. 5S, 151.

Olson W, et al. Oculocraniosomatic neuromuscular disease with "ragged-red" fibers. Histochemical and ultrastructural changes in limb muscles of a group of patients with idiopathic progressive external ophthalmoplegia. Arch Neurol (Chic). 1972;26:193–211.

Rózsa C, Fornádi L, Szabó G, Komoly S. Evidence of safety of combined immunosuppressive treatment of Myasthenia Gravis in a large patient population. Eur J Neurol. 2006;10(S1):120.

Szobor A. Egyèb autoimmun betegsègek elöfordulása mysthenia gravisban. [Concurrence of other autoimmune disorders in myasthenia gravis]. Magy Rheumatol. 1985;26:1–10.

Szobor A. Myasthenia gravis. 1st ed. Budapest: Akadèmiai Kiadó; 1990a. p. 89–96.

Szobor A, Környei E. Myasthenia gravis und dysthyreosis. Nervenarzt. 1966a;37:337–42.

Szobor A, Molnár J. Effect of thymectomy in immune diseases other than myasthenia. Acta Med Acad Sci Hung. 1985;42:101–8.

Szobor A, Samu Z. Myasthenia gravis ès amyotrophias lateralsclerosis együttes elöfordulása. [Associated occurrence of myasthenia gravis and ALS syndrome]. Ideggyógy Szle. 1984;37:241–9.

Szobor A, Bálint G, Konrádi K, Samu Z, Bozsóky S. Development of myasthenia gravis in penicillamine-treated rheumatoid arthritis patients. Hung Rheumatol. 1979;Suppl.20:28–34.

Szobor A, Simon K, Szigeti Á. Dárdzscsípès utdn kialakult, halálhoz vezetö dermatomyositis ès bulbaris myasthenia. [Lethal dermatomyositis et bulbar myasthenia gravis after wasp sting]. Morphol Igazsagugyi Orv Sz. 1985;25:207–12.

Walker MB. Treatment of myasthenia gravis with physostigmine. Lancet. 1934;i:1200–1.

Walker MB. Myasthenia gravis. Case in which fatigue of the forearm muscles could induce paralysis of extraocular muscles. Proc R Soc Med. 1938;31:722–3.

Further Readings

Angyal L. Tartós agytörzsi tünetegyüttes myasthenia gravis pseudoparalytica esetèn [Long-lasting brain stem syndrome in a case of myasthenia gravis]. Gyógyószat. 1938;78:1–6.

Engel AG. Morphologic and immunpathologic findings in myasthenia gravis and in congenital myasthenic syndromes. J Neurol Neurosurg Psychiatr. 1980;43:577–89.

Engel AG, Lambert EH, Gomez MR. A new myasthenic syndrome with end-plate acetil-kolinesterase deficiency, small nerve terminals and reduced acetilkoline release. Ann Neurol. 1977;1:315–30.

Engel AG, Lambert EH, Mulder DM, Torres CF, Sahashi K, et al. A newly recognized congenital myasthenic syndrome attributed to a prolonged open time of the acetil-koline-induced ion channel. Ann Neurol. 1982;11:553–69.

Johnson CC, Kuwabara T. Oculopharyngeal muscular dystrophy. Am J Ophthalmol. 1974;77:872–9.

Lambert EH, Eaton LM, Rooke ED. Defect of neuromuscular conduction associated with malignant neoplasms. Am J Physiol. 1956;187:612–5.

Schiffter R. Die internuklearen Ophthalmoplegien. Nervenarzt. 1975;46:116–27.

Szobor A. Sclerosis multiplex ès myasthenia gravis együttes elöfordulása [Concurrence of multiple sclerosis and myasthenia gravis]. Orv Hetil. 1984a;125:1127–9.

Szobor A. Myasthenia gravis ès oculopharyngealis myopathia familiaris elöfordulása [Familial occurrence of myasthenia gravis and oculopharyngeal myopathy]. Ideggyógy Szle. 1984b;37:97–101.

Szobor A. Myasthenia gravis. Budapest: Akadèmiai Kiadó; 1990b. p. 99–100.

Szobor A, Marek P. A manifestation of myasthenia gravis simulating certain brain stem process. In: Juhèsz P, editor. Clinical experiences in brain stem disorders. Acta 25, Conv. Neuropsychiatry EEG Hung. Budapest; 1966b. p. 59–79.

Toivakka E, Hokkanen E. The aggravating effect of streptomycin on the neuromuscular blockade in myasthenia gravis. Acta Neurol Scand. 1965;41. Suppl. 13: 275–7.

The Ocular Characteristics and Differential Diagnostics of Mixed Types Eye Movement Disorders (Disorders of Ocular Neuromuscular Junction (OMG), Non Isolated Ocular Muscle Paresis and Myogenic Paresis)

60

Judit Somlai

Contents

J. Somlai, M.D.
Unit of Neuro-Ophthalmology, Department of Neurology & Stroke, Military Hospital, Budapest, Hungary
e-mail: dr@somlaijudit.hu; http://somlaijudit.hu

Ocular Myasthenia Gravis (A Neurogenic Paresis, the Disease of the Neuromuscular Junction (NMJ))

The clinical manifestations, the neurological differential diagnostics and the therapy are discussed in Chapter 60.

Myasthenia gravis (**MG**) represents an autoimmune disorder. The etiopathomechanism is characterized by the decrease in the number of acetylcholine receptors, and consequently the blockade of the neuromuscular synapse. The process is elicited by autoimmune process, during which the antibodies produced against the stem cells of the thymus cross react with the acetylcholine receptors. However, the dysfunction of the neuromuscular junction can be brought about by endo- and exotoxins and paraneoplastic processes with different pathomechanisms. Approximately 90 % of myasthenic patients complain about eye-related symptoms, the first of which is usually an eye movement disorder. The ocular myasthenia gravis (OMG), when the neuromuscular dysfunction predominantly afflicts the ocular muscles leading to eye symptoms, does not represent a separate entity but may predictor a systemic disorder (Table 60.1).

J. Somlai, T. Kovács (eds.), *Neuro-Ophthalmology*, DOI 10.1007/978-3-319-28956-4_60

Table 60.1 The summary of the so called mixed type eye movement disorders

The summary of mixed type eye movement disorders
Ocular myasthenia gravis (a neurogenic paresis, the disease of the neuromuscular junction)
Non-isolated ocular muscle palsies
Intraaxial brainstem syndromes
Extraaxial – non-isolated ocular muscle palsies
Ocular muscle palsies due to basilar skull lesions
Extraaxial pareses due to lesions of the apex of the pyramid and its surrounding structures
Cavernous sinus syndromes leading to ocular muscle palsies
Cerebrovascular diseases
Ocular muscle palsies due to diseases of the apex and the superior fissure of the orbit.
Eye muscle diseases due to intraorbital processes
Myogenic paresis
Myopathies
Congenital or primary myopathies
Secondary myopathies of metabolic origin
Secondary myopathies due to endocrine disorders
Ocular myositis

The most important features of myasthenia gravis (MG)

- Progressive fatigue and exhaustion of the most frequently afflicted (ocular, facial, masticatory and bulbar) muscles.
- Daily fluctuation of the symptoms.
- Periodic course: remissions are interspersed with relapses.
- The cholinesterase inhibitory diagnostic drug (edrophonium chloride=Tensilon, Camsilon) results in instant improvement.
- EMG examination reveals the typical myasthenic reaction, which is characterized by the decrease in the amplitude of contractions upon repeated stimuli.
- The presence of antibodies against the acetylcholine receptor, although seronegativity does not exclude the diagnosis.

Ocular Symptoms

- Ptosis: Dysfunction of the levator palpebrae superioris, which can be isolated or associated with the functional impairment of other extraocular muscles.
- Most frequently the elevator muscles are afflicted.
- In the morning, the symptoms are less pronounced, they become more conspicuous by the evening.

Methods of Examination

- **Endurance testing with upward gaze**: Asking the patient to sustain an upward gaze, due to the fatigue of the levator palpebrae superioris, the ptosis becomes more apparent, and a parallel droop of the gaze can also be noticed due to dysfunction of the elevators.
- **Enhancement of ptosis**: Raising the eyelid on the more affected side may be increased ptosis on the contralateral side.
- **Cogan's sign** ("**palpebral jitter**"): the patient is asked to look down for 10–20 s, then he is instructed to look straight ahead. In myasthenia, changing the fixation can be accompanied by a characteristic jitter: first the eyelid elevates then falls back with some jitters to the original position.
- **Eyelid retraction**: Upon raising the ptotic eyelid, the opposite one may be retracted. On the ptotic side, it can be tested together with Cogan's sign. A more severe form of the latter is, when during Cogan test, the retraction of the eyelid gets delayed.

Paresis of the Extraocular Muscles and the Eye Movement Systems

In ocular MG, any muscle can be afflicted either in an isolated manner or in combinations, with or without ptosis. It can lead to intermittent diplopia.

- However, **muscle weakness is not typical of either in paresis of any cranial nerve** or in central eye movement disorders. By the differential diagnosis help us, this fact: the myasthenic origin should be considered if simultaneous dysfunction of several eye muscles innervated by different cranial nerves can be noticed. Another important observation in clinical practice, that the pupillomotoric functions is spared, in most of cases of OMG.

- **Gaze paresis**: similar as true vertical and/or horizontal gaze palsies. However, in contrast with the true ones, they disappear immediately but temporarily, like all myasthenic pareses upon the administration of Camsilon, i.e., Tensilon injection.
- **Pseudo-internuclear paresis (pseudo-INO)**: In 1966, Glaser suggested the term of pseudo-internuclear ophthalmoparesis to describe the frequent adduction weakness of myasthenia gravis. True INO appears in the form of uni- or bilateral adduction weakness due to the dysfunction of the longitudinal fascicle. However, in myasthenia the syndrome is imitated by the disorder of the neuromuscular junction. The syndrome can also be accompanied by vertical disorder. Then on adduction, when the patient turns his eye towards the nose, his gaze is also drooping, which is known in the literature as "downshoot phenomenon". Camsilon administration promptly resolves it.
- **Pseudo "one and a half" syndrome**: Like in the case of the neurogenic form, only one eye can be abducted in the horizontal plane, further lateral movements cannot be carried out.
- Upon Camsilon administration it also disappears (Fig. 60.1).
- **Disorder of the saccadic eye movements**: The pathological changes to the fast eye movements, like the saccades, therefore, the fast components of the nystagmuses, too, represent the earliest and most sensitive indices of the weakness of extraocular muscles. In myasthenia, the saccade is properly initiated, but the movement slows down and frequently it stops. Therefore, the patient is unable to move his gaze to a given, point and the saccades become prolonged. Therefore, during sleep, the REM phase also becomes longer. In the clinical practice, during the examination of optokinetic nystagmus, the fast component becomes longer. Upon Camsilon administration, the saccades normalize, even they can get hypermetric, and lead to oscillopsia (see Chap. 58).

Note

The international neuro-ophthalmologic literature frequently tags the eye movement disorders evoked by ocular myasthenia with the "pseudo" prefix. It reflects that the muscular disorder may imitate the typical syndromes elicited by the disease of specific neural pathways. ***The symptoms of OMG may overlap with those of neurogenic disorders but are related to the dysfunction of the neuromuscular junction (NMJ). The ocular symptoms of myasthenia gravis, therefore, represent a synaptic disorder, which mimics the classical signs of neural conduction problems or the dysfunction of those CNS nuclei, which relay the impulses of specific neural pathways.***

For Instance

According to present knowledge, the pathomechanism of uni- or bilateral internuclear ophthalmoplegia (INO) is related to the dysfunction of the medial longitudinal fasciculus. However, a similar disorder characterized by adduction weakness can be elicited by the neuromuscular disease of the ocular muscles, which is referred to in the literature as pseudo-internuclear-paresis. In both cases there exist neurogenic disorders but not at the same level of the motor unit.

The same terminology helps us make a distinction between upward gaze palsy elicited by the true Parinaud's syndrome (evoked by upper brainstem compression) and pseudo-Parinaud's syndrome of the eye muscles elicited by the disease of the NMJ.

Nystagmus

On abducting, i.e., temporally looking, eye dissociated pseudo-nystagmus, which is to be observed in pseudo-internuclear ophthalmoplegia, can be noticed. In myasthenia, due to the rapidly

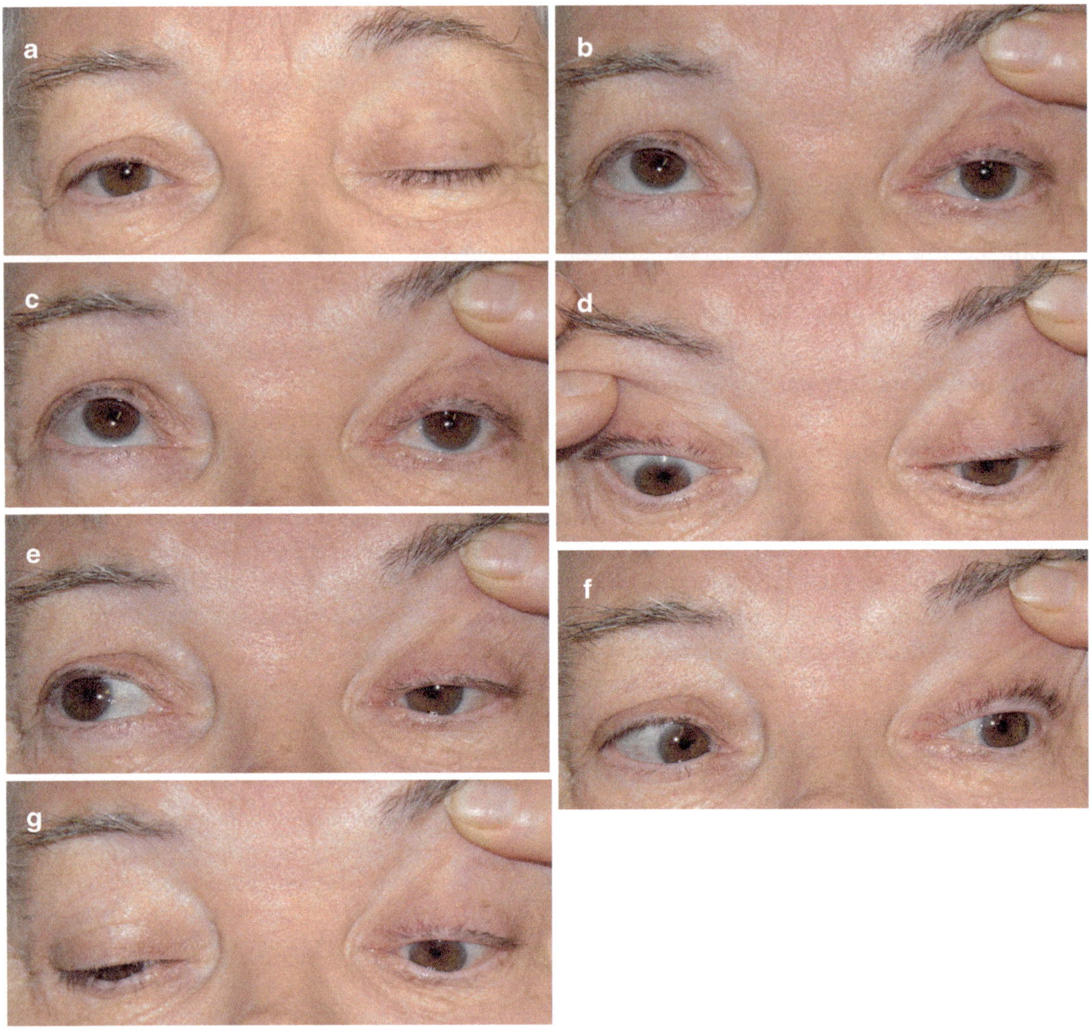

Fig. 60.1 Typical signs of the Ocular Myasthenia Gravis (OMG): (**a**) In primary position: left complete ptosis. (**b**) in primary position:-lifted ptosis: the left hhypophoria. (**c**) upon right upward: left-sided vertical gaze paresis. (**d**) convergence paresis. (**e–**, **+f**) Horizontal eye movements are without disorders; (**g**) convergentia paresis on the right side

developing fatigue of the ocular muscles, asking the patient to look temporally and upward, gaze-evoked pseudo-nystagmus develops.

Dysfunction of the Orbicularis Oculi Muscle

The dysfunction of the orbicularis oculi muscle can be demonstrated in the following two ways. On forced closure of the eyelids, the examiner tries to open the eyes. In MG, a forceful attempt reveals the relative weakness on the affected side. This sort of muscle weakness leads to another typical symptom. By the evening, fatigue of the orbicularis oculi muscle becomes more apparent. Therefore, upon relaxed closure, the palpebral fissure remains slightly open. At the first sight, it resembles a scarred outward turn, i.e., ectropion, which exposes a portion of the sclera. This sign is known in the literature as "peek" phenomenon.

Pupillary Signs and Accommodation

Myasthenia gravis does not disturb the function of the pupillary muscles. However, one component (convergence) of the accommodation triad (miosis, convergence, and the actual accommodation of the lens) relies on the external ocular muscles. It may also show hypo- (exophoria) or hyperactivity (spasm). This can cause reading difficulties, sudden onset of diplopia, or blurred vision. Upon Camsilon-Tensilon administration, the accommodation symptoms also completely resolve.

Diagnostic Options to Confirm or Exclude Ocular Myasthenia, the Camsilon (Tensilon) Test

When the characteristics of ptosis and the dysfunction of the extraocular muscles will change upon the administration of Camsilon/Tensilon, myasthenia gravis should be considered as an underlying disorder. It can be quantified by measuring the paralytic angle of strabismus, since the changes of the eye movements are frequently not evident enough. The change of milder weakness of adduction and convergence can be monitored, followed or excluded by a Hess screen or Maddox wings (regarding the methods, the reader is referred to Chapter 60). In a similar manner, the diagnosis of ocular myasthenia gravis, which imitates the nuclear and supranuclear eye movement disorders, can only be confirmed by exact measurements before and after Camsilon/Tensilon administration. The latter has practical significance in the differential diagnosis of the extraocular eye muscle pareses which are not accompanied by ptosis.

The disorder of saccadic eye movements can be checked by the diagnostic arsenal of the optokinetic nystagmuses. The sensitive, standard method for the registration of nystagmuses is photo-electronystagmography, in that case together with the administration of Camsilon/Tensilon. The test may return false positive results in ocular myositis, botulinus intoxication, orbital apex syndrome and polymyositis.

Ocular EMG and laboratory and neurological differential diagnostics are discussed in detail in Chap. 59.

The Differential Diagnostic Options in Ocular Myasthenia Gravis

The Treatment of Ocular Myasthenia Gravis (OMG)

The treatment of OMG follows the general therapeutic regime of myasthenia gravis, which relies on the alternated administration of pulse boluses and maintenance **doses of steroids**. However, in the case of myasthenic crises, besides the standard **Mestinon and/or steroid therapy**, **plasmapheresis** must be commenced, immediately and later the treatment should be complemented with **immunosuppressive** drugs. It is also recommended to look for and **extirpate** the underlying **thymoma**, which can be the culprit in the generalized forms with ocular involvement. The therapy should be started in neurological centers which are specialized in the treatment of myasthenia, in order to properly manage, prevent and nurse other muscle symptoms and complications. Diseases like demyelinization and cerebrovascular disease require the team work of neurologists, ophthalmologists, neuro-ophthalmologists and electrophysiologists.

Ocular myasthenia gravis can appear alone as the first sign of the disease. As the activity of the underlying disorder usually fluctuates, so does the bewildering pattern of the ocular symptoms. In some cases only do the ocular symptoms persist. However, the condition can rapidly change. Facial, bulbar and trunk muscles may follow, which represent a much more alarming situation. *Ocular myasthenia gravis can mimic any sort of (either central or peripheral) neurogenic paresis. Not only these cases, but also any other eye movement disorder, presentation of which is not typical of the isolated dysfunction of a given cranial nerve, or conditions which involve muscles innervated by several oculomotor nerves, should make the physician consider the diagnosis of ocular myasthenia.* **Myasthenia gravis can mimic all types of eye movements disorders**! (**Prof. Y. Goldhammer**)

When the patient is diagnosed in time, and he/she receives proper treatment, severe complications can be prevented. Therefore, in the early diagnosis, which makes the treatment of the disease possible at the beginning of its course, eye-related symptoms provide indispensable help (Table 60.2).

Non-isolated Ocular Muscle Palsies

This group consists of eye movement disorders which present with the symptoms of the external eye muscles and/or the pupils due to simultaneous paralysis of two or all three oculomotor nerves. The damage can affect the brainstem section of the pathway of the given cranial nerve, or peripherally in the fascicular part. The lesion is **intraaxial and non-isolated**, when the nucleus and/or the axons of the oculomotor nerve suffer injury together with a long pathway of the brainstem. **Extraaxial non-isolated** eye muscle palsies consist of disorders in which the simultaneous damage of the oculomotor cranial nerves and consequent paresis develops in the skull base, the cavernous sinus, the apex of the orbit or the orbit itself. Intraaxial brainstem syndrome usually develops due to cerebrovascular disorders, but multiple sclerosis, gliomas of the brainstem or external compressive processes can also elicit it. Since on the ipsilateral side of the lesion, ocular muscle palsy, while on the contralateral side, long neural pathway symptoms can be observed due to the impairment of the crossing long pathway, and the syndrome is also known as alternating syndrome. The type of axonal impairment also indicates the level of injury.

The Intraaxial Non Isolated Ocular Muscle Palsies

See Table 60.3.

The Extraaxial Non Isolated Ocular Muscle Palsies

Extraaxial non-isolated eye muscle palsies consist of disorders in which the simultaneous damage of the oculomotor cranial nerves and consequent paresis develops:

Table 60.2 The differential diagnosis of neurogenic pareses and the so-called myopathy-related pseudopareses

	Neurogenic paresis	Neuromuscular pareses	Myopathies, pseudopareses
Clinical characteristics	The paresis becomes more severe, symptoms according to the localization of the plegia	Daily fluctuations – the fatigue can imitate any paresis forms	+/– orbitopathy pseudo-abducens pseudo-Parinaud paresis
Pupillmotor functions	Generally: +	–	Lesion of the sympathetic fibers
Neurological symptoms	Generally: +	Bulbar, pharyngeal pareses – Life threatening!	Disease – : In endocrine cases + : When systemic autoimmune
Systemic diseases	–	Autoimmune diseases (RA, SLE, Sjögren's syndrome) Paraneoplasia (lung, liver, colorectal cc.)	Hashimoto's thyroiditis autoimmune disease +/– Neurological syndromes
Cranial or orbit CT Chest-CT, MR	Etiology specific + –	– Thymoma: +	Orbito–, myopathy:+ –
Tensilon test	–	+	–: Except with OMG
EMG	–	+	+/–

Abbreviations: *RA* rheumatoid arthritis, *SLE* systemic lupus erythematosus, *EMG* electromyography, *OMG* ocular myasthenia gravis, *cc* carcinoma

Table 60.3 Summary of the intraaxial brainstem syndromes

Intraaxial brainstem syndromes	Causes	Eye-related symptoms
Dorsolateral medullary syndrome (Wallenberg's syndrome)	Cause: the circulatory disorder of the vertebral artery (VA) and the posterior inferior cerebellar artery (PICA)	Central Horner's syndrome, ipsilateral ocular tilt reaction, OTR
Ventrocaudal pontine syndrome (Millard–Gubler or Foville's syndrome)	Cause: occlusion of the circumferential branches (anterior inferior cerebellar artery (AICA) of the basilar artery (BA)	Ipsilateral abducens paresis and/or peripheral, partial facial paresis, ipsilateral Horner's syndrome
Paramedian midbrain syndrome (Benedikt's syndrome)	Cause: The occlusion of the interpeduncular branches of the basilar artery (BA) or the posterior cerebral artery (PCA)	Ipsilateralis nervus oculomotorius paresis
Cerebral peduncle syndrome (Weber's syndrome)	Cause: The occlusion of the interpeduncular perforating branches of the posterior cerebral artery (PCA) and/or the (AchP)	Ipsilateral oculomotor nerve paresis
Nothnagel's syndrome	Cause: occlusion of the posterior cerebral artery (PCA)	Uni- or bilateral oculomotor nerve paresis
Parinaud's syndrome	Cause: occlusion of the long circumferential branches of the P1 segment of the posterior cerebral artery (PCA)	Up and/or downward gaze palsy

- in the skull base
- in the cavernous sinus
- in the orbital apex
- or in the orbit itself

These conditions lead to the dysfunction of two or all three oculomotor nerves. After leaving the brain, the fascicles of the oculomotor nerve (n. III) runs on the skull base between the posterior cerebral artery and the superior cerebellar artery, then around the posterior communicating artery and finally joining the trochlear, the trigeminal and the abducens nerves, and it enters the *cavernous sinus*. The three oculomotor nerves get to the orbit, together with the 1st branch of the trigeminal nerve (n.V/1) through the *superior orbital fissure*. From clinical point of view, the anatomical situation that the abducens nerve crosses the dura between the clinoid process and apex of the pyramid is of great significance. According to the anatomical localization, the extraaxial lesions of the oculomotor nerves can be classified as follows (Table 60.4).

Ocular Muscle Palsies Due to Basilar Skull Lesions

The injury to the fibers, which run ***on the skull base***, can lead to monosymptomatic conditions:

Table 60.4 Summary of the extraaxial brainstem syndromes

Extraaxial non-isolated ocular muscle palsies
Ocular muscle palsies due to basilar skull lesions
Ocular muscle palsies due to the diseases of the surroundings and the apex itself of the pyramid
Gradenigo's syndrome
Thrombosis of the lateral sinus
Carcinomas of the sinuses and/or the nasopharynx
Cavernous sinus syndromes leading to ocular muscle palsies
Cerebrovascular diseases
Ocular muscle palsies due to the disorders of the apex and the superior fissure of the orbit
Ocular muscle palsies due to intraorbital processes

- Direct compression by the aneurysm of the posterior communicating artery: heavy pain with Argyll-Robertson pupil sign
- Aneurysm of the posterior cerebral artery may less frequently bring about monosymptomatic disease of one cranial nerve.
- Transtentorial herniation: In progressing hemispheric processes, the uncus gyri hippocampi is squeezed under the tentorium and compresses the oculomotor nerve (*more details in* Chap. 50).
- In childhood, increased intracranial pressure usually leads to central herniation. Tumors of the posterior scale or the ventricles result in hydrocephalus, symmetrical dilation of the ventricles, then downward displacement of the brainstem and unior bilateral abducens nerve palsy together with severe neurological symptoms.

Dysfunction of all three oculomotor cranial nerves, i.e., a multisymptomatic condition can be observed in the following skull base processes:

- meningitides (bacterial, tuberculotic, fungal, or carcinomatous)
- direct tumor progression (from the sinuses and the nasopharynx)
- systemic disorders (sarcoidosis, herpes zoster, Guillain–Barre syndrome)
- dilation and ectasia of the aneurysm of the basilar artery
- tumors of the skull base (chordoma, carcinoma)
- basilar skull fracture

Ocular Muscle Palsies Due to the Diseases of the Surroundings and the Pyramidal Apex Itself

The abducens nerve penetrates the dura between the clinoid process and the apex of the pyramid. Its unilateral injuries are caused most often by the following conditions.

Gradenigo's Syndrome

Otitis media progressing toward the pyramid or mastoiditis can cause inflammation not only in the bone itself, but it can also lead to thrombosis of the petrosal sinus.

Symptoms and signs: severe pain, beside abducens nerve palsy, the facial, the trigeminal and the vestibulocochlear nerves will also be affected.

Differential diagnosis: Ramsay–Hunt syndrome type II, herpes zoster infection of the geniculate ganglion (vesicular rashes on the ear, facial nerve palsy).

Other reasons: cerebellopontine syndrome, acoustic neurinoma, meningioma of the pyramid, cholesteatoma, chordoma, neurinoma, sarcoma.

Thrombosis of the Lateral Sinus

Due to mastoiditis: rapidly progressing increase in intracranial pressure can be observed due to the impairment of the circulation in the venous sinus. It may be difficult to differentiate it from the abscess of the posterior scale.

Carcinomas of the Sinuses and/or the Nasopharynx

The processes of the ambient tissues progressing to the apex of the pyramid present with pain with sudden onset and abducens palsy.

Benign, transient abducens palsies of childhood as the complications of infections. The results of modern imaging techniques and the short and benign course of the disease help the differential diagnosis.

Cavernous Sinus Syndromes Leading to Ocular Muscle Palsies

The three oculomotor nerves run together in the venous channel of the cavernous sinus. Their injuries can be classified according to topographic aspects, such as:

Cavernosus sinus	Localization	Cranial nerve lesions
Lesion of the **anterior cavernous sinus**	Disease of the region spanning *between the cavernous sinus and the superior orbital fissure*	n. III., n. IV., n. VI., n. V/1.
Diseases of the **middle portion cavernous sinus**	The disease of the *middle and posterior thirds of the cavernous sinus*	n. III., n. IV., n. VI., n. V/1., n. V/2.

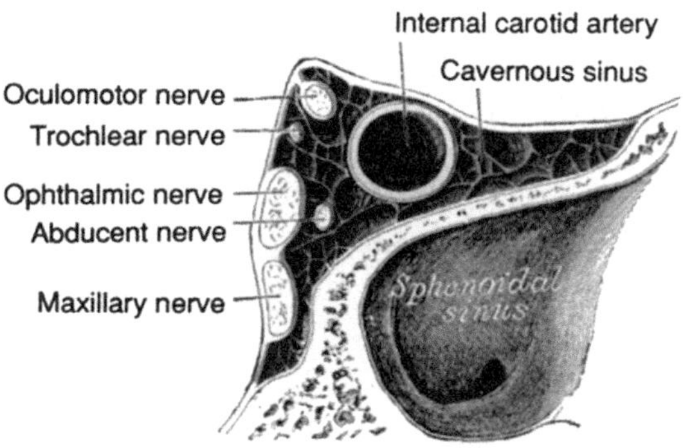

Fig. 60.2 The sagittal section of the cavernous sinus: the location of the internal carotid artery and the oculomotor cranial nerves

Cavernosus sinus	Localization	Cranial nerve lesions
Diseases of the **retrocavernous region**	*Beside the cavernous sinus*, the *optic chiasm* and the *retrochiasmal region* are affected	Optic nerve – n. III. – n. IV. – n. VI. n. V/1. – n. V/2. – n.V/3.

To help understanding the eye movement disorders related to the diseases of the cavernous sinus see the attached anatomical illustration on next page (Fig. 60.2)

Reasons of Cavernous Sinus Syndromes +/– Ocular Muscle Palsies

Tumors

- *Pituitary tumor* of lateral progression or hemorrhagic infarction of tumor
- *meningeoma of the tuberculum sellae*
- *intracavernous meningeoma*
- *intracavernous aneurysm*: the acute symptoms follow
  - a sudden hypertension episode
  - palpebral edema and exophthalmos
  - abrupt loss of vision
  - oculomotor nerve palsy
  - pain with sudden onset + paresis abducens nerve (progresses toward the retrocavernous region)
- trigeminal neurinoma
- tumors progressing upwards from the skill base: chordoma, metastatic carcinoma.

Inflammation

Tolosa–Hunt syndrome: Granulomatous inflammation in the cavernous sinus, which in severe cases involves the retroocular tissues of the orbits. Often it is the precursor of an autoimmune disease.

Its ocular symptoms: retrobulbar pain, diplopia, increased sedimentation rate, exophthalmos, eye movement disorder, remission with steroid treatment, relapsing course.

Vascular Disorders Leading to Extraaxial, Non-isolated Ocular Muscle Palsies

- *thrombosis of the cavernous sinus*
- *aneurysm of the internal carotid artery (ICA)*
- *carotid–cavernous fistula (CCF)*

Thrombosis of the cavernous sinus is usually the consequence of infectious conditions as the suppurative processes of the face or the paranasal sinuses progress to the skull.

Ocular symptoms:

- exophthalmos,
- edema of the eyelids
- abducens nerve paresis
- pain

Carotid–cavernous fistula (CCF) represents a pathological shunting between the cavernous sinus and the internal carotid artery (ICA), which crosses the cavernous sinus (*see* Fig. 60.2). This arteriovenous shunting can be spontaneous, but in 80 % of the cases, it develops due to traumatic skull injuries, which disrupt one of the branches of the internal carotid artery (ICA) or the ICA itself. It is characterized by, besides progressive headache, orbital pain, blurred vision and diplopia, a typical, pulse-synchronous "machine-like murmur", which can be heard not only by auscultation over the bulb but also by the patient himself. The modern neuroradiological procedures help to recognize this atypical syndrome, which can soon result in loss of vision.

Ocular symptoms: (*usually they are bilateral*):

- progressive **loss of vision**, due to
  - the increased intraocular pressure and
  - the venous congestion, venous stasis elicited retinopathy
- **papilledema** leads to "bigger blind spot" syndrome of visual field
- **high ocular pressure**: hardly can be influenced by pharmacological means
- progressive simultaneous **paralysis of the oculomotor, trochlear and**
- **abducens nerves**; total external ophthalmoplegia.
- **edematic**, **swollen eyelids**, the superficial veins of the skin are tortuous and palpable
- **severe conjunctival edema** (**chemosis**), which can be of such extent that the patient cannot close his eyes (see Fig. 60.3)
- Congestional hyperemia of the conjunctiva ("**red eye**", which mimics inflammation). It develops due to overflow of the conjunctiva by arterialized venous blood
- Uni- or bilateral severe **exophthalmos**, which can reach even 8–10 mm
- **pulse-synchronous "locomotive murmur"**
- fundoscopy: congestion of the retinal veins due to disturbance of back-flow, **papilledema**, **perivenous striated bleedings**, **tortuous retinal veins** then **maculopathy** develops (see Fig. 60.4).

Treatment Local, symptomatic treatment and *neurosurgical endovascular operation* with closure of the afflicted blood vessel (*see* Chap. 9).

The **arteriovenous malformations** and the **arteriovenous shunts of the dura** should be separated from the condition. The latter is presumed to develop due to pathological shunting of arterial blood to the venous sinuses of the dura. It causes headache, blurred vision and diplopia.

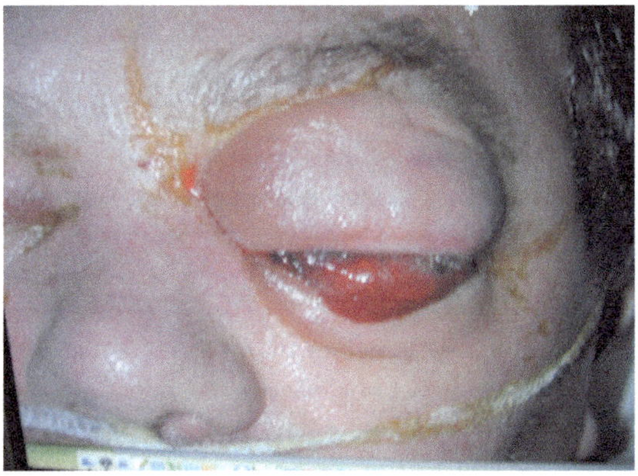

Fig. 60.3 Typical external ocular signs of CCF: bilateral, severe conjunctiva and palpebral edema and chemosis

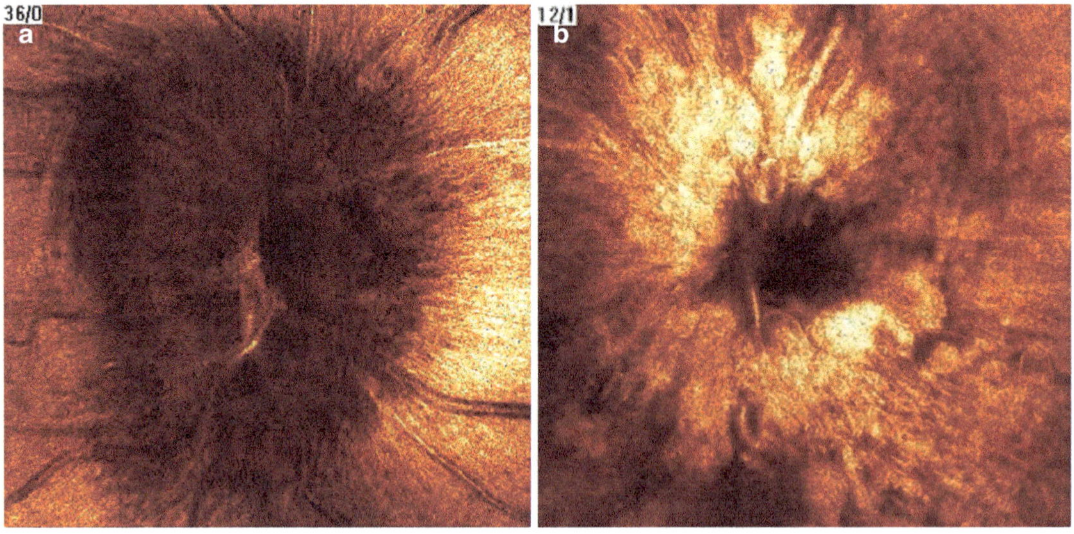

Fig. 60.4 Fundoscopic images of carotid–cavernous fistula. (**a**) Unilateral severe papilledema due to venous congestion. (**b**) Impending unilateral renal vein thrombosis due to the progressive impairment of venous efflux

Ocular Muscle Palsies Due to the Disorders of the Apex and the Superior Fissure of the Orbit

- disorders progressing toward the apex or the superior fissure of the obit (inflammation, injury or tumor)
- dysfunction of all three cranial nerves
- the lesion of the n. V/1 branch (corneal reflex- hypaesthesia),
- when the orbital apex is affected the syndrome is complemented by the symptoms of optic nerve dysfunction.

Causes and ocular signs:

- carcinoma metastasis directly propagating to the orbit – proptosis, rapidly developing eye-muscle pareses
- benign orbital tumor – slowly progressing proptosis, mild visual impairment, sometimes diplopia
- pseudotumor of the orbit – Tolosa-Hunt syndrome, endocrine myo- and/or orbitopathy
- superior orbital fissure syndrome – optic nerve is spared, exophthalmos, only eye muscle paresis.
- orbital vascular tumors and arteriovenous malformations (*see* Chap. 62).

Ocular Muscle Palsies Due to Intraorbital Processes

The pathological volume expansion in the closed compartment of the intraorbital–retroocular tissue leads to exophthalmos. The most frequent groups of diseases:

- tumorous processes of the orbit;
- inflammations;
- circulatory disorders;
- traumas;
- endocrine myo- and orbitopathies.

Tumors of the orbit can be benign, semimalignant and malignant, but the tumors of the surrounding structure can also progress to the orbit. These processes, preceding or following the impairment of the optic nerve, lead to exophthalmos and diplopia. As the extent and character of the functional impairment and the nature of the underlying disorder have been clarified, surgical and oncotherapeutical interventions are at the disposal of the therapeutic team (see Chap. 62).

Inflammatory diseases of the orbit are usually accompanied by besides edema of the eyelids, chemosis, exophthalmos, eye muscle disorders. These processes, however, show regression upon causal therapy. The most important forms are associated with cellulitis, abscess, mucokele, and pyokele. They also appear, as a part of other local and systemic disorders, in the form of pseudotumor, i.e., granulomatous inflammation of the orbit.

Among **the vascular processes of the orbi**t, thrombosis of the orbital veins and the cavernous sinus, varices of the orbit, carotid-cavernous fistula bring about exophthalmos and eye muscle palsy leading to marked diplopia.

Traumatic damages of the orbit are frequent complications of the injuries of skull base and the facial bones among neurosurgical patients. By the weaponry of modern neuroradiological equipment – usually by CT – the injuries to the soft structures of the orbit and the ocular muscles, pinching of the motor apparatus and involvement of the ambient tissues can be soon clarified beside the examination of visual functions.

Myogenic Pareses

MYOPATHIES
Congenital or primary myopathies
Secondary myopathies of metabolic origin
Secondary myopathies due to endocrine disorders
OCULARIS MYOSITIS (Table 60.5)

The **myogenic pareses**, which can be brought about by the isolated disease of the ocular muscles or may develop as the consequence of systemic disorders like the neurogenic disease, usually present with visual impairment and progressive diplopia in the everyday practice. The functional impairment in these cases develops primarily to myogenic reasons. This phenomenon is called pseudoparesis and leads to the actual disorder of impulse conduction causing

Table 60.5 Diplopia caused by non – neurogenic disorders

Disorders	Etiology – pathomechanism	Ocular +/– other symptoms	Characteristic signs of EMG
MYOTONIA **Dystrophia myotonica**	Diffuse destruction of muscle cells Autosomal Recessive – dominant inheritance	*Ptosis* *Myotonic facies* *"Swan neck" deformity* ***cataract, DPR prolonged relaxation in the skeletal muscles***	*Voluntary contraction* *High frequency potentials* *"Dive bomber" sound*
MYOPATHY-1 endocrine myopathy *thyrotoxic, myxedema-related, acromegaly-related*	Slowly progressing muscle atrophy	*Muscle cramps muscles weakness*	*Decreased innervation* *Small amplitude* *Short potentials*
MYOPATHY-2 **Mitochondrial–encenphalo–myopathies** **Kearns–Sayre syndrome**	Damage to the mtDNA Pathological proteins Mitochondrial dysfunction Oxidative injuries to the muscle and neuronal tissues "ragged red fibers"	*Ophthalmoplegia Externa Progressiva (OEP) Retinitis pigmentosa (RP) arrhythmias*	*Decreased innervation* *Small amplitude* *Short potentials*
MYOSITIS *Dermato– and polymyositis* *Rheumatoid arthritis*	Capillary necroses in the muscles Inflammatory signs Inclusion bodies	*Severe dysphagia myasthenia-like symptoms*	*The frequency increases by voluntary contraction*

mtDNA mitochondrial DNA, RA rheumatoid arthritis, RP retinitis pigmentosa, EMG electromyography, OEP Ophthalmoplegia externa progressiva

neurogenic paresis like gaze disorder and diplopia. Myogenic paresis can accompany local or systemic inflammatory processes.

Myopathies

Congenital or primary myopathies
Secondary myopathies of metabolic origin
Secondary myopathies due to endocrine disorders

Congenital or Primary Myopathies

Congenital muscular dystrophies, which are accompanied by ***ptosis*** and/or the ***impairment of the extraocular muscles***:

- **Duchenne muscular dystrophy** –the facial muscles + extraocular muscles also affected
- **Fascioscapulohumeral dystrophy** (Landouzy–Dejerine) ***ptosis*** with ***marked facial paresis***
- ***Thomsen's myotonia congenita*** – ptosis is also accompanied by facial paresis
- ***Progressive ocular myopathy*** - part of the oculopharyngeal muscular dystrophy:
  - dominant or sporadic inheritance
  - both genders are equally affected
  - progressive ptosis,
  - compensatory posture of the head
  - upward gaze pseudoparesis.

Additional symptoms and signs: retinitis pigmentosa, loss of vision, endocrine disorders, cardiac abnormalities and cerebellar functional impairment.

- **Kearns–Sayre syndrome**: a rare, but important disease, which is related to the damage of the mitochondrial DNA. It starts before the age of 20 and characterized by **progressive extraocular**

Table 60.6 The summary of secondary, metabolic or endocrine myopathies

Secondary myopathies due to metabolic reasons:	
Hypercalcemia *Hypocalcemia*	*In extremely rare instances it can affect the function of the extraocular eye muscles Besides tetanic spasms, papilledema can also develop*
Secondary myopathies due to endocrine disorders: (*see* Chap. 61)	
Diseases of the thyroid gland	The hyper- or hypofunction of the thyroid gland and/or Hashimoto's thyroidits may precede or follow the ocular signs
Eye muscle disorders caused by thyroid functional disorders	Ocular myasthenia gravis +/– thyreotoxicosis endocrine myo- and/or orbitopathy (the ocular muscles are infiltrated by lymphocytes and plasma cells) caused by autoimmune pathomechanism
Ocular symptoms	Dalrymple sign: wider palpebral fissure (palpebral retraction) Conjunctiva hyperemia – chemosis Diplopia – eye movement disorder Uni- or bilateral, exophthalmos
Complications of the worsening ocular symptoms	Inflammation and contracture of the inferior rectus and/or the internal rectus muscle scarring of the ocular muscles – consequence of myositis upward and outward gaze pseudoparesis: fixated diplopia therapy resistant corneal ulceration: keratitis e lagophthalmo (progressive exophthalmos)
Optic nerve lesion	The inflammation in the ocular muscles -, the intraorbital tissue result in exophthalmos and compression of the intraorbital part of the optic nerve
Therapeutic recommendations	Treatments of the thyroid disorders: pharmacological treatment, surgical intervention, radiotherapy optic nerve decompression (see Chaps. 9 and 61).

eye muscle palsies, retinitis pigmentosa, cerebellar ataxia and mental retardation.

Secondary Myopathies of Metabolic Origin

See in Table 60.6.

Secondary Myopathies Due to Endocrine Disorders

See in Table 60.6, Fig. 60.5.

Ocular Myositis

In its acute form, beside conjunctival hyperemia, frustrating double vision can be observed. In the chronic stage, the diplopia becomes fixated due to scarring of muscles. The granulomatous inflammation involves the whole length of the muscle from its origin till its insertion, and the process is accompanied by palpebral hyperemia and chemosis. It is usually the consequence of autoimmune diseases and quickly responds to steroid treatment.

In endocrine myopathy, the belly of muscle is infiltrated by lymphocytes and plasma cells, and the tendons remain spared. The impairment of an ocular muscle (see the serial photograph of Fig. 60.4).

- Among systemic myositidis: it can be a rare complication of the polymyositis or polymyalgia rheumatica in association with temporal arteritis.
- Locally: as a component of inflammatory processes of the orbit. Myositis besides periscleritis and perineuritis in the form of pseudotumor or granuloma with autoimmune process in the background. Good response to steroids.

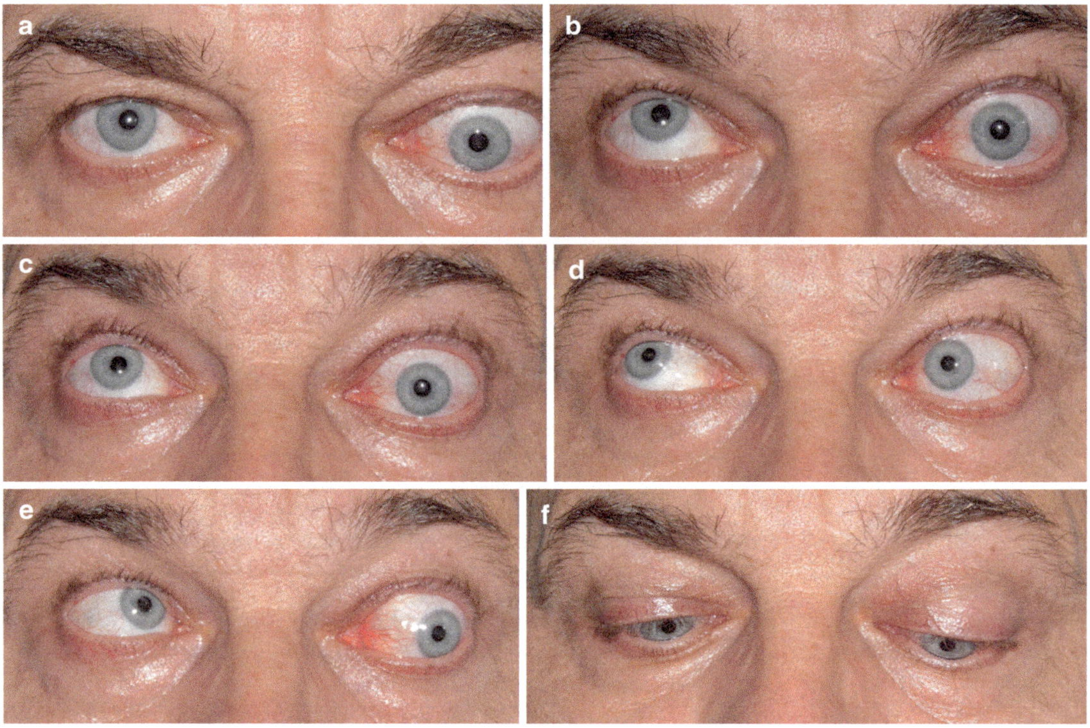

Fig. 60.5 Endocrine myopathy: consequencies of the myositis of the inferior rectus muscle: pseudoparesis upward. (**a**) in primary position: left hypophoria- left eye assumes deeper position. (**b**) Upon upward gaze, pseudoparesis of the left eye. (**c**) Forced upward gaze the upward gaze weakness of the left eye results in marked Graefe's sign. (**d**) Right-upward gaze:, left hypophoria in the left eye in adduction. (**e**) Left-upward gaze: pseudoparesis of the left eye in abduction (caused by left muscle rectus inferior myositis). (**f**) Downward gaze :the left eye is in deeper position as right eye due to the contracture of the inflamed muscle

Further Readings

Arruga J, et al. Chronic isolated trochlear nerve palsy produced by intracavernous internal carotid artery aneurysm. J Clin Neuroophthalmol. 1991;11(2):104–8.

Baker RS, et al. Vertical ocular motility disturbance in pseudotumor cerebri. J Clin Neuroophthalmol. 1985; 5:41–4.

Borchert MS. Priciples and techniques of the examination of ocular motility and alignment. In: Miller NR, Newman NJ, editors. Walsh & Hoyt's: clinical neuro-ophthalmology. Philadelphia: Lippincott Williams & Wilkins; 2005. p. 887–906.

Brandt T, et al. Different types of skew deviation. J Neurol Psychiatry. 1991;54:549–50.

Brandt T, et al. Skew deviation with ocular torsion: a vestibular brainstem sign of topographic diagnostic value. Ann Neurol. 1993;33:528–34.

Burde RM, et al. Clinical decisions in neuro-ophthalmology. St Louis: Mosby; 1985.

Calvert PS. Disorders of neuromuscular transmission. In: Miller NR, Newman NJ, editors. Walsh & Hoyt's: clinical neuro-ophthalmology. Philadelphia: Lippincott Williams &Wilkins; 2005. p. 1041–84.

Cogan D. Neurology of the ocular muscles. Springfield: CH Thomas; 1956.

Davis SL. Modeling Uhthoff s phenomenon in MS patients with internuclear ophthalmoparesis. Neurology. 2008;70(13_ Part_ 2):1098–106.

Dieterich M, Brandt T. Vestibular syndromes and vertigo. In: Bogousslasky J, Caplan L, editors. Stroke syndromes. Cambridge/New York: Cambridge University Press; 2001. p. 129–43.

Dietrich M, et al. Wallenberg's syndrome: lateropulsion, cyclorotation and subjective visual vertical in thirty-six patients. Ann Neurol. 1992;31:399–408.

Dietrich M, et al. Ocular torsion and tilt of subjective visual vertical use sensitive brainstem signs. Ann Neurol. 1993;33:292–9.

Frohman EM, et al. The utility of MRI in suspected MS. Report of the Therapeutics and Technology Assessment Subcommittee of the American Academy of Neurology. Neurology. 2003;61:602–11.

Guy JR, et al. Paraneoplastic downbeating nystagmus (a sign of occult malignancy). J Clin Neuroophthalmol. 1988;8(4):269–72.

Halmágyi GM, et al. Tonic contraversive ocular tilt reaction due to unilateral meso-diencephalic lesion. Neurology. 1990;40:1503–9.

Herzau V. Myasthenia gravis. Supplementum of course of strabismus and neuroophthalmology on IXth Congress of the European Society of Ophthalmology. Brussels; 1992.

Jay WM, et al. Pseudo-internuclear ophthalmoplegia with downshoot in MG gravis. J Clin Neuroophthalmol. 1987;7(2):74–6.

Kawasaki A. Disorders of pupillary function, accomodation, lacrimation. In: Miller NR, Newman NJ, editors. Walsh & Hoyt's: clinical neuro-ophthalmology. Philadelphia: Lippincott Williams & Wilkins; 2005. p. 739–805.

Keane JR. Internuclear ophthalmoplegia: unusual causes in 114 of 410 patients. Arch Neurol. 2005;62(5): 714–7.

Kennard C. The supranuclear control of eye movements. Supplement of IXth EUPO Course. 1992.

Korányi K, et al. Az ophthalmoneurológiai diagnosztika ès a szemèszeti terápia MG ès endocrin ophthalmopathia együttes elöfordulásakor [Diagnostics in ophthalmology and ophthalmological therapy in concomitant MG and endocrine ophthalmopathy]. Szemeszet. 1986;123:132–8.

Pierrot-Deseilligny C. Eye movement abnormalities. In: Bogousslasky J, Caplan L, editors. Stroke syndomes. Cambridge/New York: Cambridge University Press; 2001. p. 76–86.

Sargent JC. Nuclear and infranuclear ocular motility disorders. In: Miller NR, Newman NJ, editors. Walsh & Hoyt's: clinical neuro-ophthalmology. Philadelphia: Lippincott Williams &Wilkins; 2005. p. 907–68.

Somlai J. Az agytörzsi eredetü szemmozgászavarok vizsgálatának új irányzatai [New trends in examining eye movement disorders of brainstem origin]. Ideggyógy Sz. 1999;52:5–6.

Szobor A. Myasthenia gravis. Budapest: Akadèmia Kiadó; 1990.

Szobor A, et al. Myasthenia gravis: Plasmapheresis kezelès hatása [Myesthenia gravis: the effect of plasmaheresis]. Ideggyogy Sz. 1983;36:385–90.

Szobor A, et al. Myasthenia gravis: thymectomia eredmènye 550 betegen [Myasthenia gravis: the effect of thymectomy in 550 patients]. Orv Hetil. 1990;131(46): 2519–24.

Zee DS, Newman-Toker DE. Supranuclear and internuclear ocular motility disorders. In: Miller NR, Newman NJ, editors. Walsh & Hoyt's: clinical neuro-ophthalmology. Philadelphia: Lippincott Williams & Wilkins; 2005. p. 907–68.

61 Endocrine Myopathy and Orbitopathy

Csaba Balázs

Contents

Abbreviations

antibodies against Tg	Antibodies against (thyroglobulin)
antibodies against TPO	Antibodies against (thyroid peroxidase)
antibodies against TSH-R	Antibodies against thyroid stimulating hormone receptor
CTL4	Cytotoxic T lymphocyte-associated molecule-4
FT3	Free triiodothyronin
FT4	Free thyroxin
GAG	Glucoseaminoglycan
GO	Graves' Orbitopathy
Gy	Gray
IFN-γ	Interferon γ (?)
IL-1	Interleukin-1
IL-1RA	IL-1 receptor antagonist
IL-6	Interleukin-6
PPAR-α	Peroxisome proliferator activated receptor-α
PPAR-γ	Peroxisome proliferator activated receptor-γ
Th-1	T helper 1 lymphocyte
Th-2	T helper 2 lymphocyte
TNF-α (?)	Tumor necrosis factor α(?)

Graves–Basedow (GB) disease represents an autoimmune endocrinopathy, with a bewildering constellation of diverse symptoms, among which the most important ones are goiter, hyperthyroidism, orbitopathy and pretibial myxedema. Although orbitopathy represents a separate clinical entity, but even though it most frequently is associated with the autoimmune disorders of the thyroid gland, thus, in the English literature, instead of endocrine ophthalmopathy, Thyroid Associated Orbitopathy, TAO, and Graves orbitopathy (GO) are the most common denominations (Bartalena et al. 2002; Goh et al. 2005; Ludgate et al. 2004; Prabhakar et al. 2003). Previously, orbitopathy was considered a most dreaded, extra-thyroid complication of GB

C. Balázs, M.D.
Department of Internal Medicine–Endocrinology, Budai Hospital of Hospitaller Brothers, Budapest, Hungary
e-mail: drbalazscsaba@gmail.com

J. Somlai, T. Kovács (eds.), *Neuro-Ophthalmology*, DOI 10.1007/978-3-319-28956-4_61

disease, which frequently proved to be resistant to therapy. Due to recent advances in research, we know considerably more about the pathomechanism of the disease, the chances of the patients are much better and the emphasis has been shifted to prevention (Bartalena et al. 2002, 2004; Wiersinga et al. 2002; Wiersinga 2005).

Epidemiology, Clinical Features

GO develops in 50% of GB disease patients in the subclinical from. The incidence of the condition is 13.9/100,000/year (women 16/100,000/year, men 2.8/100,000/year). The clinical symptoms (conjunctivitis, periorbital edema, proptosis, visual impairment, diplopia) appear in 20% of the patients before the development of hyperthyroidism, and in 30% in the euthyroid stage after the treatment of the underlying disorder. The disorder typically afflicts two age groups (women between 40–44 and 60–64 years of age, in men between 45–49 and 65–69 years of age). In 3–5% of the patients, severe infiltrative orbitopathy develops, which ultimately leads to visual impairment or even blindness. In a significant number of the patients, the disease causes not only cosmetic problems, but it also decreases the quality of life if the patient does not receive special treatment. GO can be associated with other autoimmune diseases (e.g., myasthenia gravis, other autoimmune thyroiditides, and diabetes mellitus) (Bartalena et al. 2004; Wiersinga et al. 2002; Hatton et al. 2002). The clinical symptoms can show different pattern depending on the afflicted individual and the stage of the disease. At the beginning, the inflammatory signs dominate the clinical picture: light sensitivity, lacrimation, headache, sensation of foreign body; later more and more objective signs appear: periorbital edema, conjunctivitis, visual impairment, blurred vision and diplopia. A conspicuous sign is proptosis, the consequent retraction of the eyelids ("lagophtalmos"), the lack of convergence and the damage of the cornea. In the first phase, the inflammatory signs predominate (the so-called "wet phase", Fig. 61.1a), then degenerative, fibrotic processes take over (Fig. 61.1b). The characteristic clinical symptoms are classified and grouped into stages according to severity. These ATA (American Thyroid Association) criteria make possible to establish the clinical status of the eyes (Table 61.1) (Wiersinga et al. 2002; Pinchera et al. 1992). However, the classification was proved to be clinically impractical, therefore, to assess the activity of the disease, another scale was suggested (the "clinical activity score", Table 61.2) (Wiersinga et al. 2002; Wiersinga 2005; Pinchera et al. 1992; Mourits et al. 1997). The main advantage of such classifications is that, besides recording the given stage, they make possible to follow the effectiveness of the applied treatment. If, despite the characteristic symptoms the disease is not recognized in time, the patient is treated against conjunctivitis of unknown origin or allergic eye disease. Therefore, the earliest possible diagnosis is of vital importance regarding the outcome as the activity varies and the severity fluctuates. The chances of healing are the best, when the treatment is initiated in the active phase, because later only severe scarring can be observed, which cannot be treated by conservative treatment (Wiersinga 2005).

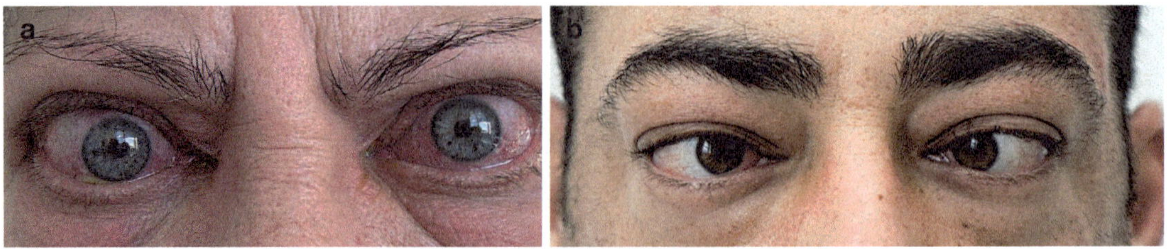

Fig. 61.1 (**a**) Inflammatory ("wet") orbitopathy. (**b**) Orbitopathy leading to deterioration of vision and diplopia

Table 61.1 The classification of the eye-related symptoms according to the criteria of the American Thyroid Association (ATA)

Stages	Changes
0	Symptom free
1	Only signs
2	Involvement of the periorbital soft tissue
0	No
a	Minimal
b	Moderate
c	Marked
3	Proptosis
0	<23 mm
a	23–24 mm
b	25–27 mm
c	>28 mm
4	Involvement of the retrobulbar muscles
0	No
a	Limitation of the eye movements
b	Apparent restriction of motion
c	Fixation of the bulbs
5	Involvement of the cornea
0	No
a	Minimal (corneal stippling)
b	Ulceration
c	Perforation
6	Loss of vision
0	No
a	Minimal (blurred vision, form 20/20 to 20/60)
b	Moderate (20/70–20/200)
c	Severe (20/200 or blindness)

Table 61.2 The activity score reflecting the severity of the orbitopathy

Changes	Score
Pain upon eye movements	1 point
Retrobulbar oppressive feeling on up-or downward gaze	1 point
Edema of the eyelids	1 point
Hyperemia of the eyelids	1 point
Hyperemia of the conjunctiva	1 point
Chemosis of the conjunctiva	1 point
Inflammation of the caruncle and/or the plica	1 point

The score is the clinical activity score (CAS) maximum 7 points

Pathomechanism

The exact target of the autoimmune process has not been completely clarified yet. Several autoantigens have been demonstrated capable of eliciting the disease. Previously the antibodies targeted against thyroglobulin were regarded the culprits, but it could not be confirmed. Some years ago, antibodies which are targeted against the external ocular muscles derived from the plasma of the patients were demonstrated by histological methods. First, these antibodies were considered to belong exclusively to the IgG group, but later research also detected antibodies of the IgA type on the surface of the eye muscles (Fig. 61.2a, b) (Hatton et al. 2002; Kaczur et al. 2003; Kekow et al. 1998). However, the direct cytotoxic activity of these antibodies is not substantiated. They seem to bring about the inflammatory reaction together with cellular components (antibody dependent cell mediated cytotoxicity). One group of the autoantibodies bind to the retrobulbar fibroblasts, that is, the TSH receptors expressed on their surface, then elicit glucoseaminoglycan (GAG) production (Bartalena et al. 2002; Balázs 2002; Cawood et al. 2004). In the production of GAG, Th-1 cytokines (TNF-a, IL-1, interferon-y) play a definite role evoking the expression of MHC II and GAG molecules. GAG molecules, being very hydrophylic, bring about swelling of the retrobulbar tissue, then the inflamed tissue mass presses froward the bulbs (proptosis) leading to exophthalmos, blurred vision, diplopia, corneal ulceration and in the most severe cases blindness due to impairment of the optic nerve. As the inflammation progresses, more and more Th-2 cytokines are produced, which gradually leads to scarring (Prabhakar et al. 2003; Wiersinga 2005). One group of the retrobulbar fibroblasts, due to the action of the cytokines, differentiates into adipocytes. Adipogenesis and stimulation of TSH-R expression is brought about by the PPAR-a and PPAR-y activators such as the fenofibrate. Therefore, thiazolidinedione derivative antidiabetics like pioglitazone, which possess similar activity profile, result in the eye-related symptoms of the patients, therefore, their administration is contraindicated. As TSH-R proved to be expressed

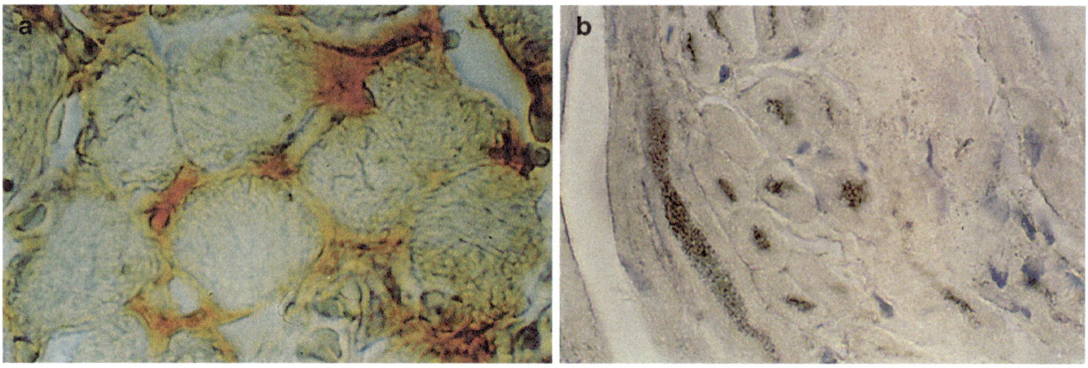

Fig. 61.2 (**a**) Binding of IgG type auto antibodies to the ocular muscles (to the perimysium and the endomysium). Indirect staining: the secondary antibody is peroxidase-linked and developed against human IgG; chromogen: aminoethyl-carbazole; nuclear staining: hematoxylin-eosin (magnification: 1250×). (**b**) Binding of IgA type auto antibodies to the ocular muscles (longitudinal and cross sections). Streptavidin immunogold indirect staining: the secondary antibody is developed against human IgA Fab2; as well (Wiersinga 2005). chromogen: silver(I)-ion; nuclear staining: hematoxylin-eosin (magnification: 1250×)

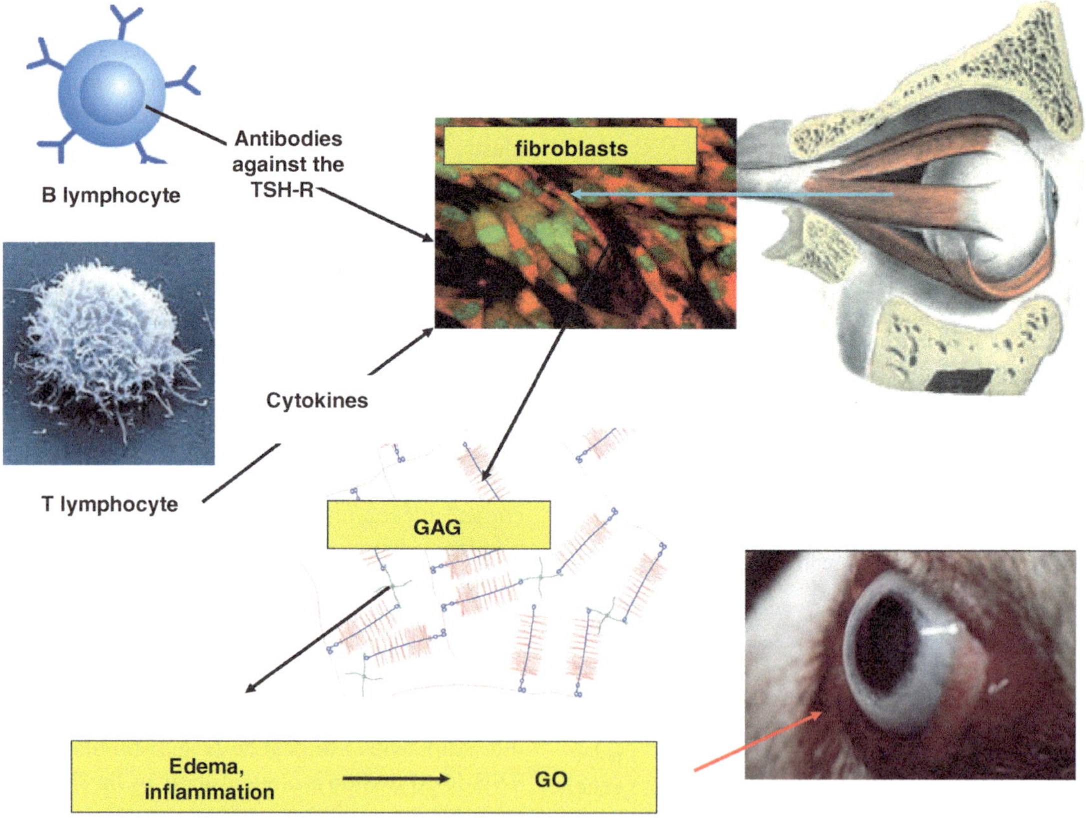

Fig. 61.3 The pathomechanism of GO

in a significant amount on the surface of the external ocular muscles and fibroblasts, its seems to play a vital role in the generation of GO (Fig. 61.3). In the pathogenesis of the disease, both genetic and environmental factors are important. Twin studies demonstrated that the concordance rate of GB in monozygotic twins is 40–50 % (Wiersinga et al. 2002). The genetic background is further confirmed by increased predisposition of individuals expressing HLA A1, B8 or DR3 haplotypes, and the course of the disease of these carriers is more severe (Kaczur et al. 2003; Davies et al. 2005; Farid et al. 1998; Stenszky et al. 1985). The analysis of polymorphism of the CTL4 molecule also revealed that some isoforms are more frequent in the sufferers of GB and GO. A/G polymorphism of the 1st exon and the C/T polymorphism of the 1st intron of the CTL4 are frequently associated with GO (Vaidya et al. 2003). Since the genetic variability of the histocompatibility and TSH-R genes per se did not provide sufficient explanation for the increased susceptibility, the epigenetic environmental factors have also been scrutinized. The epigenetic factors represent transmittable modulators of genetic expression which are not coded in the DNA.

Nucleosomes, which represent DNA and histone containing unit of the chromatin, can be "switched on" or "off". The enzymes of DNA methylation and histone modification are responsible for that the aforementioned susceptibility genes are expressed or not. Changes in epigenetic control (such as pathological DNA methylation) can lead to autoimmune processes (Egger et al. 2004). How do the genetic studies help the everyday work of a clinician? Since the genetic studies have not been localized yet the exact locus of GO, but the genetic propensity is unequivocally confirmed. Since both the frequency and the severity of the symptoms are increased in patients with given genetic traits, family history represents an indispensable part of the diagnosis. Besides the genetic factors, the causative role of more and more environmental factors have been substantiated in the development of GO. Among smokers, the incidence of GO is significantly higher, especially in patients who have positive family history for autoimmune diseases (Wiersinga et al. 2002; Balázs et al. 1990; Eckstein et al. 2003). Although several studies investigated the effect of smoking on the immune system and the function of the thyroid gland, so far the causative agent has not been identified. One explanation argues for the role of hypoxia brought about by smoking, which is a well-known factor in the production of free radicals and therefore, may contribute the development of GO. A further important factor is that the disease develops in smokers who have lower IL-1 receptor antagonist (IL-1RA) level in their plasma (Cawood et al. 2004). GO represents a rather frequent complication of the radioiodine treatment of the thyroid gland. First, it seemed, that the most feasible explanation is the strong immunogenic stimulus because of the increased release of autoantigens. The reactivation of the autoimmune processes was observed after the administration of iodine containing (amiodarone) drugs (Wiersinga 2005).

Diagnosis

Detailed case history provides indispensable information for the proper diagnosis. Obviously, when GB disease can be found in the case history, the diagnosis is much easier to be set up. From the hormonal assays, TSH, FT3, FT4 levels are absolutely necessary but not sufficient data. They shed light only on the actual activity of the endocrine status of the patient, but not on the etiopathogenetic process itself. The autoantibodies against the TSH-R, Tg and TPO do reveal the activity of the autoimmune process. Besides the characteristic stimulatory antibodies, the blocking antibodies also represent diagnostic significance (Bartalena et al. 2002; Ludgate et al. 2004; Prabhakar et al. 2003; Zhang et al. 2006). The demonstration of the binding of the IgA and IgG type antibodies to the eye muscles also help the diagnosis. The increase in the circulatory levels of GAG, TNF-α, IL-6, the soluble TNF-α -receptor (sTNF-αR), and sIL-6R corresponds to the activity of the autoimmune inflammation. This finding is also confirmed by some publications which demonstrated the significant decrease of the aforementioned cytokines and their receptors after successful therapy (Bartalena et al. 2005; Marcocci et al. 2007). Specialists have a complete arsenal of imaging techniques at their disposal, which can provide tremendous help in differential diagnosis.

Mainly in the case of unilateral GO, some of these methods help exclude the presence of retrobulbar tumors, but in some of the cases, they can indicate the activity of the inflammatory process.

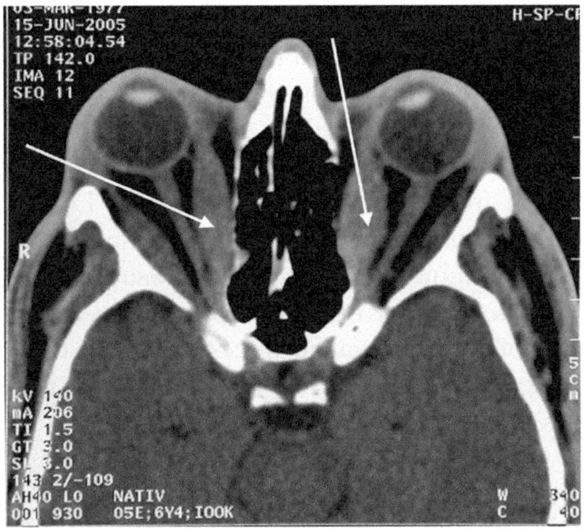

Fig. 61.4 CT examination of the orbit (*arrows* point to the thickened eye muscles)

Ultrasound has also gathered ground in this territory. Color-coded ultrasound provides information about the extent of hyperemia in the affected external ocular muscles. Such studies unveiled the strong relationship between the level of hyperemia and the intensity of the inflammatory process (Alp et al. 2000; Nèmet et al. 2005; Szücs-Farkas et al. 2003). Sometimes the CT and MR are indispensable for the exact visualization of the external eye muscles, the volume of the retrobulbar space and even some aspects of the inflammatory process itself (Fig. 61.4) (Gupta et al. 2001). In the last few years, octreotide and gallium scintigraphy gained popularity. They represent two pronged diagnostic tools, the main advantage of which is that they reflect not only the severity of the inflammation but also the effectiveness of the treatment. However, they are expensive, which impedes their spread in the clinical practice (Krassas et al. 1999).

Treatment

The therapy of severe GO represents a formidable challenge even today. In the case of this disease, it is especially true that the conservative therapy can be successful only if it is initiated in time, in the early ("active", "wet eye") stage. The pharmaceutical therapy targets the inhibition of the autoimmune process and the production of cytokines. This goal can be achieved by different strategies. The largest amount of information has been accumulated regarding steroid therapy in our practice (Bartalena et al. 2005; Ebner et al. 2004). The previously favoured local (subconjunctival and periocular triamcinolone) steroid treatment proved to be less efficient than the systemic one. In the beginning, large doses of steroid were administered orally. I meant 100 mg/day prednisolone for 5–6 months with gradual tapering. However, this therapeutic regime was accompanied by several side effects: Cushing's syndrome (85 %), glucose intolerance (20 %), gastritis (10 %), hypertension (5 %), and depression (5 %). Further, cessation of the steroid therapy leads to relapses in 35–50 % of the cases (Wiersinga 2005; Bartalena et al. 2005). Therefore, recently, intravenous administration of large methylprednisolone boluses has become the widely accepted therapy. In our surveys, this pulse therapy has been compared to the traditional oral treatment. Data of approximately 800 patients revealed that cyclic methylprednisolone treatment (15 mg/kg 3–4 times, then 7.5 mg/kg 4–6 times during two periods of 2–3 weeks) was much more effective and the number of side effects was much more limited (for instance Cushing's syndrome 12 %, hepatitis 1 %). When the therapy was commenced in time, it proved to be successful in 90 % of the cases. It is important to emphasize that the treatment should be carried out with utmost care, and the doses should be determined individually, which requires considerable therapeutic experience and additional laboratory data. The frequently noted failure and side effects of steroid treatment urged researcher to develop the retrobulbar irradiation therapy. The underlying idea of this is that the applied irradiation destroys the radiosensitive autoreactive lymphocytes. The state-of-theart treatment performed with the help of linear accelerators proved to be effective according to the literature (Bartalena et al. 2005; Marcocci et al. 2007). During the individual sessions, every other day, 2 Gy are applied. In this way, the total dosage does not exceed 20 Gy, since greater doses do not provide better results either. However, in some cases, the irradiation may lead to severe complications, therefore, its application should be reserved for certain cases. The association of GO with diabetes mellitus represents the most troublesome condition, in which diabetic retinopathy means an absolute contraindication of irradiation. Several authors have achieved better results with the combination of the pharmacological and irradiation approaches (Marcocci et al. 2007). Previously somatostatin (SS) analogues seemed to solve the therapeutic difficulties, since SS receptors (SSR) can be detected (by the Octreoscan) both on the surface of the ocular muscles and the activated lymphocytes, and the results strongly correlate with the activity of the clinical symptoms. So far about 100 GO sufferers have been treated by the SS analogue LAR ("long acting release"). The treatment regimes were different, most often 30 mg SS-LAR was administered, every 4th week for 16 weeks. After the initial publications, which had hailed the treatment, several papers questioned the efficacy of this therapeutic approach (Bartalena et al. 2005; Marcocci et al. 2007; Krassas et al. 1999). Immunoglobulin in large doses (400 mg/kg/day) was also reported to exert beneficial effects. This effect may be attributed to the ability of immunoglobulins to bind and neutralize the autoantibodies (such as the antibodies against the TSH-R), but its widespread application is delayed due to financial reasons. The etiopathogenetic role of TNF-a called for the administration of such drugs, which are able to inhibit the production of this cytokine. Pentoxifyllin has been demonstrated to inhibit the production of both TNF-a and GAG, which improves both the inflammation and the proptosis (Balázs 2002; Bartalena et al. 2005; Balázs et al. 1997, 1998; Finamor et al. 2004). In the future, the biological approach can provide better solutions such as the TNF-a binding soluble receptor (etanercept), even the first clinical trials of which have already returned impressive results. PPAR-y agonists (such as the glitazone derivatives) increase the proliferation of adipocytes, but the PPAR-y antagonists appear to inhibit the development of the eye-related symptoms. However, further clinical studies are needed to confirm these initial hypotheses (Pasqual et al. 2004; Valyasevi et al. 1999; Zhang et al. 2006). Previous publications have all recommended that during the immune modulating treatment of GO the euthyroid state is also a desirable goal, which should be achieved by thyreostatic therapy (Bartalena et al. 2002; Marcocci et al. 2007). Earlier therapeutic guidelines recommended that total thyroidectomy should have been performed in GO, based upon the hypothesis that this intervention decreases the number of both the TSH-Rs and the antibodies against the TSH-Rs. In the beginning, it seemed that the procedure is beneficial, but later several publications questioned the efficacy of the treatment. The debate is still pending, nevertheless, the removal of a large goiter may still be recommended, and it may be effective in GO (Bartalena et al. 2002; Hatton et al. 2002). In the severe and progressive instances of GO, orbital decompression surgery is still used (one or two walls of the orbit is removed). Of course, it does not influence the underlying disorder. Its main goal is to prevent the persisting or permanent damage to the eye muscles and the optic nerve. Only in those cases can the orbital decompression be the first choice of therapy, when despite conservative therapeutic efforts, optic neuropathy has not improved (Goh et al. 2005; Marcocci et al. 2007; Krastinova-Lolov et al. 2006). In the "burnt out" phase, eye surgery can help a lot in the treatment of diplopia, while cosmetic surgery may provide better quality of life (Krastinova-Lolov et al. 2006).

Prevention

Today it seems obvious that even the most up-to-date therapeutic approaches cannot be as effective as the efforts in the prevention of the disease. In the development of GO, besides the known predisposing factors which cannot be influenced, some known factors can be indeed avoided. Among them, now radioiodine therapy represents only relative contraindication (Bartalena et al. 2002; Wiersinga et al. 2002; Davies et al. 2005). However, smoking is a completely different kettle of fish, since it has already been proven that sufferers of GB disease have to give up smoking immediately

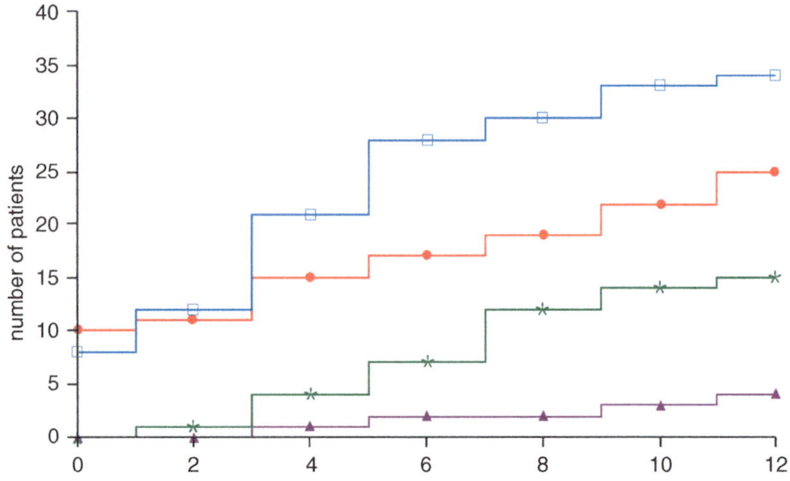

Fig. 61.5 Manifestation of GO in patients treated either with pentoxifyllin or placebo. *Blue square* patients with moderately severe GO in the control group, *green stars* patients with severe GO in the control group, *red dots* patients with moderately severe GO in the pentoxifyllin treated group, *purple triangles* patients with severe GO in the pentoxifyllin treated group

after establishing the diagnosis; even passive smoking should be avoided (Wiersinga et al. 2002). Previous studies demonstrated smoking as an independent risk factor, which increases the risk of orbitopathy, without susceptible genetic background. Ptx treatment, however, proved to be preventive in a prospective study, which revealed that in treated patients, the risk of the development of the disorder significantly decreased (Fig. 61.5). Therefore, the drug is recommended for prevention, together with thyreostatic treatment, in GB patients who are not willing to quit smoking. In the prevention and patient's care, Europe-wide the TED groups play a leading role (TED: Thyroid Eye Disease). These groups help the patients obtain information about the healing process, the therapeutic alternative, and the possible ways to improve their quality of life (Wiersinga et al. 2002).

References

Alp MN, et al. Colour Doppler imaging of the orbital vasculature in Graves' disease with computed tomographic correlation. Br J Ophthalmol. 2000;84:1027–30.

Balázs CS. Pentoxiphylline in the management of Graves' orbital disease. In: Dutton MD, editor. Thyroid eye disease. New York: Marcel Dekker, Inc.; 2002. p. 443–9.

Balázs C, et al. Association between Graves' ophthalmopathy and smoking. Lancet. 1990;336:754–5.

Balázs C, et al. Beneficial effect of pentoxifylline on thyroid associated ophthalmopathy (TAO): a pilot study. J Clin Endocrinol Metab. 1997;82:1999–2002.

Balázs C, et al. Inhibitory effect of pentoxifylline on HLA-DR and glycosaminoglycan synthesis of retrobulbar fibroblasts induced by interleukin-1, tumor necrosis factor alpha and interferon gamma. Horm Metab Res. 1998;30:496–9.

Bartalena L, et al. Graves' ophthalmopathy: a preventable disease? Eu J Endocrinol. 2002;146:457–61.

Bartalena L, et al. Relationship between management of hyperthyroidism and course of the ophthalmopathy. J Endocrinol Invest. 2004;3:288–94.

Bartalena L, et al. An update on medical management of Graves' ophthalmopathy. J Endocrinol Invest. 2005;28:469–78.

Cawood T, et al. Recent development in thyroid eye disease. Br Med J. 2004;329:385–90.

Davies TF, et al. Thyrotropin receptor-associated diseases: from adenomata to Graves' disease. J Clin Invest. 2005;115:1972–83.

Ebner R, et al. Treatment of thyroid associated ophthalmopathy with periocular injection of triamcinolone. Br J Ophthalmol. 2004;11:1359–60.

Eckstein A, et al. Impact of smoking on the response to treatment of thyroid associated ophthalmopathy. Br J Ophthalmol. 2003;87:773–6.

Egger G, et al. Epigenetics in human disease and prospects for epigenetic therapy. Nature. 2004;429:457–63.

Farid NR, et al. The genetics of thyroid associated ophthalmopathy. Thyroid. 1998;8:407–9.

Finamor FE, et al. Pentoxifylline (PTX) – an alternative treatment in Graves' ophthalmopathy (inactive phase): assessment by a disease specific quality of life questionnaire and by exophthalomometry in a prospective randomized trial. Eur J Ophthalmol. 2004;14:277–83.

Goh MS, et al. Orbital decompression in Graves' orbitopathy: efficacy and safety. Intern Med J. 2005; 35:586–91.

Gupta MK, et al. Effect of 131 iodine therapy on the course of Graves' ophthalmopathy: a quantitative analysis of extraocular muscle volumes using orbital magnetic resonance imaging. Thyroid. 2001;11:959–65.

Hatton MP, et al. The pathophysiology of thyroid associated ophthalmopathy. Ophthalmol Clin North Am. 2002;15:113–9.

Kaczur V, et al. Evolution of the thyrotropin receptor: a G protein coupled receptor with an intrinsic capacity to dimerize. Mol Genet Metab. 2003;78:275–90.

Kekow J, et al. Intravenous immunoglobulins and transforming growth factor-β. Lancet. 1998;351:184–5.

Krassas GE, et al. Somatostatin receptor scintigraphy before and after treatment with somatostatin analogues in patients with thyroid eye disease. Thyroid. 1999;9:47–52.

Krastinova-Lolov D, et al. Surgical strategy in the treatment of globe protrusion depending on its mechanism. Plast Reconstr Surg. 2006;117:553–64.

Ludgate M, et al. Inducing Graves' ophthalmopathy. J Endocrinol Invest. 2004;27:211–5.

Marcocci C, et al. A treatment strategy for Graves' orbitopathy. Nat Clin Pract Endocrinol Metab. 2007;3:430–6.

Mourits MP, et al. Clinical activity score as a guide in the management of patients with Graves' ophthalmopathy. Clin Endocrinol (Oxf). 1997;146:751–7.

Nèmet J, ès mtsai. Szemèszeti daganatok színkódolt ultrahang-vizsgálatdnak èrtèkelise a szövettani eredmèny tükrèben [Assessment of color-coded US scan results in eye tumors considering histology findings]. Magy Onkol. 2005;49:35–41.

Pasqual D, et al. Fenofibrate increases the expression of high mobility group AT-hook 2 (HMGA2) gene and induces adipocyte differentiation of orbital fibroblasts from Graves'ophthalmopathy. J Mol Endocrinol. 2004;33:133–43.

Pinchera A, et al. Classification of eye changes of Graves' disease. Thyroid. 1992;2:235–6.

Prabhakar BS, et al. Current perspective on the pathogenesis of Graves' disease and ophthalmopathy. Endocr Rev. 2003;24:802–35.

Stenszky V, et al. The genetics of Graves' disease: HLA and disease susceptibility. J Clin Endocrinol Metab. 1985;61:735–40.

Szücs-Farkas Z, et al. Using morphologic parameters of extraocular muscles for diagnosis and follow-up Graves' ophthalmopathy: diameters, areas or volume? Am J Roentgenol. 2003;179:1005–10.

Vaidya B, et al. CTLA4 gene and Graves' disease: association of Graves' disease with CTLA4 exon 1 and intron 1 polymorphisms, but not with the promoter polymorphism. Clin Endocrinol (Oxf). 2003;58:732–5.

Valyasevi RW, et al. Differentiation of orbital preadipocyte fibroblasts induces expression of functional thyrotropin receptor. J Clin Endocrinol Metab. 1999;84:2557–62.

Wiersinga WM. The philosophy of Graves' ophthalmopathy. Orbit. 2005;24:165–71.

Wiersinga WM, et al. Epidemiology and prevention of Graves' ophthalmopathy. Thyroid. 2002;12:855–60.

Zhang L, et al. Biological effects of thyrotropin receptor activation on human orbital preadipocytes. Invest Ophthalmol Vis Sci. 2006;47:5197–203.

Part VI

Diseases of the Orbit

62 Diagnostics and Therapy of Diseases of the Orbit

Katalin Korányi

Contents

The orbit is an independent anatomical structure that, besides its independence, is in close relation to the adjacent regions. It means that some of its conditions respect and do not exceed the boundaries of the orbit, whereas others spread into the surrounding regions (paranasal sinuses, retromaxillary space, intracranial space). They do it in part through anatomical openings (superior and inferior orbital fissures, optic canal) and in part by destroying the bones. On the contrary, some of them spread from the surroundings into the orbit.

A wide range of conditions may occur in the orbit. Of the conditions that cause exophthalmos, endocrine orbitopathy is by far the most common. Making the diagnosis, indicating surgery, and performing the surgery in the case of primary, secondary and metastatic tumors present a serious challenge to the orbital surgeon or the surgical team including an ENT specialist and a neurosurgeon too. Vascular lesions range from congenital capillary hemangiomas that do not require surgery to cavernous hemangiomas, the surgery of which can be elegantly performed through different orbitotomies, to carotid-cavernous fistulas that require an endovascular intervention. The diagnostics and treatment of localized and diffuse orbital inflammations (orbital pseudotumor) is challenging. The orbit may be the primary site of the development of various systemic diseases. The treatment for fractures and hematomas due to injury, and the removal of penetrating foreign bodies may be tasks of the orbital surgeon but, often, cooperation between related specialties is required.

Clinical Symptoms of Diseases of the Orbit

Since the boundaries of the orbit on the four sides and at the back are formed by bones, any enlargement of the orbital contents or an increase in the

K. Korányi, M.D.
Neuro-Ophthalmology Section,
Hungarian Ophthalmological Association,
National Institute of Oncology, Budapest, Hungary
e-mail: koranyi.katalin@oncol.hu

J. Somlai, T. Kovács (eds.), *Neuro-Ophthalmology*, DOI 10.1007/978-3-319-28956-4_62

intraorbital pressure will always push the orbital contents forward. The clinical symptom of this is *exophthalmos*, the most common symptom of diseases of the orbit. The presence of exophthalmos must be considered a pathognomonic sign as well: where there is exophthalmos, there is an intraorbital space-occupying lesion. Conditions located within the muscle cone cause axial exophthalmos. Extraconal and extraperiorbital diseases of the orbit *dislocate* the eyeball. The direction of the globe displacement is opposite to the location of the abnormal mass. A *swollen eyelid* may be a symptom of inflammatory conditions and malignant tumors. *Hyperemia* rather suggests inflammation. Swelling of the temporal third of the upper eyelid or an S-shaped deformity of the eyelid edge is usually caused by a condition of the lacrimal gland (Table 62.1).

The extraperiorbital and extraconal lesions located in the anterior part of the orbit, lacrimal gland conditions, dermoid cyst, mucoand pyoceles, are *palpable*. The conditions of the orbit may cause *restricted eye movements* in different ways: mechanically, or through the infiltration and scarring of the ocular muscles (myogenic palsy), or via peripheral paresis of the oculomotor nerves (neurogenic palsy). A large space-occupying lesion stretches and dislocates the ocular muscles. Malignant conditions of rapid progression (tumors or inflammatory conditions) cause diplopia, whereas in case of a slowly growing tumor, e.g., the benign pleomorphic adenoma of the lacrimal gland, the patient does not complain of double vision even if there is a significant bulbar dislocation. A trauma may cause an eye movement disorder associated with double vision through the injury, hematoma or due to entrapment of the muscle (blow out fracture).

Table 62.1 Clinical symptoms of diseases of the orbit

Exophthalmos
Globe displacement
Swelling of eyelid, hyperemia
Finding on palpation
Restricted eye movements, double vision
Resistance to retropulsion
Decrease in visual acuity
Retinal folds, impression on the eyeball
Inflammatory symptoms
Dilated episcleral vessels, pulsatile bruit

A condition that infiltrates the eye muscles may be of inflammatory origin (acute and chronic myositis, infiltrative and fibrotic stages of endocrine orbitopathy), or may be due to tumorous infiltration (breast cancer metastasis, rhabdomyosarcoma).

Conditions located in the orbital apex, the superior orbital fissure and the skcull base (the cavernous sinus) cause peripheral neurogenic palsy. These may include primary, secondary and metastatic tumors, inflammatory conditions or carotid-cavernous fistula. *Resistance to retropulsion of the globe* can always be observed in case of orbital space-occupying lesions. Since usually one eye is affected only, there is an apparent difference between the two sides when an attempt is made to reposition the eyeball into the orbit by placing our thumbs simultaneously on the two bulbs. When accompanied by enophthalmos, this is a clinical symptom characteristic to breast cancer metastasis. In endocrine orbitopathy, a considerable difficulty repositioning accompanied by mild exophthalmos is a sign of poor prognosis because it may predict compressive optic nerve lesion. *Decreased visual acuity* is caused by rapidly progressing malignant tumors and inflammatory conditions, and traumatic or spontaneous orbital hematomas. The same conditions may also lead to papilledema by compression of the optic nerve. Benign tumors that dislocate or compress the optic nerve, e.g., hemangioma, neurinoma, meningioma, may also decrease visual acuity in case of prolonged presence, primarily when they are located in the orbital apex. Persistent compression may also result in optic nerve atrophy and discoloration of the papilla.

Benign and malignant tumors may cause *retinal folds* if they lie against the sclera immediately behind the eyeball, and make an impression on the posterior pole of the bulb. Inflammatory conditions, pyocele, and endocrine orbitopathy may lead to folds on the posterior pole by considerably increasing the intraorbital pressure. If the folds go through the macula, and the retrobulbar pressure is persistent, there may be a severe loss of vision. This is the situation in those cases of endocrine orbitopathy where the increase in intraorbital pressure due to the autoimmune inflammatory condition is resistant to therapy, i.e., it cannot be decreased by either conservative or surgical therapy. In case of *inflammatory symptoms*– blepharal, conjunctival hyperemia, chemosis and pain—, inflammatory, granulomatous conditions must be considered. Von Graefe's symptom (lid lag sign) is a sign of endocrine orbitopathy.

Dilated episcleral vessels accompanied by a pulse-synchronous bruit over the bulb indicate the presence of a carotid-cavernous fistula.

Diagnostics and Differential Diagnostics of Diseases of the Orbit

A careful *history-taking* may help establish whether the condition is tumorous or inflammatory, or whether the tumor is benign or malignant. A long history and the presence of normal functions indicate a benign tumor. An exophthalmos or bulbar dislocation of gradual progression often remains unnoticed even by the people around the patient for a long time. Looking at old photographs may help decide when the exophthalmos may have started. A short history, a decrease in visual acuity, and double vision indicate a rapidly progressing, clinically malignant condition (tumor, hematoma, vascular condition or endocrine orbitopathy).

The evaluation of *clinical symptoms* was described in the previous chapter (Table 62.2).

Forced duction test is a simple and quick method to differentiate between paretic lesions and restrictive motolity defects. In neurogenic palsy, the forced duction test is negative, whereas it is positive in restrictive motility defects. —In the latter case the eyeball cannot be moved because of the fibrosis and shortening of the antagonistic muscle. The forced duction test is positive in case of granulomatous conditions, endocrine orbitopathy (muscle involvement) and blow out fractures. *Laboratory tests* may help in making the diagnosis of systemic diseases, and inflammatory and autoimmune conditions. In case of conditions that involve the paranasal sinuses, or intracranial spread, *related specialties* are asked to help establish the nature and extension of the condition.

Table 62.2 Diagnostics of disease of the orbit

History
Clinical symptoms (inflammatory signs, globe
Dislacement, finding on palpation, resistance to
Retropulsion, pulsation, auscultation, fundus: choked
Disc, retinal folds, intrusion of the posterior pole)
Exophthalmometry (according to Kestenbaum, Hertel)
Forced duction test
Laboratory tests, related specialties
Radiography, ultrasound, isotope scintigraphy
CT, MRI, MR angiography and venography
Biopsy

Radiograms have rarely been ordered since the introduction of imaging procedures. In lack of these, however, radiography may be useful for orientation purposes. It allows us to establish whether the paranasal sinuses are filled with air or fluids. Bone destruction due to a malignant condition and fractures are also well visible on radiograms. An enlarged optic canal is caused by an optic nerve tumor. A deepened sella turcica indicates the presence of a pituitary tumor. An enlarged bony orbit observed on an image acquired due to exophthalmos suggests a congenital, benign orbital tumor.

An *ultrasound scan* is used to visualize the intact and abnormal structures in the anterior third of the orbit. It also enables to measure and monitor the degree of and the change in muscle thickening in patients with endocrine orbitopathy. *Bone scintigraphy* confirms or rules out the bone manifestation of conditions with multiple locations (carcinoma, malignant melanoma, multiple myeloma).

The introduction of *imaging procedures* resulted in a qualitative change in the diagnostics and therapy of diseases of the orbit. The direct visualization enabled a more accurate localization of the pathological lesion and a mapping of its relationship with the surrounding structures, the eye muscles and the optic nerve. The quality of the contour of the pathological lesion and whether it is enhanced by the contrast agent—especially when assessed with various MRI sequences—give answers to differential diagnostic questions and may also provide a qualitative diagnosis. In general, benign tumors have well-defined contours, show homogeneous enhancement, and may dislocate the adjacent structures but can be distinguished from them.

The contour of malignant lesions, on the contrary, is irregular, they are attached to adjacent structures, and they infiltrate and surround them. They show heterogeneous enhancement, and contain hypodense or hypointense areas indicating necrosis. Tumors with high blood flow show intense contrast enhancement. Examples for this are cavernous hemangioma and, especially, hemangiopericytoma. Cystic lesions like mucoceles and pyoceles, and also lymphangiomas and hematomas can be easily recognized (Table 62.3).

Lymphomas, granulomas and metastatic tumors, however, can be differentiated not easily.. In these cases, the accurate evaluation of the history and the clinical symptoms may help. It must be emphasized that however easy it becomes to make the diagnosis and plan the surgery with the use of imaging diagnostics, imaging test results must always be evaluated in conjunction with clinical symptoms. *Biopsy* is required if the tumor cannot be removed in its entirety and the histological examination has therapeutic consequences. For diagnostic purposes, biopsy is performed most often if lymphoma is suspected, but it may also be required to distinguish between lymphoma and granuloma. Biopsy is contraindicated in the pleomorphic adenoma of the lacrimal gland. The practice varies in case of embryonal rhabdomyosarcoma, either biopsy or complete tumor removal is performed, and then chemotherapy follows.

Table 62.3 Differential diagnostics of tumors of the orbit

Benign tumors
Long history
Slowly progressing, unilateral exophthalmos
Eye functions remain intact for a long time
Choked disc and discolored papilla, retinal folds only in case of a long history
No pain
Imaging procedure: well-defined lesion, the orbital structures can be differentiated
Malignant tumors
Short history
Rapidly progressing exophthalmos
Swollen, hyperemic eyelid, chemosis
Eye movement disorder, decreased vision
Choked disc, retinal folds, retinal protrusion also in case of a short history
Pain may occur
Imaging procedure: diffuse lesion with ill-defined contour, the orbital structures cannot always be differentiated

Table 62.4 Disease of the orbit

Tumors of the orbit (primary, secondary and metastatic)
Inflammatory conditions, endocrine ophthalmopathy
Vascular lesions
Systemic diseases
Trauma

Diseases of the Orbit

The diseases of the orbit include the primary, secondary and metastatic tumors of the orbit, vascular lesions, inflammatory conditions, endocrine orbitopathy and other systemic diseases, skull base tumors and traumatic lesions. Tumors of the orbit may be classified based on various aspects: their location and spread, histological origin, and biological behavior (Table 62.4).

The histological classification is useful for didactic purposes, the classification according to biological behavior has a prognostic value, whereas the anatomical location is important for planning the surgery. Common diseases of the orbit important from the point of view of clinical practice are listed taking these aspects into account.

Layers of the Orbit

The different diseases of the orbit, in most cases, are typically located in specific layers of it.

1. The *layer between the bony wall and the periorbital region* is the typical location for inflammations and tumors spreading from the paranasal sinuses into the orbit. A severe disease, which usually occurs during childhood, is orbital cellulitis with subperiosteal abscess developed as a consequence of ethmoiditis. It requires urgent ethmoidectomy and antibiotic

therapy, and if it does not improve, a surgery on the orbita may also be needed. Inflamed pyoceles and mucoceles also require urgent surgery performed with the help of an ENT specialist. This is the place for tumors spreading from the paranasal sinuses into the orbit, and the primary and secondary bone conditions. Of the systemic diseases, plasmocytoma and eosinophilic granuloma also occur here.

2. The lacrimal gland is located in the *layer between the periorbital region and the eye muscles* (*extraconal space*), and therefore its conditions occur here. Cavernous hemangiomas may be extraconal *or* intraconal, whereas capillary hemangiomas and lymphangiomas are mostly extra- *and* intraconal. Hemangiopericytoma, lymphomas, sarcomas, plasmocytoma, and plexiform neurofibroma may also be found in this and the following layer. Tumors in the first and second layers are usually well palpable beneath the eyelid, and they dislocate the eyeball.
3. Conditions located *within the muscle cone* (*intraconal space*) cause axial exophthalmos. This is the typical location of cavernous hemangioma, lymphangioma and neurinoma. Other conditions that occur here include varicose veins, the already mentioned hemangiopericytoma, as well as the pseudotumor and the lymphoma.
4. Conditions of the optic nerve sheath and the optic nerve form a separate group. These include the inflammatory and tumorous conditions of the optic nerve and the optic nerve sheath. Typical tumors are optic nerve glioma and optic nerve sheath meningioma.
5. In the *space between Tenon's capsule and the bulb*, inflammatory conditions (scleritis, tenonitis) may occur, and this is the predilection site of malignant tumors (retinoblastoma, choroidal melanoma) that penetrate the bulb.

Tumors of the Orbit

Primary Tumors of the Orbit

Primary tumors of the orbit are developed in the orbit, they may be congenital or acquired, and—in accordance with their biological properties—they stay within or exceed the boundaries of the orbit. The majority of tumors of the orbit is benign and can be usually cured with surgery on the orbit.

Secondary tumors of the orbit are tumors that spread from the adjacent regions (the paranasal sinuses, the skull, the eyelids, the conjunctiva, the lacrimal sac and the eyeball) into the orbit. Most of these are malignant. The extension and the boundaries of the tumor and its relationship with the adjacent structures must be established with the highest accuracy possible using imaging techniques. If the tumor is operable, the surgery is performed by an orbital surgeon, with or without the help of an ENT specialist or a neurosurgeon, depending on the extension of the disease.

Metastatic tumors of the orbit had an incidence of about 7 %. Breast cancer metastasis is by far the most common, and it is followed by metastases from prostate cancer and malignant melanoma. During childhood, it is neuroblastoma that gives metastasis to the bony orbit.

Primary, Benign Tumors of the Orbit

Capillary hemangioma is a congenital lesion that occurs in the region of the eye, the skin of the eyelids or the conjunctiva as a smaller or larger, round or irregular spot that is slightly elevated from the surface. In the orbit, it has an extra- or intraconal location and may cause considerable exophthalmos. Capillary hemangiomas in the skin are often multiple, and may be found in different regions of the body. Its natural course is that it is growing during the first months of life and then, after 6–12 months of gradual regression, it heals almost completely. It rarely requires surgical intervention but local steroid therapy may facilitate the healing process. *Cavernosus hemangioma* is the most common benign tumor in adults, which mostly affects middle-aged women. Typically, it has an intraconal location and causes axial exophthalmos but it may occur in any layer of the orbit. It stems from tissue elements already present at birth, and usually grows very slowly. The degree of the exophthalmos, compared with the size of the tumor, is often unproportionately low. In case of prolonged presence, it may compress and dislocate the optic nerve, decrease vision, and cause papilledema or papillary decoloration. If the tumor is located close to the back surface of the bulb, it produces an impression on the posterior pole of the eyeball. The prominence in the posterior pole and the retinal folds are well visible fundoscopically. The impression on the eyeball may cause hyperopia, which must be differentiated from a decrease in visual acuity. Unilateral, acquired hyperopia may indicate an intraorbital condition that compresses the bulb. Small, asymptomatic, incidentally detected hemangiomas do not need to be removed. Large tumors with an disfiguring exophthalmos that compromises or distorts vision, however, should be removed. The removal of a detached hemangioma usually presents no difficulties. If the tumor is not detached but strongly attached to its surroundings it cannot be removed using blunt preparation. In this case, the benefits of partial removal must be considered in order to avoid loss of function. Bleeding from the orbital apex usually presents a serious risk. *Lymphangioma* is a lymphatic, congenital hamartoma, and usually affects the skin and the subcutaneous connective tissue. It is rarely developed within the orbit, and its symptoms occur during childhood. Most often, it is revealed by an acute bleeding. It fills and, characteristically, dilates the bony orbit. It has an extra- and intraconal location, and may surround the optic nerve. It spreads into the eyelids, infiltrates the conjunctiva, may also appear on the hard palate, and it thickens the facial tissues by infiltrating them. On CT and MR images, it covers the orbital structures, and it has irregular contours and structure. On T1-weighted MR images, the characteristic cysts are well visible. The tumor typically has a tendency to bleed, causing acute exophthalmos of varying degree, eye movement disorder and, possibly, a decrease in visual acuity. The clinical picture resembles that of a malignant tumor in this case. The differential diagnosis is based on the careful evaluation of clinical symptoms, and the cysts filled with fresh blood and the enlarged orbit visible on the acquired images. The surgery has serious risks due to the potential bleeding during the procedure and the permanent functional impairments that may be caused with the coagulation device. A surgical solution is required in case of a bleeding that causes severe exophthalmos and subconjunctival hemorrhage, which compromise vision, but in lack of these—because of the serious risk of surgery—monitoring the patient is recommended only.

Dermoid cyst is the most common benign, congenital tumor in children. It is a flexible, mobile mass that can be palpated beneath the upper eyelid, medially, or in the region of the lacrimal gland. Over years, it causes a slow, progressive exophthalmos, and dislocates the eyeball downwards. It forms a bony sinus, and the CT image shows a characteristic cyst with hypodense contents without contrast enhancement. In case of a long history, it may spread within the bones like the fingers of a glove, and its removal is more difficult in this case. If a sterile inflammation is developed around it, the symptoms become more pronounced and the affected skin area becomes hyperemic. During the surgery, a sebaceous content and possibly strands of hair may be found within its capsule. It is important to completely remove the capsule, otherwise it may recur.

Neurinoma is a circumscribed tumor that stems from the Schwann cells and shows moderate contrast enhancement. It is capsular and of dense consistency, and it has a tendency to become attached to its surroundings; its complete removal—without risking the integrity of the functions—is more difficult than that of hemangiomas. The recommended surgical technique involves intracapsular reduction and the careful removal of the capsule.

Neurofibromas occur in solitary or plexiform form in the orbit. The plexiform form grows along the peripheral nerves, consists of multiple sausage-shaped, flexible structures, and has an extra- and intraconal location. It may spread into the orbital apex, onto the base of the skull, as well as towards the parasellar or retromaxillary region. It is biologically benign, and it cannot always be removed radically.

Fibromas are rare tumors, which may recur after removal, and are to be considered potentially malignant.

Osteomas in the orbit primarily present a cosmetic issue, but they should be removed if they occlude the paranasal sinuses. *Optic nerve sheath meningioma* is a rare disease that affects middle-aged women. It stems from the cells in the arachnoid layer of the optic nerve sheath, and spreads in the subarachnoid space. Its initial symptoms are moderate exophthalmos and eyelid swelling. Vision remains intact for a long time but later shows gradual deterioration. A characteristic finding on the CT and MR images is the tubular or fusiform thickening of the nerve sheath, but it may also show an eccentric growth once it perforates the dura. The optic nerve sheath infiltrated by the tumor shows contrast enhancement, and the hypodense line of the optic nerve is usually well visible within it—this is the so-called tram-track sign, which is a characteristic radiological sign of optic nerve sheath meningioma. In von Recklinghausen's disease, it may occur as part of multiple meningiomatosis. A surgical intervention, while sparing the function of the optic nerve, is possible only in the case of eccentric growth.

Optic glioma is a tumor proper to the optic nerve. It consists of astrocyte elements, and its growth results in the concentric thickening of the optic nerve. It has two, fundamentally different forms: it either affects one of the optic nerves alone or occurs as part of von Recklinghausen's disease type 1. In the latter case, it is bilateral, and it also infiltrates the intracranial parts of the visual pathway. The two types differ not only in their clinical and radiological presentation but also in their prognosis. The solitary type causes a progressive, unilateral exophthalmos of considerable degree in the early years of life, and the upward gaze is usually restricted on the affected side. Vision quickly deteriorates or is rapidly lost completely. A moderately choked disc or discoloration of the optic disc can be observed on the fundus. The CT and MR images show a fusiform tumor in the location that corresponds to the optic nerve, and the optic nerve is unrecognizable. The tumor may become narrower in the orbital apex, or spread into the optic canal and widen it. It may continue in the intracranial segment, infiltrating the chiasm. If the tumor terminates before the orbital apex, and if the vision is already lost, the tumor may be removed through the orbit after cutting the optic nerve infiltrated by the tumor behind the bulb and in the apex of the orbit to eliminate the disfiguring exophthalmos and to prevent progression. Transfrontal surgery is required if the tumor has spread into the optic canal or the chiasm. The goal is to remove the optic nerve infiltrated by the tumor by transecting it at the border between the intact and the affected part.

The optic glioma developed as part of the autosomal dominant von Recklinghausen's disease type 1 is usually bilateral, and noticed later in life. It does not always cause severe exophthalmos but there have been such cases as well. The vision remains intact for a long time, or there is a persistent, moderate vision loss or visual field defect. Central scotoma and visual field defect characteristic to chiasm lesion are typical symptoms. There may be a significant difference between the two sides both in the exophthalmos and the severity of dysfunction. The acquired images show a tubular, thickened optic nerve, which is enlarged not only in its width but also in its length. The original 'S'-shaped curve of the optic nerve becomes multiple curves. The infiltration of the chiasm is not uncommon but the optic tract and the optic radiation may also be affected. Besides the persistent lesion, there is a progressive, more malignant form. Although radical surgery is not possible, a pressure-relieving shunt may be inserted if there is an increase in the intracranial pressure.

Primary, Malignant Tumors of the Orbit

Malignant tumors of the orbit—except for embryonal rhabdomyosarcoma—affect the elderly. Almost fifty percent of lymphomas, and secondary and metastatic tumors occur in the last third of life.

Rhabdomyosarcoma is the most common malignant soft tissue tumor in children. It may occur anywhere in the body where there is striated muscle tissue, although it does not necessarily stem from the muscle but presumably from residual embryonal mesenchyma. It has several histological types, the most common being the embryonal type. About 10 % of all cases of primary rhabdomyosarcoma are developed in the orbit. It typically occurs in male children under the age of 6 years. Its clinical symptoms include a rapidly (over days or 1–3 weeks) progressing, severe exophthalmos, eyelid swelling and eye movement disorders. It is most often located in the upper part of the orbit and, therefore, it dislocates the bulb downwards but it may start from any other part of the orbit and the eyelid as well. It has an extraconal location and an irregular shape on the CT image, it does not cause bone destruction, and shows intense enhancement. On T1-weighted MR images, it is hypointense compared with the adipose tissue, whereas on T2-weighted images, it shows intense contrast enhancement. Children with rhabdomyosarcoma have a better prognosis if the tumor starts from the orbit, compared with those cases where it starts from other regions. The likely reason for this is that the clinical symptoms (exophthalmos, eyelid swelling) caused by a sarcoma that starts from the orbit can be noticed immediately and, therefore, these patients are diagnosed and treated adequately earlier. In addition, the embryonal type that has a better prognosis is more common in the orbit than the alveolar type, the prognosis of which is worse. The modern treatment involves the complete removal of the tumor (or performing biopsy only) through orbitotomy, which is followed by cytostatic therapy and radiotherapy as per the protocol. The 5-year survival rate is very good, ranging between 80 and 90 % according to different statistics. In case of recurrence, another tumor resection and follow-up treatment are recommended. If the tumor recurs a second time, radical surgery, orbital exenteration is recommended. Each recurrence of the tumor decreases the chance of survival.

Lymphomas have become more and more common in the past years. They mainly affect older adults—according to US statistics, almost one-fourth of the tumors of the orbit that occur above the age of 60 years are lymphomas. They may be primary but may also occur as part of a systemic disease. They include a wide range of diseases, with non-Hodgkin B-cell lymphomas being the most common in the orbit. Their degree of malignancy varies. Since lymphatic tissue is found in the conjunctiva and the lacrimal gland only, lymphomas are most commonly developed in these two regions, although they may occur in any of the layers of the orbits. Characteristic, salmon-colored infiltration is formed beneath the conjunctiva, and the tumor is flexible and sausage-like to the touch in the eyelid. Progression depends on the degree of malignancy. The intraorbital form causes exophthalmos, eyelid swelling, possibly eyelid and conjunctiva hyperemia, chemosis and restricted eye movements. The acquired images show varying images, and there is no bone destruction. Instead of dislocating the orbital structures, it rather surrounds them. Since it spreads along the septums of the orbit, it has a characteristic, straight-line caudal border. A bilateral occurrence indicates a systemic disease. The diagnosis is based on biopsy. Biopsy is followed by staging and, depending on its result, local irradiation or cytostatic therapy.

Hemangiopericytoma is a rare, semi-malignant tumor, which is prone to recurrence, and stems from the pericytes that cover the post-capillary veins. Since it is highly vascularized, there is strikingly intense contrast enhancement on the CT and MR images, which may be a differential diagnostic sign. The tumor is attached to its surroundings and, therefore, it is not easy to remove completely. Radiation therapy is recommended after the surgery.

Primary orbital melanomas are rare. Around fifty percent ofthe cases occur starting from an Ota nevus. The clinical picture includes rapidly progressing exophthalmos, chemosis and eye movement disorders. Ota nevus, or blue nevus, is a congenital pigmentation developed along one or more branches of the trigeminal nerve. There is bluish skin discoloration on the eyelid, and characteristic, multiple blackish spots can be observed primarily in the eyelid folds. The choroidea, the orbital tissues, the ocular muscles, the bones of the orbit and the arachnoid of the cranial base may also be pigmented. A special emphasis is put on this condition because malignant transformation may occur in any area but usually in a circumscribed region only. The melanoma malignum developed in this way is biologically less malignant than spindle cell melanoma. Its surgical removal—exenteration is not feasible because of the extensive pigmented area —may ensure a survival of several years. In case of melanomas that are not developed starting from Ota nevus, exenteration is recommended.

Conditions of the Lacrimal Gland

The diagnosis and treatment of lacrimal gland conditions require a high level of attention and carefulness. Clinical and radiological symptoms must be known accurately in order to decide which of the various possibilities applies and what to do. Many times, making the diagnosis is not easy or obvious even for an experienced orbital surgeon.

The *pleomorphic adenoma* (*benign*, *mixed-cell tumor*) of the lacrimal gland is a benign tumor that may, however, go through malignant transformation after a long history. Exophthalmos, downward bulbar dislocation and a palpable mass in the region of the lacrimal gland are characteristic symptoms. It may be diagnosed only years after its development: the slow progression may remain unnoticed even by people in the patient's environment. The CT and MR images show a round or oval lesion of sharp contours in the lateral upper part of the orbit, in the area that corresponds to the lacrimal gland. The tumor is hypointense on T1-weighted images, and hyperintense on T2-weighted images. The lacrimal fossa may be deepened but there is no bone destruction. It is treated with immediate surgery—the tumor is removed completely, with its capsule and the bony tumor bed. Biopsy must not be performed, the prognosis is good, recurrence is rare and late.

The *malignant mixed-cell tumor* is the transformation of the benign tumor. The procedure is similar, postoperative radiation therapy is recommended.

Adenoid cystic carcinoma (*cylindroma*) is a malignant tumor of the lacrimal gland. The history is short and it is characterized by local pain. The clinical picture is less peaceful, the eyelid swelling may be more pronounced, and the palpable mass is larger, stiffer, firmer and tender to pressure. On the CT and MR images, it may be similar to the previous condition but the shape of the tumor is less regular. It shows heterogenous enhancement, and may contain calcified and hypodense areas. Within the orbit, it may spread backwards along the lateral rectus muscle. The recommended surgical procedures include radical tumor removal after prior biopsy, exenteration, or 'en bloc' resection with the adjacent bone. After the surgery, radio-chemotherapy is recommended. Unfortunately, there is no good solution—according to the reports, the chance of survival is independent of the surgical technique. The prognosis is poor, the tumor usually recurs within 2–3 years. Dissemination may occur without local recurrence, and a local recurrence may spread also into the intracranial space. The rare long survival is presumably not related to the surgical technique but to the individual immunological relationship between the tumor and the host.

The *adenocarcinoma* of the lacrimal gland, after prior histological confirmation, should be treated with primary exenteration. The prognosis is poor.

Other conditions of the lacrimal gland include granuloma, lymphoma, leukemia, Hodgkin's disease, lymphosarcoma and plasmocytoma. If the condition is part of a generalized, known systemic disease, surgery is not required, and if a diagnosis has not been made yet, a biopsy will ensure it.

Secondary Tumors of the Orbit

These are tumors that spread from the surrounding regions into the orbit. Basalioma may spread from the eyelids, and retinoblastoma or choroidal melanoma from the eyeball into the orbit. From the paranasal sinuses, carcinoma, sarcoma, papilloma, inverted papilloma, angiofibroma, esthesioneuroblastoma may spread into the orbit; from the lacrimal sac, carcinoma; from the intracerebral space, meningioma or glioma. The majority of these tumors are malignant, and they are often diagnosed when already inoperable. The surgical treatment—in case of operable tumors—requires teamwork.

Metastatic Tumors of the Orbit

The most common is the orbital metastasis of *breast cancer*. As already mentioned, it causes enophthalmos and, due to the dense, scirrhous infiltration of the orbital content, marked resistance is felt when repositioning the eyeball. It involves the eye muscles, causing eye movement disorders and double vision. In case of a positive history, the syndrome almost certainly indicates a breast cancer metastasis, but it is indicative even in the absence of a positive history. *Prostate cancer, melanoma, and lung and kidney cancer* may also give metastasis to the orbit. In children, *neuroblastoma* usually causes a bilateral orbital bone metastasis, which may occur before the primary tumor is detected, and is typically accompanied by eyelid hematomas. If an orbital metastasis is suspected, the most important task is to look for the primary tumor if it is unknown. In addition, the symptoms due to the metastasis must be alleviated with palliative therapy. It may be done with radiation therapy, partial or complete blepharorrhaphy, or local treatment of the eyeball for the risk the cornea is exposed to because of the exophthalmos and the lagophthalmos.

Inflammatory Conditions of the Orbit

Orbital granuloma, or orbitalpseudotumor, is a non-specific, localized or diffuse, acute, subacute or chronic inflammatory condition. Inflammatory conditions of the adjacent paranasal sinuses may have a role in inducing this condition, but the cause usually cannot be found. The *localized form* affects one or more eye muscles, the lacrimal gland, the optic nerve sheath or Tenon's capsule. It is accompanied by pain and hyperemia in the affected region. In case of acute myositis, the conjunctiva is hyperemic, and the eye movement, when gazing in the working direction of the affected muscle, is painful and restricted. In case of dacryoadenitis, the lacrimal gland is enlarged, painful and tender to pressure, and the upper eyelid is swollen and hyperemic. The granulomatous condition of the optic nerve sheath may cause a choked disc, and may severely deteriorate vision. In case of myositis, the acquired images show thickening of the muscle, which may also involve the tendinous part. Perineuritis causes an irregular broadening of the optic nerve sheath.

The *diffuse form* resembles an orbital tumor, hence the name 'orbital pseudotumor.' It causes exophthalmos, hyperemia of the eyelids and the conjunctiva can be observed, and it is accompanied by restricted eye movements and marked difficulty repositioning. Typical cases present no diagnostic difficulties. However, if the inflammatory symptoms are not pronounced, and the patient does not complain of pain, it is hard to tell a diffuse granuloma or a granuloma localized to the lacrimal gland apart from lymphomatous infiltration or other systemic diseases (multiple myeloma, Mikulicz's disease). Many times, the result of imaging procedures is also unclear. In case of a systemic disease, the lacrimal gland condition may be a part of it. If the underlying disease is unknown, biopsy should be performed or steroid therapy should be administered, the success of which is indicative of granuloma. The course of the disease is unpredictable. The long-term use of steroids may result in remission without recurrence, but more often, the disease flares up after shorter or longer symptom-free periods.

Tolosa-Hunt syndrome is an inflammatory condition that occurs in the cavernous sinus. Its signs and symptoms include slight exophthalmos, moderately restricted eye movements, double vision, pain, and a widened cavernous sinus on the images acquired. All non-specific inflammatory conditions are treated with steroids. Before this, if required, paranasal conditions must be treated. A prolonged steroid therapy with a high loading dose should be administered. If the disease recurs, the steroid dose must be increased again, and then a long-term maintenance dose must be used. Radiation therapy of the orbit may also help.

Endocrine orbitopathy is also an inflammatory condition, and forms part of the Graves-Basedow disease. It is caused by an autoimmune inflammation that occurs in the retrobulbar connective tissue elements and the ocular muscles. Cytokines that have a role in the progression and maintenance of inflammation, and hydrophilic glycosaminoglycans accumulate in the retrobulbar space. These induce proliferation of the retrobulbar connective tissue (primarily the adipose tissue), and an inflammation inside the extraoclar muscles resulting in a considerable thickening of them.

Its *clinical course* is characterized by an *active* phase accompanied by infiltrative, inflammatory symptoms and a fibrotic, *inactive* phase. Symptoms of the early, active phase include periorbital edema, hyperemia of the eyelid and the conjunctiva, and chemosis. The first sign may be von Graefe's sign, i.e., retraction of the upper eyelid. Exophthalmos and restricted eye movements occur. The patient complains of a feeling of pressure, and a pulling feeling and pain on gazing in the direction of the restricted eye movement—typically upwards. It is important to know that the function of the affected ocular muscles is restricted on gazing not in the direction of action but in the opposite direction. The most often affected muscle is the inferior rectus, followed by the medial rectus. After the active, inflammatory phase, the muscles enter a fibrotic stage, and the eyeball is locked in a downward- and/or inward-gazing position. The forced head posture opposing the position of the eyeballs is a characteristic sign. The acquired images show a characteristic, fusiform thickening of the ocular muscles, which does not affect the tendinous part of the muscles. In the inactive phase, the inflammatory symptoms go away, and the exophthalmos may decrease in euthyroid patients. In cases after the definitive treatment, where replacement therapy is used, eyelid myxedema may occur, and the exophthalmos often increases.

The most severe complication of endocrine orbitopathy is the compression of the optic nerve, which is due to the thickened ocular muscles in the orbital apex (crowded orbital apex syndrome). It is treated with high doses of steroid, and if it fails, orbital decompression surgery must be performed.

In the past years, there has been an increase in the number of endocrine orbitopathy cases in Hungary. This is another reason why the early detection and treatment of the disease is so important. Because of their eye symptoms, these patients are handicapped both in their family and in the society. Broken family relationships and lost jobs may be the consequences of the cosmetically unfavorable appearance. It is also true conversely—employers do not willingly employ people who have reached a definitive state with residual eye symptoms, but who are otherwise healed, because of their appearance. The prevention of the development of a severe state and the surgical rehabilitation may also resolve the social situation of the patients.

Quitting smoking and starting pentoxifylline therapy have an important role in prevention. In the active phase, steroid therapy according to different schemes, retrobulbar radiation therapy and local treatment should be used. Surgical rehabilitation is performed in the inactive phase. Corrective surgery (retroposition) of the fibrotic ocular muscles is performed to eliminate the extremely bothersome diplopia. The cosmetically unacceptable exophthalmos is reduced with orbital decompression surgery. In our practice, two-wall (lateral and medial wall) decompression is performed by removing the required amount of retrobulbar adipose tissue through an incision on the upper eyelid fold and with a transcaruncular approach ('hidden scar').

Vascular Conditions of the Orbit

Varicose veins and arteriovenous malformations cause intermittent exophthalmos. The degree of exophthalmos increases in the Trendelenburg's position and under other conditions that increase venous pressure, but otherwise it is absent or even enophthalmos may be present. The bulb can be repositioned easily. The radiograms and CT images of the orbit show *phleboliths* developed due to the slow circulation. A direct surgical solution is usually not feasible, occlusion with an endovascular sclerotizing agent may be an option.

A *carotid-cavernous fistula* is a spontaneous or traumatic opening on the intracavernous segment of the internal carotid artery. It leads to an increased pressure in the cavernous sinus, the flow is reversed in the ophthalmic vein, and blood of arterial pressure flows towards the orbit. Hyperemia is observed on the eyeball: the characteristic dilation of the episcleral vessels is a striking symptom. Exophthalmos, eyelid edema and, in case of a persisting condition, paresis of the cranial nerves III., IV., and VI may occur. A secondary increase in intraocular pressure, congested veins on the fundus and a choked disc may also occur. There is a pulse-synchronous bruit over the bulb on auscultation.

If spontaneous thrombosis occurs in the ophthalmic vein, there may be bleeding on the fundus, and the vision deteriorates. The typical syndrome, once it is fully developed, presents no diagnostic difficulty. In mild cases, when there is persistent pink eye or temporary double vision, it is important to differentiate between dilated episcleral vessels and diffuse conjunctival hyperemia. The former is characteristic to arteriovenous fistulas, whereas the latter is observed in conjunctivitis. The fistula is treated with endovascular occlusion.

Orbital *hematomas* are developed spontaneously or due to a trauma. Traumatic hematomas do not require too high an impact for their development. In the background of their occurrence, a pre-existing vascular malformation may be assumed, although this can be rarely confirmed with the histological examination. They usually appear in the upper part of the orbit, extraperiorbitally, and cause a high degree of exophthalmos, bulbar dislocation, and later chemosis, eye movement disorders and decreased vision. The condition that potentially leads to impaired function is treated with immediate surgery.

Systemic Diseases in the Orbit

Tumors of the orbit are rarely observed as part of a systemic disease. The first manifestation of a systemic disease, however, may occur in the orbit. In this case, biopsy and histological examination of the orbital space-occupying lesion helps make the correct diagnosis. A bilateral and rapidly progressing condition accompanied by other general symptoms (fever, poor general condition, enlarged lymph nodes, elevated erythrocyte sedimentation rate, blood count abnormalities and positive immunological tests) indicates a systemic disease.

Of the conditions that belong to this group, the relatively common ones are listed in this section.

In case of *eosinophil granuloma*, a type of Langerhans cell histiocytosis, there is proliferation of Langerhans cells in the bone marrow, which destroys the bone. It primarily affects children and young adults, it most often occurs in the skull, and it is not uncommon in the bones of the orbit. The irregular-shape or round bone loss is characteristic already in the radiogram, and the CT images provide a more accurate picture. Eyelid swelling and eyelid hyperemia may occur. These three symptoms together are of diagnostic value; however, a histological confirmation is required. It is treated with radical removal, follow-up treatment is rarely needed. Solitary *plasmacytoma* rarely occurs in the bones—it is more commonly developed as part of multiple myeloma. Multiple myeloma is a malignant hematological disease characterized by a clonal proliferation of plasma cells in the bone marrow. Its incidence increases with age. It causes bone destruction but it also has a solid part. Round, osteolytic bone defects on the skullcap are characteristic findings on radiograms and CT images. After histological confirmation, the therapeutic options are chemotherapy and, possibly, bone marrow transplantation. The prognosis is poor.

Boeck's sarcoid is a granulomatosis of unknown origin that affects multiple organ systems and usually occurs in young adults. Enlarged lymph nodes appear in the lung hila. Its characteristic histological property is that the granuloma is non-caseating. In the orbit, it may infiltrate the lacrimal gland; the diagnosis is made based on a biopsy sample.

Hodgkin's disease is a tumorous, chronic disease of unknown origin that affects the lymphatic system. The tumor growth has a mixed structure (lymphatic cells, histiocytes, monocytes, plasma cells, white blood cells). Its characteristic cells are the large, polynuclear Sternberg-Reed giant cells. The diagnosis is made based on the detection of these. The prognosis depends on the histological type. Usually, a stable disease can be achieved with medical treatment (cytostatic agents). Its predilection site in the orbit is the lacrimal gland.

Wegener's granulomatosis is an immune vasculitis of unknown origin. Pathologically, it is a necrotizing, granulomatous small-vessel inflammation. Clinically, it most often affects the respiratory tracts and, in its generalized form, the kidneys. In the orbit, the picture corresponds to diffuse necrotizing granulomatosis. It should be treated with immunosuppressants; the prognosis is poor.

Necrotizing vasculitis is also an immune disease. It may cause corneal ulceration, necrosis and perforation, and may attack the lacrimal gland. It is also treated with immunosuppressant drugs.

Injuries of the Orbit

Isolated fractures of the bones that form the orbit are rare, they are more commonly injured together with the adjacent bones and soft tissues (orbital content, paranasal sinuses, base of skull). Soft tissue injuries may be direct or due to orbital wall fracture, or traumatic hematomas or foreign bodies that penetrate the orbit. Its symptoms include eyelid edema, hematoma, ptosis, emphysema, laceration or palpable foreign body. Injuries may cause exophthalmos (hematoma, foreign body), enophthalmos (orbital wall fracture) or bulbar dislocation (extraperiorbital space occupying lesion).

The injuries may also lead to severely decreased vision by way of direct lesion of the optic nerve or an injury to the eyeball. In case of a perforating injury, the first task is to provide care for the injured eyeball. In case of a traumatic optic nerve lesion, the function usually cannot be improved. Megadose steroid therapy may be administered; the surgical decompression of the optic canal usually does not help.

Of the orbital wall fractures, the inferior wall blow out fracture is the most common. As a consequence of a blunt impact to the eyeball or the inferior margin, the thin inferior bony wall fractures, and the inferior margin remains intact, with or without entrapment of the inferior rectus muscle. It is indicated by a swollen lower eyelid (edema, hematoma, emphysema), enophthalmos, restricted upward (or downward) gaze, and maxillary nerve lesion. In case of a 'trapdoor' fracture, the eyeball cannot move upwards because the inferior rectus muscle is pinched between the closed fractured ends. If the fracture on the inferior wall is wide, there is no muscle entrapment, and there is no double vision either, but enophthalmos may occur. If the patient develops double vision, surgery is required; however, if there is no double vision but enophthalmos is present, it is a relative indication for surgery.

The purpose of the surgery is to release the entrapped muscle and to attach it to the mini-plates that replace the bone defect. A medial wall fracture may cause emphysema, whereas a lateral wall fracture usually does not result in dysfunction. In case of a superior wall fracture, the floor of the frontal sinus is fractured, and the trochlea may also be injured, causing double vision, which requires reconstruction. Any hematoma due to the injury must be evacuated immediately, in accordance with the principles already mentioned. In case of a penetrating foreign body, organic materials—such as wood—must be removed, whereas inorganic materials—such as glass or a projectile—require removal only if there is functional impairment.

Surgery of the Orbit

The *indication* for surgical removal of tumors of the orbit may be cosmetic, or it may be aimed at preserving or improving the decreased function. The surgery may be of diagnostic purpose or vital indication. The surgery is *cosmetic* if the purpose is to eliminate the disfiguring unilateral exophthalmos or bulbar dislocation in case of benign tumors that do not cause functional impairment. A tumor must be removed if it causes *impaired function*: decreased visual acuity, visual field defect or double vision. During surgeries of *diagnostic* purpose, biopsy is performed for histological examination in order to determine further actions. We speak of *vital indication* in case of malignant tumors. In this case, it must be removed completely, regardless of functions and cosmetic result.

The *direction of surgical exposure* is from where the tumor is easiest to access without the injury of the structures along the way. The approach may be extraperiorbital, pre- and transseptal, transconjunctival or transcaruncular. In case of an extraperiorbital approach, the direction of the surgical incision is the orbital margin, and the periorbital space is opened after the periosteum is detached with a blunt technique. The skin incision, depending on the location of the tumor, may be medial or lateral. If the approach is preseptal, the bony margin is approached through an incision made along the upper or lower eyelid sulcus. Transseptal exposure means an approach through the orbital septum. In case of transconjunctival approach, the orbit is entered through the superior or inferior conjunctival fornix. The transcaruncular exposure involves halving the lacrimal caruncle, and the surface of the medial orbital wall is approached in the epibulbar space, behind the lacrimal crest.

Tumors located in the orbital apex, above the plane of the optic nerve and in the optic canal may only be removed via a *transfrontal* (frontotemporal or superciliary) approach.

Urgent orbital surgery is required in case ofa condition that causes a vision-threatening, acute or rapidly progressing exophthalmos, such as spontaneous or traumatic orbital hematoma, or rapidly progressing malignant tumors (lymphoma, melanoma).

Orbital *exenteration* is performed in case of primary malignant tumors that do not exceed the bony borders, intraocular malignant tumors that have penetrated the orbit, tumors spreading from the eyelid into the orbit, in cases of local recurrence following enucleation and recurrence of embryonic rhabdomyosarcoma, and, as palliative therapy, in case of intolerable pain, bleeding or infection, or a cosmetic status that excludes social relations.

Transfrontal surgery is *contraindicated* in case of a malignant tumor that does not exceed the boundaries of the orbit, in case of non-sterile conditions, and when biopsy is to be done (Figs. 62.1, 62.2, 62.3, 62.4, 62.5, 62.6, 62.7, 62.8, 62.9, and 62.10).

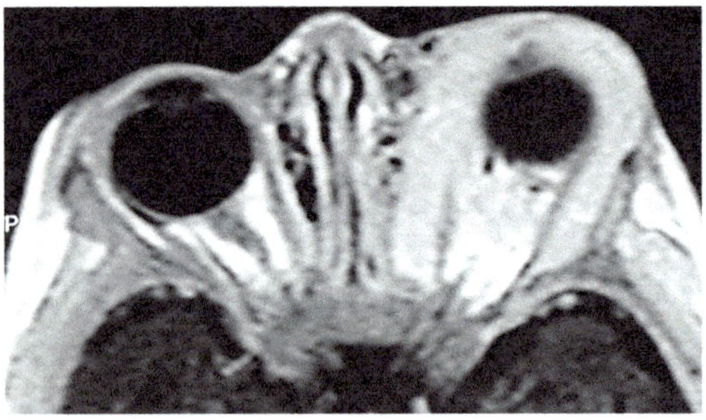

Fig. 62.1 MR image of a capillary hemangioma with extra- and intraconal location in the left orbit

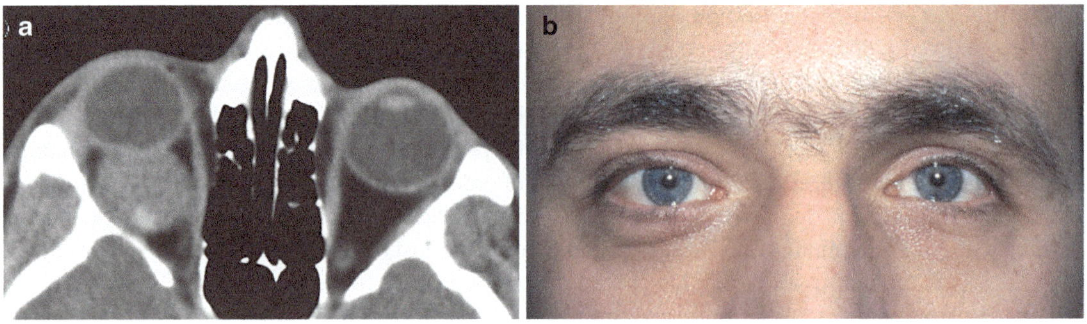

Fig. 62.2 (**a**) CT image: right-siged cavernous hemangioma causing axial exophthalmos and showing calcification. (**b**) Facial photography

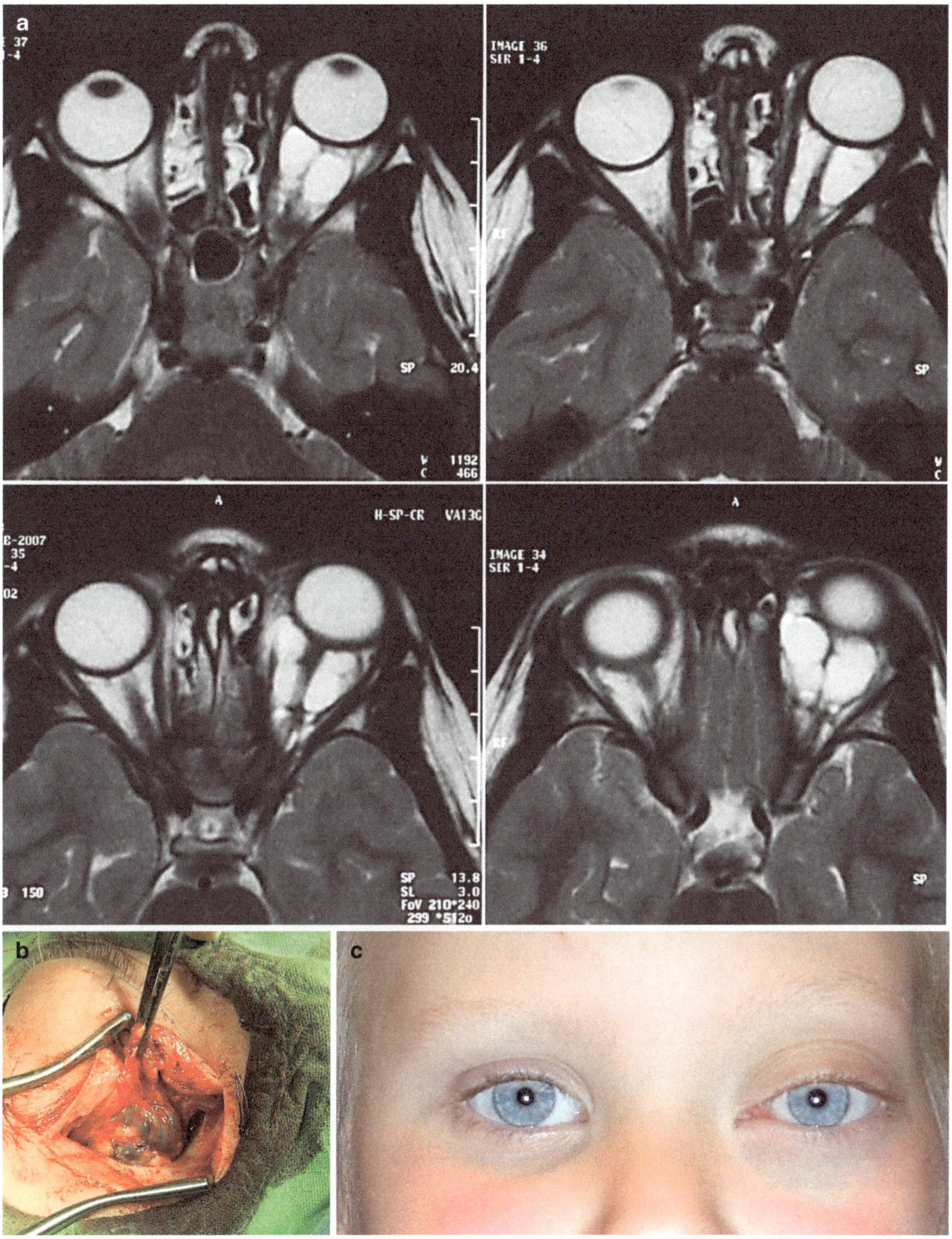

Fig. 62.3 Hemorrhagic lymphangioma in the left orbit. (**a**) MR images. (**b**) Intraoperative photography. (**c**) Facial photography

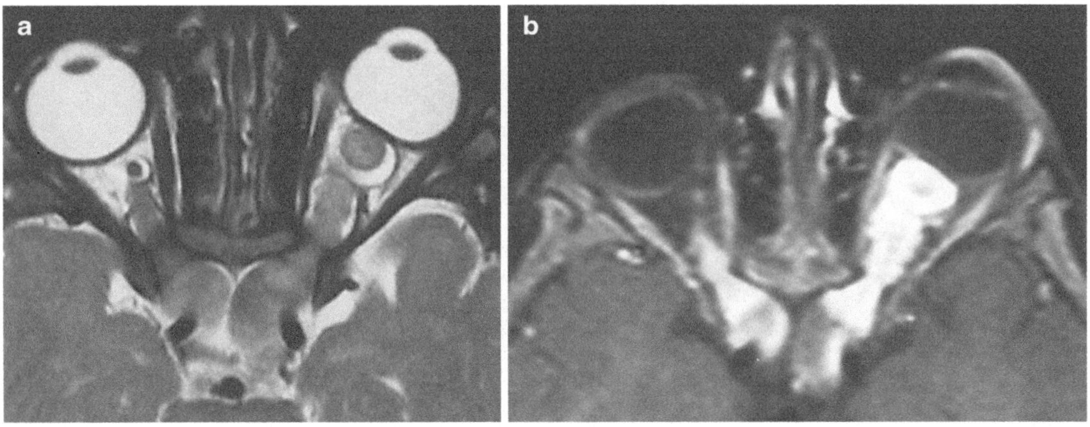

Fig. 62.4 Von Recklinghausen's disease. MR picture o bilateral optic nerve and chiasm glioma on T1- (**a**) and T2-weighted (**b**) images

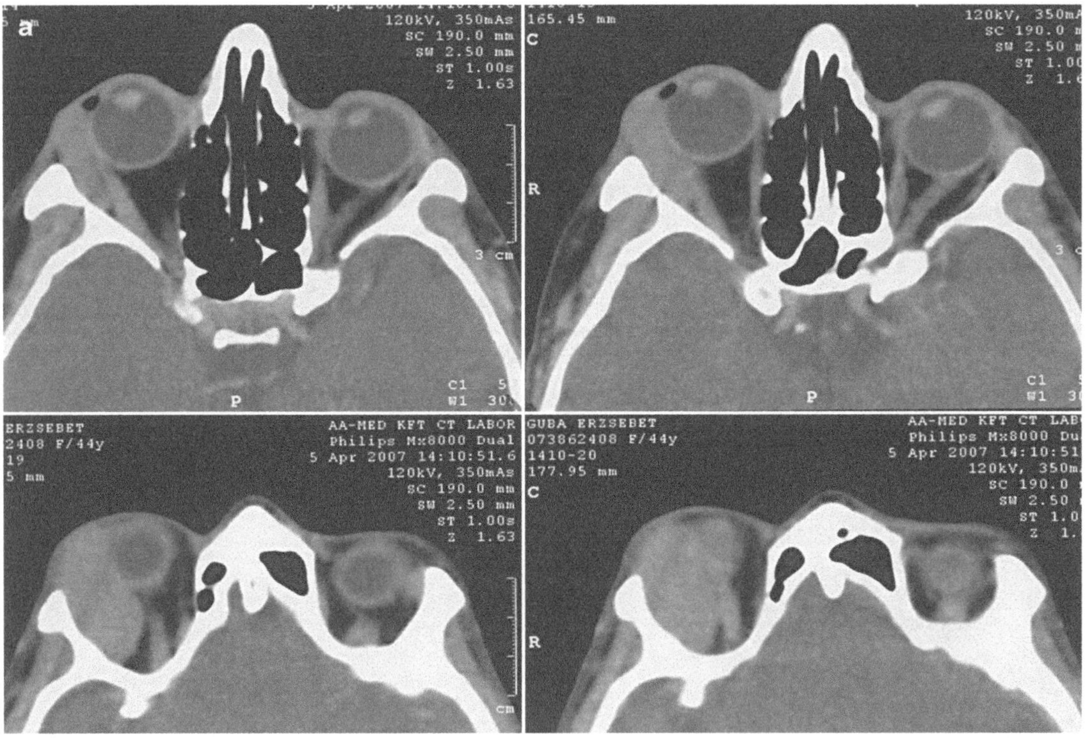

Fig. 62.5 Malignant lymphoma in the region of the right lacrimal gland (**a**) CT images. (**b**) Facial photography. (**c**) Swollen eyelid lobe

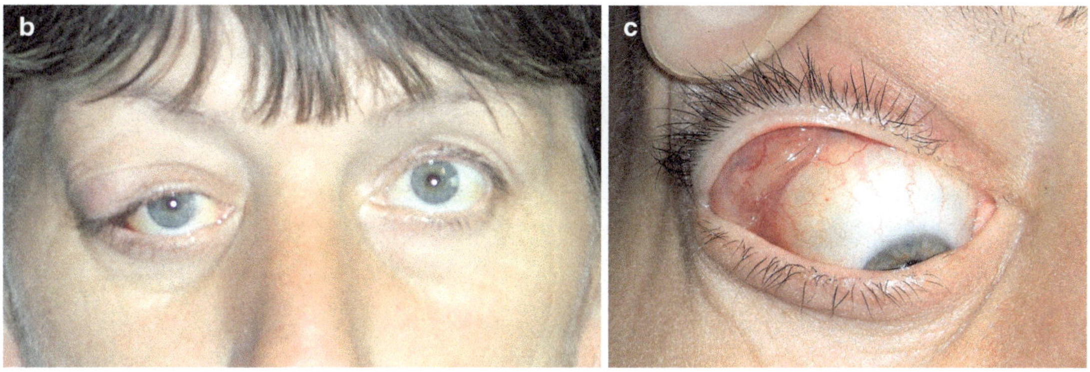

Fig. 62.5 (continued)

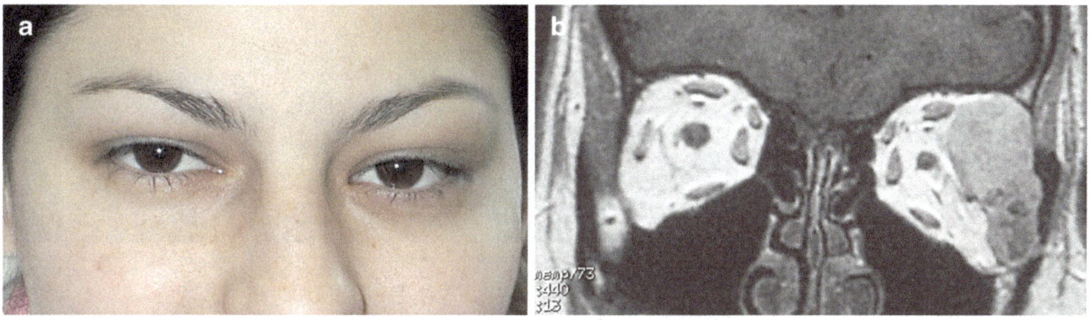

Fig. 62.6 *Adenoid cystic carcinoma of the lacrimal gland in the left orbit*. (**a**) Facial photography; (**b**) coronal MR image. The tumor shows striking heterogeneous enhancement

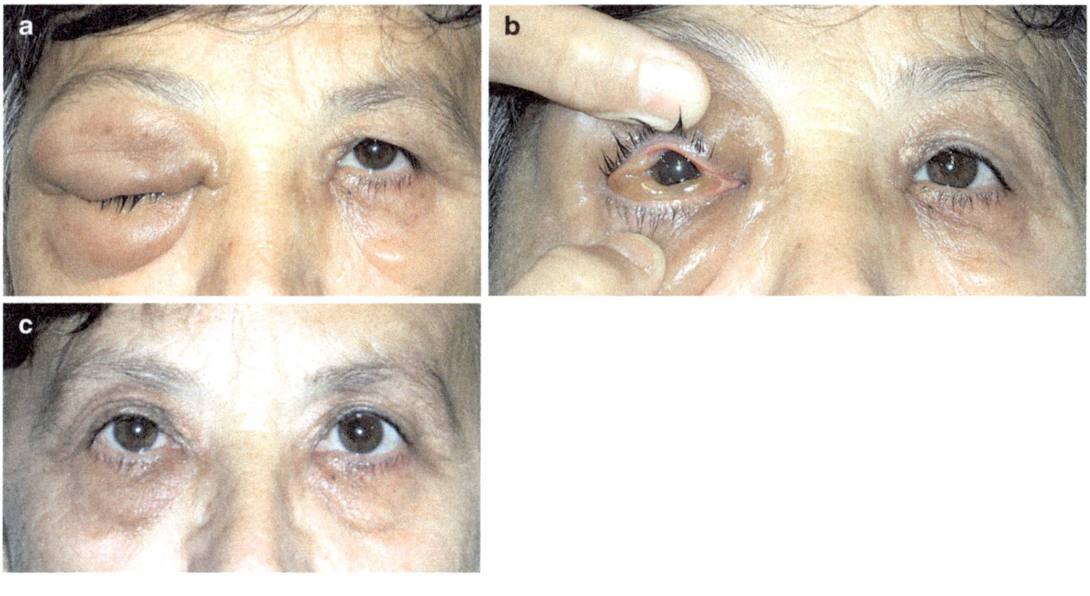

Fig. 62.7 (**a**–**c**) Acute, diffuse inflammation in the right orbit before and after steroid therapy

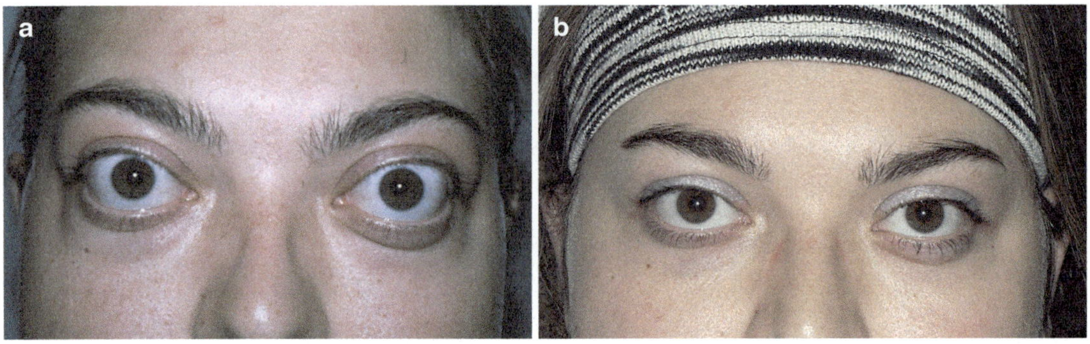

Fig. 62.8 Endocrine orbitopathy before (**a**) and after (**b**) decompression surgery

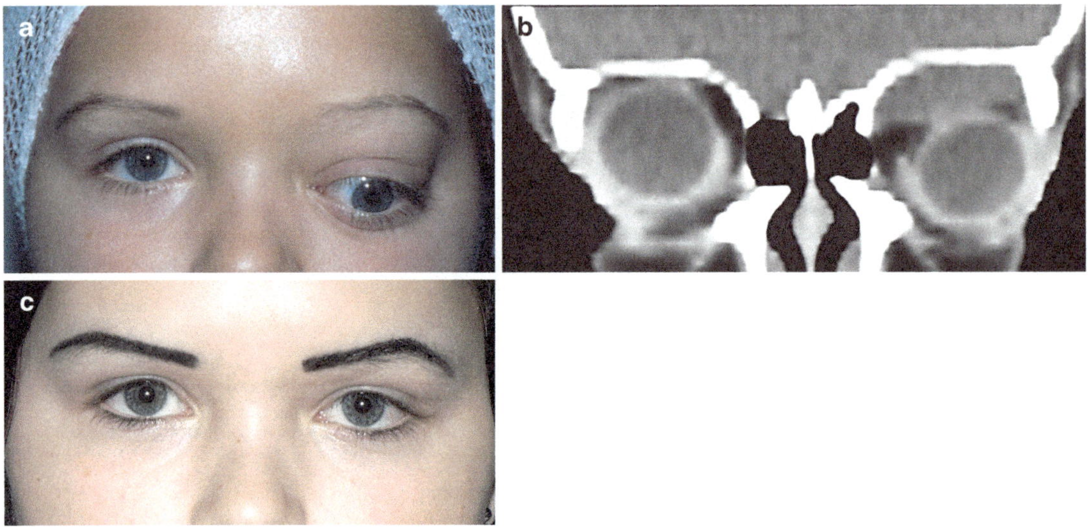

Fig. 62.9 (**a**–**c**) Traumatic hematoma in the left orbit. Facial photography before the surgery, CT image, facial photo after the surgery

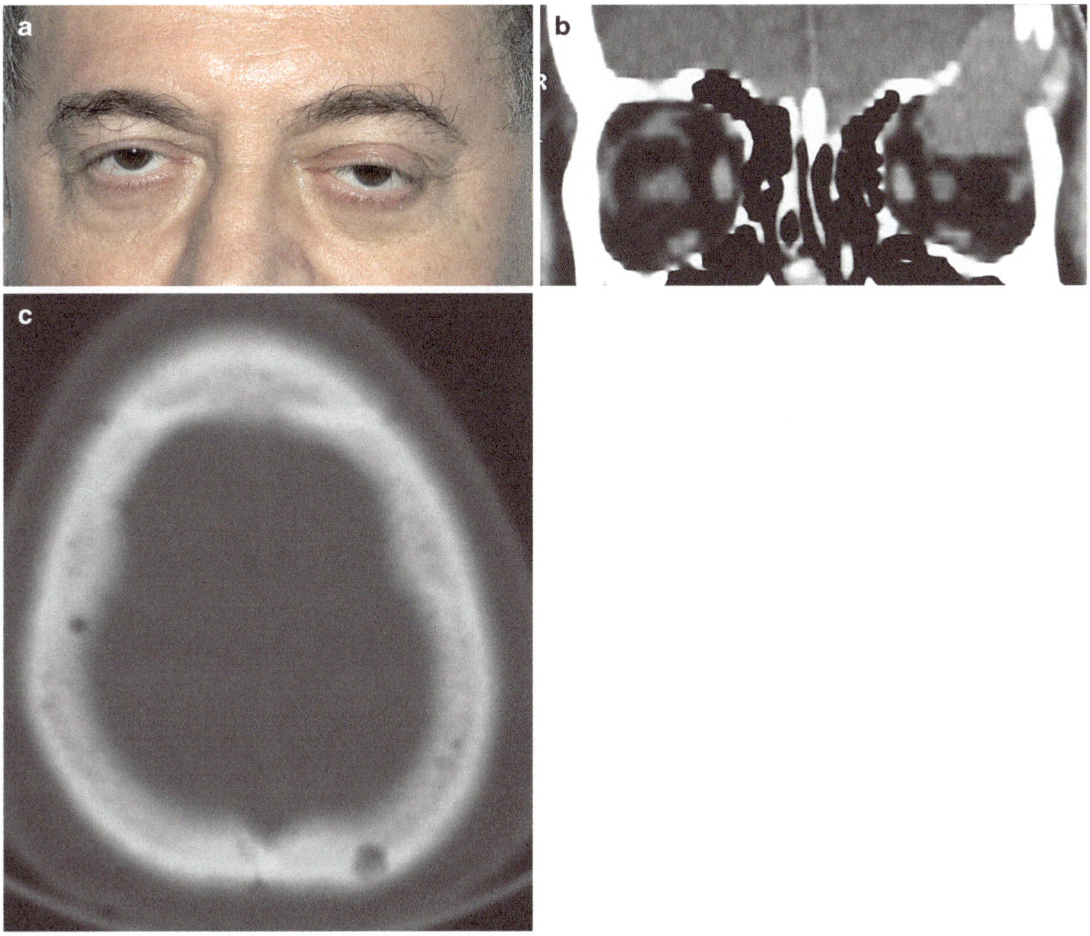

Fig. 62.10 (**a–c**) Multiple myeloma. (**a**) Facial photography; (**b**) CT image of the tumor that causes bone destruction and spreads intracranially; (**c**) multiple lesions in the bones of the skull

Traumatic Injuries of the Orbit

63

György Pulay

Contents

In case of a traumatic injury to the orbit, it is extremely common that the immediate or late vision defect of the patient is not caused by the damage to the eyeball but is due to the injury of the bones. If it remains unnoticed or not diagnosed early, it may cause severe or even irreversible vision or eye movement complications in the future. This is why we consider it important that, in addition to the ophthalmological examination of the patient, a specialist with experience in the diagnostics and therapy of the bony orbit participate in the primary (clinical, radiographic and CT) assessments, to allow an intervention, if required, as soon as possible after the treatment plan is agreed on. The objective of this chapter is to demonstrate the importance of the time factor by presenting each bone injury in the orbital region.

G. Pulay, M.D
Outpatient Department, Accident Center,
Budapest City Council Péterfy Sándor Street Hospital,
Budapest, Hungary
e-mail: office@trauma.sote.hu

Primary Reconstruction

At our department, we intend to achieve primary, definitive reconstruction in terms of both function (vision, masticatory ability) and aesthetics by providing newly injured patients with management of bone injuries (or defects) and with treatment for soft tissues in accordance with plastic surgery principles. The immediate or early delayed surgery may mean, from a professional aspect, the accurate repositioning of the fractured ends and, regarding function and aesthetics, a much easier and more effective soft tissue care, preserving viable bone fragments and a fast and distortion-free healing of the patient (instead of living, out of necessity, with a permanent defect). This is especially true for bone injuries that dislocate the eyeball or restrict eye movements.

Zygomatic Bone Fracture

The zygomatic bone forms a significant portion of the orbital frame. Its fracture, depending on the direction and degree of the dislocation, may be accompanied by vision disorders (eye movement, diplopia) and facial asymmetry (Figs. 63.1, 63.2, 63.3 and 63.4). An early diagnosis is extremely important because the treatment method and the end

J. Somlai, T. Kovács (eds.), *Neuro-Ophthalmology*, DOI 10.1007/978-3-319-28956-4_63

result often depend on the time factor. Recent cases (with a history of 3–6 days) may be repositioned using a closed approach, with a surgical hook inserted percutaneously below the base of the zygomatic bone.

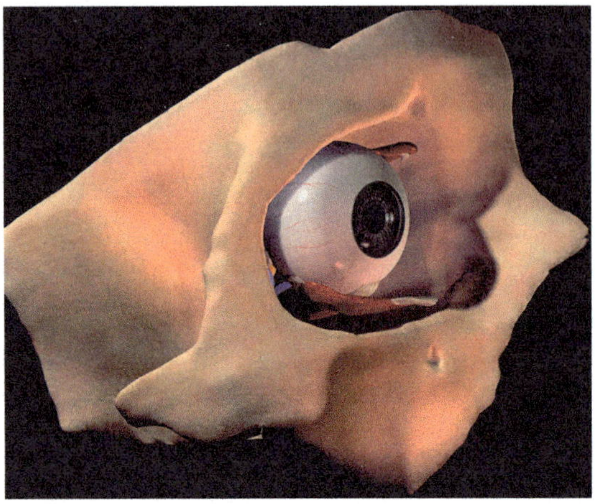

Fig. 63.1 The role of the zygomatic bone in maintaining the level of the eyeball, and its relationship with the interior rectus and inferior oblique muscles

In many cases, this minimally invasive method may eliminate diplopia, eye movement restriction due to muscle pinching, and facial asymmetry (Figs. 63.5, 63.6 and 63.7).

In case of late treatment (the fracture has a history of 1–2 weeks), besides repositioning, plate fixation of the orbital margin may also be required because an unstable position may be present after repositioning due to the rounding of the fractured ends and the incipient fibrosis

Blowout Fracture

A direct blunt-force impact on the eyeball may, most often, cause an injury on the paper-thin bone plate of the orbital floor, leaving the stronger bones of the orbital frame intact (Fig. 63.8). The diplopia and eye movement complaints of

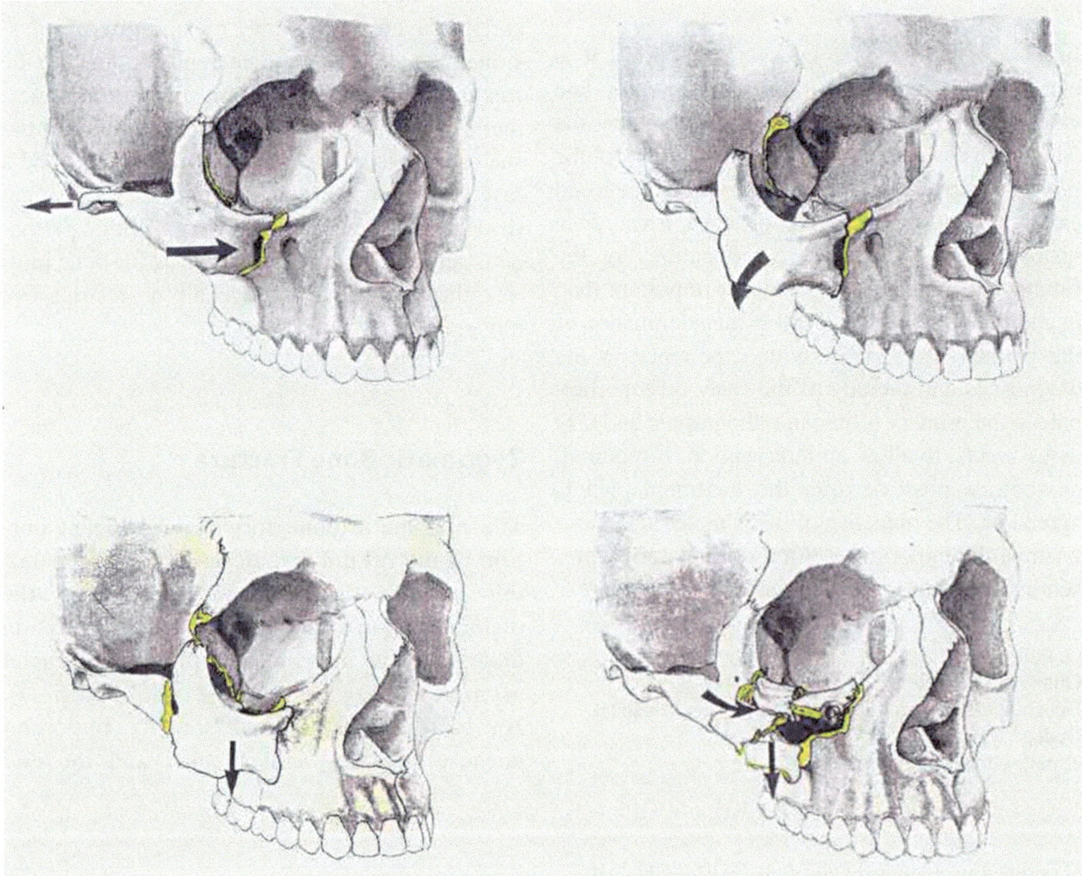

Fig. 63.2 Directions of dislocation in case of fractured zygomatic bone body

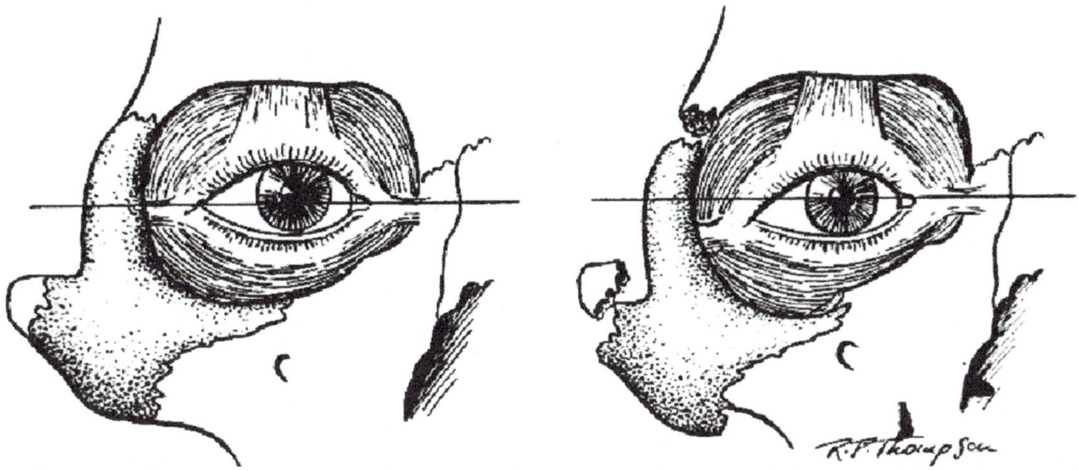

Fig. 63.3 Fracture scheme: a caudally dislocated zygomatic bone fracture is accompanied by depression of the eyeball

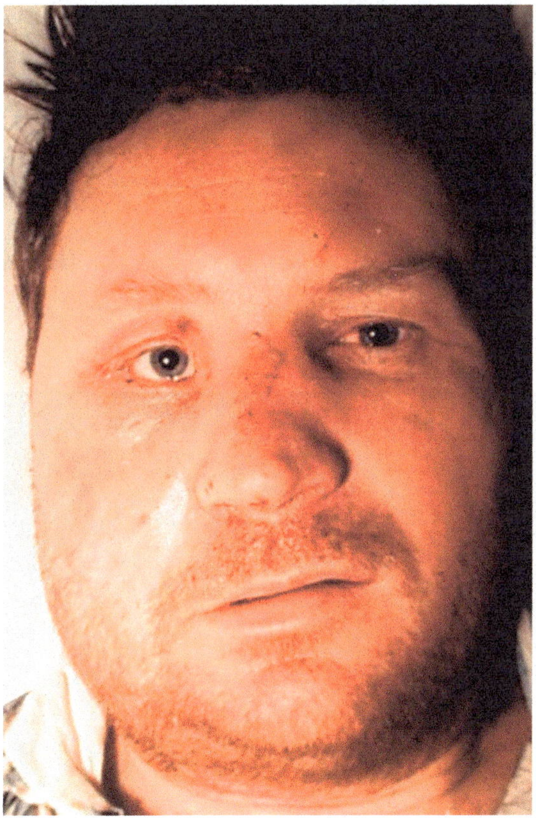

Fig. 63.4 The same, in vivo: impression of the right half of face, difference in bulbar level = diplopia

the patient, despite a normal radiogram, present a serious diagnostic challenge. The injury of the orbital floor (even herniation of peribulbar adipose tissue or muscles towards the maxillary sinus) can be confirmed with a coronal CT scan (Figs. 63.9 and 63.10). In an ideal, recent case (with a history of 3–6 days), the door wing-like fracture of the bone plate can be successfully restored from the direction of the maxillary sinus by repositioning the eyeball, after eliminating any herniation (Figs. 63.11 and 63.12).

If the orbital floor fracture is fragmented/comminuted, a direct exposure is required. This way, an attempt may be made at replacing the fragments but, many times, reconstruction with a titanium mesh is required because no loadable fragments can be achieved with replacement or because of the extension of the defect. (See also: "Comminuted Fractures") (Figs. 63.13, 63.14, and 63.15).

The implanted mesh is shaped in three dimensions based on the curves of the intact parts of the orbital floor. Once the mesh is smoothed onto the defect, the outer edge of the L-shaped mesh modeled to fit the orbital frame is secured with screws.

Comminuted Fractures

If a simultaneous injury occurs to the orbital frame, the orbital floor and the adjacent bones, even in severely dislocated, possibly fragmented cases that require treatment from both functional and aesthetic aspects, an immediate or early delayed procedure is required (6–10 days after the injury), using a direct surgical approach that depends on the type of injury but respects the aes-

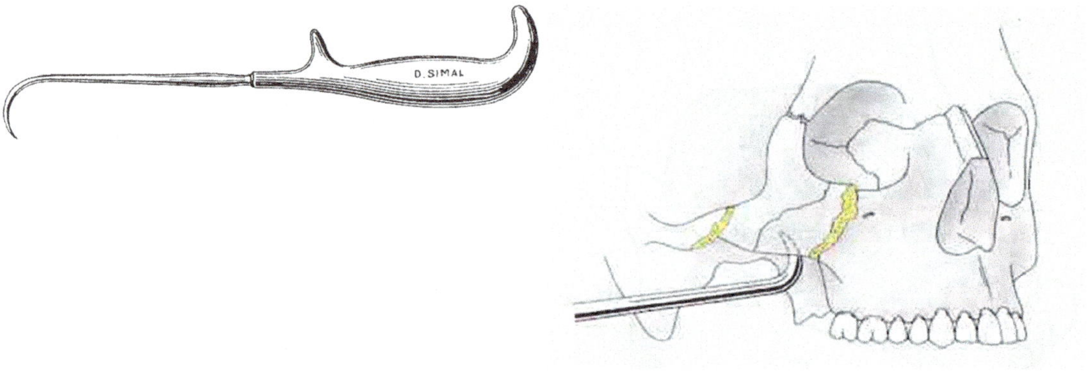

Fig. 63.5 Percutaneous, closed repositioning method with a surgical hook

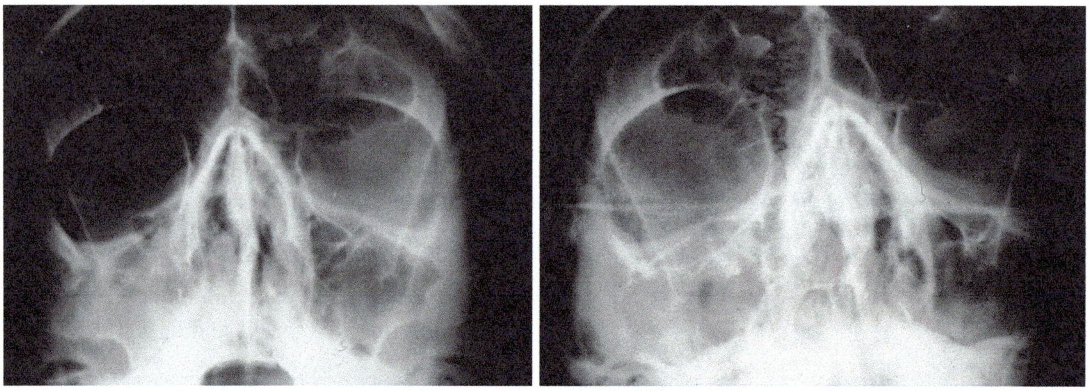

Fig. 63.6 Closed elevation of the zygomatic bone with manual repositioning of the fragment of the infraorbital margin: the eye movements become unrestricted

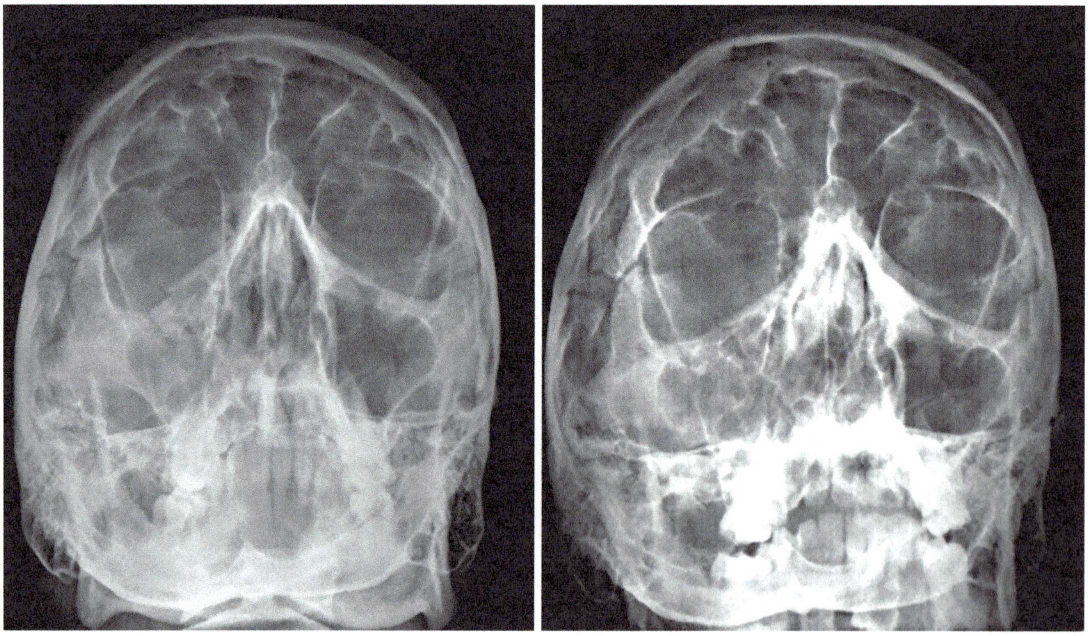

Fig. 63.7 Caudally dislocated zygomatic bone fracture. Repositioning with a hook and replacing the inferior orbital margin that shows fragmented fracture. Diplopia is gone

thetic aspects. For the reconstruction of the infraorbital margin or the orbital floor, a subciliary approach is used that does not impair the circulation and function of the lower eyelid, whereas the reconstruction of the orbital roof and the frontal sinus involves an incision made along the curve of the eyebrow. After exposure and reposition, first, the (fragmented) fracture of the orbital frame is fixed with titanium miniplates and screws, and then, if required, the orbital floor defect is replaced (after prior elimination of any soft tissue herniation) with a modeled 3D titanium mesh that follows the bone contour and which is laid onto the restored orbital margin and secured with screws there, checking the correct position of the eyeball (Figs. 63.16, 63.17, and 63.18). The percutaneously inserted surgical hook is required here as well for the replacement of the zygomatic bone body and the fragments. The unstable repositioning is fixed with osteosynthesis from a direct approach.

All this can be performed with a primary approach in unconscious **polytraumatic** patients if appropriate images are acquired, in such a way that they do not even experience the vision disorder due to the obvious bulbar dislocation observed on admission (Figs. 63.19 and 63.20).

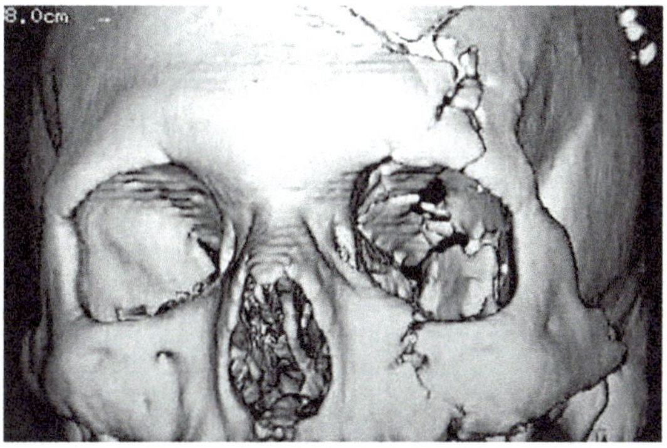

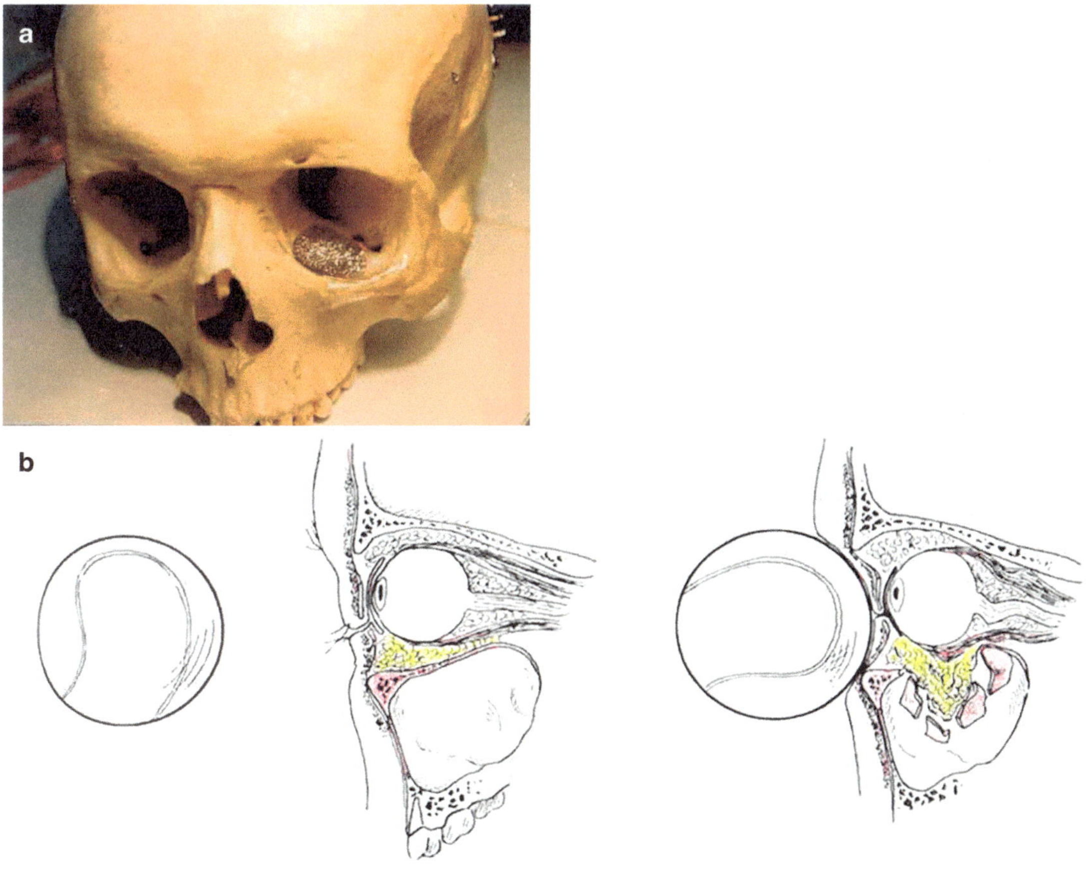

Fig. 63.8 (**a**) Intact orbital frame, defect on the orbital floor; (**b**) typical mechanism of injury

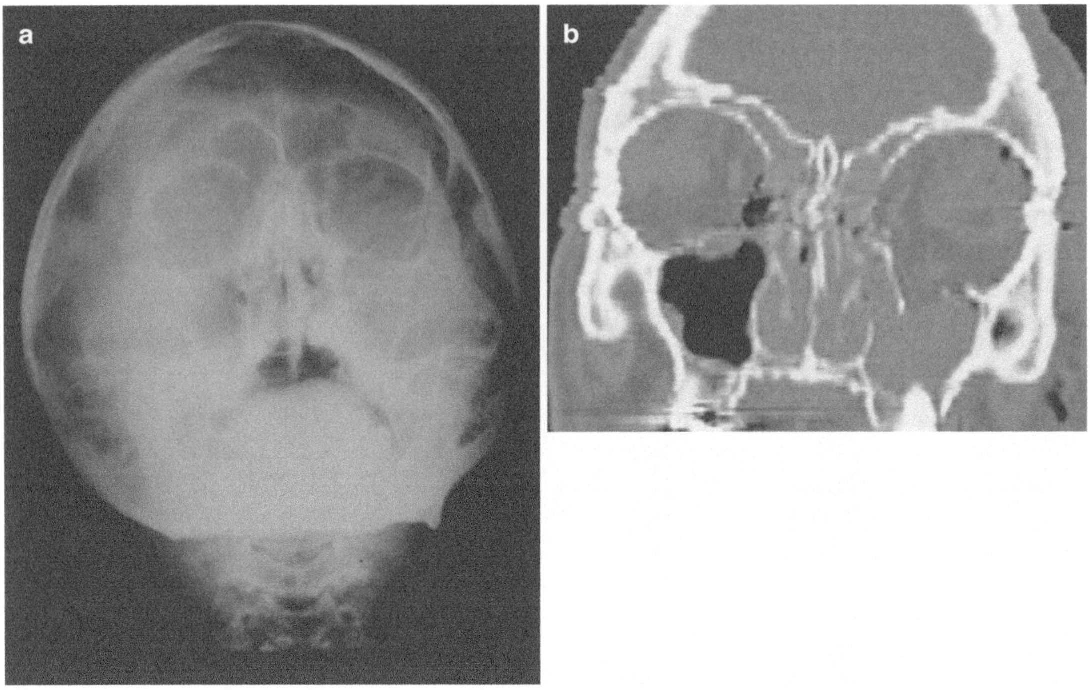

Fig. 63.9 (**a**) Plain radiogram without abnormalities. (**b**) CT image on the right: door wing-like orbital floor fracture (diplopia)

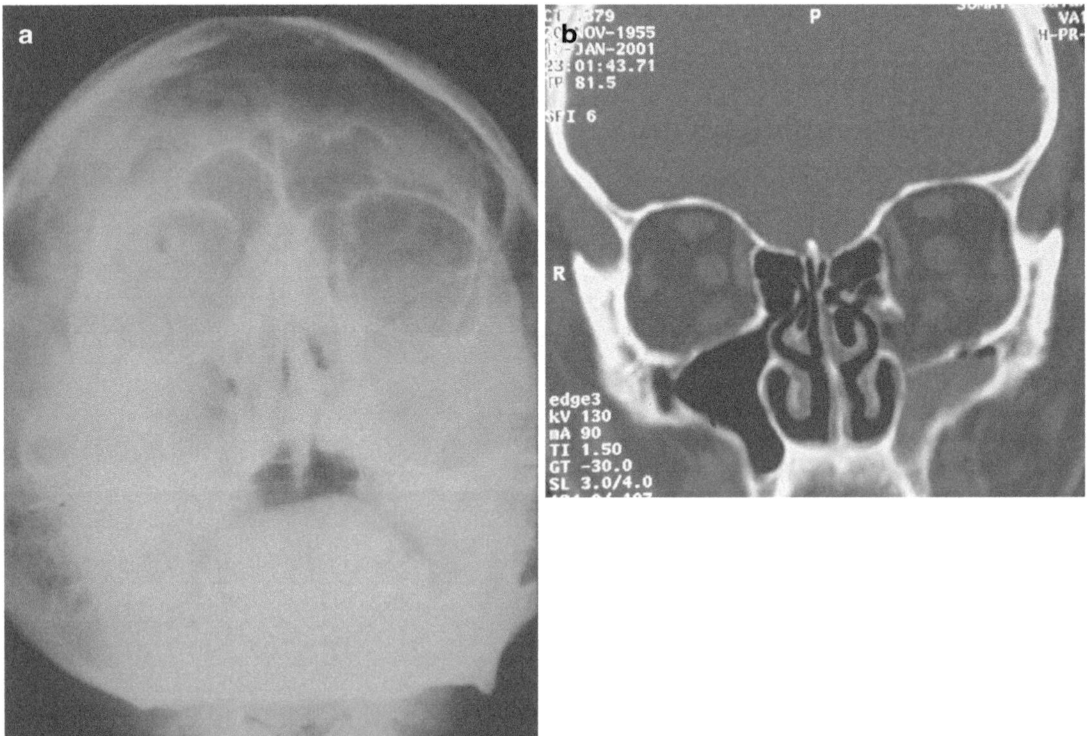

Fig. 63.10 (**a**) Radiogram—the orbital frame is intact but there are eye symptoms: diplopia and restricted eye movements. (**b**) The coronal CT image shows a similar lobular bone defect with a lateral 'shaft'

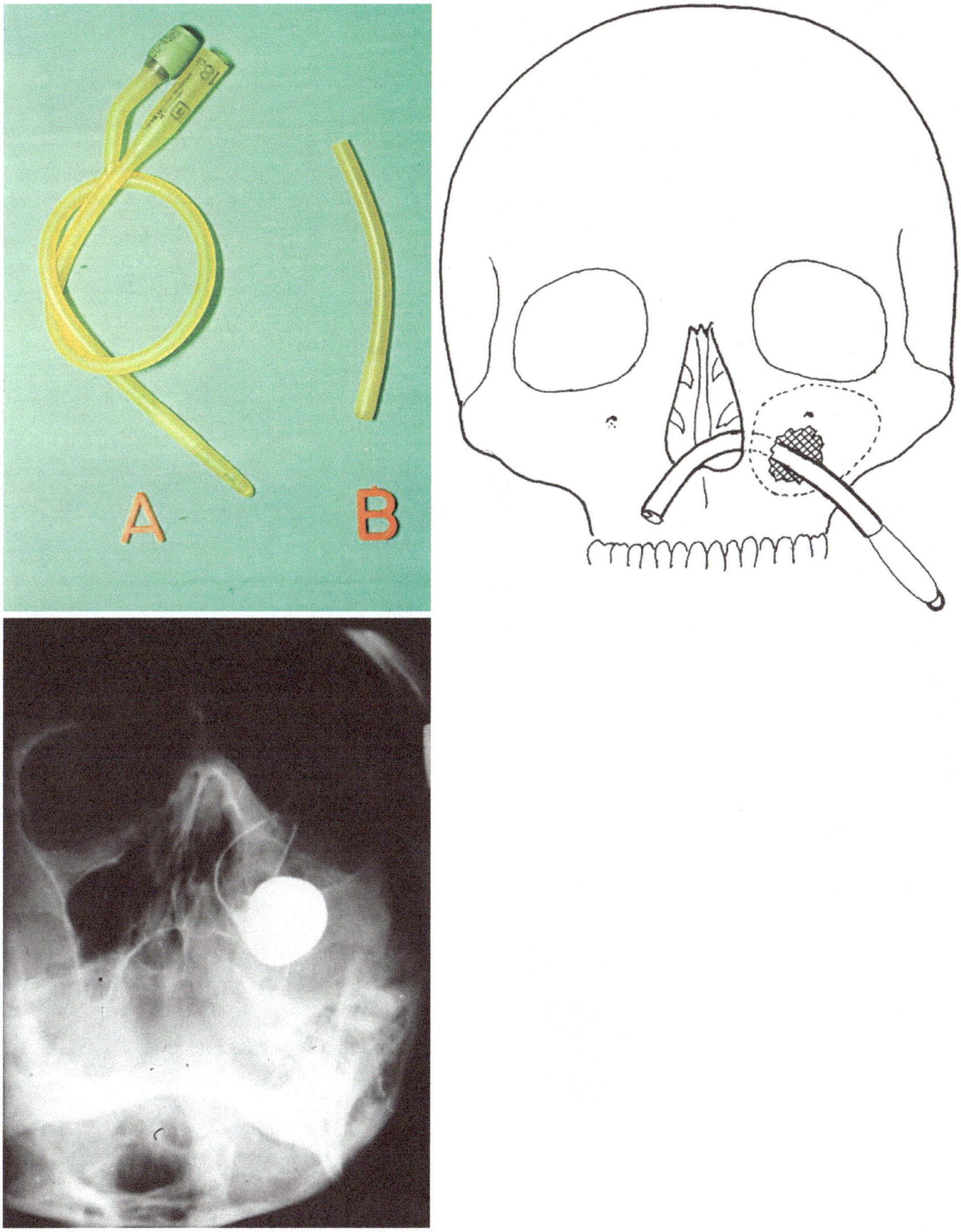

Fig. 63.11 During the surgery, after making an intraoral window on the maxillary sinus, the eyeball and the bone plate are repositioned, with a ballooncatheter support until fixation

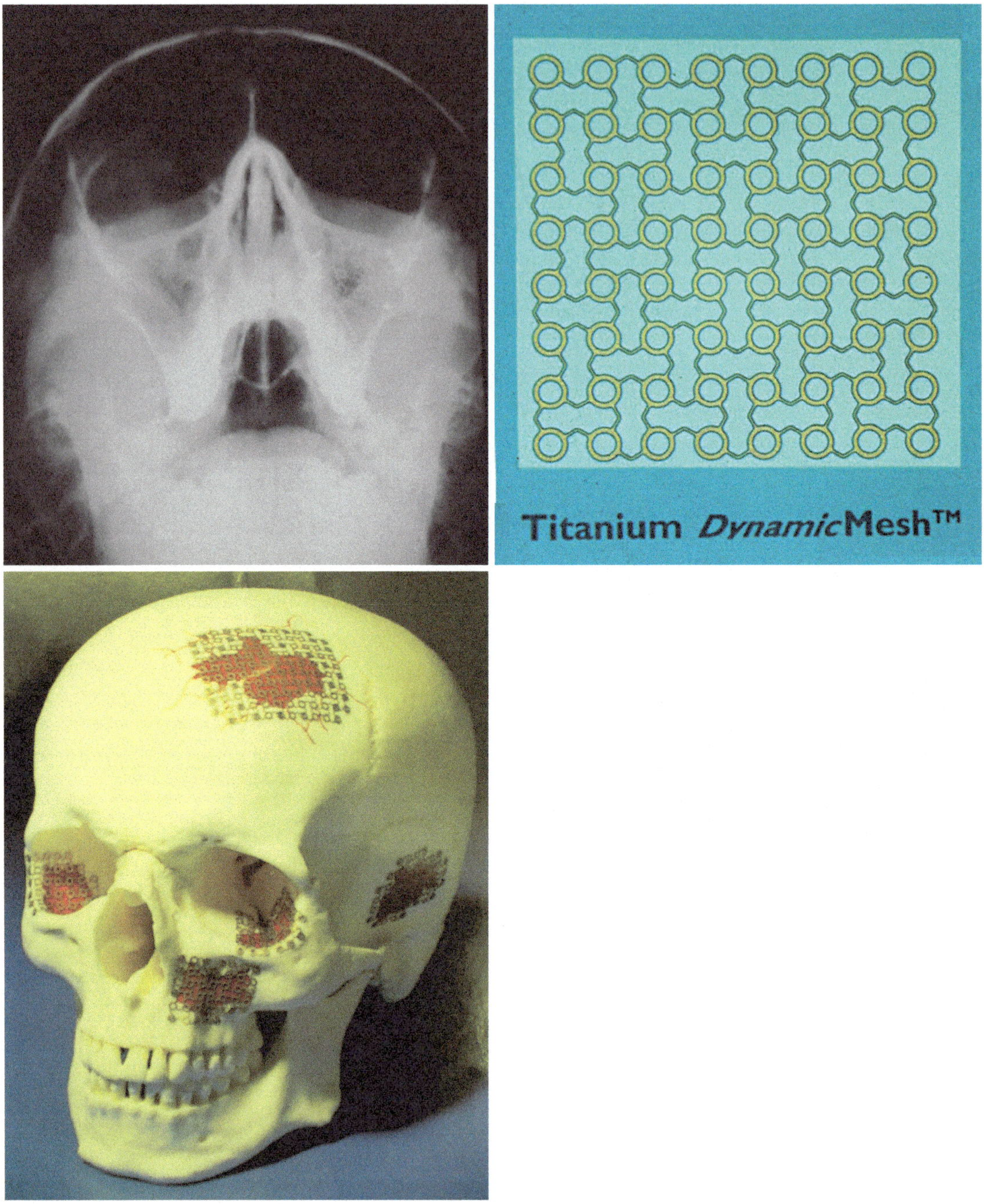

Fig. 63.12 To maintain the position of the inserted balloon, the window on the sinus is closed with a titanium mesh and screws; the mesh is also indispensable for the treatment of orbital floor, midface, frontal bone, etc. defects, and consists of a material that can be shaped in three dimensions and which is available in different thicknesses

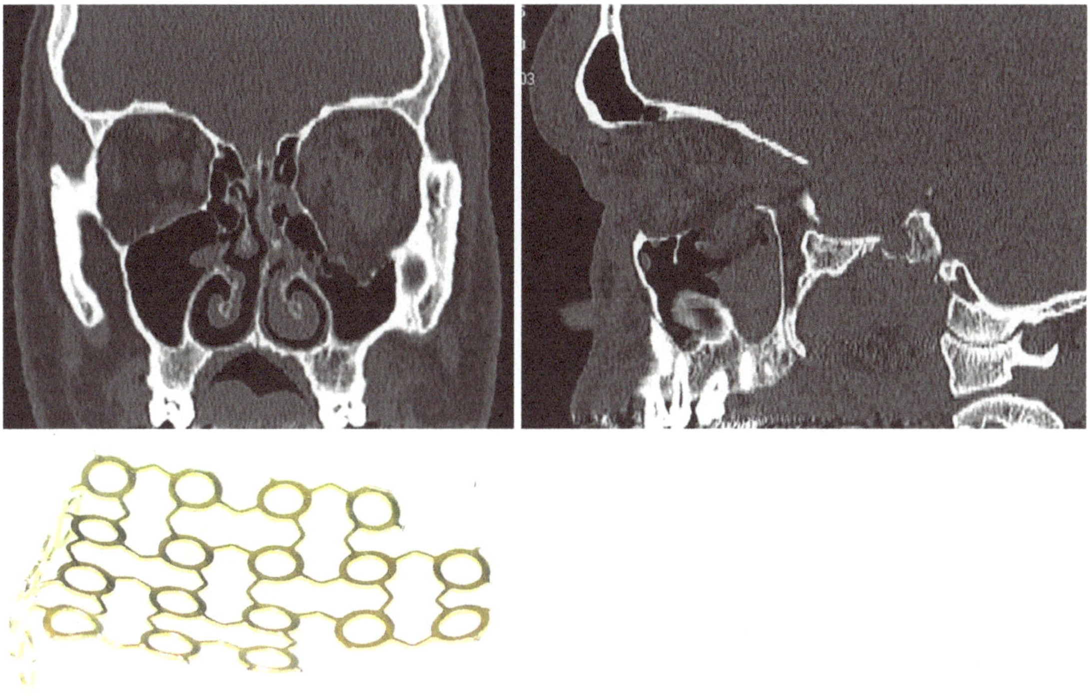

Fig. 63.13 Extremely large orbital floor defect and modeled titanium mesh

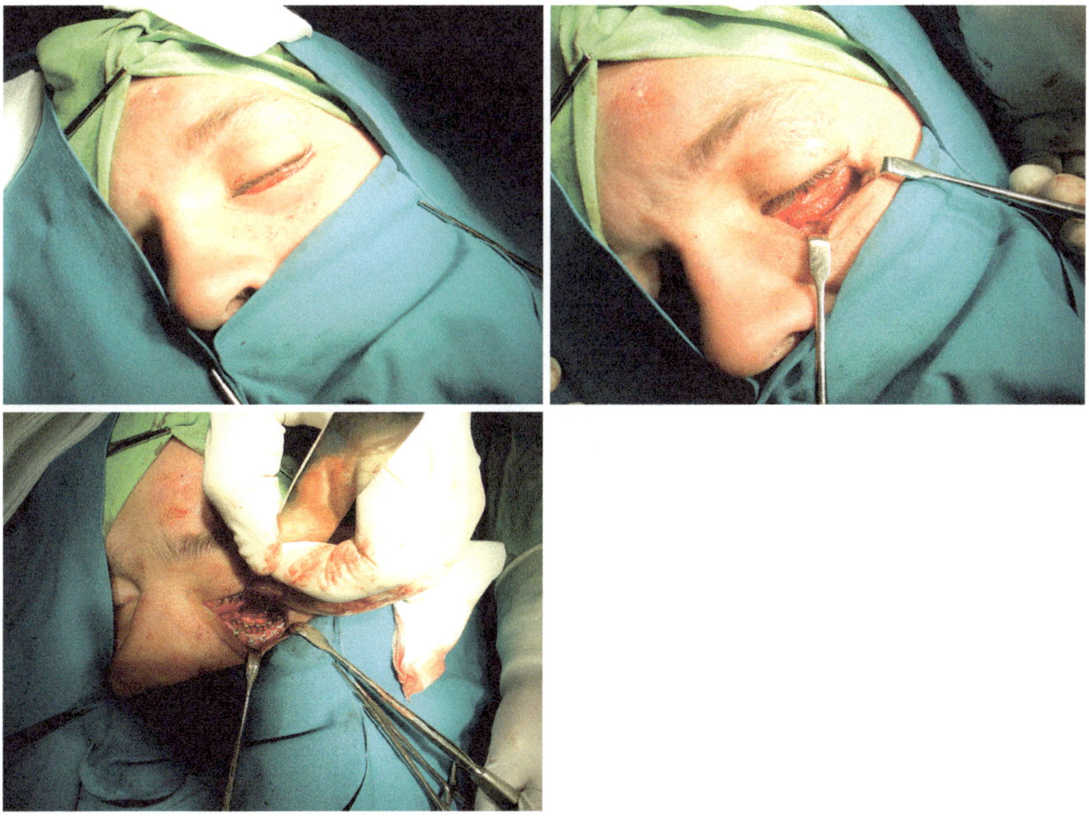

Fig. 63.14 Subciliary approach and the implant in place

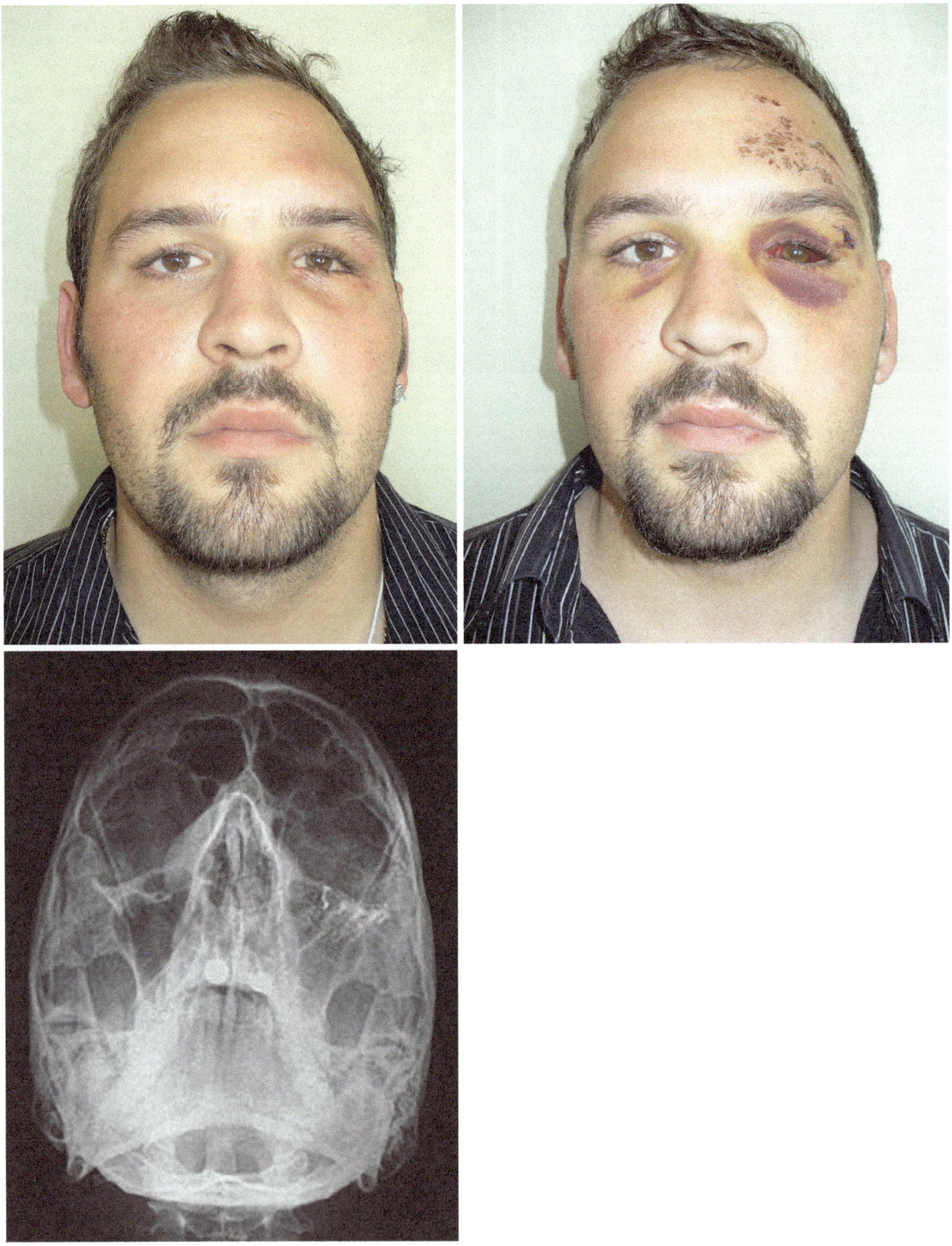

Fig. 63.15 The level of the eyeball is restored

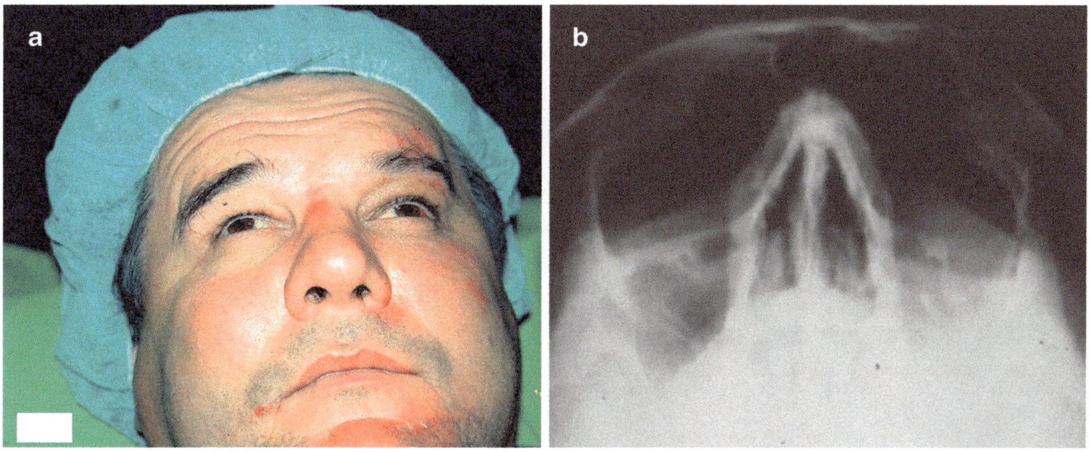

Fig. 63.16 (**a**) Fractured facial bones, difference in the level of the eyeballs. (**b**) Radiogram: fragmented zygomatic bone, orbital frame and orbital floor fracture (diplopia)

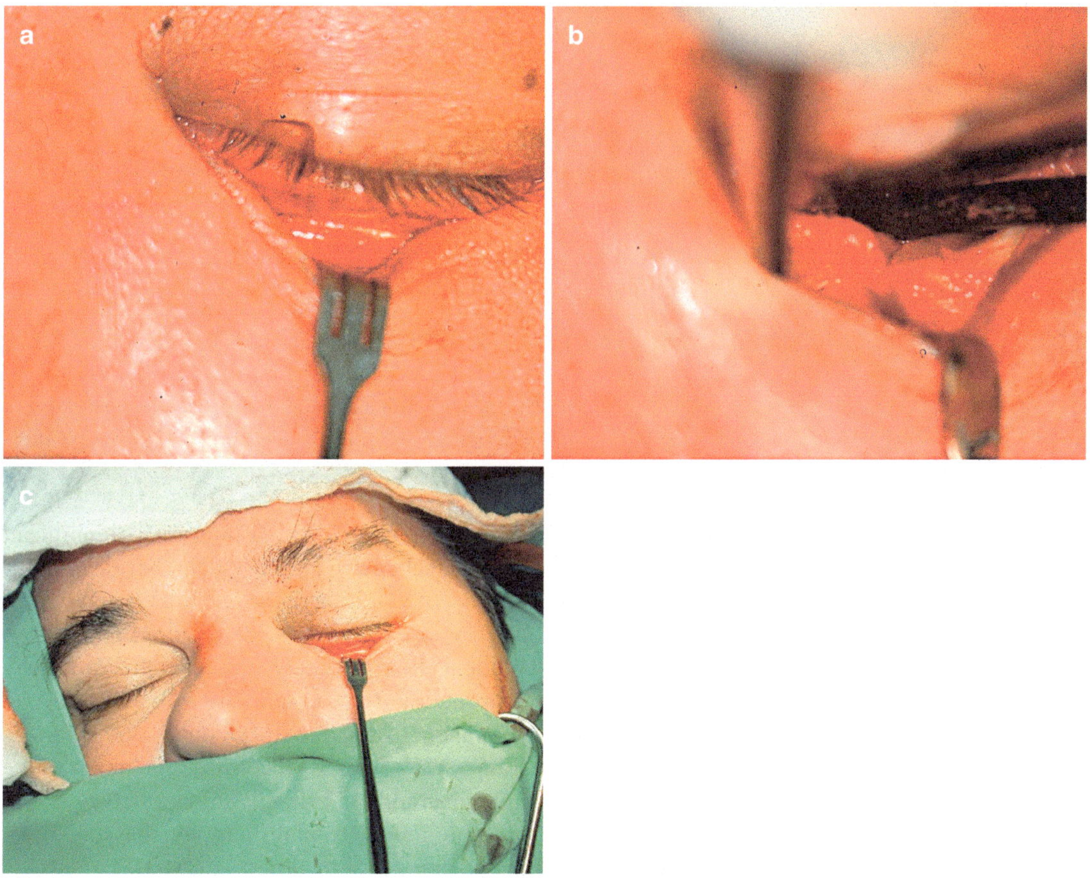

Fig. 63.17 (**a**) Surgical exposure; (**b**) fragment and step formation on the lower orbital margin; (**c**) repositioning the zygomatic bone with a hook

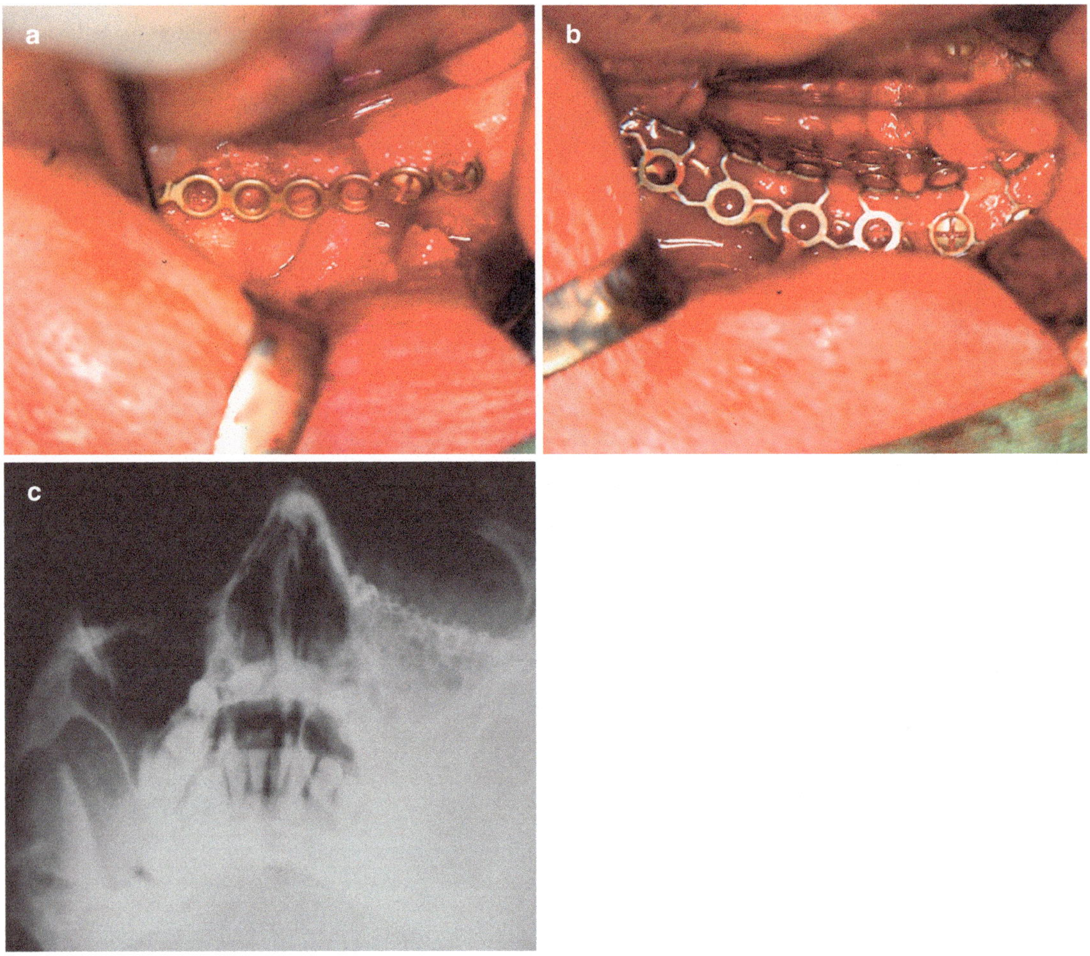

Fig. 63.18 (**a**) Fixation of the lifted zygomatic bone and the fragment with a titanium miniplate; (**b**) replacement of the orbital floor defect with a titanium mesh; (**c**) postoperative radiogram (the diplopia and facial asymmetry are gone)

During the surgery of **the frontal bone, the frontal sinus, and the lateral and upper orbital margins**, the eye movement functions must be preserved or restored. After the removal of nonviable fragments only, the orbital contour can be reconstructed more safely from functional and aesthetic aspects with fixation of the bone fragments that can be repositioned properly, simultaneously with the replacement of any remaining bone defect (Figs. 63.21, 63.22, 63.23, 63.24 and 63.25

In case of a **conjunct defect fracture of the orbit and the maxilla**, the eyeball can supported simultaneously with the reconstruction of the facial wall of the maxillary sinus with a primary approach.

Because of a panfacial injury with significant bone defect due to a car accident, besides stabilization of the midface, the left orbital and maxillary sinus defects also required treatment. Without an early reconstruction, the extremely dislocated left eye could have suffered a severe, permanent impairment due to fibrosis (Fig. 63.26). (The 3D reconstruction image of the first-generation CT image shows a defect also in the region of the frontal sinus, which is an artifact due to large slice thickness (Fig. 63.27)).

Consequences of a superficial primary clinical examination and the lack of imaging procedures (Figs. 63.28, 63.29, 63.30, 63.31, 63.32, 63.33, and 63.34):

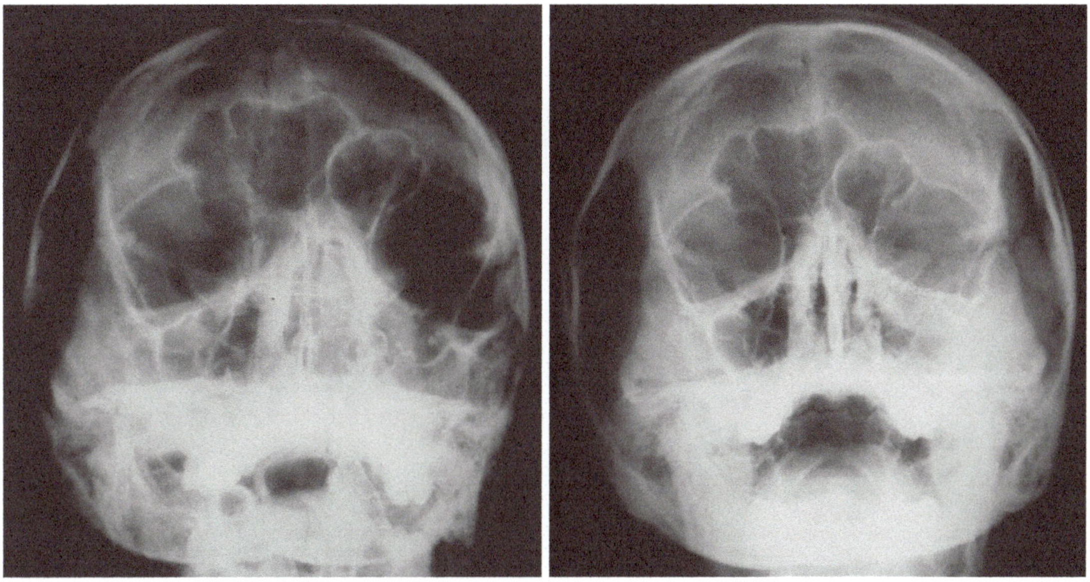

Fig. 63.19 Severely dislocated zygomatic bone body fracture with orbital floor defect. Closed repositioning of the zygomatic bone, plate fixation of the orbital frame, titanium mesh to replace the orbital floor

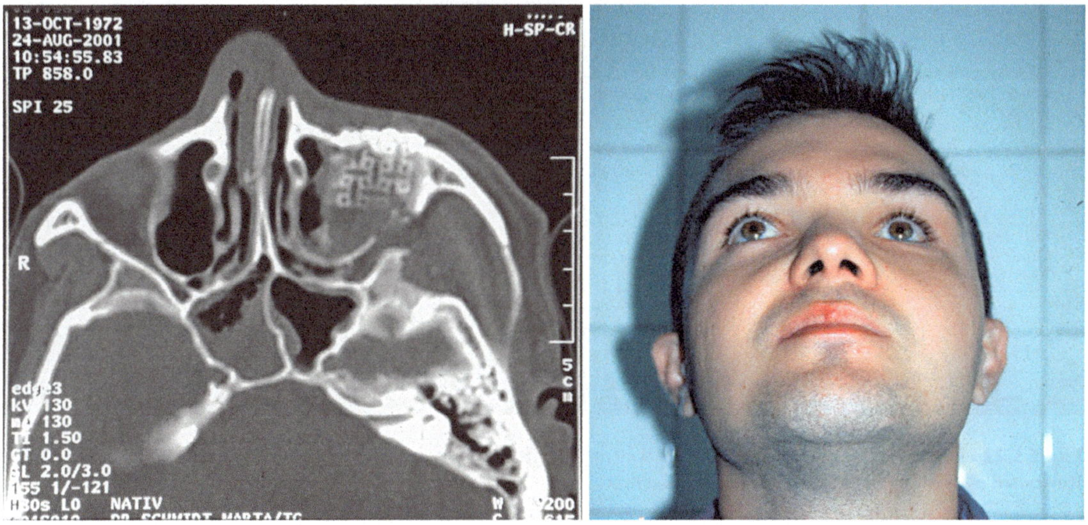

Fig. 63.20 Axial CT image with the implants in place. Postoperative photography: symmetric face, no diplopia

In lack of a proper reconstruction of the zygomatic bone and the orbital frame and, therefore, due to the incorrect position of the placed titanium mesh, a severe difference in bulbar level and diplopia occurred, which could not be helped with the implanted autologous bone graft either (Fig. 63.34).

Late Reconstruction

The surgical technical advantages of a proper primary, definitive treatment, the rapid healing of patients with, many times, considerably fewer complications and dysfunctions (fibrosis etc.), and their return to their previous life as soon as possible have already been mentioned. This is

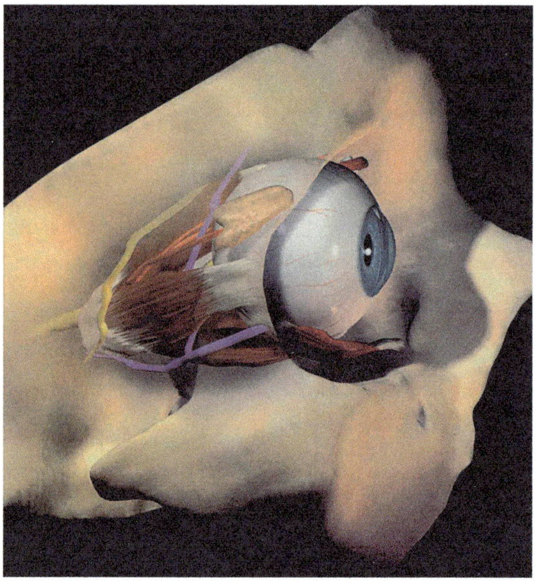

Fig. 63.21 Injuries to the lateral and upper orbital walls may result in dysfunction of the lateral and superior rectus muscles

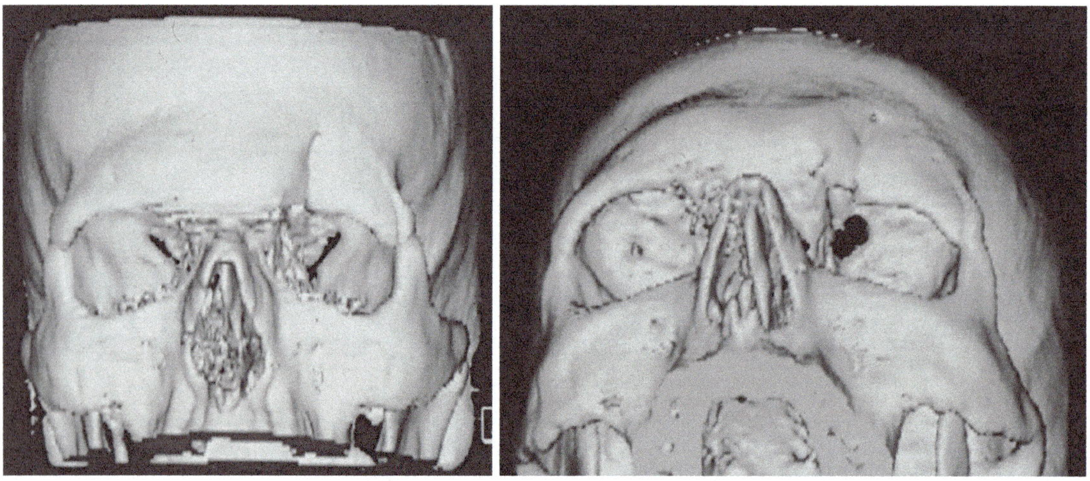

Fig. 63.22 Impression fracture of the facial wall of the frontal sinus, with caudal dislocation of the orbital roof. Restricted eye movements (superior rectus muscle?)

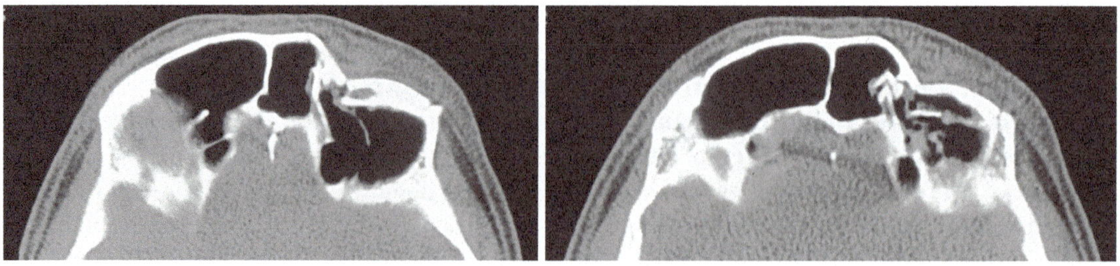

Fig. 63.23 The axial CT image taken of the patient shows the fragments of the lateral wall of the frontal sinus

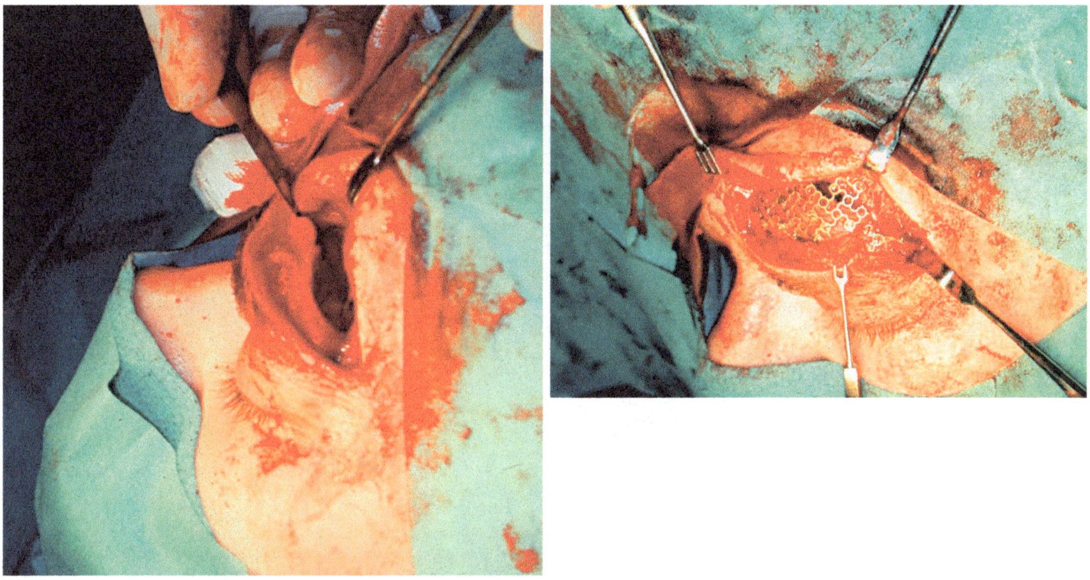

Fig. 63.24 Exposure along the eyebrow, removal of bone fragments. Frontal reconstruction with titanium mesh, repositioning and plate fixation of the orbital roof

especially true for injuries to the orbit and adjacent bones since, as already demonstrated, an inveterate fracture due to inadequate or incorrect primary treatment and the consequential function loss are significantly harder to treat later, and they may result in a permanent injury. Without a detailed description of late reconstructive procedures used earlier, we may establish that, in great majority of the cases, they did not meet or hardly met the aesthetic requirements or the need for restoration or improvement of vision. It is noted that, based on the experience, the autologous bone graft method recommended for this region, despite being a biologically beneficial technique, is objectionable from both functional and aesthetic aspects because of shapeability issues and the risk of absorption and rejection.

CAD-CAM Method

The advance of computer technology and the widespread use of CT imaging have enabled the use of the CAD-CAM (COMPUTER AIDED DESIGN–COMPUTER AIDED MANUFACTURING) method employed for numerous other purposes as well (architecture, car industry, etc.) in the planning and implementation of restorations for skull defects. It helps create implants of extremely accurate shape and size. Since 1995, we have been using a software of our own development that utilizes and filters the CT data to plan the implant first layer by layer and then on a 3D image (Fig. 63.35).

It is made of polyethylene (authorized by the Hungarian Institute of Medical and Hospital Engineering for acetabular cups, for example). Its benefits, besides being cheap, are good shapeability and mechanical protection. It resists high temperature, and its thickness can be adjusted in accordance with the needs (to avoid dead space). It is easy to make (minimal) corrections to it, if required, during surgery, e.g., thinning at the edges or wedging in according to the defect, or adjusting the fixation points as needed. It is tissue-neutral, accepted by the adjacent soft tissues, and fixed by connective tissue. It is translucent on radiograms. The surgeries were performed with case-by-case financing from 1995 to 1999, and since then, they have been financed from the annual financial budget provided by the National Health Insurance

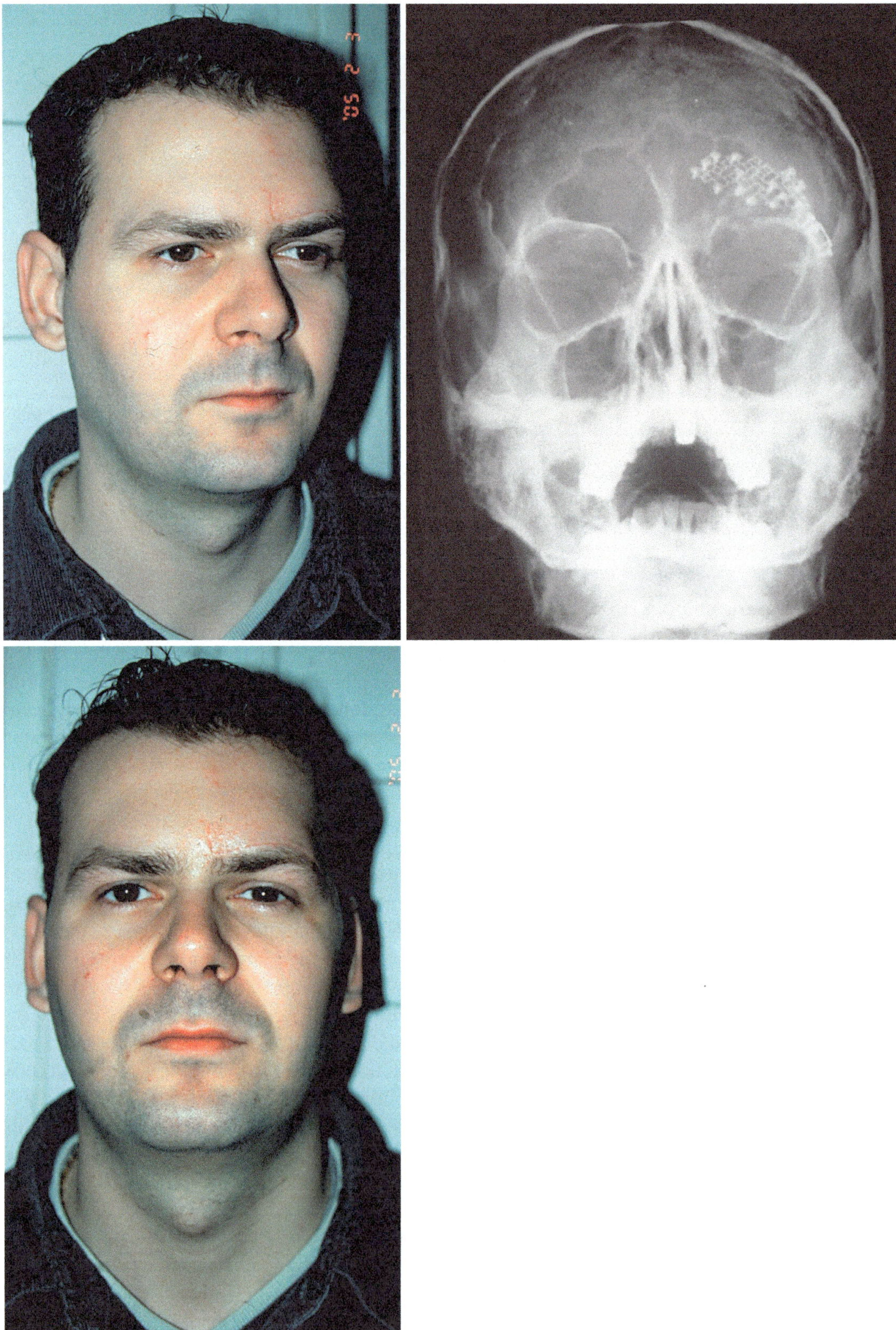

Fig. 63.25 Unrestricted eye movements, symmetric forehead

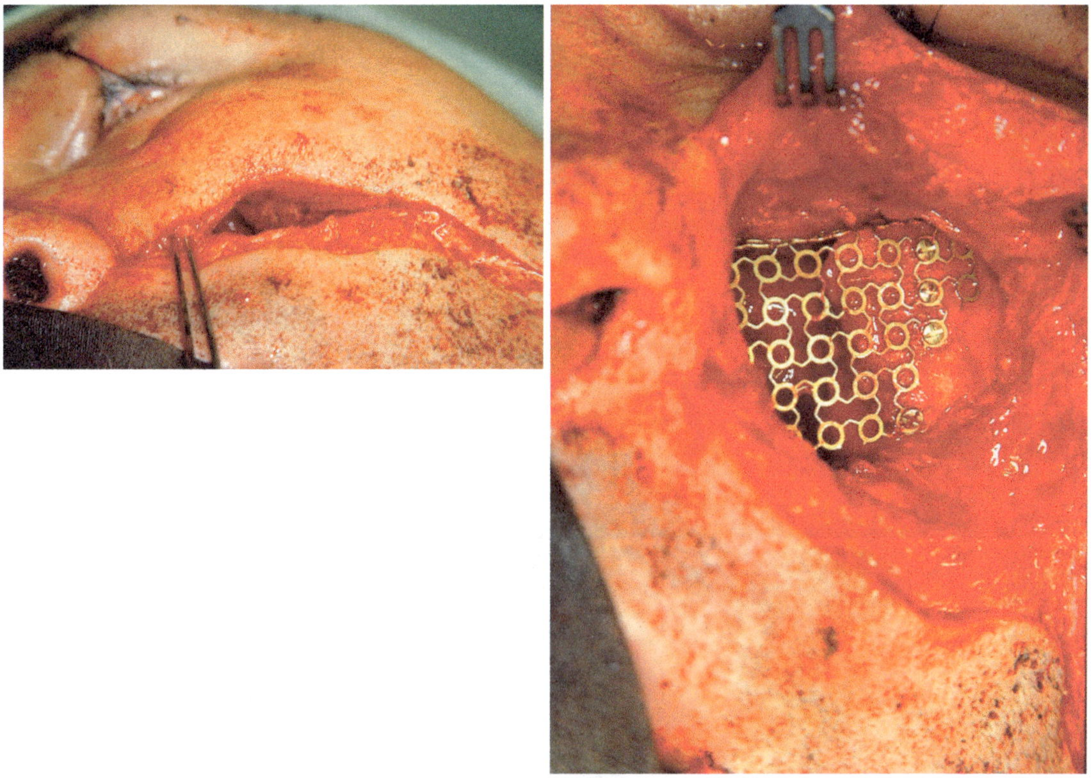

Fig. 63.26 Severe maxillary and orbital defects—the left eyeball sunk into the maxillary sinus. Reconstruction with an L-shaped titanium mesh, with exposure through the nasolabial soft tissue injury

Fund. To date, more than 100 injured patients have been treated with satisfactory functional and aesthetic results. No complications have been observed.

The possibility to achieve the required thickness can be utilized well in case of the facial bones and, especially, in the region of the orbit. This way, the eyeball can be positioned correctly, and symmetry can be achieved. A fixation that is planned based on prior bone thickness measurement is extremely important for stabilizing the restoration and for the overall appearance. The inadequacies of the primary management represent the most serious problem of late orbital reconstruction. If there is a residual bone defect of any degree and a proper (under the circumstances) eyeball reposition is not performed, a later repositioning may be almost prevented by the late fibrosis of the muscles and soft tissues (Fig. 63.36).

The defect hidden for decades behind a mop of hair was not accompanied (not) by visual disorders but lifestyle and personality problems in this case (Figs. 63.37 and 63.38).

The aesthetic incision line, the careful selection of fixation points and the design of the implant edges resulted in a hidden incision and an impalpable implant (Fig. 63.39).

The nasal root and left orbital defect in the region of the frontal bone affects both walls of the frontal sinus. Because of the soft-tissue fibrosis, a high level of patience is required during the exposure to maintain the integrity of the dura. The adequate thickness of the implant ensures the restoration of the symmetry of the forehead and the brow ridge. The almost completely missing superior orbital margin was shaped based on the intact contralateral orbit (Figs. 63.40, 63.41, 63.42, 63.43, 63.44, 63.45, and 63.46).

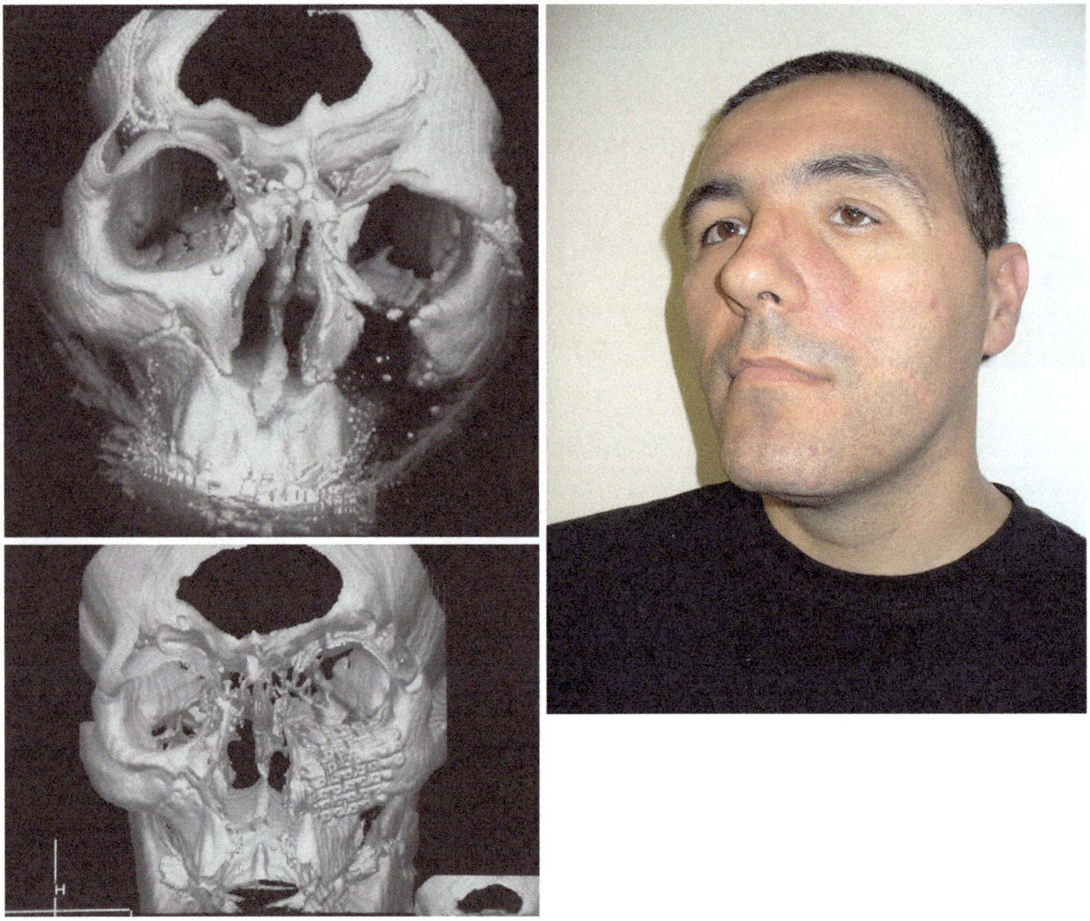

Fig. 63.27 Unrestricted eye movements, no diplopia

Combined Management

The dislocated, fragmented fracture of the left orbital frame and the zygomatic bone due to a high-impact injury was reconstructed with **immediate** surgery. The defect in the temporal region was restored later, with intact visual functions.

In lack of a primary management for the orbital and zygomatic bone body fracture, the aesthetic result of the proper forehead and orbital roof reconstruction performed in a patient who presented 6 months after the injury is only a half success because of the permanent vision disorder due to the considerable difference in the level of the eyeballs. The patient **chose** to live with diplopia!? (Fig. 63.47, 63.48, 63.49, 63.50, 63.51, 63.52, 63.53, and 63.54).

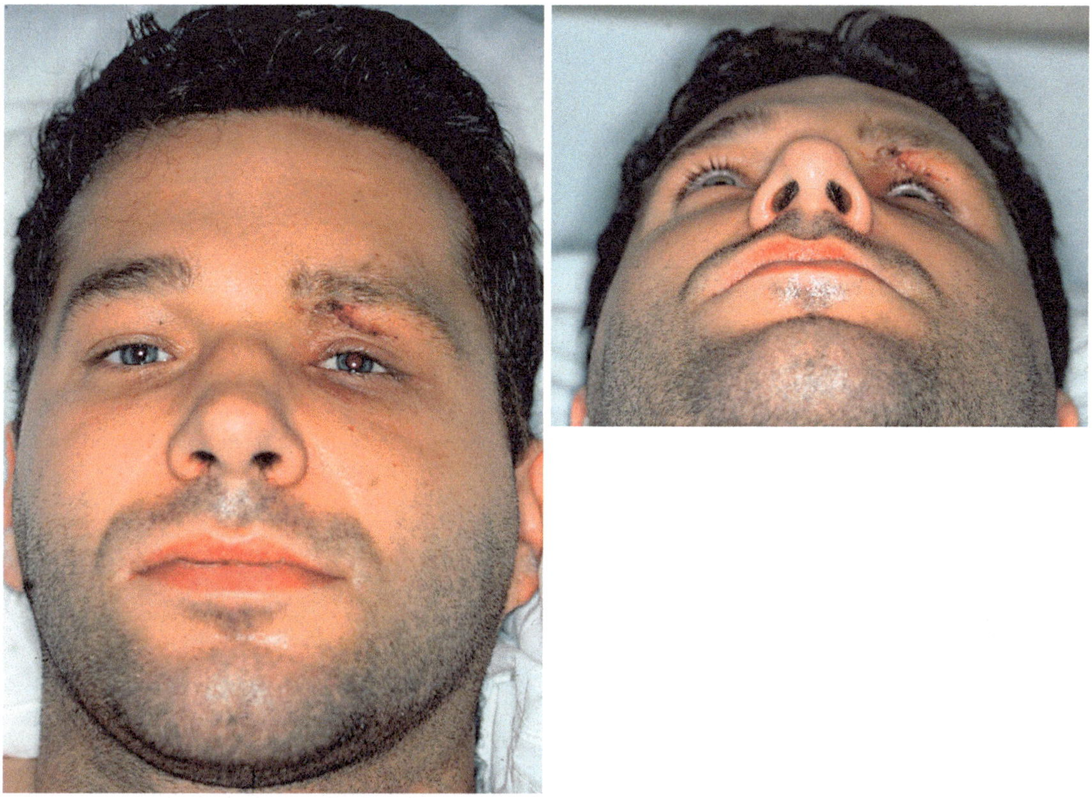

Fig. 63.28 The patient treated with three eyelid sutures at another institution presented with double vision

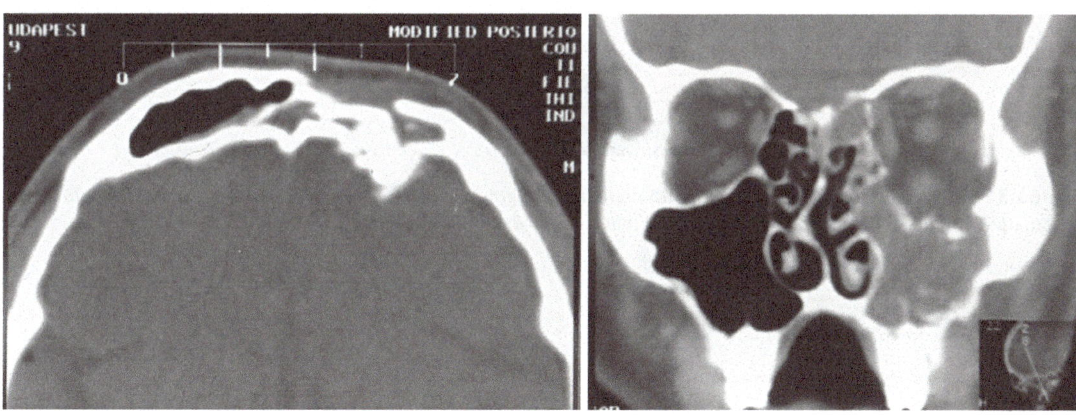

Fig. 63.29 Axial CT image: fragmented fracture of both walls of the left frontal sinus Coronal CT image: dislocated fracture of the inferior orbital wall and the zygomatic bone

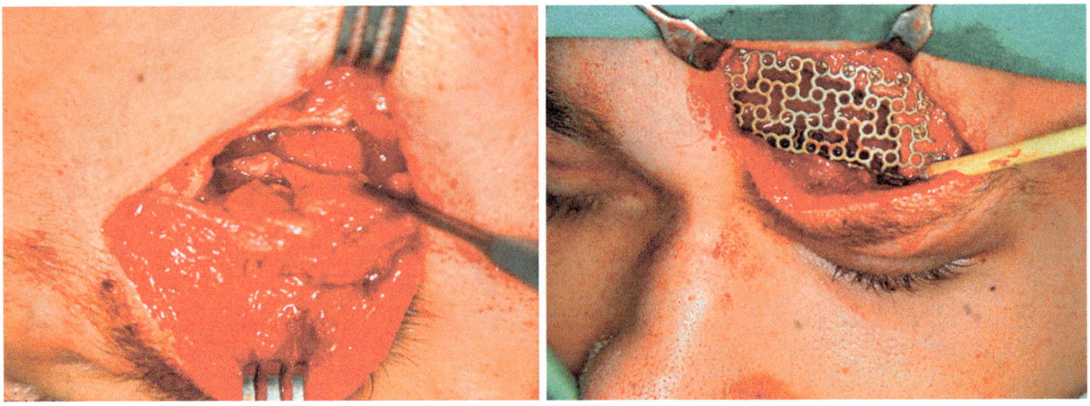

Fig. 63.30 The cranial wall fragments of the frontal sinus did not injure the dura; the forehead and the orbital roof defect were reconstructed with a titanium mesh after removal of the bone fragments

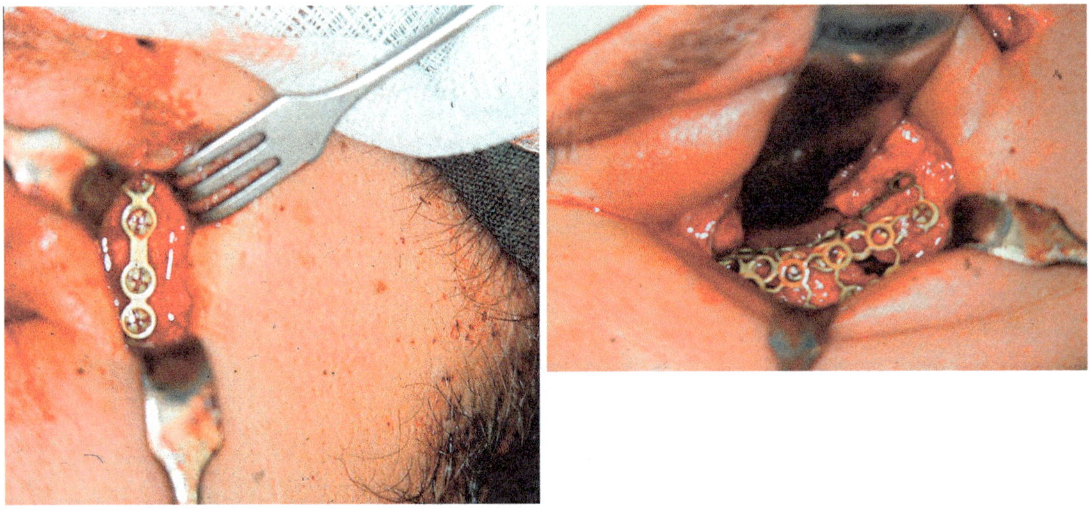

Fig. 63.31 After the closed reposition of the dislocated zygomatic bone, plate fixation was performed along the zygomatico-frontal suture and on the infraorbital margin, and the orbital floor defect was covered with a titanium mesh.

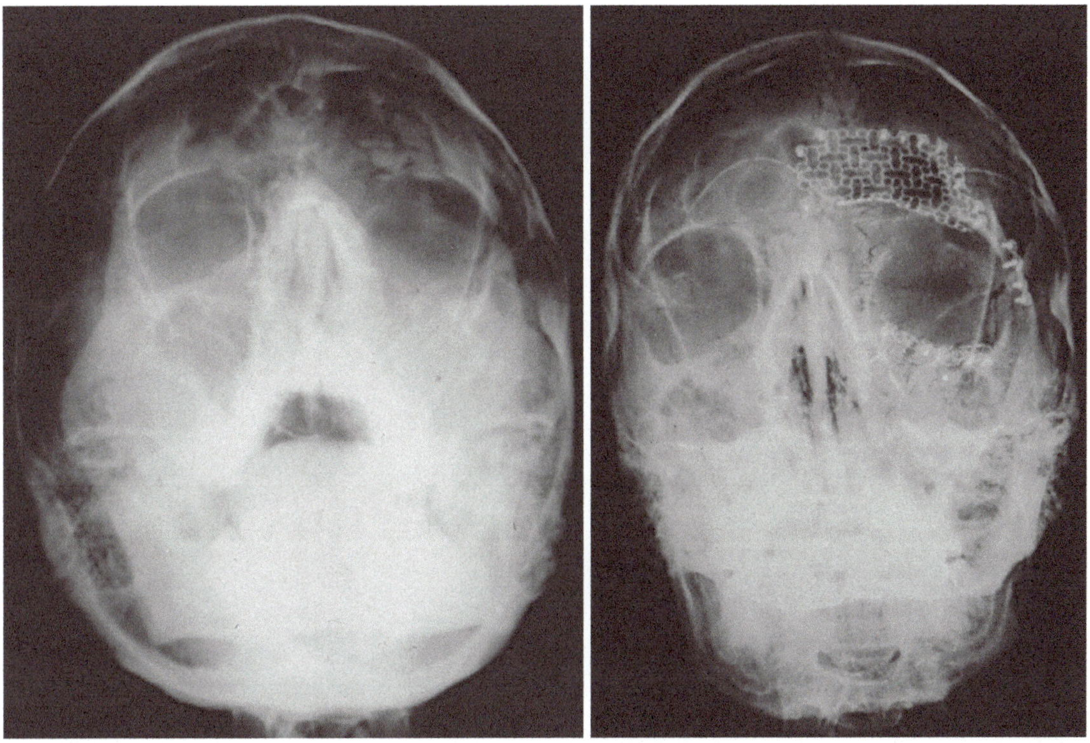

Fig. 63.32 Pre- and postoperative radiograms

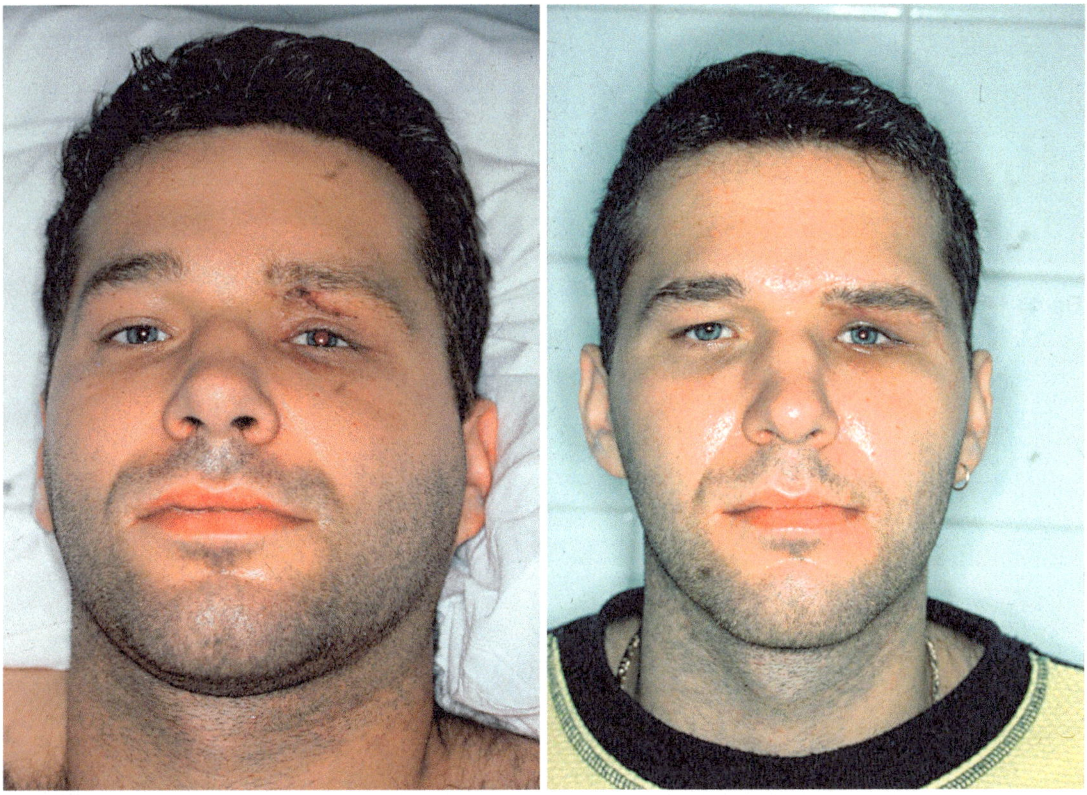

Fig. 63.33 Pre- and postoperative photographs: the diplopia is gone, the eye movements are unrestricted, the face is symmetric

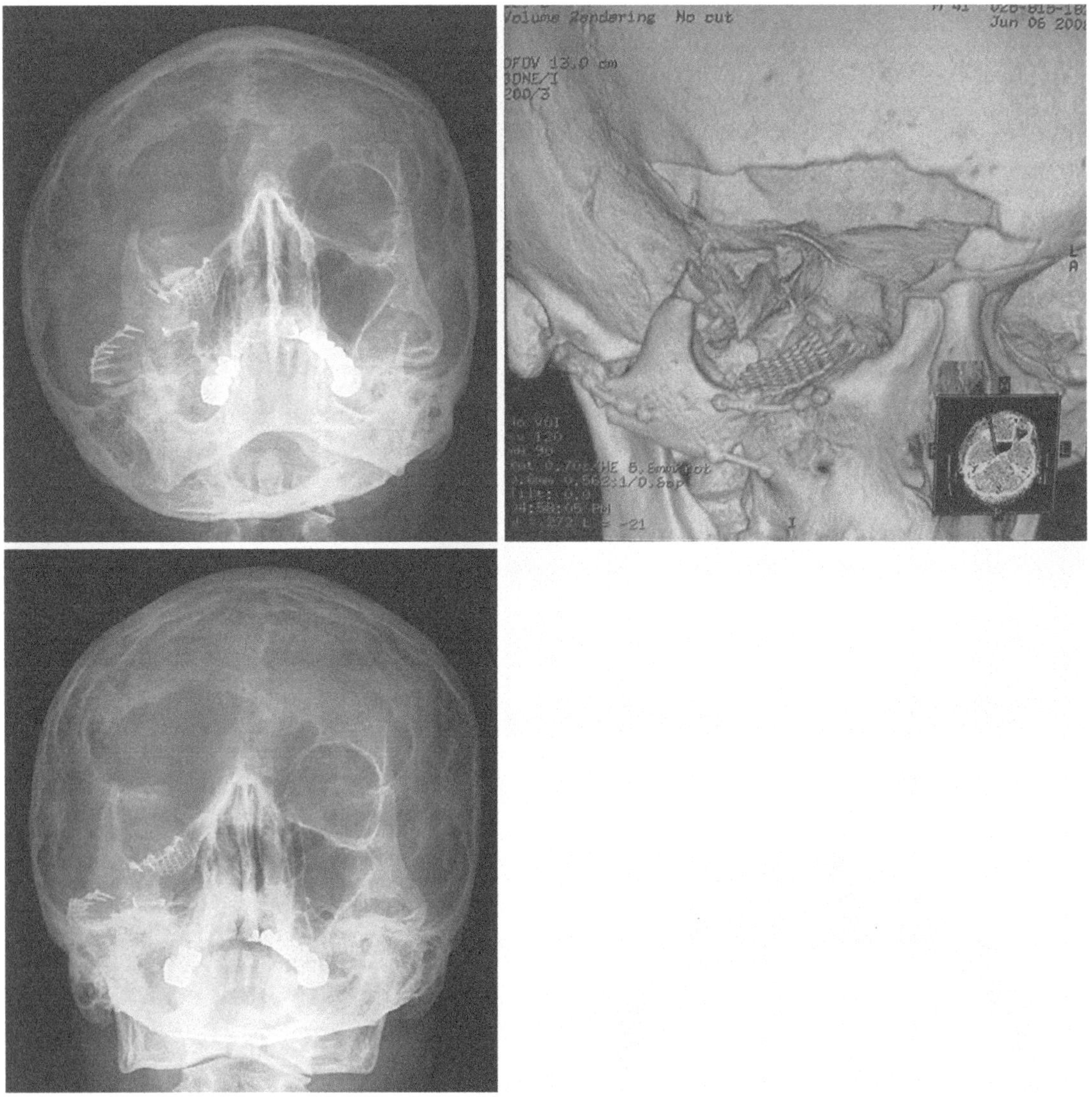

Fig. 63.34 Patient referred for consultation

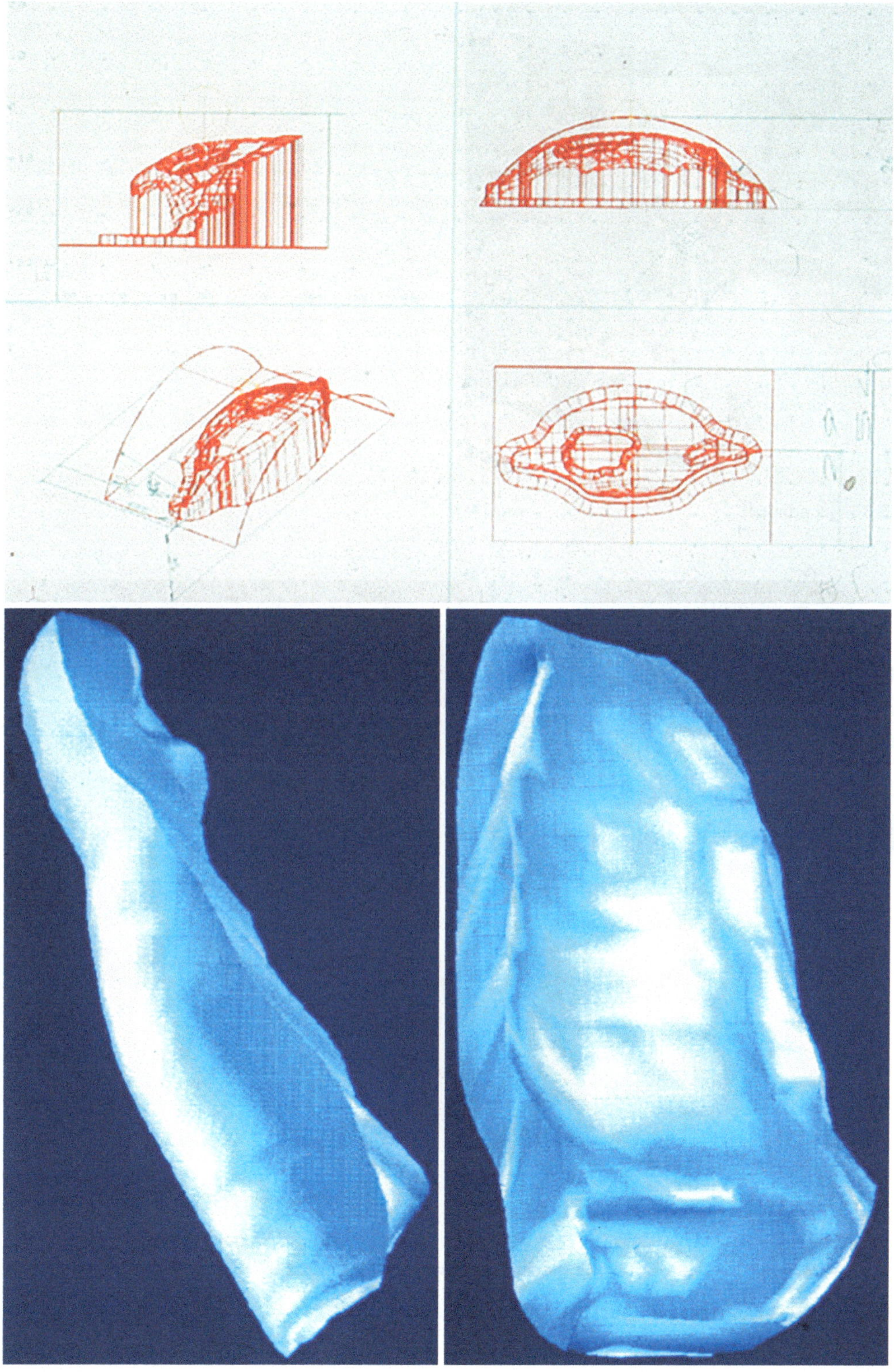

Fig. 63.35 The final restoration is created with a special precision program–milling machine based on a milling plan

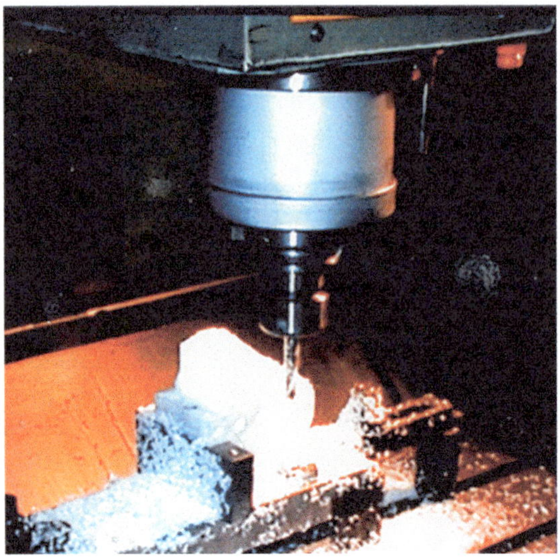

Fig. 63.35 (continued)

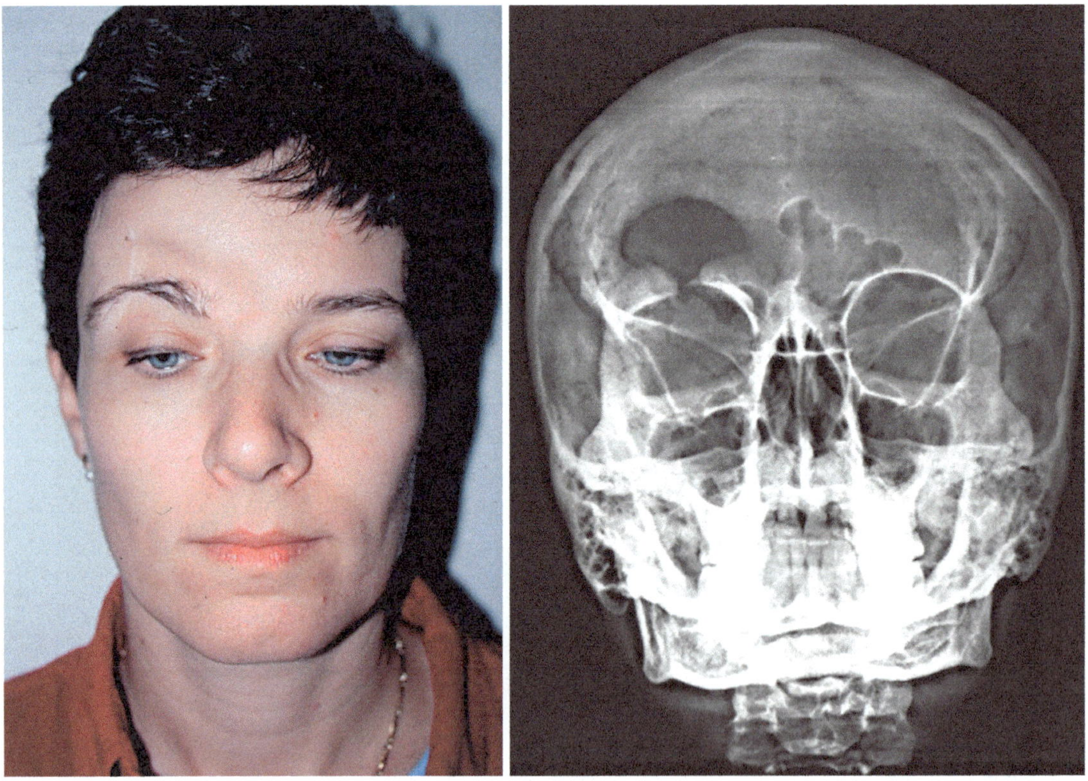

Fig. 63.36 Frontal, nasal root and right brow ridge bone defect

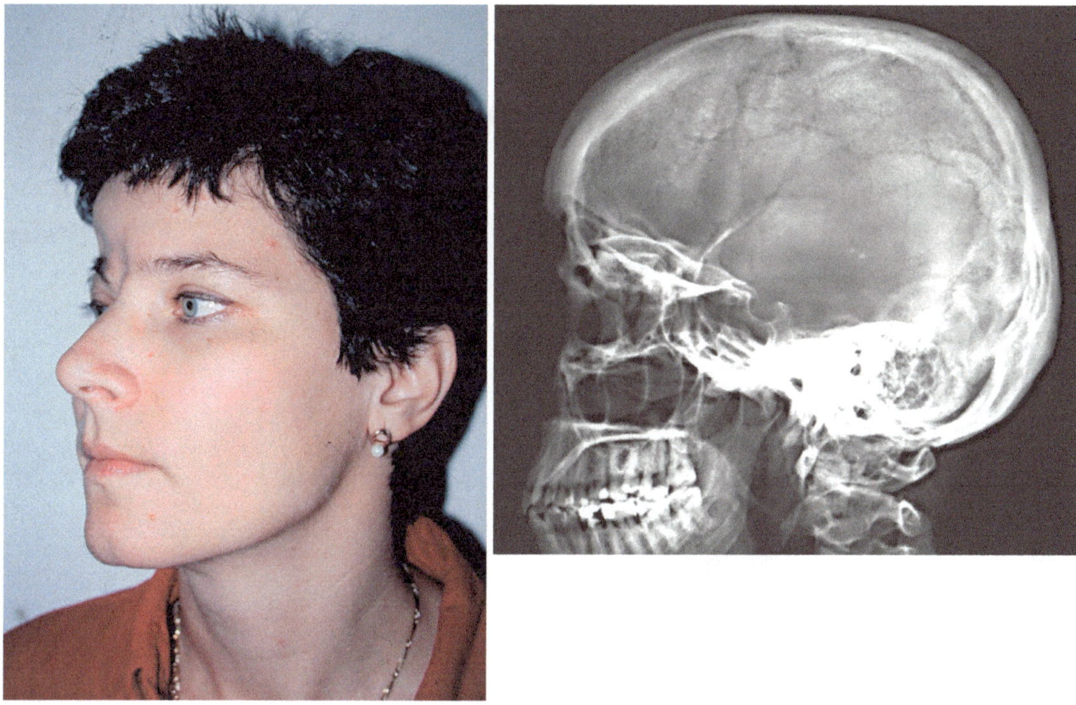

Fig. 63.36 (continued)

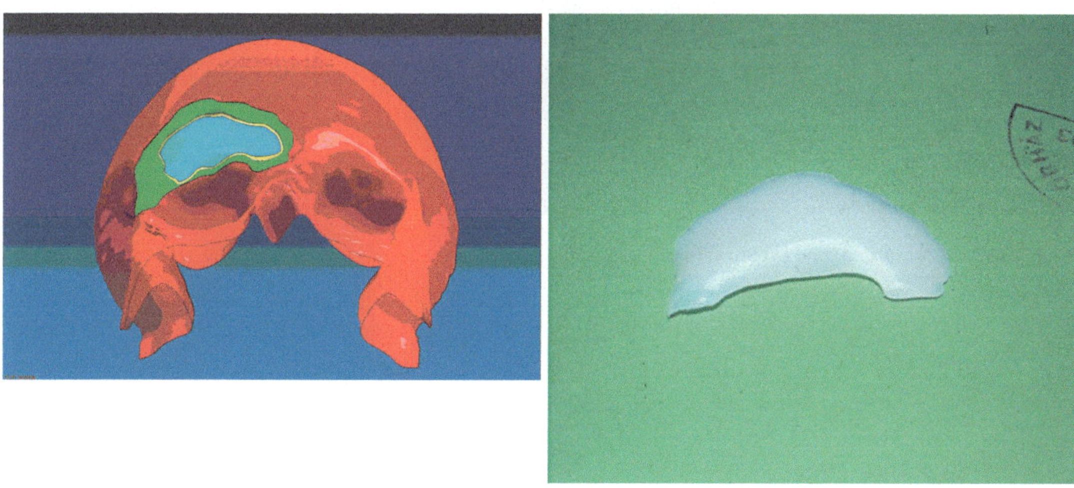

Fig. 63.37 Surgical plan and created (finished) implant

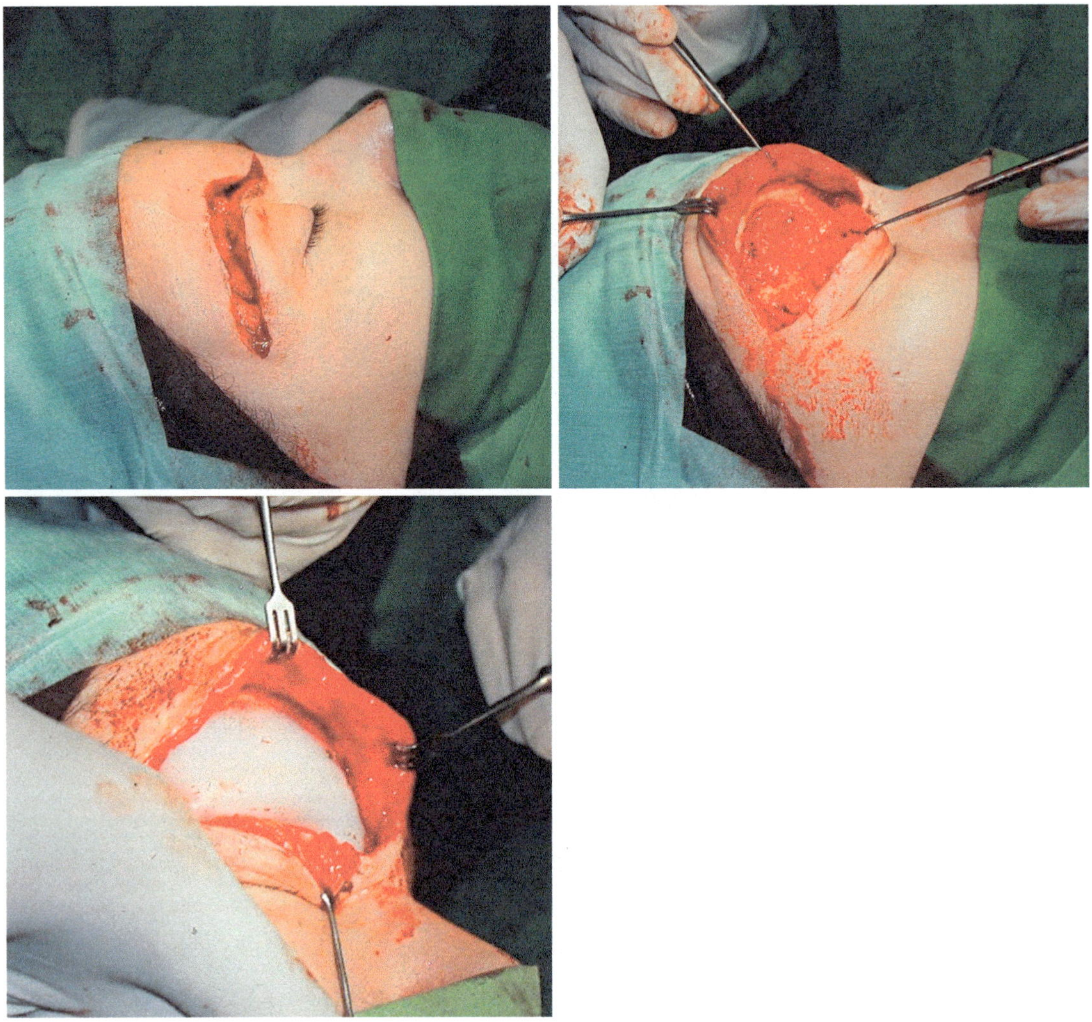

Fig. 63.38 Exposure along the eyebrow, placement of the restoration

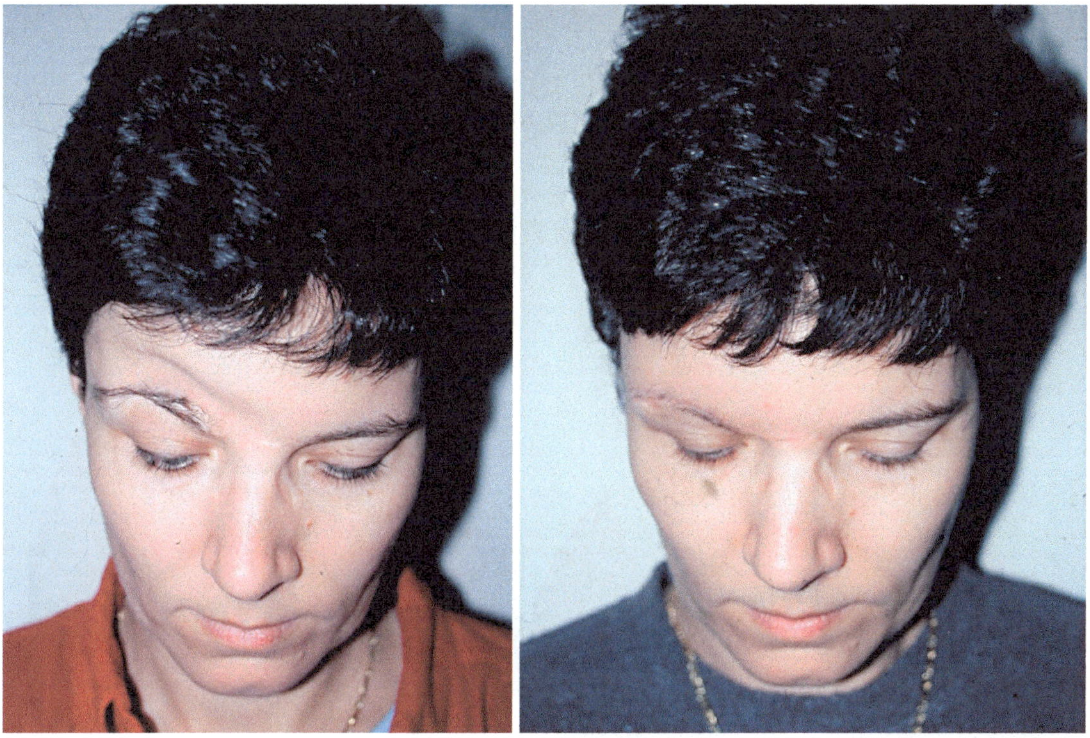

Fig. 63.39 The harmony of the face is restored

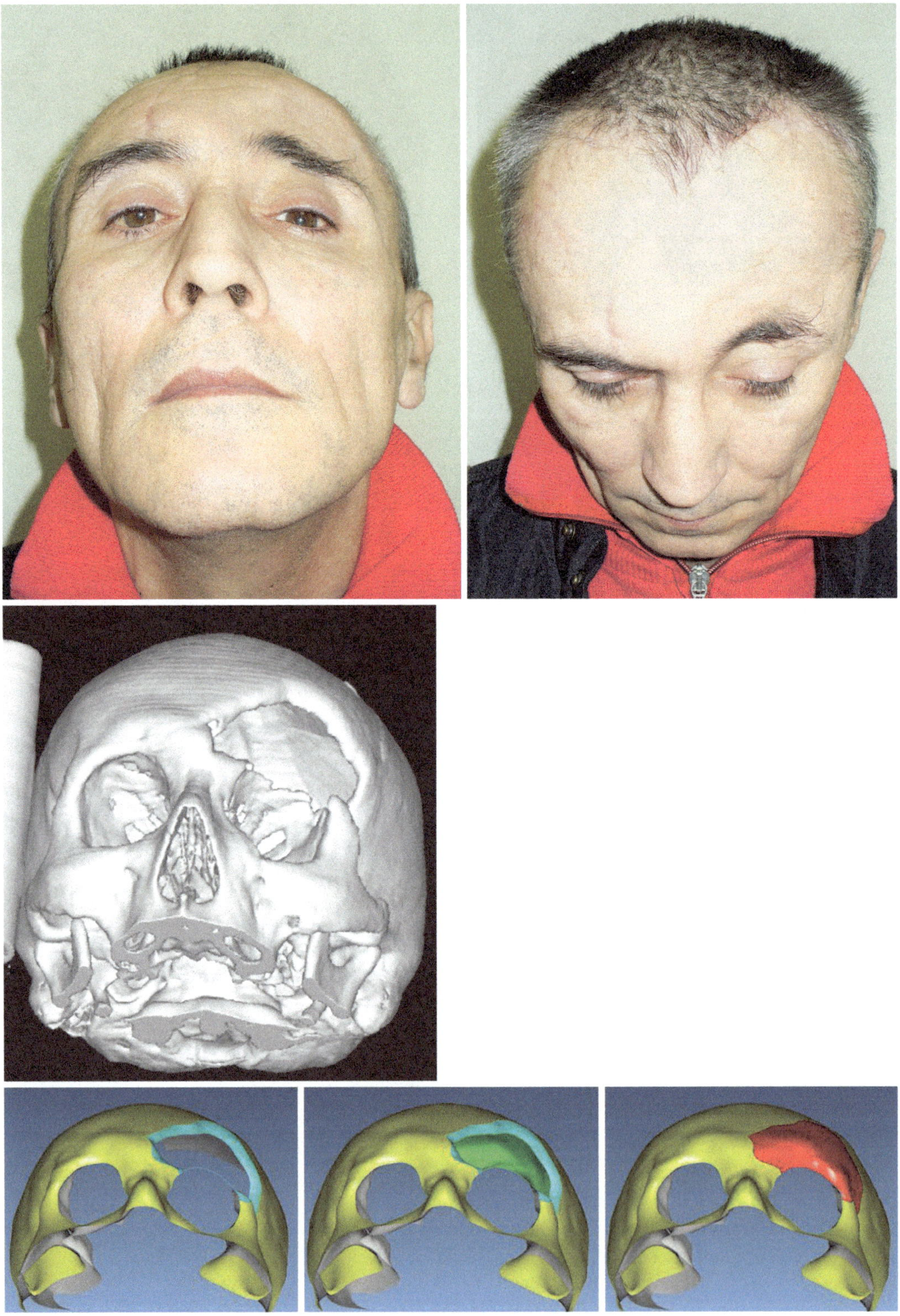

Fig. 63.40

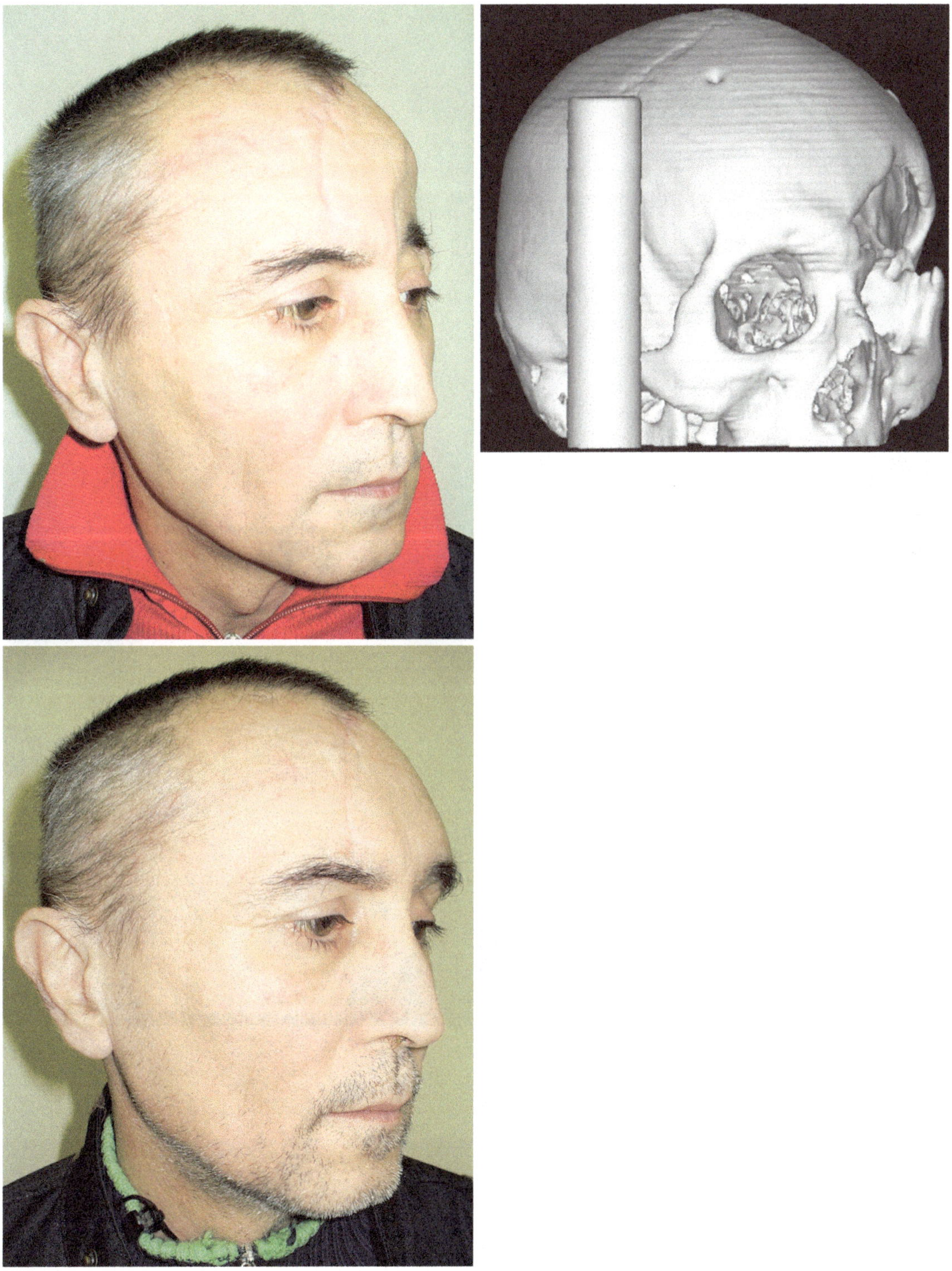

Fig. 63.40 (continued)

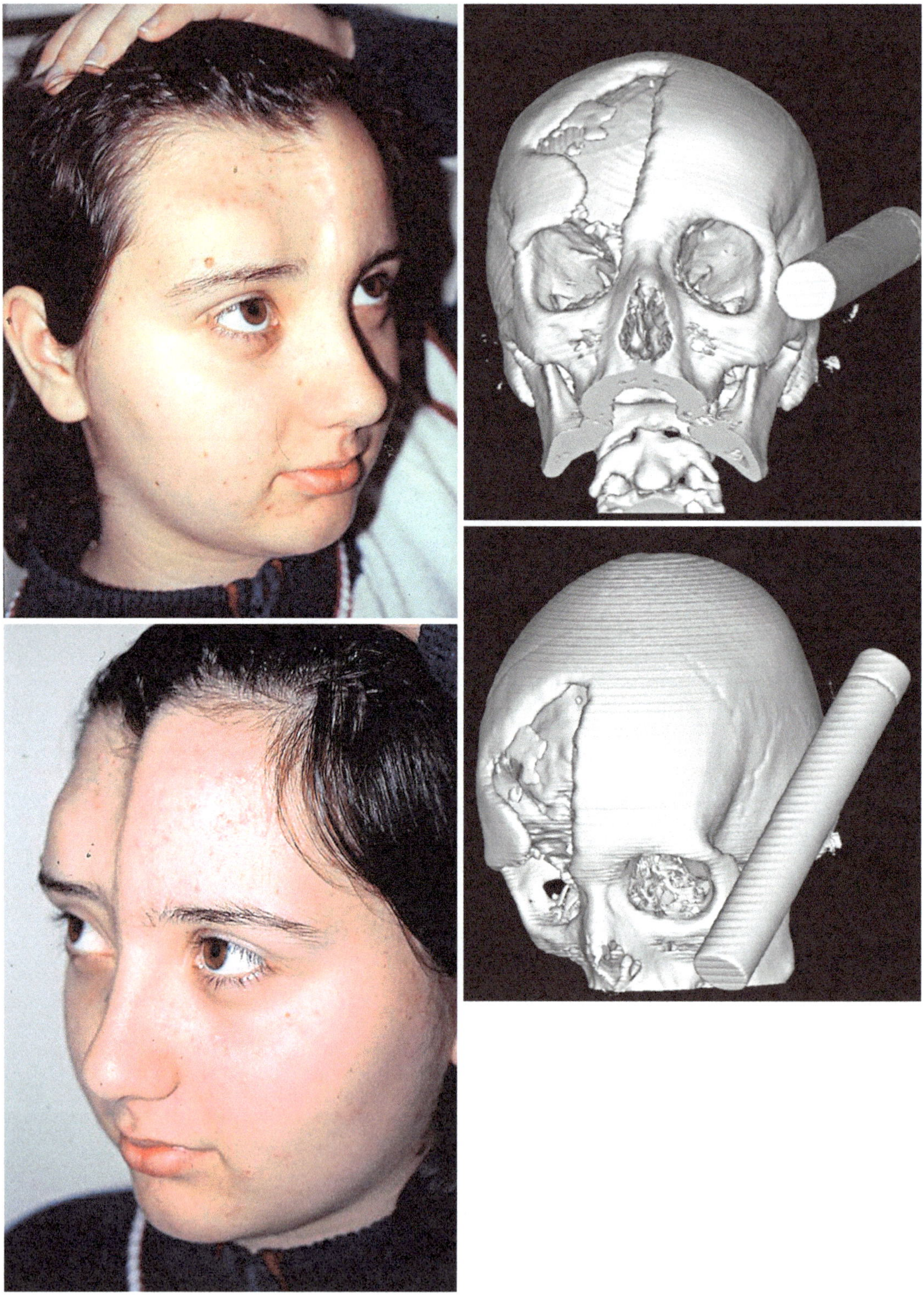

Fig. 63.41 Unilateral forehead and orbital roof defect

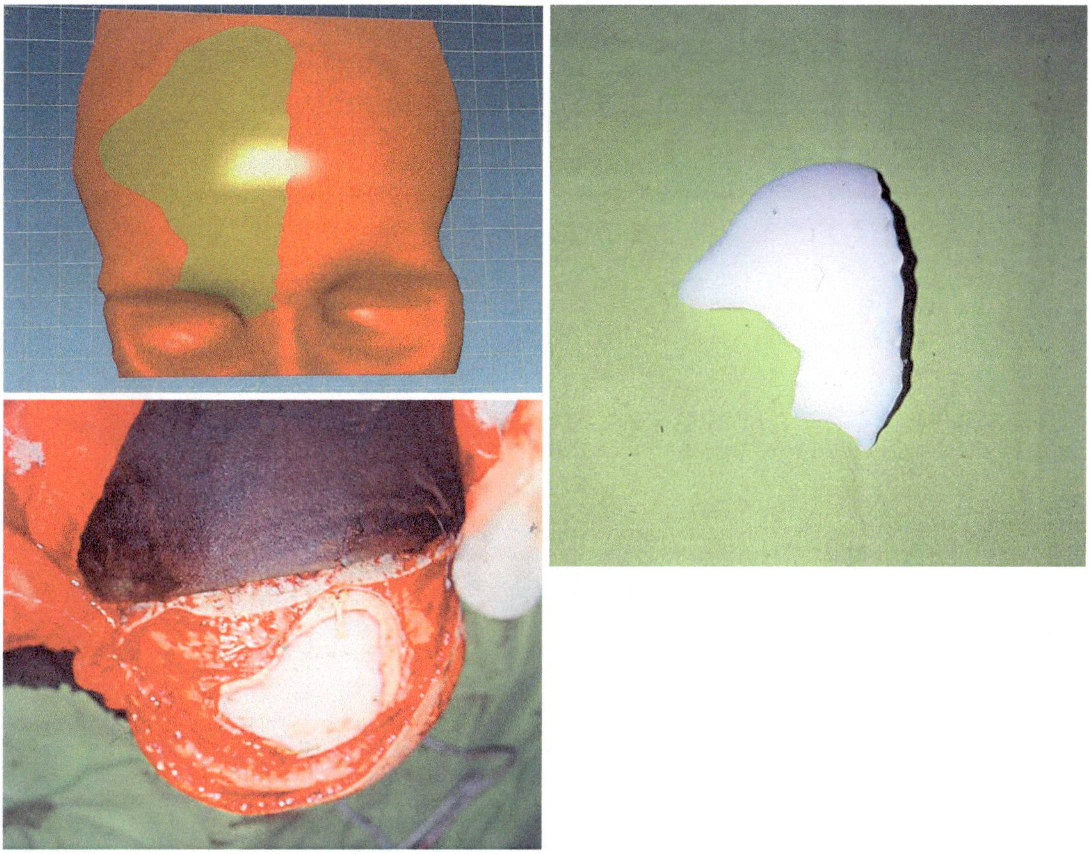

Fig. 63.42 Surgical planning, the (finished) created implant and its fixation in the bone defect

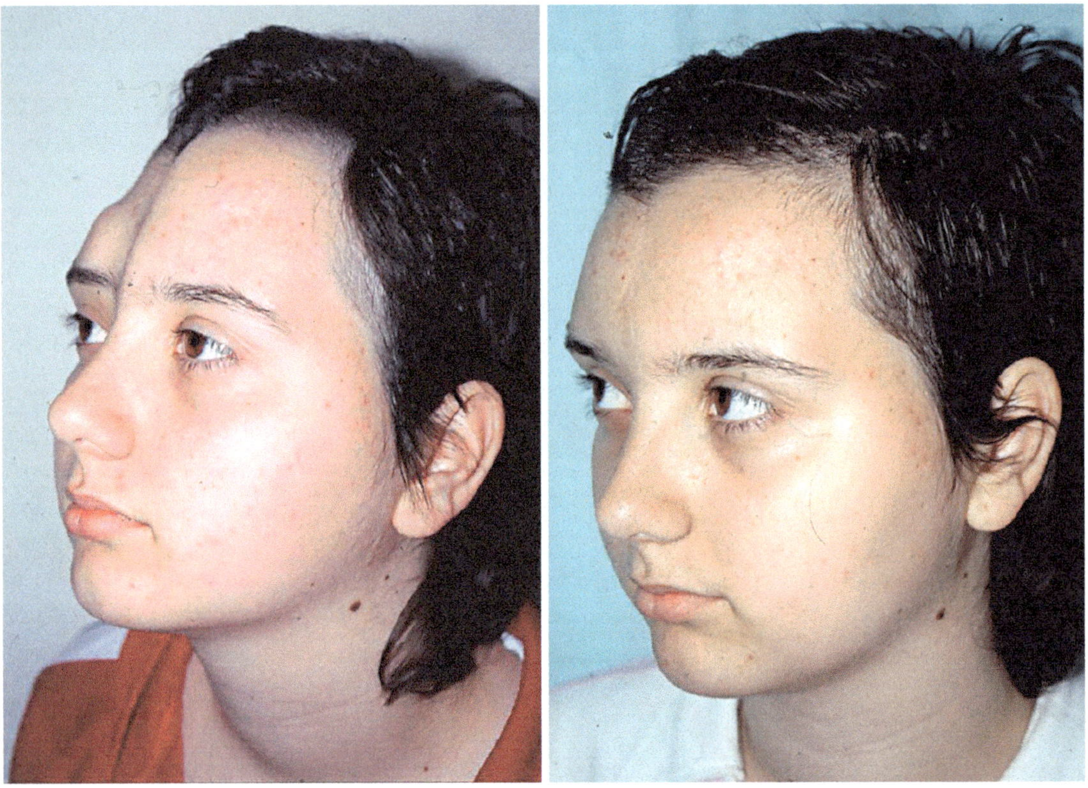

Fig. 63.43 Pre- and postoperative image of the curvature of the forehead

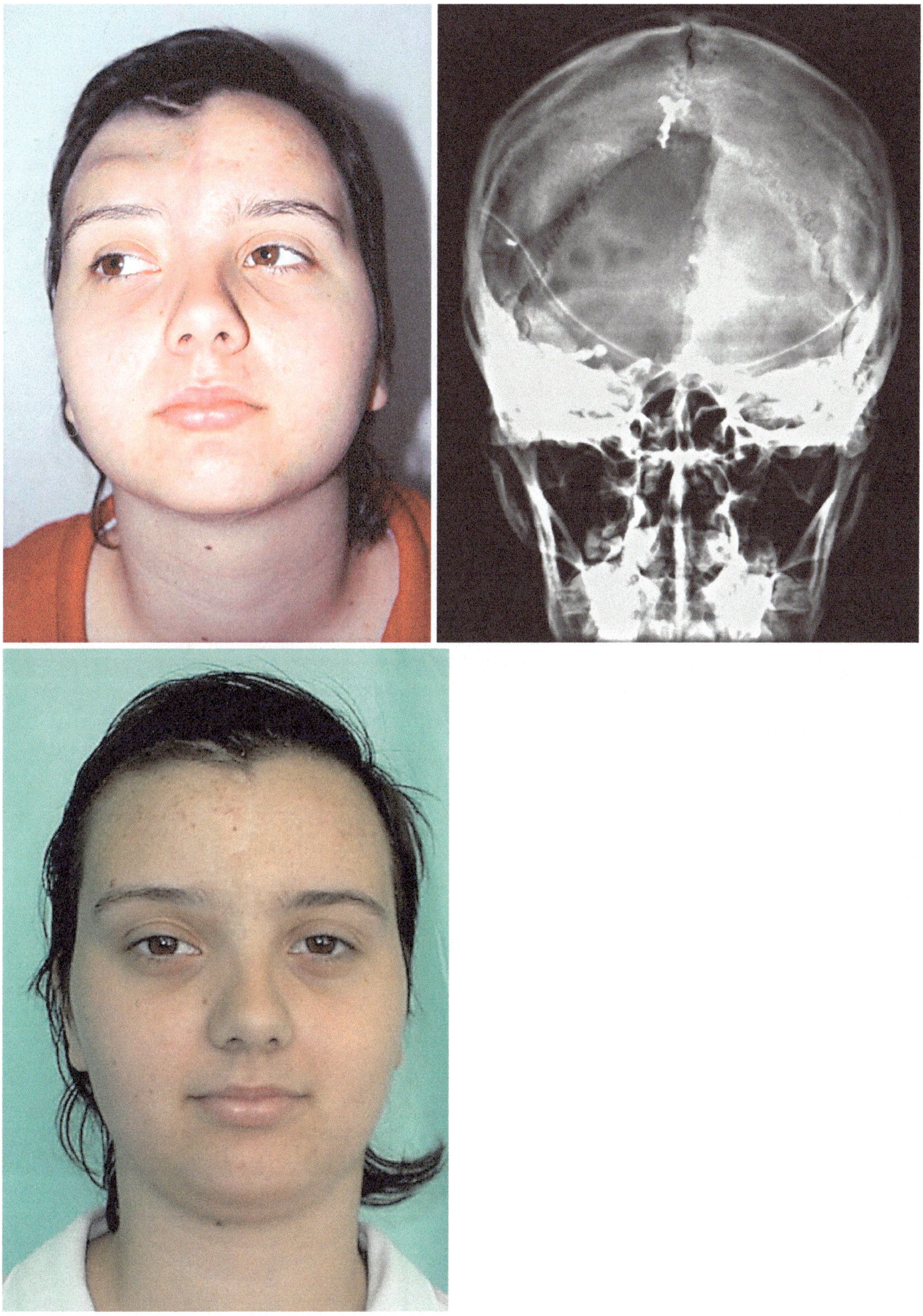

Fig. 63.44 The restored facial symmetry

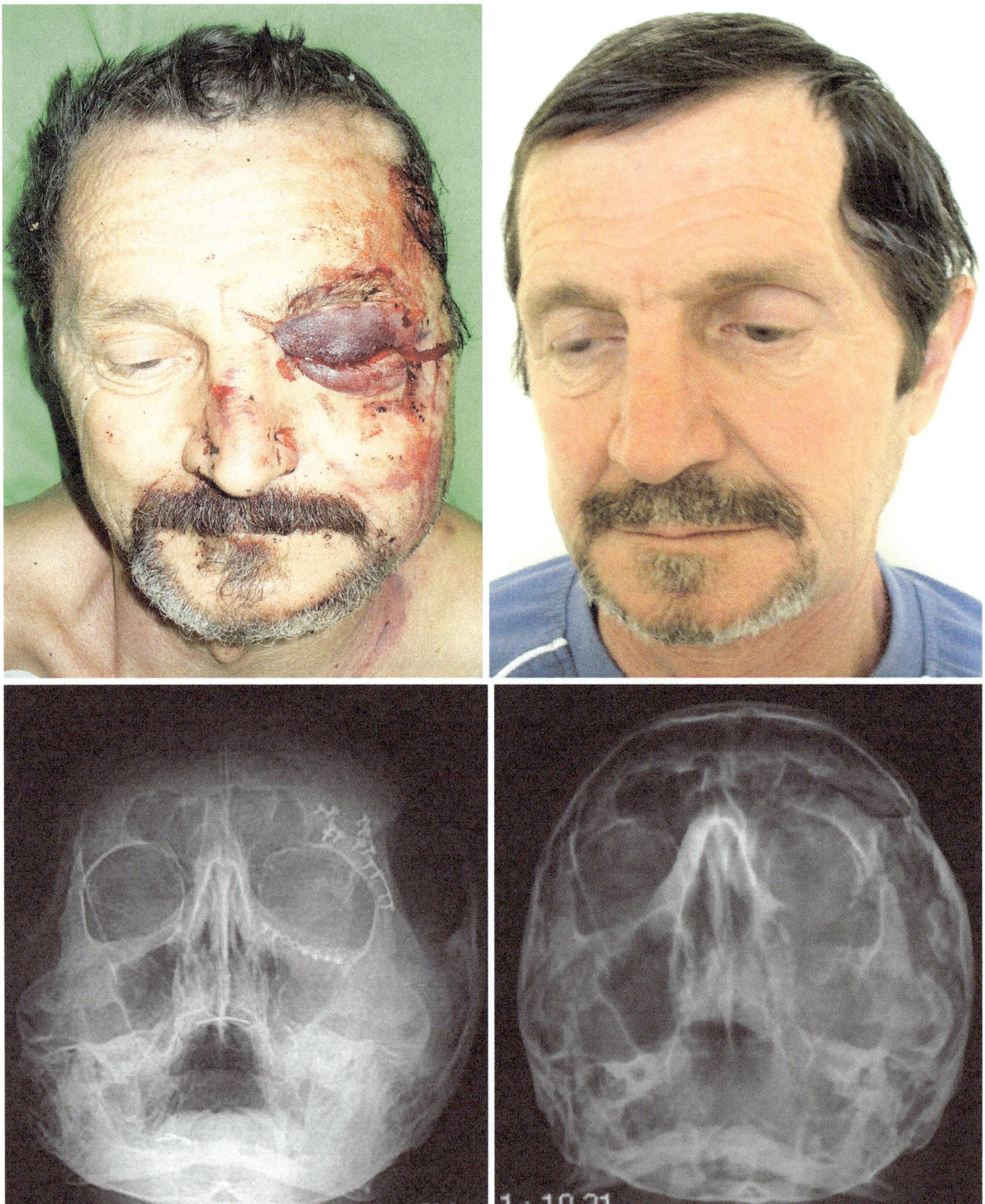

Fig. 63.45 Primary zygomatic bone and orbital reconstruction

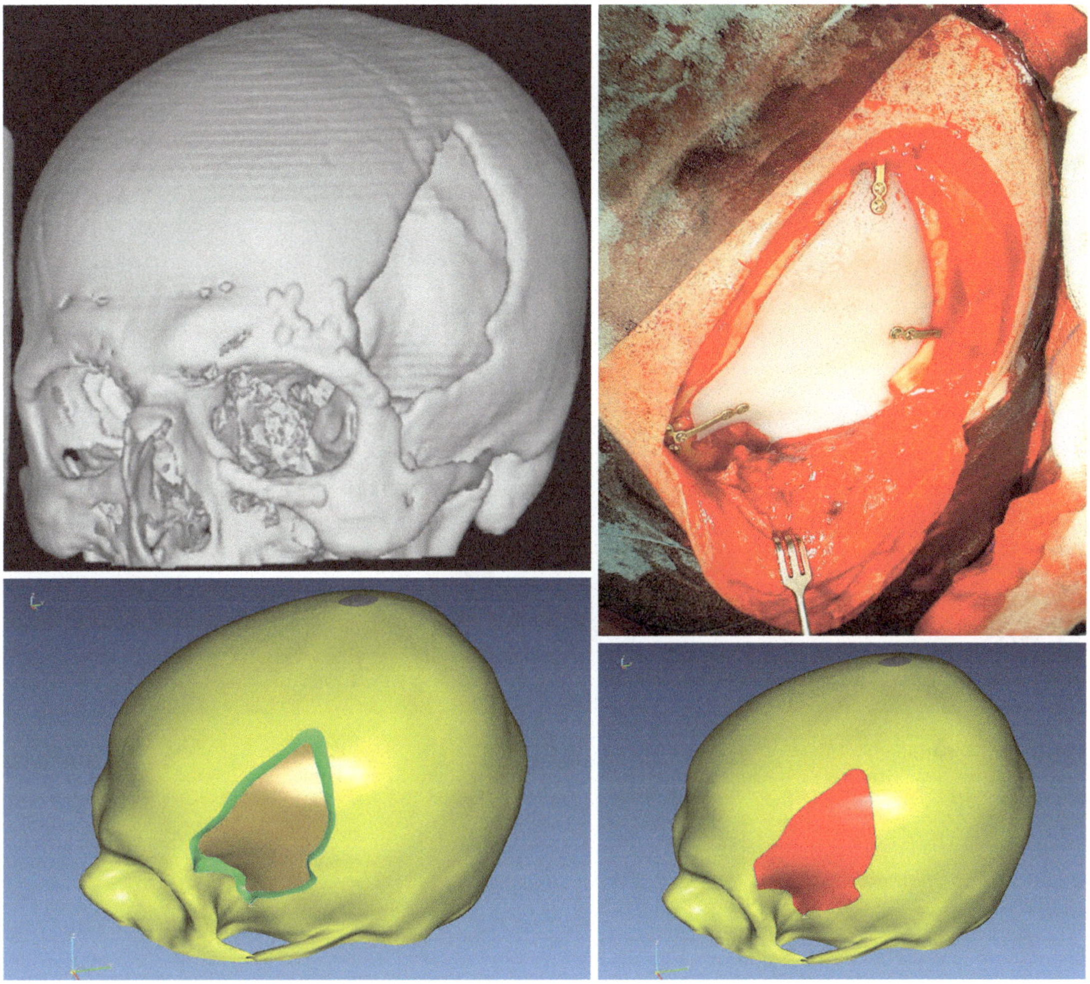

Fig. 63.46 After the simultaneous evacuation of a subdural hematoma, the residual left fronto-temporo-parietal bone defect was reconstructed with the CAD-CAM method

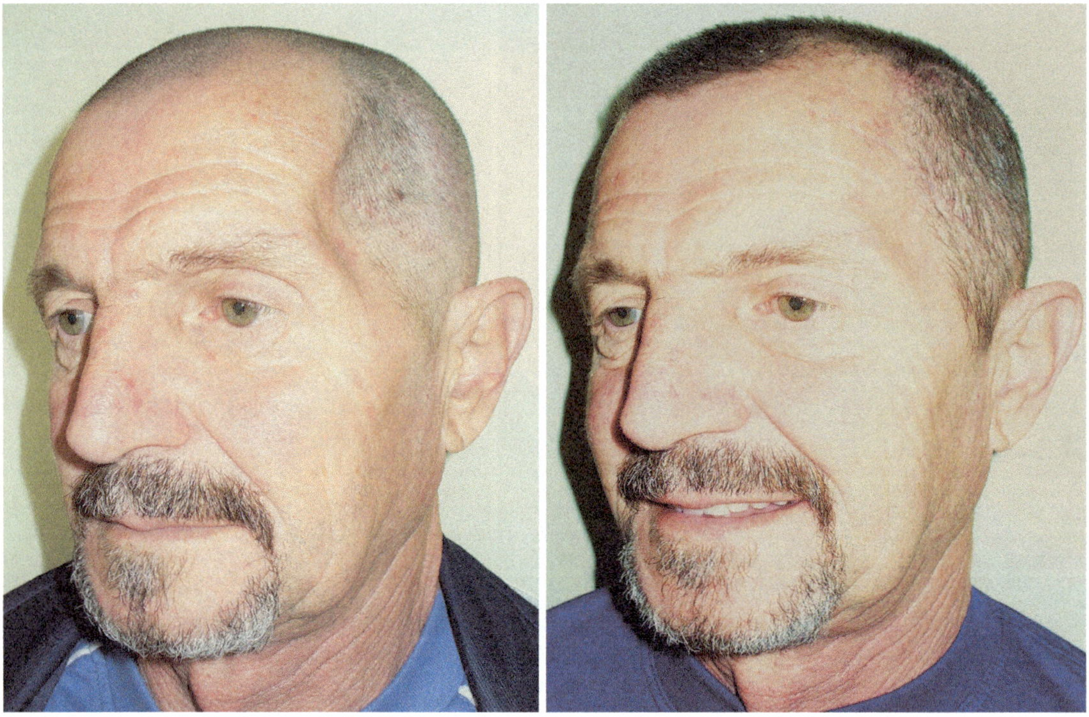

Fig. 63.46 (continued)

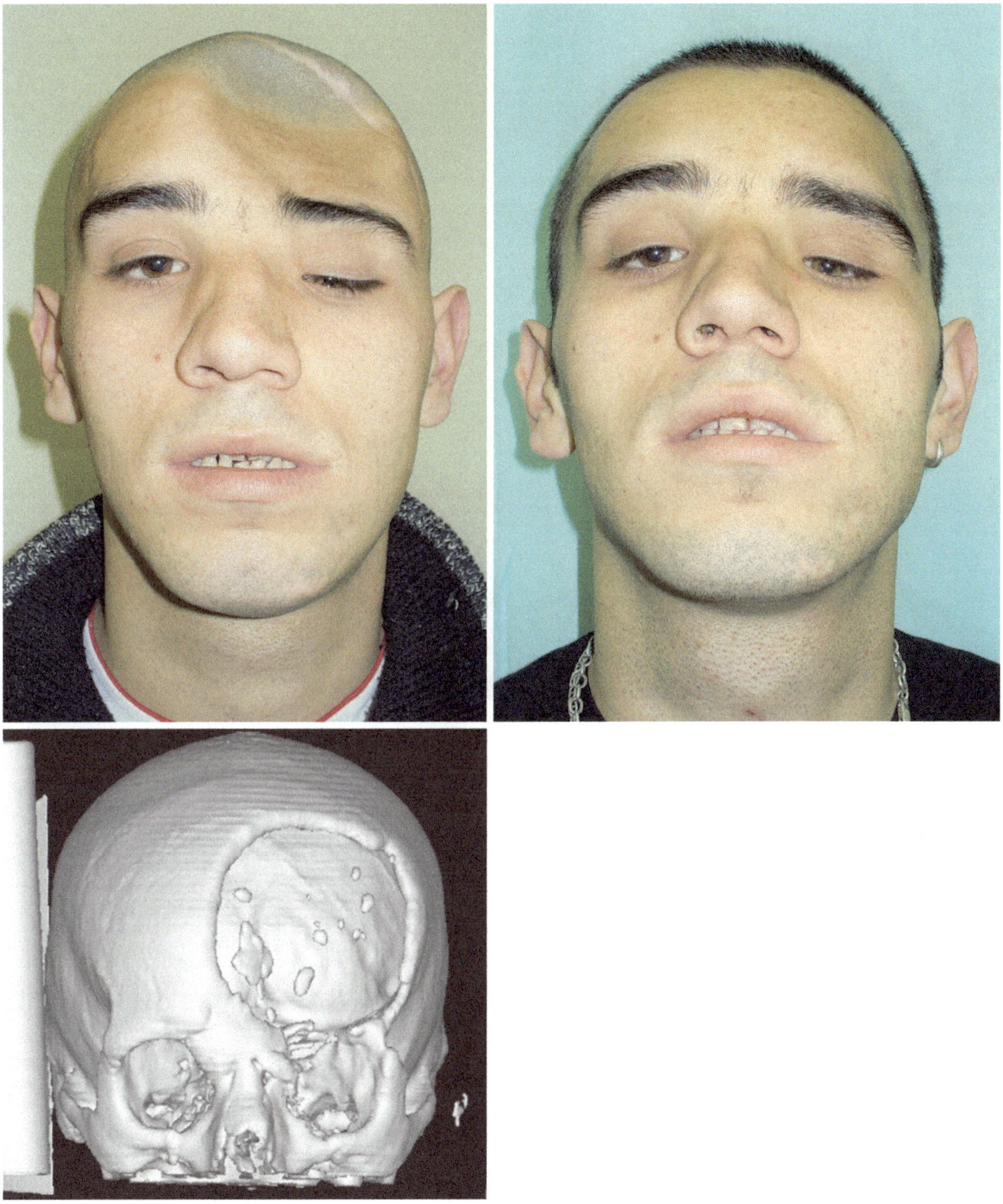

Fig. 63.47 Orbital and zygomatic bone body injury with a significant frontal bone defect. The bones forming the floor of the orbit were not repositioned (compare with the previous patient)!

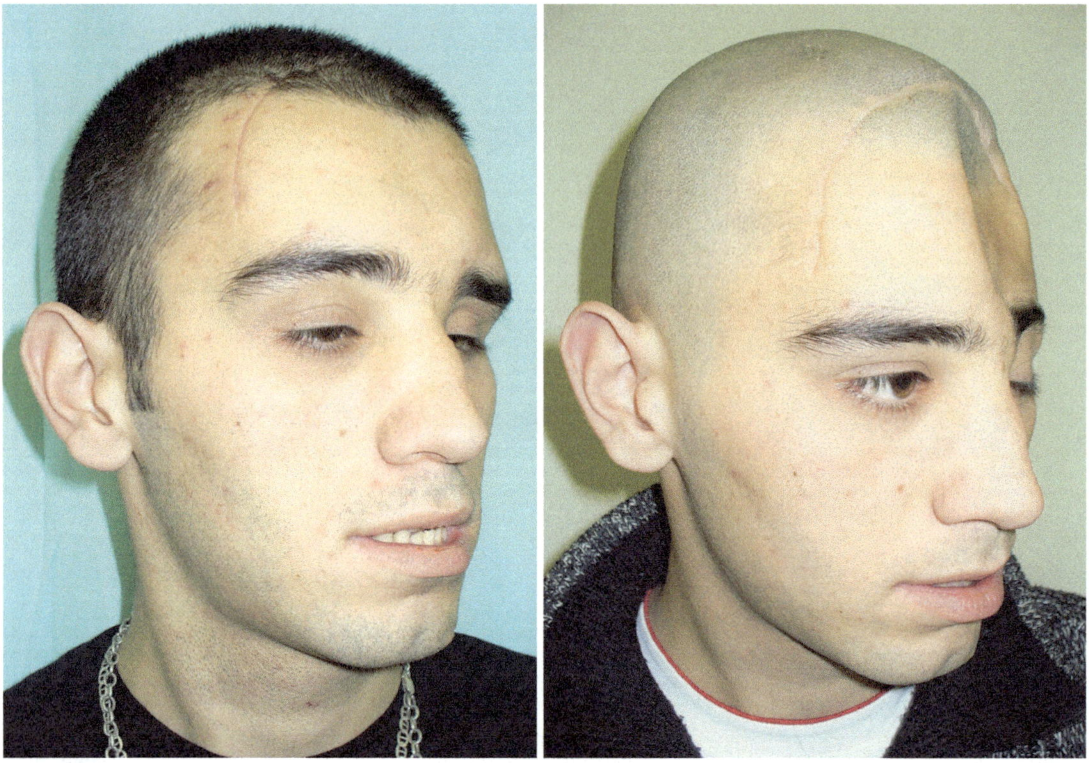

Fig. 63.48 After the CAD-CAM reconstruction of the frontal bone defect, the patient refused the late reconstruction of the orbital floor (which is much more difficult than the immediate restoration)

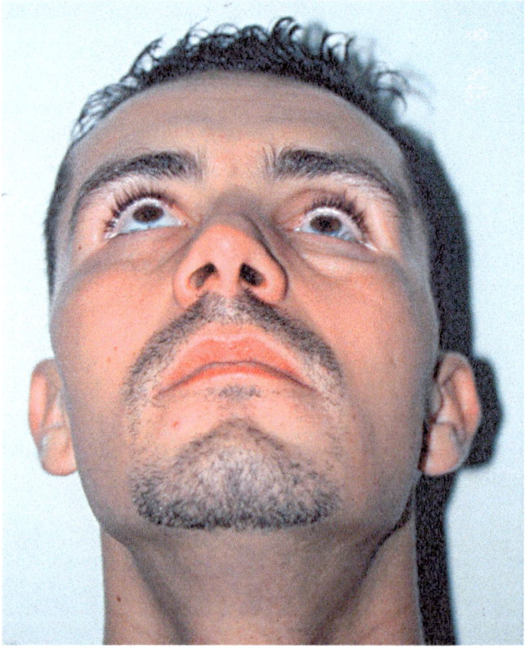

Fig. 63.49 Unsatisfactory surgical reconstruction of the left zygomatic bone and inferior orbital margin

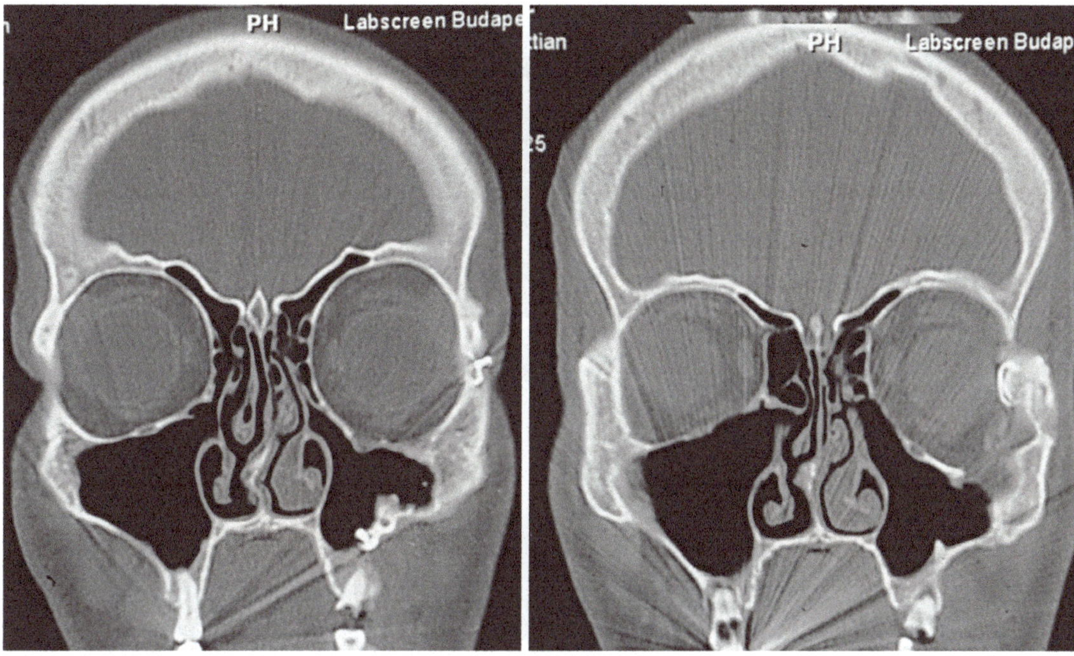

Fig. 63.50 Coronal CT: severe orbital floor defect and zygomatic bone dislocation

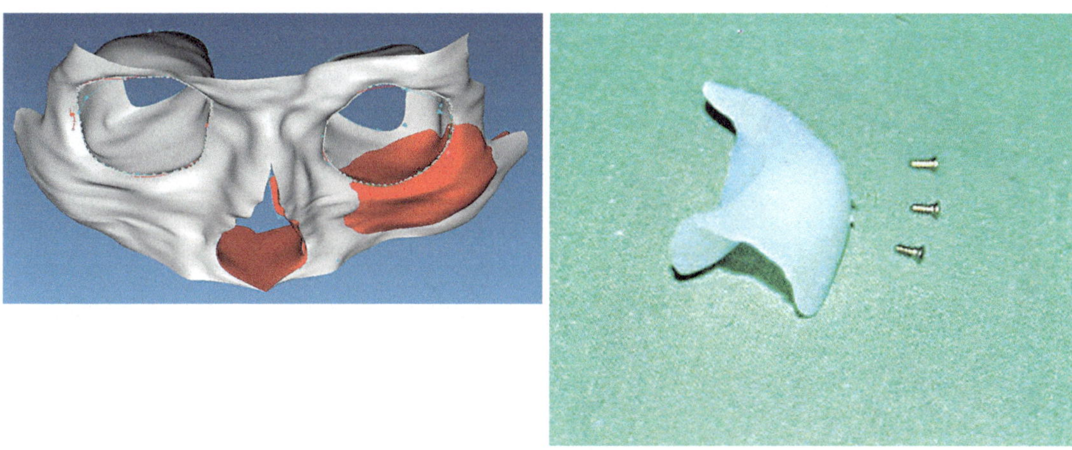

Fig. 63.51 Plan and implant for eyeball repositioning, to lift the left side of the face and restore the orbital floor defect

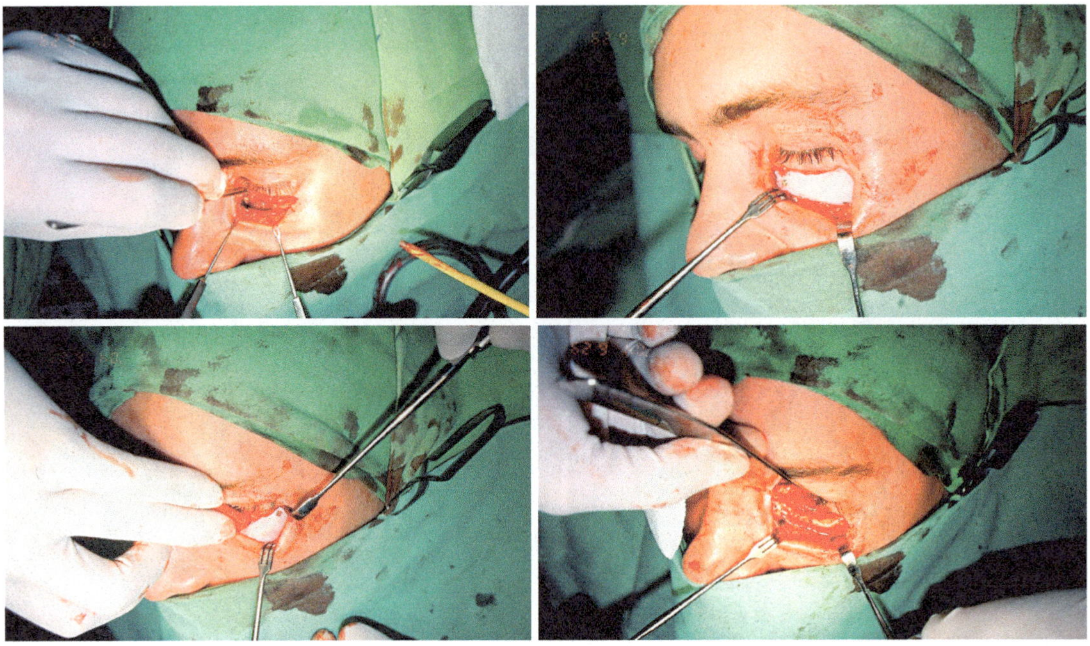

Fig. 63.52 Removal of the orbital plate and screws that fix the dislocated position are visible behind the soft tissues. Placement of the implant

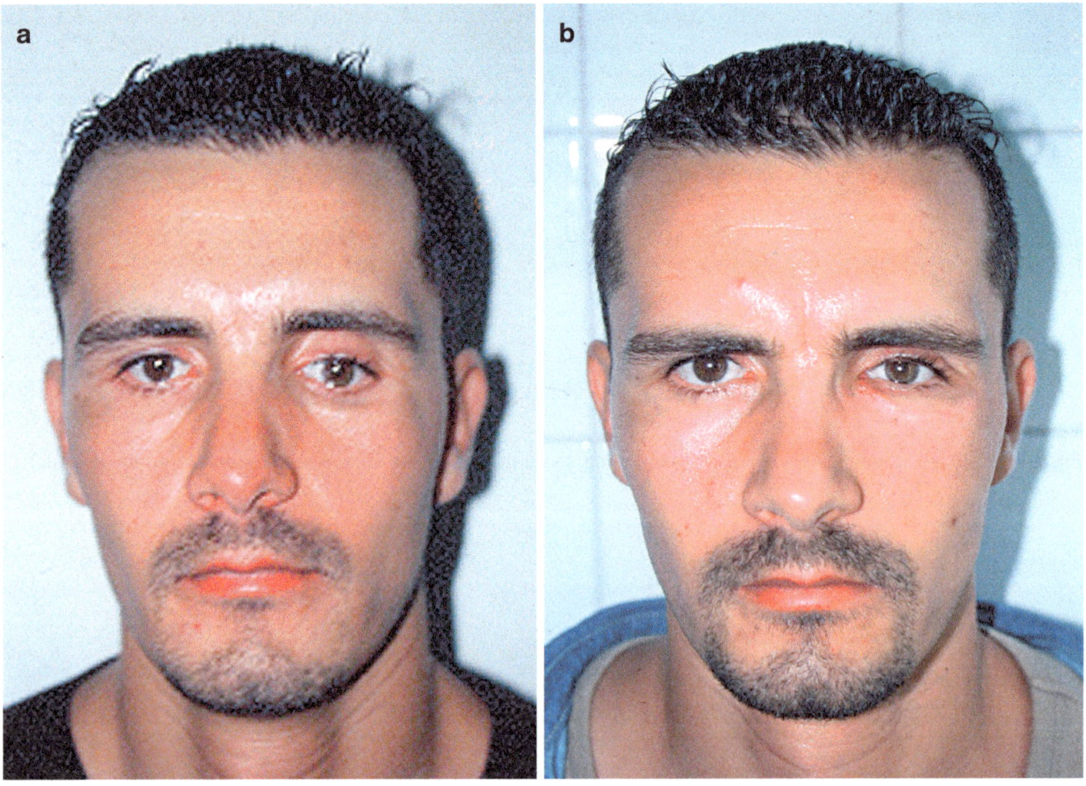

Fig. 63.53 Pre- and postoperative photographs: the face is symmetric and the diplopia is gone

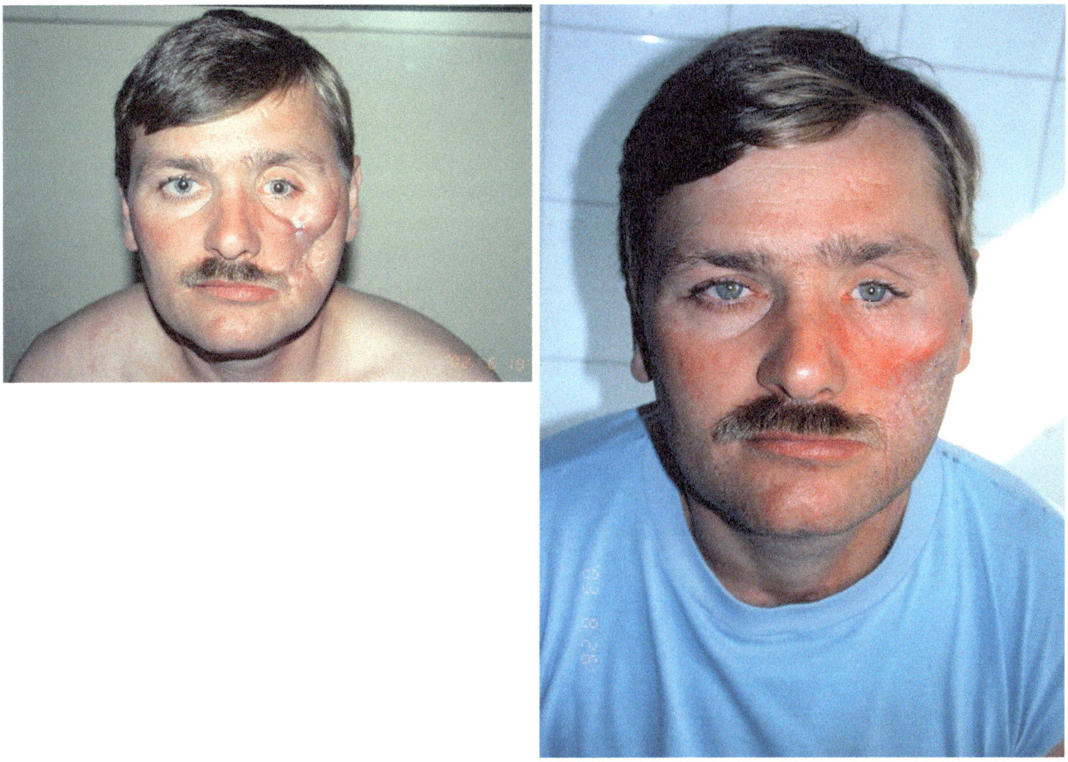

Fig. 63.54 Gunshot wound with extensive orbital floor and maxillary defect. The 'bridging' plate placed without supporting the eyeball perforated the soft tissues. After removing the plate, performing fistuloplasty and reconstructing the buccal soft tissues, a CAD-CAM implant is placed. The diplopia is gone and the contours of the face are restored.

Part VII

Neuro-Ophthalmological Considerations of the Facial Nerve

64 Tumor Lesions of the Facial Nerve

Ildikó Gádor

Contents

Muscles and motor nerves of the facial mimics, the facial nerves are important tools of non-verbal communication in human relationships. Functional disorder of this nerve – in addition to organic and esthetic disadvantages – significantly affects the psychic condition of the patient as well. Therefore, maintaining the function of the nerve and potential restoration of nerve function are responsible roles of the physician. Dysfunction of the facial nerve leads to a characteristic abnormality of the anterior segment of the eye, "keratoconjunctivitis or lagophthalmic keratitis". The ophthalmologist not only has to protect and treat disorders of eye closure with local treatment, but otorhinolaryngology consultation has to be requested in order to explore potential origin of the consequent symptoms. Determining the reason for the condition and the treatment of it may be performed with interdisciplinary cooperation (Figs. 64.1 and 64.2).

I. Gádor, M.D
Unit of Otoneurology, Department of Otorhinolaryngology, National Institute of Neurology, Budapest, Hungary
e-mail: gadorildi@gmail.com

Anatomy

Te facial nerve is a mixed nerve. Its main function is to provide motor innervation for the mimic muscles, the posterior belly of the digastric muscle, the stylohyoid muscle, and the stapedius muscle. Trough the intermediate nerve, the facial nerve plays a role in gustatory sensation of the anterior two thirds of the tongue, the secretory innervation of the lacrimal gland, smaller salivary glands of the nose and palate, the submandibular gland, and the sublingual glands, and sensation of a small area of the skin of the external auditory canal (**Hitselberger's sign**).

Motor fibers originate from the motor nucleus in the pons; the fibers bypass the abducens nucleus ("inner knee of the facial nerve"), exit at the inferior part of the pons and form the intermediofacial nerve with the fibers of the intermediate nerve. This nerve enters the inner auditory canal (**meatal segment**) above the transverse crest, and continues laterally between the anterior semicircular canal and the cochlea till the hiatus canalis nervi

J. Somlai, T. Kovács (eds.), *Neuro-Ophthalmology*, DOI 10.1007/978-3-319-28956-4_64

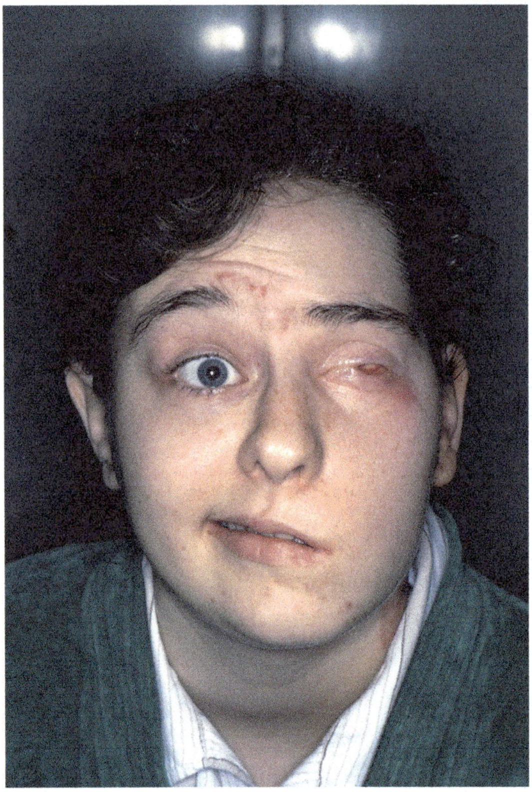

Fig. 64.1 Late postoperative stage of a large cerebellopontin angle tumor occurring in early childhood, leading to facial paralysis with consequent keratoconjunctivitis

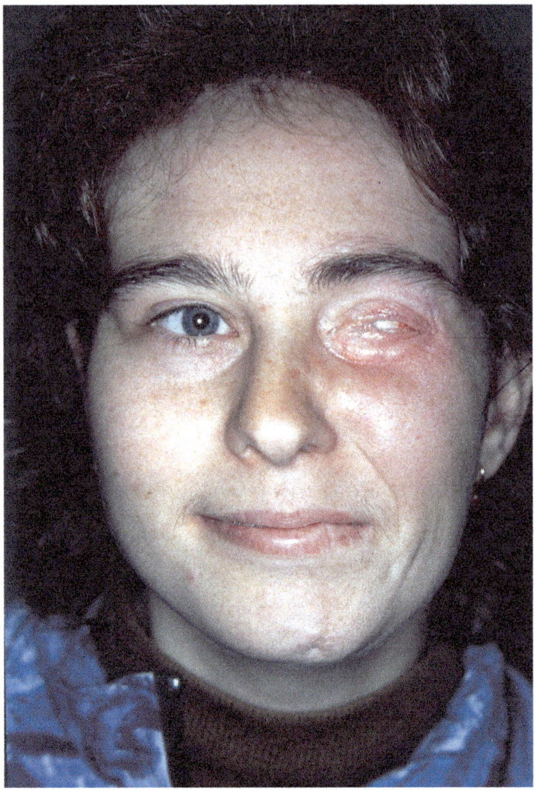

Fig. 64.2 Three years afer the VII–XI anastomosis, voluntary movement of the face commenced, the neuroophthalmologic status is irreversible

petrosi majoris, where the superior greater petrosal nerve branches of (**labyrinthine segment**).

The facial nerve makes a sharp turn in the level of the geniculate ganglion ("external knee" of the facial nerve), and it passes above the oval window (**tympanic segment**), then continues below the horizontal semicircular canal, and exits the stylomastoid foramen (**mastoid segment**) from the petrosal bone behind and laterally to the styloid process. It has various branches in the soft tissues in anterior and superior directions with a curved course between the superficial and greater deep lobe of the parotid gland. Te rostral facial nucleus is innervated by the left and right precentral gyrus, and the caudal nucleus is innervated only by the contralateral gyrus, therefore, in case of central paresis, the function of the frontal branch is intact, while in case of nuclear or peripheral paresis, the function of all three branches is impaired.

Diagnostics

Te type of paresis has to be determined first in the diagnosis of the dysfunction of the facial nerve:

- supranuclear
- nuclear
- infranuclear

In addition to neurologic examinations, CT and MRI are available to diagnose supranuclear and nuclear lesions. In addition to physical examination, gustometry, audiology examination, and tympanometry, especially examination of the stapedius refex, are performed in the diagnosis of infranuclear paresis. Schirmer's test is performed to measure tear production, and electronystagmography, photoelectronystagmography, Stenvers' projection, and if necessary, cranial CT examination or MRI are performed in case of suspected meatal lesions.

Electrophysiology is of great help in all types of facial nerve paresis. There are three various degrees of injury of peripheral nerves.

- **neurapraxia**: conduction disorder developing without the disruption of the continuity of the axon (reversible).
- **axonotmesis**: injury of the axon with intact endo-, epi-, and perinerium (not completely reversible).
- **neurotmesis**: complete tear of the nerve, without surgical fusion, the injury of the nerve is irreversible.

Location and extent of the injury and the expected prognosis and regeneration may be determined with electro diagnostic tests. Te most commonly used test is electromyography (EMG). With a needle electrode, it gives detailed information about the function of the nerve-muscle unit. It quantitatively determines the myogenic and neurogenic damage, degeneration, and regeneration. In case of a **Nerve Excitability Test** (**NET**), the nerve is stimulated with a millisecond long square impulse, and the diference between the threshold of the intact and injured side is evaluated. If the latter value is below 3.5 mA, the prognosis of paresis is good, if the value is above 3.5 m or is increasing, it suggests axonotmesis, and the prognosis is unfavorable. Currently, this is the most widely used electrophysiological test. Regarding prognostic value, **Maximal Stimulation Test** (**MST**) and **electroneuronography** (**ENoG**, **EEMG**) are more reliable methods. Te latter test examines the triggered response of the muscles innervated by the facial nerve with superfcial electrodes.

Blink Reflex It is a valuable tool in detecting changes in the function of the trigeminofacial reflex pathway.

The presence of a tumor should be suggested if facial paresis occurs slowly or facial paresis is recurring. A tumor may be in the background of facial tics and spasm as well. Rarely, facial paresis of tumor origin may occur suddenly as well. Te most common **tumors** affecting the facial nerve:

Benign Tumors

neuroma, meningeoma, hemangioma, paraganglioma, congenital cholesteatoma, lipoma, hamartoma, arachnoid cyst, etc.

Malignant Tumors

lymphoma, leukemia, neuroblastoma, rhabdomyosarcoma, chordoma, metastasis in the intratemporal region, adenocystic carcinoma most commonly in the parotid gland, mucoepidermoid carcinoma, undifferentiated carcinoma, anaplastic carcinoma, Hodgkin disease, etc.

Radical surgical removal of malignant tumors usually involves the removal of the facial nerve as well. Most recently, maintaining function is our goal as well as creating opportunities for subsequent reconstructive surgery, if it does not endanger ablasticity. The most common benign tumor is the **neuroma of the statoacoustic nerve**, which originates usually from the vestibular, or less commonly from the acoustic fibers. It may lead to tinnitus, decreased hearing, dizziness, facial paresis, trigeminal or lower cranial nerve symptoms, congestion, and visual impairment. Facial paresis is a rather late symptom, but small, intrameatal tumors may also cause early functional disorder in the facial nerve by compressing the vessels of the inner auditory tube. In case of a small tumor it surgery is performed in the so called otological phase, the chance of preserving the function of the facial nerve is greater (Figs. 64.3 and 64.4).

Neuroma of the facial nerve is significantly less common. Miehlke and Pulec have collected 58 and 98 publications respectively regarding intratemporal neuroma of the facial nerve. Rejtő has described one, Székely four, and Piffkó three cases in the national literature. In our Institute, seven patients were diagnosed with facial neuroma in the last 20 years. Its first symptom is the slowly progressing peripheral facial paresis developing usually in some years. Growth of the tumor may destroy the inner ear, and lead to deafness, vestibular disorders, and may grow into the tympanic cavity, may be seen through the tympanic membrane, or may appear in the external

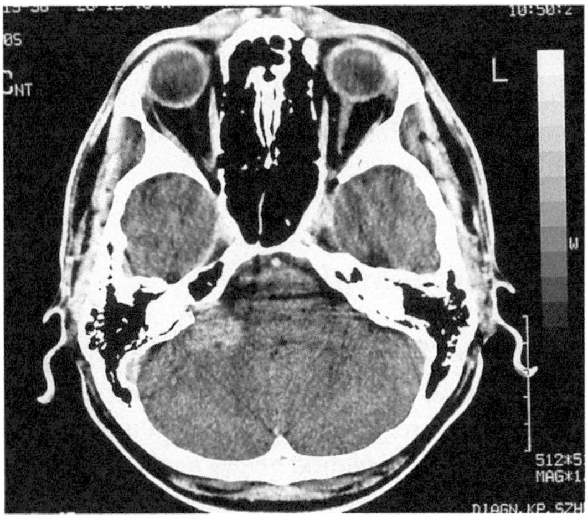

Fig. 64.3 CT image of an acoustic neuroma on the right side leading to facial nerve paresis

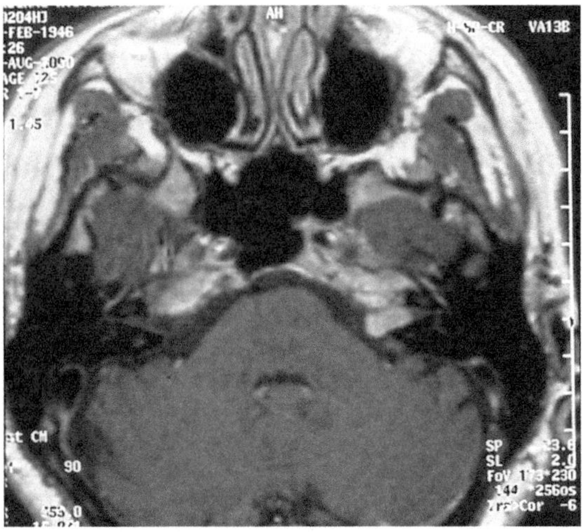

Fig. 64.4 MR image of an acoustic neuroma on the right side leading to facial nerve paresis

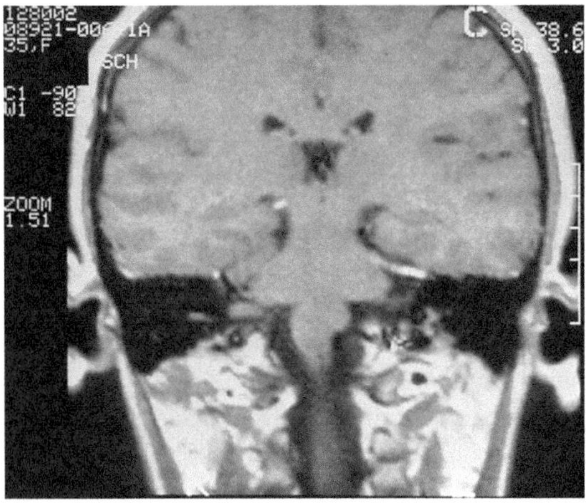

Fig. 64.5 MR image of a patient with facial neuroma on the left side

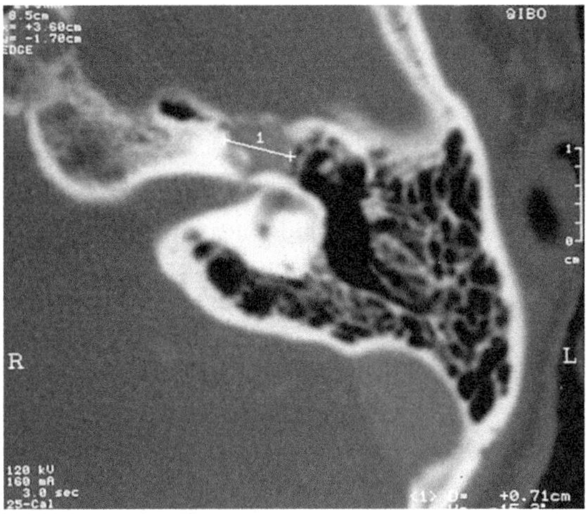

Fig. 64.6 CT image of a facial neuroma causing pyramidal destruction

auditory canal imitating a polyp. **Extratemporal facial neuromas** are less common, although 4–6 cm large neuromas have been described in the parotid grand (Figs. 64.5, 64.6, and 64.7).

The prognosis of neuroma is good. It does not pose direct threat to life, and it is usually treated with microsurgery.

An other, by now well accepted treatment for neuroma is radiosurgery (Linear accelerator/ LINAC/, gamma knife/GK/, cyber knife/CK/. The essence of radiosurgery is to stop the progression of the tumor with a single CT- or MR-guided stereotactic irradiation. The GK treatment prescription is 12–13 Gy at the 50 % isodose line, to achieve the best result in maintaining the function of the facial and acoustic nerves.

Meningeoma of the petrous pyramid apex may lead to facial nerve lesion while growing. It leads to slowly progressing hearing impairment,

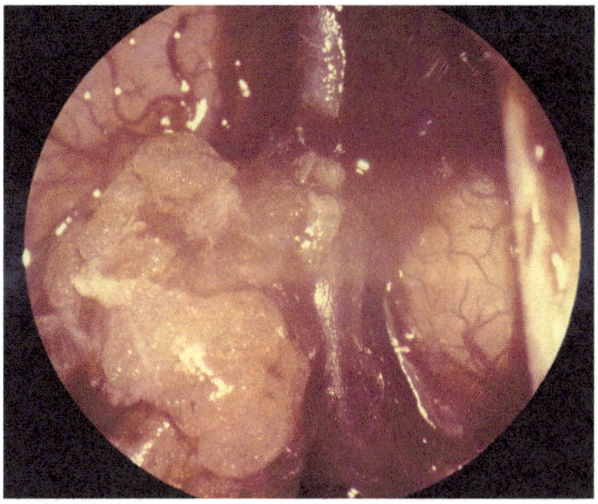

Fig. 64.7 Intraoperative microscopic image of the facial neuroma

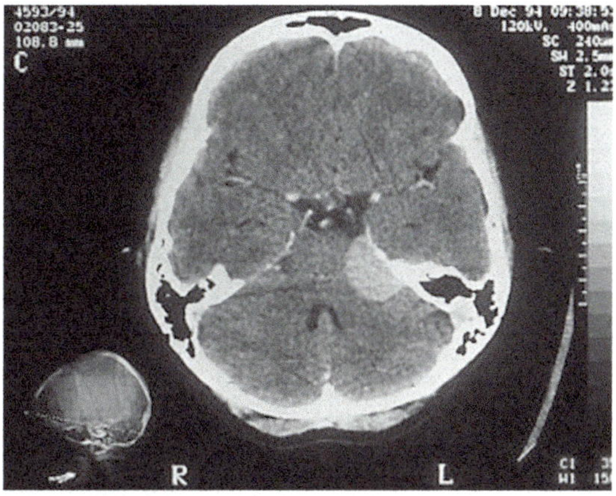

Fig. 64.8 CT image of a meningeoma in the pyramidal apex

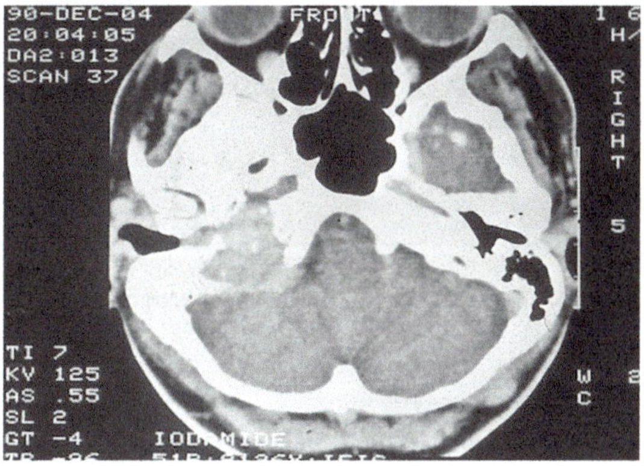

Fig. 64.9 CT image of a chemodectoma causing pyramidal destruction and consequent facial nerve lesion

tinnitus, and sometimes facial paresis as described above. Its therapy is similar to that of the acoustic neuroma (Figs. 64.8 and 64.9).

The purpose of the surgical removal of benign tumors – especially if the function of the nerve was intact before the surgery – is to remove the tumor and maintain the anatomy and function of the nerve. In such cases subtotal removal of the tumor poses smaller risk to the patient compared with the potential functional disorder of the facial nerve. However, during surgical removal of highly vascularized chemodectomas, epidermoid tumors, or recurrent pleomorphic adenomas of the parotid gland, maintaining the integrity of the facial nerve may be difficult, or sometimes impossible.

In such cases, **reconstructive surgery of the nerve** is performed:

1. **Nerve suture**: End to end microsurgical anastomosis of the prepared nerves with 2–3 epineural sutures (10/0, monofilament).
2. **Re-routing procedure**: If there are few millimeters between the nerves endings to be anastomosed, anastomosis of the nerves may be prepared more easily by lifting the nerves from the bony canal, for example by bypassing the tympanic cavity.
3. **Free transplantation**: a graft is transplanted between nerves located far from each other (such as the great auricular nerve, sural nerve, or lateral femoral cutaneous nerve graft).
4. **Dott's surgery**: Intra-extracranial surgery. Looking for the stump of the facial nerve in the angle between the cerebellum and the pons, then fusing the central stump with a graft from the sural nerve, which is subsequently rerouted to the skull base. Here the graft is reanastomosed with the previously cut and freed trunk, by the stylomastoid foramen, of the facial nerve.

If, in the posterior scala, the injured nerve cannot be sutured, during the removal of an acoustic neuroma, **anastomosis surgery** is performed.

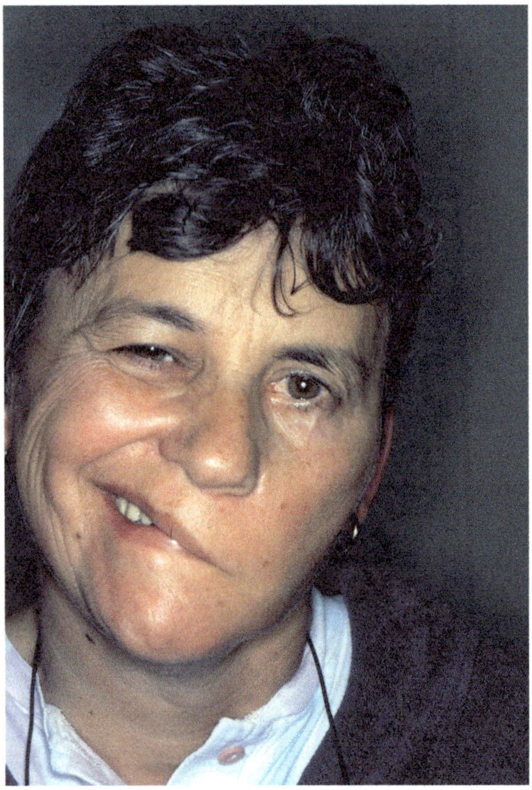

Fig. 64.10 Postoperative palsy of the facial nerve after surgery of an acoustic neuroma on the left side

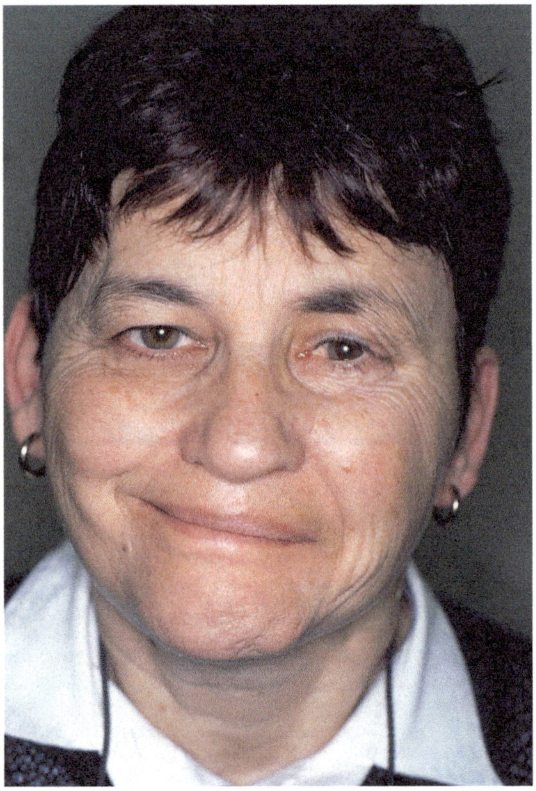

Fig. 64.11 Status after the anastomosis surgery

5. Anastomosis surgeries:
   Facio- Hypoglossal Anastomosis
   The surgical technique is known since 1904! For the preservation of tongue function, modified techniques are the most popular crossover operations in use today.
   Facio-Accessorius Anastomosis
   A modification: accessorius nerve's-**sternocleidomastoid/SCM/branch** is used to the suture. Using this technique, impaired shoulder movement is avoidable. We performed this method in our Institute (Figs. 64.10 and 64.11).

Facio-Facial Cross-Face Graft Scaramella has recommended, and subsequently Fisch, Conley, Anderl and others have modified a technique to fuse the facial nerve on the injured side with a graft prepared from the sural nerve bypassed above the lips and/or eyes with branches of the facial nerve on the contralateral side.

Only This Method Is Able to Restore Mimetic Spontaneous Smiling!

In case of nerve transplantation and anastomosis, regeneration can be expected to occur even 3–6 months after the surgery, but final results occur only 2–3 years later. Careful care of residual symptoms (such as lagophthalmos), regular physiotherapy, constant practicing and good psychic condition are essential.

Surgery of the facial nerve is a difficult and responsible task, but in case of success, the patient's quality of life improves and physicians can feel content.

Further Readings

Anderl H. Cross-face nerve transplant. Clin Plast Surg. 1979;6:433–49.

Bauer M. Intrameatalis acusticus neurinomák. Fül-orr-gégegyógyászat. 1976;22:65–77.

Conley J. Perspectives in facial reanimation. In: May M, editor. Te facial nerve. Stuttgart, New York: Tieme Verlag; 1986. p. 645–63.
Cornelius F, Sauvagat E, Tran Ba Huy P, George B. Surgical treatment of facial nerve schwannomas. Prog Neurol Surg. 2008;21:119–30.
Dott NM. Facial nerve reconstruction by graft bypassing the petrous bone. Arch Otolaryngol. 1963;78(426).
Duss P. Topical diagnosis in neurology. Stuttgart, New York: Tieme Verlag; 1983. p. 107–13.
Fickinger JC, Kondziolka D, Niranjan A, Lunsford LD. Results of acoustic neuroma radiosurgery: an analysis of 5 years' experience using current methods. J Neurosurg. 2001;94(1):1–6.
Hudgins WR. Patiens attitude about outcomes and the role of gamma knife radiosurgery in the treatment of vestibular schwannomas. Neurosurgery. 1994;34: 459–65.
Iwai Y, Yamanaka K, Shiotani M, Uyama T. Radiosurgery for acoustic neuromas: results of low-dose treatment. Neurosurgery. 2003;53(2):282–7.
Madhok R, Kondziolka D, Flickinger JC, Lunsford LD. Gamma-knife radio-surgery for facial schwannomas. Neurosurgery. 2009;64:1102–5.
Matthies C, Samii M. Management of 1000 Vestibular Schwannomas/Acoustic Neurinomas/clinical presentation. Neurosurgery. 1997;40:1–9.
May M. Te facial nerve. Stuttgart, New York: Thieme Verlag; 1986. p. 455–67.
Miehlke A. Surgery of facial nerve. München, Berlin, Wien: Urban and Schwarzenberg; 1973. p. 98–108.
Myrseth E, Moller P, Pedersen PH, Lund-Johansen M. Vestibular schwnnoma: surgery or gammaknife radiosurgery? Aprospective nonrandomized study. Neurosurgery. 2009;64(4):654–61.
Piffkó P (1980) Fül-orr megbetegedések határterületi problémáiról.Referátum. Magyar Fül-Orr-Gégeorvosok Kongresszusa, Szeged, Kongresszusi Kiadvány.
Poe DS, Scher N, Panje WR. Facial reanimation by XI–VII anastomosis without shoulder paralysis. Laryngoscope. 1989;99(10 Pt 1):1040–7.
Pulec JL. Facial nerve neuroma. Laryngoscope. 1972;82: 1160–76.
Régis J, Roche P-H (eds) (2008) Modern management of acoustic neuroma. Prog Neurol Surg Basel, Karger. 21:119–30
Rejtő A. Fall eines vom Gesichtsnerven ausgehenden Tumors. Mschr Ohrenhk. 1939;73:615.
Sabi HI, Bordi LT, Symon L, Compton JS. Facio-hypoglossal anastomosis for the treatment of facial palsy after acoustic neuroma resection. Br J Neurosurg. 1990;4(4):313–7.
Samii M, Matthies C. Indication, technique and results of facial nerve reconstruction. Acta Neurochirurgica (Wien). 1994;130:125–39.
Székely T (1969) Az extra-és intratemporalis arcidegsebészet alapjai. Referátum. Societas Medic.Otorhino-laryng. Hungary. Miskolc. Kongresszusi Kiadvány.
Székely T. Anmerkungen zur Chirurgie des Nervus facialis. Otorhinolaryngol Nova. 1991;1:53–5.
Taylor A, Clark PL (1906) Results of facio-hypoglossal anastomosis for facial palsy. Jama. XLVI(12):856–62.
Neuro-Ophthalmol (editors: Judit Somlai & Tibor Kovács).

Part VIII

The Neuro-Ophthalmological Aspects of Headaches

Neuro-Opthalmological Aspects of Headaches from the Neurologist's Aspect

65

Csaba Ertsey

Contents

Since the publication of the first edition of the present Neuro-ophthalmology book, our knowledge about headaches has broadened considerably, new diagnostic methods and categories have been introduced and the number of therapeutic options has also increased. **Jelencsik Ilona**, one of the authors of the first edition came to an untimely end since then, but her thought is still valid:

> Beside everyday clinical practice headache research also requires the close cooperation of neurologists and neuro-ophthalmologists which disciplines heavily and so obviously rely on each other.

Headache is the seventh most frequent complaint of patients, who attend physicians in the United States. Since those structures which are usually responsible for the development of headache are closely associated with the visual system, numerous patients are referred to the ophthalmologist due to headache, periocular pain or headache-related visual disturbances. Headache is probably the most frequent reason for the collaboration between the ophthalmologist and the neurologist: several forms of headache are accompanied by visual disturbance or eye-related symptoms, while some diseases of the eye go with pain, which, beside the globes, can have frontal, retrobulbar or temporal localization.

The main difficulty of the proper investigation of headaches is that a plethora of diseases are accompanied by this symptom. The International Classification of Headache Disorders (ICHD), the diagnostic handbook of the International Headache Society (IHS) distinguishes 176 types of headache (Headache Classification Subcommittee of the International Headache Society 2004). Most of the patients suffer from the so called primary headaches such as migraine, tension headache, the so called trigeminal autonomic cephalalgias and numerous rare headache variants. The common denominator of these diseases is that the pain results from the dysfunction of the otherwise morphologically intact nervous system. They are characterized by recurring stereotyped attacks, which spontaneously resolve after a characteristic

C. Ertsey, M.D, PhD
Department of Neurology, Semmelweis University, Budapest, Hungary
e-mail: csaba.ertsey@gmail.com

J. Somlai, T. Kovács (eds.), *Neuro-Ophthalmology*, DOI 10.1007/978-3-319-28956-4_65

period of time. The attacks are accompanied by symptoms, which are typical of the given form of headache. The secondary headaches (i.e., those that are caused by other underlying disorders) are less frequent: the severe conditions (brain tumors, stroke), which usually distress the patients, can very rarely be found in the background. The secondary headaches consist of those painful processes, which involve the eyes, the ears, teeth, sinuses and other organs of the head and the neck. But, the headaches related to head and neck traumas, diseases of the cranial and cervical blood vessels and other intracranial disorders (space occupying processes, changes in the pressure of the cerebrospinal fluid, etc.) also belong to them. Further, this group comprises the headaches, which accompany infections, homoeostatic disorders, abuse or withdrawal of certain chemical drugs, and psychiatric diseases.

Anatomical Considerations

Although the brain tissue itself does not contain nerve endings for pain sensation, the meninges and cerebral blood vessel are richly innervated by such fibers. The intracranial pain sensitive structures are innervated mostly by the first branch of the trigeminal nerve (i.e., the ophthalmic nerve, n. V/1), but the infratentorial items are innervated by either by the glossopharyngeal, the vagus or the upper three cervical ganglia. The cerebral blood vessels and those neuronal structures, which innervate them, form the trigeminovascular system (Mayberg et al. 1981); this notion grabs the close bidirectional relationship between the vascular and neuronal structures. The primary pain sensitive neurons synapse in the nucleus descendens of the trigeminal nerve and caudally in the dorsal horn of the C I—II segments. Attention should be paid to the fact, that nuchal and upper cervical fibers also converge to these centers, which explains the occipital—cervical localization of certain primary pain conditions (Angus-Leppan et al. 1997; Hoskin et al. 1999). The secondary sensory neurons of the nucleus descendens then project to the ventral posteromedial nucleus of the thalamus (VPM). The thalamocortical connections, however, are not completely clarified yet.

The eye-ball and the orbit are also innervated by the ophthalmic nerve (n. V/1) via the nasociliary fibers. This way the painful sensations from both the orbit and the supratentorial intracranial structures are transmitted by the ophthalmic nerve, which explains the periorbital localization of several primary headaches and the radiation of the pain of certain diseases of the eye beyond the boundaries of the orbit. Disorders accompanied by periocular pain are summarized in Table 65.1.

It is essential to know the autonomic innervation of the eye and the periorbital region in the management of both eye diseases and primary headaches. The first neuron of the parasympathetic innervation can be found in the superior salivary nucleus (Spencer et al. 1990). The efferent fibers leave the central nervous system together with the facial nerve and synapse via the geniculate ganglion in the sphenopala-

Table 65.1 Syndromes accompanied by periocular pain

Optic neuritis
Optic Disc Edema with Macular Star (ODEMS)
Giant cell arteritis
AION of non arteritic origin
Pseudotumor cerebri
Transient loss of vision
Orbital pseudotumor
Orbital myositis
Trauma of the orbit (blowout trauma)
Pathological process of the cavernous sinus
n.III. schwannoma (painful n.III. paralysis)
Proptosis
Ethmoiditis
Tolosa–Hunt-syndrome:
Benign episodic unilateral mydriasis
Ophthalmoplegic "migraine"
Migraine (either with or without aura)
Cluster headache and other trigeminal-autonomic cephalalgias
Tension headache (usually bilateral)

Adapted from Lee and Brazis (2003)
AION anterior ischemic optic neuropathy, *n. III.* oculomotor nerve

tine and carotid "mini" ganglia. The postganglionary fibers originating there supply the cerebral blood vessel, the lacrimal glands and the glands of the nasal mucous membranes. The parasympathetic fibers contain numerous neurotransmitters (acetylcholine, vasoactive intestinal polypeptide (VIP), helodermin, helospectin I and II, peptide histidin-isoleucin (PHI) and pituitary adenylate cyclase activating peptide (PACAP)). The parasympathetic system exerts a vasodilatory effect. According to animal studies, the stimulation of the trigeminal nerve leads to parasympathetic activation; the phenomenon is called trigeminal-parasympathetic or trigeminal-autonomic reflex. The afferent pathway is the ophthalmic nerve, while the efferent pathway is the lesser petrosal nerve; the connection is established by the collateral fibers of the secondary trigeminal axons, which run from the caudal nucleus of the trigeminal nerve to the thalamus.

The sympathetic innervation of the brain, the meningeal blood vessels, the skin of the eyes and the forehead is supplied by the superior cervical ganglia. The postganglionary fibers run on the surface of the internal carotid artery and get to the skull via the carotid canal. The sympathetic fibers ramify in the cavernous sinus. The sympathetic fibers, which innervate the eyes and the forehead run with the ophthalmic nerve, those supplying the levator palpebrae accompany the oculomotor nerve, and the branches, which innervate the veins and sinuses run together with the tentorial nerve. The innervation of the internal carotid artery and its main branches are provided by the carotid plexus. Norepinephrine and neuropeptide Y (NPY) are the most important transmitters of the sympathetic fibers (Edvinsson and Uddman 2005).

Primary Headaches

In the majority of patients suffering from recurring episodes of headache, neither the detailed internal, neurological and ophthalmological investigations, nor the accidentally performed imaging tests reveal alterations. In these cases, presumably a primary headache is responsible for the complaints. However, the diagnosis of primary headaches can be set up when according to the clinical characteristics, the case unequivocally fits in to a given primary headache category and any other neurological syndromes can be excluded. Therefore, the detailed case history, which describes the localization, intensity, character, distribution in time, accompanying symptoms and the results of the previous therapeutic efforts, is an indispensable part of the diagnostic algorithm. It requires the strong cooperation and meticulous approach of both the examiner and the patient. The group of primary headaches comprises migraine, tension headache, trigeminal autonomic cephalalgias and numerous other rare conditions.

MIgraine

Migraine appears in attacks: its lifelong prevalence is about 10—17 % in the developed countries (Bigal and Lipton 2009). Although most of the migraine sufferers experience 2—3 attacks per a month, it is not a well known fact that about 3 % of the population suffers from chronic migraine (more than 15 attacks in a period of 3 months). Migraine affects the active population: its prevalence is the highest in the age group between 20 and 60 years. In women it is three times as frequent as in males. A migraine attack lasts for 4—72 h without intervention Usually it represents a unilateral throbbing or pulsating headache, which gradually increases in intensity and significantly interferes with or completely prohibits the patient's daily activities The attack is accompanied by nausea/vomiting, photo-, phono- and osmo/olfactophobia (hypersensitivity to strong lights, sounds and odors) Physical activity or, bending over increase the intensity and often makes the pain pulsating. (The diagnostic criteria of migraine can be found in Table 65.2) A migraine episode is much longer than the length of the headache itself. In several patients (according to different resource in 20–80 %), half or 1 day before the actual attack (prodromal phase) "heralding" symptoms

Table 65.2 The diagnostic criteria of migraine (Headache Classification Subcommittee of the International Headache Society 2004)

A. At least five attacks, which fulfill B–D criteria
B. Headache attacks, which last for 4–72 h (when untreated in adults)
C. Headache has at least two of the following characteristics::
1. Unilateral
2. Pulsating quality
3. Moderate or severe pain intensity[a]
4. Aggravation by or causing avoidance of routine physical activity (walk, walking stairs)
D. During the headache, at least one of them are present:
1. Nausea and/or vomiting
2. Photophobia and phonophobia[b]
E. Not attributable to another disorder

Comments:
[a]Intensity of pain:
Moderately strong pain: It inhibits work or other activities;
Strong pain; It prohibits work or other activities
[b]Photo – or phonophobia are not sufficient alone, (without nausea/vomiting) to diagnose migraine

develop: mood fluctuation, irritation, hypo- or hyperactivity, pica, etc. In 20–25 % of migraine sufferers, the attack is preceded by characteristic neurological symptoms, which develop in 5–20 min, last for maximum 60 min and refer to the functional disorder of a given cortical region.

It is the so called migraine aura, which is most frequently accompanied by visual (scintillations, scotoma), other sensory (paresthesia) or motor symptoms (paresis). In typical cases, the headache follows the aura in 60 min. The last phase of the migraine attack is the restitution; the pain has already disappeared but the patients have not regained their ability to work: fatigue, general weakness, attention and memory deficit can be observed.

The frequency of migraine attacks is variable, usually 1–6 attacks/month, which individually depend on the provoking factors. When the number of attacks is low, the therapy focuses on the alleviation of the headache and the accompanying symptoms (attack therapy). Some patients' headache can be relieved by treatments based on simple or combined (e.g., caffeine) NSAID derivatives, while others respond only to specific abortive migraine medications (triptans, ergot derivatives). Both the traditional and the specific abortive substances can be used only for maximum 10 days per month, because their prolonged administration can lead to the development of chronic migraine and/or medication overuse headache. Therefore, frequent and long-lasting migraine attacks always require the introduction of a prophylactic treatment regimen as well (Ertsey et al. 2009).

Photophobia in Migraine

A characteristic feature of the migraine attacks (even one of its diagnostic criteria) is the hypersensitivity to environmental stimuli. Moreover, according to the current classification of the IHF photo- or phonophobia represents indispensable diagnostic criteria of migraine. Although it is not a separate diagnostic criterion, osmophobia (hypersensitivity to olfactory stimuli) is also a frequently noted symptom. Surveys based upon larger representative samples reflect that the frequency of photophobia can exceed 80 % in the patients (Olesen 2010). The developmental mechanism of photophobia has recently been described by Noseda and his colleagues (Noseda et al. 2010). Using retrograde tracing, they have unveiled that some ganglion cells of the retina project to the ventral posterior (VP) nucleus of the thalamus, which plays a very important role in pain sensation. These ganglion cells belong to a separate (intrinsic photosensitive (ip)) cell population, which are independent from the cone and rod cells. These ganglion cells also supply the suprachiasmatic nucleus (the "internal clock") of the hypothalamus to entrain our internal rhythm to the daily light–dark cycles. According to the findings of Noseda's group, the photic stimulation of the ganglion cells will change the firing pattern of the thalamic VP cells.

The anatomical studies were complemented by functional ones carried out on visually impaired human subjects. In those migraine sufferers, who could not see at all (for example, due to enucleation), stimulation by light during the attack did not worsen the headache. However, those visually impaired subjects, who could see at least light (e.g., retinitis pigmentosa, progressive rod—cone degeneration) such stimulation aggravated the condition. Therefore, presumably the migraine related photophobia is associated with the activity of the ip ("non-image-forming") ganglion cells.

The Migraine Aura

Although it is a well-known feature that migraine attacks may be introduced by cortical dysfunction, which most frequently presents with visual disturbances, the aura itself does not represent a diagnostic criterion of migraine. In 75–80 % of the patients, the headache is not preceded by a cortical dysfunction, which would reach the individual's threshold. Further even those patients, who experience aura, may have attacks without it. Sometimes the typical aura is not followed by a headache (*aura sine hemicrania*), in those cases, however, other ophthalmological and neurological causes of transient visual impairments should be excluded. The migraine aura consists of focal neurological signs, which typically develop in 5–20 min and disappear in 60 min. Among the symptoms of auras, visual, other sensory, motor symptoms, rarely dysphasia or brainstem dysfunctions can be observed.

The most frequent type is the visual disturbance. The majority of the patients complain about positive ("plus") symptoms: flashing lights (scintillation), bright or colorful zigzag lines, which sometimes imitate the layout of a medieval castle ("fortification spectrum") The disturbance usually moves inside the visual field and/or increases; the positive phenomena can be accompanied by the transient loss of a certain part of the visual field (Fig. 65.1).

The aura can present with blurred vision, blind spots, scotomas and tunnel vision. Sometimes complex auras were also described, which suggested the dysfunction of the para- and peristriate areas (the image rotates, its outlines undulate, palinopsia). Complex auras (which involve several cortical regions) typically start with visual

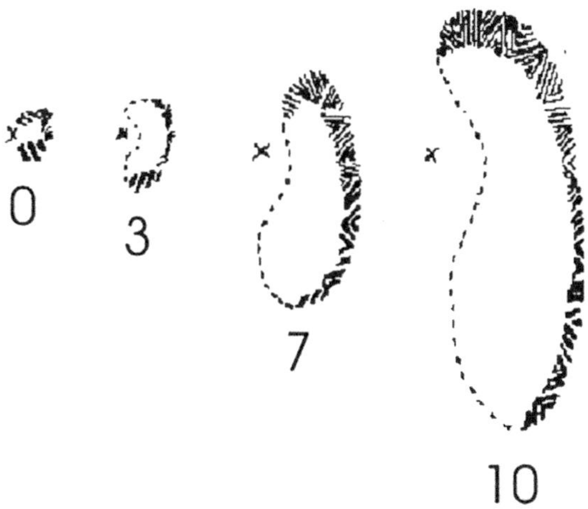

Fig. 65.1 Lashley's observation on his own aura (Lashley 1941). The point of fixation is marked by x in the figure. It is easy to follow that over time (in minutes), the size of the scintillating scotoma increases and it moves to the periphery from the point of fixation (Redrawn after Lashley (1941)

disturbance, which is followed by other sensory impairments (usually paraesthesias), and then motor symptoms appear (paresis, motor aphasia). The frequency of the given symptoms is inversely proportional to the distance from the occipital lobe. The complex auras have great differential diagnostic value.

The auras which involve only a smaller circumscribed cortical areas (especially if it is the first attack) may suggest transient ischemic attack, but the above-mentioned progressive character implies that the disorder crossed the border of different blood supply regions, therefore, the possibility of vascular origin is minimal (Silberstein et al. 1998).

Very rarely, the migraineous visual impairment may persist for weeks or months without accompanying EEG or MRI alterations (Liu et al. 1995). The SPECT analysis of these persistent visual disturbances (migraine aura status) may reveal occipital hypoperfusion (Chen et al. 2001).

In the differential diagnostics of migraineous auras, beside the aforementioned circulatory disorders, the occipital space occupying processes and the visual disturbances due to arteriovenous malformations should be considered. However, in the above conditions, usually the visual impairment is of sudden onset, and it appears always in the same region of the visual field (according to the localization of the space occupying process), whereas the typical migraine aura may develop in both visual fields with different frequency, though. The investigation of migraine auras had a major impact on the hypotheses regarding the pathomechanism of migraine. Lashley, based upon his observations (Fig. 65.1) (Lashley 1941) has concluded that the aura is evoked by a functional disorder of the cortex, which progresses in the occipital lobe at a speed of 3 mm/s. Further, Leao has recognized that, in animal studies, the stimulation of the cortex leads to spreading activation and transient depression, at the same speed of propagation (Leao 1944). Later with regional blood flow studies, progressive hypoperfusion was described in the affected area, which did not respect the borders of regions blood supply. Recently, functional MRI studies have verified the pathological activity of the cortex, which spreads from the occipital region into frontal direction; this phenomenon could have been observed even in migraines without preceding aura (Hadjikhani et al. 2001).

The Pathomechanism of Migraine

The widespread but outdated theory describes migraine as a vascular headache, which should be treated by vasodilator or circulation enhancing drugs. The hypothesis was based upon such observations as the throbbing character of the pain, the increased temporal arterial pulsation noted is some patients, the aura symptoms and the effectiveness of certain vasoactive substances. It was also supported by some data of transcranial Doppler studies and functional alterations of the platelets obtained from migraine patients. However, the investigations of the past 30 years have unambiguously verified that the migraineous attack actually starts well before the development of the pain and circulatory alterations and several features of it cannot be explained by the putative dysfunction of the cerebral blood vessels. Several studies proved that the brain function of migraine sufferer is different from that of the control patients even in the interictal periods. While in healthy controls repetitive visual and acoustic stimulations elicit less and less response (habituation), in migraine patients the habituation is deficient. Furthermore, migraine patients complain about mild photo- and phonophobia even in the interictal periods. Migraine patients have less cellular energy store (ATP and other macroergic phosphate) than the healthy counterparts. Therefore, migraine is considered a chronic disorder, which is accompanied by episodic bout of symptoms i.e., attacks (Bigal and Lipton 2008).

Therefore, at present, migraine is classified as a neurovascular headache. The common feature of these diseases is that the pain is related to the activation of the trigeminal nerve, and the changes in the diameter of the blood vessels are secondary phenomena, the consequences of the activation of trigeminal autonomic reflex loop. In the different subtypes of the neurovascular headaches, the process is triggered by separate mechanisms. In migraine, according to the most widely accepted theory, a primary cortical dysfunction initiates the process. Sufficient external and/or internal stimuli trigger the functional alteration of the occipital cortex, which in some of the cases lead to the development of an aura (Fig. 65.1). The trigeminal activation is presumably elicited by the subsequent depolarization of the free nerve endings of the trigeminal nerve in the pia mater of the occipital lobe.

Retinal Migraine

Retinal migraine (RM) belongs to disease entities which represent distinct ideas for different specialists. Galezowski, one of Charcot's colleagues was the first to describe that migraine could be accompanied by monocular visual disturbance, which he called "ophthalmic megrim" (Galezowski 1882). The concept of retinal migraine was introduced by Carroll in 1970. In his publication, he reported about 15 patients who complained about monocular, transient or persistent visual disturbance. Nevertheless, the term is rather puzzling since none of the patients complained about headache (Carroll 1970). Later several papers published cases as retinal migraines, which had actually only one common denominator, the monocular visual impairment. Some of the cases featured transient or persisting disturbance, with or without a headache. Finally, the ambiguous syndrome was correctly characterized by the first IHS classification of headaches in 1988, which exactly determined the criteria of retinal migraine, as well. (The diagnostic criteria of migraine can be found in Table 65.3.) Retinal migraine is very rare. In 2007, Hill et al. re-evaluated the data of 142 patients, who had been published as RM cases, according to the IHS criteria (Hill et al. 2007). Altogether, only 16 cases corresponded to the IHS definitions and merely five cases were definitive RM. However, the authors remarked that several patients corresponded to having RM.

Sometimes, retinal migraine develops following the visual aura of the migraine attack. Circulatory disorder of the retina might be suspected in these cases. One published case of an ophthalmologist, who worked at the Mayo clinic, deserves special attention. During the investigation of an episode of his monocular visual disturbances, the test did not reveal either retinal embolism or vasospasm (Robertson 2008). The development of RM is explained by the spreading of the depression in the retina, which was discussed in the chapter on the pathomechanism of migraine.

Table 65.3 The diagnostic criteria of retinal migraine (Headache Classification Subcommittee of the International Headache Society 2004)

A. at least two attacks fulfilling criteria B–C
B. Fully reversible monocular positive and/or negative visual phenomena (e.g., scintillations, scotoma or blindness) confirmed by a specialist's examination during an attack or (after proper instruction) by the patient's drawing of a monocular field defect during an attack
C. Headache fulfilling criteria B–D for 1.1 Migraine without aura begins during the visual symptoms or follows them within 60 min
D. Normal ophthalmological examination between attacks
E. Not attributed to another disorder 1

Note: Appropriate investigations exclude other causes of transient monocular blindness (such as TIA, dissection, ION)

The diagnosis of RM can be established when the patient repeatedly observes migraine attacks accompanied by monocular visual disorder. The visual impairment can manifest itself as scintillation, scotoma or temporary blindness. The diagnosis of retinal migraine is difficult since many patients whose complaints suggest monocular visual impairment actually experience binocular disorders, which, however, occupies the same region of the visual field (homonymous disturbance). Nevertheless, even the patients can distinguish between the two conditions by more thorough self-observations based upon the instructions received during the first visit. The lack of specific diagnostic tools raises further difficulties. Actually, retinal migraine represents a diagnosis of exclusion. Careful examination is needed to rule out the cerebrovascular conditions (amaurosis fugax) especially, when the patient observes transient monocular visual impairment of sudden onset, which resembles a descending curtain into the field of vision. Non-migraineous headache, which is accompanied by visual disturbance, does not exclude the presence of circulatory disorders or other organic alterations.

Ophthalmoplegic "Migraine"

Previously it was regarded as a separate, very rare migraine variant, but in the 2004 classification, this entity is dealt with in a different chapter (Chap. 13), and the "migraine" name is in quotation marks. These changes reflect that the syndrome at present is not regarded migraine. "Ophthalmoplegic migraine" is characterized by recurring headaches, accompanied by the transient paralysis of one of the oculomotor cranial nerves, most commonly the oculomotor nerve. The episode of the headache, however, can be much longer, it may even last for a week. Ophthalmoplegia can start during the attack or in a 4-day interval after the onset of the headache. The diagnostic criteria require the exclusion of lesions, which affect the parasellar region, the orbital fissure and the posterior scale. In some cases, the cisternal part of the affected nerve accumulates gadolinium, which suggests that the syndrome is actually the consequence of demyelinization.

Headache Accompanied by Trigeminal and Autonomic Activation

Although Nicolas Tulp and Gerhard van Swieten had already reported male patients suffering from strictly unilateral, periorbital headaches, it was in the last 30 years that several headache syndromes with combination of unilateral pain localized to the innervation area of the trigeminal nerve and ipsilateral autonomic symptoms were described. The importance of this recent knowledge is represented in the new revision of the ICHD, which grouped these entities together in a completely new, separate chapter, called trigeminal autonomic cephalalgias (TACs). In the development of trigeminal autonomic cephalalgias the C-fibers of the trigeminal nerve, which innervate the dural blood vessels, play a crucial role. The autonomic symptoms are the consequence of the activation of trigeminal-parasympathetic connections and partially the transient dysfunction of the cranial sympathetic pathways. The drugs, which affect the aforementioned systems, especially the receptors of the trigeminal nerve, can abolish the pain and the accompanying symptoms. The pathomechanism of the trigeminal, autonomic, cephalalgias clearly represents that neurological dysfunctions may lead to specific, circumscribed symptoms according to the anatomical borders of innervation. The restoration of function, with adequate treatment, will lead to the cessation of the symptoms.

The most important representative of trigeminal autonomic cephalalgias is cluster headache (CH). CH represents one of the most excruciating pain syndromes: The unbearably painful bouts are unilateral and are accompanied by local autonomic symptoms. The name itself refers to the accumulation and grouping of headache episodes in time. During one cluster episode, the daily attacks may appear regularly for some weeks or months. With the end of the episode, the patient becomes symptom-free for months or even years. A CH attack is strictly unilateral; usually it is localized around the eye, the temporal region, the forehead, but may involve, the upper teeth, the face and the maxilla. The pain is severe, usually splitting, or rarely spasmodic, burning or throbbing. The attacks during a cluster episode uniformly affect the same side, the headache is accompanied by characteristic ipsilateral symptoms They reveal partly the activation of the parasympathetic structures (lacrimation, rhinorrhea, nasal congestion, dilation of the conjunctival and the extracranial blood vessels) and partly the dysfunction of the sympathetic system (miosis, Horner's triad). The headache and the autonomic symptoms have a sudden onset, but in some instances, parasympathetic symptoms may precede the pain. Moreover, the cluster headache can also be accompanied by symptoms (nausea, vomiting, photo-, phonophobia) which strongly resemble those of the migraine (Bahra et al. 2002). Recent observations have confirmed that even a CH can be preceded by aura, but it is rarely visual in nature. Patients usually experience somato-sensory sensation before the attacks (Silberstein et al. 2000). (The diagnostic criteria of CH can be found in Table 65.4)

Therefore, at present, CH like migraine is classified as a neurovascular headache. This hypothesis is strongly supported by the finding that during spontaneous or nitroglycerine

Table 65.4 The diagnostic criteria of cluster headache

A. At least five attacks fulfilling criteria B–D
B. Severe or very severe, unilateral, orbital, supraorbital and/or temporal pain lasting 15–180 min if untreated
C. Headache is accompanied by at least one of the following:
1. Ipsilateral conjunctival injection and/or lacrimation
2. Ipsilateral nasal congestion and/or rhinorhhea
3. Ipsilateral eyelid oedema
4. Ipsilateral forehead and facial sweating
5. Ipsilateral miosis and/or ptosis
6. A sense of restlessness or agitation
D. Attacks have a frequency from one every other day to 8 per day
E. Not attributed to another disorder

evoked attacks of CH, the plasma level of some markers (e.g., CGRP and VIP) of the trigeminal and parasympathetic activation increases in the ipsilateral external jugular vein. The accumulation of attacks may be related to a certain hypothalamic dysfunction, which could be verified by functional imaging methods (May et al. 1998).

Further Trigeminal Autonomic Cephalalgias

Although the symptoms of cluster headache were described hundreds of years ago, the correct diagnostic criteria were established only in 1962. However, since then several similar headache syndromes have been described, which present with similar symptoms, but their length, frequency or therapy is different from those of the CH. Since these syndromes feature similar clinical entities, the International Headache Society, assuming a similar underlying pathomechanism, classifies them as a separate group entitled "Trigeminal autonomic cephalalgias" (Table 65.5).

Paroxysmal hemicrania was described by Sjaastad and Dale (Sjaastad and Dale 1974). The length of the attacks is between 2 and 30 min The daily frequency is usually higher than 5 but even 40 attacks have already been reported. The accompanying symptoms correspond to those of cluster headache. Paroxysmal hemicrania affects males and females in equal proportion (Sjaastad and Dale 1974). Its characteristic feature and prerequisite for the diagnosis as well is that the attacks disappear upon chronic administration of indomethacin. If left untreated, paroxysmal hemicrania typically runs a chronic course. It persists for a minimum of 1 year, and the interictal periods usually do not exceed 2 weeks. Nevertheless, very rarely, patients with episodic paroxysmal hemicrania were also reported. The **SUNCT syndrome** ("Short-lasting Unilateral Neuralgiform headache with Conjunctival injection, Tearing, sweating and rhinorrhea") received its name from the short attacks of unilateral neuralgiform headaches, which are accompanied by ipsilateral autonomic symptoms (Sjaastad et al. 1989). Among the trigeminal autonomic cephalalgias, this syndrome presents with the shortest attacks: according to the definition, it may last for 5–240 s but more frequently for 15–120 s. The pain is unilateral and may radiate to the innervation area of n. V/1 and n. V/2. The onset is sudden, but the intensity does not change over time; heavy or moderately strong, but in the majority of the cases, it is not unbearable (unlike the cluster headache). The accompanying symptoms correspond to those of the cluster headache. Frequently the attacks group into episodes, the duration of which may be between some days and months. This can be misleading in the evaluation of the therapeutic response. The disease is much more frequent in male patients. Unlike paroxysmal hemicranias, it can be triggered by touching the face, chewing, swallowing, blowing the nose, movements of the head, even strong light or walking on hard surfaces. It can be differentiated from trigeminal neuralgia as in SUNCT the pain is less severe, the attacks are longer and the autonomic symptoms can also be noticed at the beginning of the attack and accompany even milder bouts. Indomethacin and other drugs against cluster headache or trigeminal neuralgia are usually ineffective in the treatment of SUNCT. However, lamotrigine and topiramate treatment proved to be successful in some instances. SUNCT-like symptoms were described in ipsilateral cerebellopontine arterio-

Table 65.5 The most important representative of trigeminal autonomic cephalalgias is the cluster headache (CH)

Cluster headache and other trigeminal-autonomic cephalalgias	
3.1	Cluster headache
3.1.1	Episodic cluster headache
3.1.2	Chronic cluster headache
3.2	Paroxysmalis hemicrania
3.2.1	Episodic paroxysmal hemicrania
3.2.2	Chronic paroxysmalis hemicrania
3.3	SUNCT syndrome (Short-lasting Unilateral Neuralgiform headache attacks with conjunctival injection and tearing)
3.4	Probable trigeminal autonomic cephalalgia
3.4.1	Probable cluster headache
3.4.2	Probable paroxysmal hemicrania
3.4.3	Probable SUNCT syndrome

Table 65.6 The characteristics of trigeminal-autonomic cephalalgias

Type of headache	Duration (min)	Frequency of attacks (daily)	Triggers	Therapy (effective)
CF	15–180	0.5–8	Alcohol, histamine	Sumatriptan, 100 % O_2
EPH	2–30	3–30	Alcohol	Inhalation, indomethacin
CPH	2–30	1–40	Alcohol	Indomethacin
SUNCT	0.25–2	3–100	Alcohol, touch, other sensory	Unresolved

CH cluster headache, *EPH* episodic paroxysmal hemicrania, *CPH* chronic paroxysmal hemicrania, *SUNCT* short-lasting unilateral neuralgiform headache with nasal congestion and tearing
Common characteristics:

venous malformations, pontine cavernous angiomas, compression of the trigeminal nerve and the pons due osteogenesis imperfecta and venous vasculitides of the orbit. Among our patients in the Neurology Clinic, from five cases, with apparent SUNCT syndrome based on their clinical symptoms, two sufferers proved to have ipsilateral neurovascular compression of the trigeminal nerve according to MR-angiography. Due to the high incidence of headaches of SUNCT-like symptoms, cranial MRI is always recommended in such cases.

Probable trigeminal autonomic cephalalgia headache attacks are believed to be a subtype of trigeminal autonomic cephalalgia, but do not quite meet the diagnostic criteria for any of the subtypes described above (Table 65.6).

Headaches Associated with Diseases of the Eye

The classification of headaches of the International Headache Society deals with the eye disorders in Chap. 11 ("Headache or facial pain attributed to the disorder of cranium, neck, eyes, ears, nose, sinuses, teeth, mouth or other facial or cranial structures"). The first edition of the classification discussed only the painful conditions related to acute glaucoma, refractive errors and heterophoria. However, the second revised edition of 2004 also involved the headaches attributed to inflammatory diseases of the eyes. The lay patient very frequently tries to connect his headache to the disorder of every structure (including the eyes) which is discussed in Chap. 11, due to topographic proximity, even though they develop with considerable gap in time. Therefore, a detailed case history, careful investigation of the given eye disorder and meticulous final evaluation are necessary to establish the putative causal relationship between the disease of the eye and the accompanying pain. Although it does not represent a *sine qua non* of the causal relationship (since in primary headaches the placebo response can reach 30 %), the diagnostic criterion of "headache attributed to disorders of the eyes" requires that the effective treatment of the eye disease also resolves or ceases the headache. The *acute glaucoma attack* is orbital, periorbital or retroorbital severe bout, which may involve the whole head and is accompanied by unilateral, abrupt and progressive deterioration of vision. The patient may observe rainbow like halos around light sources due to the changes in the refraction of the cornea. During the attack, the eyes become hyperemic due to vasodilation of conjunctival blood vessels, the cornea becomes blurred, the pupil gets irregular, and the attack may be accompanied by lacrimation. The eyeball is hard and it is painful upon pressure. The pain can be accompanied by vomiting. The acute glaucoma attack is considered to be a case of emergency. First the pressure of the eye should be decreased, and then follows the causal therapy. The *headaches attributed to refractive errors* are usually mild bilateral conditions localized in the frontal, periorbital or rarely the occipital region. The pain is absent on awakening, it develops due to prolonged visual tasks and increases as the day progresses. Usually it is not accompanied by other symptoms apart from a mild burning sensation of the eyes. To establish the diagnosis, the uncorrected or miscorrected refractive error must be proven. Such headaches are more frequent when the two eyes considerably differ in refractive characteristics or the patient suffers from astigmatism as well. The headache is most frequent between the ages of 40 and 50, when presbyopia develops. When appropriate correction does not resolve the pain, the most frequent reason for primary headaches, the tension headache may be responsible for the complaints. The headache attributed to *heterophoria, or heterotropia* (latent or manifest squinting) recurrent, constant (non-pulsatile), mild or moderately severe, frontal headache. Diagnostic criterion is the demonstration of heterophoria or heterotropia (intermittent blurred vision, diplopia, difficulty in adjusting focus from near to distant objects, for instance) and that the headache develops or worsens during tiring visual tasks. Another criterion is that the headache is relieved or improved on closing one eye. The cause of the headache is the difficulty of retinal image fusion (the image of a fixed point should project to the identical points of the two retinas), which requires the strenuous efforts of the ocular muscles in the case of heterophoria. Therefore, the headache appears on performing exhausting visual tasks, which can be accompanied by blurred vision, diplopia and light sensitivity. Heterophoria can be recognized by covering either eye alternately (cover test). Heterotropia does not necessarily accompany the headache. In those cases, which are present from childhood, headache is rare, while heterotropias which develop later (e.g., due to eye muscles paralysis) headache is common. Tiring of the eyes (prolonged visual task, bad illumination conditions, etc.) may worsen the headache The *headaches attributed to ocular inflammatory disorders* are of orbital, retro- or periorbital localization. The pain develops during the inflammatory process; the inflammation of different structural components (iritis, iridocyclitis, chorioditis) ofthe eyes can be responsible for it. The diagnosis is based upon that the diagnosis and causal treatment of the ocular inflammation also resolve the headache.

Painful Ophthalmoplegia

The syndrome of painful ophthalmoplegia develops in days or weeks, and it is usually caused by processes involving the anterior part of the cavernous sinus or the superior orbital fissure. It can be caused by tumors (primary intracranial tumors, metastases) vascular diseases (aneurysms, dissection of the carotid artery, carotid-cavernous fistula) inflammatory disorders (pseudotumor of the orbit, giant cell arteritis, sarcoidosis, Tolosa–Hunt syndrome) and infections (mycobacterial and fungal processes). Moreover, it can also be related to ophthalmoplegic "migraine" or microvascular infarctions due to diabetes. The careful investigation of painful ophthalmoplegia helps the recognition of conditions which can lead to severe complications or even death without adequate therapy The causes of painful ophthalmoplegia are summarized in Table 65.7.

Table 65.7 The causes of painful ophthalmoplegia

Vascular reasons
Aneurysm of the posterior cerebral artery
Aneurysm of the posterior communicating artery
Intracavernous carotid aneurysm
Thrombosis of the cavernous sinus (septic–aseptic)
Carotid–cavernous fistula
Temporal arteritis
Diabetes: oculomotor nerve mononeuropathy
Pituitary apoplexia
Neoplastic processes
Pituitary adenoma
Pericavernous meningeoma
Tumors of the orbit
Nasopharyngeal tumor with orbital or intracavernous progression
Inflammatory and infectious causes
Tolosa–Hunt-syndrome:
Pseudotumor of the orbit
Sinusitis
Mucocele
Herpes zoster
Mucormycosis
Sarcoidosis
Idiopathic hypertrophic cranial pachymeningitis
Others
Ophthalmoplegic "migraine"

According to Ropper and Brown (2005) with modifications

Tolosa-Hunt-Syndrome

The most important feature of the Tolosa-Hunt syndrome (THS) is the recurrent, unilateral, peri- or retroorbital painful attack, which is accompanied by ipsilateral ocular muscles palsy and responds well to steroid treatment. According to histological studies THS is caused by an aspecific granulomatous inflammatory process of the superior orbital fissure (Tolosa 1954). The paresthesia of the periorbital branch of the trigeminal nerve refers to an intracavernous inflammatory process; orbital localization may result in the loss of vision due to optic nerve compression. The inflammatory alterations can be verified by MR-examination, which also belongs to the diagnostic criteria (Table 65.8).

However, the evaluation of larger sample of cases unveiled that from patients of typical clinical presentation only 35 % had MRI findings typical of THS, 31 % showed different alteration and 33 % was negative (La Mantia et al. 2006). The sedimentation rate was generally high. At the beginning of the symptoms, even the white blood cell count could be increased. The treatment of THS is based upon the administration of corticosteroids (125–500 mg of methylprednisolone orally for 4–5 days, and then those should be tapered); rapid improvement in 1–2 days supports the diagnosis of THS, but does not necessarily exclude other alternatives.

Table 65.8 The diagnostic criteria of Tolosa–Hunt-syndrome (Headache Classification Subcommittee of the International Headache Society 2004)

A. One or more episodes of unilateral orbital pain persisting for weeks if untreated
B. Paresis of one or more of the third, fourth and/or sixth cranial nerves and/or demonstration of a granuloma by MRI or biopsy
C. Paresis coincides with the onset of pain or follows it within 2 weeks
D. Pain and paresis resolve within 72 h when treated adequately with corticosteroids
E. Other causes have been excluded by appropriate investigations

Comments: Some reported cases of Tolosa–Hunt syndrome had additional involvement of the trigeminal nerve (commonly the first division) or optic, facial or vestibulocochlear nerves. Sympathetic innervation of the pupil is occasionally affected. The syndrome was caused by granulomatous material in the cavernous sinus, superior orbital fissure or orbit in some biopsied cases. Careful follow-up is required to exclude other possible causes of painful ophthalmoplegia

Pseudotumor of the Orbit

The syndrome implies a more extended form of the idiopathic granulomatous inflammation and swelling of the external eye muscles. The process frequently involves the globe or other structures of the orbit. The orbital pseudotumor can be accompanied by conjunctival injection and proptosis, which are absent in Tolosa–Hunt syndrome. Rarely can it be accompanied by ipsilateral loss of vision (optic compression). The ultrasound and CT examinations of the orbit reveal enlargement of the ocular muscles and other structures of the orbit. The therapy is based upon corticosteroid administration.

Arteritis Temporalis (Giant Cell Arteritis)

Giant cell arteritis is an immune mediated disorder characterized by the granulomatous inflammation of the middle and large arteries. It is the most frequent systemic vasculitis which usually afflicts patients above 50. Its incidence is about 3–9/100,000 people/year, but above the age of 50, the incidence is 17, and above the age of 80, it is 156 out of 100,000. Although it is a systemic disorder, it selectively affects certain blood vessels: the cranial form involves the temporal artery, the type which afflicts the great vessels involves the aorta, the axillary and the subclavian artery.

Beside the inflammation of the blood vessels, temporal arteritis is frequently accompanied by signs of systemic inflammation, and polymyalgia rheumatica is also a frequent accompanying disease. In this chapter, due to its neuro-ophthalmological aspects, temporal arteritis is discussed. The leading symptom of temporal arteritis, that is the permanent or transient, uni- or bilateral headache of temporal localization, can be found in 70–90 % of the patients. Further, symptoms comprise swollen, tender scalp arteries of decreased pulsation (60 %) polymyalgia rheumatica (25 %), ischemic pain (claudication) of the masticatory muscles (25–40 %), fever, anorexia, weight loss (50%). Diplopia (15%) due to the ischemia of the external eye muscles – amaurosis fugax (36%) or blindness owing to anterior ischemic optic neuropathy (15%) may also develop. The untreated systemic vasculitis may also lead to stroke, sudden loss of hearing, myelopathy, neuropathy, myocardial infarction and aortic aneurysm. The elevated sedimentation rate (>50 mm/h in 90% of the patients) may not be explained by other reasons. The level of C-reactive protein is almost unexceptionally high. Anemia and increased platelet count are also common features. Biopsy of the temporal artery may confirm the diagnosis, but the sensitivity of the histological examination is only 58%, therefore, negative findings cannot exclude the disorder. More precise histological studies require bigger samples or serial biopsies.

The diagnosis can also be supported by the MRI or ultrasound investigation of the thickened temporal arteries. The treatment of temporal arteritis has to be commenced even if the diagnosis is highly probable but not yet confirmed. Currently, the most widely accepted therapeutic regime suggests a large initiating dose of methylprednisolone (15 mg/body weight in kg) for 3 months. Then the maintenance dose is 40 mg/day orally, which should be gradually tapered according to the laboratory parameters. Complementing therapy with anti-aggregation drugs can decrease the risk of ischemic complications. Methotrexate alone is ineffective, but its administration can help decrease the doses of steroids.

References

Angus-Leppan H, Lambert GA, Michalicek J. Convergence of occipital nerve and superior sagittal sinus input in the cervical spinal cord of the cat. Cephalalgia. 1997;17:625–30.

Bahra A, May A, Goadsby PJ. Cluster headache. A prospective clinical study with diagnostic implications. Neurology. 2002;58:354–61.

Bigal ME, Lipton RB. Concepts and mechanisms of migraine chronification. Headache. 2008;48:7–15.

Bigal ME, Lipton RB. The epidemiology, burden, and comorbidities of migraine. Neurol Clin. 2009;27:321–34.

Carroll D. Retinal migraine. Headache. 1970;10:9–13.

Chen W-T, Fuh J-L, Lu S-R, Wang S-J. Persistent migrainous phenomena might be responsive to lamotrigine. Headache. 2001;41:823–5.

Edvinsson L, Uddman R. Neurobiology in primary headaches. Brain Res Rev. 2005;48:438–56.

Ertsey C, Afra J, Berky M, Bozsik G, Szok D, Tajti J, Valikovics A, Vècsei L. Az elsödleges fejfájások klasszifikációja, a migrèn epidemiológiája, a fejfájásban szenvedö betegek kivizsgálási stratègiája, az elsödleges fejfájások kezelèsènek protokollja, a fejfájás centrumok kritèriumai [Classification of primary headaches, the epidemiology of migraine, examination strategy for patients suffering from headaches, the protocol of primary headache therapy and the criteria of centers for patients with headache] (2. kiadás). Cephalalgia Hungarica. 2009;13(19):27–68.

Galezowski X. Ophthalmic megrim: an affection of the vasomotor nerves of the retina and retinal centre which may end in a thrombosis. Lancet. 1882;1:176–9.

Hadjikhani N, Sanchez Del Rio M, Wu O, et al. Mechanisms of migraine aura revealed by functional MRI in human visual cortex. Proc Natl Acad Sci U S A. 2001;98:4687–92.

Headache Classification Subcommittee of the International Headache Society. (2004) The International Classification of Headache Disorders. Cephalalgia. 24(Suppl 1):1–160.

Hill DL, Daroff RB, Ducros A, et al. Most cases labeled as "retinal migraine" are not migraine. J Neuroophthalmol. 2007;27:3–8.

Hoskin KL, Zagami AS, Goadsby PJ. Stimulation of the middle meningeal artery leads to Fos expression in the trigeminocervical nucleus: a comparative study of monkey and cat. J Anat. 1999;194:579–88.

La Mantia L, Curone M, Rapoport AM, Bussone G. Tolosa–Hunt syndrome: critical literature review based on IHS 2004 criteria. Cephalalgia. 2006;26: 772–81.

Lashley K. Patterns of cerebral integration indicated by scotomas of migraine. Arch Neurol Psychiatry. 1941; 46:331–9.

Leao AAP. Spreading depression of activity in the cerebral cortex. J Neurophysiol. 1944;7:359–90.

Lee AG, Brazis PW. Clinical pathways in neuroophthalmology. 2nd ed. New York: Thieme; 2003. p. 1–486.

Liu GT, Schatz NJ, Galetta SL, et al. Persistent positive visual phenomena in migraine. Neurology. 1995;45: 664–8.

May A, Bahra A, Buchel C, Frackowiak RS, Goadsby PJ. Hypothalamic activation in cluster headache attacks. Lancet. 1998;352(9124):275–8.

Mayberg M, Langer RS, Zervas NT, Moskowitz MA. Perivascular meningeal projections from cat trigeminal ganglia: possible pathway for vascular headaches in man. Science. 1981;213(4504):228–30.

Noseda R, Kainz V, Jakubowski M, Gooley JJ, Saper CB, Digre K, Burstein R. A neural mechanism for exacerbation of headache by light. Nat Neurosci. 2010;13:| 239–45.

Olesen J. A neural pathway for photophobia in migraine. Nat Rev Neurol. 2010;6:241–2.

Robertson DM. I am a retinal migraineur. J Neuro-Ophthalmol. 2008;28:81–2.

Ropper AH, Brown RH. Adams and Victor's principles of neurology. 8th ed. New York: McGraw-Hill; 2005. p. 145.
Silberstein SD, Lipton RB, Goadsby PJ. Headache in clinical practice. Oxford: Isis Medical Media; 1998. p. 61–90.
Silberstein SD, Niknam R, Rozen TD, Young WB. Cluster headache with aura. Neurology. 2000;54(1):219–21.
Sjaastad O, Dale I. Evidence for a new (?) treatable headache entity. Headache. 1974;14:105–8.
Sjaastad O, Saunte C, Salvesen R, Fredriksen TA, Seim A, Roe OD, et al. Short lasting unilateral neuralgiform headache attacks with conjunctival injection, tearing, sweating, and rhinorrhea. Cephalalgia. 1989;9(2):147–56.
Spencer SE, Sawyer WB, Wada H, Platt KB, Loewy AD. CNS projections to the pterygopalatine parasympathetic preganglionic neurons in the rat: a retrograde transneuronal viral cell body labeling study. Brain Res. 1990;534(1–2):149–69.
Tolosa E. Periarteritic lesions of the carotid siphon with the clinical features of a carotid infraclinoidal aneurysm. J Neurol Neurosurg Psychiatry. 1954;17:300–2.

Part IX

Rehabilitation

Viewing Down from the Top: Visual Impairments Developing as a Consequence of Cortical Injury

66

Anna Verseghi and Zita Snagy Nagy

Contents

Problems of Consideration: Attention–Eye Movement

Do we see the same things when we look at the object in the environment while going up the hill (to the top) or in case we come down from the top? Is the view the same when we, for example, go to work from home and when we go home? If the view is the same, it is very strange, as we see the environment from different angles of view, however, if we see different things, it is also very interesting, as usually these object are the same along the way. Is it only the location of an object or person in space that determines how we see this object or person? Do only the actual angle of view, our distance from the objects, the speed of our movement, light conditions, changes in the weather, our partners on the road, and changes of animals and moving objects determine what we see at a certain time?

We live our life controlled by our needs, experience, knowledge, and purposes, and they change with age. We always have to be able to highlight those elements from the several pieces of information around us that take us closer to our purposes (for example, tramway number 6), and to use these items as intended (for example, getting on the tramway, holding on, traveling). And then if we realize that we have achieved what we wanted (for example, the proper stop), we have to be able to get away from the item that was so important before (taking off). Then we have to be able to choose–for example, by controlling our look–our next target. In this process, we describe the same object the same way, although it has different meanings and importance for us depending on our actual purpose. We are not living in a meaningless, senseless world. We try to make it meaningful. Let's read the following text.

A. Verseghi, M.D. (✉)
Rehabilitation Unit for Patients with Skull and Brain Injury, National Medical Rehabilitation Institute, Budapest, Hungary
e-mail: averseghi@rehabint.hu

Z.S. Nagy
Department for Multiprofile Rehabilitation of Locomotor Diseases, National Medical Rehabilitation Institute, Budapest, Hungary

Institute of Psychology, Eötvös Lóránd University, Budapest, Hungary
e-mail: snagy.zita@chello.hu

J. Somlai, T. Kovács (eds.), *Neuro-Ophthalmology*, DOI 10.1007/978-3-319-28956-4_66

A XI O M
Re mis
F ed o to be
able to cHo o se: fromwh OM and wha
t todep endon.

We fragmented the translation of an axiom of Akos Fodor. (Hopefully the poet will not get angry because of this.) We can cope with the chaotically looking pattern with some effort. The effort our dear reader experienced shows the power of looking for a meaning, to form an understandable world, "whole items", so called "Gestalt"-s ("Shapes") with meaning from the fragments. Visual perception is an active process including bottom-up (perception) and top-down (guided attention[1] and interpreting organizing perception) processing (Czigler 1999). For detailed information on the complex regulating system of the attention directed to the extrapersonal space described by ***Mesulam*** (1981, 2009), see the chapter on neglect. Regarding this topic, it should be emphasized that active, target oriented, even consciously controlled organization of visual perception is performed by the finely tuned operation of the frontal, primarily the prefrontal cortical regions–among others. Therefore, as a consequence of the injury of the prefrontal structures, a severe perception disorder may occur even if basic perception (bottom-top) processes are normal, so no real visual agnosia (special disorder of visual perception) is present. Functional disorder of the prefrontal lobe leads to difficulty in correct recognition of an object if the view is complex; therefore, processing it requires preliminary analysis and organization. This special neuropsychological disorder is called **pseudoagnosia** (Luria 1966). A patient with symptoms of pseudoagnosia gives opinion about the object he/she sees based on superficial impression, without critical analysis. Someone may say to Fig. 66.1 that it is a "goose with a coach"–considering the poultry photographed from the side to be a coach as it has a baseball cap; considering the upper part of the open beak and the top of the head to be a cap, the patient explained this way where he/she saw the coach. In case of pseudoagnosia, perception is impulsive. Active searching eye movements are decreased in patients with brain injury, and corrective, self-controlling elements are missing from the description of the view as well.

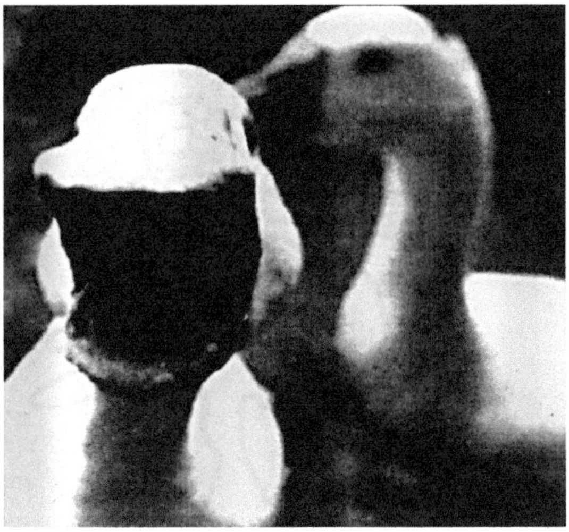

Fig. 66.1 Poultry illustrated in unusual perspective

Therefore, the ability of self-induced, voluntary examination of objects and related selective, active attention are damaged, and this problem is expressed and easily seen in the eye movements of the patient (Luria 1975; Verseghi 2005). The more complex a visual view or scene, the more likely it is that the patient will detect–without visual organization–in fragments, impulsively, superficially, not in accordance with reality, controlled by details. However, a patient with brain injury may combine parts that are not connected, the patient contaminates perception: exceeds borders of separate items or does not respect them, and combines them in one perception. For example, in case of a Poppelreuter's figure (see Fig. 66.2), when the patient's task is to name the object seen in the image, it is not a surprising answer to say that "a fish is boiling in a cauldron, and its blood is pouring here". This type of answer is not always abnormal, it may be a sign of being original, which is the basis of creativity in an adaptive and constructive

[1] Naturally, perception is not organized and modified only by conscious and controlled attention. For example, the first step of perception, detection (noticing) depends on automatic, unconscious processes (orientation reaction) as well enabled by saccadic eye movements (Sekuler and Blake 2000).

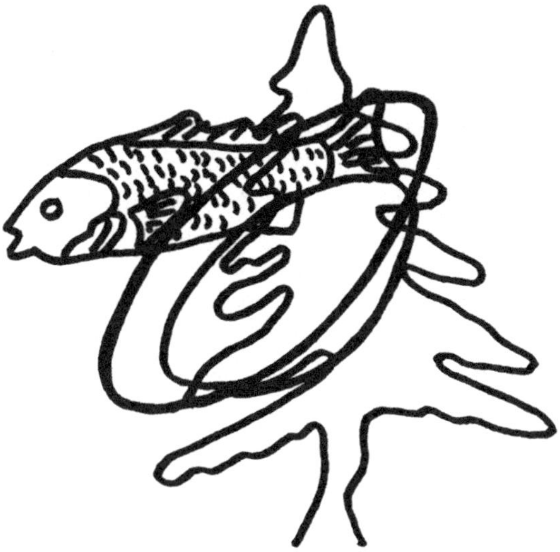

Fig. 66.2 Poppelreuter's figure to test visual impairments

form, and which assumes a high degree of imagination. Imagination, fantasy, certain processes of visual thinking, visual projecting, and designing function may also be injured in case of the damage of the prefrontal area. The role of the frontal (prefrontal) region of both hemispheres is significant in the planning process, but the right hemisphere is the dominant in visual, visual-spatial functions. The problem of the organization of visual information is not present only in case of objects and images, but in the perception of "interpersonal space" as well. In case of prefrontal dysfunction, the patient with brain injury may not be able to properly understand facial expressions, metacommunication of others; the patient often misinterprets the other's intentions. In this case, determining other person's mental condition is impaired (Stuss et al. 2001), and besides the fact that the patient with brain injury has no facial recognition disorder, he/she will easily get lost in social environment, as he/she misunderstands other people, and he/she may easily get into a conflict by unexpected, improper, impulsive reactions if the patient's surrounding has no knowledge of the background mechanism of the problem.

Visual perception may be impaired not only as a consequence of the disorder of highly organized, active attention organization, but due to the dysfunction of other aspects of the attention process. During active perception, look has to be oriented towards the most important objects in our continuously varying, complex visual environment. This may be performed, for example, via the saccadic scanning eye movements controlled on various levels (Sekuler and Blake 2000). Following saccadic eye movements is a well-established method of examining visual attention function in measuring oculomotor activity, and this test is effective in differentiating disorders developing as a result of for example, frontal and parieto-occipital injuries (Karpov et al. 1968). **Simultaneous agnosia** is a characteristic disorder of controlling visual attention from one point to another that is continuous scanning (Luria 1959, 1966; Farah 1990; Luria et al. 1963; Rizzo and Robin 1990; Coslett and Saffran 1991; Nyffeler et al. 2005).

Simultaneous agnosia is a visual attention disorder in case of which the person is unable to notice the details of the surrounding visual world simultaneously. Elementary visual functions are intact, but the patient recognizes only one element of the complex image irrespective of its size, as if the patient had tunnel vision. For example,, if the patient enters a noisy room, he hears that there are a lot of people there, but the patient is able to see only one person at a time, although he/she has no visual field disorder. Simultaneous agnosia may be of various severity, and although it occurs rarely, the patient usually has severe problems in everyday life. For example, the patient may be unable to draw as he/she sees only the paper or only the pencil, and he/she is unable to combine these two objects. In the neuro-ophthalmologic examination, Ishihara tables may be well used in addition to the examination of saccadic eye movements (EOG) in diagnosing simultaneous agnosia. Persons with brain injury have difficulty in naming numbers, although they recognize the colors well (Brasis et al. 1998). (Naturally, naming the numbers may be difficult due to another disorder, for example, aphasia as well. Be careful, and ensure not to confuse various types of symptoms that may be similar in appearance.)

The disease has two forms (Farah 1990): ***dorsal*** simultaneous agnosia develops in case of bilateral parieto-occipital injury, the ***ventral*** form occurs in case of the injury of the left inferior occipito-temporal area. Dorsal simultaneous agnosia may occur alone, but may be accompanied by two characteristic symptoms, ocular apraxia (psychic paralysis of gaze) and optic ataxia (see later).

The three symptoms together are called **Balint's syndrome** (Newcombe and Ratcliff 1989; Vertfaellie et al. 1990; Baylis and Baylis 2001), which develops as a consequence of bilateral lesion of the parieto-occipital area. This syndrome is rarely seen in the clinical practice, but case reports of rehabilitation of patients with such symptoms can be found in the literature (Rosselli et al. 2001). The syndrome was described by ***Rezso Bdlint*** in 1907; the group of symptoms was named after him (Husain and Stein 1988). Two symptoms of the syndrome, simultaneous agnosia and optic ataxia will be described in detail below in this chapter. About the third symptom, ocular apraxia, also called as psychic paralysis of gaze, it should be noted that the essence of the problem is that the patient with brain injury cannot switch his look to the new object appearing in the periphery via the foveal system (Watson and Rapcsak 1989). Although eye movements are intact, attention cannot be switched to objects appearing in the periphery.

Real Visual Agnosia

Visual Analysis and Its Disorders

We described the visual disorders developing as a consequence of lesion of higher levels of ***attention processes*** of vision above in detail. Dysfunctions of the visual ***perception*** system are described below; these can be considered to be real visual agnosia, a disorder of processing the "input visual pattern". Visual perception alone, without the closely related attention network, has several levels. A complex image arrives to the brain from the eye, and this image has to be broken down to elements and has to be analyzed in order to be processed. This analysis is performed along some characteristic visual features (such as brightness, color, direction, depth, movement) in the visual cortex (Sekuler and Blake 2000; Csatho 2008; Kovács 2003). Most common consequence of the disorder of visual analysis is the disorder of color perception (dyschromatopsia, achromatopsia), disorder of direction perception, disorder of depth perception (astereopsis), and disorder of movement perception (akinetopsia).

Dyschromatopsia and **achromatopsia** (Farah 1990; Csatho 2008; Zeki 1992; Short and Graff-Radford 2001) may develop as a consequence of the injury of the occipito-temporal, lingual, and fusiform gyri. In this case, besides the fact that basic color vision of the rods is intact in the retina, these people are unable to detect certain colors (dyschromatopsia) or in more severe cases, they are unable to detect colors, they see the colorful world as black and white or in the shades of gray (achromatopsia). In case of unilateral brain damage, disorder of color perception affects only one side (contralateral to the injury) (hemidyschromatopsia, hemiachromatopsia). During neuropsychological examination of the disorder, the patient is asked to name the color of cards, threads, and objects, and to group them according to colors. Using the two examinations together makes differentiating color agnosia and color anomia possible. Color agnosia affects the perception of the color, so the patient has difficulty in naming and grouping colors as well. In case of color anomia, the patient detects the colors, but he/she is unable to pair the proper word to them, so the patient is unable to name the color, but grouping according to colors is normal. The effect of cortical color blindness on the everyday life is well represented by the case report of a painter, Oliver Sachs (1999), who became color blind. In case of the **disorder of determining directions** (Benton et al. 1975; Hamsher et al. 1992), the person is unable to properly determine the spatial direction of lines in an image. The *"looking for parallel lines"* test is an excellent tool to examine the phenomenon (Vilkki 1984). The examined person has to find lines that are parallel to the one circled in the middle in Fig. 66.3 (we usually ask the examined person to number the lines). The figure represents the solution of a person who has not only diffi-

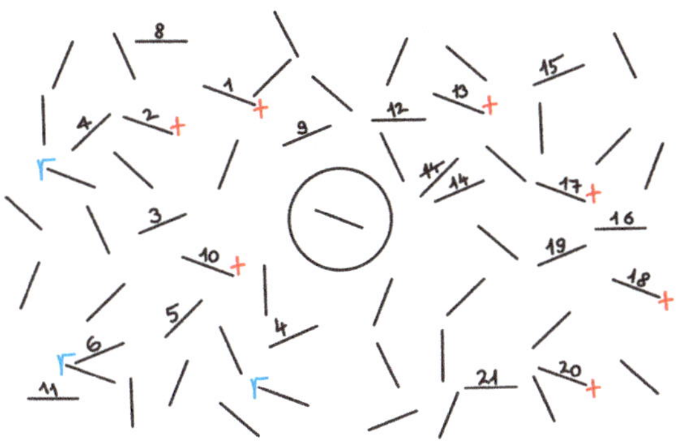

Fig. 66.3 Visual search for parallel lines test– reduced sized. Numbered parallel lines. Not numbered parallel lines

culty in determining directions, but neglect symptom as well as seen from the lines missed on the left side.

In the everyday life, patient with brain injury and disorder of determining directions has difficulty in for example, reading the clock. However, proper perception of the direction of various lines may be the basis of contour detection as well (detecting the edge of images, objects), so its dysfunction may cause problems in higher levels of object recognition as well (Csatho 2008).

In case of **astereopsis** (Newcombe and Ratcliff 1989; Csatho 2008; Benton et al. 1975), depth perception is damaged. Although binocular vision is intact, perception and estimation of the depth and distance of objects are abnormal, which may cause problem in higher levels of vision as well. For example, in everyday life, the patient may reach next to the objects (before of behind it) or try to pull the soup on the table closer till they cover themselves with the soup. These phenomena are very similar to the symptoms of optic ataxia (see later). However, in case of depth perception disorders, problems occur only in the dimension of depth of visually controlled activities, but not in horizontal or lateral direction. The disease is most commonly caused by the injury of the right hemisphere.

Akinetopsia (Csatho 2008; Zeki 1992) is a special visual deficiency when the patient does not see movements and he/she cannot interpret the movements seen. This patient recognizes static objects well, but moving objects are invisible for this patient, while auditory and tactile perception of movement remains intact.

A patient with akinetopsia is significantly disturbed by situations with more than one moving object. For example, being in a large company and traveling with high speed pose great difficulty to the patients, because a lot of people are moving at the same time, so social events often lead to anxiety for these patients. Akinetopsia is caused by the injury of the prestriatal area called V5, as the cells of the cerebral area V5 respond to movement, the majority of these cells are sensitive to the direction of moving as well. Visual perception of movement may be injured alone independent from the injury of the visual perception of objects and the space. It is important to note that disorder of perception of depth or movement is not always apparent. These visual cortical dysfunctions may lead to uncertain feelings in the person, which make moving in the physical space and being in social environment fearful. All these factors slow down relearning in rehabilitation, and it may occur as "incomprehensible" hesitation in visually controlled processes of self-sufficiency. Practical problems are often misinterpreted, especially if visual dysfunctions affect a diagnostic blind spot and remain hidden and untreated. Phobia may be suspected due to the emotional expressions and the behavior of the person with brain injury. It is recommended, for example, to think of real visual disorders (examine this disease) in the background of fear and withdrawal in persons treated with agoraphobia.

Visual Integration and Its Disorders

After visual analysis, the brain reintegrates the individual elements. This integration process is performed in two parallel pathways, as visual perception is characteristic of having (at least) two neural subsystems:

(**1**) ***ventral (occipito-temporal) pathway,*** (**2**) ***dorsal (occipito-parietal) pathway.***[2] Although

[2] For details of mechanism of parallel information processing in the visual system, see the chapter of this book written by György Benedek.

the two cortical pathways of visual perception have been known for a long time, regarding the main functions of the pathways, certain authors consider different locations to be of primary importance (Kovács 2003). The purpose of this chapter is not to describe it in details, and the extent of this book does not allow it either. In order to better understand visual disorders, we briefly described ***Goodale's and Milner's action-perception hypothesis*** (Goodale and Milner 1992; Milner and Goodale 2008) below.[3] If you think about it, visual perception may have two essential functions for a living being: (1) to know what it sees, (2) to know where it is that it sees, and as a consequence, to know how to approach, get, or avoid it. For the former, characteristics of visual perception (size, shape, color, etc.) have to be processed, and for the latter, spatial location and position of the object have to be processed with related information regarding moving. The former function can be connected to the ventral pathway system, its function enables the development of the image representation of an object, therefore ***object recognition.*** The latter function can be connected to the dorsal pathway which is the basis of ***visually controlled movement regulation.*** As a consequence, the injury of the ventral visual pathway leads to object recognition disorders, while the injury of the dorsal visual pathway causes problems in the regulation of visual-motor activities. **Neglect syndrome** (for details see the next chapter) is a complex disorder that may affect spatial perception, spatial attention, and regulation of spatial movement, so the dorsal visual pathway, but object recognition, that is the ventral pathway as well. It should be emphasized that several factors may be in the background of object recognition disorders, such as pseudoagnosia, neglect, apperceptive, or associative agnosia (see later), these disorders may be differentiated by qualitative neuropsychological analysis. In vision development, the ventral pathway is considered to be phylogenetically younger and it is thought to develop later in ontogenesis compared to the dorsal pathway (Kovács 2003). Accommodating to this developmental order, first, visual integration disorders that may be linked to the dorsal visual pathway will be described, and then disorders connected to the ventral system will be presented.

Integration Disorders of the Dorsal System

Optic ataxia (Damasio and Benton 1979; Levine et al. 1978) is the disorder of hand movement toward an object (or any movement toward a target) controlled by visual information with intact primary visual sensory-motor and somato-sensory functions. Although patients are able to accurately localize the position of the object, if they want to touch it, they miss them when reaching for them. However, movements toward a target that are not controlled by visual information are not impaired. For example, in case of a standard neurological examination, finger-to-nose tests are performed properly. It is suggested that integration of visual stimuli and proprioceptive movement information is damaged in this disease. Optic ataxia is the dysfunction of the connection of the parieto-occipital and premotor areas. In case of bilateral injuries, disorders are significant, and can be detected in case of both hands. In the everyday life, continuous writing of these persons may be slightly irregular; however, if they write with block letters, their writing becomes almost unrecognizable, as they lift the writing tool, they cannot continue at exactly the sample place, where they stopped, and therefore their drawings are very chaotic.

Patients see that they are unsuccessful, and try to correct themselves. Missing when reaching and sensory-motor coordination problem decrease or even disappear, if the patient with optic ataxia writes (can write) or draws (can draw) without lifting the pen. If the patient with brain injury is asked to circle scattered numbers in a paper and link them in order during the examination of optic ataxia, the patient can perform this test only after several attempts. An example, of this is seen in Fig. 66.4.

[3] The theory of Mishkin et al. (1983) is the consequence of the action-perception hypothesis. According to the theory, there are two basic visual system, the What (ventral) and the Where (dorsal) systems.

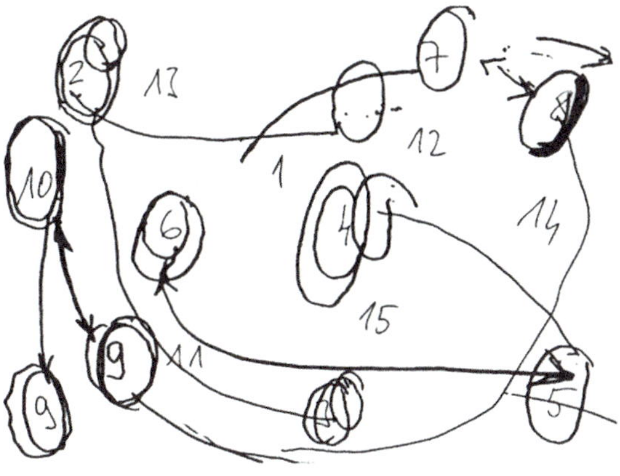

Fig. 66.4 Performance of a patient having optic ataxia in connecting and circling numbers

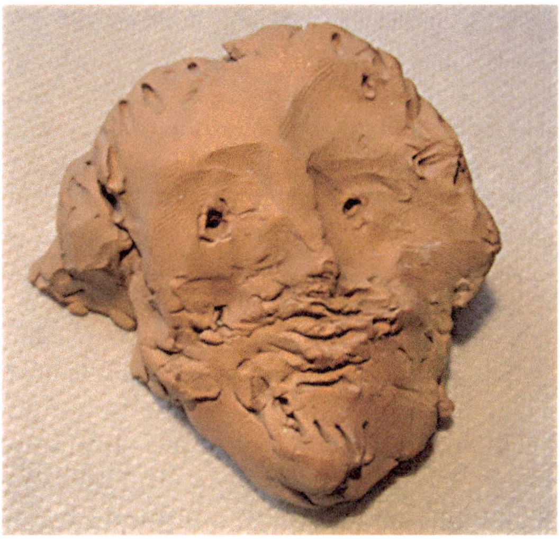

Fig. 66.5 Sculpture performed by a patient with optic ataxia

The same patient prepared a clay sculpture, as a result of the continuous movement, a head shape is recognizable (Fig. 66.5). Parts that can be prepared with a single movement–such as the eyes–are relatively successful. Where the movement had to be interrupted to elaborate it, and the work had to be restarted (for example, in case of preparing the mouth), the patient missed the target and besides several attempts, this part of the sculpture became almost unrecognizable.

Disorder of spatial orientation (Newcombe and Ratcliff 1989) can be discovered in some "wandering" patients. For example,, the patient is unable to tell someone the way home or show it in a map, and the patient is unable to navigate in a new environment.

This symptom may be part of a visual spatial memory disorder, posttraumatic amnesia, general disorientation, or dementia. It may develop alone as well, or may occur with or accompany the disorder of the direction, depth, and/or movement perception.

Integration Disorders of the Ventral System

Arranging primary information with visual modality is the first step of integration after visual analysis in the process of object recognition, during which the actual perception is complemented by visual information stored in related memory. For example, the image of a table may be complemented by the visual image of the currently not seen, covered parts present in the memory, so the complete spatial visual representation of the table develops in our brain. At the next level of integration, the actual visual representation is compared with object representations stored in the memory, therefore it gets meaning, and the object can be identified. As a final step of integration, linguistic representation is connected to the meaning of the image, and naming the object becomes possible (Csatho 2008). Disorder of object recognition is the inability to identify objects and the disorder is not the consequence of a significant visual problem (decreased visual acuity, blindness) or other cognitive injuries (difficulty finding words, attention disorder, general intellectual deterioration). There are two basic forms of object recognition disorders[4] (Karpov et al. 1968; Séra 2008; Juhász 2000), these are the consequences of the injury of differ-

[4] Humphreys and Riddoch believe that a patient having problems with several object recognition problems are difficult to classify according to Lissauer's dual (apperceptive and associative agnosia) classification, therefore, a more detailed classification is recommended. They differentiate shape, integrative, and transformational agnosia within apperceptive agnosia and divide associative agnosia into semantic and semantic access agnosia (Juhász 2000; Séra 2000).

ent levels of the above described integration process (Csatho 2008).

1. **Visual apperceptive agnosia** is the consequence of an injury in the first level of integration; in this case, stable visual representation cannot develop during perception.
2. In case of **visual associative agnosia,** visual perception is normal, but the patient does not recognize the meaning of the object, so in this case, access to semantic knowledge is injured.

How can visual apperceptive and visual associative agnosia be differentiated? Qualitative neuropsychological analysis is necessary for the differential diagnosis, as the abnormalities are not seen in the amount of mistakes but in the quality of the mistakes. In the following section, the different neuropsychological characteristics of the two visual agnosias will be described.

In case of **visual apperceptive agnosia** (Karpov et al. 1968; Séra 2008; Grossman et al. 1997), recognition of visually introduced objects or images of objects is injured despite the fact that primary sensory processes are normal. A characteristic of apperceptive agnosia is that not only recognition, but the ability to copy (image, text), write, read may be damaged in the patient with brain injury, as well as matching objects with same meaning, for example, the patient is unable to categorize two combs in the same group. Patient with severe symptoms of apperceptive agnosia for example, thought the clock to be a circle and the numbers in it to be black spots.

About the apple, the patient said: "This is red, as if it was an apple." The patient considered the scissors to be two cap-shapes and a longitudinal form. The same patient had difficulty in writing and drawing as well (Fig. 66.6).

In certain cases of apperceptive agnosia, the patient detects objects and images presented in the usual way accurately. However, if the image is presented in an unusual perspective (Fig. 66.1) or only the silhouette of the object is illustrated (Fig. 66.7), the patient makes a mistake (Séra 2008). For a healthy person, it is not a problem to recognize the same object in different or unusual spatial positions to be the same, the size of the object is not influenced by the different distance, and the color of the object is not affected by illumination. This is the significance of object constancy, which may be impaired in case of apperceptive agnosia, and therefore these patients

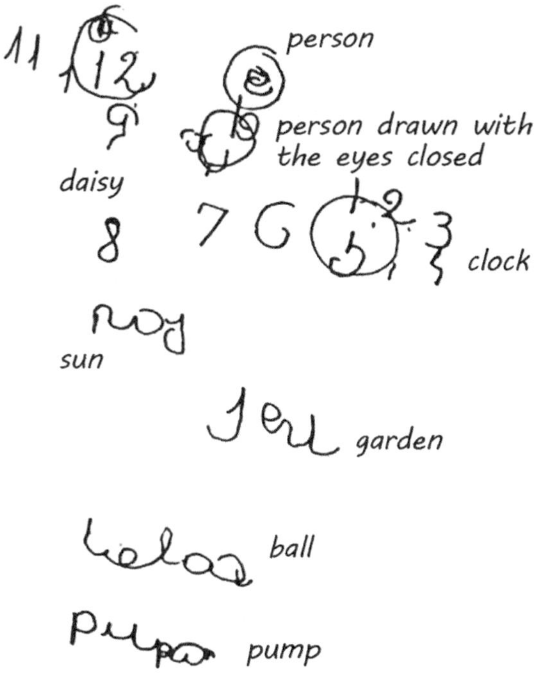

Fig. 66.6 Drawing and writing to dictation of a patient with apperceptive agnosia

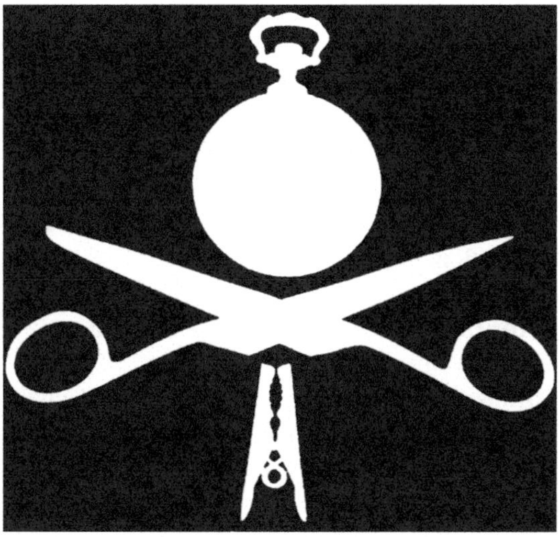

Fig. 66.7 Examination to test silhouette recognition

have poor results in recognizing images with unusual perspectives (Séra 2000).

The patient with apperceptive agnosia makes characteristic mistakes in line drawing using the Poppelreuter figure (see Fig. 66.2) as well, as the patient is so disturbed by the overlapping lines that he/she is often not able to follow the contour of each object (compare the performance of the following patient with associative agnosia in line drawing using the Poppelreuter figure).

Visual associative agnosia (Farah 1990; McCarthy and Warring ton 1986; Mack and Boller 1977) is present if recognition may be possible in the level of perception, but the patient is unable to access the meaning of the object. In case of visual associative agnosia (contrary to visual apperceptive agnosia), patients use formal characteristics of the objects in recognition, patients are able to align, able to draw the objects they do not know what they are, they even copy shapes or complex figures well without knowing their meaning. Objects with similar shape and form are most often confused. Patient with associative agnosia can recognize the overlapping drawings of objects (the fish, the plate, and the pine–see Fig. 66.2), but as the meaning of the objects do not activate, the patient is unable to name them. "I can see it, but I do not know what it is" described this problem very expressively a patient with associative agnosia. A sign of compensation may be that the patient tries to give meaning to something that he/she sees based on formal similarity, for example, he/she believes the plate to be a hat. This confusion should not be confused with optic aphasia, in which the meaning is attached to the object, but naming the visually presented object is damaged (Iorio et al. 1992). For the sake of illustration, but not as a case report, we present M. T., 15-year-old female patient having symptoms of associative agnosia. The patient is right handed and has brain injury. Her performance is seen in some tests during neuropsychological examination 4–5 months after the traumatic brain injury. The injury mainly affected the left hemisphere temporally and occipitally (based on CT and MRI). The neuro-ophthalmologic examination showed right-sided homonymous hemianopsia caused by excessive lesion in the left optic radiation and showed left lower quadrant quadrantopia. The patient was aware of her difficulties. Her first symptom was that "I do not know what is what", "I do not know what does each food like, only if they tell me that". In comparison, she gave the following response to Fig. 66.1 presented before (image from an unusual perspective): "it is surely a person, at least it looks like one"–said the patient about the animal shown from the front–"and this looks like a horse"–pointed the girl to the goose at the back. Uncertainty can be observed in her answers ("looks like"), and her complaints can be explained by the apparent difficulty. Persons with symptoms of pseudoagnosia do not have this kind of uncertainty when performing the tests, they do not describe their problem, and they often have no complaints. Figure 66.8 shows that M. T. drew a colored line around the forms that she thought to be single shapes–we asked to use one

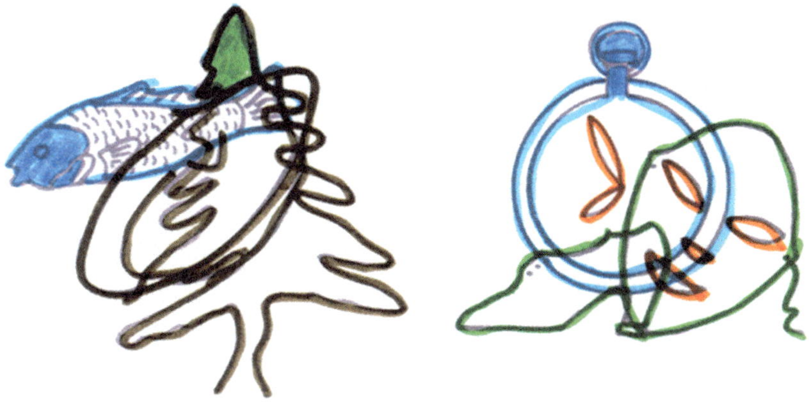

Fig. 66.8 Solutions of M. T. for the task of drawing the lines in the Poppelreuter's figures

color for each shape–in the test performed with Poppelreuter figures (see the baseline in Fig. 66.2). Based on the test, it can be seen that she formed "good whole figures" perceptually. Essentially, she differentiated the real forms in the drawing well, however, it can be seen that she organized forms in the same unit that were part of different figures based on perceptual similarity–see drawings with orange.

While performing the test, the patient was unable to tell us what she drew around. M. T. identified the colors practically well, although she could not name them. In addition, she performed well in copying tests requiring eye movement coordination. In the reduced line following test shown in Fig. 66.9, the patient has to say which letter he/she reaches if he/she starts from a number on the left side and follows each line. M. T. solved this test without any mistake, which shows that primary perceptual organizational processes that made her able to solve this rest successfully were intact, so she was able to discriminate and follow complex mix of lines.

Figure 66.10 shows drawings of M. T. prepared for the request of the examiner. From the left to the right in order: circle, triangle, square, cube, glass, table, in the 2nd line: apartment, tree, man. It can be noted that the patient is able to form linear and round lines, and to connect them, so she has the basic visual-motor abilities required for drawing. The apartment, tree and man drawings are strange as these "items" have characteristics that are illustrated properly, but are combined with parts that are not correct or not exactly correct regarding the real characteristics of the object (mental representation).

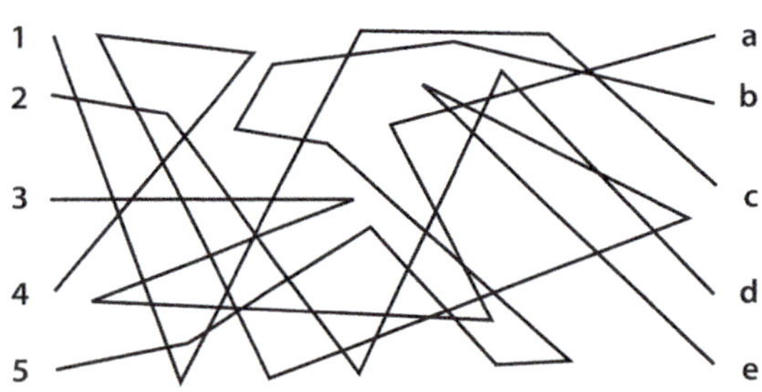

Fig. 66.9 Following lines–one of Rey's tests (reduced)

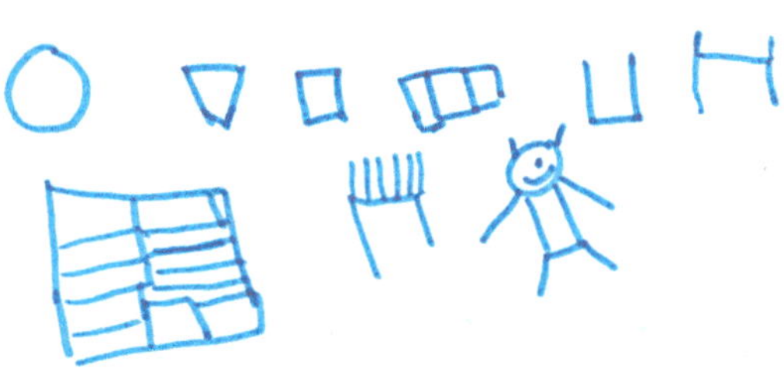

Fig. 66.10 Drawings of M. T.

For example, the man has an eye in the middle, and it cannot be defined if there are two horns in the head or the two lines represent the ears. M. T. could not name ordinary objects, such as the telephone, if she only saw it or only touched it with her hand. However, when the examiner helped her by telling her to listen to the "lifted" part of the object–receiver–as soon as she heard the humming sound, she recognized and named the telephone from its sound. M. T. had general difficulty in naming objects, and it meant even larger problem to identify animals, cars, and faces of people. It can be said that recognizing the meaning of living (whether it is coming towards or away from her) and moving objects with seemingly continuously changing shapes was almost impossible for her. She was unable to memorize the names of the pets around her. She had difficulty reading as well. Regarding her memory, she had difficulty remembering verbs and images verbally, although she recognized visually seen objects easily, when she had to select them from images.

Neuropsychological examination of M. T. was very detailed, and followed her condition (improvement) for several years, although currently, due to limited space, we have to be content with the presented examples. Regarding rehabilitation, she had to relearn "meaning field" of the world around her, somewhat like when a small child gets to know the world, but it was a little different, as she had clear concepts in her head, she used the language properly, she was able to talk, and to perform abstract thinking. She needed an individual, experimental, developing path for her individual problem, her family, friends, school, and therapists accompanied her in this path. There was no previously manufactured "therapeutic uniform package" for her that could have been given to her after her accident.

Patients with difficulties of **prosopagnosia** (Sekuler and Blake 2000; Farah 1990; Séra 2008; De Haan et al. 1992; Ettlin et al. 1992; Busigny et al. 2010; Sacks 2008) have visual recognition disorder specifically affecting faces. Patients with brain injury and facial recognition disorder often recognize their acquaintances only from their voices or other characteristic feature (such as a tattoo), and/or are unable to remember new persons based on their faces. During their examination, it is often seen that these patients are unable to accurately determine the similarity and difference of faces shown simultaneously. The problem is caused by bilateral injury of the temporal area or injury of the temporal area on the right side. It is a basic question in the literature whether prosopagnosia is a special disorder alone or a symptom of a general dysfunction of visual recognition. There are several reports and examinations analyzing various types of facial recognition problems, their connections and forms of dissociations with more and more differentiated methods (Delvenne et al. 2004; Anaki et al. 2007). Appearance of prosopagnosia may be classified based on whether the problem is in processing the visual pattern of the face (like apperceptive agnosia) or activation of the meaning of the face (whose face) (like in case of associative agnosia, when the meaning of the objects cannot be mobilized). In the previous case, the patient is unable to recognize the difference and similarity or identity of the faces due to discrimination, transformation, or integration difficulties. In the latter case, the person is unable to recognize familiar faces or faces of famous people. In the clinical practice, prosopagnosia may be suggested based on the complaints of the relatives, for example, the patient isolates from his/her relatives and does not recognize them. However, it is not sure that prosopagnosia is in the background of such problems, it may be Capgras syndrome. The patient with symptoms of Capgras syndrome considers familiar faces to be foreign, while the patient recognizes faces well. For example, the patient refuses to be with his/her closest relatives, as he/she thinks that they have been replaced with substitutes who are imitators (Draaisma 2009). Sometimes patients consider their relatives to be aliens. The patient may be so afraid of an attack that he/she may cause injuries for the person wrongly perceived to be foreign. It is important to differentiate neurological (neurodegenerative–Lewy body dementia) and other types of problems (such as so called paranoid psychotic conditions) in the background of the disorder (Joseph 2007). Fregoli's symptom (Lykouras et al. 2002; Tényi et al. 1999) may appear with Capgras syndrome or alone, in this case, the patient considers unknown people to be familiar, for example, he/she thinks that the roommates in the hospital are relatives or friends. Fregoli's delusion most often occurs in case of schizophrenia, schizoaffective disorders, but may occur after organic injury (such as cerebral contusion) or in case of disorientation. Capgras and Fregoli phenomena occur in emotional conditions, in case of alienation or in case of making foreign faces familiar, the facial recognition problem usually occurs in case of an emotional condition.

Consciousness, Acknowledgement and Visual Perception

"Do You See It? Don't You See It? You See It!"

In case of the above described Capgras syndrome and Fregoli symptom, and the previously mentioned neglect syndrome, patients are usually not aware of their problems. Anton's syndrome (McDaniel and McDaniel 1991; Argenta and Morgan 1998) is a similar, but perhaps more unbelievable phenomenon, in case of which the patient denies cortical blindness. Cortical blindness may be caused by the extensive bilateral injury of the occipital lobe (complete injury of Brodmann areas 17, 18, 19). In this case, the patient with brain injury has no visual experience, however, the anterior visual pathways are intact[5] (Celesia et al. 1991). Patient with Anton's syndrome are often looking for excuses why they

[5]Celesia et al. (1991) describes the criteria of cortical blindness as follows: (1) lack of every visual experience, (2) loss of the oculo-palpebral reflex, (3) intact pupil reactions when looking at the distance and at a close object too, (4) normal fundus, (5) no disorder is seen in the function of extraocular eye movements.

are not able to see at the moment (for example, there is not enough light) or they are asserting that they can see so much that they threaten their physical integrity (for example, they the bump into the wall). Anton syndrome is a type of missing acceptance of the disease (anosognosia) which is usually accompanied by dementia, but it may occur in case of local injury of the brain or severe bilateral disorder of the frontal lobe (Argenta and Morgan 1998). Anton syndrome seems to be more special if we consider the close relationship between vision and consciousness (awareness) that is expressed so variously in our language (such as "see through", "realizes", "glimpses", "I believe it if I can see it", "does not believe his eyes").

Blind vision is another strange phenomenon related to cortical blindness (Sekuler and Blake 2000; Gulyás et al. 2003). Patients with cortical blindness may have certain visual abilities left. They may be able to determine the location of a stimulus with larger possibility compared to coincidence, realize motion, or differentiate direction of lines or simple forms (such as an X- or O-shape) besides the fact that the patient has no experience about visual information. It can be suggested that the brain–supposedly via the superior colliculus–process visual information below the cortex as well, therefore, this unconscious performance resembling vision is possible. In case of blind vision, detection does not become perception, but the nervous system uses the information. As the patient may respond to the unconscious, but still used information as a reflex (for example, turning towards the stimulus), the patient's environment may doubt the severity of the patient's blindness. The responsibility of the professionals is especially important in this case, to explain the background of the phenomenon to the relatives in detail, as they may have unreal expectations to the future of the recovery of the patient thinking of "blind vision" as a ray of hope.

In case of Anton's syndrome, the patient, or in case of blind vision, the relatives and friends may have problems with disease acknowledgement. If the visual disorders occur with problems of disease awareness, rehabilitation becomes more complicated. The goal of rehabilitation is to change, so it is based on willingness and ability to change. However, only those problems can be willingly changed that we are aware of, so one of the driving forces of rehabilitation is awareness. Therefore, in case of ability disorders accompanied by anosognosia, it is not enough to therapeutically develop the missing ability, but awareness of the patient has to be supported first (Verseghi et al. 2010). This awareness process should be performed by a neuropsychologist, or psychologist trained in the field, as organic disorders of awareness can easily be misunderstood as a preventing mechanism driven by psychic self-protection superficially. The two problems require different therapeutic approach.

Overview

This chapter reviews information collected during neuropsychological examination and rehabilitation of adults having brain injury and related literature. We would like to emphasize that injury of the visual perceptive processes in children with brain injury has different characteristics. Psychic structure of the perceptive process changes with age and by learning the language, concepts fixed in the language give new opportunities for perception (Luria 1975). We may say that little children think and remember the same way as they notice, however, an adult recognizes as he/she thinks and remembers. As the frontal lobe (prefrontal regions) matures, we become more and more able to consciously organize our impressions top-down, change, renew again and again, and cure with empathy (Verseghi et al. 2010). The above subtitle receives meaning only from this higher, more abstract level.

Carefully check, whether you understand what you saw above. You received an insight into the higher organized top-down processes of the visual system, and now, while reviewing the last lines, you may find out whether you are able to read between the lines, and whether the presented concept is clear and our field of vision increases or not.

SEE you later.

References

Anaki D, Kaufman Y, Freedman M, Moscovitch M. Associative (prosop)agnosia without (apparent) perceptual deficits: a case-study. Neuropsychologia. 2007;45:1658–71.

Argenta PA, Morgan MA. Cortical blindness and Anton syndrome in a patient with obstetric hemorrhage. Obstet Gynecol. 1998;91:810–2.

Baylis GC, Baylis LL. Visually misguided reaching in Balint's syndrome. Neuropsychologia. 2001;39:865–75.

Benton AL, Hannay HJ, Varney NR. Visual perception of direction in patients with unilateral brain disease. Neurology. 1975;25:907910.

Brasis PW, Graff-Radford NR, Newman NJ, Lee AG. Ishiara color plates as a test for simultanagnosia. Am J Ophthalmol. 1998;126(6):850–1.

Busigny T, Graf M, Mayer E, Rossion B. Acquired prosopagnosia as a face-specific disorder: ruling out the general visual similarity account. Neuropsychologia. 2010;48:2051–67.

Celesia GG, Bushnell D, Cone Toleikis S, Brigell MG. Cortical blindness and residual vision: is the "second" visual system in humans capable of more than rudimentary visual perception? Neurology. 1991;41:862–9.

Coslett HB, Saffran E. Simultanagnosia. To see but not to see. Brain. 1991;114:1523–45.

Csatho Á. A vizuális észlelés neuropszichológiája. In: Bevezetés a neuropszichológiába [Neuropsychology of visual perception In: Introduction to neuropsychology] (Kállai J, Bende I, Karádi K, Racsmány M szerk.) Budapest: Medicina; 2008. P. 115–62.

Czigler I. Figyelem és percepció. [Attention and perception]. Debrecen: Kossuth Egyetemi Kiadó; 1999.

Damasio AR, Benton AL. Impairment of hand movements under visual guidance. Neurology. 1979;29:170–8.

De Haan EHF, Bauer KM, Greve KW. Behavioural and psychological evidence for covert face recognition in a prosopagnosic patient. Cortex. 1992;28:77–95.

Delvenne JF, Seron X, Coyette F, Rossion B. Evidence for perceptual deficits in associative visual (prosop)agnosia: a single-case study. Neuropsychologia. 2004;4:597–612.

Draaisma D. Kizökkent elmék. [Disrupted minds]. Budapest: Gondolat Kiadó; 2009.

Ettlin TM, Beckson M, Benson DF, Lang fitt JT, Amos EC, Pineda GS. Prosopagnosia: a bihemispheric disorder. Cortex. 1992;28:129–34.

Farah MS. Visual agnosia. Disorders of object recognition and what they tell us about normal vision. Cambridge: The MIT Press; 1990. p. 7–30.

Goodale MA, Milner AD. Separate visual pathways for perception and action. Trends Neurosci. 1992;15(1):20–5.

Grossman M, Galetta S, D'Esposito M. Object recognition difficulty in visual apperceptive agnosia. Brain Cogn. 1997;33:306–42.

Gulyás B, Kovács Gy, Vidnyánszky Z. A vizuális tudat. In: Kognitív idegtudomány [The visual consciousness. In: Cognitive neurology.] (Pléh Cs, Kovács Gy, Gulyás B szerk.). Budapest: Osiris Kiadó; 2003. P. 620–49.

Hamsher K, Caproso DX, Bemon A. Visuospatial judgement and right hemisphere disease. Cortex. 1992;28:493–5.

Husain M, Stein J. Rezső Bálint and his most celebrated case. Arch Neurol. 1988;45:89–93.

Iorio L, Falanga A, Fragassi NA, Grossi D. Visual associative agnosia and optic aphasia. A single case study and review of the syndromes. Cortex. 1992;28:23–37.

Joseph KA. Capgras syndrome and its relationship to neurodegenerative disease. Arch Neurol. 2007;64(12):1762–6.

Juhász LZ. BORB, egy új tesztbatéria a vizuális tárgyfelismerés zavarainak vizsgálatára. [BORB, a new test battery to examine disorders of visual object recognition]. Magyar Pszichológiai Szemle. 2000;4:375–87.

Karpov BA, Luria AR, Yarbuss AL. Disturbances of the structure of active perception in lesions of the posterior and anterior regions of the brain. Neuropsychologia. 1968;6:157–66.

Kovács I. Az emberi látás fejlődése. In: Kognitív idegtudomány [Development of human vision. In: Cognitive neurology] (Pléh Cs, Kovács Gy, Gulyás B szerk.) Budapest, Osiris Kiadó; 2003. P. 273–84.

Levine DN, Kaufman KJ, Mohr JP. Inaccurate reaching associated with a superior parietal lobe tumor. Neurology. 1978;28:556–61.

Luria AR. Disorders of "simultaneous perception" in a case of bilateral occipito-parietal brain injury. Brain. 1959;82(3):437–49.

Luria AR. Higher cortical functions in man. New York: Basic books; 1966. p. 451–61.

Luria AR. Válogatott tanulmányok. [Selected studies]. Budapest: Gondolat; 1975.

Luria AR, Pravdina-Vinarskaya EN, Yarbuss AL. Disorders of ocular movement in a case of simultanagnosia. Brain. 1963;86(2):219–28.

Lykouras L, Typaldou M, Gournellis R, Vaslamatzis G, Christodoulou G. Coexistence of Capgras and Fregoli syndromes in a single patient. Clinical, neuroimaging and neuropsychological findings. Eur Psychiatry. 2002;17:234–5.

Mack JL, Boller F. Associative visual agnosia and its related deficits: the role of the minor hemisphere in assigning meaning to visual perceptions. Neuropsychologia. 1977;15:345–9.

McCarthy RA, Warring ton EK. Visual associative agnosia: a clinicoanatomical study of a single case. J Neural Neurosurg Psychiatry. 1986;49:1233–40.

McDaniel KD, McDaniel LD. Anton's syndrome in a patient with posttraumatic optic neuropathy and bifrontal contusions. Arch Neurol. 1991;48:101–5.

Mesulam MM. A cortical network for directed attention and unilateral neglect. Ann Neurol. 1981;10:309–25.

Mesulam MM. Neglect syndrome and the spatial attention network. In: Adelman G, Smith B, editors. Encyclopedia of neuroscience. Amsterdam: Elsevier; 2009. p. 37–41.

Milner AD, Goodale MA. Two visual system re-viewed. Neuropsychologia. 2008;46:774–85.

Mishkin M, Ungerleider LG, Maczkó KA. Object vision and spatial vision: two cortical pathways. Trends Neurosci. 1983;6:414–7.

Newcombe F, Ratcliff M. Disorders of Visuospatial analysis. In: Boller F, Grafman J, editors. Handbook of neuropsychology, vol. 2. Amsterdam: Elsevier; 1989. p. 333–56.

Nyffeler T, Pflugshaupt T, Hofer H, Baas U, Gutbrod K, von Wartburg R, Hess CW, Muri RM. Oculomotor behaviour in simultanagnosia: a longitudinal case study. Neuropsychologia. 2005;43:1591–7.

Rizzo M, Robin DA. Simultanagnosia: A defect of sustained attention yields insights on visual information processing. Neurology. 1990;40(3):447–55.

Rosselli M, Ardila A, Beltran C. Rehabilitation of Balint's syndrome: a single case report. Appl Neuropsychol. 2001;8(4):242–7.

Sachs O. Antropológus a Marson. [Antropologist on the Mars]. Budapest: Osiris Kiado; 1999. p. 19–59.

Sacks O. A férfi aki kalapnak nézte a feleségét. [The man who considered his wife to be a hat]. Budapest: Park Könyv Kiadó; 2008.

Sekuler R, Blake R. Észlelés. [Perception]. Budapest: Osiris Kiadó; 2000.

Séra L. A tárgykonstancia és neuropszichológiai vizsgálatai. [Object constancy and its neuropsychological examinations]. Magyar Pszichológiai Szemle. 2000;4:389–401.

Séra L. Tárgy és arcfelismerési zavarok. In: Bevezetés a neuropszichológiába [Disorders of object and facial recognition. In: Introduction to neuropsychology] (Kállai J, Bende I, Karádi K, Racsmány M szerk.) Budapest: Medicina; 2008. P. 217–48.

Short RA, Graff-Radford NR. Localization of hemiachromatopsia. Neurocase. 2001;7:331–7.

Stuss DT, Gallup Jr GG, Alexander MP. The frontal lobes are necessary for "theory of mind". Brain. 2001;124: 279–86.

Tényi T, Ábrahám I, Trixler M, Lénárd K. Frégoli-tünet és szexuális magatartás – a kognitív neuropszichológia megközelítése. [Fregoli symptom and sexual behavior – approach of cognitive neuropsychology]. Psychiatr Hung. 1999;14(2):307–10.

Verseghi A. Kapcsolatban lenni. In: Tanulmányok az afázia témaköréből [Being in a relationship. In: Studies about aphasia.] (Kraszárné Erdős F, Feketéné Gacsó M szerk.) Budapest: Eötvös József Kiadó; 2005. P. 94–117.

Verseghi A, Nagy Zita S, Köteles F. Tudatában lenni. A tudatosság problematikája a neuropszichológiai rehabilitációban. [Being aware. Problems of awareness in neuropsychological rehabilitation]. Rehabilitáció. 2010; 1:28–36.

Vertfaellie M, Rapcsak SZ, Heilman KM. Impaired shifting of attention in Balint syndrome. Brain Cogn. 1990;12:195204.

Vilkki J. Visual hemi-inattention after ventrolateral thalamotomy. Neuropsychologia. 1984;22:399–408.

Watson RT, Rapcsak SZ. Loss of spontaneous blinking in a patient with Balint's syndrome. Arch Neurol. 1989; 46:567–70.

Zeki S. Vizuális kép az elmében és az agyban. [Visual image in the mind and in the brain]. Tudomány. 1992;8:25–32.

Ignored World Without Missing It Neglect

67

Anna Verseghi and Zita Snagy Nagy

Contents

The Phenomenon of Neglect: "Ambiguous"

When we see that a person looks continuously to the right, and not at us while talking to us, if we take a closer look, we might see that his/her hair is combed on the right side, but messy on the left side, or–if this person is male–the right side of his face is fairy properly shaved, while the left side is stubbly, or small unshaved spots may be seen on this side, or the eyeglass is placed one-sidedly, only on the right ear, we have to consider that this person may have brain injury in the right hemisphere, and symptoms of *neglect* are seen. In case of further examination, it may be seen that the patient's clothes are asymmetric, as if he/she has not finished dressing up on the left side (for example, the trousers or skirt is not completely adjusted at the wrist, or the sleeve of the dress is twisted on the left arm) and it seems that the patient is not disturbed by these. During everyday activities, it may also be seen that for example, the patient left the meal on the left side of the plate, or the patient sleeps in the bed asymmetrically (for example, on the right side of the bed or on the left side, almost hanging on the bed), his/her left arm and leg bump into objects while walking, the patient obviously does not evade the objects. Can so many various phenomena be caused by one basic problem? According to *Heilman's* (1979) classic definition, *neglect syndrome* means the *neglect of stimuli* on the opposite side of the injury, patients do not recognize, and do not orient towards information from this direction. These symptoms occur although all basic perception processes are normal. These symptoms are most commonly seen in case of the injury of the right hemisphere, and means that the left side of the environment and body are *neglected.* A characteristic of the syndrome is that if the patient's attention is drawn to the neglect, they are able to recognize the symptoms at that moment.

A. Verseghi, M.D. (✉)
Rehabilitation Unit for Patients with Skull and Brain Injury, National Medical Rehabilitation Institute, Budapest, Hungary
e-mail: averseghi@rehabint.hu

Z.S. Nagy
Department for Multiprofile Rehabilitation of Locomotor Diseases, National Medical Rehabilitation Institute, Budapest, Hungary

Institute of Psychology, Eötvös Lóránd University, Budapest, Hungary
e-mail: snagy.zita@chello.hu

J. Somlai, T. Kovács (eds.), *Neuro-Ophthalmology*, DOI 10.1007/978-3-319-28956-4_67

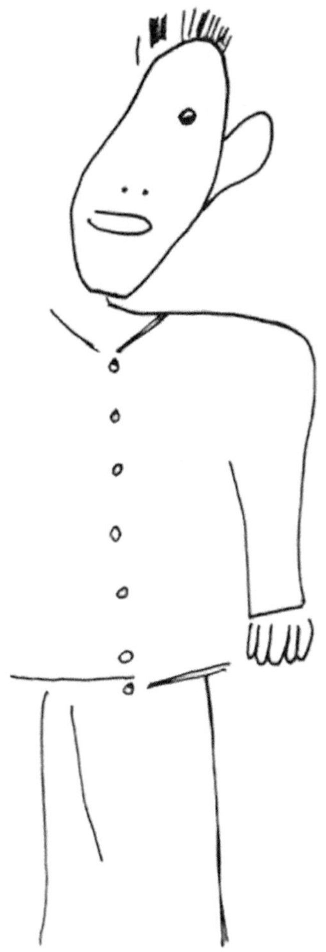

The above–seemingly simple–definition does not reflect the variability of this behavioral syndrome. From the above description it can be concluded that symptoms of neglect may be various. Neglect may affect the *personal space (own body)* or the *extrapersonal space (environment noticed by vision, hearing)* (Karádi 2008). Neglect may affect one modality or the disorder may occur affecting a combination of various modalities–visual spatial, auditory, somatosensory, olfactory -, or may even be global (Heilman et al. 1985). If the neglect is global and affects the personal space (own body), it can be seen that the patients do not pay any attention to the left side of their body, for example,–as described before–they do not take care of this side of the body, do not dress up the affected extremities, or sit on or lie on their left hand, or may cause injuries to the left side of their body without noticing it. Sometimes these patients confidently say that someone is lying next to them on the bed and touches them, although this is only an illusion from the proprioceptive-kinetic feedbacks of their own extremities (Sacks 2004). Ignoring proprioceptive-kinetic feedback information may be a reason for having balance problems in walking, starting to walk, and patients are usually unable to correct these problems. Standing vertically usually feels like leaning towards one side, they try to correct it, and as a result, they loose their balance. A general experience is that movement rehabilitation of hemiplegic, hemiparetic patients is usually longer if the patient has neglect problem (Fehér et al. 1988). *Laplane* and *Degos* (1983) specifically emphasizes a special form of personal neglect, when the patient do not use the extremities on the affected side as it would be possible regarding muscle strength or sensibility, this is called motor neglect.

Recent research suggests that *egocentric and allocentricforms of extrapersonal neglect* should be differentiated (Ota et al. 2001). The basis of this concept is a wide-spread cognitive framework stating that the extrapersonal space is processed by two methods: egocentrically, by comparing them to ourselves, and allocentrically comparing them to an external object (Vogeley and Gereon 2003). In case of egocentric neglect, the person ignores stimuli from the opposite side of the brain affected by brain injury (usually from the left side). In case of allocentric neglect, in case the stimulus is on the right side or on the left side of the patient having injury, the patient will ignore the respective side of the stimulus contralateral to the side of the brain injury. Therefore a patient sees 33 instead of 88 in case of a brain injury on the right side. Marsch and Hillis (2008) think that these two types of neglect–irrespective of modality–often dissociate and may be linked to the injury of various regions in one hemisphere. These manifestations will be presented later in some of the figures. Regarding rehabilitation (see later), it cannot be ignored which modality is affected by neglect, and whether it affects the patient's own body and/or the extrapersonal space and whether neglect is egocentric, allocentric, or both in the person with brain injury. The patient's attention can be called to look to the left, but this instruction is less helpful if the neglect is allocentric.

Neurological Background of Neglect

Although neglect is a very widely examined phenomenon of neuropsychology (Bisiach et al. 1986; Calvanio et al. 1987; Ishiai et al. 1987; Feinberg 1990; Marshall and Halligan 1993; Halligan and Marshall 1993; Ládavas et al. 1994; Storrie-Baker et al. 1997; Rossetti et al. 1998; Maddicks et al. 2003; Snagy Nagy 2008), and several publications were published in this topic from the second half of the 70s, we are still almost astonished with it.

Based on an almost complete, detailed, comprehensive review of Heilman et al., it is clear that neglect syndrome may be caused by the dysfunction of several regions of the right hemisphere or isolated function of some of these regions–although temporary and less severe neglect of the right side of the space may rarely occur in case of the injury of the left hemisphere (Heilman et al. 1985). The hypothesis of Mesulam (1981; 2009) is especially attractive, as it is comparable with our practical experience. Mesulam considers neglect of the extrapersonal space to be caused by a disorder in processing spatial information. In his model in Fig. 67.1, he convincingly connects various cerebral regions with basic components of *the* control of attention towards the extrapersonal space.

In order to recognize an object in our environment, it is inevitable to be able to detect it (to see, hear, smell, etc. it in the space). So it is important that regions of the brain responsible for perception be intact, the *posterior parietal region* primarily responsible for spatial vision should be emphasized. Important stimuli should be able to be highlighted from the several neutral stimuli around us. Information from the sensory area arrives in the *thalamus*–among others–where this screening takes place (Reep and Corwin 2009).

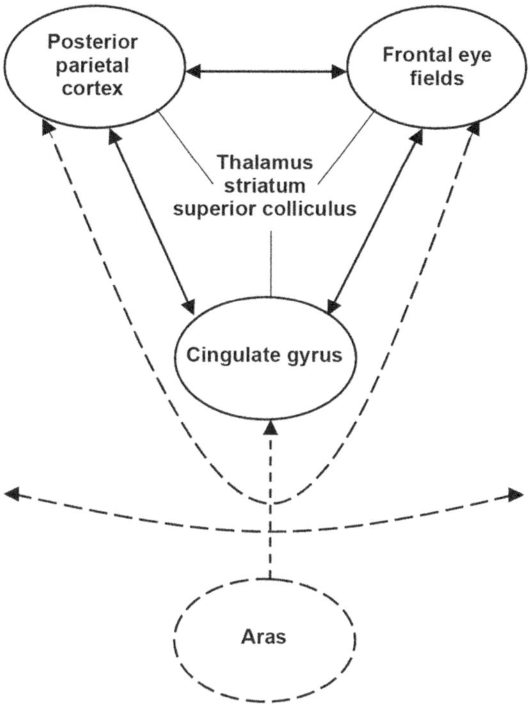

Fig. 67.1 The main components of the (neural) network taking part in controlling spatial attention according to Mesulam

The process of stimulus screening is regulated by areas of the frontal lobe. Effective regulation of the direction of attention and motor programming of exploration (searching, directing, fixating) can be linked to the *frontal lobe* as well. Our motivation is also important in noticing a stimulus. Although everyone has experienced that he/she wanted to copy something, but could think of a nearby copier, but while going home, there is a copier in every corner, or something similar. The *cingular cortex* provides the neural background for the motivational component of spatial attention. Finally, our attention is basically influenced by how alert or tired we are. The regulation of the level of activation-alertness can be linked to the *reticular formation* in the brain stem. Mesulam thinks that integrative function of these cerebral regions play a role in regulating the attention towards the extrapersonal space.

This hypothetic network assumes that the extrapersonal space has at least three complementary and interacting representations: *a sensory representation in the posterior parietal cortex, a scheme for distributing exploratory movements in the frontal cortex, and a motivational map in the cingulate cortex.* Depending on which part of the system is injured, neglect is expressed with other symptoms. In the following section, various but typical behaviors and problem solving methods of persons with neglect will be presented with some useful examinations.

Examination of Neglect Syndrome

The examination of neglect–as every neuropsychological examination–focuses not only on how successful a person is in a certain test, but on *how* the person achieved the certain result, so quantitative analysis is complemented by *qualitative analysis.* Clarifying the background mechanism of neglect syndrome is inevitable in every patient for rehabilitation, as to create individual, problem oriented developing strategies, it is important to know which part of information processing is impaired and how in a certain individual. In addition, it is useful if the neuropsychological examination involves identifying symptoms of neglect and accompanying symptoms as well in patients (for example, dressing up apraxia, construction apraxia, alloesthesia, visual apperceptive agnosia, pseudoagnosia, attention and memory disorder, disorientation, and lack of disease awareness). Analytic description of individual cognitive patterns may give important clues for individual practical rehabilitation and from a theoretical point of view, it may be important to better know the structure of the cognitive processes.

To avoid misunderstanding, it should be noted that syndrome analysis does not simply mean preparing and identifying a list of symptoms, but–as mentioned before–quantitative analysis of error of various symptoms, detection of how impaired functions connect to each other in their own way (for more information about syndrome analysis, see Verseghi, (2008). This chapter is primarily about the diagnosis of the visual form of neglect, which is especially important as patients with neglect are often not aware of the deficiency (anosognosia) (compared to complete hemianopsia), and this may endanger them while moving. The disease is not always easy to differentiate from real hemianopsia, as these disorders may occur simultaneously. In addition to extinction tests performed with a perimeter, the following neuropsychological procedures may also help in the differential diagnosis.

Ophthalmologic Examinations (Grüsser 1986; Kanath and Hartje 1987; Mayyuchi et al. 1985; Meienberg et al. 1986)

The role of the ophthalmologist is to determine the symptom of *attention hemianopsia*=**hemianopia** in case neglect syndrome is suspected, and it should be differentiated from *real hemianopsia*=**hemianopia** developing as a consequence of injuries of the visual pathway with any other origin (bleeding, tumor, trauma).

After the routine ophthalmologic examinations (visual acuity, fundus, eye movements), so called *extinction visual field examination* should be performed. The essence of this examination is that the visual fields of the two eyes are examined *simultaneously and with confrontational examination,* **which may even be performed as a bedside examination without any device.** In this case, **we sit in front of the patient and the examiner fixate the examination to a certain point of the patient's face, for example, the tip of the nose, then** the examiner presents two stimuli in the homologous points of the visual fields, one in each visual field simultaneously (for example, move fingers) for the patient. In case of neglect syndrome, the patient does not detect the stimulus on the other side compared to the brain injury (usually the one in the left visual field), the patient detects only the stimulus presented on the side of the lesion (Feinberg 1990). As a consequence of spatial attention disorder, the stimulus on the intact side "cancels" the effect of the stimulus presented on the affected side, therefore, this procedure is called *extinction.* After the extinction visual field test, the borders of the visual field have to be determined in both eyes separately using **any available method**

suitable to examine the visual field, with a perimeter. If the borders of the visual fields are complete with monocular examinations that is in case of examining the eyes separately with perimetric visual field tests, but the confrontational, binocular extinction examination shows the deficit of the left side, neglect syndrome is likely. In this case, the patient would be able to detect the left visual field, but he/she ignores, neglects it. Naturally, in case of the injury of the optic tract or the optic radiation, homonymous hemianopsia detected with a perimeter may mask the extinction. Therefore in this case, there is no point in performing the extinction test, and it may lead to difficulties in differential diagnosis.

From the 1990s (Hornak 1992; Karnath and Huber 1992; Fanthome and Lincoln 1995), more systematic analysis of the eye movements and visual scanning is more common in the literature regarding neglect syndrome. These methods, although they would be effective tools for patient examination–for example, to measure the suitability to drive a car, predict the risk of an accident -, are not in the everyday practice of routine diagnosis. The neuropsychologist may help in the differential diagnosis of neglect syndrome in addition to the neuro-ophthalmologic examination by using neuropsychological test procedures. Extinction test may not only be performed in case of visual modality. In case of the tactile extinction test, the right and/or left side of the patient's body is touched at various points, one after the other, and then simultaneously. Simultaneous stimulation–like in case of the visual examination–may trigger the extinction of the stimulus applied on the left side. However in some patients with brain injury, so called *alloesthesia* may occur. If two sides of the patient is stimulated simultaneously but asymmetrically (for example, the right elbow and the left shoulder are touched at the same time), the patient may feel the stimuli on both sides, but the stimulus applied on the left side is usually misplaced towards the location of the stimulus felt on the right side (in the above example,, the patient feels stimuli in both elbows). The following section describes some specific visual exercises routinely used in the clinical practice that triggers the symptoms of neglect, but it should be noted that in case of any spatial-visual tests and real-life situations, signs suggestive of neglect may occur.

Neuropsychological Procedures

The Phenomenon of Classic Neglect

The *line bisection test* is a classic test in the examination of neglect of one side of the space, and it has several variations -(such as Bisiach (1983). The examined persons are asked to bisect 2, 4, 6, and 8 cm long lines (in a 3×4 pattern) in the variant developed and used by us. Egocentric and allocentric neglect of the extrapersonal space may be differentiated with this test as well. Solutions of K. M, a 55 year old right-handed male patient are seen in Figs. 67.2, 67.3, 67.6, and 67.7. K. M. had an extensive ischaemic vascular lesion in the right hemisphere (CT), and as a consequence, he had left hemiparesis and neglect affecting the left side as main symptoms. Rehabilitation was performed after acute care. The following drawings were performed in the neuropsychological examination 5 months after the onset of the disease. A common mistake is seen in Fig. 67.2, both types of neglect can be recognized. The patient completely ignored the stimuli on the left side, which suggests egocentric form of neglect. However, it is well seen that the examined person performed the line bisections asymmetrically (the left segments are considerably longer) which suggests allocentric neglect. Interestingly, in the last, 2 cm long line, the right segment is longer, which may be a sing of the *compensatory mechanism* of the person; it

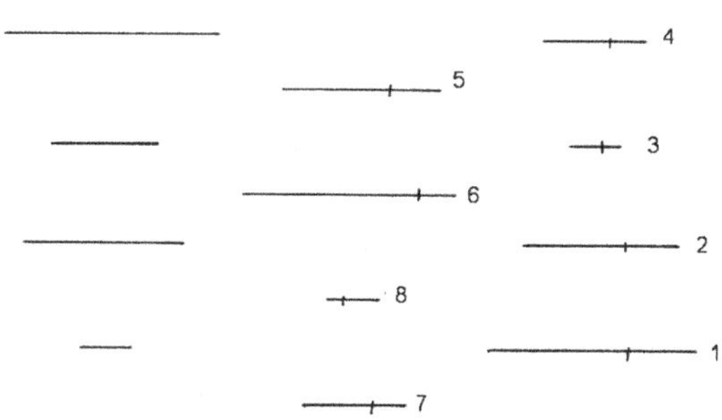

Fig. 67.2 A version of Line bisection test (A. Verseghi)

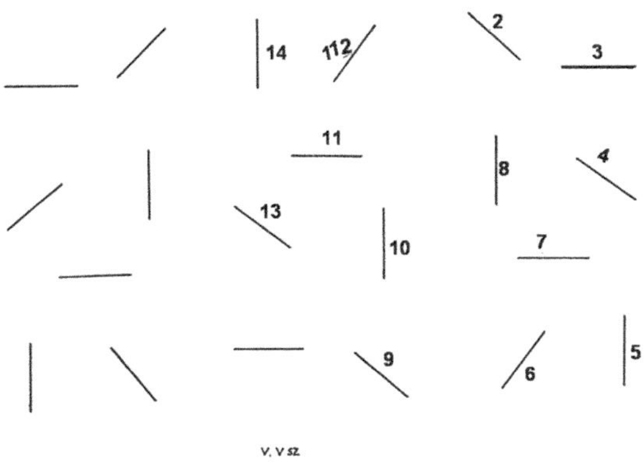

Fig. 67.3 Numbering lines

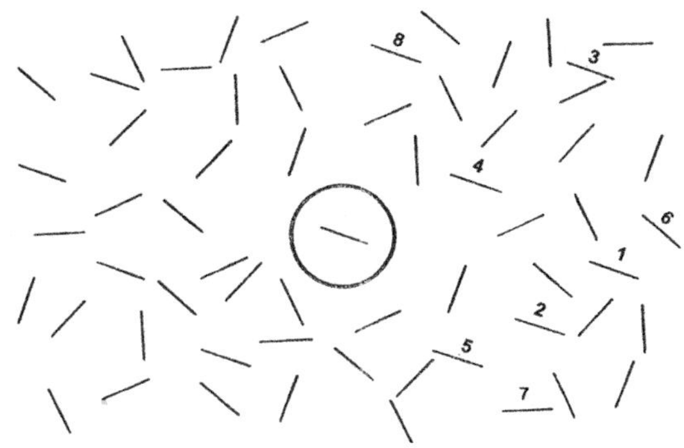

Fig. 67.4 Visual search for parallel lines

may be unconscious or conscious as well. (It may be very helpful to notice the compensatory efforts, strategies of the patient, as these may be the bases of individual rehabilitation.)

Neglect of one side of the space can be examined most easily by "searching" exercises, during which the person has to find different stimuli in a sheet. In case of the previously mentioned line bisection test, it is very informative if the order of bisections is recorded. Therefore, numbering the bisections can be a "searching" situation in addition to following the process. There are several "searching" exercises in the clinical practice and in the research, such as: Bells' (Gauthier et al. 1989), Albert's test with crossing out lines (Albert 1973), and crossing out stars (Halligan et al. 1991). In *Verseghi's* (1986) *line numbering* test, the person is asked to number the lines in the sheet (the lines are 3 cm long in the original test).

In Fig. 67.3, the test result of K. M. is seen in the line numbering test, he did not detect the stimuli on the left side of the sheet. Patients should be asked to number the items in the "searching" tests, as although the test is somehow modified, numbering enables recording the direction of visual "scanning". This method enables the display of "spatial information processing in neglect" as a method of operation. Healthy, right handed patients start discovering stimuli from left to write, as in case of reading, irrespective of whether they use vertical or horizontal searching strategies. Persons with neglect often start to explore the surrounding space from right to left, irrespective of whether they are left or right handed. Therefore, if we see that the person with brain injury reviews the whole sheet– that is quantitatively neglect is not present -, but the person does it from right to left, it may be considered to be a symptom of neglect, but the person uses a successful compensation strategy in this simple test. It should be mentioned that this test is very useful in diagnosing visual agnosias as well. Right to left vertical or chaotic numbering suggests visual apperceptive agnosia or pseudo-agnosia, this hypothesis has to be confirmed or excluded by other targeted exercises.

Allocentric neglect may manifest in "searching" tests as well, for example,, it may be seen that the patient numbers a certain stimulus twice. The reason for this may be that while doing the test, the patient does not detect the number he/she wrote on the left side of the stimulus later, and he/ she writes a new number next to it (see number 1 and 12 next to the same line in Fig. 67.3). One of the most sensitive "searching" tests is the *"Visual search for parallel lines"* (Vilkki 1984). The examined person has to find lines that are parallel with the line circled in the middle in Fig. 67.4– the lines are 2 cm long in the original test. The test often confirmed visual neglect even if neglect of the left side was not seen before. In addition to neglect (attention component), it may be detected with this test whether the spatial information processing system, such as direction detection is affected or not. Thus, it can be seen in Fig. 67.4 that the person performing this test had slightly injured direction detection as well. It can be seen that two of the eight numbered lines are not parallel with the target stimulus.

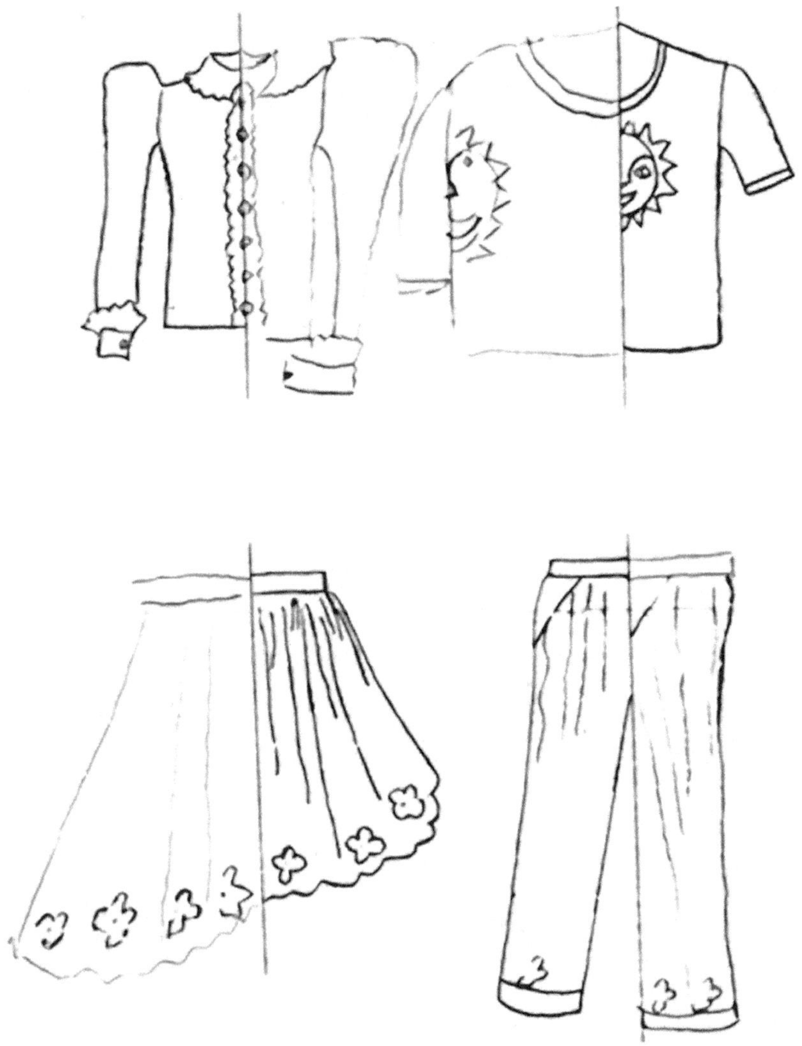

Fig. 67.5 Symmetrical-figures complementation task

The Space Becomes Asymmetric

In case of neglect syndrome, in addition to simple neglect, it is often seen that symmetric spatial perception is impaired, the *Symmetrical-figures complementation task (Verseghi)* is especially sensitive to this. In this test, the examined person has to draw the other half of the unfinished drawing.

Figure 67.5 shows characteristic mistakes suggesting that the space has become asymmetric: size differences between the right and left side of the figures, difficulties in mirroring, and a specific symptom, *allochiria* (Becchio and Bertone 2005). The patient started drawing with the figures on the right side, and the patient drew the wrinkles and the flowers of the skirt on right side–not detected consciously–to the trousers while completing the trousers. The reason for this may be that in case of neglect syndrome, basic perception processes of the patient with brain injury are intact, so the patient "would be able to recognize" the stimulus on the affected side as well, but he/she does not recognize it. However, stimuli on the left side may unconsciously be processed. A most commonly known example, of this phenomenon was described by Marshall and Halligan (1988). The authors showed figures of houses drew with lines to their patient with neglect, in one of the drawings; smoke was present on the left side. The patient thought that–visually–there was no difference between the two houses, however when the patient was asked which house he/she would move into, the patient chose the house with no smoke. Another good example, of the above described behavioral characteristics of neglect is that if the patients are asked to draw or copy simple symmetric objects, forms (daisy, sun with rays, clock, person from the front–as seen in the illustration at the beginning of the chapter), or are asked to simply write something. Performances in case of these exercises show well that neglect does not simply mean the ignorance of the "left side" but in general, the space and the objects in it become disproportionate, and commonly this only worsens by "over expressing" the left side as a result of compensation efforts.

Drawings of Figs. 67.6 and 67.7 were prepared by the same patient, whose results in the line bisection and numbering test are seen on Figs. 67.2 and 67.3. In the drawings and writings in Fig. 67.6, neglect can be recognized, primarily its egocentric form, the space and symmetrical figures became asymmetric, and perseveration is often seen in solutions of patients with neglect (Menyes and Verseghi 2008) which may have very special manifestations in case of drawing the outlines of a figure in Fig. 67.7. In this exercise, the patient (green color) had to draw the outline of the simple figures of the examiner (orange lines). The examiner drew the next figure when a drawing was finished. It is very strange that while the right side of the figure is prepared well, on the left side, the patient perseverates the left side of the previous figure or the figure is unfinished. As if typical examples of disorders of inhibition and control processes were seen in front of us.

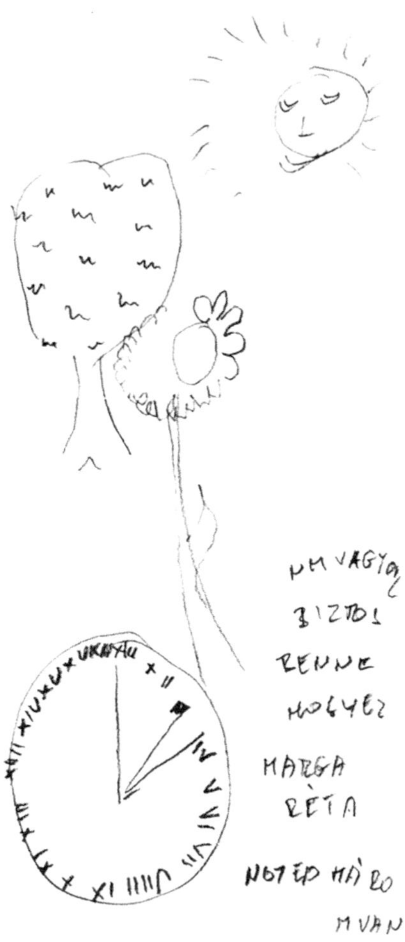

Fig. 67.6 Drawing symmetrical *"I am not sure that this is a daisy. It is quarter past two"*

Interpretation, Giving Meaning

The above described specific space perception disorder may have additional severe consequences as well. Person with symptoms of neglect naturally reacts to events detected by the person. As information from perception is incomplete, consequences of this perception will be false as well. Phenomenon of "completion" of incomplete perception is seen based on partial information if the patient with brain injury is shown complex or unclear images (*Verseghi*, Fig. 67.8), and the patient is asked to tell us what he/she sees in detail.

Patients often give separate meaning to the part of the figure seen on the right side without integrating it to the other parts of the figure. Therefore, person with brain injury may say that a woman performing an exercise is seen in the figure represented in Fig. 67.8, and the woman is leaning forward and is placing her head between her legs (the patient thinks that her arms are legs).

Naturally, the process of giving meaning may be impaired or not depending on whether the person checks if the detected and thought image may

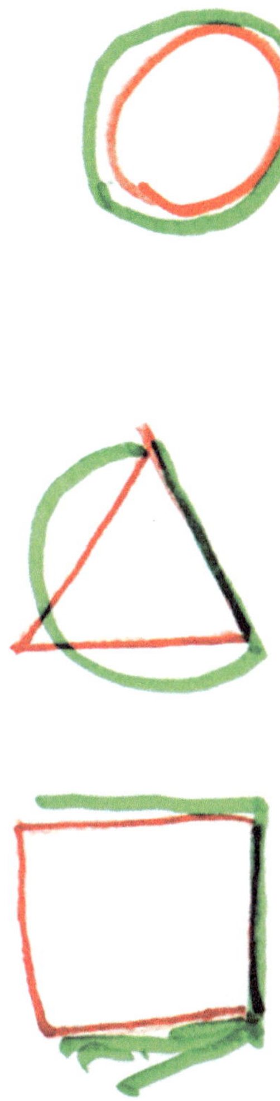

Fig. 67.7 Perseveration characteristics of a patient with Neglect

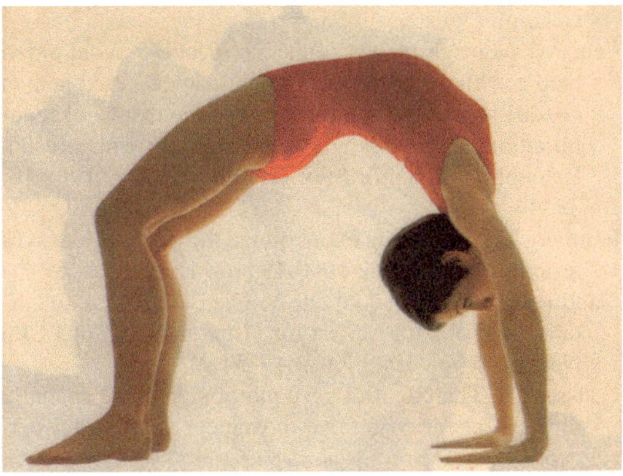

Fig. 67.8 Unusual image from our examination album

represent the reality or not. However, suspicion that something is not right should be present. Although one of the most severe characteristics of the phenomenon of neglect is that the patient with brain injury does not recognize that the seen image does not represent the reality. Therefore neglect syndrome may be called *the lack of sense of loss* (Verseghi 2005). So the first step of rehabilitation should be to make the patient accept that from now on, he/she *cannot believe his/her eyes.* This is one of the most difficult things, as during our life, we learn to believe our eyes. The right action is based on correct, accurate perception. Therefore, it is difficult for persons with brain injury and symptoms of neglect to accept what and how many things the patient does not recognize around him/her, while those things are apparent for their alert environment. Therefore, the responsibility of the professional is great in calling the attention of the person with symptoms of neglect and the person's family that while the symptoms are present, the patient should not walk in crowded streets alone and should not the drive a car as it is dangerous. The following section briefly describes the most important considerations of the rehabilitation of neglect.

Rehabilitation

Treatment of neglect syndrome is a basic area of *cognitive rehabilitation,* as it affects the bases of everyday activities. The phenomenon is more wide-spread than it is thought. According to *Diller* and *Weinberg* (1977), 40 % of patients with brain injury on the right side have some form of this phenomenon.

The first step of therapy is–as we mentioned before–to make the person aware of the problem and its consequences. Azouvi et al. (2003) have created a simple method for the quantitative detection of anosognosia (lack of disease awareness) using the Catherine Bergego Scale (CBS). CBS ask questions regarding symptoms suggestive of neglect that occur in the everyday life–described in the introduction. If the scale is completed by the therapist and the patient as well, the difference between their answers shows the severity of anosognosia. The study of Azouvi et al. shows that the more severe the neglect is, the more severe the lack of disease awareness is. Therefore, the therapy of neglect and disease awareness cannot be separated. Making the patient read is one of the most suitable methods to treat the two problems together, as in case the patient ignores either the left side of the words or the left side of the text, the patient will not understand it, and it is a clear indicator that something is wrong. Although the desire to understand the text may be the basis of compensation, as it makes the person find the beginning of the words and the lines. If the neglect is not severe, this may be performed automatically, therefore, reading is a good therapeutic tool, but less sensitive in diagnostics. Unfortunately, the fact that the patient with neglect knows what his/her disease means, it does not mean that the patient will be able to compensate it. This is most often possible only after long-term training. Ideally, this is based on the co-operation of the ophthalmologist, neuropsychologist, movement therapist, and the environment of the patient, as the general principle of therapy is, in order to enhance awareness, the immediate feedback of any symptoms of neglect and not only during therapy but in the everyday life as well (Wilson and Manly 2003).

Training is the most effective if patients with neglect have to turn their attention to the contralateral side in several various situations. This may be performed by movement exercises (such as slalom, ball exercises), visual, searching, or auditory, sound localization exercises and in case of hobbies such as drawing, painting, modeling, embroidery, puzzles, etc. In the international clinical practice, there are various pursuits to reduce neglect, such as vestibular stimulation, stimulating the extremities, using a prism (Storrie-Baker et al. 1997; Rossetti et al. 1998; Maddicks et al. 2003). However, introducing and describing these rehabilitation attempts and procedures go far beyond the scope of this chapter.

The more we understand about neglect syndrome, the more capable we become to see the similarities of various symptoms, that is why neglect is called a *syndrome* in neurologic (broader) and neuropsychological (narrower) sense as well. However, the main question asked by a patient with neglect practically remains unanswered. *How should I notice what I cannot see?*

There may be general tricks, rehabilitation guidelines, but only long work performed with full effort can lead to results. There are only individual answers for each person, situation, teams, and families at the moment, developing a response always needs great attention. *Attention is essential for improvement.* Attention is the gate to knowledge and consciousness, and consciousness is the basis of the active effort to make a person be active in his/her recovery.

References

Albert ML. A simple test of visual neglect. Neurology. 1973;23:658–64.

Azouvi P, et al. Behavioral assessment of unilateral neglect: study of the psychometric properties of the Cathrine Bergego Scale. Arch Phys Med Rehabil. 2003;84:51–7.

Becchio C, Bertone C. The ontology of neglect. Conscious Cogn. 2005;14:483–94.

Bisiach E. Line bisection and cognitive plasticity of unilateral neglect of space. Brain Cogn. 1983;2:32–8.

Bisiach E, et al. Unilateral neglect: personal and extrapersonal. Neuropsychologia. 1986;24:759–67.

Calvanio R, Petrone PN, Levine DN. Left visual neglect is both environment-centered and body-centered. Neurology. 1987;37:1179–83.

Diller LA, Wenberg J. Hemi-inattention in rehabilitation: the evolution of a rational remediation program. Adv Neurol. 1977;18:63–82.

Fanthome Y, Lincoln NB. Eye movements in patients with visual neglect following right hemisphere stroke. Clin Rehabil. 1995;9:347–53.

Fehér M, Verseghi A, Osmanné SJ. A jobb és a bal oldali hemiparetikus betegek rehabilitációs eredményei közötti különbség. [Differences of the results of rehabilitation of patients with right and left hemiparesis]. BalneológiaRehabilitáció Gyógyfürdőügy. 1988;10: 39–44.

Feinberg TE. Ipsilateral extinction in the hemineglect syndrome. Arch Neurol. 1990;47:802–4.

Gauthier L, Dehaut F, Joanette Y. The Bells test: a quantitative and qualitative test for visual neglect. Int J Clin Neuropsychol. 1989;XI(2):49–54.

Grüsser OJ. The effect of gaze motor signal and spatially directed attention on eye movements and visual perception. Prog Brain Res. 1986;64:391–403.

Halligan PW, Marshall JC. Homing in on neglect: a case study of visual search. Cortex. 1993;29:167–74.

Halligan PW, Cockburn J, Wilson BA. The behavioral assessment of visual neglect. Neuropsychol Rehabil. 1991;I(2):5–32.

Heilman KM. Neglect and related disorders. In: Heilman KM, Valenstein E, editors. Clinical neuropsychology. New York: Oxford University Press; 1979. p. 268–307.

Heilman KM, et al. The neglect syndrome. In: Frederiks JAM, editor. Clinical neuropsychology. Amsterdam: Elsevier; 1985. p. 153–83.

Hornak J. Ocular exploration in the dark by patients with visual neglect. Neuropsychologia. 1992;30(6):547–52.

Ishiai S, Furukawa R, Tsukagoshi H. Eye-fixation patterns in homonymus hemianopsia and unilateral spatial neglect. Neuropsychologia. 1987;25:675–9.

Kanath HO, Hartje W. Residual information processing in the neglected visual halffield. J Neurol. 1987;234: 180–4.

Karádi K: A téri hemineglekt neuropszichológiája. In: Bevezetés a neuropszichológiába [Neuropsychology of spatial hemineglect. In: Introduction to neuropsychology] (Kállai J, Bende I, Karádi K, Racsmány M szerk.) Budapest: Medicina; 2008. P. 195–216.

Karnath H-O, Huber W. Abnormal eye movement behaviour during text reading in neglect syndrome: a case study. Neuropsychologia. 1992;30(6):593–8.

Ládavas E, Carletti M, Gori G. Automatic and voluntary orienting of attention in patients with visual neglect: horizontal and vertical dimensions. Neuropsychologia. 1994;32:1195–208.

Laplane D, Degos JP. Motor neglect. J Neurol Neurosurg Psychiatry. 1983;46:152–8.

Maddicks R, Marzilier SL, Parker G. Rehabilitation of unilateral neglect in the acute recovery stage: the efficacy of limb activation therapy. Neuropsychol Rehabil. 2003;13(3):391–408.

Marsh EB, Hillis AE. Dissociation between egocentric and allocentric visuospatial and tactile neglect in acute stroke. Cortex. 2008;44:1215–20.

Marshall JC, Halligan PW. Blindsight and insight in visuo-spatial neglect. Nature. 1988;336:766–7.

Marshall JC, Halligan PW. Imagine only the half of it. Nature. 1993;364:193–4.

Mayyuchi O, Posteraro L, Nuzzi G, Parma M. Unilateral visual agnosia. Cortex. 1985;21:309–16.

Meienberg O, Harrer M, Wehren C. Oculographic diagnosis of hemineglect in patients with homonym hemianopia. J Neurol. 1986;233:97–101.

Menyes C, Verseghi A. Akaratlan ismétlések – perszeverációk. [Involuntary repetitions – perseverations]. Rehabilitáció. 2008;18(4):168–75.

Mesulam MM. A cortical network for directed attention and unilateral neglect. Ann Neurol. 1981;10:309–25.

Mesulam MM. Neglect syndrome and the spatial attention network. In: Adelman G, Smith B, editors. Encyclopedia of neuroscience. Amsterdam: Elsevier; 2009. p. 37–41.

Ota H, Fujii T, Suzuki K, Fukatsu R, Jamadori A. Dissociation of body-centered and stimulus-centered representations in unilateral neglect. Neurology. 2001;57:2064–9.

Reep RL, Corwin JV. Posterior parietal cortex as part of neural network for directed attention in rats. Neurobiol Learn Mem. 2009;91:104–13.

Rossetti Y, Rode G, Pisella L, Farne A, Li L, Boisson D, et al. Prism adaptation to a rightward optical deviation rehabilitates left hemispatial neglect. Nature. 1998; 395:166–9.

Sacks O. A férfi aki kalapnak nézte a feleségét és más történetek. [The man who considered his wife to be a hat and other stories]. Budapest: Park Könyvkiadó; 2004. p. 85–6.

Snagy Nagy Z. Neglektes személyek funkcionális testsémájának vizsgálata. [Examination of the functional body image of persons with neglect]. Rehabilitáció. 2008;18(4):176–82.

Storrie-Baker HJ, Segalowitz SJ, Black SE, Mclean JAG, Sullivan N. Improvement of hemispatial neglect with cold-water calorics: an electrophysiological test of the arousal hypothesis of neglect. J Int Neuropsychol Soc. 1997;3:394–402.

Verseghi A. Kapcsolatban lenni. In: Tanulmányok az afázia témaköréből [Being in a relationship. In: Studies about aphasia.] (Kraszárné Erdős F, Feketéné Gacsó M szerk.) Budapest: Eötvös József Kiadó; 2005. P. 94–117.

Verseghi A. Kvalitatív megközelítések a neuropszichológiában. In: Bevezetés a neuropszichológiába [Qualitative approaches in neuropsychology. In: Introduction to neuropsychology.] (Kállai J, Bende I, Karádi K, Racsmány Mszerk.) Budapest: Medicina; 2008. P. 19–44.

Verseghi A. Rehabilitation of patients with neglect syndrome. Models of brain injury rehabilitation. London; 1986.

Vilkki J. Visual hemi-inattention after ventrolateral thalamotomy. Neuropsychologia. 1984;22:399–408.

Vogeley K, Gereon RF. Neural correlates of the first-person-perspective. Trends Cog Sci. 2003;7(1):38–42.

Wilson FC, Manly T. Sustained attention training and errorless learning facilitates self-care functioning in chronic ipsilesional neglect following severe traumatic brain injury. Neuropsychol Rehabil. 2003;13:537–48.

Introducing Tools and Services Helping Life of People with Impaired Vision

68

Mihaly Szuhaj and Peter Szatmari

Contents

The twenty-first century is the era of the spreading of informatics; our lives cannot be imagined without using a computer today. In Hungary, as all over the world, informatics has become available for persons with visual impairment over the last decade. The computer equipped with special softwares has become the tool of the rehabilitation of blind people and persons with impaired vision as well. It significantly helps learning, entertainment, obtaining information, and working. It erases communication problems, and greatly increases the independence of people with impaired vision. If a blind person is able to read a newspaper, letter, or book–either paper-based or electronic–alone with a computer, the person almost regains a part of his/her lost vision and independence.

Informatics–in addition to transport and orientation–is the most popular service of primary rehabilitation centers. Special informatics devices of people with impaired vision should be introduced for this reason as well. It should be known that the extremely high price of the special hardware and the software makes wide spread use of these devices difficult. Besides the continuously increasing range of devices, the National Health Insurance Fund (Orszagos Egeszsegugyi Penztar, OEP) contains only some white canes in the list of medical aids for blind people as devices that

M. Szuhaj (✉) • P. Szatmari
Computer Programmer Mathematician, "Informatics for people with visual injury" Foundation, Budapest, Hungary
e-mail: szuhaj.mihaly@infoalap.hu; szatmari.peter@infoalap.hu; http://www.infoalap.hu

J. Somlai, T. Kovács (eds.), *Neuro-Ophthalmology*, DOI 10.1007/978-3-319-28956-4_68

are available with subsidy. Therefore, people with visual impairment can access IT complementary devices necessary for them primarily with tenders and individual supporting actions.

Using the Computer

Screen reader softwares read the pressed keys and information on the screen aloud with a sound card and a speaker or headset.

General services of screen reader programs:

- reading text aloud (characters, words, paragraphs, and the whole text),
- reading websites, emails, menus, submenus, icons, dialog boxes aloud,
- continuous reading out or reading highlighted sections aloud,
- changing speech features (pitch, speed, volume).

Blind users need screen reader softwares to use the computer. In Hungary, JAWS for Windows screen reader program is the most common screen reader program. This program was introduced in Hungary by "Informatika a latasserultekert" Alapitvany (IT Foundation for the visually impaired), the program has Hungarian built-in speech synthesizer. Furthermore NVDA, an open source screen reader program is also available in Hungarian, which is used–according to a research–by approximately one fifth of the users.

Blind people do not use a mouse when using the computer, as they do not see what they click on. They have to use the keyboard alone, and it should be known that all common operating systems (such as Windows XP and Windows 7, 8, 8.1) can be effectively used only with the keyboard. The knowledge of several shortcuts is necessary for this–informatics education of blind people consists mostly of teaching these shortcuts and practicing them with the blind people. Naturally, there are primarily websites or special programs that require a mouse. Blind users cannot use these programs; these programs have to be modified to be suitable for the disabled.

From the point of view of informatics, people with visual impairment are those who have difficulty, but can read the text on the screen of the monitor. Although as impaired vision always means some individual ophthalmologic problem, informatics help cannot be unified either: it means a huge difference whether the patient has difficulty in seeing something in a short distance or something in a long distance, whether increased brightness disturbs or helps the person, as in each case, different help (in our case: settings) is required.

Hardware Tools

Monitor

For better overview, the size of the monitor should be at least 19″, unless the person with visual impairment has impaired visual field (for example, tunnel vision), in this case, a larger monitor size may make finding the information on the screen more difficult. The range of brightness and contrast settings should be as wide as possible.

Keyboard

Thorough knowledge of the keyboard and learning the regular touch typing are especially important in case of blind users. Replacing the regular QWERTY keyboard with a Braille keyboard is technically possible, however, the first one can be perfectly used by people with visual impairment, and the Braille keyboards are especially expensive and not wide-spread. Keyboards are available in various colors (for example, black keyboard with yellow labels or conversely) with larger buttons and labels for users with impaired vision. The labels of normal sized keyboards may be replaced with large labels as well.

Speaker and Headphone

For blind users, mainly in order not to disturb others around them, a good quality headphone is very important in addition to the speaker. Types developed for call center employees suitable for long-term, continuous use should be selected. A wireless device should be selected for home use, as the user will not get caught in or pull the wire when carrying or packing the devices. Comfortable volume control is important as well, and the headset should be able to be connected to the speaker (not to the back of the computer, where it is difficult to access). So the user can easily switch between the speaker and the headset.

Braille Displays

In addition to various acoustic solutions, Braille displays that can be connected to the computer are useful alternative options. The benefit of these displays is that they can be used without disturbing others. These touchable displays use a so called piezoelectric method and display the Braille characters after each other based on the text appearing on the screen. There are devices with twenty, forty, and eighty cells, but several European companies have other variants (with 8, 24, 32, 64 cells). Most Braille displays can be connected to the computer with a USB port or via Bluetooth connection, and are controlled by softwares reading text (however, reading function may be switched off in this case).

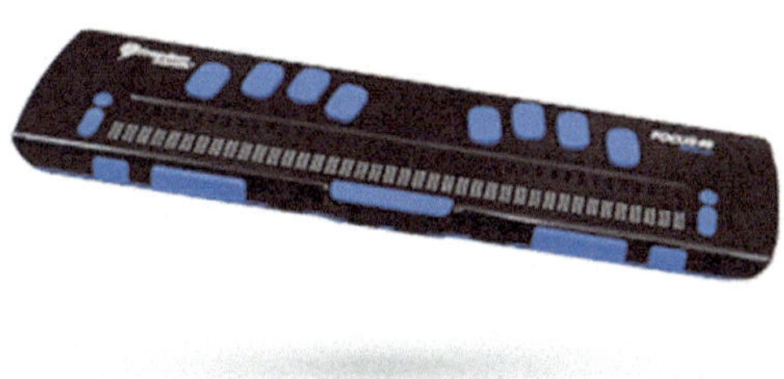

Softwares

Screen Reader Softwares

JAWS for Windows

The JAWS (Job Access With Speech) for Windows developed by the American Freedom Scientific is one of the best screen reader programs providing the most services, the first Hungarian version was introduced in March 2003. As a result of localization, messages, help menu, and the manual of the program are available in Hungarian language. The software can be installed from CD, and the installation is facilitated by sound information as well. The program automatically starts after the system is initiated; therefore, it provides auditory support from the beginning. The JAWS program is compatible with almost all popular computer softwares, but it does not replace them. The JAWS is prepared to be used with the most common applications used in Windows, for example, with Word, Excel, Internet Explorer, Firefox, or Outlook. Using these programs is not only possible but specifically comfortable with the special services.

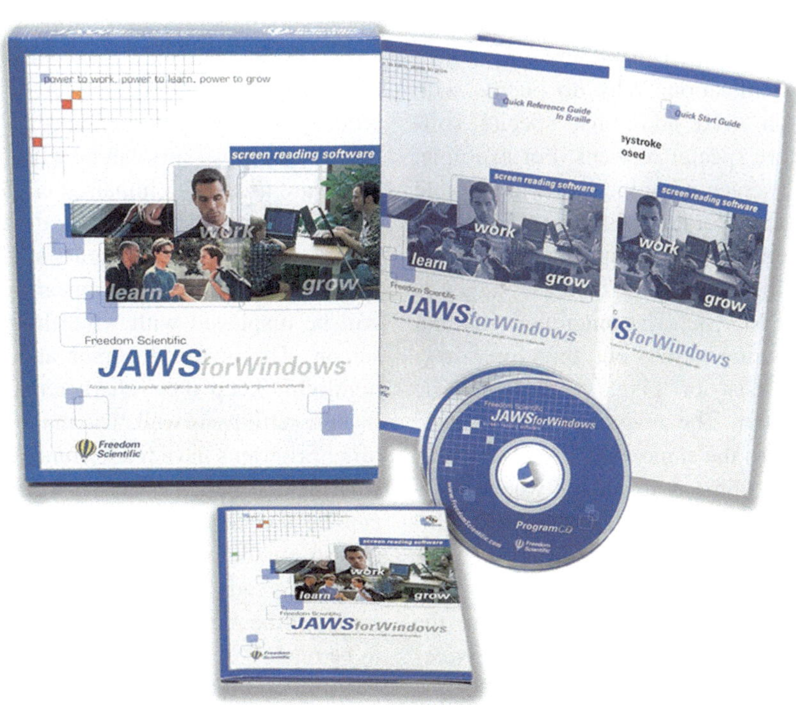

In order to operate the system, knowledge of the keyboard shortcuts to control each program is essential–blind users do not use the mouse at all, in addition, the JAWS program can be easily used with Braille display as well.

Besides JAWS for Windows, NVDA (Non Visual Desktop Access) screen reader program is popular as well. NVD is a free of charge, open source software for Microsoft Windows operation system. Its services are fairly similar to those of JAWS for Windows. The basic difference between the two is that NVDA provides primarily basic services. For those who use the computer for everyday tasks or just get acquainted with it, it is fairly enough. Professional users on the other hand prefer JAWS. Further aspect is that although users have to pay for JAWS for Windows, between 2002 and 2014 Hungarian visually impaired people could have it free in the framework of different calls. Support from the distributor is provided, as e.g. personal helpdesk, or helpdesk via phone or e-mail.

Screen Magnifier Softwares

The user interface of all operation system can be thoroughly adjusted for individual needs. Individual colors and font size can be adjusted, and the operating systems have special additional options as well. For example, the magnifier service of Windows 7, which enables magnifying up to 16 fold magnification. Why do people with impaired vision need additional special softwares? For more special services. For example, the MAGic 11 screen magnifier software is able to magnify up to 36 fold magnification. There are three stages between single and double zoon in Windows Zoom, the number of these stages is nine in case of MAGic. The magnifier does not smooth the magnified letters out; therefore, these letters will consist of pixels, while MAGic smooths them out. The magnifier can be used with all softwares the same way, the function of MAGic can be adjusted to all softwares separately. Other settings may be used for text editing, table processing, e-mail writing, or browsing.

Another important difference is that the screen magnifier softwares have speech services as well with the built-un speech synthesizer. The MAGic and the ZoomText screen magnifier contain for example, the same Hungarian speech synthesizer as the JAWS for Windows screen reader program for blind users. In addition, it is important that the user does not overload his/her vision with reading a long email or article, and is able to listen to it. In addition, loss of vision is gradual, so understanding the speech synthesizer and using it gives transition and time to get to know the screen reader programs the person may need after losing his/her vision. The most commonly used screen magnifier softwares in Hungary are the MAGic and the ZoomText programs.

The MAGic Screen Magnifier Program

The MAGic screen magnifier program magnifies the screen with one of the five available types of magnification (full screen, lens shaped, magnification with fixed corners, dynamically changing magnification and divided screen magnification). With the MAGic screen magnifier program, the user may change the enhancement (color), size, opacity, and duration of visibility of the cursor and the mouse cursor. In both cases, setting up various frames and crosshairs may help focusing. These modifications make following the cursor easier while writing or modifying the text. Naturally its form and color can be selected individually as well. Opacity and thickness of the frames and crosshairs can be adjusted separately. There are users with impaired vision who benefit from color contrast in reading, therefore, the program enables inverse mode settings as well, which means that the text appearing on the screen will be displayed with white letters on a black screen. The adjusted cursor and mouse cursor highlights keep their characteristics in case of inverse settings as well. The majority of the magnifier programs have reader function as well considering the needs of users. Sound information can be switched off and on, like tracking the mouse cursor or keyboard cursor. The MAGic program reads the icons, menus, etc. on the screen if the mouse cursor is placed over the area to be read.

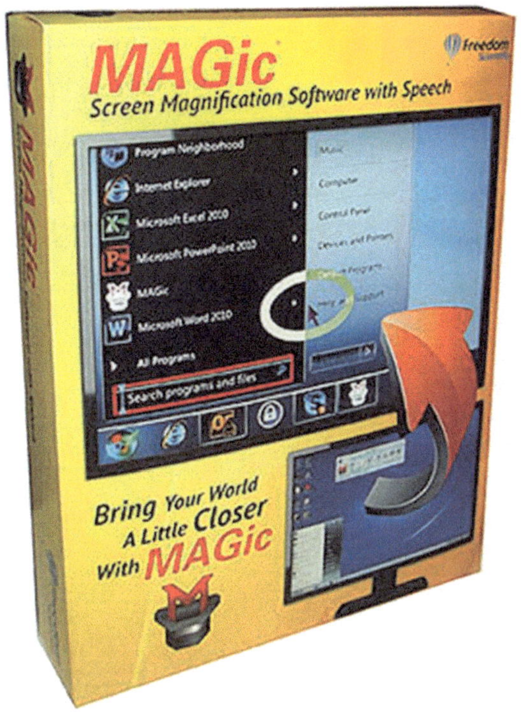

Optical Character Recognition

For patient with visual impairment, in addition to available digital information, the importance of paper based documents are still significant problems, as they cannot read them. Optical character recognition technology gives a solution for this. OCR (Optical Character Recognition) softwares convert scanned printed documents into text formats (these programs are not able to recognize handwriting yet). Recognition can be started by scanning the text, PDF documents or image files (JPG) can be used as well. In this case, the arrangement of the several tiny points creating the image is used to form letters, numbers and punctuation marks. During text recognition, the software reviews the arrangement of each image point and determines which letter, number or punctuation mark they form. The result is a text that can be edited by the computer and can be processed by any text editor programs. Books, newspapers, contracts, faxes, letters and promotional literature, etc. can be converted into digital form rapidly and in a user friendly way with the optical character recognition softwares. Therefore, printed documents are available with other tools as well, can be edited, and blind users may use screen reader programs to read and understand them.

Plustek OpticBook 3800 book scanner should be known as well, it was developed specifically to scan books, and therefore, it is especially beneficial for people with visual impairment. Any book can lay flat completely and smoothly on the glass surface of the device using SEE (Shadow Elimination Element) technology. The result is an image that has no shadows in the middle of book pages and the lines are not distorted. With this technology, damaging the edge of the book can be prevented, and optical character recognition is more effective.

In Hungary, the two most commonly used optical character recognition programs are the ABBYY FineReader and the Nuance Omnipage. Both softwares are of good quality, able to perform thorough recognition, and keep the form and structure of the original software. Some of the individual technical features of the program are presented below.

ABBYY FineReader Optical Character Recognition Software

Main features:

- Recognizes 186 languages (including Hungarian)
- Grammar checking is available in 39 languages (including Hungarian)
- Menu interface that can be used in 19 languages (including Hungarian)
- Hungarian manual
- Handling multilingual texts
- Automatically separates pages in case of books
- Rapid processing method
- It can be started directly from the Word text editor program
- Has a built-in medical and legal dictionary

Poet Compact Reader Device

Poet Compact is a computer with a built-in scanner which can be used to scan printed texts after pressing a button and reading it, the user does not need to learn the instructions for use. No computer knowledge is necessary to use it. Every component is placed in a designed house and is integrated with some operating buttons.

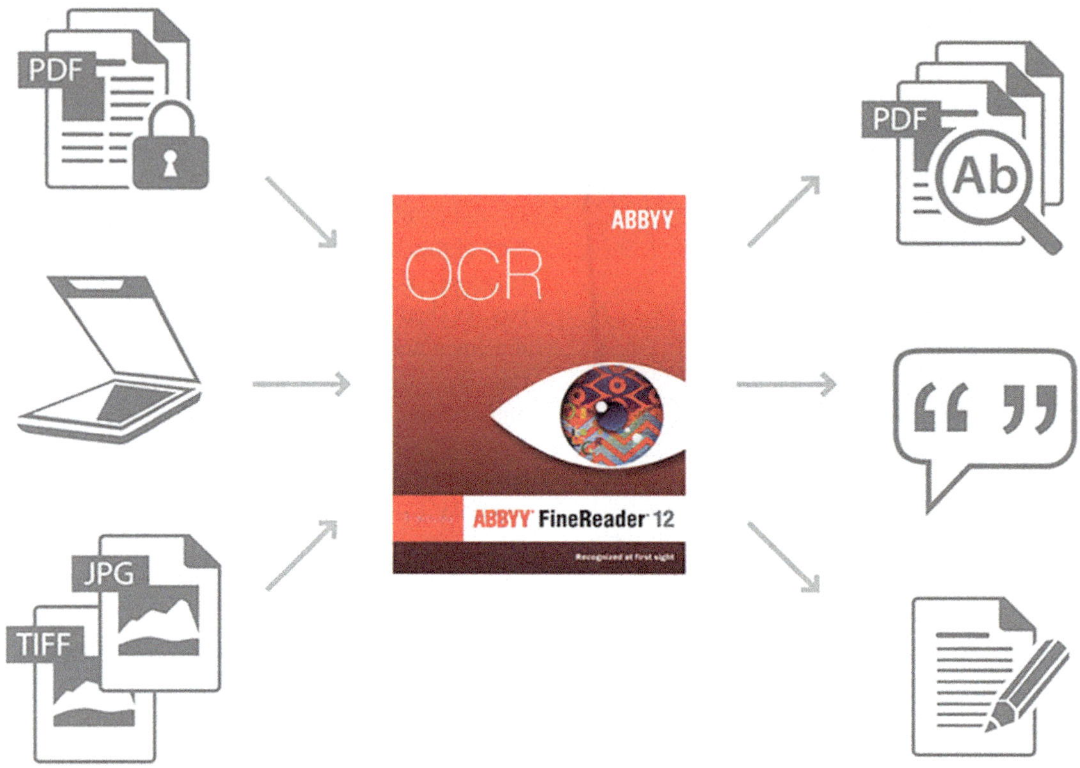

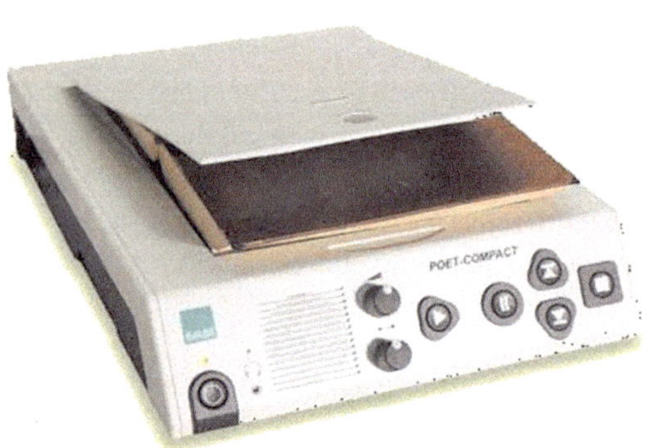

The device automatically recognizes the direction of the document placed in the device, it translates the text and then reads the information clearly and understandably. Speech speed may be decreased or increased; the language of reading may be English, German, Italian, or Hungarian. The device has a significantly large memory, the built-in memory may store large amount of saved texts that can be found and read again rapidly.

Talking Linux

The majority of the programs listed above cost money, as IT devices generally. However there is a branch in IT, which is free of charge, it is the world of open source softwares. It is not our aim here to introduce open source softwares, but it is worth mentioning that they are free for everyone, either for home or for professional work, their usage is somehow less easy, and these are not well known softwares. This is true not only for operation systems (Windows–Linux), but for office programs as well (Microsoft Word, Excel–Open Office Writer, Calc).

Open source softwares are available for visually impaired people via Talking Linux (BeLin), which can be an alternative for Microsoft Windows and Microsoft Office. Talking Linux (BeLin) is a version of Ubuntu Linux, and has been developed according to the special needs of visually impaired people. From the beginning screen reading and screen magnifying softwares are available, as well as an open source office software pack, which is called OpenOffice. It consists of a text editor, a spreadsheet application, etc.

Talking Linux is published by IT foundation for the visually impaired. The 4.0 version of BeLin was published in October, 2014, and can be downloaded from the website of the foundation.

Everyday Devices

Mobile Phones

Nowadays, mobile phones can be used for several more things than simply talking and sending SMS. Websites may be accessed; emailing, music playing, taking and looking at images and videos are also possible. People with visual impairment could not use basic functions as the phonebook or the SMS before. They made calls by typing in the numbers or with preprogrammed shortcuts. However, devices enabling the use of external programs have occurred as well, so the screen reader or screen magnifier programs could be installed to them. Telephone screen reader softwares read the pressed buttons and the messages on the screen just like the related computers. As these can be installed only to modern smart phones, people with visual impairment usually choose these more expensive devices and they can use previous functions (phone book, SMS), and new, special function (internet, email, listening to the music) as well.

Different screen reader and magnifier programs are available for almost every smart phone internationally. Nokia Symbian, Google Android, BlackBerry, iPhone or Windows Phone may be selected and used by people with visual impairment. In Hungary, the situation is worse due to the lack of knowledge of languages: Hungarian screen reader program is available for telephone with Nokia Symbian operating system, with Android and from 4th generation iPhone devices. However, new smart phones are touch screen devices, and although touch screen devices may be used by blind people, many of them find it very uncomfortable. In Hungary, visually impaired people used telephones with Nokia Symbian operating system, Android and iPhone roughly in the same proportion in 2014.

Nuance Talks&Zooms

The Talks&Zooms program tells the information displayed on the screen of the telephone to the person with visual impairment in Hungarian. This solution makes possible to use the function of the telephone with a Symbian (S60 and S80) system, such as the phonebook, handling of SMS, or browsing the internet. Parameters of speech, such as the volume and speed can be adjusted freely as the user wants. Text labels may be prepared for icons with the figure describing function; therefore, applications may be accessed more easily. The function to read the name of the caller may be switched on in the telephone, so the caller may be identified before picking up the phone, and the program reads the received SMS as well. The Zooms screen magnifier program enables that in addition to reading the content of the screen, the display is seen with 16× magnification for elderly users or people with impaired vision. The software makes automatic scrolling of the magnified image possible, color settings and inverting may be performed as well.

Digital Manual Magnifier Devices

The digital manual magnifiers are portable devices helping people with impaired vision in several everyday situations in reading captions, short texts, invoices, maps, time-tables, or TV programs, and sign documents. The devices are small, fit comfortably in one hand, operate from battery, and several color schemes may be used. These devices can easily be used by those who are inexperienced in informatics.

RUBY Portable Digital Magnifier

The RUBY is the smallest portable magnifier with the largest amount of individual settings. It can be placed in an upright position, and can be used with greater safety to sign a document or prepare brief notes. The non-slip cover prevents slipping in the hand, on the counter, desk, or smooth surface. The function to prepare a still image helps "taking a picture" of and comfortably viewing a distant text, for example, in a high place.

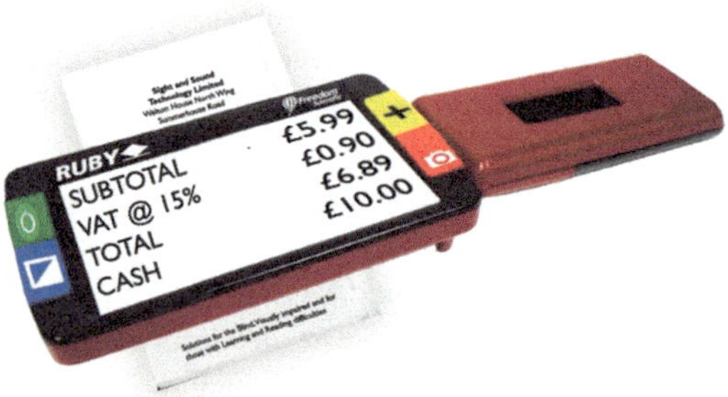

Magnification Range: 2–14 Fold

Camera: Complete color mode and 4 highlighted contrast for reading: black text with white background, white text with black background, yellow text with blue background or yellow text with black background. Display: 10.2 cm, 4:3 ratio Weight: 280 g

Zoomax Snow Digital Manual Magnifier

The device guarantees excellent picture with 19 fold magnification. It is compact with a styled design. Reading is helped by 10 different modes and 16 magnification scales. Weight: only 205 g

Reader Televisions

TV desktop readers make typed letters, handwriting, and small details easier to read. The sheet below the camera can be moved easily, then magnification, contrast, color settings, etc. can be adjusted individually as necessary. Typical areas of use:

- fine print of a contract
- telephone numbers in a phonebook
- descriptions of medications
- product labels
- crossword
- managing telephones and remote controls
- reading newspapers and booklets

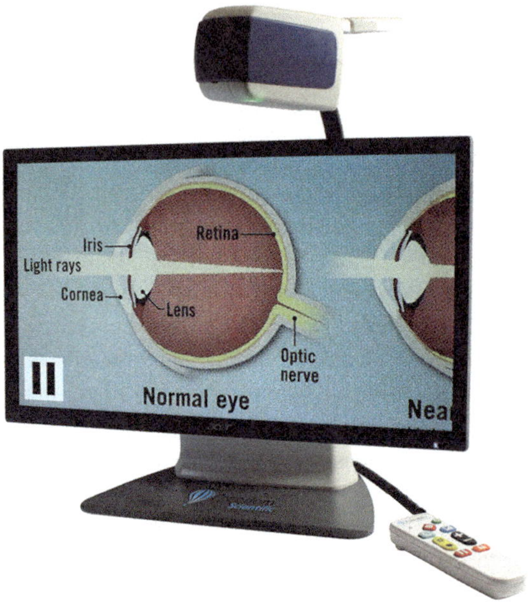

ONYX Deskset

The ONYX deskset is a flexible video magnifier. The camera does not have to be touched after proper setup thanks to the remote control. The device is portable; it can easily be moved from one workplace, classroom or room to another. The camera can be configured in several adjustable positions as required individually, even for work with three-dimensional objects. The camera enables even 100-fold magnification of the original size in case of a large screen television. Three different views may be configured: distant, document, and own view with real reflection. The lock makes it possible for the user to work freely below the camera on a detailed, magnified image of an object without unintended focusing on the user's hand or the device.

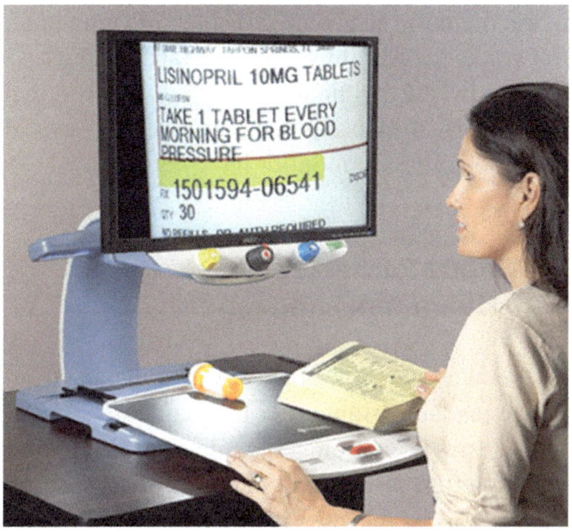

Topaz Reader Television

The TOPAZ desktop reader television is available with a 20, 22 or 24″ monitor or without a monitor. The built-in camera of the device is 21.5 cm above the reader desktop, so there is large space to work, write, and perform activities such as tightening small screws in a glass frame, threading the needle for sewing and sewing.

The main features are: 16 magnification levels, individual color contrast settings, automatic focus, extra large reader page, push button control, positioning to determine the position of the document.

Egérszem ("Mouse Eye") Device

Common feature of the various Egerszem ("Mouse eye") devices is that a mouse-like IT device has to be moved above the selected page and the image seen by the camera placed in the device and seen on the monitor or television may be viewed with magnification. The features of the device may be different in case of each Egerszem ("Mouse eye") devices, but these are usually the following:

- color or black and white image
- simple way to move the device above the image to be displayed
- standard connection options for television or monitor
- the extent of magnification may vary from three to eight fold
- contrast and brightness are adjustable
- low energy consumption, small size, easily portable

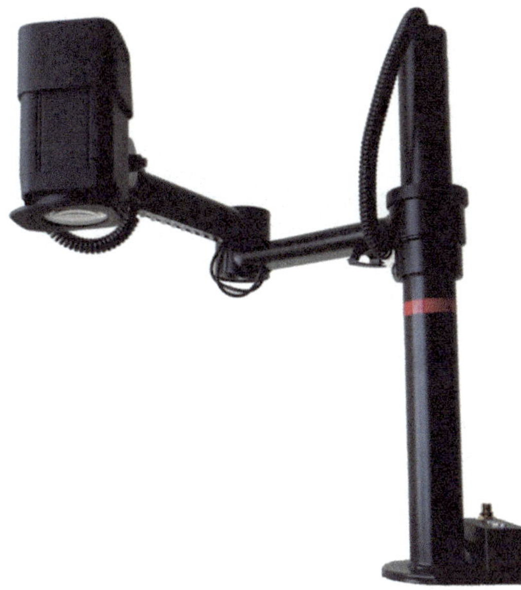

Sasszem ("Eagle Eye") and Bagolyszem ("Owl Eye") Devices

Devices manufactured in Hungary have similar parameters as reader televisions manufactured abroad, these are the following:

- easy handling
- may be used to read and write, the table may be moved
- automatic focus
- the extent of optical magnification may vary from 1 to 40 fold
- LCD monitor may be connected
- adjustable contrast and brightness
- positive and inverse colors may be used
- the two camera versions may be well used by students to view the desk and the board.

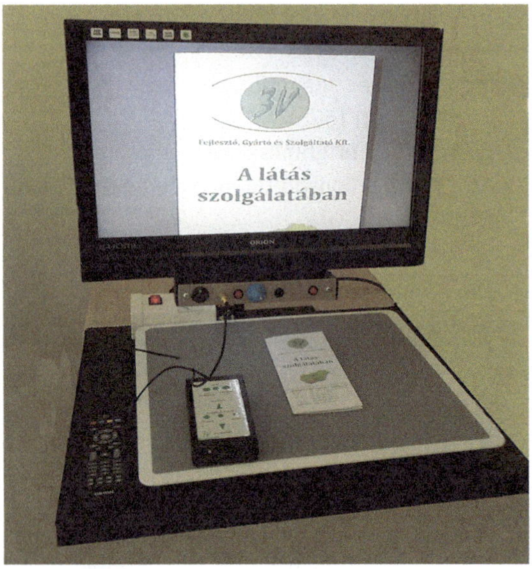

Additional Useful Devices

Naturally, in addition to the above described devices, there are several various electronic devices for people with impaired vision; some of these are described below:

SE7000 Talking Blood Pressure Monitor

An electronic blood pressure monitor that can be applied on the upper arm was complemented with a talking unit which tells the user the data (measured values, low battery life, result stored in the memory, etc.) on the display in Hungarian, the voice is a female voice. The talking unit was placed in the original device so the original parameters, measuring accuracy and services of the blood pressure monitor have not changed.

SPW-1002 Packet Watch with Hungarian Language

The device announces the exact time in clear, understandable Hungarian language after pressing a single button. Specific characteristics: single button setting and handling, the information is told to the user in a clear, human voice, time, date announcement, alarm function, notification that can be set at four time points, for example, to take medicines, administer insulin, automatic handling of daylight-saving time, small size that can be easily held by the hand, can be attached to the bag, belt, or neck.

DKS-1055 Hungarian Talking, Flat Glass Kitchen Scale

The device is a kitchen scale complemented with a talking unit that tells the user the data appearing on the display in a pleasant female voice (measured values, low battery life, overload, etc.). The talking unit was placed in the original device so the original parameters, measuring accuracy and services of the scale have not changed.

Contact information of the distributors		
Distributors	Distributed products	Contact information
"Informatika a latasserultekert" (Informatics for people with visual injury) Foundation	JAWS for Windows screen reader software	1145 Budapest,
	MAGic screen magnifier software	Bacskai u.29/b.
	ZoomText screen magnifier software	Telephone: +36(1) 273–3180
	Focus Blue 14, 40 and 80 Braille display	Fax: (1) 273–3189
	Plustek OpticBook 3800 book scanner	E-mail: ertekesites@infoalap.hu
	ABBYY FineReader optical character recognition software	Website: http://www.infoalap.hu

Contact information of the distributors

Distributors	Distributed products	Contact information
	RUBY digital manual magnifier	
	TOPAZ reader television	
	ONYX deskset digital camera	
Labrador Bt.	Poet Compact reader device	1115. Budapest,
	Zoomax Snow digital manual magnifier	Tetenyi u. 49. Telephone: +36 30 248 6641 E-mail: labrador.bt@gmail.com Website: http://www.labrador-bt.hu
3 V Fejleszto,	Mouse eye magnifier aid	7622 Pecs,
Gyarto es Szolgaltato Kft.	Eagle eye and owl eye magnifier device	Nagy Lajos kiraly u. 6/a. Telephone: +36 72 511 575 E-mail: a3vkft@gmail.com Website: www.latasjavitok.hu
Hangvilag Kft.	SE-7000 talking blood pressure monitor	1192 Budapest
	SPW-1002 packet watch with Hungarian language	Meszaros Lorinc utca 49/2.
		Telephone: 06-30-237-0796
	DKS-1055 Hungarian talking flat glass kitchen scale	E-mail: ugyfel@hangvilag.hu Honlap: www.hangvilag.hu

Hungarian Federation of the Blind and Partially Sighted

The Hungarian Federation of the Blind and Partially Sighted (Magyar Vakok es Gyengenlatok Orszagos Szovetsege, MVGYOSZ) is one of the oldest Hungarian organizations safeguarding interest. The National Guard Association for the Blind was founded in 1901, however, it has not been initiated by blind people, but the responsibility of the contemporary society. Employing workshops has been made, where the blind people worked for the coverage of their own supplies.

After the 1st World War, a great amount of people with impaired vision appeared in all of the society sections. In the initiative of qualified blind people, the Association for the Blind was founded in October 1918. Between the two world wars, there were two organizations working for the blind: the National Guard Association for the Blind which has been supplied by the government and the society too, and the Association for the Blind, which has been founded by the blind people themselves. The contemporary social politics were caritative, and it has favored the National Guard Association for the Blind.

In 1941, co-operation between the two organizations was established, the main reason for this was not the similarity of the activities of the organizations, but person-related, because the president of the federation was the deputy director of the National Guard Association for the Blind. In 1945, two organizations were merged in the Federation of the Blind. The constitution which has approved in 1976 already contains the name National Association for the Blind ad particularly Sighted. In 1938, the Association published its first regular journal, the World of the Blind, which provided a forum for discussion of problems of blind people.

The National Federation of the Blind and Visually Impaired is operating as an independent social organization from 1989. Its management is based on budget support, application resources and partially covered by donations. The MVGYOSZ has undergone a significant transformation in September 2005 for the last time. Since than, the members of the organization have not only been natural persons with impaired vision but mainly organizations representing these people. In 2014, the MVGYOSZ is operating in every county, and there are two member organizations in Pest

County, in Fejer County and in Szabolcs-Szatmar-Bereg County. The main decision making body of the MVGYOSZ is the Envoy Assembly, and the operative head of the organization is the chairperson and a management with seven members. The MVGYOSZ is basically an organization safeguarding interest, but it provides various services as well, primarily in Budapest, but several services are available in other parts of the country as well via the member organizations. The following section describes the most important services provided to natural persons by the MVGYOSZ.

Aid Shop

Special devices for use, medical aids, publications and softwares that make everyday life of people with visual impairment easier are available in the Aid Shop of the MVGYOSZ.

Roles of the Aid Shop:

- evaluation of membership needs
- purchase of goods at home and abroad
- selling appliances.

The Federation makes lending appliances possible for natural persons with membership card.

Braille Press

The dot-writing has spread in Hungary since 1893. With the spreading of dot-writing, the basis of the Braille-library has been set up too. The more and more equipped Braille-press created a lot of jobs, and the continuous development has reached a point where 10–14 people are necessary to ensure the coordinated work. When the computers appeared and have been involved in work, heavy physical work had become easier. With modernization, the printing processes have changed too. The Braille-press is working on the printing and delivering of publications, journals, books, and other documents. It is important in supporting literacy and providing access to information for people with impaired vision, providing Braille text books for educational facilities and accomplishing individual and external orders.

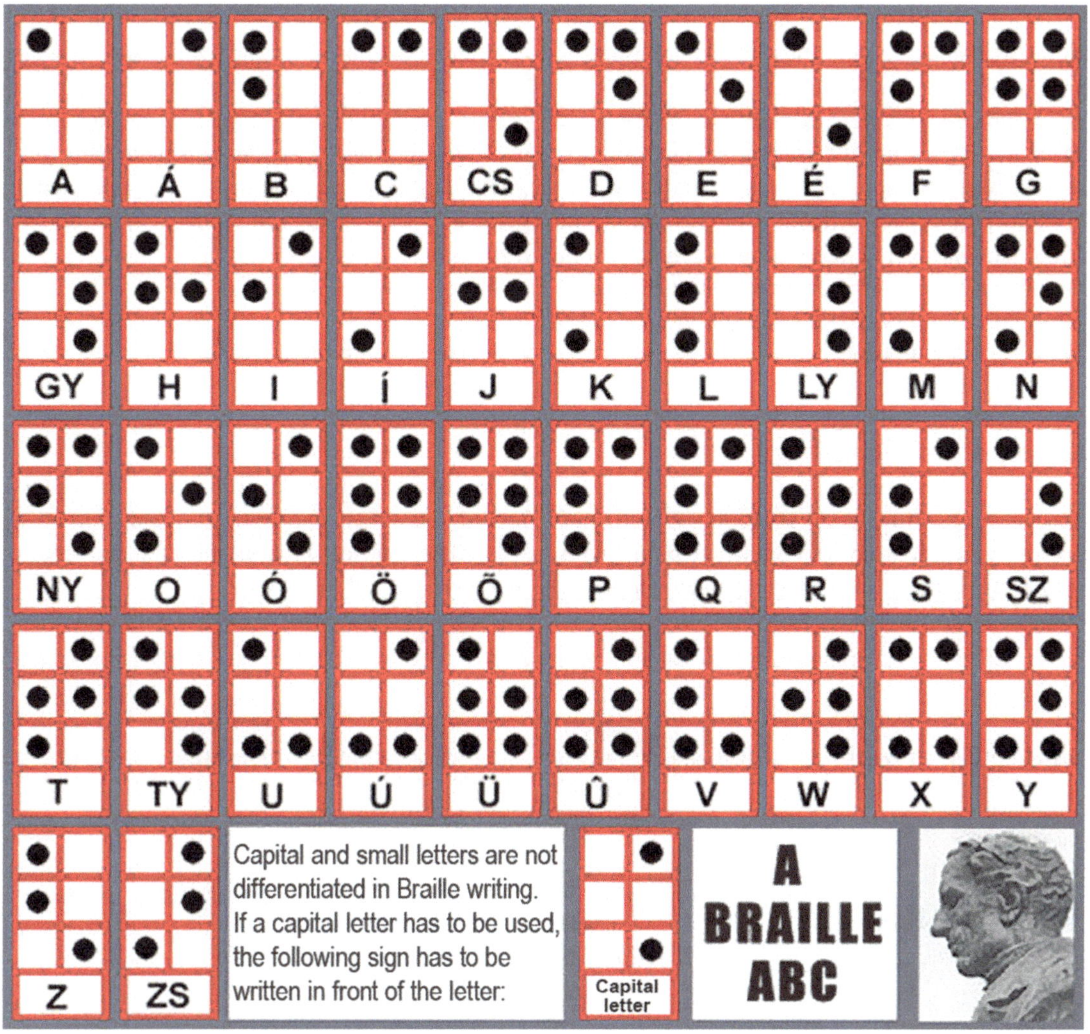
A
Á
B
C
CS
D
E
É
F
G
GY
H
I
Í
J
K
L
LY
M
N
NY
O
Ó
Ö
Ő
P
Q
R
S
SZ
T
TY
U
Ú
Ü
Û
V
W
X
Y
Z
ZS
Capital and small letters are not differentiated in Braille writing. If a capital letter has to be used, the following sign has to be written in front of the letter:
Capital letter
A BRAILLE ABC

Braille Library

The Braille Library was first opened in Budapest in 1896. It is still open today and waits for the readers. There are 900 works in the current collection of library consisting of 8500 volumes. The library has 198 registered readers. One reader reads an average of 6–12 works a year.

Roles of the Braille Library

- Giving special books containing dotted cells (Braille writing) for people with visual impairment.
- Improving reading abilities of blind children. Increasing the knowledge of blind people. Special cultural opportunities for those in need.
- Cataloguing and specifically marking new books from the press.
- Checking books returned by readers, correcting errors, replacing missing pages.
- Disposal of useless works.

Audio Library

The Audio Library of MVGYOSZ opened in 1961. Till the middle of the 70s, books that could be heard only with a reel-to-reel tape recorder were available at libraries, cassette players appeared later. For about 10 years, reel-to-reel tapes and cassettes were available in the libraries as well, and then in 1989, reel-to-reel tapes finally retired. The first book that was available in CD became part of the collection of the library in 2000. Hungarian and international novels, works of currently active modern writers, travel guides, informative books and books for children are also available in the library.

Supply of Textbooks

In accordance with Act XVII of2004, directors of primary and secondary schools where pupils with visual impairment learn may organize supply of textbooks partly with the co-operation of the National Federation of the Blind and Visually Impaired. There are more and more textbooks that are available via this organization and can be used by pupils with visual impairment every year. These textbooks are modified and can be used by person with visual impairment without any limitation.

Types of textbooks:

- electronic textbook,
- mp3 textbook,
- Braille textbook.

Magnified and black and white copies of textbooks and other publications are available as well. The service is available for the county members of the MVGYOSZ.

Applicant's name	Region	Country	Address:	Availability	Name of the head of the organization	Name of the contact person
Vakok Allami Intezete (National Institution for Blind People)	Central Hungary	Budapest	1146 Budapest Hermina ut 21.	Telephone: +36 1 383 2589 Fax: +36 1 383 2589 titkarsag@ vakokintezete.hu	Mrs. Berta Iren Szabone	Ingrid Lengyel
Kiemelkedoen Kozhasznu Feher Bot Alapitvany (White Cane Non-profit Foundation)	Northern Great Plain	Hajdu-Bihar	4087 Hajdudorog Nanasi ut 4.	Telephone: +36 52 389 246 Fax: +36 52 232 313 szab o .m@kkfba@ axelero .hu	Dr Miklos Szabo	Dr Miklos Szabo
Siketvakok Orszagos Egyesulete (Hungarian Deafblind Association)	Central Hungary	Pest	1146 Budapest	Telephone: +36 1 209 58 29 Fax: +36 1 209 5829 kedveseda@gmail. com	Tamas Gangl	Eda Kedves
			Ajtosi Durer sor 39.			
Kreativ Formak Alapitvany (Creative Forms Foundation)	Southern Great Plain	Csongrad	6726 Szeged	Telephone: +36 30 825 30 03 Fax: same ferenc@ santa.hu	Ferenc Santa	Ferenc Santa
	Region		Leda u. 8.			
Ki-Latas Kozhasznu Alapitvany (Perspective Public Foundation)	South-Transdanubian Region	Somogy	7400 Kaposvar Fo u. 63.	Telephone: + 36 82 319 229 Fax: + 36 82 319 229 danyadine_b@ t-online.hu	Mrs. Cecilia Danyadine Molnar	Mrs. Cecilia Danyadine Molnar

Applicant's name	Region	Country	Address:	Availability	Name of the head of the organization	Name of the contact person
Vakok es Gyengenlatok						
Gyor-Moson-Sopron Megyei Egyesulete (Organization of the Blind and Visually Impaired in Gyor-Moson-Sopron County)	West-Transdanubian Region	Gyor-Moson-Sopron	9024 Gyor Bartok Bela ut 23. Fsz. 4.	Telephone: +36 96 528 805 Fax: +36 96 528 805 info@gyorivakok.hu	Mrs. Laczi Tamasne	Mrs. Laczi Tamasne
Buzavirag Alapitvany (Buzavirag Foundation)	North-Hungaria Region	Borsod-Abauj-Zemplen	3941 Vamosujfalu Kossuth u. 42/A	Telephone: +36 47 594 004 Fax: +36 47 594 004	Mrs. Olah Tibor Istvanne	Marta Nemeth
Latasserultek Regionalis	Central Transdanubian Region					
Kozhasznu Egyesulete (Regional Non-profit Organization of People with Impaired Vision)		Fejer	8000 Szekesfe-hervar Balatoni u. 15. 1/3.	Telephone: +36 22 318 700 Fax: +36 22 318 700	Zsolt Szoko	www.larke.hu

Elementary and Occupational Rehabilitation of People with Impaired Vision

69

Marta Tolnayne Csattos and Laszlo Joszt

Contents

M.T. Csattos, M.D. (✉)
Head of National Institution for Blind People
Tiflopedagogist, Rehabilitation Instructor,
National Institution for Blind People,
Budapest, Hungary
e-mail: vercs@vakokintezete.hu;
tolnaynecsattosmarta@gmail.hu

L. Joszt
Social Worker, Rehabilitation Instructor of Visually
Impaired Patients Physical Accessibility Expert,
National Institution for Blind People,
Budapest, Hungary
e-mail: laszlojoszt@gmail.com

The right to rehabilitation is constitutional right of every Hungarian national. The service of elementary and the vocational rehabilitation together form the rehabilitation process which gives the desired result like the **Rehabilitation Clockwork model.** It may only be affected by the motivation and individual determination of the person. The person participating in the rehabilitation, so the person who became visually impaired "orders" the rehabilitation service and "contracts" for the offered services. The "Customer" has every important and up-to-date piece of information required to use the rehabilitation services with maximal autonomy. The person with visual impairment will contract with the service provider that is the representative of the institution providing elementary rehabilitation for the offered services and rehabilitation components that improve and support abilities the person wishes to improve. This contract specifies the undertaken rights and obligations in writing for both parties, creating the bases for working together.

In the last decades, only few people knew that there is a professional workgroup providing elementary rehabilitation service in Hungary since 1980 the purpose of which is to provide a "fresh start" in an altered life situation for persons with visual impairment developing in adulthood.

For a long time, the information relevant and important for a lot of people could spread difficulty and under reduced circumstances. Professionals tried to spread the information about the service

J. Somlai, T. Kovács (eds.), *Neuro-Ophthalmology*, DOI 10.1007/978-3-319-28956-4_69

from several directions. For example, they contacted ophthalmologists personally all over the country, Clinics operating in the country and used their personal relationships in ophthalmology; in events and in case of media requests, they tried to take every opportunity to invite decision makers and experts in healthcare. The strongest and most authentic channel to the persons involved is the opinion of persons having visual impairment and life experience in this matter. Various components of the elementary rehabilitation service try to rebuild the motivational system in a complex way by setting and achieving newer purposes. In addition, significant efforts have been made by healthcare and social professionals in order to change it. A common goal is to inform primarily the persons concerned and relatives, as well as professionals working in this field. A great step was when the head of the Department of Ophthalmology, University of Semmelweis and special educations teachers in the Hungarian Deafblind Association started negotiations about the development of an advisory office which was considered to be unique in the country after a study trip in England. The office started in September 2005 with a full-time special education teacher and a voluntary social worker (László 2006). The elementary and vocational rehabilitation service network operated as a regional center in Hungary can be mentioned among the results of professional work performed in the spirit of interprofessionalism. The network was the result of slow but persistent work. Actual contact information of elementary rehabilitation centers available in Hungary for people with visual impairment can be found online under the following menu: Rehabilitation/Complex rehabilitation of people with visual impairment on the *website of Equal Opportunities of Persons with Disabilities Non-profit Ltd. (Fogyatékos Személyek Egyesélyegyenlőségéért Közalapítvány, FSZK).* The service is provided by the Hungarian Government and the civil society as well. The service of elementary rehabilitation is a bridge between medical and vocational rehabilitation. With this service, the person with visual impairment learns new information, and with this information, he/she can become a self-governing individual again who builds personal relationships and moves towards new goals. The following case report reflects the effective co-operation of additional components of Healthcare (Medical Rehabilitation) and complex rehabilitation, and gives an insight into the large variety of the components and devices of elementary rehabilitation.

Peter M. (32-year-old) male patient comes from the western part of the country; he is working in the enterprise of his father in the building industry. He has always performed hard physical work, although he has detected visual problems for years, but he neglected them. He lived in a relationship in the capital. He had a driving license, but he has not driven for a long time. In 2007, Peter went to the Specialty Out-patient Clinic of Ophthalmology, and then he had different examinations.

His treating ophthalmologist diagnosed optic nerve atrophy. In June 2007, the ophthalmologist contacted the advisory office of the clinic to ask about rehabilitation options for Peter. Six months later, after the scheduled ophthalmologic check-up visit, Peter called the advisory social worker and asked for information about the possibilities, as he felt that his condition in fact gradually worsened. He had more arguments in his relationship, as he could not provide the previous quality of life, and it was officially confirmed (by the expert opinion of the National Institute of Medical Experts) that he has visual impairment (disability which is also a status in Hungary) and he could not continue his previous work. Peter realized that he has to learn and he needs help to proceed and return to his work. Peter started to receive Elementary Rehabilitation service in January 2008 in the Rehabilitation Center for the Blind (Vakok Elemi Rehabilitációs Csoportja, VERCS) *in the Department of Institute for the Blind.*

Available forms of elementary rehabilitation services

1. living-in system
   - providing complete education or
   - partial education
2. attending system
   - providing complete education or
   - partial education or
3. out-patient care, or
4. home teaching

Living-in System

Clients choosing living-in education usually live far from the center providing elementary rehabilitation service. This form may be indicated based on social environment or individual considerations. The living-in education is performed in courses, in small groups or in the form of individual activities. In addition to scheduled lessons, healthcare is provided as well, but team building programs, free time activities are available as well. The clients may participate in partial or complete education depending on their abilities. In partial education, the client can or wants to learn only part of the information available in courses providing complete education. Those clients will receive complete education who are able to and would like to learn all information available based on the evaluated abilities and needs.

Formal benefits of living-in service:

- professional therapeutic and living environment
- planned pedagogic work of specialized colleagues
- in small group education, activities of the clients motivate each other, therefore, the efficacy of pedagogic work increases
- after the courses, clients may practice together, increase the acquired knowledge during free time activities

Disadvantages:

- the client is away from the original family and his/her usual environment
- institutional conditions are ideal for the client

Attending Service

This form of education is available for people with visual impairment who visit the facility individually or with the help of an institution (support services), who therefore do not need accommodation. Clients receiving complete education are very motivated, and would like to and are able to understand and learn all the available activities. People with visual impairment receiving partial education are able to and/or would like to learn only certain parts of the available knowledge.

Benefits of attending education:

- the client meets the family members daily
- does not have to leave his/her usual family environment
- professionals in the institution participate in handling conflicts occurring in the altered situation

Disadvantages:

- daily traveling is physically burdening and decreases efficacy
- practicing is not performed in a protected, safe environment
- the client lacks the ability to hide in a group, and enhancing effects of group dynamic are missing as well

Out-patient Client Care

Clients receiving out-patient care receive only certain services of elementary rehabilitation, or wish to learn a few selected activities. According to the education plan, clients visit the facility on certain days and receive service. Activities are always performed based on an individual plan irrespective of the direction of education. Clients may participate in this form of education for more than once, and the course may be repeated to obtain new information. Clients may participate in several programs simultaneously as well.

Benefits of out-patient care:

- accommodation is not required
- workers do not have to leave their job
- it may be performed in the form of a few hours long service
- the service may be repeated if necessary

Disadvantages:

- physically inconvenient daily traveling may decrease efficacy
- practicing is not performed in a protected, safe environment
- the client lacks the ability to hide in a group
- capacity of professionals decreases during individual trainings, therefore, it is expensive

Home Teaching

Home teaching is the oldest service of elementary rehabilitation (Ponchillia and Ponchillia 1996). The professional visits the person with impaired vision at home, and teaches him/her the required knowledge. This form of education is usually applied in case of elderly patients or clients with multiple diseases. Adaptation training is performed at home as well, which means that the clients participating in the course receive adaptation service at home. Information learnt and exercised during education will be adjusted and used under local conditions with adaptation. If possible, living environment and tools should be accessible.

Benefits:

- training is performed in the patient's own environment
- older people or persons with less good physical condition may participate

Disadvantages:

- isolation
- several rehabilitation directions remain unknown
- the client does not familiarize with other devices
- there is no group effect, which means reduced efficacy (Mrs. Marta Tolnayne Csattos 2007)

Components of Elementary Rehabilitation

Psychological Rehabilitation

Forms of physiological rehabilitation

The role of the ***rehabilitation psychologist*** is to enhance reintegration of the personality, reduce subsequent stress, and provide effective support in the treatment of negative social effects. The activity has two basic forms:

- individual advisors, supporter, and psychotherapeutic discussions, and
- in the form of group therapy.

Individual difficulties of processing trauma may be significantly reduced by the acceptable, empathic situations of individual dialogues, and group dynamic processes experienced in group therapy. These processes enhance integration and harmonization of the person via internal psychic experience and strengthening positive self-protective mechanisms (elaboration, sublimation, identification) regarding accommodation to external needs and requirements. An evaluating questionnaire is used at the end of the group exercises.

Special Education Rehabilitation

The rate of utilization and quality of the patient's vision is evaluated from practical considerations during the ***functional visual examination.*** Part of the examinations may be performed with manual devices, other examinations require computer programs. Elements of the examinations are the same as those of the ophthalmologic examination.

The purpose of ***functional visual training*** performed during basic rehabilitation is that clients can practice "vision" under optimal circumstances and the clients may interpret and process the seen objects more effectively with this training. We try to find the most suitable optical equipment and method for those in need so that they are able to use and interpret several visual stimuli to the greatest extent. The professional performing the functional visual test often meets the phenomenon that the person shows worse performance than expected based on ophthalmologic data and opinion of the ophthalmologist. Using the learnt techniques results in significant changes in quality of life in case of relatively good functional vision as well. The role of visual training in these cases is to improve localization, change gaze, follow a standing and moving stimulus with the eye and search regarding the nature of the visual problem (for example, good scanning ability helps in compensating for the narrowing of the visual field or blind spots in the visual field, fixation and localization exercises improve decreased vision, and the ability to follow standing and moving stimuli improves mobility skills). Color and shape detection, visual attention, memory, eye-body, eye-hand coordination can be improved with using vision techniques. Functional vision training is the newest, still developing branch of neurorehabilitation, it provides new rehabilitation options for people with cortical visual impairment.

Orientation and Mobility Training

The purpose of orientation and mobility training is to make the individual capable of traveling alone in the altered situation. With teaching and using special and adapted equipment and techniques, the person will become able to get to another place alone. Other purposes include developing techniques and abilities necessary for safe and independent orientation and mobility in closed and open space, known and unknown environment, in different parts of the day and under varying weather conditions regarding the abilities of the individual. There are special techniques and equipment for people with low vision, partially sighted people and blind people supporting independent orientation and mobility, these techniques are sophisticated.

With this activity, the person with visual impairment is expected to learn the information and abilities necessary for safe and independent orientation and mobility and to adapt these abilities in the situation with impaired perception. Orientation and mobility with a long white cane and/or vision supporting equipment under different visibility, on terrains and in situations of various difficulties. The activity is performed by tiflo-pedagogues specialized in orientation and mobility training. Mobility training with a guide dog is not part of the elementary rehabilitation service. Several people practice mobility with a dog regarding their life situation or personality (Figs. 69.1 and 69.2).

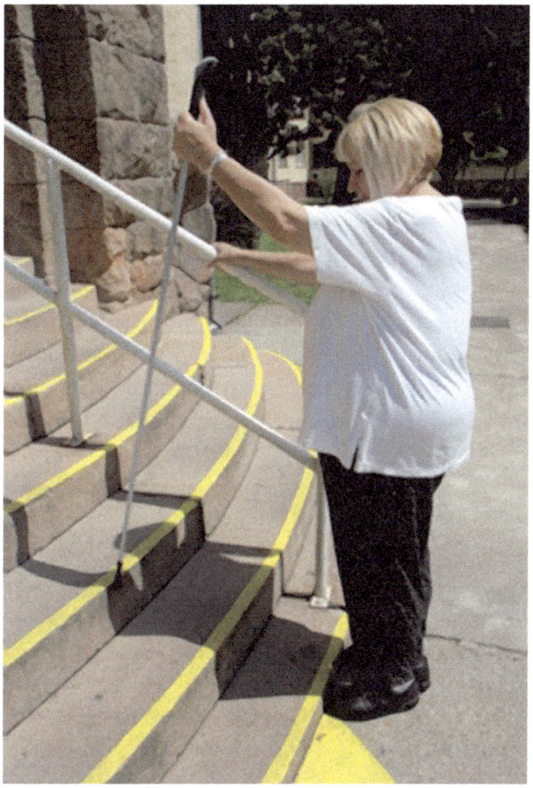

Fig. 69.1 Orientation and mobility training using special and adapted equipment

Teaching and Re-teaching Daily Living Skills

In daily living skills, person having visual impairment as an adult are taught and made to practice those special techniques he/she performed with visual control for even years or decades. While performing each task, the belief is given that the client is able to perform simple or more difficult tasks in the new life situation as well. The activity from planning through teaching, practicing, and performing tasks alone is determined by the personality, needs, and requirements of the client. The purpose is that every person with visual impairment becomes more independent and confident in daily living skills regarding their own abilities and possibilities. New techniques may be learned in personal hygiene (manicure, makeup, shaving, beard care); in organizing and indicating clothes, documents, kitchen equipments; and in performing work in and around the house and meaningful passing of free time as required.

Teaching How to Use Devices That Help Daily Living Skilly

Using various adapted and special devices may make daily living easier in the altered life situation for a more independent life. When selecting from the list of available devices, the extent of visual impairment, perception abilities, interests, needs, financial status, and prioritization of devices should be considered (Fig. 69.3).

Re-teaching Free Time Activities

Meaningful and cultural passing of free time is very important in our daily living skills in everyday life. A large portion of people with impaired vision sits in the armchair and listens to the radio all day. If we ask them, they do not know what this activity is, as they only pass time in the changed situation without any purpose. Participants of the service may learn several free time activities available for people with impaired vision as well, these activities provide joy and decrease stress, such as the currently popular and much liked patch-work, bead weaving, or preparing jewelry, gardening, or bricolage.

The rehabilitation process is individual: the professional providing the service selects devices and technique regarding the interest and age of

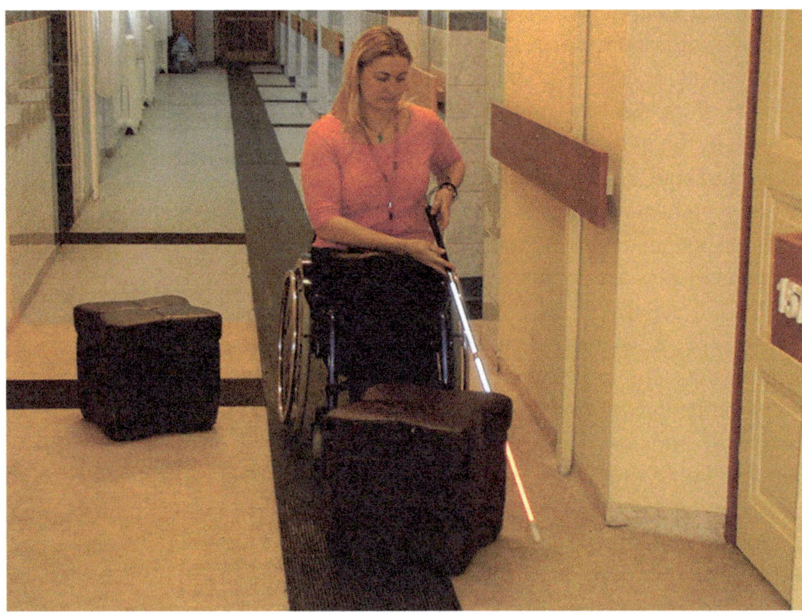

Fig. 69.2 Orientation training with vision supporting equipment under different visibility and on terrain and in situations of various difficulty

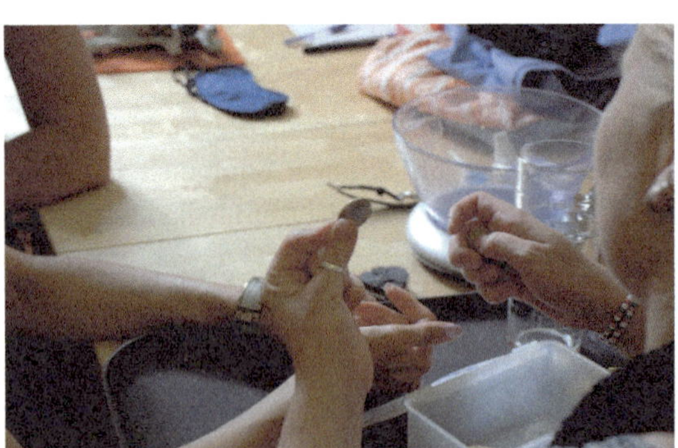

Fig. 69.3 Teaching how to use devices that help daily living skills

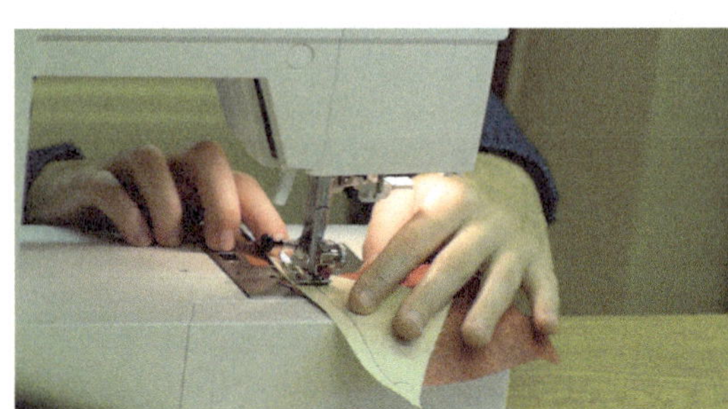

Fig. 69.4 Re-teaching free time activities

the person with visual impairment and the extent and quality of the injury (Fig. 69.4).

Teaching Tactile Writing and Reading

Its purpose is to re-teach the option of reading and writing and show the technique of tactile writing and reading for people losing vision at adulthood or adults having visual impairment. Our colleagues often meet persons who have difficulty in learning Braille writing and reading. The age of the person and health problems may be in the background. Difficulty of tactile discrimination (recognition and differentiation with palpation), abstracting ability, memory problems, and tactile sensation disorders of persons with diabetes mellitus, limited information collection of the finger tips due to sensory neuropathy may make learning Braille writing and reading requiring fine tactile abilities impossible (Figs. 69.5 and 69.6).

By teaching linear communication techniques, older, cumulatively injured people and people with visual impairment having somatic diseases as well may also learn writing and reading more easily. Our aim is to increase the number of available services that can be learned regarding the abilities of the clients, providing a teaching plan regarding individual needs in teaching cultural techniques (connection and mode the individual and his/her surrounding interact, and flow of information develops).

Communication and Using Computer

We live in the world of informatics devices, using these devices is part of our everyday life now. However, using these devices requires a new way of thinking, which does not represent a problem for young people today, but some middle-aged persons and the majority of the elderly population find it difficult. As information technology (IT) based devices may return lost independency to people with visual impairment in several fields in large extent, participants of elementary rehabilitation services should learn how to use them and what the bases of their operation is. Decreasing the feeling of vulnerability and requiring the help of partners with normal vision may significantly improve the mental status of the person with impaired vision.

Social Work Based on Individual Case Management

Persons with impaired vision participating in elementary rehabilitation services are followed up and supported by a social worker as a case manager from the time the person indicates to require the service till vocational rehabilitation. As a consequence, needs, social situation, family relationships and relationships with friends may be better understood, improving activities provided for these persons may be more coordinated. In addition, the social worker may help in resolving problems, conflicts occurring during

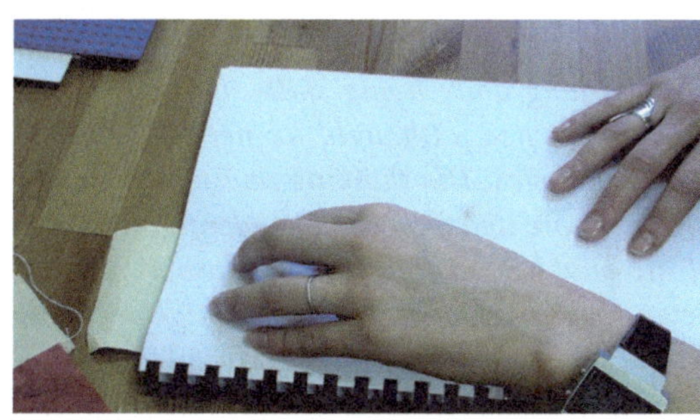

Fig. 69.5 Teaching tactile writing and reading

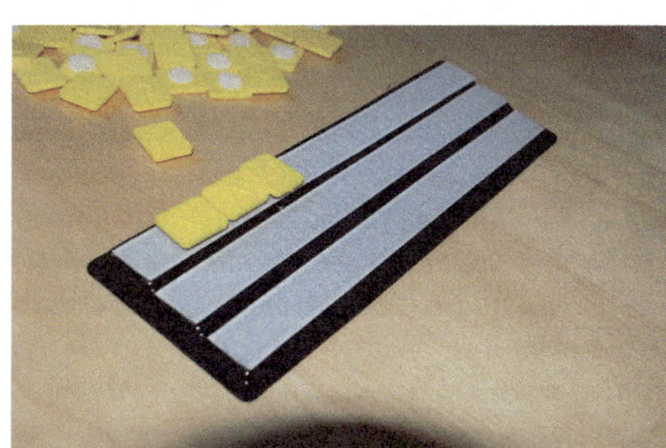

Fig. 69.6 Teaching device to teach the ability to write and learn for persons with multiple injuries

the rehabilitation process, creating the conditions enhancing independent living, benefiting from conditions supporting individual living.

Peter received continuous visual training after functional vision test, additional elements of the service were planned according to the results. For Peter, functional vision significantly influenced the planning and learning process while learning orientation and mobility. Functional vision further deteriorated during rehabilitation, and the patient told us that he hopes that development of medicine will soon resolve his problem and he will be able to see as he did before. Increasing informatics knowledge seemed to be inevitable for Peter, as he had previous knowledge and he considered informatics as a potential future profession, mainly as he was interested in the technical field. He learned how to use the screen magnifier and screen reader programs in the computer as well. With increasing informatics knowledge, Peter started to feel more confident that he did not want to understand and learn tactile writing and reading systems, that is the Braille writing.

Regarding daily living skills, he had significant experience, although, he needed to learn safe techniques. His thinking and motivation to become more and more independent in all areas of life enabled a rapid learning process. First, Peter was skeptic regarding mental hygienic services, and then he strongly refused to participate. Regarding spiritual experience, his interest increased inversely, and alternative medicine became one of his areas of interest seeing it as a potential solution to stop the deterioration of his vision or to reverse the process. Peter received elementary rehabilitation services while living in the institution, he soon found his place and those fellow patients he had similar interests with and with whom they could help each other day by day in the 10–14 member groups. He learnt to ask for help and to accept it. Peter participated in the VERCS intensive (living-in) training twice subsequently, and six month later, he applied to receive treatment in the rehabilitation facility of the National Institute for Blind People, where the institution provides living-in and additional rehabilitation improving services in accordance with a contract made for a certain amount of time. Learning and working are especially important for Peter from the beginning; therefore, professionals helped him to reach this purpose within vocational rehabilitation. Recently, he enrolled in the evening course of a secondary school in Budapest where he is learning successfully. Real subjects pose some difficulties for him, but the developing pedagogues of the institution help him in his advancement. He considers learning in higher education, but he is uncertain of changing specialization. Peter has been working as a sales representative in a Company where people with visual impairment are employed as call-center employees. He is content with his work, as he became closer to his concepts to become an active member of the open job market. He has been living in the rehabilitation section of the institution for two years, he has fitted in relatively rapidly, as during the months spent in the VERCS; he has met several fellow clients living in the facility. He has no conflicts regarding living together. With his quiet but not withdrawn personality, he created good relationship with people with impaired vision and professionals working in the Institution. He contacts professional groups of the Institution less and less frequently for help, which leads to the conclusion that he can manage his life more independently. He participates in a savings program, in order to resolve living alone. According to Peter, his alcohol consumption habits have changed, as he used to drink alcohol regularly, but nowadays, he drinks alcohol rarely and rather only during the holidays. His friends responded to the change in his life situation exceptionally well, as they actively support him since they found out that Peter has to live with visual impairment. As he helped his friends a lot before, they return this favor now, and support him on weekdays. This is of great importance, as based on our experience; our clients often lose these important human relationships. His relationship deteriorated, he ended it, and let a new perspective in. Currently, Peter does not feel that his visual impairment is worsening; however several (healthcare) professionals warn him that his condition leads to complete blindness. This makes psychic processing difficult, as Peter is currently waiting for a "life changing" operation. On the whole, Peter has made a significant improvement on his own decision, from the moment his ophthalmologist informed him about his visual impairment. In addition to Peter's personality and the ability to improve his personal abilities, his ophthalmologist played an important role in the success of his rehabilitation by informing him about the potential outcome of his visual impairment at the beginning, and encouraging him to contact rehabilitation professionals and ask for rehabilitation services.

All these factors helped Peter that his current life situation is continuously developing with "his own work" in the spirit of self-determination.

References

Jose RT. Understanding low vision. New York: AFB.

László J. Tanácsadó szolgálat a látássérültekért [Advisory service for persons with impaired vision]. Szemészet folyóirat. 2006.

Márta C. Az elemi rehabilitáció magyarországi története, szolgáltatási formák [History of elementary rehabilitation in Hungary, forms of services] (Látássérült személyek elemi rehabilitációja IV. ELTE GYFK Budapest). 2007.

Ponchillia PE, Ponchillia SV. Foundations of rehabilitation teaching with persons who are blind or visually impaired. New York: American Foundation for the Blind; 1996.

70 The Importance of Rehabilitation and the Options of a Neuro-ophthalmologist

Judit Somlai

Contents

> The eternal dilemma concerning which is harder:
> to imagine a world one has never seen
> or
> to lose a world that has once been familiar with
> and
> to accept that it will never return?
> We must never decide, just let empathy guide us.

Neurosurgical and neurologic diseases–perhaps more often at a young age–may be accompanied by severe and irreversible visual loss. A cranial injury caused by an accident, bleeding caused by rupture of an aneurysm or stroke take place in a fraction of moments, and cause loss of consciousness in most cases. Patients often do not notice that they have lost their vision after regaining consciousness. The real tragedy for the patient and for the ophthalmologist begins when the injury of the visual pathway is so severe that only a small visual field or nothing is left or returns. First, the ophthalmologist has to do everything not to diagnose partial or complete blindness affecting both eyes and not to tell the patient such a diagnosis. However, if it is the case, we have to be partners in the complex rehabilitation of the patient as in determining the problem.

The role of the ophthalmologist:

- record the status detected in the acute phase accurately
- perform complementary examinations (neurology, neurosurgery, neuroradiology) if necessary
- evaluate the progression of the process in long-term care–if necessary, life-long care

The role of the neuropsychologist:

- after determining the cognitive deficiency, the extent of sensory involvement and the presence of visual neglect for example, with basic examinations:
- long-term psychotherapeutic treatment starts individually, tailored to the person and the disease

J. Somlai, M.D.
Unit of Neuro-Ophthalmology,
Department of Neurology and Stroke,
Military Hospital, Budapest, Hungary

Neuro-Ophthalmology Section,
Hungarian Ophthalmological Association,
Budapest, Hungary

Trustee, NOSZA Foundation (for the Prevention and Screening of Ocular Storke), Budapest, Hungary
e-mail: dr@somlaijudit.hu; http://somlaijudit.hu

J. Somlai, T. Kovács (eds.), *Neuro-Ophthalmology*, DOI 10.1007/978-3-319-28956-4_70

The Role of Informatics in Reconfiguring the Management of the Lives of People with Impaired Vision

Primary Education

Primary education for children with impaired vision is, as far as I know, excellent, a more distressing fact is the narrow range of learning opportunities in higher education. *(See detailed in* Chap. 69.*)*

Treating Visual Field Impairment with a Computer

At a European neuro-ophthalmological congress, the International Neuro-ophthalmological Society (INOS), German colleagues presented a procedure they have been using for years. They have published this procedure for several times since. The essence of the procedure is that in case of center halving homonymous hemianopsia, the patient participates in re-fixation training. This reveals 5–10 % of the central visual field by making the patient fixate in a new region near the center. This way, central visual field defect caused by visual field impairment is eliminated.

Speech Synthesizer and Reading Computer Programs

A special program converts the scanned text into speech, which creates a **"window to the world"** for people with impaired vision. In an exemplary manner, there are several so called talking programs in Hungary. These programs are free for several hundreds of people with impaired vision, a foundation and the inventor of the program, ***Mihdly Szuhaj*** "opened a window to the world". The Man of the Year in 2003, Mihaly Szuhaj informatics and informatics teacher helps people with congenital and acquired impaired vision with their life and regarding work opportunities by making invisible information of informatics audible, and giving the opportunity not only to learn and collect new information, but work, change career, and create human relationships. He gives a set of tools to the people with impaired vision being in a seemingly irresolvable situation that makes the impossible possible, and gives new meaning to life, to start over, he gives these people a powerful force. *(See detailed in* Chap. 68.*)*

Mihály Szuhaj (37-year-old informatics) became practically blind to both eyes, so he became amaurotic for having a serious disease at a late stage at the age of 10. With sacrificing help from his family, he finished high school with excellent results, and then he graduated in the Faculty of Informatics and Informatics Teacher in the Eötvös Lóránd University (ELTE), and created a software with Recognita RT that received a *3rd prize in the World Competition in the EU in Brussels*. He not only made this program available, but started the career of more than 500 persons with impaired vision with a foundation operated by a national informatics network. He is an exemplary person. It is not a coincidence that the Hungarian newspaper called *Magyar Hírlap* chose him to be the ***Man of the Year in 2003***. An exemplary figure of the young generation can still do a lot of things to help people with visual impairment who cannot expect any more medical help from us, doctors.

In Chap. 68, he thoroughly described the modern methodical possibilities with his colleagues, as well as those tools that may help and are essential for patients with visual impairment.

The role of our doctor colleagues is to carry on possibilities and knowledge and to promote complete rehabilitation of people with impaired vision all over the country, and help these people fit back into the "seeing society"–much more effectively as before.

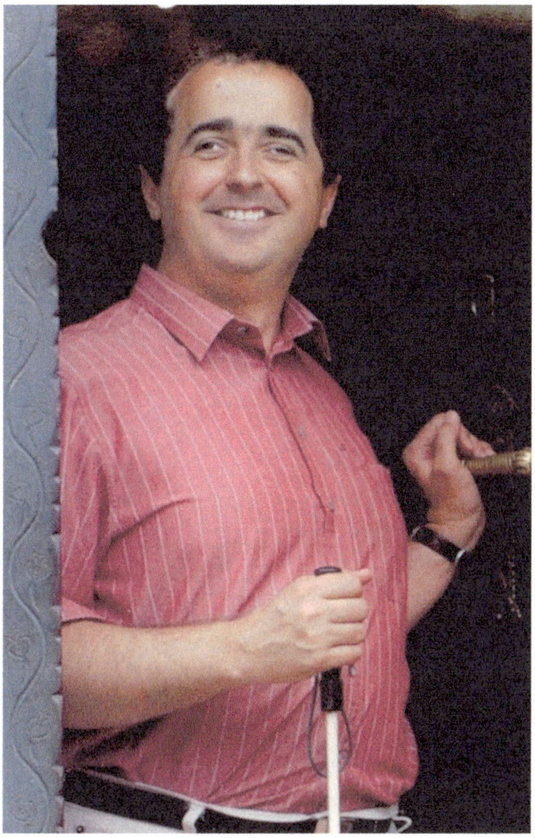

Appendix: Colour Scheme of the Book Content

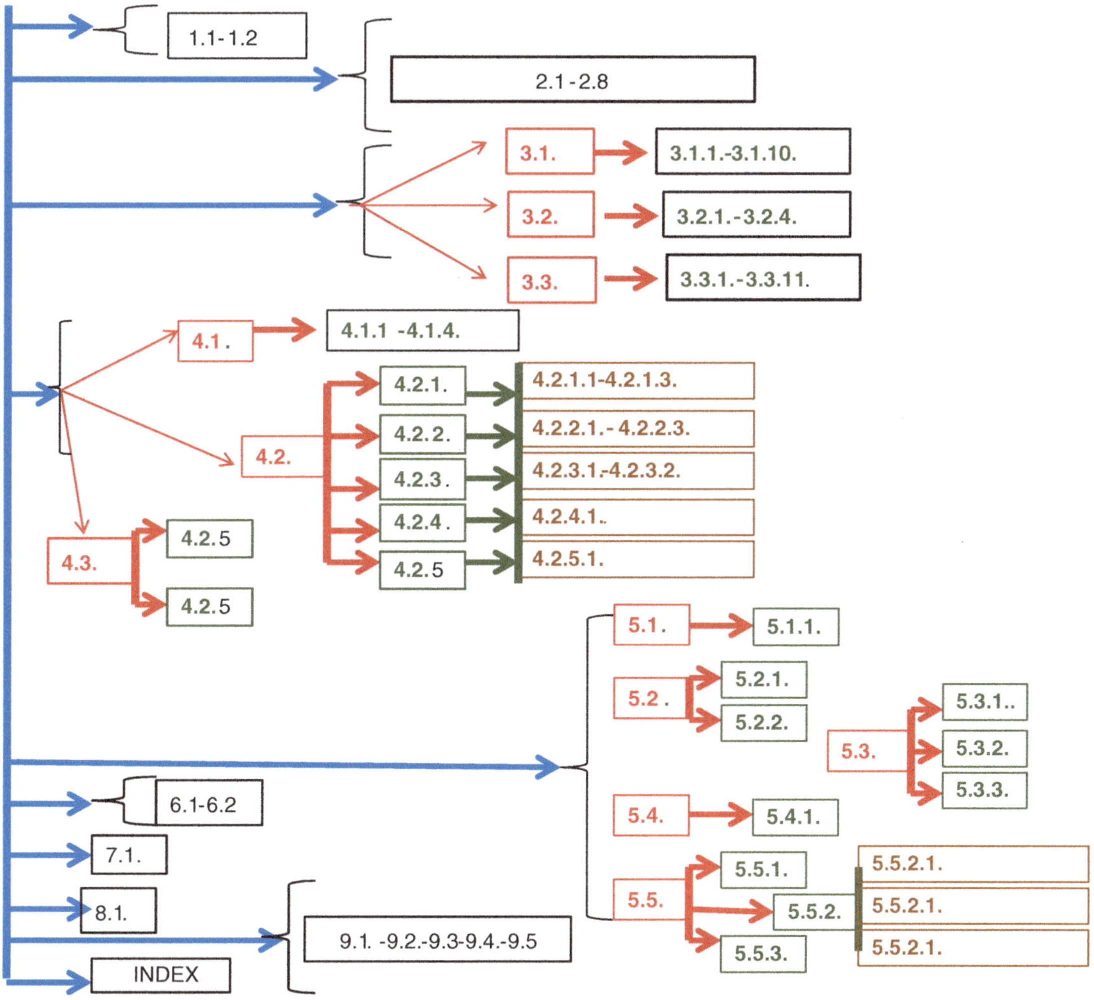

J. Somlai, T. Kovács (eds.), *Neuro-Ophthalmology*, DOI 10.1007/978-3-319-28956-4

Index

J. Somlai, T. Kovács (eds.), *Neuro-Ophthalmology*, DOI 10.1007/978-3-319-28956-4

D

E

F

Q

R

S

Printed by Printforce, the Netherlands